AF734631

MedOne

# Access the additional media content with this e-book via Thieme MedOne.

## Access additional media now!

With three easy steps, unlock access to the additional media for this title via MedOne, Thieme's online platform.

1. Note your access code below:

2. Scan the QR code or enter your access code at **MedOne.thieme.com/code**

3. Set up a username on MedOne and sign in to activate your access to the e-book and its additional online media.

## Quick Access

After you successfully register and activate your code, you can find your book and additional online media at

**medone.thieme.com/9783132427518**

or with this QR code.

## Important Notes

- Use of this product is restricted to the buyer or, for library copies, authorized users.
- Sharing passwords is not permitted. The publisher has the right to take legal steps for violations.
- Access to online material is solely provided to the buyer for private use. Commercial use is not permitted.

Connect with us on social media

Thieme

AOTRAUMA

Michael Blauth, Stephen L Kates, Joseph A Nicholas

# Osteoporotic Fracture Care

Medical and Surgical Management

AOTRAUMA

Michael Blauth, Stephen L Kates, Joseph A Nicholas

# Osteoporotic Fracture Care

## Medical and Surgical Management

More than 1,000 high-quality x-rays, clinical photographs, and illustrations

Library of Congress Cataloging-in-Publication Data is available from the publisher.

**Hazards**

Great care has been taken to maintain the accuracy of the information contained in this publication. However, the publisher, and/or the distributor, and/or the editors, and/or the authors cannot be held responsible for errors or any consequences arising from the use of the information contained in this publication. Contributions published under the name of individual authors are statements and opinions solely of said authors and not of the publisher, and/or the distributor, and/or the AO Group.

The products, procedures, and therapies described in this work are hazardous and are therefore only to be applied by certified and trained medical professionals in environments specially designed for such procedures. No suggested test or procedure should be carried out unless, in the user's professional judgment, its risk is justified. Whoever applies products, procedures, and therapies shown or described in this work will do this at their own risk. Because of rapid advances in the medical sciences, AO recommends that independent verification of diagnosis, therapies, drugs, dosages, and operation methods should be made before any action is taken.

Although all advertising material which may be inserted into the work is expected to conform to ethical (medical) standards, inclusion in this publication does not constitute a guarantee or endorsement by the publisher regarding quality or value of such product or of the claims made of it by its manufacturer.

**Legal restrictions**

This work was produced by AO Foundation, Switzerland. All rights reserved by AO Foundation. This publication, including all parts thereof, is legally protected by copyright.

Any use, exploitation or commercialization outside the narrow limits set forth by copyright legislation and the restrictions on use laid out below, without the publisher's consent, is illegal and liable to prosecution. This applies in particular to photostat reproduction, copying, scanning or duplication of any kind, translation, preparation of microfilms, electronic data processing, and storage such as making this publication available on Intranet or Internet.

Some of the products, names, instruments, treatments, logos, designs, etc referred to in this publication are also protected by patents and trademarks or by other intellectual property protection laws (eg, "AO", "ASIF", "AO/ASIF", "TRIANGLE/GLOBE Logo" are registered trademarks) even though specific reference to this fact is not always made in the text. Therefore, the appearance of a name, instrument, etc without designation as proprietary is not to be construed as a representation by the publisher that it is in the public domain.

Restrictions on use: The rightful owner of an authorized copy of this work may use it for educational and research purposes only. Single images or illustrations may be copied for research or educational purposes only. The images or illustrations may not be altered in any way and need to carry the following statement of origin "Copyright by AO Foundation, Switzerland".

Check hazards and legal restrictions on www.aofoundation.org/legal

Copyright © 2018 by AO Foundation, Clavadelerstrasse 8, 7270 Davos Platz, Switzerland

Distribution by Georg Thieme Verlag, Rüdigerstrasse 14, 70469 Stuttgart, Germany, and Thieme New York, 333 Seventh Avenue, New York, NY 10001, USA

ISBN: 9783132427518
e-ISBN: 9783132427525

1 2 3 4 5 6

# Foreword

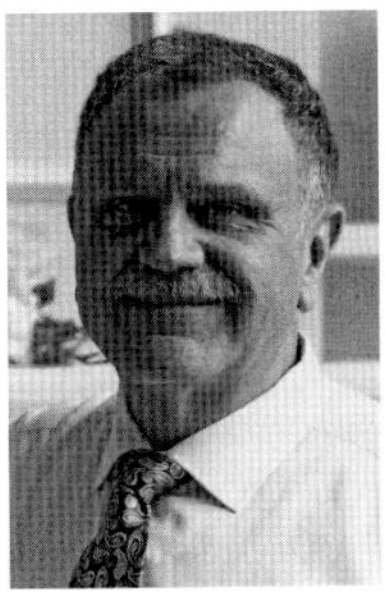

**Steven A Olson**, MD
Professor in Orthopaedic Surgery
Duke University School of Medicine
Durham, NC 27710
USA

When Dr Kates asked me if I was interested in writing a foreword for the *Osteoporotic Fracture Care* book, I could not refuse. Having worked with Dr Kates on issues involving insufficiency fracture care as both a colleague and friend, I understand the passion and commitment that has been brought to this textbook.

The care of the young male high-energy trauma patient often dominates the focus of trauma education. The care of the older adult with osteoporotic fractures often seems to be of less interest in both trauma education and research. This AO book entitled *Osteoporotic Fracture Care* provides an important reminder of why this area is of key importance in healthcare today for all of us. A recent report found the burden of hospitalization of women over age 55 in the US for osteoporotic fractures is greater than the hospitalization burden for myocardial infarction, stroke, or breast cancer [1].

Multiple important topics are covered in this textbook including societal impact of the clinical problem of osteoporotic fractures as well as important current perspectives in all aspects of patient care.

The outline of the book spans the entire scope of care including basic pathophysiology, clinical assessment, patient-specific considerations in determining treatment, and specific recommendations for pre-, intra-, and postoperative care; it also covers templated order sets to facilitate the care of the osteoporotic fracture patient and strategies for secondary osteoporotic fracture prevention. This is a thorough and well-written reference work for all musculoskeletal care providers who treat patients with osteoporotic fractures. I hope you find this textbook a useful reference.

Durham, November 2017

1. **Singer A, Exuzides A, Spangler L, et al.** Burden of illness for osteoporotic fractures compared with other serious diseases among postmenopausal women in the United States. *Mayo Clin Proc.* 2015 Jan;90(1):53–62.

# Preface

The inspiration for this textbook comes from the vibrant AOTrauma Care of the Geriatric Fracture Patient courses held across the world, as orthogeriatric care education has been pushed to the forefront for orthopedic surgeons, medical physicians, and other care teams involved in care of the fragility fracture patient. These innovative and interactive courses were launched in Rochester, NY, USA, in 2006 under the leadership of Dr Stephen Kates and Dr Daniel Mendelson and introduced into the AO Courses in Davos in December 2007 by Drs Michael Blauth, Stephen Kates, and Daniel Mendelson as the first truly interdisciplinary course in AO followed by a worldwide rollout. They continue to provide the best in evidence-based medicine, geriatric principles, and clinical experience to promote better care for older adults undergoing orthopedic surgery. From an academic standpoint, these courses bring together some of the most prominent orthopedic and geriatric medicine faculty in this emerging field. From an educational and clinical standpoint, these courses are inspirational and invigorating, designed for clinicians to share current experiences, learn new fracture reduction and fixation techniques, consider the unique physiology of geriatric patients, and begin to design systems of care that dramatically improve patient outcomes and reduce system costs. The content of these courses inevitably changes the way the faculty and the attendees practice. This textbook aims to capture the essential evidence and clinical principles so well identified during these courses.

In order to develop innovative teaching methods for these truly interdisciplinary courses, AO launched an Orthogeriatric Task Force that is still active. Another product that came out of this task force is an Orthogeriatric App about the management of osteoporosis, delirium, pain, and anticoagulation that can be downloaded free of charge.

Optimal outcomes for fragility fracture patients depend on excellent surgical care of osteoporotic bone, incorporation of geriatric medicine into the routine care pathways, and construction of new systems of care. To address these areas, this book is organized into three sections:

The *Principles* section outlines the unique medical, surgical, and anesthesia needs of fragility fracture patients; these chapters focus on practical approaches to the most common and important clinical issues facing the geriatric fracture patient. We aim to create a basic understanding of why older adult patients benefit significantly from an adapted management and environment compared to younger adult patients, analogous to the approach to pediatric patients.

In the section *Improving the system of care*, physicians and administrators present chapters with local, regional, and national health delivery changes that are necessary to optimize patient outcomes.

The majority of the textbook is devoted to *Fracture management*; this section is focused on expert and specific surgical management of the wide array of fragility fractures as they present to most physicians and hospitals worldwide.

The impact of the dramatic demographic shift of the world's population and the explosion in fragility fractures demands that health systems and physicians be willing to update their clinical approaches, improve their understanding of the needs of older adults, and develop interprofessional and interdisciplinary systems to manage complex and frail patients safely and efficiently.

We hope this textbook will support the necessary revolution in care for orthogeriatric patients, their families, and the clinicians caring for them.

Michael Blauth, MD
Stephen L Kates, MD
Joseph A Nicholas, MD

# Acknowledgments

It would not have been possible to produce and publish the *Osteoporotic Fracture Care* textbook without the dedication and support of an extensive list of contributors. From hard-working AO surgeons donating their time and expertise, to colleagues volunteering case notes and images, to our staff within our own medical institutions, and to the teams at AOTrauma and AO Education Institute, we thank you for assisting us in developing this publication.

While there are many people to thank, we would especially like to mention these individuals:

- Members of the AOTrauma Education Commission for recognizing the importance and significance of this educational opportunity and for approving the development of this publication.
- Urs Rüetschi, Robin Greene, and Michael Cunningham from the AO Education Institute for their guidance and expertise and for enabling extensive resources and staff to prepare this publication and make it into the best publication possible.
- The authors, our colleagues from around the world, who provided chapters, cases, and images.
- Steven Olson for writing the Foreword to this book.
- Carl Lau, Manager Publishing, and Katalin Fekete, Project Manager for this project, plus Michael Gleeson, Amber Parkinson, Irene Contreras, Jecca Reichmuth, and Vidula Bhoyroo for their professional support.
- Tom Wirth from Nougat who was responsible for the overall layout of this book and for taking in the many rounds of editorial corrections.
- And lastly, to our families for their unwavering support and encouragement throughout this project.

Michael Blauth, MD
Stephen L Kates, MD
Joseph A Nicholas, MD

# Contributors

## Editors

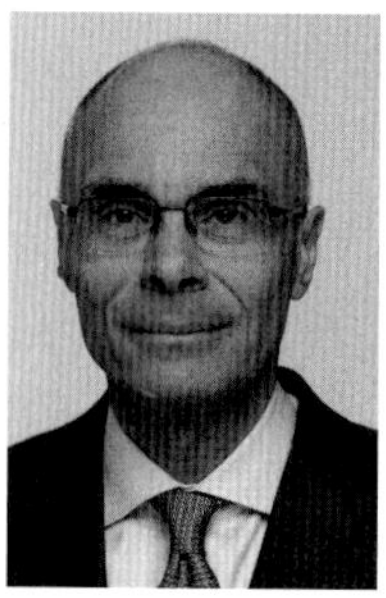

**Michael Blauth**, MD
Professor and Director
Department for Trauma Surgery
Medical University Innsbruck
Anichstrasse 35
Innsbruck 6020
Austria

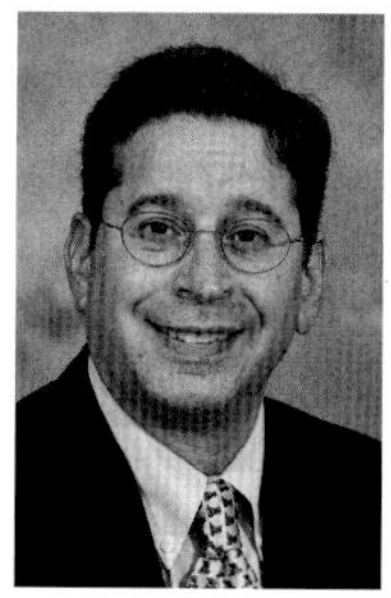

**Stephen L Kates**, MD
Professor and Chair of Orthopaedic Surgery
Virginia Commonwealth University
Department of Orthopaedic Surgery
1200 E. Broad St
Richmond, VA 23298
USA

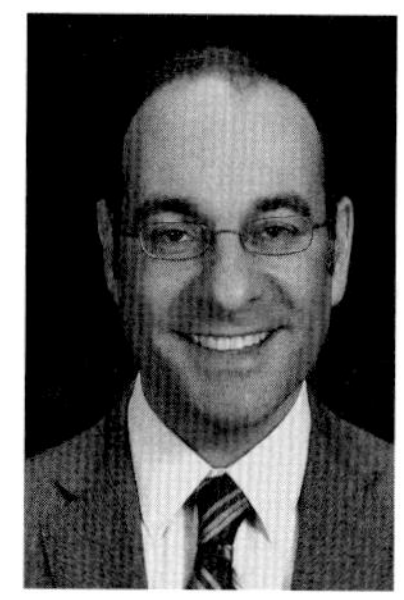

**Joseph A Nicholas**, MD, MPH
Associate Professor of Medicine
Geriatrics Division
University of Rochester
Highland Hospital
Rochester, NY 14620
USA

## Authors

**Rohit Arora**, PD Dr med
Associate Professor
Deputy Director Department of Trauma Surgery
Medical University Innsbruck
Anichstrasse 35
6020 Innsbruck
Austria

**Reto Babst**, Prof Dr med
Vorsteher Department Chirurgie
Chefarzt Unfallchirurgie
Klinik Orthopädie und Unfallchirurgie
Luzerner Kantonsspital
6000 Lucerne 16
Switzerland

**Peter Brink**
Benzenrade 15c
6419 PG
Heerlen
The Netherlands

**Adeela Cheema**, MD
Geriatrics Fellow
Section of Geriatrics & Palliative Medicine
5841 S. Maryland Ave
Chicago, IL 60637
USA

**Colin Currie**
17 Merchiston Gardens
Edinburgh EH10 5DD
UK

**Nemer Dabage**, MD FACP
Program Director at Blake Medical Center
2020 59th Street West
Bradenton, FL 34209
USA

**Christian CMA Donken**, MD, PhD
Department of Orthopedic Surgery
Sint Maartenskliniek
Hengstdal 3
P.O. Box 9011
6500 GM Nijmegen
The Netherlands

**Simon Euler**, PD Dr med
Facharzt für Unfallchirurgie
Klinik für Unfallchirurgie und Sporttraumatologie
Medizinische Universität Innsbruck
Anichstrasse 35
6020 Innsbruck
Austria

**Susan M Friedman**, MD, MPH, AGS
Associate Professor of Medicine
University of Rochester School of Medicine and Dentistry
Department of Medicine
Highland Hospital
1000 South Avenue, Box 58
Rochester, NY 14620
USA

**Elizabeth B Gausden**, MD, MPH
Orthopaedic Surgery Resident
Hospital for Special Surgery
535 E 70th St
New York, NY 10021
USA

**Andrea Giusti**, MD
ASL3
Department of Locomotor System
Via Casaregis 24/19
16129 Genoa
Italy

**Lauren J Gleason**, MD, MPH
Assistant Professor of Medicine
University of Chicago Medicine
5841 S. Maryland Avenue, MC 6098
Chicago, IL 60637
USA

**Claudia M Gonzalez Suarez**, MD
Thompson Health Family Practice Macedon
350 Parrish Street Canandaigua, NY 14424
1033 State Route 31
Macedon NY 14502-8218
USA

**Markus Gosch**, Dr med univ
Professor and Medical Director
Department for Geriatrics
Paracelsus Medical University Nuremberg, Germany
Nuremberg Hospital North
Prof.-Ernst-Nathan-Str. 1
Nuremberg 90419
Germany

**Michael Götzen**, Dr med, PhD
Univ.-Klinik für Unfallchirurgie
Zentrum Operative Medizin
Anichstrasse 35
6020 Innsbruck
Austria

**Clemens Hengg**, PD Dr med
Facharzt für Unfallchirurgie und Sporttraumatologie
Univ.-Klinik Innsbruck
Anichstrasse 35
6020 Innsbruck
Austria

**Alexander Hofmann**, Dr med
Professor, Chefarzt
Klinik für Unfallchirurgie und Orthopädie 1
Westpfalz-Klinikum GmbH
Hellmut-Hartert Strasse 1
67655 Kaiserslautern
Germany

**Timothy J Holahan**, DO, CMD
Senior Clinical Instructor of Medicine
University of Rochester Medical Center
Highland Hospital
1000 South Avenue
Rochester, NY 14620
USA

**Hans-Christian Jeske**, Prof Dr med
Univ.-Klinik für Unfallchirurgie und Sportmedizin
Medizinische Universität Innsbruck
Anichstrasse 35
6020 Innsbruck
Austria

**Herman Johal**, MD, MPH, Phd(c) FRCSC
McMaster Orthopaedics
Centre for Evidence-based Orthopaedics
293 Wellington Street North, Suite 110
Hamilton, Ontario
Canada L8L 8E7

**Peter Kaiser**, Dr med univ, PhD
Univ.-Klinik für Unfallchirurgie
Zentrum Operative Medizin
Medizinische Universität Innsbruck
Anichstrasse 35
6020 Innsbruck
Austria

**Christian Kammerlander**, PD Dr med
Vice Director
Ludwig Maximilian University Munich
Department for General, Trauma- &
Reconstructive Surgery
Marchioninistrasse 15
81377 Munich
Germany

**Alexander Keiler**, Dr med
Univ.-Klinik für Unfallchirurgie
Anichstrasse 35
6020 Innsbruck
Austria

**Marco Keller**, Dr med
Department of Trauma Surgery
Medical University Innsbruck
Anichstrasse 35
6020 Innsbruck
Austria

**Rashmi Khadilkar**, MD
Senior Instructor of Medicine
Department of Medicine
Highland Hospital
1000 South Avenue, Box HH 58
Rochester, NY 14620
USA

**Joon-Woo Kim**, MD, PhD
Assistant Professor
Department of Orthopedic Surgery
School of Medicine
Kyungpook National University Hospital
130, Dongduk-ro, Jung-gu
Daegu, 41944
South Korea

**Franz Kralinger**, PD Dr
Abteilungsleiter Unfallchirurgie
und Sporttraumatologie
Wilhelminenspital
Montlearstrasse 37
1160 Vienna
Austria

**Dietmar Krappinger**, PD, MD, PhD, MBA
Head of Pelvic and Acetabular Surgery
Head of Bone Reconstruction Surgery
Senior Consultant Spine Surgery
Department of Trauma Surgery
Medical University Innsbruck
Anichstrasse 35
6020 Innsbruck
Austria

**Malikah Latmore**, MD
Assistant Professor of Clinical Anesthesiology
Mount Sinai St. Luke's and Mount Sinai West
Hospitals
1111 Amsterdam Ave
New York, NY 10025
USA

**Richard A Lindtner**, MD, PhD
Consultant
Department of Trauma Surgery
Medical University of Innsbruck
Anichstrasse 35
6020 Innsbruck
Austria

**Björn-Christian Link**, Dr med
Leitender Arzt
Klinik für Orthopädie und Unfallchirurgie
Luzerner Kantonsspital Luzern
Spitalstrasse
6000 Lucerne 16
Switzerland

**Frank A Liporace**, MD
Chairman and Vice President
Chief Orthopedic Trauma and Adult Reconstruction
Jersey City Medical Center
RWJ Barnabas Health Orthopedic Group
(Jersey City)
377 Jersey Ave
Suite 280-A
Jersey City, NJ 07302
USA

**Dean G Lorich**, MD
Associate Director of the Orthopedic Trauma Service
Hospital for Special Surgery
535 E 70th St
New York, NY 10021
USA

**Justinder Malhotra**, MD
QueensCare Health Center
150 North Reno St
Los Angeles, CA 90026
USA

**Edgar Mayr**, Dr med, Dr h.c.
Professor and Head of Trauma, Orthopaedics,
Plastic and Hand Surgery
Klinikum Augsburg
Stenglinstrasse 2
86156 Augsburg
Germany

**Iain McFadyen**, MBChB, MRCS (Ed), FRCS (Tr & Orth)
Consultant Orthopaedic Surgeon
University Hospitals of North Midlands
Newcastle Road
Stoke-on-Trent
Staffordshire ST4 6GQ
UK

**Simon C Mears**, MD, PhD
Department of Orthopaedic Surgery
University of Arkansas for Medical Services
4301 W Markham St
Little Rock, AR 72205
USA

**Daniel A Mendelson**, MS, MD
Konar Professor, Division of Geriatrics
University of Rochester
Associate Chief of Medicine, Director of Palliative Care & Co-Director of Geriatric Fracture Center
Highland Hospital
1000 South Avenue
Rochester, NY 14620-2733
USA

**Paul J Mitchell**, BSc (hons), CChem, MRSC
Adjunct Senior Lecturer
School of Medicine
Sydney Campus
The University of Notre Dame Australia
140 Broadway
Chippendale NSW
Australia

**Jennifer D Muniak**, MD
Senior Instructor of Medicine
Department of Medicine
Highland Hospital
1000 South Avenue
Rochester, NY 14620
USA

**Carl Neuerburg**, PD Dr med
Oberarzt, stellv. Leiter Alterstraumatologie
Klinik für Allgemeine-, Unfall- und Wiederherstellungschirurgie
Facharzt für Orthopädie und Unfallchirurgie
Klinikum der Universität München
Campus Grosshadern
Marchioninistrasse 15
81377 Munich
Germany

**Chang-Wug Oh**, MD
Professor
Department of Orthopedic Surgery
School of Medicine, Kyungpook National University
Kyungpook National University Hospital
130 Dongdeok-ro, Jung-gu
Daegu 41944
South Korea

**Jong-Keon Oh**
Director, Department of Orthopaedic Surgery
Korea University College of Medicine
Guro Hospital
97 Gurodong-gil, Guro-gu
Seoul 152-703
South Korea

**Vajara Phiphobmongkol**, MD
Department of Orthopedic Sugery
Bangkok Hospital
2 Soi Soonvijai 7, New Petchburi Rd.
Huai Khwang
Bangken, Bangkok, 10310
Thailand

**Giulio Pioli**, MD, PhD
Geriatrics Unit
Department of Neuromotor Physiology
ASMN – IRCCS Hospital
Viale Risorgimento, 80
42100 Reggio Emilia
Italy

**Philippe Posso**, med pract
Luzerner Kantonsspital
Spitalstrasse 16
6000 Lucerne
Switzerland

**Andrew J Pugely**, MD
Assistant Professor of Orthopedics and Rehabilitation
Office: 01025 John Pappajohn
University of Iowa
200 Hawkins Drive
Iowa City, IA 52242
USA

**Herbert Resch**, Prof Dr med
Dean, Paracelsus Medical University
Strubergasse 21
5020 Salzburg
Austria

**Bernardo Reyes Fernandez**, MD
Associate Director Internal Medicine Residency and Director of Geriatrics and Palliative Care
Charles E. Schmidt College of Medicine
Florida Atlantic University
777 Glades Road
Boca Raton, FL 33431
USA

**Pol M Rommens**, Dr med, Dr h.c.
Professor, Direktor Zentrum für Orthopädie und Unfallchirurgie
Director Department of Orthopaedics and Traumatology
Universitätsmedizin der Johannes Gutenberg-Universität Mainz
Langenbeckstrasse 1
55131 Mainz
Germany

**Krupa Shah**, MD, MPH
Associate Professor of Medicine
Highland Hospital
1000 South Avenue
Department of Medicine, Box 58
Rochester, NY 14620
USA

**Ali Shariat**, MD
Clinical Assistant Professor of Anesthesiology
The Mount Sinai Hospital
Mount Sinai St. Luke's and Mount Sinai West Hospitals
1111 Amsterdam Ave
New York, NY 10025
USA

**Darby Sider**, MD
Vice-Chair, Department of Internal Medicine, Cleveland Clinic Florida
Program Director, Internal Medicine Residency, Cleveland Clinic Florida
2950 Cleveland Clinic Blvd
Dept of Internal Medicine
Weston, Florida 33331
USA

**Kerstin Simon**, Dr med univ
Trauma Surgery Resident
Department of Trauma Surgery
Medical University Innsbruck
Anichstrasse 35
6020 Innsbruck
Austria

**Katrin Singler**, PD Dr med, MME
Geriatric Department
Associate Professor
Klinikum Nürnberg Nord
Prof. Ernst Nathan Strasse 1
90419 Nürnberg
Germany

**Christoph Sommer**, Dr med
Kantonsspital Graubünden
Chefarzt Allgemein- und Unfallchirurgie
Departement Chirurgie
Loëstrasse 170
7000 Chur
Switzerland

**Karl Stoffel**, Prof Dr med, FRACS (Orth), FAOrth (Tr)
Co-Chefarzt Orthopädie und Traumatologie
Kantonsspital Baselland
Teamleiter Hüft/Beckenchirurgie und
Leiter Traumatologie
Facharzt für Orthopädie und Traumatologie
des Bewegungsapparates
Fellow Royal Australasian College of Surgeons
Kantonsspital Baselland
Standort Bruderholz
4101 Bruderholz
Switzerland

**Susanne Strasser**, Dr med, PhD
Univ.-Klinik für Unfallchirurgie
Medizinische Universität Innsbruck
Anichstrasse 35
6020 Innsbruck
Austria

**Julie A Switzer**, MD
Department of Orthopaedic Surgery
Associate Professor, University of Minnesota
Director, Geriatric Trauma Program, Regions Hospital
640 Jackson St
Mail stop: 11503L
St Paul, MN 55101
USA

**Joshua Uy**, MD
Associate Professor of Clinical Medicine
Geriatric medicine fellowship program director
Medical Director, Renaissance Healthcare &
Rehabilitation Center (formerly Park Pleasant)
University of Pennsylvania
Ralston-Penn Center
3615 Chestnut Street
Philadelphia, PA 19104
USA

**Steven Velkes**
Head of Orthopedic Surgery
Rabin Medical Center
Petah Tikva 49100
Israel

**Michael HJ Verhofstad**, Dr med
Professor
Chair of trauma and orthopedic trauma surgery
Department of Surgery
Erasmus MC, University Medical Center Rotterdam
P.O. Box 2040
3000 CA Rotterdam
The Netherlands

**Richard S Yoon**, MD
Director, Orthopaedic Research
Division of Orthopaedic Trauma and
Adult Reconstruction
Department of Orthopaedic Surgery
Jersey City Medical Center – RWJBarnabas Health
377 Jersey Ave, Suite 280A
Jersey City, NJ 07302
USA

# Abbreviations

| | |
|---|---|
| **AAOS** | American Academy of Orthopaedic Surgeons |
| **ABCDE** | airway, breathing, circulation, disability, exposure/examination |
| **ACC** | American College of Cardiology |
| **ACCP** | American College of Chest Physicians |
| **ACE** | angiotensin-converting enzyme |
| **ACEI** | angiotensin-converting enzyme inhibitors |
| **ACL** | anterior cruciate ligament |
| **ADL** | activity of daily living |
| **AF** | ankle fracture (chapter 3.17 Ankle) |
| **AF** | atrial fibrillation |
| **AFF** | atypical femoral fracture |
| **AFN** | antegrade femoral nail |
| **AGS** | American Geriatrics Society |
| **AHA** | American Heart Association |
| **ANZHFR** | Australian and New Zealand Hip Fracture Registry |
| **AO** | Arbeitsgemeinschaft für Osteosynthesefragen |
| **AOCID** | AO Clinical Investigation and Documentation |
| **AP** | anteroposterior |
| **APL** | abductor pollicis longus |
| **aPTT** | activated partial thromboplastin time |
| **ARIF** | arthroscopy-assisted reduction and internal fixation |
| **ARB** | angiotensin receptor blockers |
| **ASA** | American Society of Anesthesiologists |
| **ASBMR** | American Society for Bone and Mineral Research |
| **ASIS** | anterior superior iliac spine |
| **ASLS** | angular stable locking system |
| **ATE** | arterial thromboembolism |
| **ATLS** | advanced trauma life support |
| **AVN** | avascular necrosis |
| | |
| **BGS** | British Geriatrics Society |
| **BIPAP** | biphasic positive airway pressure |
| **BMD** | bone mineral density |
| **BMI** | body mass index |
| **BOA** | British Orthopaedic Association |
| **BP** | bisphosphonate |
| **BPF** | best practice framework |
| **BPT** | Best Practice Tariff |
| | |
| **CAD** | coronary artery disease |
| **CAM** | Confusion Assessment Method |
| **CCD** | caput-collum-diaphyseal (angle) |
| **CCI** | Charlson Comorbidity Index |
| **C-clamp** | compression clamp (for pelvis) |
| **CGA** | comprehensive geriatric assessment |
| **CGC** | clinical practice guidelines |
| **CHF** | congestive heart failure |
| **CI** | confidence interval |
| **COPD** | chronic obstructive pulmonary disease |
| **CPG** | clinical practice guidelines |
| **CPM** | continuous passive motion |
| **CRP** | cardiopulmonary resuscitation |
| **CRPS** | complex regional pain syndrome |
| **CSF** | cerebrospinal fluid |
| **CT** | computed tomography |
| **CVA** | cerebrovascular accident |
| **CVD** | cardiovascular disease |
| | |
| **DASH** | Disabilities of the Arm, Shoulder and Hand |
| **DECT** | dual-energy computed tomography |
| **DEXA** | dual energy x-ray absorptiometry |
| **DFF** | distal forearm fracture (chapter 3.6 Distal forearm) |
| **DFF** | distal femoral fracture (chapter 3.12 Distal femur) |
| **DFR** | distal femoral replacement |
| **DHF** | distal humeral fracture |
| **DFN** | distal femoral nail |
| **DHS** | dynamic hip screw |
| **DM** | diabetes mellitus |
| **DOSS** | Delirium Observation Screening Scale |
| **DRF** | distal radial fracture |
| **DRG** | diagnosis-related group |
| **DRUJ** | distal radioulnar joint |
| **DSM-V** | Diagnostic and Statistical Manual of Mental Disorders |
| **DUF** | distal ulnar fracture |
| **DVT** | deep vein thrombosis |
| | |
| **EF** | external fixator |
| **EFD** | elbow fracture dislocation |
| **EPL** | extensor pollicis longus |
| | |
| **FAITH** | Fixation using Alternative Implants for the Treatment of Hip fractures |
| **FCR** | flexor carpi radialis |
| **FCU** | flexor carpi ulnaris |
| **FDA** | Food and Drug Administration |
| **FFN** | Fragility Fracture Network |
| **FFP** | fragility fracture patient (all chapters except 3.7 Pelvic ring) |
| **FFP** | fragility fracture of the pelvic ring (only in chapter 3.7 Pelvic ring) |

| | |
|---|---|
| **FLS** | fracture liaison service |
| **FRAX** | Fracture Risk Assessment |
| **FSF** | femoral shaft fracture |
| **FWB** | full weight bearing |
| **FWBAT** | full weight bearing as tolerated |
| **GA** | general anesthesia |
| **GAF** | geriatric acetabular fracture |
| **GI** | gastrointestinal |
| **GCS** | Glasgow Coma Scale |
| **GORU** | geriatric orthopedic rehabilitation unit |
| **GP** | general practitioner |
| **GT** | greater tuberosity (chapter 3.1 Proximal humerus) |
| **GT** | greater trochanter (chapter 3.13 Periprosthetic fractures around the hip) |
| **HBR** | home-based rehabilitation |
| **HO** | heterotopic ossification |
| **HRQoL** | health-related quality of life |
| **HSA** | head-shaft angle |
| **HTN** | hypertension |
| **HU** | Hounsfield Unit |
| **IADL** | instrumental activity of daily living |
| **ICD** | implantable cardioverter defibrillator |
| **ICU** | intensive care unit |
| **IGF** | insulin-like growth factor |
| **IKS** | International Knee Score |
| **IL** | interleukin |
| **IM** | intramedullary |
| **INR** | international normalized ratio |
| **IOF** | International Osteoporosis Foundation |
| **IPCD** | intermittent pneumatic compression devices |
| **IQR** | interquartile range |
| **IR** | internal rotation |
| **IRF** | inpatient rehabilitation facility |
| **ISP** | Infraspinatus (muscle/tendon) |
| **ISS** | Injury Severity Score |
| **IU** | International units |
| **IV** | intravenous |
| **IVC** | inferior vena cava |
| **K-wire** | Kirschner wire |
| **KSS** | Knee Society Score |
| **LAP** | locking attachment plate |
| **LBD** | local bone density |
| **LBQ** | local bone quality |
| **LC-DCP** | limited-contact dynamic compression plate |
| **LCP-DF** | reversed distal femoral locking compression plate |
| **LCL** | lateral collateral ligament |
| **LCP** | locking compression plate |
| **LHB** | long head of the biceps |
| **LHS** | locking head screw |
| **LISS** | less invasive stabilization system |
| **LMWH** | low-molecular-weight heparin |
| **LOS** | length of hospital stay |
| **LP** | locked plating |
| **LT** | lesser tuberosity (chapter 3.1 Proximal humerus) |
| **LT** | lesser trochanter (chapters 3.13 Periprosthetic fractures around the hip, 3.14 Periprosthetic fractures around the knee) |
| **MCD** | minimum common dataset |
| **MCL** | medial collateral ligament |
| **MET** | metabolic equivalent |
| **MGF** | mechano growth factor |
| **MI** | myocardial infarction |
| **MIPO** | minimally invasive plate osteosynthesis |
| **MIPPO** | minimally invasive percutaneous extraperiostally plate osteosynthesis |
| **MIS** | minimally invasive surgery |
| **MNA** | Mini-Nutritional Assessment |
| **MRI** | magnetic resonance imaging |
| **MVA** | motor vehicle accident |
| **NA** | neuraxial |
| **NHFD** | National Hip Fracture Database |
| **NHFS** | Nottingham Hip Fracture Score |
| **NHS** | National Health Service |
| **NICE** | National Institute for Health and Care Excellence |
| **NMS** | New Mobility Score |
| **NOAC** | new oral anticoagulant |
| **NPWT** | negative-pressure wound therapy, also called vacuum-assisted wound closure (VAC) |
| **NRS** | numerical rating scale |
| **NSAIDs** | nonsteroidal antiinflammatory drugs |
| **NOF** | National Osteoporosis Foundation |
| **OGU** | Orthogeriatric unit |
| **ONJ** | osteonecrosis of the jaw |
| **ONS** | oral nutrition supplements |
| **ORIF** | open reduction and internal fixation |
| **OTA** | Orthopaedic Trauma Association |
| **PACU** | postanesthesia care unit |
| **PADL** | personal activity of daily living |
| **PCA** | patient-controlled analgesia |
| **PCC** | prothrombin complex concentrate |

| | |
|---|---|
| **PCM** | perioperative cardiac morbidity |
| **PDCA** | plan-do-check-act |
| **PDPH** | postdural puncture headache |
| **PE** | pulmonary embolism |
| **PET-CT** | positron emission tomography combined with computerized tomography |
| **PFN** | proximal femoral nail |
| **PFNA** | proximal femoral nail antirotation |
| **PHF** | proximal humeral fracture |
| **PHILOS** | proximal humerus internal locked system |
| **PMMA** | polymethylmethacrylate |
| **POMA** | performance-oriented mobility assessment |
| **PROM** | patient-reported outcome measure |
| **PPHF** | periprosthetic hip fracture |
| **PPI** | proton pump inhibitors |
| **PPKF** | periprosthetic fractures around the knee |
| **PPS** | prospective payment system |
| **PROM** | patient-reported outcome measures |
| **PRWE** | Patient-Rated Wrist Evaluation |
| **PSIS** | posterior superior iliac spine |
| **PTF** | proximal tibial fracture |
| **PTH** | parathyroid hormone |
| **PTS** | postthrombotic syndrome |
| **PWB** | partial weight bearing |
| **PWBAT** | partial weight bearing as tolerated |
| **QALY** | quality-adjusted life year |
| **RA** | regional anesthesia |
| **RCRI** | Revised Cardiac Risk Index |
| **RCT** | randomized controlled trial |
| **ROI** | region of interest |
| **ROM** | range of motion |
| **RSA** | reverse shoulder arthroplasty |
| **SAHFE** | Standardized Audit of Hip Fracture in Europe |
| **SD** | standard deviation |
| **SERM** | estrogens, selective estrogen receptor modulator |
| **SHA** | shoulder hemiarthroplasty |
| **SNF** | skilled nursing facility |
| **SPPB** | short physical performance battery |
| **SQ** | subcutaneous |
| **SSC** | subscapularis |
| **SSP** | supraspinatus (muscle/tendon) |
| **TAD** | tip-apex distance |
| **Tc** | technetium |
| **TEA** | total elbow arthroplasty |
| **TENS** | transcutaneous electrical nerve stimulation |
| **TFCC** | triangular fibrocartilaginous complex |
| **TFN** | trochanteric femoral nail |
| **THA** | total hip arthroplasty |
| **TIA** | transient cerebral ischemia attack |
| **TKA** | total knee arthroplasty |
| **TNF-α** | tumor necrosis factor α |
| **TSF** | tibial shaft fracture |
| **TSH** | thyroid-stimulating hormone |
| **TUG** | Timed Up and Go test |
| **UCS** | Unified Classification System |
| **UFH** | unfractionated heparin |
| **UTI** | urinary tract infection |
| **VAS** | Visual Analog Scale |
| **VDS** | Verbal Descriptor Scale |
| **VTE** | venous thromboembolism |
| **WBAT** | weight bearing as tolerated |
| **WHO** | World Health Organization |

# Online AO Educational Content

Abundant online educational offerings from across AO are accessible through the QR codes printed on each chapter title page. Using a QR code scanner on a mobile device, readers will be taken to specific chapter microsites that contain supplemental AO educational content curated by the book editors specifically for that chapter topic.

Links to supplemental AO educational content include:

- AO Surgery Reference
- Webinars and webcasts
- Lectures
- Teaching videos
- eLearning modules
- Mobile apps

As the array of online AO educational resources evolves and develops, the offerings in the chapter microsites will be regularly reviewed and updated by the book editors. This will ensure that readers are linked to the latest in AO education.

# Table of Contents

# Section 1
# Principles

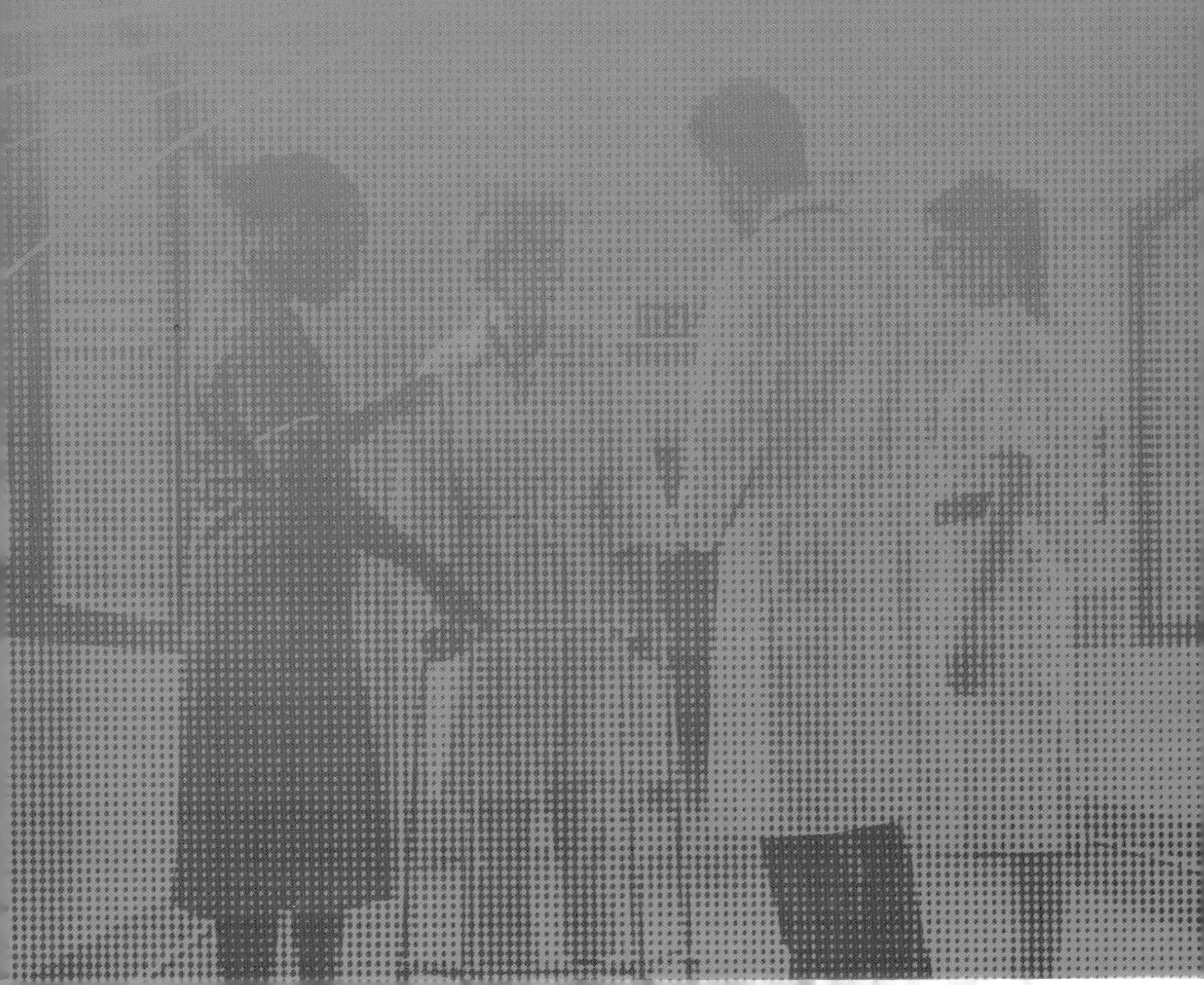

# Section 1
## Principles

# 1.1 Principles of orthogeriatric medical care

Joseph A Nicholas

## 1 Introduction

Despite the large amount of surgical care delivered to older adults [1], perioperative practice remains inappropriately anchored to the surgical experience of more robust and less comorbid patients. At best, many common and accepted approaches to specific illnesses are ineffective in older adults, and at worst, these practices contribute to serious morbidity and mortality [2, 3]. The negative impact of usual medical and surgical care is most pronounced in frail and medically complicated patients [4, 5].

The typical fragility fracture patient (FFP) is emblematic of patients for whom usual medical care is often the wrong care. To those who treat and research this population, it is not surprising that superior postoperative outcomes have been found through unique clinical and systems approaches to the geriatric patient [6, 7], strategies that often diverge from the types of medical investigations and treatments used in most care settings.

Fortunately, there is growing evidence that improved clinical outcomes can be obtained in frail older adults with osteoporotic fractures through the incorporation of a relatively small number of standard approaches and clinical pathways [8]. The major barriers to implementing these approaches are not technological or financial but involve an understanding and commitment to creating systems and expertise that focus on standardizing care, avoiding adverse events, and adapting treatments to the unique physiology and prognosis of the older adult.

While the details of such care will change as the evidence base expands, we expect the basic strategies outlined in this book to remain relevant for years to come. In the chapters that follow, readers will be introduced to the principles and specifics of caring for the typical FFP, based on the improved outcomes produced by orthogeriatric comanagement in organized fracture center programs. To set the stage, there are a number of principles that are important to recognize.

## 2 Key principles

### 2.1 Older adults are not simply adults with more illnesses

Compared with younger adults, older adults have unique physiologies, regardless of the presence or absence of specific comorbidities [9, 10]. Aging results in biological changes that render the older adult more susceptible to the harms of immobility, diagnostic tests, and medication effects. For this reason, many common medical practices can be ineffective or harmful in older adults. Examples include exaggerated hypotension in the presence of anesthetics and blood loss, low thresholds for delirium, complications due to polypharmacy, and rapid functional decline with immobility. This general decreased ability to respond to physiological stress is best described as frailty [11].

### 2.2 Hip fracture surgery can be performed safely and effectively even on frail patients

High-performing hip fracture centers produce low short-term mortality rates (ie, less than 2%), even in populations with high degrees of frailty and comorbidity [6, 12]. Advances in anesthesia, implant technology allowing for early weight bearing as tolerated, orthopedic procedural improvements, and orthogeriatric comanagement all contribute to rapid, safe, and effective repair of the overwhelming majority of hip fracture patients. Urgent surgery in the optimized patient is now standard care to avoid the short-term harms of ongoing pain, blood loss, and immobility.

### 2.3 Age is not the most important indicator of risk or prognosis in hip fracture patients

While age is a general predictor for outcomes and complications, it is more helpful to base risk assessments and treatment decisions on functional status, cognitive status, and comorbidity [13]. Asking patients about their day-to-day life can help estimate operative risk, recovery potential, and life expectancy better than disease-based assessments.

## 2.4 Surgical delay and immobility leads to irreversible muscle loss in the older adult

Early surgery is superior [14] and essential for frail and comorbid patients. The medical and surgical team must constantly weigh the impact of functional decline and operative delay against operative risk. Even the frailest patients can usually be optimized quickly, repaired, and begin immediate full weight bearing and rehabilitation [15].

## 2.5 Get the patient moving as soon as possible

Because rapid loss of muscle mass and function is a fundamental issue resulting in poor overall outcomes [16], all care pathways should be optimized to support early mobility and rehabilitation. While surgical delay and bed rest orders are obvious factors, polypharmacy, excessive testing, frequent subspecialty consultation, and inadequate pain control are all common barriers to mobilization that need to be minimized. Early mobility provides the necessary physical and emotional stimulation [17] for healing and recovery and helps minimize skin breakdown, constipation, and neuromuscular wasting. Mobility can be the difference between rapid recovery and prolonged hospitalization.

## 2.6 Less is often more

Most FFPs have multiple comorbidities and abnormalities on diagnostic testing, many of which are chronic, clinically irrelevant, or unable to be improved. Unfortunately, this often results in excessive testing and consultation, overdiagnosis, and polypharmacy. Organized programs work hard to avoid these distractions, and focus instead on key areas like hemodynamic stability, pain control, prompt fracture reduction, and mobilization [18].

## 2.7 Many surgeons, internists, and specialists do not understand typical geriatric medical physiology

Regardless of professional training, unique geriatric responses to therapies are not adequately emphasized in most medical school and postgraduate training programs [19, 20]. Clinical experiences in geriatrics often fail to focus on acute care approaches, and subspecialty training in many medical and surgical disciplines does not typically promote adaptation of clinical expertise to frail older adults [21]. Competency in acute geriatric care does not require formal fellowship training, but can be achieved with a continuing medical education approach. Attending a course, viewing educational media, or visiting an established geriatric fracture program can help develop competency in caring for older adults.

## 2.8 Many geriatricians, internists, and specialists do not understand acute perioperative medicine

Current medical training offers little focus on the perioperative period. Other than performing outpatient preoperative risk assessments in relatively robust patients or planning an elective procedure, most internists, subspecialists, and geriatricians do not gain expertise in acute stabilization, optimization, and recovery of patients undergoing urgent surgery. Approaches to common medical issues are different in perioperative patients from those in typical medical admissions [22].

## 2.9 Very little high-quality evidence is applicable to the care of older adults

Most medical and surgical evidence is based on adults that are very different from the geriatric fracture patient [23]. Geriatric populations do not experience the same balance of benefits and harms younger, healthier, and more robust adults do. Rather than trying to comply with multiple disease-specific guidelines, high-performing geriatric fracture centers create strategies based on general geriatric principles, like avoiding polypharmacy, anticipating and managing delirium, and rapid restoration of mobility.

## 2.10 Recognize failing patients at the end of life

For many patients, falls and fragility fractures are the result of decompensated medical illnesses and frailty, and many will have a life expectancy of less than 6 months [24]. Failing patients do not respond well to usual medical care, suffering more harm than benefits from hospitalization, testing, and treatment. Early recognition of failing patients is important to identify achievable goals, set realistic expectations for the family and the clinical team, and to focus future care appropriately on end of life. Orthopedic surgery plays an essential role in pain control and quality of life. All clinicians involved in the care of FFPs need to have an ability to recognize the failing patient (ie, frailty).

## 2.11 Organized fracture programs work

There is no single surgical technique, preoperative risk assessment tool, or standard medical consultation that will produce ongoing results as good as an organized approach to the FFP. Investments in an organized program with geriatric comanagement will yield improvement in outcomes, costs, and both patient and physician satisfaction [8, 25]. Organized programs are becoming the standard of care in many medical and surgical communities [26], and even for other surgical problems [27, 28].

## 3 References


1. **Centers for Disease Control and Prevention.** Number of discharges from short-stay hospitals, by first-listed diagnosis and age: United States, 2010. Available at: www.cdc.gov/nchs/data/nhds/3firstlisted/2010first3_numberage.pdf. Accessed April 15, 2017.
2. **Gerstein HC, Miller ME, Byington RP, et al.** Effects of intensive glucose lowering in type 2 diabetes. *N Engl J Med.* 2008 Jun 12;358(24):2545–2559.
3. **Mossello E, Pieraccioli M, Nesti N, et al.** Effects of low blood pressure in cognitively impaired elderly patients treated with antihypertensive drugs. *JAMA Intern Med.* 2015 Apr;175(4):578–585.
4. **Odden MC, Peralta CA, Haan MN, et al.** Rethinking the association of high blood pressure with mortality in elderly adults: the impact of frailty. *Arch Intern Med.* 2012 Aug 13;172(15):1162–1168.
5. **Mosquera C, Spaniolas K, Fitzgerald TL.** Impact of frailty on surgical outcomes: The right patient for the right procedure. *Surgery.* 2016 Aug;160(2):272–280.
6. **Friedman SM, Mendelson DA, Bingham KW, et al.** Impact of a comanaged Geriatric Fracture Center on short-term hip fracture outcomes. *Arch Intern Med.* 2009 Oct 12;169(18):1712–1717.
7. **Kammerlander C, Gosch M, Blauth M, et al.** The Tyrolean Geriatric Fracture Center: an orthogeriatric co-management model. *Z Gerontol Geriatr.* 2011 Dec;44(6):363–367.
8. **Friedman SM, Mendelson DA, Kates SL, et al.** Geriatric co-management of proximal femur fractures: total quality management and protocol-driven care result in better outcomes for a frail patient population. *J Am Geriatr Soc.* 2008 Jul;56(7):1349–1356.
9. **Cheitlin MD.** Cardiovascular physiology-changes with aging. *Am J Geriatr Cardiol.* 2003 Jan–Feb;12(1):9–13.
10. **Walston J, Hadley EC, Ferrucci L, et al.** Research agenda for frailty in older adults: toward a better understanding of physiology and etiology: summary from the American Geriatrics Society/National Institute on Aging Research Conference on Frailty in Older Adults. *J Am Geriatr Soc.* 2006 Jun;54(6):991–1001.
11. **Fried LP, Tangen CM, Walston J, et al.** Frailty in older adults: evidence for a phenotype. *J Gerontol A Biol Sci Med Sci.* 2001 Mar;56(3):M146–M156.
12. **Brauer CA, Coca-Perraillon M, Cutler DM, et al.** Incidence and mortality of hip fractures in the United States. *JAMA.* 2009 Oct 14;302(14):1573–1579.
13. **Semel J, Gray JM, Ahn HJ, et al.** Predictors of outcome following hip fracture rehabilitation. *PM R.* 2010 Sep;2(9):799–805.
14. **Lefaivre KA, Macadam SA, Davidson DJ, et al.** Length of stay, mortality, morbidity and delay to surgery in hip fractures. *J Bone Joint Surg Br.* 2009 Jul;91(7):922–927.
15. **Keehan R, Rees D, Kendrick E, et al.** Enhanced recovery for fractured neck of femur: a report of 3 cases. *Geriatr Orthop Surg Rehabil.* 2014 Jun;5(2):37–42.
16. **Visser M, Harris TB, Fox KM, et al.** Change in muscle mass and muscle strength after a hip fracture: relationship to mobility recovery. *J Gerontol A Biol Sci Med Sci.* 2000 Aug;55(8):M434–M440.
17. **Kalisch BJ, Lee S, Dabney BW.** Outcomes of inpatient mobilization: a literature review. *J Clin Nurs.* 2014 Jun;23(11–12):1486–1501.
18. **Nicholas JA.** Preoperative optimization and risk assessment. *Clin Geriatr Med.* 2014 May;30(2):207–218.
19. **Monette M, Hill A.** Arm-twisting medical schools for core geriatric training. *CMAJ.* 2012 Jul 10;184(10):E515–E516.
20. **Sedhom R, Barile D.** Teaching our doctors to care for the elderly: a geriatrics needs assessment targeting internal medicine residents. *Gerontol Geriatr Med.* 2017 Jan–Dec;3:2333721417701687.
21. **Potter JF, Burton JR, Drach GW, et al.** Geriatrics for residents in the surgical and medical specialties: implementation of curricula and training experiences. *J Am Geriatr Soc.* 2005 Mar;53(3):511–515.
22. **Braude P, Partridge JS, Hardwick J, et al.** Geriatricians in perioperative medicine: developing subspecialty training. *Br J Anaesth.* 2016 Jan;116(1):4–6.
23. **Tinetti ME, Bogardus ST Jr, Agostini JV.** Potential pitfalls of disease-specific guidelines for patients with multiple conditions. *N Engl J Med.* 2004 Dec 30;351(27):2870–2874.
24. **Neuman MD, Silber JH, Magaziner JS, et al.** Survival and functional outcomes after hip fracture among nursing home residents. *JAMA Intern Med.* 2014 Aug;174(8):1273–1280.
25. **Kates SL, Mendelson DA, Friedman SM.** The value of an organized fracture program for the elderly: early results. *J Orthop Trauma.* 2011 Apr;25(4):233–237.
26. **Fisher AA, Davis MW, Rubenach SE, et al.** Outcomes for older patients with hip fractures: the impact of orthopedic and geriatric medicine cocare. *J Orthop Trauma.* 2006 Mar;20(3):172–178; discussion 179–180.
27. **Tadros RO, Faries PL, Malik R, et al.** The effect of a hospitalist comanagement service on vascular surgery inpatients. *J Vasc Surg.* 2015 Jun;61(6):1550–1555.
28. **Montero Ruiz E, Rebollar Merino A, Rivera Rodriguez T, et al.** Effect of comanagement with internal medicine on hospital stay of patients admitted to the Service of Otolaryngology. *Acta Otorrinolaringol Esp.* 2015 Sep–Oct;66(5):264–268.

# 1.2 Principles of orthogeriatric surgical care

Michael Blauth

## 1 Introduction

Fragility fracture patients (FFPs) represent up to 40% of patients in many orthopedic trauma units worldwide. This trend is increasing. As a consequence, over the last decade, refined surgical care approaches have been developed from growing experience and close collaboration with geriatricians in order to improve patient outcomes and lower healthcare expenses.

Similar to fracture care in children, geriatric fracture care also differs in many aspects from the standard treatment of middle-aged adults. Due to the relative paucity of randomized trial data for many treatments, many of the following recommendations represent expert opinions with some based on biomechanical or clinical investigations.

The four AO Principles certainly apply to the care of fragility fractures and should be carefully adhered to:

1. Fracture reduction and fixation to restore anatomical relationships
2. Stability by fixation or splinting, as the personality of the fracture and the injury requires
3. Preservation of blood supply to soft tissues and bone by careful handling and gentle reduction techniques
4. Early and safe mobilization of the part and the patient

## 2 Goal setting

The entire patient must be considered including his/her medical problems, medications, living situation, and goals for care. Overall, the following issues assume prominence in care of FFPs:

- Pain relief
- Prevention of functional decline
- Maintenance of independence
- Prevention of complications, such as reoperations, pneumonia, pressure sores, urinary tract infection, and delirium

Making the right therapeutic decisions is much more complex than with younger patients. Fragility fracture patients are functionally and physiologically variable (from nonambulatory "No-goes" to ambulatory "Go-goes") that the benefits and risks of treatment are not as clear as in younger patients. Therefore, it is essential to establish a consensus for the treatment goals among all of the team members.

Defining individual goals for each FFP is an important step which should be established and agreed upon as early as possible by the interdisciplinary team. The individual goals influence diagnostic and therapeutic surgical and medical measures and should be clearly communicated. Goal setting avoids unnecessary steps and streamlines the treatment. Goals may be adjusted during the treatment process.

First, treatment goals should be very specific, clear and easy. Second, if you cannot measure it, you cannot manage it. Third, a goal needs to be attractive and acceptable to the patient and the clinical team. Fourth, the goal should be realistic, meaning achievable or "doable". Fifth, the timeline to achieve the goal should be considered by setting a time frame.

It is useful to find short-term as well as long-term goals. Usually, the long-term goal is the expected outcome in several weeks or months, like to live independently or to walk without using a walking aid. When approaching a long-term goal, you need different short-term goals for each problem, like walking with a rolling walker after the first week, or removing a urinary catheter within 2 or 3 days after surgery.

The goals may be modified due to medical or surgical complications or if patients become unwilling or unable to continue or if they progress more slowly or quickly than expected. Goal setting should be integrated in the regular team meetings.

## 3 Time matters

Most studies suggest that performing surgery within the first 24–48 hours of admission decreases the number of complications and mortality. Delays longer than 72 hours are associated with an increased risk of multiple complications and mortality.

Surgical fixation reduces pain and blood loss significantly. It is also unethical to unnecessarily delay surgery.

The earlier surgical stabilization is performed, the better. This guiding principle is often violated because of the patient condition, patient consent, or hospital system barriers. The system of care must be optimized to avoid delay and iatrogenic problems.

The operating time should be as short as possible to reduce the stresses of surgery and its burdens on the patient.

The decision-making process regarding the definitive treatment in complex situations or relative indications is often delayed for multiple reasons. Goal setting and standardized communication pathways help to avoid unnecessary delay and expedite treatment.

## 4 Soft-tissue conditions

The musculoskeletal system of older patients is more vulnerable to problems and less tolerant of stress:

- Skin may be thin and less elastic due to atrophy or malnutrition and making pressure sores and degloving injuries more common. Wounds in older adults may also heal poorly for similar reasons. During positioning and draping, the surgeon must remember that the older patient's skin is fragile and can tear or be avulsed with minimal shear stresses. Shear forces from manual traction, removal of surgical drapes or localized pressure by splints and traction devices must be avoided (**Fig 1.2-1**). In surgery, meticulous positioning helps avoid skin breakdown.

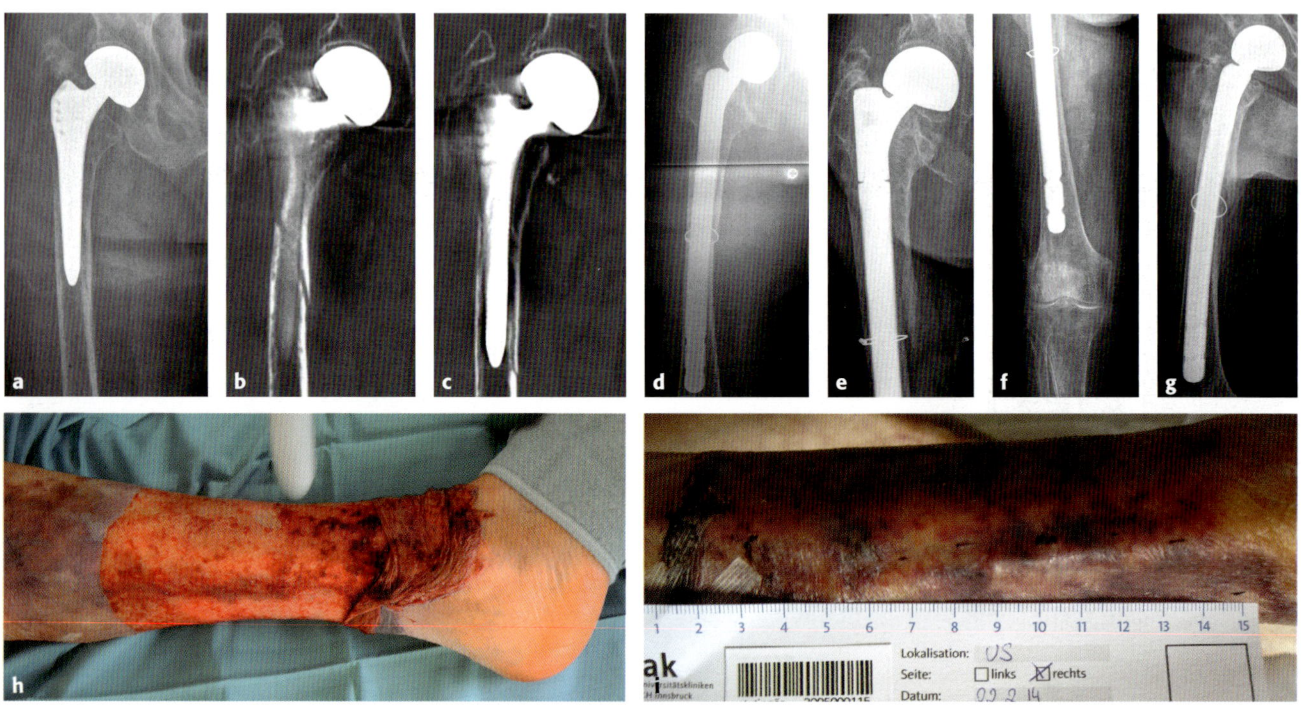


**Fig 1.2-1a–i**
**a–c** An 88-year-old woman with a type B2 periprosthetic femoral fracture.
**d–g** Revision hemiarthroplasty (**d**), follow-up at 2 months (**e–g**).
**h** After removing the covers, a degloving of the lower leg skin by gentle traction for intraoperative reduction became apparent.
**i** Uneventful healing after 10 days.

- Trophic changes: Arterial disease may result in ischemic changes and poor healing while venous hypertension produces edema, ulcers, and chronic skin changes. Using minimally invasive surgical (MIS) techniques may help to reduce problems.
- Hematoma: Surgeons must take great care to lose as little blood as possible. Meticulous hemostasis helps avoid tipping the patient out of equilibrium. Subcutaneous hematoma should be evacuated even with active anticoagulation to avoid rapid skin breakdown.
- Muscles are frequently atrophied and weaker than in younger patients (sarcopenia). Any manipulations during surgery should be carried out gently. Minimally invasive procedures are generally preferred.

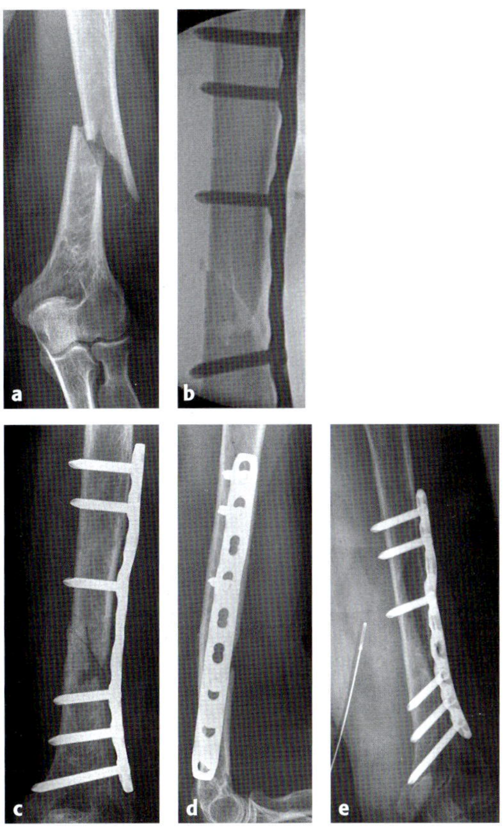

**Fig 1.2-2a–e**
**a** A 76-year-old woman with a simple 2-part fracture of the left humerus.
**b** After anatomical reduction, a 3.5 mm titanium lag screw was used to provide absolute stability (not displayed). After tightening the screw just a little bit too much, a multifragmentary situation emerged. The reduction was challenging and a bridging type of construct was chosen.
**c–e** Uneventful healing after 2 months (**c, d**) and 5 months (**e**). The patient did not even have osteopenia.

## 5 Bone quality

Bony quality varies substantially from the typical wide osteoporotic tube with thin cortices to a thickened but brittle cortex in atypical fractures. Thus, cortex perforation or other iatrogenic damage generated by clamps or lag screws is more likely to occur than in normal bone (**Fig 1.2-2**). Forceful reduction maneuvers and aggressive handling of bone may result in extension of the injury beyond the original pattern. The use of clamps must be performed cautiously to avoid additional damage (**Fig 1.2-3**). Avoid the use of crushing reduction forceps helps avert worsening the comminution. Fracture patterns are often complex, with impaction occurring in the setting of a low-energy trauma.

Interestingly, the impact of osteoporosis as a standalone factor on "mechanical failures" of implants could not be shown in several clinical studies. Quality of reduction and implant placement are obviously even more important [1, 2]. In a retrospective study of proximal humeral fractures, it was shown that the risk for mechanical failure increases significantly with the combination of several negative factors [3].

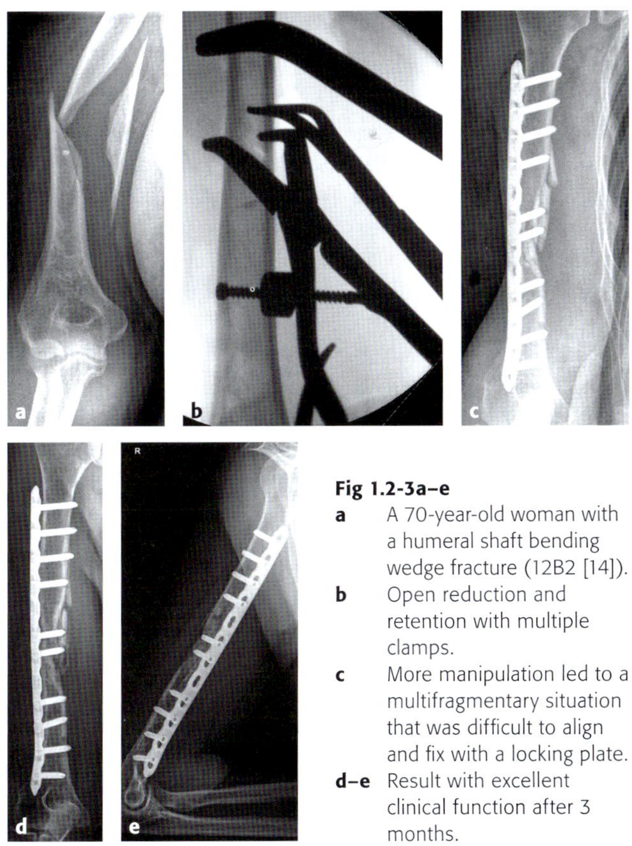

**Fig 1.2-3a–e**
**a** A 70-year-old woman with a humeral shaft bending wedge fracture (12B2 [14]).
**b** Open reduction and retention with multiple clamps.
**c** More manipulation led to a multifragmentary situation that was difficult to align and fix with a locking plate.
**d–e** Result with excellent clinical function after 3 months.

## 6 Bone deformation

Anterior and lateral bowing of the femur have a clinical impact in geriatric fractures and may make it very challenging to use standard intra and extramedullary implants [4]. A recent report also found that a significant increase in the lateral and anterior bow of the femur was associated with low-energy femoral shaft fractures. Therefore, the increased bowing of femoral shaft should be recognized as an important risk factor of this injury [5].

Specifically, lateral bowing of the femoral shaft may be increased in older adults as well as in younger patients with decreased bone mineralization.

Osteoporosis or osteomalacia induce a varus or bowing of the femur. The lateral femoral shaft is subjected to tensile strains during a variety of physical activities; walking has the strongest impact. This effect will be pronounced with bowing in osteoporotic patients [6]. Preexisting advanced varus knee osteoarthritis, with shifting the mechanical axis medially, has been considered as a minor reason for bowing of the femoral shaft.

Although atypical femoral fractures have been associated with long-term use of bisphosphonates (BPs), it was also noted that these fractures may develop without BPs use, especially in patients of Asian descent. In 2013, the Task Force of the American Society for Bone and Mineral Research revised the definition of atypical femoral fracture, removing specific diseases and drug exposures as one of the association from the minor features [7]. According to this definition, stress fractures caused by femoral bowing deformity may also be classified as atypical femoral fractures.

Despite being the most commonly recommended implant choice, intramedullary (IM) nails can be difficult to insert, as the curvature of IM nail is different from that of the radius of bowed femur. In cephalomedullary nailing, the distal end of nail may break or penetrate the anterior cortex of femur in the distal segment.

Reaming is often difficult as well and must be performed gently due to the narrow medullary canal and the brittle nature of the bone.

Also, the nailing may cause an inadvertent fracture or malreduction with a bony gap on the medial aspect of the bone, especially in the atypical femoral shaft fractures with bowing [8]. This effect may result in impaired fracture healing or even nonunion.

Plate fixation can be a solution in bowed femoral fractures. In such cases, the plate may need to be contoured before fixation, considering the contralateral, noninjured leg. Otherwise, the proximal or distal end of plate will step off the bone, and it may be a source of malreduction when screws are tightened [4].

## 7 Classification

Classification of fragility fractures is often challenging because of different fracture patterns. Osteoporotic fractures often occur in patterns not described in the currently used classification schemes. This frustrates attempts to classify the fractures and may result in incorrect procedure or implant selection. The AO/OTA Fracture and Dislocation Classification is useful for many, but not all, fragility fractures.

## 8 Indications for fixation

Most fractures of the lower extremity should be surgically managed. In a small group of bedridden, terminal patients, nonoperative palliative management of hip and other lower leg fractures may be adequate. Those decisions should be team decisions made with the geriatrician, patient, family, and medical team.

For the upper extremity, the need to preserve function should be considered to allow the patient to accomplish activities of daily living like eating, self-care, grooming, and ambulation. Attaining these goals may involve taking more surgical and overall risk. Therefore, surgical treatment may only be indicated if it will result in a significant improvement in function. In the proximal humerus, olecranon, and distal radius, nonsurgical management often leads to an acceptable functional result [9–11].

Some nonsurgical approaches are not tolerated as well as in younger individuals. Casts interfere with functionality and increase the risk of falls. Immobilization may render old patients immediately dependent for basic activities like eating and grooming, and promote accelerated functional decline. In a sense casts are also tethers that patients have difficulties to deal with. The cast will prevent a patient from accomplishing daily activities like walking, and the patient may therefore require placement in a nursing home. Casts and braces tend to exacerbate delirium in older adults (**Fig 1.2-4**).

Complete recovery after trauma is typically the goal of treatment below the age of 60 years. This does not apply to FFPs. In this age group, we focus on the restoration of individual functional needs. Decision making can be difficult due to the variable physiological and functional nature of older patients. It is often necessary to individualize treatment approaches with the consensus of the orthogeriatric team and patients' family.

## 9 Positioning

Correct intraoperative positioning avoids pressure sores and skin damage: It is essential to carefully position the patient on the surgical table. Avoidance of pressure sores is of particular importance as sores significantly interfere with recovery and take an extended time to heal. An infected pressure sore may actually result in sepsis and death in the older fracture patient.

In most cases, the supine position is preferred to allow for overall care by the anesthetist. When under regional anesthesia, the patient can breathe easier when supine and this position is usually more comfortable.

## 10 Single shot surgery

It is obvious that any kind of revision surgery must be avoided because of the limited patient reserves necessary to tolerate and recover from surgery and functional decline. The choice of treatment should be influenced by this principle. Hemiarthroplasty instead of fracture fixation for femoral neck fractures and other primary joint replacement surgeries are good examples.

## 11 Weight bearing as tolerated and functional aftertreatment

Usually, the surgeon's attention is focused on the intraoperative and immediate perioperative treatment period. Postoperatively, if the wound healing is progressing normally and x-rays are satisfactory, limited attention is paid to rehabilitation options and progress. The communication among surgeons, staff nurses, and physiotherapists regarding mobilization issues is often poor.

Early postoperative mobilization and unrestricted weight bearing as tolerated are important principles for a multitude of reasons. Prolonged bed rest or "sitting mobilization" are not adequate options because of the following consequences:

- Loss of muscle mass represents an independent risk factor for new falls and fractures in older adults.

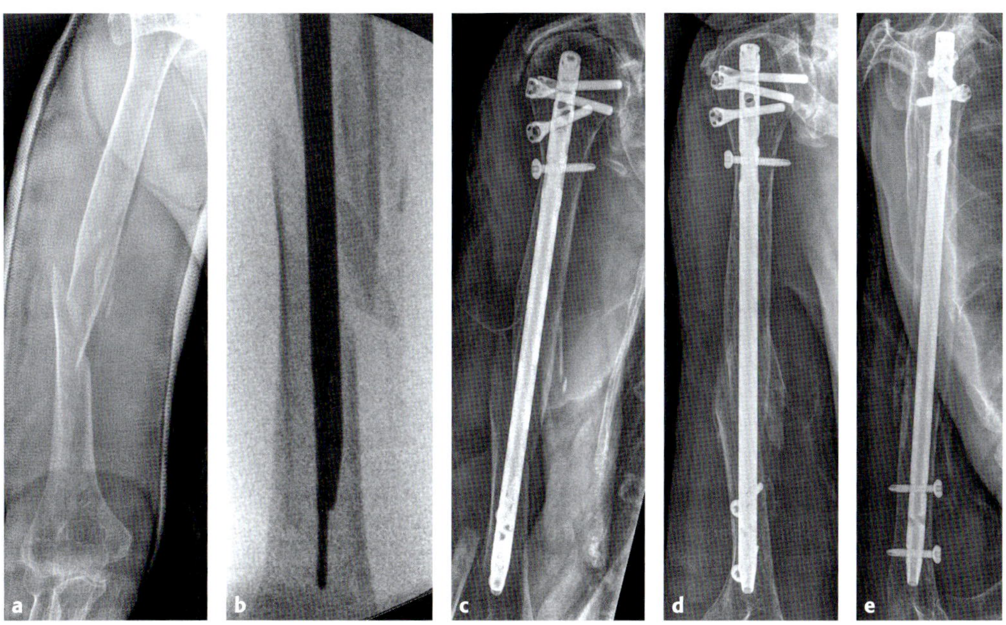


**Fig 1.2-4a–e**
**a** A 92-year-old woman with a humeral fracture (12B3). Bracing was not tolerated well.
**b–c** After 10 days close reduction and fixation with a long multilock nail.
**d–e** Uneventful healing after 3 months. The function reached the preinjury level.

- Restriction of weight bearing inflicts a significant physiological burden on the geriatric patient. The energy expenditure for ambulation without full weight bearing increases fourfold, leading to rapid exhaustion [12].
- Fragility fracture patients are often physically unable to perform partial weight bearing due to sarcopenia, lack of proprioception and weakness in the arms; or they are admitted with an already impaired functional deficit in upper and lower extremities, preventing them from using crutches or walkers in a way that the affected lower extremity is effectively spared.
- Patients develop unnecessary fear and get anxious about their inability to return to their preinjury functional status. Consequently, motivation may drop. The altered gait mechanism needs cognitive input and may lead to complaints of overload or low back pain.
- Many FFPs have some degree of cognitive impairment. They may not understand (or rapidly forget) instructions and instead follow their own impulses.
- Partial weight-bearing protocols are not evidence-based but often the result of the surgeon's own uncertainty.
- Even for patients on adequate pain medication, pain will typically guide the patient to use the appropriate weight bearing and safely progress with ambulation. Patients with severely impaired cognitive function are more prone to fall, but they have the same self-protective mechanisms as cognitively normal patients.

Early weight bearing can promote fracture healing and union of the fracture without increasing loss of fixation [13, 14]. Immobilization of joints is poorly tolerated in many older patients; early functional range of motion prevents joints from stiffening. The daily loss of muscle mass during periods of bed rest is dramatic. Modern surgical procedures and implants permit immediate unrestricted weight bearing for most fractures.

Temporary external transarticular fixation can be a unique solution in fractures around the knee if internal fixation does not seem to be stable enough for immediate mobilization, if soft tissues have to settle down or if there is no chance to apply implants directly to the bone (**Fig 1.2-5**) [15].

## 12 Fixation techniques

The major technical problem the surgeon faces is the difficulty producing secure fixation of the implant to the bone. There is less cortical and cancellous bone for the screw threads to engage and the pullout strength of implants is significantly lower in osteoporotic bone.

Bone mineral density correlates linearly with the holding power of screws. If the load transmitted at the bone-implant interface exceeds the strain tolerance of osteoporotic bone, microfracture and resorption of bone with loosening of the

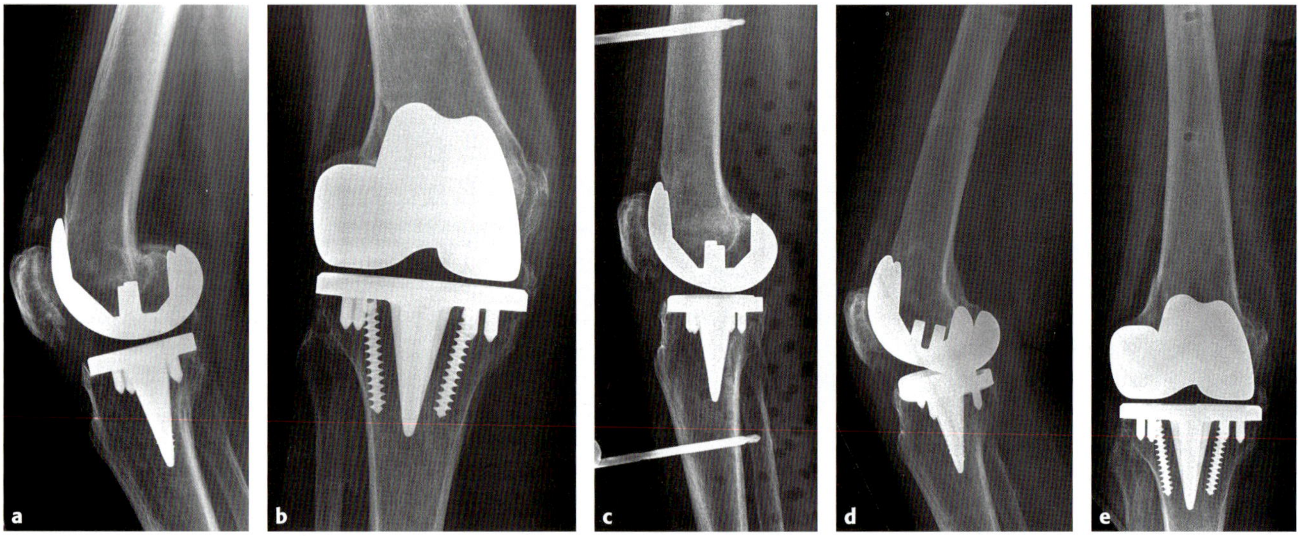


**Fig 1.2-5a–e**
**a–b** A 75-year-old woman with low periprosthetic fracture after total knee arthroplasty (TKA) and severe comorbidities.
**c** Temporary transarticular fixation for 8 weeks.
**d–e** Bony healing after 3 months. Final range of motion 0–10–100°.

implant and secondary failure of fixation will occur. The common mode of failure of internal fixation in osteoporotic bone is bone failure rather than implant failure.

Internal fixation must take the local bone mineral distribution into account. This varies with fracture location, age, and gender.

Proper preoperative planning, implant choice, fixation technique, and understanding of the biomechanical principles are essential.

The general principles of fracture management are applicable to most fragility fractures, but the decrease in bone strength requires some adaption to decrease the risk of failure.

### 12.1 Minimally invasive surgery

Minimally invasive surgery (MIS) techniques feature multiple "traditional" advantages that are even more helpful in FFPs than in younger patients. Many older adults are anticoagulated and suffer already from muscle weakness. Technically, MIS is easy to perform as soft-tissue layers can be separated easily. For more details, see Blauth et al [16].

Specifically designed instruments for MIS are available. It is important to develop a familiarity with their use.

### 12.2 Relative stability

Thin cortices cannot withstand the compressive forces that are needed to create absolute stability. Tightening lag screws a little too much may create iatrogenic fractures that worsen the situation significantly (**Fig 1.2-2, Fig 1.2-3**). In osteoporotic bone it may not always be possible to obtain and maintain anatomical reduction and compression with absolute stability because the weakened cortical and cancellous bone may fail under compression. It is essential not to mix the principles of relative and absolute stability in one fracture fixation.

As a simple rule, intramedullary devices are preferred over extramedullary devices if fracture patterns and soft tissues allow for it. Unfortunately, for metaphyseal fractures around the knee, locking options are not yet optimized for osteoporotic bone and thus nails are often not applicable.

Short plates with every screw hole filled will cause concentration of forces, which may exceed the strain tolerance of osteoporotic bone. Basic rules have been previously established in the literature [17, 18]:

- Simple transverse fractures are best addressed by intramedullary implants. If this is not possible, the fracture gap must be closed as much as possible, ie, bone contact must be achieved. Three to four holes should be left free and three to four bicortical locking head screws (LHSs) in each main fragment are needed.
- Spiral-type 2-part fractures should be reduced and "adapted" as much as possible and preliminarily fixed with suture or hardware cerclages or cables. If screws are used, they should be tightened with caution as "reduction screws". The first plate screw should be inserted at the end of the fracture line. Three to four bicortical LHSs in each main fragment are necessary depending on the type of bone (**Fig 1.2-6**).
- In comminuted fractures, the first screws should be placed adjacent to the fracture zone. Four to five bicortical screws in each main fragment are sufficient.

### 12.3 Splinting the whole bone

Subsequent fractures adjacent to the end of plates, nails or prosthesis occur due to the stress riser between the stiff implant and the soft bone. The frequency is not clear. If possible, the whole bone should be protected at the first fixation including the femoral neck in case of the femur (**Fig 1.2-7, Fig 1.2-8**). To achieve this goal, sometimes a combination of intramedullary with extramedullary implants becomes necessary.

### 12.4 Angular stable implants and blades

Implants with locking head mechanism and fixed or variable angle between screw and plate as well as angular stable locking options for intramedullary nails all have biomechanically shown to provide superior stability in bone with reduced cortical thickness.

Locking head screws cannot be overtightened or overinserted rendering them unstable because the thread gets destroyed. They should always be used in a bicortical mode to improve their working length with thin cortices.

In addition, locking screws have a larger core diameter than conventional screws, which results in a higher pullout strength and overall strength. This is especially helpful in metaphyseal bone where intramedullary nails may fail. The holding power of the LHS can further be increased by orienting them in different directions: This method is used with the proximal humeral plate and the distal femoral and proximal tibial plates.

A blade for fixation of pertrochanteric fractures offers biomechanical advantages over a lag screw. The blade condenses the bone around the implant, while screw insertion always results in some bone loss.

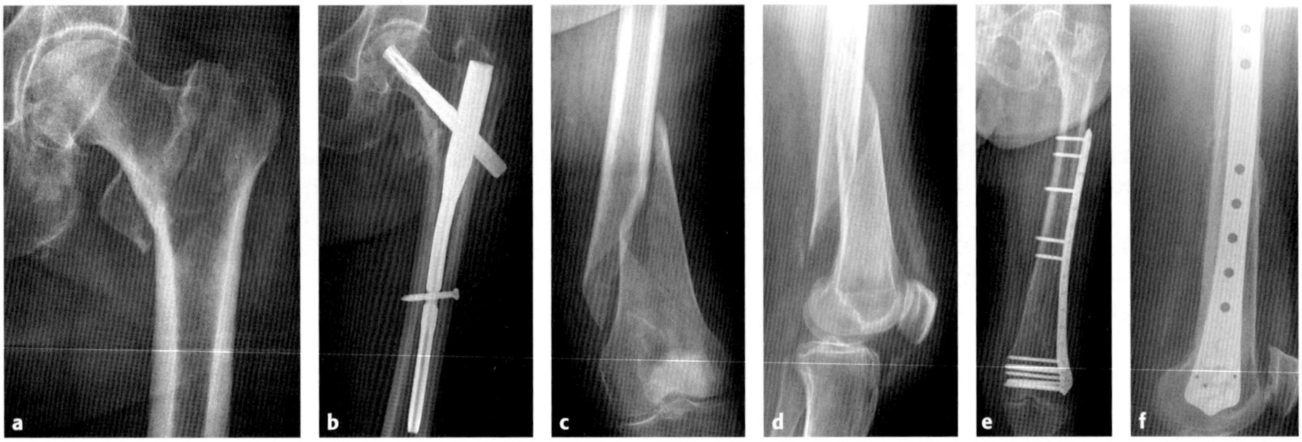

**Fig 1.2-6a–f**

**a–b** a A 77-year-old woman with a pertrochanteric fracture (31A2).
**b** Fixation with proximal femoral nail antirotation.
**c–d** The nail was removed 1.5 years later because of lateral thigh pain. Three years later, she sustained a spiral diaphyseal fracture (32A1).
**e–f** Minimally invasive reduction in lateral position and preliminary fixation with suture wire. Definitive fixation in relative stability with distal femoral plate, the first proximal screw starting at the end of the fracture and 10 cortices. Uneventful healing with small callus formation. Ideally, a longer plate to protect the whole femur would have been indicated.

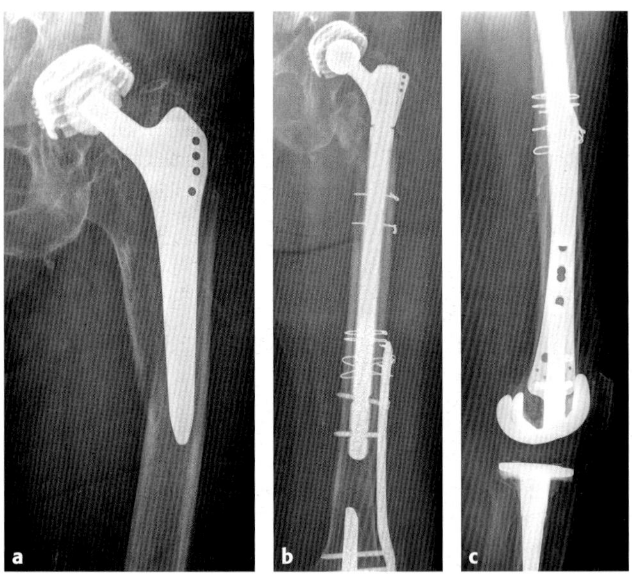

**Fig 1.2-7a–c**

**a** A 92-year-old woman with periprosthetic fracture type B2.
**b–c** Open reduction, fixation with cerclage wires and revision arthroplasty with a long-stemmed implant with locking options. Distal femoral plate to protect the bone between the two prostheses.

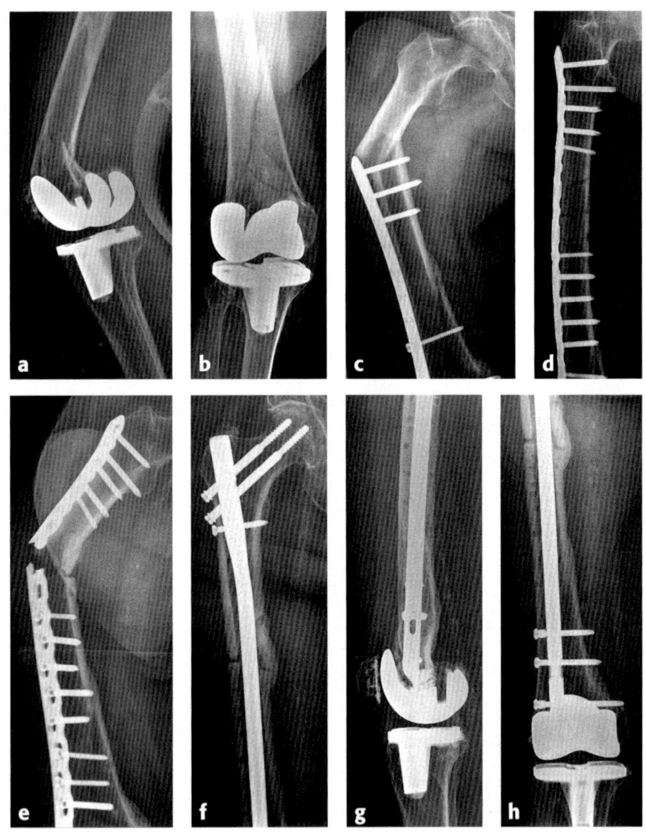

**Fig 1.2-8a–h**

**a–b** An 80-year-old woman with a periprosthetic knee fracture.
**c** Two and a half months after fixation with a distal femoral plate fracture adjacent to the proximal end of the plate.
**d** Application of a longer plate. Fixation in varus malalingment and with the fracture gap still open.
**e** The construct is too stiff and fails after another 2.5 months.
**f–h** Final solution with antegrade femoral nail. Distal locking with axial loading screws.

## 12.5 Anatomical alignment

Correct anatomical alignment represents an important prerequisite for uneventful bone healing. Fixation of osteoporotic bones is less tolerant for any deviation than in younger bone. Specifically varus malalignment should be avoided in femoral fractures.

Severe rotational malalignment is an underrecognized problem and occurs typically with very unstable proximal femoral fractures. Rotational malalignment should be avoided.

## 12.6 Bone impaction

Bone impaction at the fracture site is a key element in the surgical management of osteoporotic fractures as it reduces the risk of implant failure.

In many cases, like for example in the valgus-impacted fracture of the femoral neck, impaction is created by the trauma itself. Controlled impaction can be attained by tensioning internal fixation devices. Implants, such as the dynamic hip screw, which allow for controlled impaction of the fracture while preventing penetration of the joint by the hip screw.

## 12.7 Augmentation with polymethylmethacrylate

Fixation in osteoporotic bone can be improved by augmenting the bone with cement. Augmented purchase of the implant, in particular of screws, reduces the risk of hardware migration, cut out, cut through and pull out. It can also be used as a void filler to support the bone structure, for example, of a vertebral body or the tibial plateau, and prevent it from collapsing.

Polymethylmethacrylate (PMMA) remains the material of choice and may be used in different ways:

- For filling voids that mainly result after reduction of cancellous bone. A typical example is vertebral body compression fracture treated with closed reduction with vertebroplasty or kyphoplasty. The same principle can be applied to proximal tibial fractures; cement used as a void filler prevents the articular surface from collapsing after elevation.
- In standardized implant augmentation, the cement is typically injected with a specific cannula through perforated implants to improve the bone-implant interface by preventing high bone strain and distributing the force to the bone in a load-sharing rather than load-bearing configuration (**Fig 1.2-9**).
- In nonstandardized implant augmentation, the cement is applied via the screw hole or cortical window before or after the implant is inserted.

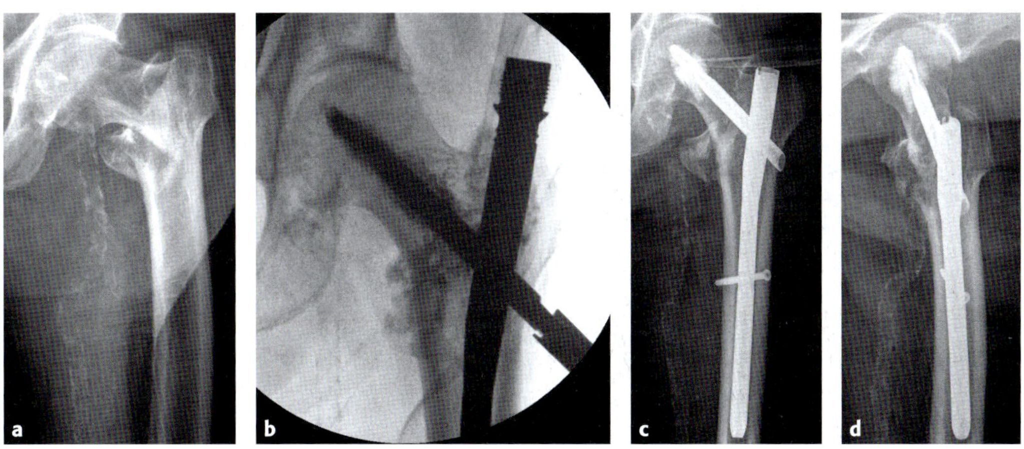

**Fig 1.2-9a–d**

**a** An 82-year-old man with a proximal femoral fracture (31A2).

**b** Close reduction with traction table. After insertion of nail and blade, the decision was taken to augment the blade because of severe osteoporosis and a very low resistance while inserting the blade. Intraoperative contrast dye test demonstrated no arthrogram, ie, no perforation into the hip joint.

**c–d** Injection of 4 mL of polymethylmethacrylate through a special cannula. Result after mobilization with center-center position of the head-neck-element and equally distributed cement.

Standardized implant augmentation has been thoroughly studied in recent years:

- Many sites have been tested biomechanically. In the proximal femur, proximal humerus, proximal tibia and sacrum, augmentation with PMMA cement improved cycles required to cause mechanical failure by ~ 100%; this applies only in osteoporotic bone.
- Small volumes of cement are sufficient. Larger quantities do not improve implant purchase significantly.
- Heat generation outside the cement does not exceed 42° C, because the metallic implant serves as a heat sink for the exothermic chemical reaction.
- No signs of cartilage damage next to the cement mass were noted in sheep experiments.
- Interference with bone healing has not been demonstrated so far.

Standardized implant augmentation with PMMA limits the negative effect of osteoporosis on implant fixation, "converting" osteoporotic bone into normal bone.

## 12.8 Autografts

Corticocancellous bone autografts to assist fracture healing and to fill gaps can also be harvested in older patients. Unless used as avoid filler, grafts should be fixed to the bone by cortical screws (**Fig 1.2-10**).

## 12.9 Allografts

Allograft bone has good mechanical properties but less osteogenic potential compared to autografts. In osteoporotic bone, allografts are used to fill metaphyseal voids and to prevent articular and other fragments from subsiding. This can be helpful in fractures of the proximal and distal humerus, distal radius and proximal tibia.

Allograft struts are also used in periprosthetic femoral fractures with poor bone quality to enhance the mechanical strength of the construct (**Fig 1.2-11**).

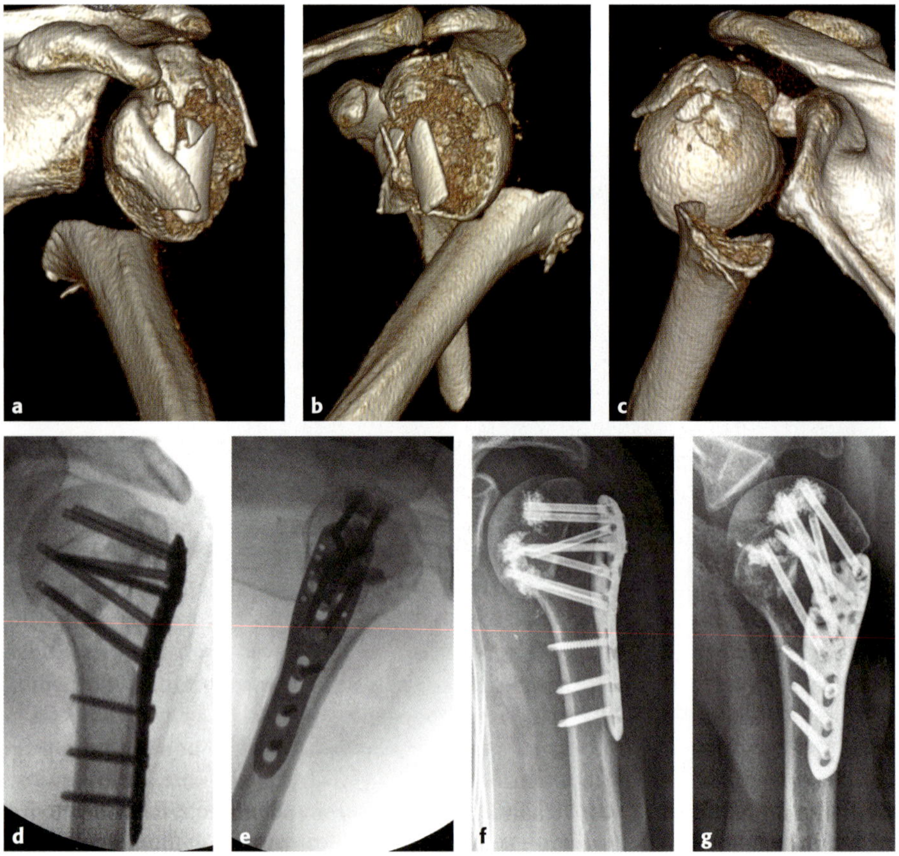


**Fig 1.2-10a–g**
**a–c** A 70-year-old woman with an unstable 3-part fracture.
**d–e** Fracture fixation was indicated despite the obvious risk for avascular necrosis because a stable reconstruction seemed to be possible. Anatomical reduction and fixation with PHILOS.
**f** Standardized implant augmentation via cannulated locking head screws with 0.5 mL of polymethylmethacrylate each to minimize the risk of mechanical failure.
**g** Injection of cement is only indicated and possible in osteoporotic bone. Follow-up after 3 months.

## 12.10 Joint replacement

Joint replacement plays an important role in older patients. It is commonly used in the proximal femur, mainly with femoral neck fractures. The indication for fracture arthroplasty is not as clear in proximal humeral fractures. A reverse shoulder arthroplasty is useful in cases where stable fixation is not possible. The use of an endoprosthesis in fractures of the distal humerus, distal radius and proximal tibia remains controversial. More rapid restoration of adequate function along with a reduced life expectancy and fewer revision surgeries are appealing arguments in favor of immediate joint replacement.

There is a paucity of published evidence to inform clinical care in this area. If the general goals of fracture treatment can be achieved without violation of the above-mentioned principles, fracture fixation is usually preferred.

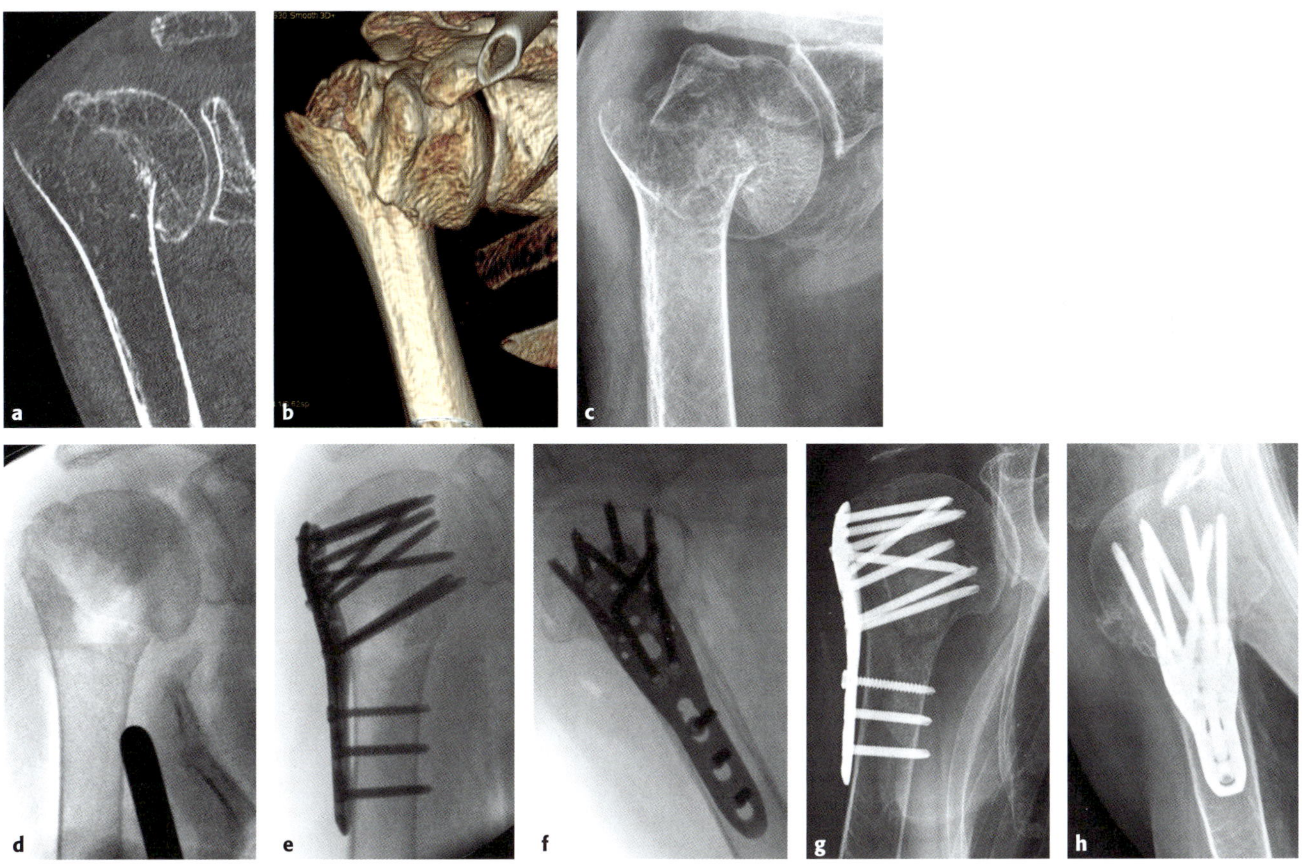


**Fig 1.2-11a–h**

**a–c** A 76-year-old woman with a displaced 2-part fracture of the proximal humerus. Severe osteoporosis with T-score lumbar spine -3.8, femoral neck -3.6 and a slender head fragment.

**d–f** Central void after open reduction (**d**) that is filled with a structural allograft from the bone bank (**e–f**).

**g–h** Follow-up after 3 months.

## 13 References

1. **Kralinger F, Blauth M, Goldhahn J, et al.** The influence of local bone density on the outcome of one hundred and fifty proximal humeral fractures treated with a locking plate. *J Bone Joint Surg Am.* 2014 Jun 18;96(12):1026–1032.
2. **Muller MA, Hengg C, Krettek C, et al.** Trabecular bone strength is not an independent predictive factor for dynamic hip screw migration—a prospective multicenter cohort study. *J Orthop Res.* 2015 Nov;33(11):1680–1686.
3. **Krappinger D, Bizzotto N, Riedmann S, et al.** Predicting failure after surgical fixation of proximal humerus fractures. *Injury.* 2011 Nov;42(11):1283–1288.
4. **Hwang JH, Oh JK, Oh CW, et al.** Mismatch of anatomically pre-shaped locking plate on Asian femurs could lead to malalignment in the minimally invasive plating of distal femoral fractures: a cadaveric study. *Arch Orthop Trauma Surg.* 2012 Jan;132(1):51–56.
5. **Sasaki S, Miyakoshi N, Hongo M, et al.** Low-energy diaphyseal femoral fractures associated with bisphosphonate use and severe curved femur: a case series. *J Bone Miner Metab.* 2012 Sep;30(5):561–567.
6. **Oh Y, Wakabayashi Y, Kurosa Y, et al.** Potential pathogenic mechanism for stress fractures of the bowed femoral shaft in the elderly: mechanical analysis by the CT-based finite element method. *Injury.* 2014 Nov;45(11):1764–1771.
7. **Shane E, Burr D, Abrahamsen B, et al.** Atypical subtrochanteric and diaphyseal femoral fractures: second report of a task force of the American Society for Bone and Mineral Research. *J Bone Miner Res.* 2014 Jan;29(1):1–23.
8. **Oh CW, Oh JK, Park KC, et al.** Prophylactic nailing of incomplete atypical femoral fractures. *Sci World J.* 2013.
9. **Duckworth AD, Bugler KE, Clement ND, et al.** Nonoperative management of displaced olecranon fractures in low-demand elderly patients. *J Bone Joint Surg Am.* 2014 Jan 01;96(1):67–72.
10. **Arora R, Lutz M, Deml C, et al.** A prospective randomized trial comparing nonoperative treatment with volar locking plate fixation for displaced and unstable distal radial fractures in patients sixty-five years of age and older. *J Bone Joint Surg Am.* 2011 Dec 07;93(23):2146–2153.
11. **Twiss T.** Nonoperative treatment of proximal humerus fractures. In: Crosby LA, Neviaser RJ, eds. *Proximal Humerus Fractures—Evaluation and Management.* Switzerland: Springer International Publishing; 2015:23–41.
12. **Westerman RW, Hull P, Hendry RG, et al.** The physiological cost of restricted weight bearing. *Injury.* 2008 Jul;39(7):725–727.
13. **Koval KJ, Sala DA, Kummer FJ, et al.** Postoperative weight-bearing after a fracture of the femoral neck or an intertrochanteric fracture. *J Bone Joint Surg Am.* 1998 Mar;80(3):352–356.
14. **Joslin CC, Eastaugh-Waring SJ, Hardy JR, et al.** Weight bearing after tibial fracture as a guide to healing. *Clin Biomech (Bristol, Avon).* 2008 Mar;23(3):329–333.
15. **Krappinger D, Struve P, Schmid R, et al.** Fractures of the pubic rami: a retrospective review of 534 cases. *Arch Orthop Trauma Surg.* 2009 Dec;129(12):1685–1690.
16. **Blauth M, Kates SL, Kammerlander C, et al.** Fragility fractures. In: Babst R, Bavonratanavech S, Pesantez R, eds. *Minimally Invasive Plate Osteosynthesis (MIPO).* 2nd ed. Stuttgart New York: Thieme; 2012:651–678.
17. **Stoffel K, Dieter U, Stachowiak G, et al.** Biomechanical testing of the LCP—how can stability in locked internal fixators be controlled? *Injury* 2003 Nov;34(Suppl 2):B11–19.
18. **Fulkerson E, Egol KA, Kubiak EN, et al.** Fixation of diaphyseal fractures with a segmental defect: a biomechanical comparison of locked and conventional plating techniques. *J Trauma.* 2006 Apr;60(4):830–835.

# 1.3 Principles of orthogeriatric anesthesia

Ali Shariat, Malikah Latmore

## 1 Introduction

This chapter examines age-related changes that render older adults susceptible to adverse events in the perioperative period and provide a summary of current best practices regarding anesthesia for fragility fracture patients (FFPs) [1]. The major complications related to anesthetic interventions in older adults include perioperative cardiovascular morbidity, eg, hypotension, arrhythmias and acute coronary syndromes, respiratory failure, kidney injury, and delirium.

Despite these risks, high-performing geriatric fracture programs report remarkably low perioperative mortality rates of less than 2%, even in highly comorbid and frail referral populations [2, 3]. This chapter reviews relevant physiological changes in older adults, the assessment and preparation of fragility fracture patients for anesthesia and surgery, and the risks and benefits of general anesthesia (GA), regional anesthesia (RA) and multimodal analgesia. Unique geriatric considerations with regard to anesthetic choice, intraoperative positioning and teamwork are also examined.

## 2 Important pathophysiological changes in older adults

### 2.1 Cardiac morbidity

Perioperative cardiac morbidity (PCM) is the leading cause of death during and after surgery and includes myocardial infarction (MI), congestive heart failure (CHF), unstable angina, serious dysrhythmia, and cardiac death [4, 5]. Stressors such as perioperative pain, blood loss, anesthesia, and fluid shifts all contribute to an imbalance between myocardial oxygen demand and supply [1]. In addition, the aging process results in specific changes to the autonomic nervous system including increased sympathetic nervous system activation, decreased parasympathetic activity, and decreased baroreceptor activity, limiting the ability of the older adult to respond effectively to surgical stress [1]. Older patients are more likely to have preexisting cardiac comorbidities, such as coronary artery disease (CAD) or congestive heart failure (CHF). These factors all contribute to a decrease in cardiovascular reserve and lower the threshold at which older adults develop cardiac complications and hemodynamic instability [4, 6].

### 2.2 Pulmonary morbidity

Normal aging results in clinically significant changes in the respiratory system, including loss of alveolar surface area, decline in intercostal muscle mass and strength, kyphotic thoracic spine changes, and calcification of rib cage cartilage [7]. These changes reduce chest wall compliance, elastic recoil of the lungs, and the strength of the respiratory muscles [8, 9]. Normal central respiratory responses to hypoxia and hypercapnia are reduced by approximately 50% in older adults [10]. The cough reflex is less forceful and effective, increasing the risk of aspiration pneumonia [9]. Older patients have increased sensitivity to the respiratory depressant effects of opioids due to an increase in the volume of distribution as well as a decrease in renal and hepatic clearance [9, 11].

### 2.3 Cognitive dysfunction

Older adults are especially susceptible to delirium in the perioperative period, and there is concern that perioperative delirium may also contribute to longer-term cognitive dysfunction [12] (see chapter 1.14 Delirium for more information on delirium). An abrupt decline in perioperative cognition is a robust predictor of increased mortality within the first 3–12 months after surgery [12–14]. Theories explaining the relationship between cognitive dysfunction and mortality include direct damage to the brain, inability of patients with cognitive impairment to care for their own health, and consideration of cognitive decline as an indirect marker of systemic organ disease [14].

Medical complications such as pneumonia, deep vein thrombosis, pressure ulcers, MI, gastric ulcers, and depression are more common in patients with postoperative delirium [15].

Since cognitive decline in the postoperative period can have an enormous impact on postoperative complications and functional recovery, minimization of delirium in the perioperative period is an important goal.

## 3 Preoperative risk assessment and preparation

Poor preoperative preparation has been implicated in 40% of deaths attributed to surgery and anesthesia [16].

Most published guidelines concerning preoperative optimization are based on patients undergoing elective surgery. Under elective conditions, preexisting systemic disease is closely investigated in order to define the disease, quantify its severity, and optimize the patient's condition for operative repair. Many of these practices and protocols can only be loosely extrapolated to urgent cases such as hip fracture, as the risks of surgical delay resulting from hemodynamic instability, delirium and immobility typically exceed the benefits of further preoperative testing.

Older age alone is no longer considered an important predictor of perioperative risk. Rather, the overall physical and functional status and the number and severity of comorbid conditions are considered more robust predictors of outcome [1]. Quantifying comorbidity and functional capacity are important tools to predict outcome. See chapter 1.4 Preoperative risk assessment and preparation for a more thorough discussion of preoperative risk assessment and preparation.

### 3.1 Functional capacity

Functional capacity is a more accurate predictor of intraoperative risk than most specific comorbid conditions or the results of extensive diagnostic testing [17].

Functional capacity can be assessed in terms of metabolic equivalents (METs) of activity. Ability to perform activities of greater than four METs is considered good functional capacity; examples of such activities include climbing up a flight of stairs, walking more than 6.4 km/h (4 mph), or doing heavy household work [18]. This threshold (> 4 METs) has been used to indicate adequate reserve for most orthopedic and other intermediate-risk surgeries.

### 3.2 Cardiac risk

While the development of robust risk assessment tools is of increasing relevance for elective surgical procedures, there remains a dearth of studies to accurately estimate risk for the typical FFP. The Revised Cardiac Risk Index [19] is the most widely studied tool for hip fracture surgery and stratifies cardiovascular risk based on the presence of six predictors of cardiac morbidity and mortality:

- High-risk surgery (typically vascular or intraperitoneal)
- History of ischemic heart disease
- History of CHF
- History of cerebrovascular disease
- Insulin-dependent diabetes
- Preoperative serum creatinine > 2 mg/dL

The presence of two or more factors identifies patients with moderate to high risk for perioperative complications. These criteria have been used during elective surgical planning as triggers to consider additional noninvasive testing, further medical therapy, and/or invasive monitoring [17, 19]. These factors are likely to also predict outcomes in the urgent surgical setting.

History of unstable angina, CHF, significant dysrhythmias, severe valvular disease, and pacemaker or an automated implantable cardioverter defibrillator (ICD) placement should be determined [18]. If a patient has a pacemaker or an ICD, a plan for perioperative management should be discussed. Information to be obtained includes the type and manufacturer of the device as well as the underlying dysrhythmia or other cardiac condition that led to the placement of the device. Perioperative management of the device must be individualized, with some devices requiring preoperative interrogation and possibly reprogramming by the cardiology team [18].

### 3.3 Procedure risk

In addition to risk stratification for patients, surgical procedures may also be classified according to risk. High-risk procedures include emergent procedures, major vascular procedures, and prolonged procedures with major fluid shifts and blood loss. They are typically defined as having adverse cardiac event risks greater than 5%. Low-risk procedures include endoscopy, breast surgery, and cataract surgery and have an adverse cardiac event risk lower than 1%. Most orthopedic procedures are considered intermediate risk and have an adverse cardiac event risk between 1% and 5% [18].

### 3.4 Routine preoperative testing

Only after clinically significant diseases have been identified on a medical history and physical examination should further testing be considered; this testing should only be pursued if it is likely to change management, improve outcomes, and provide benefits that outweigh the harms of surgical delay [18] (see also chapters 1.4 Perioperative risk assessment and preparation and 2.6 Orthogeriatric team—principles, roles, and responsibilities). In hip fracture patients, operative delay of more than 48 hours after admission increases the odds of a 30-day mortality by 41 % and a 1-year mortality by 32 % [20].

The American Society of Anesthesiologists in collaboration with the American Board of Internal Medicine Foundation recommend the following baseline preoperative laboratory tests: complete blood count, basic or comprehensive metabolic panel (ie, electrolytes, renal function and glucose), and coagulation studies for patients when significant blood loss and fluid shifts are expected [21].

In patients with established heart disease, an electrocardiogram may provide important prognostic information about short-term and long-term mortality, and provides a baseline against which perioperative changes may be judged [18].

More advanced preoperative cardiac testing (eg, transthoracic/esophageal echocardiography or cardiac stress testing) in asymptomatic, stable patients with known cardiac disease (eg, CHF or valvular disease) is not recommended and is generally not appropriate for hip fracture patients in the absence of signs and symptoms of significant active cardiovascular compromise [21, 22].

With the exception of concern for severe aortic stenosis, echocardiographic assessment of valvular function does not lead to clinically important changes in management [18].

### 3.5 Medication management

All preoperative medications must be correctly identified, recorded and considered for continuation or discontinuation during the perioperative period. The risk of intraoperative hypotension and excessive blood loss is elevated in older trauma patients, and teams must consider the potential impact of home medications on blood pressure and bleeding. Some common perioperative considerations include:

- Long-term beta-blocker therapy should be continued perioperatively due to the benefits of heart rate control and decreased myocardial oxygen consumption, and the potential harm of withdrawal when abruptly stopped [18]. In patients not receiving long-term beta-blocker therapy, beta-blockers should not be initiated prior to surgery due to the increased risk of hypotension, stroke, and death [18].
- Angiotensin-converting enzyme inhibitors (ACEIs) and angiotensin receptor blockers (ARBs) can lead to increased episodes of intraoperative hypotension and acute kidney injury, particularly when used in association with diuretics [23]. Most experts recommend discontinuation of ACE inhibitors/ARBs and diuretics preoperatively [17].
- Long-term antiplatelet therapy with aspirin, clopidogrel and other antiplatelet agents is typically stopped in the preoperative period. For patients who have undergone coronary stent implantation within the past 6 weeks, dual antiplatelet therapy with aspirin and P2Y12 platelet inhibitor should be continued unless the risk of surgical bleeding outweighs the risk of stent thrombosis [18].

Additional discussion of preoperative medication management can be found in chapter 1.4 Preoperative risk assessment and preparation. Discussion of the management of long-term anticoagulation during the perioperative period can be found in chapter 1.6 Anticoagulation in the perioperative setting.

## 4 Intraoperative anesthetic choices

General and regional anesthesia each have potential advantages and disadvantages for hip fracture patients, and anesthetic choices require a thorough understanding of the physiological changes related to trauma and the stress of surgery. As will be discussed in topic 4.1, recent systematic reviews and metaanalyses [24] do not support the superiority of one method of intraoperative anesthesia (ie, general versus regional) over the other in the urgent repair of fragility fractures; reasonable differences in practice patterns exist within institutions and worldwide.

### 4.1 Definitions and concepts

General anesthesia is typically delivered through a combination of intravenous and inhalational agents and results in loss of consciousness, lack of response to stimuli and typically requires ventilatory support.

Regional anesthesia encompasses neuraxial (NA) techniques (eg, epidural and spinal anesthesia), and peripheral nerve blockade. Regional anesthetic techniques can be combined with systemic sedatives, but do not typically involve complete loss of consciousness or the need for complete ventilator support.

The stress of surgery causes a cascade of neural and humoral mediators that trigger tachycardia, blood pressure lability, and hypercoagulability, and can lead to MI, pulmonary infection, and thromboembolism [23]. Since pain plays a central role in triggering this stress response, effective analgesia can mitigate the ensuing adverse effects on various organ systems and improve outcomes [25]. General anesthesia modulates this response through the central nervous system, while RA blocks this pathway at the level of peripheral nerves or at the spinal cord [26].

Effective management of pain in the postinjury period is crucial, as uncontrolled pain may lead to both short-term complications and chronic pain syndromes [26].

Unlike RA, adequate blockade of the surgical stress response under GA requires large doses of opioids given prior to incision [25, 27]. Large doses of opioids increase the incidence of opioid-related adverse effects such as respiratory depression, sedation, nausea, ileus, and pruritus.

The addition of epidural anesthesia blocks the perioperative increases in adrenaline, cyclic adenosine monophosphate [28], renin, aldosterone, cortisol [29, 30], and vasopressin [31]. When epidural anesthesia is begun prior to surgery and maintained for 24 hours after surgery, muscle catabolism is minimized [32].

As noted previously, some aspects of this stress may be reduced by the administration of RA [1].

### 4.2 General versus neuraxial anesthesia

General anesthesia is required for patients with contraindications to NAs (eg, coagulopathy, infection at site, increased intracranial pressure), and may be preferred by some anesthesiologists and surgeons for patient-specific or procedure-specific issues. Some literature [33] suggests that regional techniques are associated with less delirium and fewer perioperative complications, but anesthetic practice varies greatly worldwide, and there are no large randomized trials of FFP to definitively inform this question [1, 24, 34]. For fractures of or trauma to the lower extremity, spinal, epidural, nerve blocks and GA may be used to provide anesthesia and analgesia. Proximal humeral fractures typically require GA in the FFP population.

### 4.3 Neuraxial anesthesia

A number of metaanalyses have compared outcomes of NA versus GA alone in a variety of surgical procedures and patient populations, but there remains a paucity of high quality literature as it applies to FFPs. In older cohorts, NA, whether used by itself or in combination with GA, was associated with a 59% reduction in postoperative respiratory depression. In studies focused on the use of NA in elective nonorthopedic surgeries, the odds of postoperative pneumonia are reduced by 39% and pulmonary embolism by 55% [35]. The largest studies of hip fracture patients [36] suggest decreased mortality and respiratory complications with NA but are limited by their observational and retrospective nature.

Compared to intravenous opioid therapy, NAs for pain control decrease the incidence of new angina, dysrhythmia, and CHF in high-risk patients [37]. A large systematic review comparing NA to GA found a reduction of approximately 33% in the incidence of MI [35]. A further systematic review found a decrease in PCM and mortality when epidural analgesia is continued for 24 hours after surgery [38]. Improved mortality rates and decrease pulmonary morbidity has been validated in at least one large retrospective study of older patients undergoing hip fracture surgery [39]. Opinions [40, 41] differ as to the extent of benefit conferred by regional anesthetic techniques, but improved outcomes seem to be greatest for high-risk patients [37, 42].

Due to a lower volume of cerebrospinal fluid (CSF), the presence of spinal stenosis, and reduced myelination of the nerves, older patients generally have a reduced latency time, higher dermatomal level, and increased block density with spinal anesthetic than younger patients. For these reasons, local anesthetic dosage should usually be reduced when performing NA in geriatric patients [26].

The presence of anticoagulation is often a limiting factor in the consideration of NA techniques for FFP. Epidural and spinal hematomas are rare but devastating complications of NA with the most significant risk factor being the presence of anticoagulation [43]; anticoagulation is much more prevalent with the increased emphasis on perioperative thromboprophylaxis in recent years [44]. Prior to the placement of a neuraxial anesthetic, the patient's coagulation status must be assessed, as NA is contraindicated in these patients. The American Society of Regional Anesthesia and Pain Management guidelines are applied to patients receiving neuraxial interventions as well as 'deep plexus' blocks or catheters (eg, lumbar plexus block) [45].

The following regional techniques are contraindicated in anticoagulated patients:

- Neuraxial, ie, epidural or spinal
- Paravertebral blocks
- Deep plexus blocks, ie, lumbar plexus and lumbar sympathetic plexus

Although these guidelines apply to all patients, older patients are more likely to have comorbid cardiovascular disease requiring anticoagulation or antithrombotic therapy, making a focused evaluation of anticoagulation status especially relevant.

Postdural puncture headache (PDPH) is the most common complication of spinal anesthesia and is caused by delayed closure of the dura resulting in a continuous CSF leak and decreased CSF volume and pressure. The incidence of PDPH diminishes significantly with increasing age and is rare in the older adults [46].

### 4.4 Lower extremity peripheral nerve blocks

All peripheral nerve blocks that are used for surgery of the lower extremity can also be used for analgesia following traumatic injury [26]. Femoral, sciatic, lumbar plexus and fascia iliaca blocks are all possible and their selection is dependent on the location of injury, type of operation and ability to position the patient [26].

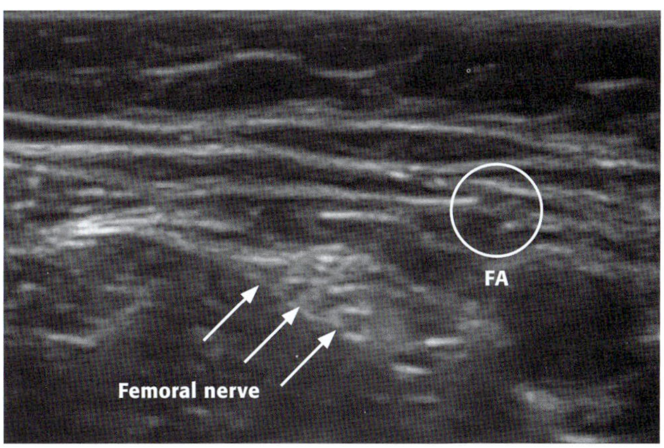


**Fig 1.3-1** Ultrasound image of the femoral nerve. Abbreviation: FA, femoral artery.

Issues to consider regarding lower extremity nerve blocks:

- The fascia iliaca block is performed in a region that is distant from vascular and other vital structures, making it relatively safe. It has been widely studied as a preoperative treatment of pain following hip fracture with reductions in acute pain and delirium [47]. Recently, however, the distribution, reproducibility, and utility of this block have come under question [48].
- The lumbar plexus block, consisting of L1–4 spinal roots with a contribution from T12, lies in the psoas muscle where these nerves can be blocked. The terminal nerves of the lumbar plexus are the iliogastric (L1), ilioinguinal (L1), genitofemoral L1/2), lateral femoral cutaneous nerve (L2/3), the femoral nerve (L2-4) and the obturator nerve (L2–4) [49].
- Femoral block is useful for trauma of the femur or patella (**Fig 1.3-1**) [49].
- The sciatic nerve block is widely used for surgery and/or pain control of the entire leg below the knee with the exception of the cutaneous distribution of the medial aspect of the lower leg [49].

### 4.5 Upper extremity peripheral nerve blocks

Issues to consider regarding upper extremity nerve blocks:

- For trauma of the shoulder, lateral clavicle, or proximal humerus, an interscalene block, performed at the level of C5 and C6 roots or the upper trunk, can provide excellent analgesia and/or anesthesia (**Fig 1.3-2**, **Fig 1.3-3**) [50]. This block can cause 100% hemidiaphragmatic paralysis either due to local anesthetic coursing towards the phrenic

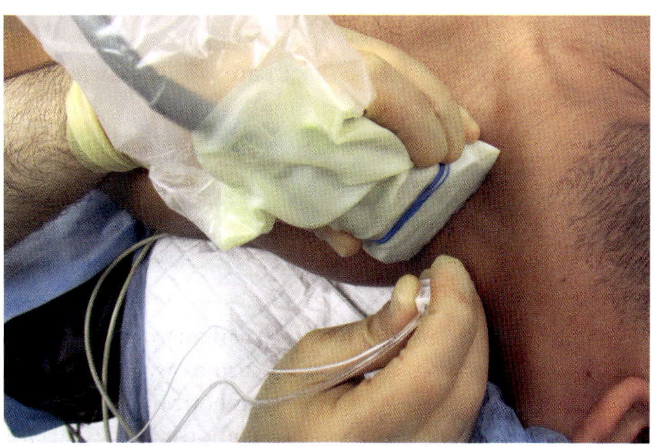

**Fig 1.3-2** Ultrasound transducer and needle position for performance of ultrasound-guided interscalene block in the out-of-plane orientation.

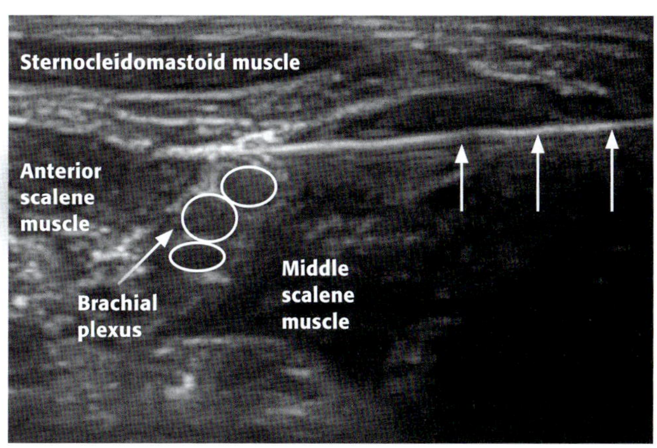


**Fig 1.3-3** Ultrasound image of interscalene brachial plexus with needle in the in-plane orientation. Arrows point to the incoming needle.

nerve or due to cephalad spread of local anesthetic towards C3–5 roots and therefore must be considered with caution in patients who have limited respiratory reserve [51]. It is contraindicated in patients with contralateral pneumothorax or pneumonectomies, contralateral phrenic nerve palsy, or contralateral recurrent laryngeal nerve palsies [52]. In such cases, GA is the preferred method of anesthesia.

- For more distal injuries, supraclavicular, infraclavicular, or axillary blocks may be used [26]. In trauma patients, the cervical spine must often be cleared prior to removal of the cervical collar and placement of an interscalene block [26].
- Supraclavicular blocks also carry a risk of phrenic nerve paralysis, albeit less than with the interscalene approach. Pneumothorax is a risk when performing either supraclavicular or infraclavicular blocks [26]. Due to a decrease in nerve myelination in older patients, greater diffusion of local anesthetics is possible utilizing lower volume. Therefore, as with NA, effective doses of local anesthetics should be reduced when performing peripheral nerve blocks in geriatric patients [1].

### 4.5.1 Nerve injury and peripheral nerve blocks

Nerve injury can result from a number of factors related to the patient (eg, preexisting trauma and/or neuropathy), surgery (eg, mechanical, tourniquet), or the nerve block and most often involves a combination of factors [53]. Neural injury resulting from a nerve block is rare, occurring with a frequency of 0.4 per 1,000 blocks [54] but can result from direct mechanical trauma of the needle, neurotoxicity from the local anesthetic, or an intraneural injection of local anesthetic [53]. According to the double crush hypothesis, patients with preexisting nerve injury or neural disease are at greater risk of developing a clinically significant neuropathy if a nerve is subsequently injured at a second location along the neural pathway [55]. For this reason, nerve blocks following traumatic injury should be approached with caution and include a robust assessment of risks and benefits as well as discussion with the patient and the surgical team. Age-related changes in the somatic nervous system include peripheral nerve deterioration and decreased myelinated nerve fiber conduction [1].

It is unclear whether such changes increase the older patient's susceptibility to nerve injury due to the performance of RA. However, preoperative assessment and documentation of preexisting neural compromise are important.

### 4.5.2 Compartment syndrome

Treatment of pain following a traumatic injury to an extremity with RA carries the risk of masking the pain of compartment syndrome [56]. Performing RA after traumatic injury therefore remains a controversial topic with early case reports indicating a delay in the diagnosis of compartment syndrome [57, 58]. However, more recent case reports show that breakthrough pain in the presence of a regional block is not masked by peripheral nerve blocks [56, 59]. Moreover, the emergence of breakthrough or crescendo pain, together with edema of the affected extremity, in the presence of a continuous nerve catheter has been suggested as evidence of compartment syndrome [60]. This topic remains controversial and requires an assessment of risks and benefits and close communication between the orthopedic and anesthesia teams.

### 4.5.3 Effects of sedation

There has been some emerging evidence that patients who are more heavily sedated under RA have an increased risk of postoperative delirium and may even have an increased risk of mortality after 1 year than those who are more lightly sedated [61, 62]. However, these studies have not established a causative relation between anesthetic depth and mortality, have not been confirmed by other studies [63], and their validity has been questioned [64]. Due to the susceptibility of the geriatric population to postoperative delirium, heavy sedation is likely not ideal in this population.

## 4.6 Multimodal analgesia

Multimodal analgesia involves the use of a variety of analgesic agents, each with different mechanisms, to treat pain [26]. The use of multimodal analgesia has become a mainstay of perioperative pain management in order to reduce opioid use and related adverse effects including respiratory depression, sedation, nausea, ileus, and pruritus [65, 66]. Moreover, when opioids are used as a single modality, higher doses are required, increasing the risk of adverse effects [67–69]. These adverse effects may be more pronounced in older adults due to impaired pharmacodynamics and pharmacokinetic handling of the drugs [70]. While opioid-sparing therapies are of potential benefit to older adults, the risks of other pharmacological agents are not particularly well studied. Many nonopioid analgesic agents have limiting adverse effects, particularly in the clinically unstable FFP.

Specifically, nonsteroidal antiinflammatory drug use is limited in the immediate perioperative period due to concerns with gastrointestinal bleeding and renal injury in the hemodynamically tenuous older adult. Caution should also be taken with the use of gabapentinoids due to dose-related adverse effects such as sedation and dizziness, especially given the goals of early ambulation.

Recently, intravenous acetaminophen has become available in the United States and has produced promising results and few adverse effects. In patients having hip and knee arthroplasties, reduced morphine consumption and improved Visual Analog Scale pain scores have been noted with the inclusion of acetaminophen [71]. The cost of intravenous acetaminophen limits its use in many centers. Additionally, the N-methyl-D-aspartate antagonist ketamine has profound analgesic properties and has been shown to be an effective component of a multimodal analgesic regimen by diminishing opioid use, decreasing postoperative pain, and improving time to reaching physical therapy goals in orthopedic patients [72–76]. But it requires additional study in older trauma patients due to the risk of dysphoria, sedation, hallucinations, and postoperative cognitive dysfunction.

## 5 Intraoperative positioning

Careful patient positioning is of utmost importance during the intraoperative period, particularly in patients who are deeply sedated, under GA, or have a regional anesthetic, rendering them unable to alert physicians to early signs of injury [77]. Although patient positioning is an important consideration for all patients in the operating room, special care must be taken when applied to the older patient due to increased incidence of osteoporosis, hypertension, diabetes mellitus, and peripheral vascular disease [78–81]. Ischemic stroke is an especially feared complication in the beach chair position [82]. The effect of gravity decreases venous return, reducing cardiac output and cerebral perfusion pressure. Risk factors for stroke are far more common in older patients, necessitating meticulous management of hemodynamic factors, such as maintenance of blood pressure as close as possible to the patient's baseline values [83]. For these reasons, the regular use of hypotensive anesthesia for improved visualization in arthroscopic shoulder surgery should be either avoided or used with great caution in patients with risk factors for stroke, such as hypertension or cerebrovascular disease [82]. Alternatively, the beach chair position can be avoided altogether.

## 6 Partnering with anesthesiologists

The practice of medicine in general, and anesthesia in particular, has often been compared with other high-stakes professions such as aviation where evidence has long shown that inadequate teamwork is one of the main reasons for preventable error [84]. Effective communication, mutual monitoring, and both giving and receiving feedback are all essential elements of teamwork [82, 84] (see also chapter 2.6 Orthogeriatric team—principles, roles, and responsibilities).

## 7 References

1. **Nordquist D, Halaszynski TM.** Perioperative multimodal anesthesia using regional techniques in the aging surgical patient. *Pain Res Treat.* 2014;2014:902174.
2. **Friedman SM, Mendelson DA, Bingham KW, et al.** Impact of a comanaged Geriatric Fracture Center on short-term hip fracture outcomes. *Arch Intern Med.* 2009 Oct 12;169(18):1712–1717.
3. **Kammerlander C, Gosch M, Blauth M, et al.** The Tyrolean Geriatric Fracture Center: an orthogeriatric co-management model. *Z Gerontol Geriatr.* 2011 Dec;44(6):363–367.
4. **Mangano DT.** Perioperative cardiac morbidity. *Anesthesiology.* 1990 Jan;72(1):153–184.
5. **Mangano DT, Browner WS, Hollenberg M, et al.** Long-term cardiac prognosis following noncardiac surgery. The Study of Perioperative Ischemia Research Group. *JAMA.* 1992 Jul 8;268(2):233–239.
6. **O'Hara DA, Duff A, Berlin JA, et al.** The effect of anesthetic technique on postoperative outcomes in hip fracture repair. *Anesthesiology.* 2000 Apr;92(4):947–957.
7. **Sharma G, Goodwin J.** Effect of aging on respiratory system physiology and immunology. *Clin Interv Aging.* 2006;1(3):253–260.
8. **Janssens JP, Pache JC, Nicod LP.** Physiological changes in respiratory function associated with ageing. *Eur Respir J.* 1999 Jan;13(1):197–205.
9. **Lalley PM.** The aging respiratory system—pulmonary structure, function and neural control. *Respir Physiol Neurobiol.* 2013 Jul 1;187(3):199–210.
10. **Peterson DD, Pack AI, Silage DA, et al.** Effects of aging on ventilatory and occlusion pressure responses to hypoxia and hypercapnia. *Am Rev Respir Dis.* 1981 Oct;124(4):387–391.
11. **Mann C, Pouzeratte Y, Eledjam JJ.** Postoperative patient-controlled analgesia in the elderly: risks and benefits of epidural versus intravenous administration. *Drugs Aging.* 2003;20(5):337–345.
12. **Monk TG, Weldon BC, Garvan CW, et al.** Predictors of cognitive dysfunction after major noncardiac surgery. *Anesthesiology.* 2008 Jan;108(1):18–30.
13. **Schupf N, Tang MX, Albert SM, et al.** Decline in cognitive and functional skills increases mortality risk in nondemented elderly. *Neurology.* 2005 Oct 25;65(8):1218–1226.
14. **Bosworth HB, Schaie KW, Willis SL.** Cognitive and sociodemographic risk factors for mortality in the Seattle Longitudinal Study. *J Gerontol B Psychol Sci Soc Sci.* 1999 Sep;54(5):P273–P282.
15. **Olofsson B, Lundstrom M, Borssen B, et al.** Delirium is associated with poor rehabilitation outcome in elderly patients treated for femoral neck fractures. *Scand J Caring Sci.* 2005 Jun;19(2):119–127.
16. **Holland R.** Anaesthetic mortality in New South Wales. *Br J Anaesth.* 1987 Jul;59(7):834–841.
17. **Abel RB, Rosenblatt MA.** Preoperative evaluation and preparation of patients for orthopedic surgery. *Anesthesiol Clin.* 2014 Dec;32(4):881–892.
18. **Fleisher LA, Fleischmann KE, Auerbach AD, et al.** 2014 ACC/AHA guideline on perioperative cardiovascular evaluation and management of patients undergoing noncardiac surgery: a report of the American College of Cardiology/American Heart Association Task Force on practice guidelines. *J Am Coll Cardiol.* 2014 Dec 9;64(22):e77–137.
19. **Lee TH, Marcantonio ER, Mangione CM, et al.** Derivation and prospective validation of a simple index for prediction of cardiac risk of major noncardiac surgery. *Circulation.* 1999 Sep 7;100(10):1043–1049.
20. **Shiga T, Wajima Z, Ohe Y.** Is operative delay associated with increased mortality of hip fracture patients? Systematic review, meta-analysis, and meta-regression. *Can J Anaesth.* 2008 Mar;55(3):146–154.
21. **American Society of Anesthesiologists.** Five Things Physicians and Patients Should Question. Available at: http://www.choosingwisely.org/doctor-patient-lists/american-society-of-anesthesiologists/. Accessed June 10, 2016.
22. **Douglas PS, Garcia MJ, Haines DE, et al.** ACCF/ASE/AHA/ASNC/HFSA/HRS/SCAI/SCCM/SCCT/SCMR 2011 Appropriate Use Criteria for Echocardiography. A Report of the American College of Cardiology Foundation Appropriate Use Criteria Task Force, American Society of Echocardiography, American Heart Association, American Society of Nuclear Cardiology, Heart Failure Society of America, Heart Rhythm Society, Society for Cardiovascular Angiography and Interventions, Society of Critical Care Medicine, Society of Cardiovascular Computed Tomography, and Society for Cardiovascular Magnetic Resonance Endorsed by the American College of Chest Physicians. *J Am Coll Cardiol.* 2011 Mar 1;57(9):1126–1166.
23. **Kheterpal S, Khodaparast O, Shanks A, et al.** Chronic angiotensin-converting enzyme inhibitor or angiotensin receptor blocker therapy combined with diuretic therapy is associated with increased episodes of hypotension in noncardiac surgery. *J Cardiothorac Vasc Anesth.* 2008 Apr;22(99):180–186.
24. **Guay J, Parker MJ, Gajendragadkar PR, et al.** Anaesthesia for hip fracture surgery in adults. *Cochrane Database Syst Rev.* 2016 Feb 22;2:CD000521.
25. **Liu S, Carpenter RL, Neal JM.** Epidural anesthesia and analgesia. Their role in postoperative outcome. *Anesthesiology.* 1995 Jun;82(6):1474–1506.
26. **Clark L, Robinson M, Varbanova M.** Role of regional anesthesia in orthopedic trauma. *Anesthesiol Clin.* 2014 Dec;32(4):789–808.
27. **Giesecke K, Hamberger B, Jarnberg PO, et al.** High- and low-dose fentanyl anaesthesia: hormonal and metabolic responses during cholecystectomy. *Br J Anaesth.* 1988 Nov;61(5):575–582.
28. **Engquist A, Fog-Moller F, Christiansen C, et al.** Influence of epidural analgesia on the catecholamine and cyclic AMP responses to surgery. *Acta Anaesthesiol Scand.* 1980;24(1):17–21.
29. **Brandt MR, Olgaard K, Kehlet H.** Epidural analgesia inhibits the renin and aldosterone response to surgery. *Acta Anaesthesiol Scand.* 1979 Jun;23(3):267–272.
30. **Engquist A, Brandt MR, Fernandes A, et al.** The blocking effect of epidural analgesia on the adrenocortical and hyperglycemic responses to surgery. *Acta Anaesthesiol Scand.* 1977;21(4):330–335.
31. **Kehlet H.** Epidural analgesia and the endocrine-metabolic response to surgery. Update and perspectives. *Acta Anaesthesiol Scand.* 1984 Apr;28(2):125–127.
32. **Carli F, Webster J, Pearson M, et al.** Protein metabolism after abdominal surgery: effect of 24-h extradural block with local anaesthetic. *Br J Anaesth.* 1991 Dec;67(6):729–734.
33. **Parker MJ, Handoll HH, Griffiths R.** Anaesthesia for hip fracture surgery in adults. *Cochrane Database Syst Rev.* 2004 (4):CD000521.
34. **Maxwell L, White S.** Anaesthetic management of patients with hip fractures: an update. *Continuing Educ Anaesth Critic Care Pain.* 2013;13(5):179–183.
35. **Rodgers A, Walker N, Schug S, et al.** Reduction of postoperative mortality and morbidity with epidural or spinal anaesthesia: results from overview of randomised trials. *BMJ.* 2000 Dec 16;321(7275):1493.

36. **Neuman MD, Silber JH, Elkassabany NM, et al.** Comparative effectiveness of regional versus general anesthesia for hip fracture surgery in adults. *Anesthesiology.* 2012 Jul;117(1):72–92.
37. **Yeager MP, Glass DD, Neff RK, et al.** Epidural anesthesia and analgesia in high-risk surgical patients. *Anesthesiology.* 1987 Jun;66(6):729–736.
38. **Rigg JR, Jamrozik K, Myles PS, et al.** Epidural anaesthesia and analgesia and outcome of major surgery: a randomised trial. *Lancet.* 2002 Apr 13;359(9314):1276–1282.
39. **Matot I, Oppenheim-Eden A, Ratrot R, et al.** Preoperative cardiac events in elderly patients with hip fracture randomized to epidural or conventional analgesia. *Anesthesiology.* 2003 Jan;98(1):156–163.
40. **Rawal N.** Epidural technique for postoperative pain: gold standard no more? *Reg Anesth Pain Med.* 2012 May–Jun;37(3):310–317.
41. **Roy RC.** Choosing general versus regional anesthesia for the elderly. *Anesthesiol Clin North Am.* 2000 Mar;18(1):91–104, vii.
42. **Beattie WS, Badner NH, Choi P.** Epidural analgesia reduces postoperative myocardial infarction: a meta-analysis. *Anesth Analg.* 2001 Oct;93(4):853–858.
43. **Pumberger M, Memtsoudis SG, Stundner O, et al.** An analysis of the safety of epidural and spinal neuraxial anesthesia in more than 100,000 consecutive major lower extremity joint replacements. *Reg Anesth Pain Med.* 2013 Nov–Dec;38(6):515–519.
44. **Vandermeulen EP, Van Aken H, Vermylen J.** Anticoagulants and spinal-epidural anesthesia. *Anesth Analg.* 1994 Dec;79(6):1165–1177.
45. **Horlocker TT, Wedel DJ, Rowlingson JC, et al.** Regional anesthesia in the patient receiving antithrombotic or thrombolytic therapy: American Society of Regional Anesthesia and Pain Medicine Evidence-Based Guidelines (Third Edition). *Reg Anesth Pain Med.* 2010 Jan–Feb;35(1):64–101.
46. **Dodge HS, Ekhator NN, Jefferson-Wilson L, et al.** Cigarette smokers have reduced risk for post-dural puncture headache. *Pain Physician.* 2013 Jan;16(1):E25–30.
47. **Rashiq S, Vandermeer B, Abou-Setta AM, et al.** Efficacy of supplemental peripheral nerve blockade for hip fracture surgery: multiple treatment comparison. *Can J Anaesth.* 2013 Mar;60(3):230–243.
48. **Shariat AN, Hadzic A, Xu D, et al.** Fascia Iliaca block for analgesia after hip arthroplasty: a randomized double-blind, placebo-controlled trial. *Reg Anesth Pain Med.* 2013 May–Jun;38(3):201–205.
49. **Hadzic A.** *Hadzic's Peripheral Nerve Blocks and Anatomy for Ultrasound-Guided Regional Anesthesia.* 2nd ed. New York: McGraw-Hill Professional; 2012.
50. **Fredrickson MJ, Krishnan S, Chen CY.** Postoperative analgesia for shoulder surgery: a critical appraisal and review of current techniques. *Anaesthesia.* 2010 Jun;65(6):608–624.
51. **Urmey WF, Talts KH, Sharrock NE.** One hundred percent incidence of hemidiaphragmatic paresis associated with interscalene brachial plexus anesthesia as diagnosed by ultrasonography. *Anesth Analg.* 1991 Apr;72(4):498–503.
52. **Urmey WF, McDonald M.** Hemidiaphragmatic paresis during interscalene brachial plexus block: effects on pulmonary function and chest wall mechanics. *Anesth Analg.* 1992 Mar;74(3):352–357.
53. **Lirk P, Birmingham B, Hogan Q.** Regional anesthesia in patients with preexisting neuropathy. *Int Anesthesiol Clin.* 2011 Fall;49(4):144–165.
54. **Barrington MJ, Watts SA, Gledhill SR, et al.** Preliminary results of the Australasian Regional Anaesthesia Collaboration: a prospective audit of more than 7000 peripheral nerve and plexus blocks for neurologic and other complications. *Reg Anesth Pain Med.* 2009 Nov–Dec;34(6):534–541.
55. **Upton AR, McComas AJ.** The double crush in nerve entrapment syndromes. *Lancet.* 1973 Aug 18;2(7825):359–362.
56. **Munk-Andersen H, Laustrup TK.** Compartment syndrome diagnosed in due time by breakthrough pain despite continuous peripheral nerve block. *Acta Anaesthesiol Scand.* 2013 Nov; 57(10):1328–1330.
57. **Morrow BC, Mawhinney IN, Elliott JR.** Tibial compartment syndrome complicating closed femoral nailing: diagnosis delayed by an epidural analgesic technique—case report. *J Trauma.* 1994 Nov;37(5):867–868.
58. **Hyder N, Kessler S, Jennings AG, et al.** Compartment syndrome in tibial shaft fracture missed because of a local nerve block. *J Bone Joint Surg Br.* 1996 May;78(3):499–500.
59. **Aguirre JA, Gresch D, Popovici A, et al.** Case scenario: compartment syndrome of the forearm in patient with an infraclavicular catheter: breakthrough pain as indicator. *Anesthesiology.* 2013 May;118(5):1198–1205.
60. **Cometa MA, Esch AT, Boezaart AP.** Did continuous femoral and sciatic nerve block obscure the diagnosis or delay the treatment of acute lower leg compartment syndrome? A case report. *Pain Med.* 2011 May;12(5):823–828.
61. **Sieber FE, Zakriya KJ, Gottschalk A, et al.** Sedation depth during spinal anesthesia and the development of postoperative delirium in elderly patients undergoing hip fracture repair. *Mayo Clin Proc.* 2010 Jan;85(1):18–26.
62. **Brown CHt, Azman AS, Gottschalk A, et al.** Sedation depth during spinal anesthesia and survival in elderly patients undergoing hip fracture repair. *Anesth Analg.* 2014 May;118(5):977–980.
63. **Kertai MD, Palanca BJ, Pal N, et al.** Bispectral index monitoring, duration of bispectral index below 45, patient risk factors, and intermediate-term mortality after noncardiac surgery in the B-Unaware Trial. *Anesthesiology.* 2011 Mar;114(3):545–556.
64. **Cohen NH.** Anesthetic depth is not (yet) a predictor of mortality! *Anesth Analg.* 2005 Jan;100(1):1–3.
65. **Kehlet H, Dahl JB.** Anaesthesia, surgery, and challenges in postoperative recovery. *Lancet.* 2003 Dec 6;362(9399):1921–1928.
66. Practice guidelines for acute pain management in the perioperative setting: an updated report by the American Society of Anesthesiologists Task Force on Acute Pain Management. *Anesthesiology.* 2012 Feb;116(2):248–273.
67. **Guignard B, Bossard AE, Coste C, et al.** Acute opioid tolerance: intraoperative remifentanil increases postoperative pain and morphine requirement. *Anesthesiology.* 2000 Aug;93(2):409–417.
68. **Vanderah TW, Ossipov MH, Lai J, et al.** Mechanisms of opioid-induced pain and antinociceptive tolerance: descending facilitation and spinal dynorphin. *Pain.* 2001 May;92(1–2):5–9.
69. **Bowsher D.** Paradoxical pain. *BMJ.* 1993 Feb 20;306(6876):473–474.
70. **Kruijt Spanjer MR, Bakker NA, Absalom AR.** Pharmacology in the elderly and newer anaesthesia drugs. *Best Pract Res Clin Anaesthesiol.* 2011 Sep;25(3):355–365.
71. **Sinatra RS, Jahr JS, Reynolds LW, et al.** Efficacy and safety of single and repeated administration of 1 gram intravenous acetaminophen injection (paracetamol) for pain management after major orthopedic surgery. *Anesthesiology.* 2005 Apr;102(4):822–831.

72. **McCartney CJ, Sinha A, Katz J.** A qualitative systematic review of the role of N-methyl-D-aspartate receptor antagonists in preventive analgesia. *Anesth Analg.* 2004 May;98(5):1385–1400.
73. **Jabbour HJ, Naccache NM, Jawish RJ, et al.** Ketamine and magnesium association reduces morphine consumption after scoliosis surgery: prospective randomised double-blind study. *Acta Anaesthesiol Scand.* 2014 May;58(5):572–579.
74. **Elia N, Tramer MR.** Ketamine and postoperative pain—a quantitative systematic review of randomised trials. *Pain.* 2005 Jan;113(1–2):61–70.
75. **Aveline C, Gautier JF, Vautier P, et al.** Postoperative analgesia and early rehabilitation after total knee replacement: a comparison of continuous low-dose intravenous ketamine versus nefopam. *Eur J Pain.* 2009 Jul;13(6):613–619.
76. **Remerand F, Le Tendre C, Baud A, et al.** The early and delayed analgesic effects of ketamine after total hip arthroplasty: a prospective, randomized, controlled, double-blind study. *Anesth Analg.* 2009 Dec;109(6):1963–1971.
77. **Parks BJ.** Postoperative peripheral neuropathies. *Surgery.* 1973 Sep;74(3):348–357.
78. **Zarrelli MM, Amoruso L, Beghi E, et al.** Arterial hypertension as a risk factor for chronic symmetric polyneuropathy. *J Epidemiol Biostat.* 2001;6(5):409–413.
79. **Vinik AI, Park TS, Stansberry KB, et al.** Diabetic neuropathies. *Diabetologia.* 2000 Aug;43(8):957–973.
80. **Richardson JK, Jamieson SC.** Cigarette smoking and ulnar mononeuropathy at the elbow. *Am J Phys Med Rehabil.* 2004 Sep;83(9):730–734.
81. **Welch MB, Brummett CM, Welch TD, et al.** Perioperative peripheral nerve injuries: a retrospective study of 380,680 cases during a 10-year period at a single institution. *Anesthesiology.* 2009 Sep;111(3):490–497.
82. **Rains DD, Rooke GA, Wahl CJ.** Pathomechanisms and complications related to patient positioning and anesthesia during shoulder arthroscopy. *Arthroscopy.* 2011 Apr;27(4):532–541.
83. **Pohl A, Cullen DJ.** Cerebral ischemia during shoulder surgery in the upright position: a case series. *J Clin Anesth.* 2005 Sep;17(6):463–469.
84. **Brindley PG.** I. Improving teamwork in anaesthesia and critical care: many lessons still to learn. *Br J Anaesth.* 2014 Mar;112(3):399–401.

# 1.4 Preoperative risk assessment and preparation

Joseph A Nicholas

## 1 Introduction

Skilled preoperative assessment and optimization of the geriatric fracture patient directly contributes to excellent outcomes. Although there is a paucity of relevant literature on older adults undergoing urgent surgery, best practices are heavily informed by geriatric principles combined with evidence extrapolated from other populations and settings. The perioperative medical practices supported by much of the existing literature require modification for the physiologies and vulnerabilities of older adults, and geriatric fracture care should not simply replicate practices patterns used for the stable and healthier elective surgery patient.

Medical centers using a standardized geriatric medicine approach to preoperative care have reliably demonstrated improved outcomes in mortality, length of stay and reduction in complications [1–3]. This chapter focuses on the strategies used by many of these centers in the areas of risk assessment and optimization.

Key principles and goals:

- Early surgical fixation, particularly for highly frail or comorbid patients
- Optimization by a general medical service for surgery in less than 24 hours for most patients, and many in less than 6 hours
- Pain control with parenteral opiates and regional nerve block techniques
- Anticipation of hypotension in the intra and postoperative period; liberal use of intravascular hydration, and cessation or reduction of most antihypertensive medications
- Avoidance of excessive perioperative testing, medical consultation and polypharmacy

## 2 Unique perioperative aspects

In addition to risk assessment and surgical planning, the perioperative management of older adults is focused on active efforts directed towards pain control, maintenance of hemodynamic stability and avoidance of functional decline. Early surgery is the most important way to achieve these goals, and the preoperative medical assessment needs to prioritize early surgery and early mobility over many other chronic medical issues. For these reasons, high-performing geriatric fracture centers have implemented clinical pathways that emphasize timely transition to operative repair, even in highly comorbid or frail older adults. Many notable comorbidities warranting more intensive preoperative testing and consultation prior to elective surgery are not vigorously pursued in the geriatric fracture setting.

## 3 Preoperative risk assessment

For almost all patients, the benefits of operative fracture repair, including hemostasis, pain control and mobilization, exceed the risks related to anesthesia and surgery. This is due to both the improved safety of advanced anesthetic and surgical techniques and the excessive morbidity and mortality of hip fracture patients in the absence of surgical repair. Patient-specific risks can be roughly estimated with the careful use of preoperative risk calculators, and may allow for better anticipation of patient-specific outcomes and complications.

### 3.1 Risk calculators

The Nottingham Hip Fracture Score [4] is the best-validated instrument for predicting 30-day and longer outcomes in the hip fracture population, and incorporates measures of comorbidity burden, functional status (ie, type of residence), cognitive status (ie, mini-mental test score), nutritional status (ie, albumin), and key demographic factors (ie, age, gender). Elements like institutionalization and mini-mental test score are not universally consistent across different international settings, but likely can be approximated and remain useful for estimating perioperative risk and short-term outcomes (**Table 1.4-1**, **Table 1.4-2**).

A number of additional calculators have been developed in the attempt to provide a reasonable estimate of serious complications in surgical patients; none are validated in older adults undergoing urgent orthopedic surgery. Three calculators that were examined in the most recent American College of Cardiology/American Heart Association (ACC/AHA) guidelines include the Revised Cardiac Risk Index (RCRI) [6], the Myocardial Infarction or Cardiac Arrest calculator [7], and the American College of Surgeons' National Surgical Quality Improvement Program Surgical Risk Calculator [8]. The key features of the RCRI are summarized in **Table 1.4-3**.

## 3.2 Other assessments of prognostic importance

Despite the historical emphasis on comorbidity scoring for estimating surgical risk, functional and cognitive impairment have long been recognized in geriatric medicine to predict many clinically significant perioperative complications and mortality [10]. There are several tools to quickly classify cognitive and functional status into meaningful categories; these can be easily incorporated into standard medical, surgical or nursing assessments.

### 3.2.1 Functional capacity

The Parker Mobility Score is a simple measure of function that has been derived and validated in the hip fracture setting, and evaluated in multiple settings and for multiple important outcomes (**Table 1.4-4**). More extensive functional status evaluation can be helpful in the rehabilitation phase.

| Variable | Value | Points |
|---|---|---|
| Age, y | 66–85<br>> 85 | 3<br>4 |
| Gender | Male | 1 |
| Admission hemoglobin | ≤ 10 g/dL | 1 |
| Admission mini-mental test score | ≤ 6 of 10 | 1 |
| Living in an institution | Yes | 1 |
| Number of comorbidities | ≥ 2 | 1 |
| Malignancy | Yes | 1 |

**Table 1.4-1** Nottingham Hip Fracture Score, adapted from Maxwell et al [4].

| Nottingham Hip Fracture Score | Estimated 30-day mortality, % |
|---|---|
| 1 | 1 |
| 3 | 3 |
| 5 | 7–10 |
| 7 | 16–23 |
| 10 | 45–57 |

**Table 1.4-2** Nottingham Hip Fracture Score and predicted mortality rates, adapted from Moppett et al [5].

| Risk factors | Points |
|---|---|
| High-risk surgery (intraperitoneal, intrathoracic, suprainguinal vascular) | 1 |
| Ischemic heart disease history | 1 |
| Heart failure history | 1 |
| Stroke or cerebrovascular ischemia history | 1 |
| Diabetes requiring insulin | 1 |
| Renal failure with creatinine > 2 mg/dL | 1 |

| Total points | Risk of major cardiac event, % |
|---|---|
| 1 | 1.0 |
| 2 | 2.4 |
| ≥ 3 | 5.4 |

**Table 1.4-3** Perioperative Risk Calculator: Revised Cardiac Risk Index, adapted from Devereux et al [9].

| Mobility | No difficulty | With an aid | With assistance | Not at all |
|---|---|---|---|---|
| Around house | 3 | 2 | 1 | 0 |
| Out of house | 3 | 2 | 1 | 0 |
| Shopping | 3 | 2 | 1 | 0 |

| Total (NMS) | 1-year mortality, % |
|---|---|
| ≤ 3 | 56 |
| 4–5 | 38 |
| > 5 | 15 |

**Table 1.4-4** New (Parker) Mobility Score (NMS) [11].

### 3.2.2 Cognitive assessments

Impaired cognition is significantly associated with functional dependence and poor outcomes, and by itself is a marker of increased perioperative risks and postoperative dependency [12]. For patients without a preexisting diagnosis, diagnostic assessment for dementia is often not possible during the preoperative period, due to the complicating presence of delirium. In these situations historical features can often suggest the presence of dementia; impairments in telephone use, handing of finances and medication self-administration best correlate with underlying dementia [13]. For patients without delirium, the Mini-Cog test is a validated, efficient tool with good ability to identify dementia [14]. See chapter 1.14 Delirium for further discussion.

### 3.2.3 Exercise capacity

Exercise capacity is used as a surrogate for functional capacity and physiological reserve, and has been incorporated into the ACC/AHA guidelines to discriminate high- and low-risk patients, using a threshold of 4 metabolic equivalents of task [15]. Common activities that meet this threshold include walking up a flight of stairs, walking up a hill, walking at a minimum pace of 6.4 km/h (4 mph), or heavy housework like scrubbing floors and moving heavy furniture. For patients undergoing elective surgery, these guidelines suggest that patients who can perform this level of exertion do not require additional cardiovascular testing preoperatively. This level of exercise capacity should be relatively reassuring for the geriatric fracture patient as well.

## 4 Routine preoperative testing

The standard preoperative evaluation should be limited to bedside clinical evaluation, basic blood work and essential radiographic studies. Excellent perioperative outcomes can be obtained with the following tests: radiography of the fracture, hemoglobin level and platelet count, basic serum electrolytes and renal function, and a resting electrocardiogram [3].

Recommended preoperative tests include:

- Standard:
  - Complete blood count
  - Basic electrolytes and renal function
  - Serum calcium
- Typically recommended:
  - Electrocardiogram
  - Coagulation studies
    (particularly for patients taking warfarin)
  - Albumin
    (to correct calcium and screen for malnutrition)
- Metabolic bone evaluation:
  - Vitamin D levels
  - Parathyroid hormone (PTH) levels
  - Thyroid studies

As part of a standard protocol, it may be helpful to perform metabolic bone assessments (ie, calcium and phosphorus, PTH, thyroid hormone, vitamin D levels) or help identify malnutrition (ie, albumin levels), although the results of these studies are not essential prior to proceeding to surgical fixation. Standardized order sets and protocols can help streamline this preoperative testing process and minimize inappropriate variation in care [16].

Bedside clinical evaluation should focus on the assessment of intravascular volume status and the rapid identification of the few active medical conditions that warrant surgical delay, including acute pulmonary edema, acute coronary syndrome, sepsis, unstable arrhythmias, or acute stroke.

## 5 Advanced investigations

For most fragility fracture patients there is no demonstrated benefit to routine advanced investigations such as echocardiography, noninvasive cardiovascular stress testing, or prolonged preoperative cardiac rhythm monitoring. Retrospective studies suggest that routine advanced cardiovascular testing, including echocardiography, results in significant surgical delay without clinically important changes in management [17, 18]. In addition, the preoperative care teams should carefully avoid preoperative workup of otherwise stable chronic comorbidities like chronic renal failure, chronic stable coronary disease, or chronic neurological deficits; there is no known benefit to more intensive workup and consultation prior to fracture fixation. Other routine tests of uncertain preoperative impact include routine urinalysis, chest radiography and biomarker assays, ie, B-type natriuretic peptide and troponin levels. The high incidence of asymptomatic bacteriuria in older adults, particularly women, can prompt inappropriate antibiotic use, and nonspecific biomarker elevations may lead to acute interventions that promote hypotension, bleeding and surgical delay. Until there is better prospective data supporting routine use of biomarker assays in fragility fracture patients, these should be limited in this setting to symptomatic patients.

## 6 Preoperative medical treatments

In addition to clinical assessments and risk stratification, preoperative optimization typically requires a small set of interventions to minimize surgical delay and intraoperative hypotension.

### 6.1 Intravascular volume restoration

Almost all older adults with femoral fractures suffer from acute intravascular volume depletion and require volume restoration to minimize perioperative hypotension. Initial hemoglobin assessment prior to volume restoration can significantly underestimate the degree of anemia, and blood loss will often continue until the fracture is reduced and fixed, especially in the patients with recent use of antithrombotic or anticoagulant medications.

Most published reviews support the initiation of isotonic intravenous fluids as soon as possible for patients without clinically significant acute pulmonary edema. Geriatric fracture centers typically report preoperative hemoglobin targets of 10 mg/dL, in anticipation of further blood loss during the perioperative period [19].

In general, it is easier to treat the consequences of pulmonary edema from overhydration than to manage those related to volume depletion (ie, hypotension, stroke and renal failure).

### 6.2 Pain management

Acute pain control is another cornerstone of acute preoperative care for fragility fracture patients. Inadequate pain control is associated with increased adrenergic drive and myocardial oxygen demand and contributes to a number of complications including delirium, tachyarrhythmia and myocardial infarction.

Pain control is one of the reasons that early surgical fixation is associated with improved postoperative complications. In the preoperative phase, most published protocols use standard doses of intravenous opioids to achieve adequate pain control. Morphine sulfate, hydromorphone and oxycodone have all been shown to be effective and safe when used in adjusted doses for frail older adults. In addition, there is a growing body of literature on the safety and efficacy of blocks of the femoral nerve other local nerve blocks, particularly with ultrasound guidance [20]. Successful nerve blocks can produce faster time to analgesia and result in less opioid use for the duration of the block. Intravenous acetaminophen/paracetamol has not been well studied in this population, but is expected to be helpful as well, although its use may be limited by cost in many institutions. Techniques for pain assessment and management in older adults is more thoroughly covered in chapters 1.12 Pain management and 1.7 Postoperative medical management.

### 6.3 Medication management

One of the most nuanced areas in perioperative optimization includes the management of long-term medications in older adults. Each medication should be evaluated for its potential efficacy or harm in the acute fracture setting, and determine the risk of continuation, acute cessation or, in the case of some anticoagulants, reversal. This is optimally done by a medical physician with experience in perioperative care of older adults. Additional approaches are discussed in further detail in chapter 1.13 Polypharmacy.

#### 6.3.1 Antihypertensive medications

The high risk of perioperative hypotension in the older fracture patient makes the routine continuation of long-term blood pressure medications particularly dangerous in this setting. With the exception of beta-blockers and clonidine, acute cessation of most other commonly used antihypertensive medications is not problematic.

#### 6.3.2 Beta-blockers

Perioperative beta-blocker recommendations have undergone dramatic changes over the past 10 years, and the initiation of beta-blockers in patients prior to surgery is no longer recommended [21].

Patients taking long-term beta-blockers should have them continued in this setting, although dose attenuation may be required in patients with perioperative blood pressures in the low-normal range. Other medications used for long-term heart rate control, eg, diltiazem, verapamil, may also need to be continued.

#### 6.3.3 Angiotensin-converting enzyme inhibitors and angiotensin-receptor blockers

Angiotensin-converting enzyme inhibitors (ACEIs) and angiotensin-receptor blockers (ARBs) are known to cause hypotension and acute kidney injury in the perioperative setting [22, 23], as well as contribute to acute kidney injury in hemodynamically unstable patients [24]. In the typical fragility fracture patient with increased risks for hypotension and acute renal failure, routine cessation of ACEIs/ARBs in the preoperative period is usually appropriate.

#### 6.3.4 Statins

Both the ACC/AHA and the European Society of Cardiology guidelines support the continuation of statin therapy for patients already taking them. There is no evidence for the acute initiation of statin therapy in patients undergoing urgent nonvascular surgery.

#### 6.3.5 Diuretics

In light of concern for intravascular volume depletion, all diuretics are typically held in the preoperative period.

#### 6.3.6 Noncardiovascular medications

Oral diabetic medications typically should be held preoperatively to avoid clinically significant hypoglycemia in the perioperative phase. Patients using insulin will also need attenuation of long-term insulin doses; the use of frequent blood glucose monitoring and the use of short-acting insulin is the safest approach in the dynamic perioperative period. Patients receiving long-term psychiatric medications will often need these continued, although dose attenuation or temporary cessation in the event of excessive sedation or other side effects may need to be considered. Patients on long-term opioid or benzodiazepine therapy are at risk for withdrawal with abrupt cessation, and parenteral replacement may be necessary if patients are not able to take oral medications. Patients receiving long-term opiate therapy may need to have augmented doses of opiates to overcome tolerance and achieve effective pain relief. Overall, patients require routine monitoring for acute toxicity and complications of long-term medications in the perioperative setting.

#### 6.3.7 Antithrombotic and anticoagulants

Management of anticoagulation in the perioperative setting is as much art as science, and the impact of the use or cessation of anticoagulant medication needs to be closely monitored until the patient has recovered. In the preoperative setting, almost all antithrombotic and anticoagulant medications should be held or reversed, depending on the attainment of adequate hemostasis and on the risk of thrombosis for particular indications [25]. This issue is more thoroughly covered in chapter 1.6 Anticoagulation in the perioperative setting.

## 7 Other preoperative issues

There are a number of common perioperative medical complications that impact postsurgical outcomes; many of these develop or require intervention in the postoperative period. Comanagement with a general medical service with experience with common geriatric syndromes is essential to optimal outcomes. Some of these issues emerge in the preoperative phase and are introduced here.

### 7.1 Delirium

Delirium is an acute, waxing and waning change in mental status marked by deficits in attention, and often complicated by agitation, lethargy or disorganized thinking [26]. It is common in hospitalized older adults, particularly in those with underlying cognitive disorders including dementia. Delirium can be provoked by underlying medical issues, which should always be sought. In the preoperative setting, uncontrolled pain should be strongly considered, particularly in patients with no other obvious cause. Initial attempts at management should include treating underlying clinical issues, optimizing pain control and attempting nonpharmacological supports like gentle reorientation, decreasing excessive stimulation, and restoring eyeglasses and hearing aids. For severe agitation or distress, low-dose haloperidol (0.5 mg intravenously or orally) can be administered safely in most patients. Delirium is not a contraindication to surgical fixation; fracture reduction and mobilization may be necessary to promote resolution.

### 7.2 Urinary retention

Urinary retention can be due to a number of contributing factors, including pain, delirium, and prostatic hypertrophy and is a common adverse effect of opioid medications. Bedside physical examination and ultrasonic bladder scan can assist with the diagnosis. Urinary catheterization carries risks such as infection, urinary tract bleeding and delirium, and should be used judiciously.

### 7.3 Polypharmacy

In light of the number of competing acute and chronic issues faced by older adults, polypharmacy and its effects can be viewed as a distinct clinical issue. Polypharmacy is defined as the use of six to nine medications at once and has been associated with a high likelihood of drug-drug interactions. Polypharmacy is associated with delirium, functional decline and poor surgical outcomes. In addition to avoiding poorly tolerated classes of medications like anticholinergic agents and benzodiazepines, careful reduction in the number and doses of other medications may be helpful in optimizing outcomes. See chapter 1.13 Polypharmacy for a more thorough discussion.

## 8 References

1. **Folbert EC, Smit RS, van der Velde D, et al.** Geriatric fracture center: a multidisciplinary treatment approach for older patients with a hip fracture improved quality of clinical care and short-term treatment outcomes. *Geriatr Orthop Surg Rehabil.* 2012 Jun;3(2):59–67.
2. **Fisher AA, Davis MW, Rubenach SE, et al.** Outcomes for older patients with hip fractures: the impact of orthopedic and geriatric medicine cocare. *J Orthop Trauma.* 2006 Mar;20(3): 172–178; discussion 179–180.
3. **Friedman SM, Mendelson DA, Bingham KW, et al.** Impact of a comanaged Geriatric Fracture Center on short-term hip fracture outcomes. *Arch Intern Med.* 2009 Oct 12;169(18):1712–1717.
4. **Maxwell MJ, Moran CG, Moppett IK.** Development and validation of a preoperative scoring system to predict 30 day mortality in patients undergoing hip fracture surgery. *Br J Anaesth.* 2008 Oct;101(4):511–517.
5. **Moppett IK, Parker M, Griffiths R, et al.** Nottingham Hip Fracture Score: longitudinal and multi-assessment. *Br J Anaesth.* 2012 Oct;109(4):546–550.
6. **Lee TH, Marcantonio ER, Mangione CM, et al.** Derivation and prospective validation of a simple index for prediction of cardiac risk of major noncardiac surgery. *Circulation.* 1999 Sep 7;100(10):1043–1049.
7. **Gupta PK, Gupta H, Sundaram A, et al.** Development and validation of a risk calculator for prediction of cardiac risk after surgery. *Circulation.* 2011 Jul 26;124(4):381–387.
8. **American College of Surgeons' National Surgical Quality Improvement Program (ACS NSQIP).** Surgical Risk Calculator. Available at: http://riskcalculator.facs.org/RiskCalculator/. Accessed June 2016.
9. **Devereaux PJ, Goldman L, Cook DJ, et al.** Perioperative cardiac events in patients undergoing noncardiac surgery: a review of the magnitude of the problem, the pathophysiology of the events and methods to estimate and communicate risk. *CMAJ.* 2005 Sep 13;173(6):627–634.
10. **Penrod JD, Litke A, Hawkes WG, et al.** Heterogeneity in hip fracture patients: age, functional status, and comorbidity. *J Am Geriatr Soc.* 2007 Mar;55(3):407–413.
11. **Parker MJ, Palmer CR.** A new mobility score for predicting mortality after hip fracture. *J Bone Joint Surg Br.* 1993 Sep;75(5):797–798.
12. **Seitz DP, Adunuri N, Gill SS, et al.** Prevalence of dementia and cognitive impairment among older adults with hip fractures. *J Am Med Dir Assoc.* 2011 Oct;12(8):556–564.
13. **Cromwell DA, Eagar K, Poulos RG.** The performance of instrumental activities of daily living scale in screening for cognitive impairment in elderly community residents. *J Clin Epidemiol.* 2003 Feb;56(2):131–137.
14. **Borson S, Scanlan JM, Chen P, et al.** The Mini-Cog as a screen for dementia: validation in a population-based sample. *J Am Geriatr Soc.* 2003 Oct;51(10):1451–1454.
15. **Jette M, Sidney K, Blumchen G.** Metabolic equivalents (METS) in exercise testing, exercise prescription, and evaluation of functional capacity. *Clin Cardiol.* 1990 Aug;13(8):555–565.
16. **Friedman SM, Mendelson DA, Kates SL, et al.** Geriatric co-management of proximal femur fractures: total quality management and protocol-driven care result in better outcomes for a frail patient population. *J Am Geriatr Soc.* 2008 Jul;56(7):1349–1356.
17. **Ricci WM, Della Rocca GJ, Combs C, et al.** The medical and economic impact of preoperative cardiac testing in elderly patients with hip fractures. *Injury.* 2007 Sep;38 Suppl 3:S49–S52.
18. **O'HEireamhoin S, Beyer T, Ahmed M, et al.** The role of preoperative cardiac investigation in emergency hip surgery. *J Trauma.* 2011 Nov;71(5):1345–1347.
19. **Nicholas JA.** Preoperative optimization and risk assessment. *Clin Geriatr Med.* 2014 May;30(2):207–218.
20. **Brenner S.** *Nerve Blocks for Pain Management in Patients with Hip Fractures: a Rapid Review.* Toronto: Health Quality Ontario; 2013.
21. **Fleisher LA, Fleischmann KE, Auerbach AD, et al.** 2014 ACC/AHA guideline on perioperative cardiovascular evaluation and management of patients undergoing noncardiac surgery: a report of the American College of Cardiology/American Heart Association Task Force on practice guidelines. *J Am Coll Cardiol.* 2014 Dec 9;64(22):e77–e137.
22. **Cittanova ML, Zubicki A, Savu C, et al.** The chronic inhibition of angiotensin-converting enzyme impairs postoperative renal function. *Anesth Analg.* 2001 Nov;93(5):1111–1115.
23. **Arora P, Rajagopalam S, Ranjan R, et al.** Preoperative use of angiotensin-converting enzyme inhibitors/angiotensin receptor blockers is associated with increased risk for acute kidney injury after cardiovascular surgery. *Clin J Am Soc Nephrol.* 2008 Sep;3(5):1266–1273.
24. **Onuigbo MA.** Reno-prevention vs. reno-protection: a critical re-appraisal of the evidence-base from the large RAAS blockade trials after ONTARGET—a call for more circumspection. *QJM.* 2009 Mar;102(3):155–167.
25. **Douketis JD, Spyropoulos AC, Spencer FA, et al.** Perioperative management of antithrombotic therapy: antithrombotic therapy and prevention of thrombosis, 9th ed: American College of Chest Physicians Evidence-Based Clinical Practice Guidelines. *Chest.* 2012 Feb;141(2 Suppl):e326S–e350S.
26. **Inouye SK.** Delirium in older persons. *N Engl J Med.* 2006 Mar 16;354(11):1157–1165.

# 1.5 Prognosis and goals of care

Joshua Uy

## 1 Introduction

For older adults, a hip fracture is often a life-altering event. Even after successful surgical repair, there remain significant consequences for life expectancy, impaired function, and diminished quality of life. Hip fracture outcomes vary widely, from full recovery to end-of-life decline. In addition, other fragility fractures of the spine, pelvis and ribs are also associated with similar prognostic implications, including high rates of 1-year mortality [1]. Incorporating patient-specific estimates of prognosis into routine practice can lead to better anticipation of complications, more realistic goals for rehabilitation, appropriate care of comorbidities, better patient and family communication and identification of palliative needs.

## 2 Prognostication of outcomes—general approaches

Outcome prognostication in the older adult can be very challenging, but useful estimates are possible. The literature offers many tools that can be used to adequately separate older adults who have a good estimated prognosis from those who are likely to do poorly in the immediate future. These tools range from complex calculators that incorporate 15–20 different health history and physical examination parameters to single items such as gait speed or grip strength. Generally speaking, prognostication in older adults is best achieved by routinely evaluating the three different patient factors age, comorbidities, and functional status.

### 2.1 Age

Age alone is a good but clinically insufficient predictor of life expectancy with consistent trends of decreasing life expectancy as a person ages [2]. A 65-year-old man in the United States will live an average of 18 more years compared to nearly 21 years for the typical 65-year-old woman. By age 85, life expectancy drops to 6.1 and 7.3 years for men and women in the US, respectively. Despite these general estimates, there is a wide distribution in the life expectancy at any given age [3]. For example, life expectancy for 85-year-old men can range as much as fourfold, from about 2 to 8 years. To further refine patient-specific estimates of life expectancy, it is important to also consider a patient's comorbidities and personal functional trajectory.

### 2.2 Comorbidities

As expected, patients with more comorbidities have lower life expectancies and experience more surgical complications. The Charlson Comorbidity Index (CCI) [4] is a well-known example of a pure comorbidity scale used for prognostication. The CCI assigns a weighted point value to a number of common diseases and can also be age-stratified by assigning a point for age for every decade after 40 (see **Table 1.5-1**).

Higher scores correlate with higher mortality. A hospitalized patient with a score of 0 will have a 1-year predicted mortality of 12%; patients with scores of 3–4 have a 1 year mortality of 52%, and scores greater than 5 predict an 85% 1-year mortality [4].

| Charlson Comorbidity Index | Points assigned |
|---|---|
| Myocardial infarction | 1 |
| Congestive heart failure | 1 |
| Peripheral vascular disease | 1 |
| Cerebrovascular disease | 1 |
| Dementia | 1 |
| Chronic pulmonary disease | 1 |
| Connective tissue disease | 1 |
| Ulcer disease | 1 |
| Mild liver disease | 1 |
| Diabetes | 1 |
| Hemiplegia | 2 |
| Moderate or severe renal disease | 2 |
| Diabetes with end organ damage | 2 |
| Any tumor | 2 |
| Leukemia | 2 |
| Lymphoma | 2 |
| Moderate or severe liver disease | 3 |
| Metastatic solid tumor | 6 |
| AIDS | 6 |

**Table 1.5-1** Charlson Comorbidity Index scoring (without age score).

In hip fracture patients, a CCI is also an independent predictor of 30-day mortality; patients with a CCI > 6 are more than twice as likely to die during this time frame [5].

### 2.3 Functional status

It addition to age and comorbidity assessment, it has been increasingly recognized that function is an important independent prognostic indicator in older adults. Functional debility is a common pathway for any disease, as it increases in severity and is typically easy to assess. The most common geriatric functional scale is the Barthel Index of Activities of Daily Living [6], in which patients are assessed for independence in the following daily abilities: toileting, continence (bowel and bladder), transferring, mobility, stair use, feeding, grooming, bathing and dressing. Lower scores reflect increased dependency, which is also an independent predictor of mortality (**Table 1.5-2, Table 1.5-3**).

Functional assessment is most important in the oldest patients. Function correlates more closely with mortality than comorbidities for those older than 80 years, while for those younger than 70 years comorbidities are better at predicting mortality [9]. Other studies have used function to predict survival in cancer, heart failure, surgeries and dementia [10–14].

| Activity | Scoring range (points) 0 = dependent |
|---|---|
| Toileting | 0–2 |
| Bowel continence | 0–2 |
| Bladder continence | 0–2 |
| Grooming | 0–1 |
| Feeding | 0–2 |
| Dressing | 0–2 |
| Transferring | 0–3 |
| Mobility | 0–3 |
| Stairs | 0–2 |
| Bathing | 0–1 |

**Table 1.5-2** Barthel Index of Activities of Daily Living [7].

| Performance of ADL | Median life expectancy in years |
|---|---|
| No difficulty with ADLs | 10.6 |
| Able to do all ADLs with some difficulty and bathe and walk with a lot of difficulty | 6.5 |
| Able to toilet, dress and transfer with a lot of difficulty and unable to bathe or walk | 5.1 |
| Able to perform only one ADL, unable for all others | 3.8 |
| Complete dependency in ADLs | 1.6 |

**Table 1.5-3** Median life expectancy for community adults older than 70 years, based on the Barthel Index of Activities of Daily Living assessment [8].
Abbreviation: ADL, activity of daily living.

The most valid predictors of postsurgical outcomes come from comprehensive tools that incorporate elements of age, comorbidity and function. The best studied of these in the hip fracture population is the Nottingham Hip Fracture Score (NHFS), which assigns points for age, gender, number of comorbidities, cognitive impairment, anemia, institutionalization and malignancy [15]. Patients can be grouped as low risk (NHFS ≤ 4) or high risk (NHFS > 5) with differences in survival at 30 days (96.5% versus 86.3%) and 1 year (84.1% versus 54.5%) [16]. **Table 1.5-4** summarizes the NHFS scoring.

Despite the presence of procedure-specific outcome estimates, it is critical to recognize that individual older adults will have a wide range of responses to medical and surgical treatments. Assessing age, comorbidities and function allows for a more individualized assessment and care plan.

Without individualizing care based on prognosis and frailty, the clinician is at great risk for overtreatment of some patients, and undertreatment in others. Individualizing care based on patient-specific assessment allows for a treatment plan that is tolerable, purposeful, effective, and consistent with a patient's goals of care.

## 3 Functional prognosis for hip fracture patients

In addition to significant mortality associations, hip and other fragility fractures have specific prognostic implications for functional outcomes. Understanding these implications allows patients, families and care teams to have realistic expectations for the future, and to anticipate and prepare for upcoming needs.

| Variable | Value | Points |
|---|---|---|
| Age, y | 66–85 | 3 |
| | > 86 | 4 |
| Gender | Male | 1 |
| Admission hemoglobin | ≤ 10 g/dL | 1 |
| Mini-mental test score | ≤ 6 of 10 | 1 |
| Living in an institution | Yes | 1 |
| Comorbidities | > 2 | 1 |
| Malignancy | Yes | 1 |

**Table 1.5-4** Nottingham Hip Fracture Score.

### 3.1 Mortality

About 25% of older adults with hip fractures die within the year. Mortality rates are nearly 50% higher for men than women and more than double for those older than 85 years [17]. Other factors associated with higher 1-year mortality include cognitive impairment (91% higher), prefracture gait instability (up to seven times higher), and nursing home residence (75% higher).

### 3.2 Functional outcomes

Functional outcomes may be more important than mortality to patients and families. The recovery from a hip fracture takes months and postfracture dependence can develop in more areas than just ambulation. Most patients will require rehabilitation in a nursing facility (about 60%) or an acute rehabilitation facility (about 25%) after the hospital stay. A small minority will be discharged directly home (15%) [18].

Maximum recovery of cognition (ie, resolution of delirium), depression and upper extremity activities of daily living (ADLs) is most often seen at about 4 months. Maximum recovery of gait and balance will be seen at about 9 months. Maximum recovery of lower extremity ADLs, instrumental ADLs, and social function will be seen at 11 months [19].

Some functional loss will be permanent. For many hip fracture patients, achieving complete independence is not possible. Functions that are unlikely to recover include: ability to climb 5 steps (10% achieve recovery), getting in and out of a shower (17%), getting on and off the toilet (34%) and housekeeping (38%). Functions that are more likely to recover include putting on pants (80% achieve recovery), cooking (76%), using a telephone (78%), getting in and out of a bath (69%), walking 3 meters (~ 10 feet) (60%), and shopping (58%). The consequence of this slow functional recovery is that between 15% and 33% of patients with hip fractures will still be in a nursing home 1 year after their fracture [20].

The major predictor for the degree of functional recovery is the patient's prefracture level of function [21]. For example, for a patient without preexisting disability, nearly half will experience a rapid recovery (over approximately 3–6 months). On the other hand, for those with even mild prefracture disability the prognosis changes considerably; almost none are expected to recover rapidly, half will experience a gradual recovery (over approximately 6–9 months), and half will experience little or no recovery.

The trajectory and pace of prefracture functional decline can also be a big determinate for recovery. For example, among those with moderate disability, around 87% of those experiencing a prefracture progression of disability will have no recovery compared to only 14% of those with stable disability.

Together, all this information suggests that for most patients the year after a hip fracture is highly dynamic and challenging. Patients and families may have to contend with the likelihood of a slow recovery taking place over several different systems of healthcare, with intensive financial requirements, significant risks of mortality, rehospitalization and permanent loss of function, and the redefinition of family relationships to include difficult caregiving roles and the shifting of expectations. The healthcare team at each site of care, ie, hospital, acute rehabilitation, nursing home and home health, should play essential roles in educating and preparing families for these transitions.

## 4 Identifying goals of care

Hip fractures often occur within the wider context of frailty and functional decline. As described in chapter 1.11 Sarcopenia, malnutrition, frailty, and falls, frailty is a complex state where outcomes of standard medical and surgical treatments are less predictable and typically inferior to those seen in younger, more robust patients. In frailty, therapeutic windows between harms and benefits are often smaller or nonexistent, and achieving traditional disease-specific goals may lead to actual harms.

A medical example for this is using glucose-lowering medications to obtain glycosylated hemoglobin target less than 7 in patients with diabetes, a standard recommendation that is associated with harms in frail older adults. A surgical example is attempting a functionally unnecessary surgical fracture reduction and developing a postoperative deterioration of the kidney function necessitating dialysis.

### 4.1 Value-based decisions

Because frail patients have a more problematic response to standard therapy, patients and families often have to make value-based decisions, and prioritize amongst competing treatments and outcomes. These patient-specific values and priorities are referred to as goals of care. Defining these goals with each patient helps to clarify a clinically meaningful target for all medical care. For example, a hip fracture patient who lives alone and has a high fall risk may make a decision to prioritize safety and longevity over independence by moving in with one of their children. Another patient with similar function and fall risk may prioritize independence over safety and choose to live alone. Patients and families often choose to prioritize comfort, longevity or a chance for independence differently. These priorities should inform the medical and surgical treatment plans, so that the patient has the best chance of meeting his or her individual goals.

Goals of care are best assessed with open-ended questions [22] such as "What should we consider when making decisions about your care?" Assessing goals of care is a bedside clinical skill that develops over time. Learning to ask and learning to actively listen will help guide the older adult and their family through a potentially challenging life transition.

In the setting of a hip fracture, there are several specific issues related to goals of care, including resuscitation status, acceptable functional outcomes, and willingness to endure treatment plans.

### 4.2 Resuscitation

Formal ascertainment and documentation of resuscitation wishes (ie, code status) are appropriately required in most healthcare systems. A hip fracture is a good time to verify patients' expectations and wishes about cardiopulmonary resuscitation (CPR). Here too, clinicians should have some general information about the effectiveness of CPR in this population.

The efficacy of resuscitation is significantly limited in older adults and particularly in those with frailty or functional impairment. Postcardiopulmonary resuscitation survival to hospital discharge in previously independent older adults is estimated at 13–18% with lower rates of survival in those with dependency. As many as 30% of survivors of CPR are left with new neurological impairments [23, 24]. In light of the low likelihood of independent survival, many patients may opt to forgo any attempts at resuscitation.

Resuscitation in the operating room or anesthesia areas is expected to be more successful than elsewhere in the hospital, and patients may elect to suspend "Do Not Resuscitate" during the surgical and immediate postoperative period.

The American College of Surgeons [25] supports exploring a person's goals and limits in the context of the operating room, as patients likely have different desires for attempts at resuscitation in this situation. Some tools used in resuscitation such as intubation, for instance, are already a part of surgery and may not be uniquely burdensome. Others like chest compressions or electrical cardioversion likely carry a greater potential burden and worse prognosis. No single model or protocol is appropriate for all older adults undergoing hip repair, and shared decision making between the surgeon and patient is necessary. Some recommendations for phrasing resuscitation status discussions are listed in **Table 1.5-5**.

### 4.3 Other limits of care

In addition to resuscitation, older adults may wish to place other limits on the intensity of hospital or posthospital care, to place limits on a range of interventions while they are still alive. For some patients this may mean a firm desire to avoid intensive care unit admissions, for others it may mean allowing the surgeon to operate on them as many times as it takes to have the best possible outcome. In any case, the care team should not assume that patients are willing to undergo management of any and every complication that may develop after a surgery, a concept known as surgical buy-in [27].

| **Discussing resuscitation status** | |
|---|---|
| Introduction questions: | |
| • Do you have an advance directive or a living will?<br>• I would like to ask you a question that some patients may find difficult or other do not have the answer to. | Sometimes patients have already made decisions and documented them. Simply asking is an easy way to start. For other patients, asking permission to talk about code status decreases the pressure already inherent in the question and allows the discussion to be more collaborative. |
| How to ask about code status: | |
| • If you were to die unexpectedly, would you want us to attempt to bring you back to life? | Emphasizes that a code status is only relevant when someone has actually died and that there is no guarantee of success. |
| • Do you want us to allow a natural death? | While not as relevant for a surgical code status, this can prompt a person to think about what is natural to them. |
| Phrasing to avoid: | |
| • Do you want us to do everything? | This is biased toward an affirmative answer, is very vague, and focuses on the intervention instead of the goal. |
| • Do you want to be resuscitated? | The setting is unclear (that the person is dead) and can mean everything from intravenous fluids to CPR. |
| • If your heart stops, do you want us to restart it? If you stop breathing, do you want to be on a breathing machine? | Focusing on an organ distracts from the big picture that the person has died. Asking if someone wants their heart restarted makes it sound simple and easily successful. Asking if they want to be on a breathing machine can apply while they are alive apart from a code status. |

**Table 1.5-5** Suggestions for framing discussions about cardiopulmonary resuscitation [26].
Abbreviation: CPR, cardiopulmonary resuscitation.

When older adults undergo an urgent surgery, the decision about how to manage future potential complications may not yet have been made. It is important to routinely reassess goals after an urgent surgery to prevent the potentially faulty assumption of surgical buy-in [28].

Regularly assessing limits on care is important because what a person is willing to undergo may depend on the likelihood of a patient-defined successful outcome.

## 5 Managing multimorbidity in frail patients

Finally, in addition to coming to decisions on CPR and other potential limits on interventions, the hip fracture admission is an appropriate time for the medical team to reevaluate a person's entire medical treatment plan to align with the patient's goals of care, as elicited from the patient or their surrogate decision makers. After a hip fracture, two things can change:

- Quality of life goals may take priority over continued compliance with standard therapies
- Long-term disease-specific treatment benefits may become irrelevant due to shortening overall life expectancy.

The anticipated benefits of many chronic disease therapies like in hypertension, hyperlipidemia, diabetes mellitus or coronary artery disease are typically small or nonexistent during the last years of life and can easily be overwhelmed by the harms of treatment with polypharmacy, multiple consultations and diagnostic tests as well as medicalization of life. A suggested framework for evaluating chronic disease therapies in the frail older adult is outlined in the following list:

1. Is the intervention known to be effective in older adults?
2. Is it expected to produce a patient-desired clinical end point?
3. Is the patient expected to live long enough to benefit from the therapy?
4. What is the chance of achieving the anticipated benefit of the intervention?
5. What are the potential harms of treatment (ie, adverse effects, costs, healthcare encounters, need for monitoring)?
6. Is the intervention likely to achieve the patient's goal?
7. Is it a priority among the patient's other medical problems?
8. Is there a cultural or spiritual belief that needs to be considered?

Compared to disease-specific therapies, the most efficacious approaches to multimorbidity are poorly understood. While there are guidelines to help set priorities in medically complex and frail patients [29], managing multimorbidity is often more of an art than a science. The challenge of multimorbidity is that sometimes treating one disease can cause another disease to get worse. For example, using nonsteroidal antiinflammatory drugs for osteoarthritis can worsen heartburn or congestive heart failure. While a full discussion of balancing risks and harms of medical treatments is beyond the scope of this article, an approach to prioritization of competing issues is offered in **Table 1.5-6**. As one moves up the prioritization framework from primary prevention to active symptoms, the medical problems become a bigger threat to health and mortality. It is worth focusing on lower priority issues only if the higher priority issues are resolved. For example, there is no justification for tight control of diabetes (priority 3) if the older adult is suffering from recurrent falls (priority 2). In this sense, it may be wise to reduce the intensity of diabetes treatment by minimizing medications. Lower priority items also typically have a longer time frame to clinical benefit than higher priority items. Last, the overarching priority is to individualize a plan that is consistent with the patient's own goals and values.

### 5.1 Hospice

Hospice plays an important role for patients with hip fractures, both for patients who suffer hip fractures while already receiving hospice therapy, and for the many for whom the hip fracture is either a cause or consequence of an end-of-life decline. For patients near the end of life, pain control is of utmost importance. For patients with a life expectancy of weeks to months, hip fracture repair often offers the best chance at pain control, particularly for patients who are trying to minimize the sedation associated with high doses

| Priority | Category | Clinical examples |
|---|---|---|
| Highest | Active symptoms/acute medical illness | Pain, dyspnea, nausea<br>Hip fracture, pneumonia, CHF exacerbation |
| | Syndromes affecting quality of life | Falls, weight loss, cognitive decline, functional decline, polypharmacy |
| | Secondary prevention of chronic disease complications | CHF, COPD, DM, HTN, osteoporosis |
| Lowest | Primary prevention of chronic disease | Cancer screening, dietary restrictions |

**Table 1.5-6** Prioritization framework for multimorbid patients
Abbreviations: CHF, congestive heart failure; COPD, chronic obstructive pulmonary disease; DM, diabetes mellitus; HTN, hypertension.

of opiates and other medications. It is not uncommon for some hip fracture patients to transition during the postsurgical period to hospice care, particularly if persistent delirium or dysphagia complicate the postoperative period. In order to counter a sense among clinicians and families that hospice and withdrawal of ongoing medical care is not appropriate following a successful surgical fixation, an explicit time-limited trial for recovery can be useful to negotiate a more humane and realistic treatment plan in patients with poor prognosis [28].

As palliative concepts in surgery begin to mesh more and more with palliative concepts in medicine, it is clear that even for hospice patients and patients heading toward hospice, surgery still has an important palliative, noncurative role [30].

## 6 References


1. **Gosch M, Druml T, Nicholas JA, et al.** Fragility non-hip fracture patients are at risk. *Arch Orthop Trauma Surg.* 2015 Jan;135(1):69–77.
2. **Centers for Disease Control and Prevention.** Publications and Information Products. Available at. www.cdc.gov/nchs/products/life_tables.htm. Accessed February 1, 2016.
3. **Monahan RH.** Editorial: Joint Commission on Allied Health Personnel in Ophthalmology. *Arch Ophthalmol.* 1975 Jul;93(7):471.
4. **Charlson ME, Pompei P, Ales KL, et al.** A new method of classifying prognostic comorbidity in longitudinal studies: development and validation. *J Chronic Dis.* 1987;40(5):373–383.
5. **Kirkland LL, Kashiwagi DT, Burton MC, et al.** The Charlson Comorbidity Index Score as a predictor of 30-day mortality after hip fracture surgery. *Am J Med Qual.* 2011 Nov-Dec;26(6):461–467.
6. **Mahoney FI, Barthel DW.** Functional Evaluation: the Barthel Index. *Md State Med J.* 1965 Feb;14:61–65.
7. **Collin C, Wade DT, Davies S, et al.** The Barthel ADL Index: a reliability study. *Int Disabil Stud.* 1988;10(2):61–63.
8. **Stineman MG, Xie D, Pan Q, et al.** All-cause 1-, 5-, and 10-year mortality in elderly people according to activities of daily living stage. *J Am Geriatr Soc.* 2012 Mar;60(3):485–492.
9. **Lee SJ, Go AS, Lindquist K, et al.** Chronic conditions and mortality among the oldest old. *Am J Public Health.* 2008 Jul;98(7):1209–1214.
10. **Oken MM, Creech RH, Tormey DC, et al.** Toxicity and response criteria of the Eastern Cooperative Oncology Group. *Am J Clin Oncol.* 1982 Dec;5(6):649–655.
11. **The Criteria Committee of the New York Heart Association.** *Nomenclature and Criteria for Diagnosis of Diseases of the Heart and Great Vessels.* 9th ed, Boston: Little, Brown & Co; 1994:253–256.
12. **Robinson TN, Eiseman B, Wallace JI, et al.** Redefining geriatric preoperative assessment using frailty, disability and co-morbidity. *Ann Surg.* 2009 Sep;250(3):449–455.
13. **Hamel MB, Henderson WG, Khuri SF, et al.** Surgical outcomes for patients aged 80 and older: morbidity and mortality from major noncardiac surgery. *J Am Geriatr Soc.* 2005 Mar;53(3):424–429.
14. **Sclan SG, Reisberg B.** Functional assessment staging (FAST) in Alzheimer's disease: reliability, validity, and ordinality. *Int Psychogeriatr.* 1992;4 Suppl 1:55–69.
15. **Maxwell MJ, Moran CG, Moppett IK.** Development and validation of a preoperative scoring system to predict 30 day mortality in patients undergoing hip fracture surgery. *Br J Anaesth.* 2008 Oct;101(4):511–517.
16. **Wiles MD, Moran CG, Sahota O, et al.** Nottingham Hip Fracture Score as a predictor of one year mortality in patients undergoing surgical repair of fractured neck of femur. *Br J Anaesth.* 2011 Apr;106(4):501–504.
17. **Smith T, Pelpola K, Ball M, et al.** Pre-operative indicators for mortality following hip fracture surgery: a systematic review and meta-analysis. *Age Ageing.* 2014 Jul;43(4):464–471.
18. **Bentler SE, Liu L, Obrizan M, et al.** The aftermath of hip fracture: discharge placement, functional status change, and mortality. *Am J Epidemiol.* 2009 Nov 15;170(10):1290–1299.
19. **Magaziner J, Hawkes W, Hebel JR, et al.** Recovery from hip fracture in eight areas of function. *J Gerontol A Biol Sci Med Sci.* 2000 Sep;55(9):M498–M507.
20. **Marks R.** Hip fracture epidemiological trends, outcomes, and risk factors, 1970–2009. *Int J Gen Med.* 2010 Apr 08;3:1–17.
21. **Gill TM, Murphy TE, Gahbauer EA, et al.** The course of disability before and after a serious fall injury. *JAMA Intern Med.* 2013 Oct 28;173(19):1780–1786.
22. **Mahon MM.** An advance directive in two questions. *J Pain Symptom Manage.* 2011 Apr;41(4):801–807.
23. **Abbo ED, Yuen TC, Buhrmester L, et al.** Cardiopulmonary resuscitation outcomes in hospitalized community-dwelling individuals and nursing home residents based on activities of daily living. *J Am Geriatr Soc.* 2013 Jan;61(1):34–39.
24. **Girotra S, Nallamothu BK, Spertus JA, et al.** Trends in survival after in-hospital cardiac arrest. *N Engl J Med.* 2012 Nov 15;367(20):1912–1920.
25. **American College of Surgeons.** Statement of the American College of Surgeons on Advance Directives by Patients: "Do Not Resuscitate" in the Operating Room. *Bull Am Coll of Surg.* 2014 Jan;99(1):42–43.
26. **von Gunten CF.** Discussing do-not-resuscitate status. *J Clin Oncol.* 2003 May 1;21(9 Suppl):20s–25s.
27. **Paul Olson TJ, Schwarze ML.** Failure-to-pursue rescue: truly a failure? *Ann Surg.* 2015 Aug;262(2):e43–44.
28. **Neuman MD, Allen S, Schwarze ML, et al.** Using time-limited trials to improve surgical care for frail older adults. *Ann Surg.* 2015 Apr;261(4):639–641.
29. **American Geriatrics Society Expert Panel on the Care of Older Adults with Multimorbidity.** Guiding principles for the care of older adults with multimorbidity: an approach for clinicians:. *J Am Geriatr Soc.* 2012 Oct;60(10):E1–E25.
30. **Dunn GP.** Surgical palliative care: recent trends and developments. *Anesthesiol Clin.* 2012 Mar;30(1):13–28.

# 1.6 Anticoagulation in the perioperative setting

Lauren J Gleason, Adeela Cheema, Joseph A Nicholas

## 1 Introduction

The common presence of anticoagulant and antiplatelet agents in fragility fracture patients (FFPs) presents unique challenges in the perioperative period. Management decisions typically involve balancing short-term bleeding and thrombosis risks and considering the use of bridging anticoagulant therapy. Delaying surgery to manage the effects of these medications can increase the likelihood of adverse events, such as delirium, pneumonia, pressure ulceration, and mortality [1–3]. In the immediate perioperative period, the risks of bleeding often outweigh the risks of thrombosis for most older adults.

Standards of care and published guidelines in this area vary widely throughout the world. This chapter reflects the principles for anticoagulation management in the perioperative period, with specific recommendations based on current US and European approaches. Consultation with local guidelines may be necessary to align practice with other national or regional standards.

## 2 Perioperative anticoagulant management

### 2.1 General approach

There are four considerations in the management of antithrombotic agents in the perioperative period [4]:

1. The short-term risk of acute thromboembolism if the anticoagulation/antiplatelet agent is discontinued
2. The risk of major bleeding from the procedure if the anticoagulation/antiplatelet agent is continued
3. The effectiveness, availability and safety of reversal agents (eg, plasma and vitamin K)
4. The overall need to minimize surgical delay and maximize mobility

Additionally, part of the preoperative assessment should include the procedure-specific bleeding risk, and the anticipated consequences of bleeding if anticoagulants are resumed during this time. For example, percutaneous screw fixation has a much lower risk of bleeding than that of hip arthroplasty, and the harm of continuation or early resumption of long-term anticoagulation is presumed to be lower than for patients treated with arthroplasty or implant fixation [5].

### 2.2 Anticoagulants and antiplatelet agents

Both anticoagulants and antiplatelet agents interfere with thrombus formation. Anticoagulant medications (eg, warfarin, heparin, apixaban, dabigatran, and rivaroxaban) interfere with the coagulation cascade and clotting factors, while antiplatelet agents (eg, aspirin, and clopidogrel) target platelets. While all of these agents can contribute to clinically significant blood loss, anticoagulants are generally more potent at preventing venous, arterial or intracardiac thrombosis, and are also more likely to cause serious postoperative bleeding. Specific indications and issues are detailed below. **Figure 1.6-1** shows the mechanism of action of some of these agents.

### 2.3 Reasons for use

In order to assess the risk of short-term cessation of anticoagulant or antiplatelet medications, it is important to determine the a priori indication for their use.

Older adults are often anticoagulated for various medical conditions including atrial fibrillation (AF), venous thromboembolism (VTE) (eg, hypercoagulable states, deep vein thrombosis [DVT], pulmonary embolism [PE]), and prosthetic heart valves, each of these indications having a different short-term risk of thrombosis during the perioperative period.

### 2.4 Thrombotic risk assessment by indication

After confirming the indication for anticoagulation, it is important to determine the short-term risk of thrombosis when stopping an anticoagulant. Note that the risk of thromboembolism for these indications is typically reported as an annual risk; for most patients the short-term risk during a typical perioperative period is assumed to be much lower.

### 2.4.1 Atrial fibrillation

The most common indication for anticoagulant use in the older adult population is for prevention of thromboembolic strokes in nonvalvular AF.

The risk of thromboembolism varies and can be estimated by the $CHADS_2$ and the enhanced $CHA_2DS_2$-VASC scores [6, 7]. The relevant criteria and associated risk of stroke are shown in **Table 1.6-1** and **Table 1.6-2**.

### 2.4.2 Venous thromboembolism

In those with venous thromboembolism, the risk of recurrent thrombosis, thrombus propagation, and embolization is greatest in the first 3 months after the diagnosis and initiation of therapy [8]. This risk also varies depending on whether the VTE was provoked, unprovoked, or resolved.

### 2.4.3 Mechanical heart valves

Patients with mechanical heart valves are at significantly increased long-term risk for embolic stroke. The risk varies by the type, number, and location of prosthetic valve and associated medical conditions (**Table 1.6-3**) [9].

| | Risk factor | Point value | Total score | Annual stroke risk, % |
|---|---|---|---|---|
| C | Congestive heart failure | 1 | 0 | 1.9 |
| H | Hypertension–blood pressure consistently above 140/90 mm Hg (or treated hypertension on medication) | 1 | 1 | 2.8 |
| A | Age ≥ 75 years | 1 | 2 | 4 |
| D | Diabetes mellitus | 1 | 3 | 5.9 |
| S2 | Prior stroke or TIA or thromboembolism | 2 | 4 | 8.5 |
| | | | 5 | 12.5 |
| | | | 6 | 18.2 |

**Table 1.6-1** The $CHADS_2$ can be used to estimate the risk of thromboembolism.
Abbreviation: TIA, transient cerebral ischemia attack.

| | Risk factor | Point value | $CHA_2DS_2$-VASC total score | Stroke risk, % per year |
|---|---|---|---|---|
| C | Congestive heart failure (or left ventricular systolic dysfunction) | 1 | 0 | 0 |
| H | Hypertension–blood pressure consistently above 140/90 mm Hg (or treated hypertension on medication) | 1 | 1 | 1.3 |
| A | Age: ≥ 75 years | 2 | 2 | 2.2 |
| D | Diabetes mellitus | 1 | 3 | 3.2 |
| S2 | Prior stroke or TIA or thromboembolic event | 2 | 4 | 4 |
| V | Vascular disease (eg, peripheral artery disease, myocardial infarction, aortic plaque) | 1 | 5 | 6.7 |
| A | Age: 65–74 years | 1 | 6 | 9.8 |
| Sc | Female gender | 1 | 7 | 9.6 |
| | | | 8 | 12.5 |
| | | | 9 | 15.2 |

**Table 1.6-2** $CHA_2DS_2$-VASC score and stroke risk to estimate the risk of thromboembolism.
Abbreviation: TIA, transient cerebral ischemia attack.

| Risk category | Mechanical heart valve | Atrial fibrillation | Venous thromboembolism |
|---|---|---|---|
| **High**<br>• > 10%/year risk of ATE<br>OR<br>• > 10%/month risk of VTE | • Any mechanical mitral valve<br>• Older aortic valve<br>• Recent (< 6 months) stroke or TIA | • $CHADS_2$ score of 5 or 6<br>• Recent (< 3 months) stroke or TIA<br>• Rheumatic valvular heart disease | • Recent (< 3 months) VTE<br>• Severe thrombophilia |
| **Moderate**<br>• 4–10%/year risk of ATE<br>OR<br>• 4–10%/month risk of VTE | Bileaflet aortic valve and one of the following:<br>• Atrial fibrillation<br>• Prior stroke/TIA<br>• Hypertension<br>• Diabetes<br>• Heart failure<br>• Age > 75 years | • $CHADS_2$ score of 3 or 4 | • VTE within past 3–12 months<br>• Recurrent VTE<br>• Nonsevere thrombophilic conditions<br>• Active cancer |
| **Low**<br>• < 4%/year risk of ATE<br>OR<br>• < 2%/month risk of VTE | • Bileaflet aortic valve without atrial fibrillation and no other risk factors for stroke | • $CHADS_2$ score of 0–2 (and no prior stroke or TIA) | • Single VTE within past 12 months<br>AND<br>• No other risk factors |

**Table 1.6-3** American College of Chest Physicians (ACCP) suggested risk stratification for perioperative thromboembolism.
Reproduced from Douketis et al [10] with permission of the ACCP.
Abbreviations: ACCP, American College of Chest Physicians; ATE, arterial thromboembolism; TIA, transient cerebral ischemic attack; VTE, venous thromboembolism.

### 2.5 Bleeding risk assessment

Older adults are prone to bleeding in general and many adults at relatively high risk for thrombosis also have an elevated risk for bleeding. Cardiovascular aging, comorbidity and some medications can result in friable blood vessels and prolonged postoperative bleeding after orthopedic surgery. In addition to procedure-specific risk estimates, there are different prediction tools to evaluate bleeding risk in individual patients [11–13]. The HAS-BLED score [12] evaluates 1-year risk of major bleeding (defined as intracranial bleeding, bleeding requiring hospitalization, hemoglobin decrease > 2 g/L, and/or transfusion) in patients with AF (see **Table 1.6-4**). There are no well-validated predictors for short-term bleeding risks, but the risk factors in the HAS-BLED tool are likely relevant in the perioperative setting as well.

### 2.6 Management of long-term anticoagulation in preparation for surgery

Most hip fracture surgery is considered urgent and requires reversal of anticoagulation within 24–48 hours. Approaches to preparing patients for safe fracture fixation vary by agent.

### 2.7 Warfarin

Warfarin anticoagulation results in a prolonged international normalized ratio (INR). For hip fracture repair, the INR should be reduced to a subtherapeutic threshold; most experts recommend achieving an INR of ≤ 1.5 prior to surgery [14–16].

An elevated INR prior to surgery increases the risk of intraoperative bleeding and associated complications like spinal or epidural catheter bleeding as well as wound hematoma, infection, and possible need for reoperation [17].

There are multiple options to reverse warfarin:

- Oral and intravenous (IV) vitamin K have been shown to have equivalent efficacies in reducing INR values over a 24-hour period. Oral vitamin K has been shown to be more effective than subcutaneous dosing when lowering an elevated INR value, and is typically used in doses ranging from 2.5 to 10 mg [18]. While the optimal dose of vitamin K to lower INR values is unclear, the use of 3 mg intravenously has been shown to be safe and effective in one study [19, 20]. The use of oral vitamin K over IV vitamin K is advantageous as it avoids the risk of fatal anaphylaxis, which has been reported previously with older preparations [21]. Subcutaneous and intramuscular vitamin K administration is associated with unpredictable absorption and should be avoided.
- Fresh frozen plasma is an alternative and/or adjunct to vitamin K to correct coagulopathy [22]. This is human plasma that contains many plasma proteins including coagulation factors. One proposed formula to obtain an INR of less than 1.5 recommends:
  - 1 unit for an INR of 1.5–1.9
  - 2 units for an INR of 2.0–3.0
  - 3 units for an INR of 3.0–4.0
  - 4 units for an INR of 4.0–8.0
  - More than 4 units for an INR of more than 8.0 [23]

  Each unit of plasma has a volume of 190–240 mL. The challenges with plasma include its short duration of action (ie, 4–6 hours) and risks including adverse transfusion effects (eg, infection, acute lung injury) and volume overload and the associated risk of congestive heart failure.

| | Risk factor | Point value | HAS-BLED total score | Bleeds per 100-patient years |
|---|---|---|---|---|
| H | Hypertension (systolic blood pressure > 160 mm Hg) | 1 | 0 | 1.13 |
| A | • Abnormal renal function (long-term dialysis, renal transplant, serum creatinine > 2.4 mg/dL)<br>• Hepatic function (chronic hepatitis, bilirubin > 2× upper normal with liver enzymes > 3× upper normal) | 1<br>1 | 1 | 1.02 |
| S | History of stroke | 1 | 2 | 1.88 |
| B | Bleeding (ie, major bleeding history) | 1 | 3 | 3.74 |
| L | Labile INRs (ie, therapeutic range < 60% of time) | 1 | 4 | 8.7 |
| E | Elderly (≥ 65 years old) | 1 | 5 | 12.5 |
| D | • Drugs (concomitant antiplatelet, NSAIDs)<br>• Alcohol consumption > 8 drinks/week | 1 (each) | > 5 | Insufficient data |

**Table 1.6-4** HAS-BLED score to evaluate 1-year risk of major bleeding.
Abbreviations: INR, international normalized ratio; NSAID, nonsteroidal antiinflammatory drug.

- The combination of vitamin K and fresh frozen plasma has been shown to be safe in hip fracture patients in two retrospective cohort studies [24, 25]. This approach provides both rapid reversal (plasma) and more prolonged reversal (vitamin K) of anticoagulation to minimize ongoing postoperative bleeding.
- Prothrombin complex concentrate (PCC) is another option for reversal in cases of severe bleeding. Prothrombin complex concentrates are plasma products from human donors. Four-factor PCC contains all vitamin K–dependent coagulation factors; 3-factor PCCs contain factors II, IX, and X, but relatively little factor VII. Four-factor PCC is capable of restoring individual clotting factor activity in nearly 100% of patients within minutes of administration, whereas 3-factor PCCs must be supplemented with FFP or a low dose of recombinant factor VIIa to more optimally lower the INR. Inactivated 4-factor PCC contains factors II, VII, IX, and X and is indicated for the treatment of major warfarin-associated bleeding in conjunction with vitamin K. If unavailable, FFP can be used in its place or a 3-factor prothrombin complex concentrate (missing factor VII) with a supplemental dose of FFP or recombinant activated factor VII as per the American College Chest Physicians (ACCP) guidelines 2012 [26, 27].
  Advantages of PCC use include:
  - No cross-matching required
  - Rapid INR reversal achieved in case of emergent surgery
  - Less volume administrations sometimes preferred for patients in fluid overload, acute kidney injury, and heart failure

  Disadvantages include:
  - Cost
  - Possibly thrombogenic
  - Limited high-quality studies for risks and benefits in fracture patients.
- Discontinuation of warfarin with a watch-and-wait approach is a poor option given that warfarin has a half-life of > 1.5 days (or 40 hours) and there is a wide interpatient variation with INR decrease [28]. Very often, the older and frailer a person is, the longer it will take for the warfarin to be eliminated.

Two common concerns exist when reversing anticoagulation. First, there is a potential for aggressive reversal to cause increased risk of thromboembolism and second, after reversal with vitamin K, there can be a delay in anticoagulation when warfarin is resumed postoperatively. While it may take longer to achieve a therapeutic level of warfarin after vitamin K reversal, this has not been shown to delay discharge [29].

## 2.8 Direct oral anticoagulants

In the past several years, numerous new oral anticoagulants (eg, direct thrombin and factor Xa inhibitors) have been introduced. These newer agents are often used in place of warfarin for their convenience, simplicity in dosing, and the lack of routine monitoring.

These characteristics complicate perioperative management due to the difficulty in accurately measuring the degree of anticoagulation in each patient. In addition, there are currently no well-established reversal agents available, limiting the ability to actively manage patients to expedite surgery and potentially increasing the risk of preoperative blood loss. While there are no standard guidelines for how best to manage patients on these agents who require urgent surgery, most recommendations involve balancing the risks of operative delay, the risks of bleeding, and using pharmacokinetic data to best guide therapy [30]. Patients on these agents may require hematology consultation for optimal surgical timing and preoperative planning.

### 2.8.1 Dabigatran

Key features of dabigatran:

- Direct thrombin inhibitor (**Fig 1.6-1**) typically requiring a waiting period of at least 48 hours from the last dose for adequate clearance.
- The majority of dabigatran's excretion is renal (80–85%). It typically has a half-life of 12–18 hours in those with creatinine clearance greater than 50 mL/min. However, in moderately severe renal dysfunction (creatinine clearance of 30–50 mL/min, present in most fracture patients), the half-life extends to about 18–28 hours.
- Measuring the activated partial thromboplastin time (aPTT) can be clinically useful, as an abnormal aPTT can indicate the continued presence of dabigatran. However, a normal aPTT does not exclude significant persistent anticoagulation due to dabigatran. In addition, it is important to note that aPTT elevations do not correlate well with the degree of anticoagulation, as values often plateau at high concentrations and may underestimate supratherapeutic concentrations [31, 32].
- Is potentially dialyzable in extreme situations.
- Currently, there are no official guidelines or recommendations for time to surgery for emergent or urgent procedures for patients on dabigatran; most approaches are extrapolated from elective surgery data and the need to balance the risks of bleeding from that of excessive surgical delay. Recommendations for elective procedures or surgeries with critically high bleeding are to wait 2–4 days after stopping the medication to ensure clearance [33].

For most fracture patients, a delay of approximately 48 hours after the last dose is required to minimize bleeding risks. Additionally, given that dabigatran is renally cleared, it is critical to monitor renal function and maintain adequate hydration in fracture patients presenting on this medication.

### 2.8.2 Rivaroxaban and apixaban

Key features of rivaroxaban and apixaban:

- Direct factor Xa inhibitors (**Fig 1.6-1**) with no efficient way to measure the degree of anticoagulation in current clinical practice. A waiting period of approximately 48 hours from the last dose is typically required for adequate clearance.
- There is less renal clearance than dabigatran with half-lives ranging between 9 and 12 hours, but can be longer in older adults.
- Rivaroxaban can affect prothrombin time values and this can be monitored prior to surgery. Both of these medications can have rapid onset of action like dabigatran and the same approach should be used with these patients as in dabigatran-treated patients.

### 2.8.3 Reversal agents

In a recent development, the US Food and Drug Administration has approved idarucizumab for reversal of dabigatran in emergency bleeding situations [34]. Two other agents currently under development include andexanet alfa (a potential reversal agent for Xa inhibitors and low-molecular-weight heparin [LMWH]) and ciraparantag (a potential reversal agent for several different classes of anticoagulant drugs) [35–37].

There is a paucity of clinical data to evaluate the effectiveness, risks and benefits of these agents as of this writing. Hematology consultation may be required for optimal management.

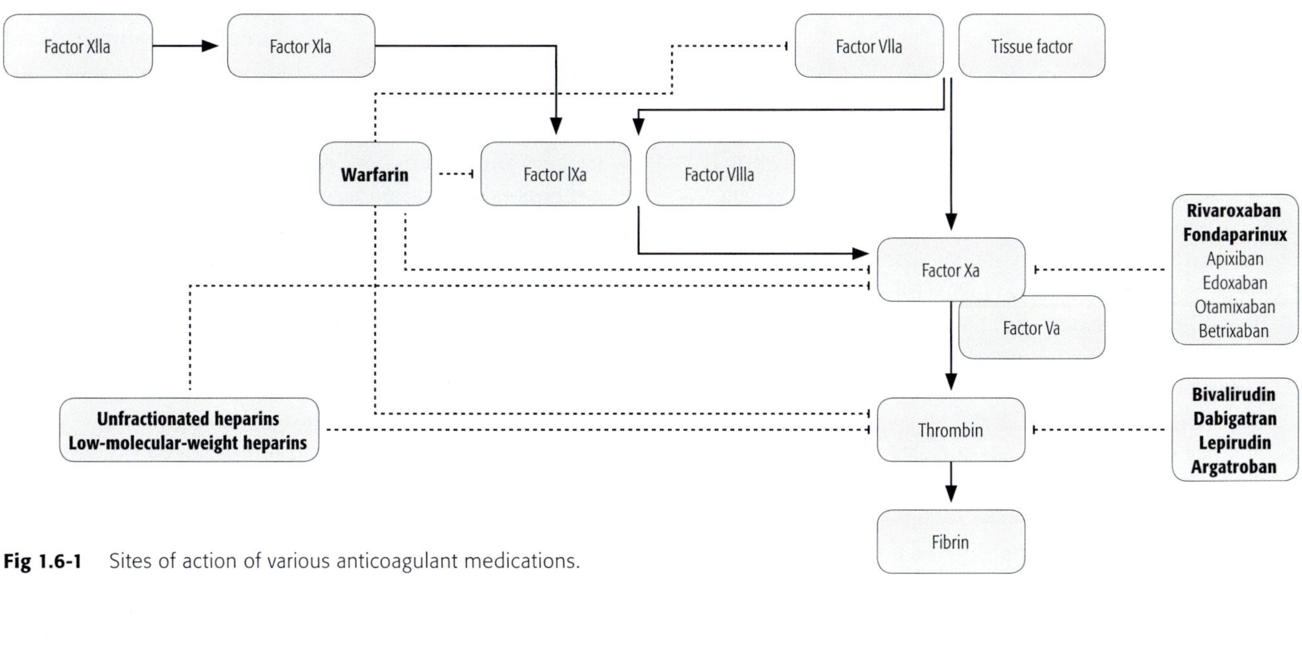


**Fig 1.6-1** Sites of action of various anticoagulant medications.

## 3 Perioperative management of antiplatelet agents

Antiplatelet agents typically have a different set of indications, potency, half-life, and bleeding risk than anticoagulants. Most older adults take these agents for preexisting vascular disease, including coronary artery disease with or without stenting, peripheral arterial disease or cerebrovascular disease. These medications are used to limit the development of local thrombosis or progression of a vascular stenosis. Rapid reversal of these agents is not typically possible or necessary in the setting of fracture repair. Recent coronary stent placement is a unique consideration where the risks and benefits of perioperative continuation of antiplatelet agents should be strongly considered.

### 3.1 Aspirin and aspirin/dipyridamole

Aspirin inhibits the production of thromboxane, which binds platelet molecules together to create a patch over damaged walls of blood vessels. Aspirin is prescribed to help prevent myocardial infarction, strokes, and blood clots. The 2012 guidelines from the ACCP recommend continuing aspirin around the time of surgery for patients at moderate to high risk for cardiovascular events who are undergoing noncardiac surgery [38].

Dipyridamole reversibly inhibits platelet aggregation with a half-life of 12 hours and duration of action of approximately 2 days after discontinuation. The combination of aspirin and dipyridamole does not substantially increase the risk of clinically important postprocedural bleeding [39].

Like other agents discussed, the decision to continue or withhold aspirin and aspirin/dipyridamole should reflect a balance of the consequences of perioperative hemorrhage versus the risk of perioperative vascular complications.

### 3.2 Clopidogrel, prasugrel, ticagrelor, and ticlopidine

Key features of nonaspirin antiplatelet agents:

- Prescribed for treatment of symptomatic atherosclerosis in acute coronary syndrome without ST segment elevation, ST elevation myocardial infarction, cerebrovascular disease, and peripheral vascular disease.
- The use of these agents has gone up with the increase in drug-eluting coronary artery stenting procedures.
- Antiplatelet agents work to block adenosine diphosphate subtype P2Y12 and prevent the activation of platelets and eventual cross-linking by the protein fibrin, thus preventing platelet aggregation and clot formation. Platelet inhibition can be demonstrated 2 hours after a single dose of oral clopidogrel, and the effect lasts for 5–9 days (ie, the entire lifespan of the platelets). Inhibiting platelet aggregation can increase the risk of serious bleeding in patients undergoing surgery.
- Because of the prolonged effect of these agents, surgical delay for medication clearance is typically not an option for the acute fracture patient. As with the anticoagulants, the risks of cessation depend on the indication.

#### 3.2.1 Thrombotic risk assessment

Patients using clopidogrel and other nonaspirin antiplatelet agents after coronary artery stent placement can be at increased risk for stent thrombosis. The risk of coronary artery stent thrombosis after the premature cessation of clopidogrel is relatively low but may be catastrophic. The ACCP recommends that for those who have had a bare metal stent within the past 6 weeks or a drug-eluting stent in the past 6 months, both aspirin and clopidogrel be continued perioperatively [38, 40].

Elective surgery should be postponed whenever possible until the minimum period of therapy with P2Y12 receptor blocker therapy is completed.

#### 3.2.2 Management for surgery

There is no reversal agent for clopidogrel and other antiplatelet agents. In general, there should be no surgical delay for patients undergoing general anesthesia, although meticulous surgical hemostasis can be helpful.

Staff managing clopidogrel for FFP should take into consideration the following:

- A single retrospective study assessed the perioperative bleeding risks and clinical outcome after early hip fracture surgery on patients taking clopidogrel. In this cohort, patients taking clopidogrel were not at substantially increased risk for bleeding, bleeding complications, or mortality. In this cohort the clopidogrel group did have a greater number of comorbidities, American Society of Anesthesiologists scores and postoperative length of stay [41].
- Due to the risk of bleeding, spinal anesthesia is often contraindicated in those taking clopidogrel.
- Perioperative platelet transfusion has been suggested, as the transfused platelets may be effective in forming a viable plug, but clinical effectiveness of this approach has not been studied. Platelet transfusions are not standard of care and should be reserved for selected very high-risk or excessively bleeding patients (see chapter 2.3 Clinical practice guidelines).

## 4 Prophylaxis against venous thromboembolism

Hip fracture patients are at high risk for VTE for multiple reasons related to Virchow's triad [42]. Venous stasis occurs after hip fracture due to immobility. At the time of fracture or surgery, vascular intimal injury may occur. Last, a hypercoagulable state may occur from the release of tissue factors.

The risk of VTE following hip fracture repair is high and reported rates often vary depending on when the study was conducted and the type of measurement used. The incidence of proximal DVT has been estimated at 27% without prophylaxis and the risk of fatal PE has been estimated at 1.9% [43, 44].

The ACCP recommends routine VTE prophylaxis in fracture patients [45]. There are several options available and should be chosen based on patient characteristics (**Table 1.6-5**). Low-molecular-weight heparin is a preferred agent and should be started 12 or more hours postoperatively. Other options include warfarin (goal INR of 1.8–2.5), low-dose unfractionated heparin (UFH), fondaparinux, and aspirin. Prophylaxis duration with pharmacological agents is recommended for up to 35 days after surgery. Furthermore, extended prophylaxis (28–35 days) with LMWH reduces the rate of VTE without excess bleeding. Aspirin was added to the list of pharmacological options in 2008. Aspirin has been shown to be effective in reducing VTE risk in hip fracture, but is less effective than LMWH and not used in most high-performing geriatric fracture centers [46]. Aspirin is usually considered for orthopedic patients who have undergone a total hip or knee replacement and are not candidates for other anticoagulants.

| Agent | Grade of evidence |
|---|---|
| Low-molecular-weight heparin, for example:<br>• Enoxaparin 40 mg SQ daily<br>• Dalteparin 5,000 units SQ daily | 1B |
| Warfarin (goal INR 1.8–2.5) | 1B |
| Fondaparinux (2.5 mg daily) | 1B |
| Low-dose UFH (5,000 units SQ 2–3 times daily) | 1B |
| Aspirin | 1B |
| Patient (some agents may require renal adjustment) | |

**Table 1.6-5** Preferred thromboprophylaxis agents for prophylaxis in the fragility fracture patients.
Abbreviations: SQ, subcutaneous; UFH, unfractionated heparin.

### 4.1 Nonpharmacological options for thromboprophylaxis

Thromboprophylaxis with intermittent pneumatic compression devices (IPCDs) have the potential advantage of reducing the incidence of VTE without the risk for increased bleeding. The ACCP guidelines list IPCDs as an alternative to pharmacological prophylaxis [45]. Intermittent pneumatic compression devices can cause skin breakdown, promote falls, and contribute to delirium in geriatric patients. Inferior vena cava (IVC) filter has historically been considered in those patients who have contraindications to both pharmacological and mechanical thromboprophylaxis, but has fallen out of favor in most circumstances. The risks of IVC filter placement include DVT at the insertion site, occlusion of the IVC due to thrombosis below the filter, migration of the filter, and failure to remove and/or complications with removal. There is no evidence that routine use in this population produces better outcomes, and the ACCP suggests against using IVC filter placement for primary prevention over no thromboprophylaxis in patients with an increased bleeding risk or contraindications to both pharmacological and mechanical thromboprophylaxis [45]. Inferior vena cava filters that are removable may have isolated use if PE or proximal DVT has occurred within the previous 4 weeks [39].

### 4.2 Bridging therapy

For patients needing to interrupt long-term warfarin therapy for surgery, the use of short-acting parenteral anticoagulation such as LMWH or UFH until long-term anticoagulation is achieved is termed bridging therapy. The use of bridging therapy reflects an attempt to minimize thrombotic complications with agents or doses that can be quickly reversed or cleared if excessive bleeding occurs. Bridging therapy can contribute to excessive perioperative blood loss, and an individualized approach to balance risks and benefits is necessary.

In terms of risk of thrombosis, the ACCP divides long-term anticoagulated patients into three categories:

- High (> 10% annual risk of arterial thromboembolism [ATE])
- Moderate (5–10% annual risk ATE)
- Low (< 5% risk ATE)

Note that the risk of thromboembolism is typically reported as an annual risk; for most patients the short-term risk during a typical perioperative period is assumed to be much lower.

High-risk groups should be considered most strongly for bridging therapy (**Table 1.6-3**) [38]. This includes:

- Artificial mitral valve replacement
- Older aortic valves (caged ball, tilting disk)
- Atrial fibrillation with $CHADS_2 \geq 5$
- Stroke or transient cerebral ischemia attack (TIA) within the past 6 months
- Rheumatic valvular heart disease
- Patients or providers unwilling to accept any risk for ATE

In moderate-risk patients the decision to use bridging therapy and the degree of intensity of bridging therapy should be individualized.

Bridging in moderate and low-risk patients should be undertaken cautiously in light of the high sensitivity of older adults to typical anticoagulant doses, and the high prevalence of renal and hepatic dysfunction and other risk factors for bleeding [47].

A large randomized, double-blind placebo control study looked at bridging patients with AF and a mean $CHADS_2$ score of 2.3, who had warfarin treatment interrupted for an elective operation or other elective invasive procedure. The study found that forgoing bridging anticoagulation was noninferior to perioperative bridging with LMWH, and associated with less bleeding. In this study, the incidence of ATE was 0.4% in the no bridging and 0.3% in the bridging group; the incidence of major bleeding was 1.3% in the no bridging and 3.2% in the bridging group [48].

There is no clear evidence to guide the exact timing or dosing for bridging. Once adequate hemostasis has been achieved, options depend on renal function and include:

- Full dose LMWH, aiming for complete therapeutic anticoagulation
- Lower dose LMWH (eg, doses often used for VTE prophylaxis)
- Unfractionated heparin to target PTT (1.5–2 normal)

Even in patients at high risk for a thromboembolic event, the relatively high risk of bleeding may outweigh a smaller risk of thrombosis occurring over the 2–3 postoperative days until hemodynamic stability and hemostasis are achieved. Clinicians should be prepared to stop bridging therapy if there is evidence of significant postoperative bleeding.

Warfarin can often be resumed the night after surgery, and almost always within 24 hours after surgery [38]. If there is no evidence of active bleeding, bridging therapy should be continued until the target INR has been reached for 48 hours.

Bridging therapy should be considered in a patient-specific fashion with the input from both the surgical and medical teams.

## 5 References


1. **Juliebo V, Bjoro K, Krogseth M, et al.** Risk factors for preoperative and postoperative delirium in elderly patients with hip fracture. *J Am Geriatr Soc.* 2009 Aug;57(8):1354–1361.
2. **Khan SK, Kalra S, Khanna A, et al.** Timing of surgery for hip fractures: a systematic review of 52 published studies involving 291,413 patients. *Injury.* 2009 Jul;40(7):692–697.
3. **Zuckerman JD, Skovron ML, Koval KJ, et al.** Postoperative complications and mortality associated with operative delay in older patients who have a fracture of the hip. *J Bone Joint Surg Am.* 1995 Oct;77(10):1551–1556.
4. **Gleason LJ, Friedman SM.** Preoperative management of anticoagulation and antiplatelet agents. *Clin Geriatr Med.* 2014 May;30(2):219–227.
5. **Marsland D, Colvin PL, Mears SC, et al.** How to optimize patients for geriatric fracture surgery. *Osteoporos Int.* 2010 Dec;21(Suppl 4):S535–S546.
6. **Gage BF, Waterman AD, Shannon W, et al.** Validation of clinical classification schemes for predicting stroke: results from the National Registry of Atrial Fibrillation. *JAMA.* 2001 Jun 13;285(22):2864–2870.
7. **Lip GY, Nieuwlaat R, Pisters R, et al.** Refining clinical risk stratification for predicting stroke and thromboembolism in atrial fibrillation using a novel risk factor-based approach: the euro heart survey on atrial fibrillation. *Chest.* 2010 Feb;137(2):263–272.
8. **Kearon C, Akl EA, Comerota AJ, et al.** Antithrombotic therapy for VTE disease: antithrombotic therapy and prevention of thrombosis, 9th ed: American College of Chest Physicians Evidence-Based Clinical Practice Guidelines. *Chest.* 2012 Feb;141(2 Suppl):e419S–e494S.
9. **Cannegieter SC, Rosendaal FR, Briet E.** Thromboembolic and bleeding complications in patients with mechanical heart valve prostheses. *Circulation.* 1994 Feb;89(2):635–641.
10. **Douketis JD, Berger PB, Dunn AS, et al.** The perioperative management of antithrombotic therapy: American College of Chest Physicians Evidence-Based Clinical Practice Guidelines (8th edition). *Chest.* 2008 Jun;133(6 Suppl):299S–339S.
11. **Gage BF, Yan Y, Milligan PE, et al.** Clinical classification schemes for predicting hemorrhage: results from the National Registry of Atrial Fibrillation (NRAF). *Am Heart J.* 2006 Mar;151(3):713–719.
12. **Pisters R, Lane DA, Nieuwlaat R, et al.** A novel user-friendly score (HAS-BLED) to assess 1-year risk of major bleeding in patients with atrial fibrillation: the Euro Heart Survey. *Chest.* 2010 Nov;138(5):1093–1100.
13. **Friberg L, Rosenqvist M, Lip GY.** Evaluation of risk stratification schemes for ischaemic stroke and bleeding in 182 678 patients with atrial fibrillation: the Swedish Atrial Fibrillation cohort study. *Eur Heart J.* 2012 Jun;33(12):1500–1510.
14. **Al-Rashid M, Parker MJ.** Anticoagulation management in hip fracture patients on warfarin. *Injury.* 2005 Nov;36(11):1311–1315.
15. **Kearon C, Hirsh J.** Management of anticoagulation before and after elective surgery. *N Engl J Med.* 1997 May 22;336(21):1506–1511.
16. **Jaffer AK, Brotman DJ, Chukwumerije N.** When patients on warfarin need surgery. *Cleve Clin J Med.* 2003 Nov;70(11):973–984.
17. **Horlocker TT, Wedel DJ, Benzon H, et al.** Regional anesthesia in the anticoagulated patient: defining the risks (the second ASRA Consensus Conference on Neuraxial Anesthesia and Anticoagulation). *Reg Anesth Pain Med.* 2003 May–Jun;28(3):172–197.
18. **Crowther MA, Douketis JD, Schnurr T, et al.** Oral vitamin K lowers the international normalized ratio more rapidly than subcutaneous vitamin K in the treatment of warfarin-associated coagulopathy. A randomized, controlled trial. *Ann Intern Med.* 2002 Aug 20;137(4):251–254.
19. **Dezee KJ, Shimeall WT, Douglas KM, et al.** Treatment of excessive anticoagulation with phytonadione (vitamin K): a meta-analysis. *Arch Intern Med.* 2006 Feb 27;166(4):391–397.
20. **Burbury KL, Milner A, Snooks B, et al.** Short-term warfarin reversal for elective surgery—using low-dose intravenous vitamin K: safe, reliable and convenient*. *Br J Haematol.* 2011 Sep;154(5):626–634.
21. **Fiore LD, Scola MA, Cantillon CE, et al.** Anaphylactoid reactions to vitamin K. *J Thromb Thrombolysis.* 2001 Apr;11(2):175–183.
22. **Schulman S.** Clinical practice. Care of patients receiving long-term anticoagulant therapy. *N Engl J Med.* 2003 Aug 14;349(7):675–683.
23. **Fakheri RJ.** Formula for fresh frozen plasma dosing for warfarin reversal. *Mayo Clin Proc.* 2013 Jun;88(6):640.
24. **Vitale MA, Vanbeek C, Spivack JH, et al.** Pharmacologic reversal of warfarin-associated coagulopathy in geriatric patients with hip fractures: a retrospective study of thromboembolic events, postoperative complications, and time to surgery. *Geriatr Orthop Surg Rehabil.* 2011 Jul;2(4):128–134.
25. **Gleason LJ, Mendelson DA, Kates SL, et al.** Anticoagulation management in individuals with hip fracture. *J Am Geriatr Soc.* 2014 Jan;62(1):159–164.
26. **Refaai MA, Goldstein JN, Lee ML, et al.** Increased risk of volume overload with plasma compared with four-factor prothrombin complex concentrate for urgent vitamin K antagonist reversal. *Transfusion.* 2015 Nov;55(11):2722–2729.
27. **Goldstein JN, Refaai MA, Milling TJ Jr, et al.** Four-factor prothrombin complex concentrate versus plasma for rapid vitamin K antagonist reversal in patients needing urgent surgical or invasive interventions: a phase 3b, open-label, non-inferiority, randomised trial. *Lancet.* 2015 May 23;385(9982):2077–2087.
28. **White RH, McKittrick T, Hutchinson R, et al.** Temporary discontinuation of warfarin therapy: changes in the international normalized ratio. *Ann Intern Med.* 1995 Jan 1;122(1):40–42.
29. **Tharmarajah P, Pusey J, Keeling D, et al.** Efficacy of warfarin reversal in orthopedic trauma surgery patients. *J Orthop Trauma.* 2007 Jan;21(1):26–30.
30. **Bell BR, Spyropoulos AC, Douketis JD.** Perioperative management of the direct oral anticoagulants: a case-based review. *Hematol Oncol Clin North Am.* 2016 Oct;30(5):1073–1084.
31. **Schulman S, Majeed A.** The oral thrombin inhibitor dabigatran: strengths and weaknesses. *Semin Thromb Hemost.* 2012 Feb;38(1):7–15.
32. **Douxfils J, Mullier F, Robert S, et al.** Impact of dabigatran on a large panel of routine or specific coagulation assays. Laboratory recommendations for monitoring of dabigatran etexilate. *Thromb Haemost.* 2012 May;107(5):985–997.
33. **Ageno W, Gallus AS, Wittkowsky A, et al.** Oral anticoagulant therapy: Antithrombotic Therapy and Prevention of Thrombosis, 9th ed: American College of Chest Physicians Evidence-Based Clinical Practice Guidelines. *Chest.* 2012 Feb;141(2 Suppl):e44S–e88S.
34. **Pollack CV Jr, Reilly PA, Eikelboom J, et al.** Idarucizumab for Dabigatran Reversal. *N Engl J Med.* 2015 Aug 6;373(6):511–520.

35. **Ansell JE, Bakhru SH, Laulicht BE, et al.** Use of PER977 to reverse the anticoagulant effect of edoxaban. *N Engl J Med.* 2014 Nov 27;371(22):2141–2142.
36. **Ansell JE.** Universal, class-specific and drug-specific reversal agents for the new oral anticoagulants. *J Thromb Thrombolysis.* 2016 Feb;41(2):248–252.
37. **Connolly SJ, Milling TJ Jr., Eikelboom JW, et al.** Andexanet alfa for acute major bleeding associated with factor Xa inhibitors. *N Engl J Med.* 2016 Sep 22;375(12):1131–1141.
38. **Douketis JD, Spyropoulos AC, Spencer FA, et al.** Perioperative management of antithrombotic therapy: antithrombotic therapy and prevention of thrombosis, 9th ed: American College of Chest Physicians Evidence-Based Clinical Practice Guidelines. *Chest.* 2012 Feb;141(2 Suppl):e326S–e350S.
39. **Baron TH, Kamath PS, McBane RD.** Management of antithrombotic therapy in patients undergoing invasive procedures. *N Engl J Med.* 2013 May 30;368(22):2113–2124.
40. **Daemen J, Wenaweser P, Tsuchida K, et al.** Early and late coronary stent thrombosis of sirolimus-eluting and paclitaxel-eluting stents in routine clinical practice: data from a large two-institutional cohort study. *Lancet.* 2007 Feb 24;369(9562):667–678.
41. **Collinge CA, Kelly KC, Little B, et al.** The effects of clopidogrel (Plavix) and other oral anticoagulants on early hip fracture surgery. *J Orthop Trauma.* 2012 Oct;26(10):568–573.
42. **Bagot CN, Arya R.** Virchow and his triad: a question of attribution. *Br J Haematol.* 2008 Oct;143(2):180–190.
43. **Geerts WH, Bergqvist D, Pineo GF, et al.** Prevention of venous thromboembolism: American College of Chest Physicians Evidence-Based Clinical Practice Guidelines (8th Edition). *Chest.* 2008 Jun;133(6 Suppl):381S–453S.
44. **Dahl OE, Caprini JA, Colwell CW Jr, et al.** Fatal vascular outcomes following major orthopedic surgery. *Thromb Haemost.* 2005 May;93(5):860–866.
45. **Falck-Ytter Y, Francis CW, Johanson NA, et al.** Prevention of VTE in orthopedic surgery patients: Antithrombotic Therapy and Prevention of Thrombosis, 9th ed: American College of Chest Physicians Evidence-Based Clinical Practice Guidelines. *Chest.* 2012 Feb;141(2 Suppl):e278S–e325S.
46. **Gent M, Hirsh J, Ginsberg JS, et al.** Low-molecular-weight heparinoid orgaran is more effective than aspirin in the prevention of venous thromboembolism after surgery for hip fracture. *Circulation.* 1996 Jan 1;93(1):80–84.
47. **Birnie DH, Healey JS, Wells GA, et al.** Pacemaker or defibrillator surgery without interruption of anticoagulation. *N Engl J Med.* 2013 May 30;368(22):2084–2093.
48. **Douketis JD, Spyropoulos AC, Kaatz S, et al.** Perioperative Bridging Anticoagulation in Patients with Atrial Fibrillation. *N Engl J Med.* 2015 Aug 27;373(9):823–833.

# 1.7 Postoperative medical management

Jennifer D Muniak, Susan M Friedman

## 1 Introduction

The early postoperative period after hip fracture repair is characterized by dynamic physiological changes in individuals with little functional reserve. Traditional approaches to postoperative care are typically poorly coordinated and primarily reactive to medical complications as they arise. These approaches put geriatric patients at risk for multiple adverse events, excessive testing and consultations, and polypharmacy (**Fig 1.7-1**) [1].

In contrast, high-performing geriatric fracture centers can lower complication rates, length of hospital stay, and mortality following hip fracture repair. Best practice strategies require collaborative surgical and medical management, standardized protocols to address common clinical issues, a focus on early mobility, and early discharge planning [2]. Frequent medical assessments enable tailored symptom control, early recognition and treatment of postoperative complications and optimal postoperative recovery.

This chapter outlines a practical approach to the postoperative period following hip fracture repair. Emphasis is placed upon proactive, collaborative care and understanding the unique challenges faced by the older adult during this vulnerable time.

Key points are:

- Postoperative care using geriatric principles is essential to optimal outcomes
- Early mobilization, pain control, restoration of adequate intravascular volume, and avoidance of iatrogenic harm are essential
- Some home medications may not be appropriate to resume during the postoperative period, particularly those that lower blood pressure
- Discharge communication and handoffs are particularly important

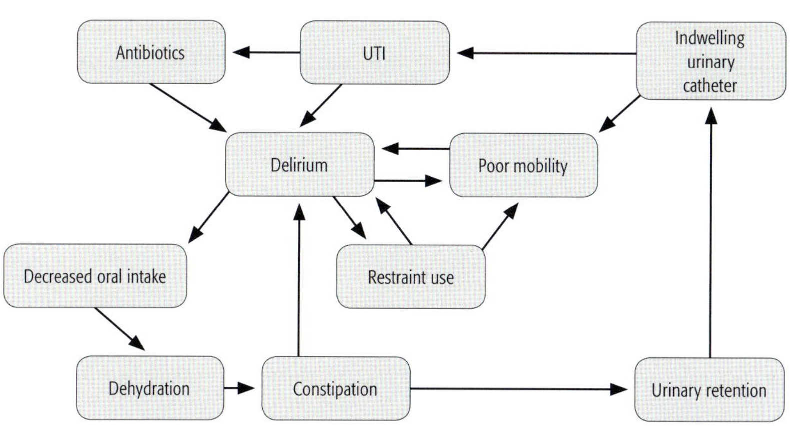


**Fig 1.7-1** Example of interrelated postoperative complications.
Abbreviation: UTI, urinary tract infection.

## 2 Management of postoperative anemia

Maintaining adequate intravascular volume is an important goal of the early postoperative period. Older adults are likely to need blood and volume resuscitation postoperatively, but the timing and the amount should be tailored to the individual based on baseline and perioperative circumstances. In the early perioperative period, the risks of hypovolemia include orthostasis and syncope, acute stroke and acute kidney injury. In the late perioperative period, edema and hypervolemia can complicate wound healing and postoperative recovery. For most patients, maintaining adequate intravascular volume to support standing blood pressure and end organ perfusion is the first priority, particularly in the first 48 hours after surgery.

### 2.1 Isotonic fluids

- Isotonic fluids, eg, 0.9% sodium chloride solution, can help maintain perioperative intravascular volume.
- Continuous fluid infusion is generally started prior to hip fracture surgery and discontinued on the first or second postoperative day, after reestablishing stable intravascular volume and resuming oral intake.
- Daily assessments of volume status and monitoring for signs of hypovolemia are necessary.

### 2.2 Blood transfusion

Standards for transfusion are in flux as emerging data has shed light on the lack of benefit and in some cases harm with liberal transfusion policies. The best data at the time of this writing comes from the FOCUS trial [3] and suggests that typical hip fracture patients can be safely managed with a transfusion blood hemoglobin threshold of 8 g/dL.

Patients in the FOCUS trial who were transfused at the 8 g/dL threshold received 65% fewer blood products than those transfused at a threshold of 10 g/dL with similar rates of death, acute coronary syndrome, and the ability to ambulate at 60 days.

Harm has also been found with liberal transfusion policies in nonhip fracture populations, though the severity of this remains largely unknown. A recent study of patients with acute gastrointestinal bleeding found significantly higher all-cause mortality at 6 weeks with a transfusion threshold of 9 g/dL compared to 7 g/dL [4]. Volume overload is the most common risk of transfusion, and this risk increases with higher volumes of infused red cells or a history of heart failure [5].

It is unlikely that a single threshold will be appropriate for all patients, and clinicians should consider the proportion and rate of blood loss in addition to the absolute hemoglobin value. Signs and symptoms due to anemia warrant transfusion regardless of threshold. Tachycardia, hypotension, altered mental status, chest pain, and dyspnea can suggest symptomatic anemia. Expected hemodynamic changes can be suppressed by comorbidity or medications, eg, beta-blocker blunting tachycardia. Higher transfusion thresholds may be needed for patients with a bleeding predisposition, those with large volume intraoperative blood loss, or higher prefracture hemoglobin levels from chronic pulmonary disease.

## 3 Early mobility

Early mobilization is a cornerstone in prevention of postoperative complications, including pressure ulcers, prolonged pain, and functional decline. Some factors may limit early mobility, such as delirium, tethers, and medical illness. All medical plans should be evaluated with mobility in mind.

Many patients will have nonmodifiable risk factors such as sarcopenia, motor weakness, gait disturbance, bradykinesia, impulsivity, poor proprioception, and low vision/blindness.

Physical therapy consultation on the first postoperative day and every day thereafter is necessary for promoting early physical recovery.

Physician orders should be written in a manner to encourage activity unless there is a special mobility consideration. A surgical repair that allows for weight bearing as tolerated will help to facilitate this process.

### 3.1 Limiting tethers and excessive monitoring

Medical equipment used for monitoring and treating hospitalized patients also "tethers" them to the bed and represent functional restraints. Tethers significantly limit mobility and can lead to complications when removed by patients. A restrained patient is more likely to develop delirium.

Clinicians should evaluate the need for such tethers on every visit and remove them as soon as possible.

More specific issues concerning common tethers include:

- Urinary catheters are most appropriate for patients awaiting hip fracture surgery in order to accurately measure urine output and provide comfort to the bedridden patient who cannot toilet himself. Postoperatively, catheters hinder mobility, lead to infection and can often be removed within the first 2 postoperative days. See topic 10.2 in this chapter for further discussion of urinary catheters.
- Continuous intravenous infusions represent a major barrier to mobility and are cumbersome for both nurses and patients, often distracting from the most important postoperative care goals. Most infusions can be stopped on postoperative day 1 or 2, once the patient is hemodynamically stable. If intravenous infusions are necessary, consider giving intermittently to avoid conflicts with activity or physical therapy sessions.
- Continuous cardiac monitoring is only indicated in patients with unstable or newly diagnosed cardiac arrhythmias and is not indicated as part of standard postoperative care.
- Supplemental oxygen should only be used to treat target signs or symptoms, and should be discontinued in patients with adequate oxygenation.
- Frequency of obtaining vital signs should weigh the usefulness of this information with the burden to the patient. If the patient is hemodynamically stable, consider abstaining from vital sign checks for an 8-hour period at night to promote sleep.
- Physical restraints should be avoided due to their ability to cause significant physical and psychological harm. Restraints do not prevent falls, and can promote agitation and cause significant injury and death as restrained individuals attempt to escape [6, 7]. Avoiding restraint use in hospitalized older adults can best be achieved through the prevention or prompt treatment of delirium see chapter 1.14 Delirium. Alternatives to physical restraints include companion or family sitters, changes to the patient's environment (eg, lighting and noise), and low-dose antipsychotic medications when necessary.

## 4 Delirium

Delirium is the most common complication of hip fracture surgery and characterized by acutely disordered thinking and altered levels of alertness, often with fluctuating severity. It is an independent predictor of in-hospital as well as postdischarge mortality [8]. Prompt recognition and treatment of delirium is important for early and effective rehabilitation as well as other aspects of recovery.

For further discussion of delirium, see chapter 1.14 Delirium.

## 5 Malnutrition

Many older patients are malnourished at the time of the hip fracture; this can negatively impact their recovery as well as 1-year mortality [9]. Not surprisingly, older adults also struggle to maintain adequate nutrition during the postoperative period. Appetite can be reduced from anesthesia-induced gut stasis. The act of eating may be hindered by lethargy, throat discomfort following intubation, lack of dentures, undesirable food choices, or new or worsened dysphagia. Poor in-hospital nutrition is associated with increased mortality and functional decline [10, 11].

It remains unclear whether optimized in-hospital nutrition can mitigate or neutralize these negative outcomes; however, optimizing in-hospital nutrition remains an important goal with at least theoretical benefits of improvements in gut motility, intravascular volume, and mood.

Older adults consume more food when diets do not impose severe restrictions in salt, refined sugar, or saturated fat [12]. Similarly, oral consumption generally improves when small, high-calorie portions are available throughout the day. Feeding conditions should be optimized and tailored to the needs of the patient (eg, meal set-up, proper positioning, hand feeding).

Nutritional supplements do not have a well-defined role in hospital care of older adults. They do not appear to reduce complications or mortality in hip fracture patients [13].

Dysphagia is relatively common in older adults, and can worsen in the perioperative period. Ensure that the appropriate diet consistency is ordered and that feeding assistance is given (ie, meal supervision is sometimes necessary). If clinicians are unsure about the safety of oral intake, a swallowing evaluation can be helpful. For further discussion of malnutrition see chapter 1.11 Sarcopenia, malnutrition, frailty, and falls.

## 6 Avoidance of pressure ulcerations

Pressure ulcers are a predictable, costly, and dangerous complication of immobility.

Frail geriatric patients are among the most likely to incur a pressure ulcer [14, 15]. Odds are high for a fragility fracture patient to develop or exacerbate a pressure ulcer, as tissue damage can occur within a few days of bed rest [16, 17]. Tenets of ulcer prevention align with other best practices of hospital care, including minimizing the total time of immobility, optimizing nutrition and maintaining adequate hygiene. Nursing staff are instrumental in recognizing at-risk patients and providing the mainstay of skin care.

Mechanical offloading of pressure from the sacrum and heels is crucial in ulcer prevention and becomes more important in a patient unable or unwilling to ambulate after surgery. Offloading is best accomplished by daily transfer to a chair in combination with frequent repositioning while in bed. Repositioning should occur at least every 4 hours, although the optimum frequency is not yet established [18]. Socks or padded boots are preferred for offloading the heels.

Skin should be kept dry and protected. Dress existing sacral ulcers to prevent contamination with urine and stool. Avoid friction and shear forces with protective dressings and careful repositioning and transferring of patients.

Nurse-administered risk assessment tools are helpful for identifying patients at high risk of developing a pressure ulcer. The scores they generate help nurses allocate resources and create effective care plans, although they have not been found to decrease the incidence of pressure ulcers [19]. The Braden Scale and the Norton Scale are the most widely used tools and both are recommended by the Agency for Healthcare Research and Quality to be used in the hospital and nursing home settings [20]. Optimal frequency of risk assessment continues to be debated but repeated assessment at least at admission and after 48–72 hours is recommended [21].

## 7 Pain management

Effective pain control facilitates early mobilization and reduces risk for delirium. Frequent assessment of pain and adequate medication dosing is essential.

Routinely scheduled acetaminophen provides a safe and well-tolerated foundation for postoperative pain control in most older adults. Consider 650–1,000 mg of acetaminophen three times daily for at least 2–3 weeks postoperatively in patients without liver dysfunction. Ensure that the patient is not taking any other acetaminophen-containing products.

Most patients will need low-dose opioid medications in the first days to weeks after hip fracture. Patients who are not chronically dependent upon opioids may only need occasional, low-dose opioid therapy, most often with activity and at night. Geriatric patients will typically tolerate a regimen of oxycodone immediate release 2.5 mg every 3 hours as needed. Encourage nursing staff to offer an opioid dose 30 minutes prior to physical therapy sessions or transfers. For further discussion of pain management, see chapter 1.12 Pain management.

## 8 Avoidance of constipation

Patients undergoing hip fracture repair are at high risk for constipation due to gut stasis from surgical stress and decreased mobility. Without careful attention to bowel function, patients are at risk for ileus and possibly fatal obstruction.

The care team should aggressively treat constipation and ensure a bowel movement has occurred prior to hospital discharge. Other aspects of postoperative care will promote return of normal bowel function, such as early mobility and oral nutrition/hydration, and limiting tethers. Polyethylene glycol is an osmotic laxative that is powerful, generally well tolerated, and has the ability to be titrated. Consider giving 17 g of polyethylene glycol orally daily or twice daily in the early postoperative period. Often, a rectal suppository is also needed to facilitate the first bowel movement following surgery.

## 9 Polypharmacy—when to stop or restart medications

The stress of surgery and rapid physiological shifts of the early postoperative period increase the patient's vulnerability to medication effects, even with medications that were well tolerated in the outpatient setting. It is wise to prescribe the fewest and lowest possible doses of usual medications in the early postoperative setting. Only a handful of medications have well-described withdrawal effects (eg, betablockers, clonidine, long-term opioids, and long-term benzodiazepines); these may need to be continued at current or attenuated doses. Otherwise patients should demonstrate a physiological need for a medication prior to it being prescribed or restarted. This strategy is likely to reduce polypharmacy and adverse medication effects. See chapter 1.13 Polypharmacy for a detailed description of polypharmacy and its management.

### 9.1 Blood pressure medications

Antihypertensive therapy is often stopped prior to hip fracture repair in anticipation of perioperative hypotension. It is reasonable to continue holding angiotensin-converting enzyme inhibitors (ACEIs), angiotensin-receptor blockers (ARBs), and diuretics in the early postoperative period as hydration status is often tenuous and renal perfusion suboptimal. When blood pressure does necessitate treatment with an antihypertensive, restart agents slowly and consider an attenuated dose.

Beta-blockers are an exception, as they are usually continued in the perioperative period for cardioprotection and to reduce the risk of rebound tachycardia. Similarly, some calcium channel blockers that are used for rate control may need to be continued in the perioperative period.

### 9.2 Anticoagulants

Following hip fracture surgery, clinicians must weigh the risk for postsurgical bleeding and transfusion with the potential benefits of antithrombotics and anticoagulants. Decision making should reflect consensus between the medical and surgical services. Prophylactic dosing of low-molecular-weight heparin is usually effective as a single agent for prevention of venous thromboembolism in the early postoperative period when the bleeding risk is highest. After hemostasis is achieved, it is reasonable to consider resumption of additional anticoagulants. For consideration of special anticoagulation needs, see chapter 1.6 Anticoagulation in the perioperative setting.

### 9.3 Diuretics

Most patients who use diuretics over extended periods will not have normal urine output until these are resumed. Most patients are able to resume diuretics by postoperative day 3–4 when the need for postoperative hydration is over and the patient is taking adequate fluid by mouth.

## 10 Avoidance of serious medical problems

### 10.1 Pneumonia

Patients at highest risk for developing pneumonia in the postoperative period are those who are older, malnourished (as defined by albumin < 3.5), dependent in activities of daily living (ADLs), have a history of congestive heart failure and those with chronic pulmonary problems such as chronic obstructive pulmonary disease [22]. Collectively, "lung expansion modalities", eg, incentive spirometry and deep breathing, have the strongest evidence base for pneumonia prevention in the postoperative setting, as found by the American College of Physicians [22], and are strongly recommended, although the magnitude and relative effectiveness of each method has yet to be elucidated. Focused efforts to achieve early mobility, adequate pain control, and head of the bed elevation are simple to do and have additional benefits.

### 10.2 Urinary tract infection

Indwelling urinary catheters place hip fracture patients at risk for developing urinary tract infection (UTI), especially when left for more than 2 days following surgery [23]. Catheters should be removed on the first postoperative day unless there is an extenuating circumstance. Urinary retention is a common barrier to catheter removal but risk of this can be mitigated by preventing constipation, early mobility, and avoidance of anticholinergic medications. If clinically significant retention persists, continued urinary catheterization may be necessary.

Clinicians should avoid screening for UTI in asymptomatic patients, and if asymptomatic bacteriuria is found in a urine sample, this does not necessitate treatment with antibiotics. Any antibiotic has the potential for adverse reactions, interactions with other medications, and *Clostridium difficile* infection.

### 10.3 Heart failure

Accurate diagnosis of postoperative heart failure can be difficult in older patients. Physical examination findings such as pulmonary crackles, elevated jugular venous pressure and peripheral edema are often nonspecific in the older adult. Often, a trial of diuresis is necessary as a diagnostic and therapeutic tool [1]. In cases of newly discovered heart failure, echocardiography and cardiology consultation may be warranted to evaluate for potentially correctable causes such as valvular problems, arrhythmia, or ischemia.

### 10.4 Hyponatremia

In the surgical setting, hyponatremia is often caused by neurohormonal stress with antidiuretic hormone release, resulting in expanded intravascular volume [24]. Usually the condition is mild and resolves without specific treatment. Consultation with nephrology is warranted in patients with falling sodium despite volume equilibration. Sodium stabilization needs to occur prior to hospital discharge.

### 10.5 Myocardial infarction and elevated troponins

Following hip fracture repair, clinically diagnosed myocardial infarction is rare. However, elevation of the cardiac biomarker troponin is relatively common and has been linked to increased cardiac and all-cause mortality at 6 months [25]. As a result, routine troponin monitoring has been proposed as a routine practice to aid in prognostication [26]. The impact of such monitoring on clinical outcomes remains unclear and needs further study to quantify the risks and benefits of this approach.

## 11 Discharge planning and safe handoffs

Successful handoffs require a proactive, coordinated team effort, especially when caring for medically complex patients. Patients undergoing fragility fracture repair are particularly vulnerable to poorly executed handoffs, which contribute to rehospitalization, adverse events, and patient dissatisfaction [27]. Fracture programs effective at reducing the length of stay have standardized protocols for discharge planning that begin on admission, anchored by automatic social work and physical therapy consultations to determine the discharge destination [2]. Discharge destination depends on both patient care needs and the services available in a specific healthcare system.

The hospitalization summary is a critical piece of medical communication to accepting care teams, especially when caring for medically complex patients. This document should be composed by a physician, physician's assistant or nurse practitioner who has an active role in the patient's care while hospitalized and should be written through the lens of facilitating effective posthospital care. The summary should be completed prior to discharge and ideally accompanied by a phone call to the accepting care provider. Standardizing the patient handoff with a checklist likely improves the quality of the communicated information [28].

Components of a proper hospitalization summary are:

- Baseline functional status and chronic medical problems
- Surgical details, ie, date, surgeon, type of procedure, and complications
- Details of postoperative complications and their treatment
- Results (summarized) of any major tests
- Names, roles and contact information of consulting physicians
- Discharge medication list, complete with doses, frequency, route, and indication:
  - Note discontinued (or dose attenuated) medications and the reason
  - Note added medications and the reason
  - Plan for osteoporosis treatment
- Instructions for the accepting care team, ie, wound care, activity level, diet
- Pending laboratory tests and dates/times of follow-up appointments
- Goals of care including resuscitation status and desires for life-sustaining therapies

Further discussion of postacute care can be found in chapter 1.9 Postacute care.

## 12 Prognostic discussions with patients and families

Anticipatory guidance is an important part of a clinician's role, especially when the patient is expected to have a change in functional trajectory. About 20% of patients with hip fracture will die within a year of repair, and 25% of community-dwelling patients will need nursing home care [29]. Still more will not regain their functional abilities, needing additional help with ambulation and ADLs [30]. Estimation of the patient's clinical trajectory is often possible early in the postoperative course, taking into account the patient's prior level of function, surgical and perioperative complications, and progress with rehabilitation. Discussing these findings with patients and families is important for framing long-term care goals and preparing them for the possibility of an adverse event or new disability. The postoperative hospital stay is an ideal time to do this, as patients are engaged in their medical care and generally open to anticipatory guidance. Further discussion of prognosis and goals of care can be found in chapter 1.5 Prognosis and goals of care.

## 13 References


1. **Nicholas JA.** Management of postoperative complications: cardiovascular disease and volume management. *Clin Geriatr Med.* 2014 May;30(2):293–301.
2. **Friedman SM, Mendelson DA, Kates SL, et al.** Geriatric co-management of proximal femur fractures: total quality management and protocol-driven care result in better outcomes for a frail patient population. *J Am Geriatr Soc.* 2008 Jul;56(7):1349–1356.
3. **Carson JL, Terrin ML, Noveck H, et al.** Liberal or restrictive transfusion in high-risk patients after hip surgery. *N Engl J Med.* 2011 Dec 29;365(26):2453–2462.
4. **Villanueva C, Colomo A, Bosch A, et al.** Transfusion strategies for acute upper gastrointestinal bleeding. *N Engl J Med.* 2013 Jan 3;368(1):11–21.
5. **Li G, Rachmale S, Kojicic M, et al.** Incidence and transfusion risk factors for transfusion-associated circulatory overload among medical intensive care unit patients. *Transfusion.* 2011 Feb;51(2):338–343.
6. **Lofgren RP, MacPherson DS, Granieri R, et al.** Mechanical restraints on the medical wards: are protective devices safe? *Am J Public Health.* 1989 Jun;79(6):735–738.
7. **Miles SH, Irvine P.** Deaths caused by physical restraints. *Gerontologist.* 1992 Dec;32(6):762–766.
8. **Witlox J, Eurelings LS, de Jonghe JF, et al.** Delirium in elderly patients and the risk of postdischarge mortality, institutionalization, and dementia: a meta-analysis. *JAMA.* 2010 Jul 28;304(4):443–451.
9. **Koval KJ, Maurer SG, Su ET, et al.** The effects of nutritional status on outcome after hip fracture. *J Orthop Trauma.* 1999 Mar–Apr;13(3):164–169.
10. **Sullivan DH, Sun S, Walls RC.** Protein-energy undernutrition among elderly hospitalized patients: a prospective study. *JAMA.* 1999 Jun 2;281(21):2013–2019.
11. **Zisberg A, Shadmi E, Gur-Yaish N, et al.** Hospital-associated functional decline: the role of hospitalization processes beyond individual risk factors. *J Am Geriatr Soc.* 2015 Jan;63(1):55–62.
12. **Dorner B, Niedert KC, Welch PK.** Position of the American Dietetic Association: liberalized diets for older adults in long-term care. *J Am Diet Assoc.* 2002 Sep;102(9):1316–1323.
13. **Avenell A, Handoll HH.** Nutritional supplementation for hip fracture aftercare in older people. *Cochrane Database Syst Rev.* 2006 (4):CD001880.
14. **Allman RM, Goode PS, Patrick MM, et al.** Pressure ulcer risk factors among hospitalized patients with activity limitation. *JAMA.* 1995 Mar 15;273(11):865–870.
15. **Houwing R, Rozendaal M, Wouters-Wesseling W, et al.** Pressure ulcer risk in hip fracture patients. *Acta Orthop Scand.* 2004 Aug;75(4):390–393.
16. **Barton A, Barton M.** *The Management and Prevention of Pressure Sores.* London: Faber and Faber; 1981.
17. **Versluysen M.** How elderly patients with femoral fracture develop pressure sores in hospital. *Br Med J (Clin Res Ed).* 1986 May 17;292(6531):1311–1313.
18. **Krapfl LA, Gray M.** Does regular repositioning prevent pressure ulcers? *J Wound Ostomy Continence Nurs.* 2008 Nov–Dec;35(6):571–577.
19. **Pancorbo-Hidalgo PL, Garcia-Fernandez FP, Lopez-Medina IM, et al.** Risk assessment scales for pressure ulcer prevention: a systematic review. *J Adv Nurs.* 2006 Apr;54(1):94–110.
20. **Agency for Healthcare Research and Quality (Quality AfHRa).** Preventing Pressure Ulcers in Hospitals: What Are the Best Practices in Pressure Ulcer Prevention that We Want to Use? Available at: http://www.*ahrq*.gov/professionals/systems/long-term-care/resources/pressure-ulcers/pressureulcertoolkit. Accessed February 19, 2015.
21. **Bergstrom N, Braden B, Boynton P, et al.** Using a research-based assessment scale in clinical practice. *Nurs Clin North Am.* 1995 Sep;30(3):539–551.
22. **Lawrence VA, Cornell JE, Smetana GW.** Strategies to reduce postoperative pulmonary complications after noncardiothoracic surgery: systematic review for the American College of Physicians. *Ann Intern Med.* 2006 Apr 18;144(8):596–608.
23. **Wald HL, Ma A, Bratzler DW, et al.** Indwelling urinary catheter use in the postoperative period: analysis of the national surgical infection prevention project data. *Arch Surg.* 2008 Jun;143(6):551–557.
24. **Lane N, Allen K.** Hyponatraemia after orthopaedic surgery. *BMJ.* 1999 May 22;318(7195):1363–1364.
25. **Ausset S, Minville V, Marquis C, et al.** Postoperative myocardial damages after hip fracture repair are frequent and associated with a poor cardiac outcome: a three-hospital study. *Age Ageing.* 2009 Jul;38(4):473–476.
26. **van Waes JA, Nathoe HM, de Graaff JC, et al.** Myocardial injury after noncardiac surgery and its association with short-term mortality. *Circulation.* 2013 Jun 11;127(23):2264–2271.
27. **Coleman EA, Boult C.** Improving the quality of transitional care for persons with complex care needs. *J Am Geriatr Soc.* 2003 Apr;51(4):556–557.
28. **Halasyamani L, Kripalani S, Coleman E, et al.** Transition of care for hospitalized elderly patients—development of a discharge checklist for hospitalists. *J Hosp Med.* 2006 Nov;1(6):354–360.
29. **Braithwaite RS, Col NF, Wong JB.** Estimating hip fracture morbidity, mortality and costs. *J Am Geriatr Soc.* 2003 Mar;51(3):364–370.
30. **Magaziner J, Hawkes W, Hebel JR, et al.** Recovery from hip fracture in eight areas of function. *J Gerontol A Biol Sci Med Sci.* 2000 Sep;55(9):M498–M507.

# 1.8 Postoperative surgical management

Michael Blauth, Peter Brink

## 1 Introduction

The postoperative period has not been a primary focus for many surgeons, at least not to the same degree as the intraoperative one. As long as wound healing is progressing normally and postoperative x-rays are satisfactory, little attention is usually paid to other important issues that impact postsurgical recovery, rehabilitation, and overall functional outcomes. The communication between surgeons, staff nurses, and physiotherapists regarding common postoperative recovery is often poor.

This is partly due to the lack of availability and application of tools that focus on functional outcomes of individual patients. In addition, surgical and medical providers may not know how to best influence the rehabilitation progress.

Postoperative management seems as important as surgical treatment in producing optimal outcomes. Surgeons' advice has an enormous influence on the patient, relatives, nurses, and physiotherapists, and can positively influence the quality of care in these areas. In this chapter we will focus on the importance of early mobility and rehabilitation, wound and skin management, and the prevention and treatment of pressure sores.

## 2 The impact of immobilization

### 2.1 Loss of muscle mass

Loss of muscle mass and muscle strength is common in older adults and is highly associated with frailty, functional decline, immobility, and falls (**Fig 1.8-1**) [1]. This age-related decline of human muscle mass and strength is known as sarcopenia (see chapter 1.11 Sarcopenia, malnutrition, frailty, and falls) and may be exacerbated by short periods of immobilization [2]:

- Wall et al [3] have generated pilot data from eight older adults demonstrating that 5 days of limb immobilization leads to a 1.5% loss of quadriceps cross-sectional area. When extrapolating this to a whole-body level, merely 5 days of bed rest would result in the loss of roughly 1 kg of muscle tissue.
- Skeletal muscle atrophy is caused by a variety of stressors including decreased external loading and neural activation (ie, disuse), inflammatory cytokines and glucocorticoids, and malnutrition [2]. A combination of unloading and reduced neural activity occurs frequently in clinical settings following limb immobilization, bed rest, spinal cord injury and partial/complete peripheral nerve damage, resulting in significant loss of muscle mass and force production [2].
- Older adults display a marked reduction in their ability to regain lost muscle tissue following a period of disuse, even with an intensive, supervised, resistance-type exercise training schedule [4–6].
- Substantial muscle atrophy occurs during short-term disuse, with higher rates of muscle loss during more prolonged disuse. This suggests that the mechanisms responsible for the early loss of muscle during disuse differ from those occurring in prolonged disuse [3].
- Older adults reduce their normal daily activity following a period of bed rest. Even with structured, supervised training, older adults spend the majority of their day completely inactive [7].

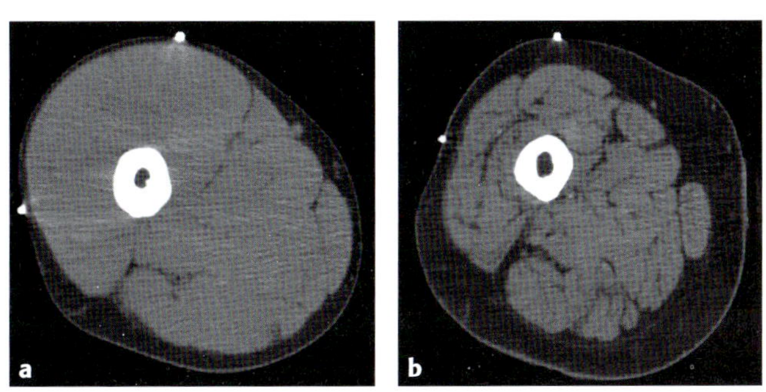


**Fig 1.8-1a–b** Difference in muscle mass of the upper leg between two men aged 25 and 81 years, matched for length and body weight.

- Structured and prolonged resistance training is effective for muscle mass gain in older adults [8, 9] and should be considered vital to their recovery. Most current clinical practice does not mandate such a rehabilitation program following a period of immobility, and older adults generally show low adherence to nonsupervised, structured resistance-type exercise training [10–12].

Composition of the slow, oxidative muscle fibers (type 1) and the fast, glycolytic muscle fibers (type 2) changes with age. Due to a natural loss of type 2 fibers, older adults are unable to react adequately to an unforeseen situation and fall easily. Both walking speed and coordination are decreased, which results in increased risk of falling and fracture. During immobilization, this process continues and the loss of fast twitch fibers progresses. Both the number and the volume of the fibers diminish.

Since there is a direct relation between muscle mass and muscle strength, this loss of muscle mass represents an independent risk factor for new falls and fractures. Restoration of muscle mass will improve performance during mobilization after fracture treatment [13].

There is clear evidence that considerable muscle atrophy occurs during the early phase of immobilization and is attributed to a rapid increase in muscle protein breakdown accompanied by a decline in muscle protein synthesis [3]. A persistent catabolic state hampers the improvement of this situation, so nutritional intake (1.25–1.5 mg of protein per kilogram of body weight per day) together with active mobilization is essential to regain muscle power and coordination. Both are a challenge in older adults.

Early mobilization by itself is not sufficient to prevent a decline in function. There is increasing evidence that strength training for the frail geriatric patient is an effective way to restore muscle function and to eliminate muscle strength asymmetry after surgery within 3 months [1].

In order to regain prefracture level of function and independence, early active mobilization with resistance exercises and adequate protein intake is essential.

## 3 Rehabilitation

Each surgical intervention in fragility fractures should enable the patient to make immediate use of the injured extremity. Undertaking the risk of surgery while still being restricted in postoperative range of motion or active mobilization often results in unacceptable overall functional outcomes.

Why are we afraid that we might overload our fracture/implant construct? Biomechanical studies show that constructs fail at distinct levels typically above physiological loads, even in cadaveric bone without soft tissue and active muscles to support the construct. We have an incomplete understanding of the in vivo forces during partial, full, and non-weight bearing as well as of forces emerging with upper extremity movements.

Surprisingly, forces in the hip joint measured in patients lying in bed and lifting their buttocks are higher than in the same hip joint during full weight bearing (FWB), using two crutches [14]. In light of these biomechanical and clinical realities, immediate weight bearing as tolerated (WBAT) using support should be promoted.

The same reasoning applies, if nonoperative treatment is chosen.

Some general remarks:

- Patients usually enjoy mobilization and use of their extremities. It makes them less dependent on help and reduces frustration noted with activity restrictions.
- Patients may be afraid of pain. It is always helpful if the surgeon assists in the early postoperative phase with moving joints, sitting and standing in front of the bed, to reassure patients about the safety of mobilization during pain.
- Walking exercises should be supervised by the surgeon to enable him/her to interpret utterances and questions with regard to pain. Never rely on reports from other healthcare providers. There is no way around a personal visit and observation of the patient.
- Giving patients individually tailored tips and tricks to safely improve mobilization may give them emotional support and be extremely helpful.
- Talking to the patients, touching their hands, and answering concerns may also help and encourage them.
- Pain management is critical. Timing, drug selection and dosage all influence patients' ability and willingness to get mobilized and to cooperate.

Patients should feel comfortable while being mobilized, and different walking aids should be offered. Canes or walking sticks are usually more difficult to use and require arm force and coordination. A walker with or without wheels may be easier to use at the beginning or even permanently but may not allow for enough independence.

### 3.1 Lower extremity

Based on traditional teaching, anecdotal information and fear of loss of reduction, many surgeons are hesitant to permit FWB after reduction and stable fixation of fractures of the pelvis and/or lower limb.

No or limited weight bearing for some time is supposed to limit forces on the reconstructed bone and fixation material and to prevent loosening, hardware failure and secondary displacement of the fracture and implant. Of course, if such an event occurs, it is a disaster for patient and physician. Traditionally, limited weight bearing only is allowed for a time span of 6, 8 or 12 weeks after surgery.

One origin of this time-based protocol for weight bearing is the *AO Principles of Fracture Management* by Müller et al [15] that advocates a limited weight-bearing recommendation with 3 months of 5–10 kg load for hip fractures, unfortunately without any support from evidence-based literature. It is remarkable that these classic protocols are still in use, while at least some evidence promoting a less restricted weight-bearing protocol has existed since the end of the last century.

Failures of fixation are mostly associated with biomechanical flaws including suboptimal reduction and/or fixation.

#### 3.1.1 Partial weight bearing is not an option

In the authors' opinions, immediate postoperative WBAT is the only reasonable option in geriatric patients with lower extremity injuries. This applies to all kinds of fixations and joint replacements. Biomechanically sound constructs and close observation of the patient are prerequisite for this regimen.

If a fixation is deemed to be 'not stable enough', it could mean weeks to months of bed rest and/or partial weight bearing (PWB) until fracture healing has taken place. Usually, bone resorption at the fracture site renders the stability of the bone-implant-construct even weaker in the first weeks.

Even though high-level evidence is lacking, the authors list a few thoughts:

- Failures typically occur between the 2nd and 3rd months after surgery, and there is no evidence that they occur more often in patients with weight-bearing permission.
- Restriction of weight bearing inflicts a significant physiological burden on the older patient. The energy expenditure for ambulation without FWB increases fourfold, which leads to rapid exhaustion [16].
- Most fragility fracture patients (FFPs) are not physically able to perform PWB due to sarcopenia, lack of proprioception and arm weakness. Many have preexisting impaired function of the upper and lower extremities which prevents them from using crutches or walkers in a way that effectively and safely spares the affected lower extremity. This makes implementation of a nonweight-bearing or PWB protocol impossible and forces the patient to prolonged bed rest and its well-known negative ramifications, predominantly a rapid loss of muscle mass. In addition, it makes non-weight bearing risky and increases the likelihood for another injury.
- Patient motivation may drop due to fear and anxiety of failure to make functional progress.
- The altered gait mechanism can lead to complaints of overload or low back pain.
- Many FFPs have cognitive impairment, and may not understand or remember weight-bearing instructions.
- Partial weight-bearing protocols are not evidence-based.
- Even in the presence of appropriate doses of pain medication, pain will guide the patient to bear weight safely and appropriately. Patients with severely impaired cognitive function typically have the same self-protective mechanisms as cognitively intact patients.
- Early weight bearing can promote fracture healing and union of the fracture without increasing loss of fixation [17–19].

There is no evidence that PWB after operative treatment of fractures of the pelvis and lower extremity has any advantages for the patient over FWB. Since there are many advantages of immediate full WBAT, this should be the standard approach. It may help to diminish adverse effects of sustaining a fracture such as loss of independence, less sarcopenia, less fear of falling and is expected to lead to a better outcome.

### 3.1.2 Recommendations

The following recommendations regarding weight bearing should serve to produce optimal outcomes for typical FFPs:

- Surgical treatment should be adapted and extended to make fixation as safe as possible. Additional implant augmentation, the use of long, splinting constructs with relative stability, and joint replacement instead of an unstable osteosynthesis requiring PWB are examples.
- Patients should be mobilized with WBAT as soon as possible after surgery. Usually, bedside sitting and standing in front of the bed with equal weight on both legs should be the initial approach.
- Use a walker to assist with WBAT. More specific walkers with support for both upper extremities and the upper part of the body make patients feel safe with regard to falling or becoming so weak that walking is no longer possible.
- Create a safe environment to improve patient confidence and reduce the risk of falling.
- Stress body awareness to help patients identify situations where overload may occur.
- For most intraarticular fractures reduced and fixed with an implant, there is no need to restrict weight bearing. Even though cartilage is damaged, anatomy is restored. Axial loading helps circulation in the joint and the cartilage and facilitates joint healing and strength.
- Surgeons should intermittently observe the postoperative patient during mobilization and ambulation and pay special attention to any barriers to rehabilitation. Little remarks, tips and encouragement from the surgeon can be extremely important for optimal outcomes.

### 3.1.3 Evidence

Literature review indicates that WBAT is safe for most post-fixation FFPs.

- Koval et al [17] demonstrated that older adults encouraged to perform FWB initiated PWB up to 50% in the first week and increased up to 87% in 3 months without any loss of fixation if they were allowed to bear weight as tolerated from day 1.
- The use of bathroom scales to instruct the patient with a biofeedback system is useful for standing but not for walking [20].
- We do not know the actual amount of axial load delivered to the implant-bone construct. We know that patient compliance to follow precise instructions is fairly low and implant constructs rarely fail. So why employ a restricted weight-bearing protocol and not shift to a protocol for weight bearing as tolerated?
- There is no solid proof for an earlier onset of osteoarthritis in general, and it is hardly an issue in this population. It is not the timing of weight bearing, but inadequate articular reduction that predicts the outcome. The few studies of early weight bearing in geriatric acetabular fracture patients showed results similar to nonweight-bearing studies with no secondary loss of reduction [21]. One should realize that in acetabular fractures most forces are exerted posteriorly during transfers and sitting while axial compression during walking transmits force to the acetabular roof which is relatively robust even in severe osteoporosis. Even nonoperatively treated acetabular fractures patients can tolerate weight bearing (**Fig 1.8-2**).
- Similar principles apply to fractures of the tibial plateau. After adequate reduction and plate fixation early weight bearing does not predict malunion or nonunion. Some physicians use locked plates and/or postoperative braces, but superiority for these have not been proven yet [22–24].

## 3.2 Immobilization

### 3.2.1 Immobilization by cast and splint

In nonoperative treatment of lower leg/ankle fractures, an external bracing technique (mostly using plaster of Paris) is used to hold the reduction, to reduce pain and to gain time for consolidation. In intrinsic stable fracture types, weight bearing is permitted if, after reduction of the swelling, a proper external immobilization is possible. In less stable fracture types the initiation of weight bearing is delayed, until signs of bone healing are detected. The well-known drawbacks of external immobilization, including muscle loss and joint stiffness, is the reason to promote internal fixation whenever possible.

External bracing using plaster of Paris or splints today is often used as an adjunct to support the construct inside in osteoporotic bone. In addition to the known drawbacks of both internal fixation and nonoperative treatment in combination, there is no evidence to support this combination management approach. Considering the additional skin and mobility issues in older adults with external bracing, the use of external fixation with plaster should be an exception and not a rule.

If internal fixation is poor due to the quality of the bone, an external fixator could be used as a temporary adjunct. Realize that when plate-screw fixation is poor, the pins for the external fixator will not hold for an extended period of time.

### 3.2.2 Immobilization by traction

Preoperative traction of lower extremity fractures is no longer common, and in the older adult traction entails specific risks. If skin traction is used, a traction weight of more than 1 kg can easily damage the skin in older adults. The use of pins has disadvantages including nerve injury, loosening, and the risk of infection. For these reasons, early definitive surgery is recommended. If the soft tissue does not allow early surgery, a temporary external fixator might be safer than traction.

## 3.3 Upper extremity

Patients are often kept in a sling for 3 weeks or more after fractures of the proximal humerus and the humeral shaft. Fractures of the olecranon and the distal humerus, dislocations and fracture dislocations of the elbow are often immobilized in a plaster despite surgical fixation. The same applies to distal radial fractures. Surgeons argue about reduced bone quality and potential wound healing problems.

Postoperative management after surgery of the upper extremity (mostly proximal humerus or distal radius) is less controversial than of the lower extremity. Again, internal fixation after reduction of the fracture, either open or closed, should not be routinely combined with immobilization. For example, plate fixation of the proximal humerus does not need an extended time of restricted functional therapy. In the operating room the stability of the construct is tested, using the image intensifier. If the surgeon can safely move the shoulder in all directions in the operating room, the patient and/or physiotherapist should be able to tolerate the same, at least using passive motion. Early mobilization is the best way to reduce pain and helps the patient to regain confidence in the injured extremity, and also applies to both the elbow and

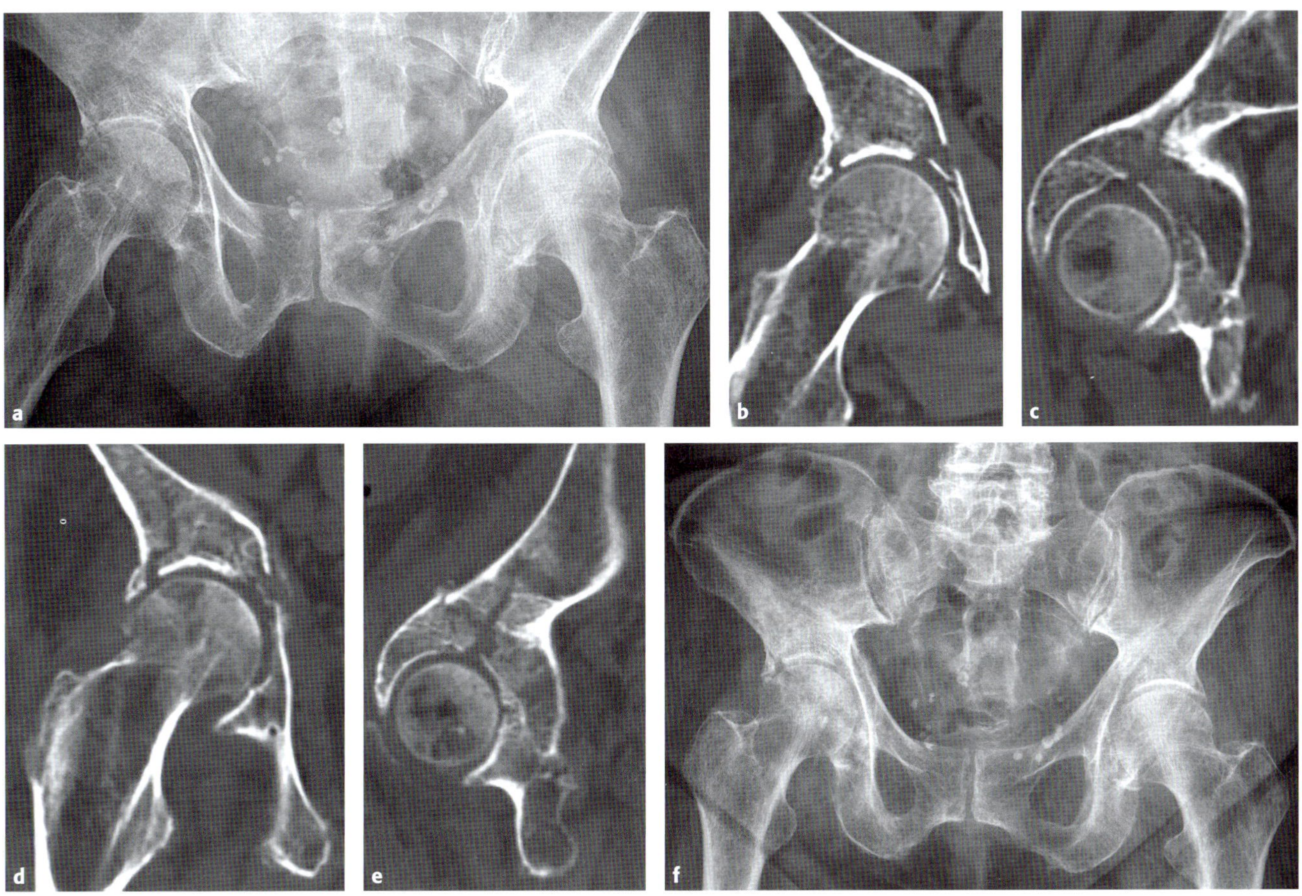


**Fig 1.8-2a–f**

**a–c** Right acetabular fracture in a 91-year-old woman. Immediate pain adapted mobilization with walker.

**d–e** After 2 months slight displacement of fracture fragments but almost pain free with callus formation.

**f** Same situation after 3 months.

distal radius. After wound healing, stimulation of movement of the fingers and wrist is only possible if the plaster is removed. Only when K-wires are used for the distal radius, which are actually contraindicated in osteoporotic bone, is a plaster of Paris mandatory for support of the construct.

### 3.4 Combined injuries

In patients with combined injuries of both the upper and lower limb, rehabilitation is especially problematic. Adaptation of the crutch on the injured side, using an elbow crutch, might be a solution if the wrist is injured. The rehabilitation program should be individualized in these patients in order to find the best way to promote early movement and preserve weight bearing.

## 4 Skin and wound management

### 4.1 Perioperative skin management

The skin of older adults is extremely fragile and vulnerable to injury compared to younger individuals. Older adults are at increased risk for degloving injuries which can occur during positioning on the operating room table by pulling the leg for hip joint reduction (**Fig 1.8-3**). In the postoperative phase, care should be taken when wound dressings have to be removed. A simple bandage instead of an adhesive wound dressing should be used in patients with fragile skin. If a superficial skin deglovement occurs, the use of small butterfly bandages are preferred instead of stitches to replace and fix the skin.

### 4.2 Wound management

Infection prevention is one of the cornerstones of postoperative care of older adults. The skin becomes more friable with age, dehydration, medication effects, malnutrition, immobility, and comorbidities.

There is no generally accepted standard for wound closure in trauma regardless of age. To prevent wound infection, adequate attention to wound closure is important. Control of obvious bleeding, limitation of dead spaces, removal of any dead soft tissue in the wound before closure are basic surgical principles, especially in older adults.

Closure is done by using staples or sutures, according to the surgeon's preference. It is not clear whether staples or sutures are better. Studies comparing staples with sutures, especially regarding hip replacement in older adults, are conflicting. One metaanalysis shows fewer infections in the sutured group compared with staples [25] while another review could not demonstrate a difference [26].

After suturing of the wound, protection of the wound using adhesive strips is one way to reduce tension on the wound. It is advisable, however, to use the strips in full length parallel to the wound instead of perpendicular. Several studies have shown that perpendicular stripping resulted in blisters in 10–41% of patients after hip surgery, which was related to postoperative swelling and increased local stress on the skin [27–29]. Dry dressings are adequate to absorb drainage of blood and fluids and will help to avoid the creation of a

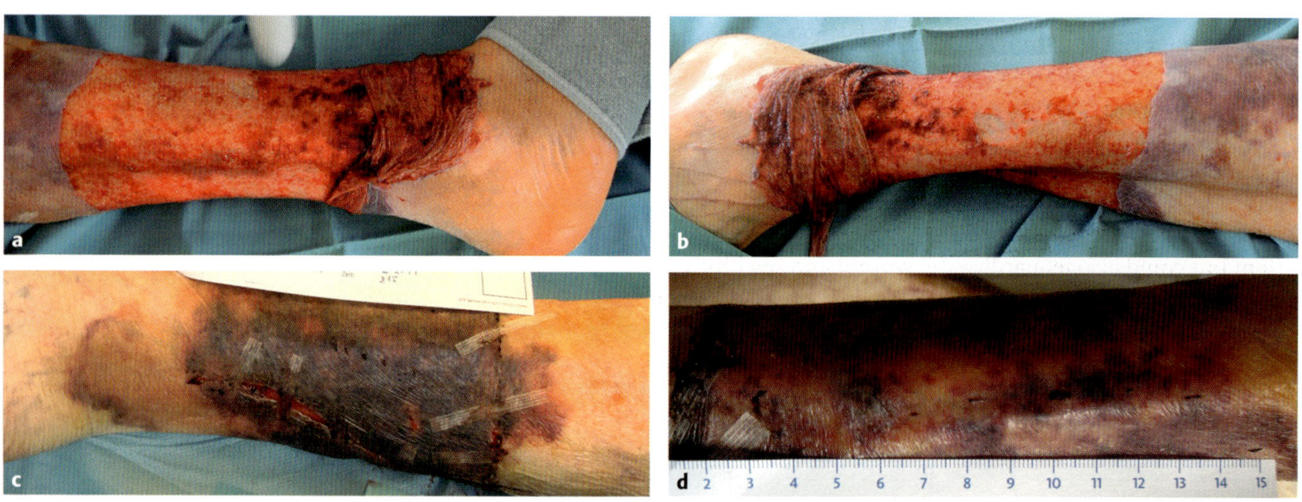


**Fig 1.8-3a–d**
**a–b** Unnoticed intraoperative degloving of the right lower leg in a periprosthetic hip fracture.
**c–d** Uneventful healing over the next weeks.

warm, high fluid-saturated environment that can promote bacterial growth. Care should be taken to avoid blister formation, which can cause pain and disrupt the skin barrier. In general, after 48 hours, bandages are not necessary to cover sutured wounds. In cases of urinary incontinence, an occlusive bandage is recommended. Keeping the wound clean and dry is the best way to prevent wound problems.

Sometimes clear exudate drains from the wound for several days. A dry sterile bandage is needed to absorb the fluid. It could be either extracellular fluid due to local or systemic edema, fat necrosis from stripping the fascia, or a sterile reaction to suture material (eg, polylactin). In some cases, this represents a suture-related pseudoinfection (ie, negative culture and positive histological samples with foreign body reaction) [30].

### 4.2.1 Wound drainage and hematoma management

To drain or not to drain, that has been a general question for many years now and is also a controversial topic in geriatric fracture care. Closed suction drainage after operative treatment of proximal femoral fractures was promoted since the early 1960s [31]. The rationale seems logical, that is to prevent wound hematomas and to decrease the risk for wound infection.

There are a small number of relevant studies of wound drainage in fracture treatment [32–34]. Varley and Milner [32] found that using two drains, high vacuum for < 48 hours did not produce statistically significant reductions in wound infections. The more recent studies [33, 34] showed no relation between hematoma formation and infection, suggesting that the use of drains is unnecessary. There is insufficient evidence from randomized trials to support the routine use of closed suction drainage in orthopedic surgery [35], so larger studies may be helpful in the future. At this time, the routine use of suction drains in hip fracture surgery is not recommended.

Subcutaneous hematoma can lead to discomfort for the patient but could also jeopardize the wound and healthy skin due to diminished circulation of the surrounding tissue (**Fig 1.8-4**). It should be noted that sterile hematoma resorption will produce inflammatory signs, including a subfebrile rise of body temperature. Opening of the wound should only be considered when inflammation is combined with laboratory signs indicating that an infection is likely.

In hip surgery, the fascia lata protects the implants but may also cover an ongoing infection for some time. Pain and raised temperature are signs to evaluate the hardware more intensively. In the case of a hematoma, evacuation is only recommended if the tension on the skin might cause skin necrosis or if it is draining. Pain can be a sign of excessively high pressure. There is no evidence that infection rates increase in closed hematomas (**Fig 1.8-4**) [33].

## 5 Prevention of thromboembolic events

Surgeons know the benefits of prophylactic anticoagulation treatment for their patients and consider this to be good clinical practice. In older adults, the fear of adverse effects of anticoagulation (ie, bleeding) might cause inappropriate underuse of these medications [36, 37]. Aging is regarded as one of the strongest and most prevalent risk factors for thromboembolic events [38]. Comorbid conditions and a lack of mobility are thrombogenic factors as well [39]. Immobilization and type of surgery both contribute to the risk for thromboembolic complications. Geriatric fracture patients may have a period of bed rest from injury until the first attempt to mobilize the patient after surgery and have a moderate risk of 10–40% developing a venous thromboembolism. A hip fracture surgery or major trauma increases this risk to 40–80% [40].

### 5.1 Venous thromboembolism prophylaxis

Venous thromboembolism (VTE) prophylaxis should be given at all ages, unless absolute contraindications exist like significant gastrointestinal, intracranial, wound or intraabdominal bleeding. In these situations mechanical prophylaxis with intermittent pneumatic compression devices or venous foot pump and/or graduate compression stockings are recommended options [40]. A comprehensive review of anticoagulation can be found in chapter 1.6 Anticoagulation in the perioperative setting.

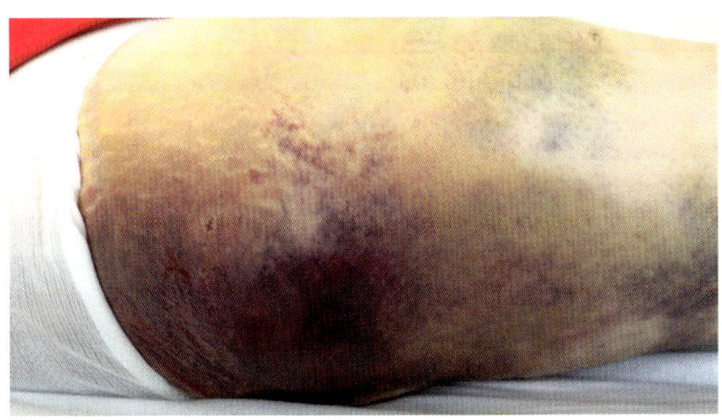

**Fig 1.8-4** Subcutaneous hematoma with skin at risk for necrosis. Evacuation should be considered.

### 5.2 Compression stockings

The use of compression stockings for geriatric patients after trauma surgery could either be indicated for prophylaxis or treatment of VTE but carry the additional risks of skin breakdown and arterial compression. Their use in geriatric patients must be done with care. Elastic compression stockings counteract the effect of increased intravenous hydrostatic pressure. The reduction of the venous pressure gradient improves the reabsorption of fluids from connective tissue.

A Cochrane review shows that graduated compression stockings are effective in diminishing the risk of DVT in hospitalized patients, especially in combination with other prophylactic therapy [41].

If compression stockings reduce the incidence of postthrombotic syndrome (PTS), particularly severe postthrombotic syndrome is still under debate. The only multicenter randomized placebo-controlled trial [42] shows no benefit, probably due to a lack of compliance.

Be careful that the stocking does not roll down, as peroneal nerve palsy due to compression may occur [43].

### 5.3 Pharmacological approaches to venous thromboembolism prophylaxis

To prevent thromboembolic complications in the FFP with a fracture of the lower limb, temporary bed rest, surgery and/or staged mobilization, consider the following pharmacological options:

- Low-molecular-weight heparins (LMWHs), subcutaneous both for intermediate and high-risk patients. The advantage of an LMWH offers the possibility to continue medication after discharge from the hospital. For typical dosage recommendations, see the Orthogeriatrics App [44] about anticoagulation and chapter 1.6 Anticoagulation in the perioperative setting.
- Factor Xa inhibitors (eg, idraparinux, fondaparinux) by subcutaneous route. Fondaparinux is very effective in the prevention of thromboembolic events but increases the chance of (mainly) surgical site bleeding [45].
- New oral anticoagulants (NOACs) (eg, rivaroxaban, dabigatran, apixaban) are tablets. Their definitive role in the prevention of thromboembolic diseases in older patients is not clear yet.

All LMWHs and fondaparinux have been proven to be safe and effective in geriatric patients [37]. For prophylaxis LMHWs are still the first choice [46]. In case of extended use of anticoagulant therapy in older patients after hip surgery, the use of vitamin K antagonists (with a target international normalized ratio of 2.0–3.0) is an alternative way to reduce the risk for thromboembolic complications, but the risk of major bleeding is a concern. Overanticoagulation should be avoided to minimize hemorrhagic complications. Be aware of the risk for major bleeding in patients already receiving antiplatelet therapy (eg, aspirin and clopidogrel). Since there is no evidence that antiplatelet therapy is superior to anticoagulant therapy, except in case of a prosthetic heart valve, it is safer to stop antiplatelet therapy temporarily.

For patients undergoing a surgical procedure for fracture reduction and fixation the authors recommend:

- For patients not undergoing immediate surgery, administer LMWH no closer to surgery than12 hours. Postoperatively, LMWH can be started 6 hours or more after fixation.
- Continue for 10–15 days and in case of hip surgery up to 5 weeks.

In case of isolated lower leg injuries requiring leg immobilization, there is no proof that anticoagulant therapy is beneficial unless the patient belongs to a high-risk group.

## 6 Management of urinary bladder disorders

Many FFPs have urinary incontinence during the perioperative period, due to preexisting urinary tract dysfunction and temporary factors including delirium, pain, positioning, constipation, and medication adverse effects. With age, bladder capacity, contractility decrease, and involuntary detrusor contractions increase. Moreover, almost 90% of all patients with a hip fracture have an acute urinary retention which could lead to overflow incontinence [47]. Immobility, the use of analgesics and opiates and increased intravenous fluid intake are all factors promoting urinary retention [47].

For this reason an indwelling urinary catheter is used perioperatively. The optimal management includes removal of the urinary catheter no more than 48 hours after surgery followed by intermittent catheterization that is repeated at regular intervals if necessary. After surgery, it is the cognitive state of the patient and not the fracture itself that is correlated with urinary retention; these cognitively impaired patients need extra attention to avoid bladder distention [48]. To avoid catheter-related urinary infections, the adapted protocol of Tenke et al [49] is recommended:

1. Catheters should be introduced under antiseptic conditions.

2. The catheter system should remain closed.
3. Unnecessary catheterizations should be avoided.
4. The duration of catheterization should be as short as possible.
5. The use of a nurse-based electronic catheter reminder system is recommended.
6. Educational programs targeting best practices for urinary catheter insertion and maintenance should be provided to all relevant staff.
7. The use of hydrophilic-coated catheters is recommended for clean intermittent catheterization.

See chapter 1.7 Postoperative medical management for further discussion on catheters and tethers.

## 7 Prevention and treatment of pressure ulcers

Pressure ulcers, also called sores, are a common problem in geriatric patients in hospitals, and the prevalence might be underestimated [50]. It is not only a burden during the hospital stay but many stage 3 and 4 pressure ulcers become chronic wounds, decreasing the quality of life [51]. Pressure ulcers might develop within several hours, but they may take years to heal. The presence of a pressure ulcer is the outcome of a multifactorial pathological condition. It is the cumulative effect of impairment due to immobility, nutritional deficiency, and chronic diseases which predisposes the aging skin to increased vulnerability [51].

Recommended actions to prevent pressure sores are:

- Prevention should start in the emergency department.
- Early use of pressure relief devices. Both dynamic support surfaces like alternating pressure mattresses, low-air loss beds, spacer mattresses, air fluidized mattresses and surface improvement like specialized foam or sheepskin have been proven to be better than a standard mattress to prevent pressure ulcers [52].
- Involvement of a multiprofessional team including nursing staff, aides, physician, dietician, occupational and physical therapist, and social worker.
- Early mobilization is the most important action to be taken while immobility is the most significant risk factor for development of pressure ulcers [53].
- The four most common external physical forces are axial pressure, shearing pressure, friction and excessive moisture [54]. Besides the treatment of the patient-related internal factors, paying attention to these external factors is extremely important.
- Frequent repositioning in bed, early mobilization, avoiding wet dressings or sheets are simple measures that can be taken by all healthcare providers.
- Patients should be encouraged to sit and walk shortly after surgery. When bed rest is unavoidable, the patient should be repositioned every 2 hours. Sliding should be prevented and the elevation of the head of the bed should be less than 30° [51].
- Daily inspection of areas at risk like sacrum, coccyx, ischium, or greater trochanter is mandatory.

Furthermore, the heels should be inspected daily and these areas should be staged, using the staging system developed by the National Pressure Ulcer Advisory Panel [55]:

| | |
|---|---|
| Stage 1 | Nonblanchable erythema: intact skin with nonblanchable redness |
| Stage 2 | Partial thickness: partial thickness, loss of dermis presenting as a shallow open ulcer with a red pink wound bed, without slough.<br>May also present as an intact or open/ruptured serum-filled or serosanguineous-filled blister |
| Stage 3 | Full thickness of skin or tissue loss: subcutaneous fat may be visible, but bone, tendon, or muscle are not exposed |
| Stage 4 | Full thickness tissue loss with exposed bone, tendon or muscle |

Stage 2 and deeper ulcers require an appropriate dressing that absorbs fluids but maintains moisture and encourages granulation tissue formation. Additives like silver ions, topical analgesics or activated charcoal to neutralize odor are available and can be used according to local practice. Treatment should be based on the stage of the pressure ulceration and may require surgical debridement (**Fig 1.8-5**).

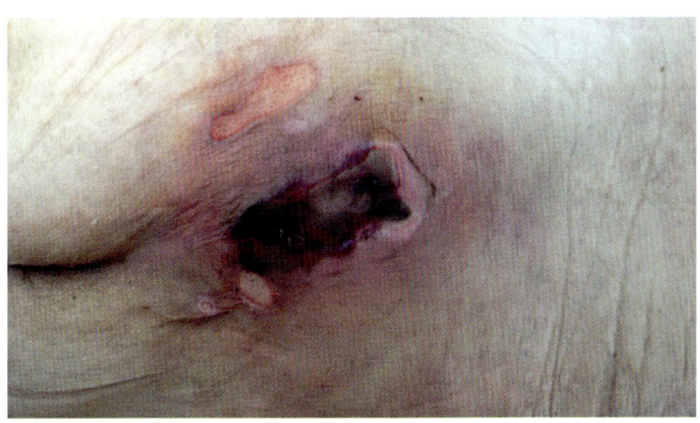

**Fig 1.8-5** Mostly stage 2 but centrally stage 3 pressure ulcer in a patient with a hip fracture and multiple comorbidities, which makes early mobilization difficult.

In case of a stage 3 or 4 pressure ulcer, debridement, starting with surgical debridement and followed by autolytic debridement, is a common technique. There is little evidence concerning best practice for cleansing of pressure ulcers [56]. The use of topical antibacterial creams does not appear to be beneficial [51]. Surgery for pressure ulcers (eg, excision of prominent/necrotic bone or flap surgery) is rarely performed in debilitated patients and will not be the solution when immobility still exists [51].

## 8 References


1. **Suetta C, Magnusson SP, Beyer N, et al.** Effect of strength training on muscle function in elderly hospitalized patients. *Scand J Med Sci Sports.* 2007 Oct;17(5):464–472.
2. **Bodine SC.** Disuse-induced muscle wasting. *Int J Biochem Cell Biol.* 2013 Oct;45(10):2200–2208.
3. **Wall BT, Dirks ML, van Loon LJ.** Skeletal muscle atrophy during short-term disuse: implications for age-related sarcopenia. *Ageing Res Rev.* 2013 Sep;12(4):898–906.
4. **Hvid L, Aagaard P, Justesen L, et al.** Effects of aging on muscle mechanical function and muscle fiber morphology during short-term immobilization and subsequent retraining. *J Appl Physiol (1985).* 2010 Dec;109(6):1628–1634.
5. **Suetta C, Hvid LG, Justesen L, et al.** Effects of aging on human skeletal muscle after immobilization and retraining. *J Appl Physiol (1985).* 2009 Oct;107(4):1172–1180.
6. **Suetta C, Frandsen U, Mackey AL, et al.** Ageing is associated with diminished muscle re-growth and myogenic precursor cell expansion early after immobility-induced atrophy in human skeletal muscle. *J Physiol.* 2013 Aug 01;591(15):3789–3804.
7. **Kortebein P, Symons TB, Ferrando A, et al.** Functional impact of 10 days of bed rest in healthy older adults. *J Gerontol A Biol Sci Med Sci.* 2008 Oct;63(10):1076–1081.
8. **Evans WJ.** Reversing sarcopenia: how weight training can build strength and vitality. *Geriatrics.* 1996 May;51(5):46–47, 51–43; quiz 54.
9. **Fiatarone MA, Marks EC, Ryan ND, et al.** High-intensity strength training in nonagenarians. Effects on skeletal muscle. *JAMA.* 1990 Jun 13;263(22):3029–3034.
10. **Dunstan DW, Vulikh E, Owen N, et al.** Community center-based resistance training for the maintenance of glycemic control in adults with type 2 diabetes. *Diabetes Care.* 2006 Dec;29(12):2586–2591.
11. **Kohler A, Kressig RW, Schindler C, et al.** Adhärenz-Raten bei Interventions-programmen zur Bewegungsförderung älterer Menschen: ein systematischer Literaturüberblick [Adherence rate in intervention programs for the promotion of physical activity in older adults: a systematic literature review]. *Praxis (Bern 1994).* 2012 Nov 28;101(24):1535–1547. German.
12. **Miller MD, Foley A, Gunn SM, et al.** Progression and adherence to an individually prescribed and supervised resistance training intervention in older adults recovering in hospital from lower limb fragility fracture. *Patient Prefer Adherence.* 2008 Feb 02;2:107–113.
13. **Verdijk LB, Snijders T, Beelen M, et al.** Characteristics of muscle fiber type are predictive of skeletal muscle mass and strength in elderly men. *J Am Geriatr Soc.* 2010 Nov;58(11):2069–2075.
14. **Schwachmeyer V, Damm P, Bender A, et al.** In vivo hip joint loading during post-operative physiotherapeutic exercises. *PLoS One.* 2013;8(10):e77807.
15. **Müller ME, Allgöwer M, Schneider R, et al.** *Manual der Osteosynthese-AO—Technik.* 2nd ed. Berlin Heidelberg: Springer-Verlag; 1977. German.
16. **Westerman RW, Hull P, Hendry RG, et al.** The physiological cost of restricted weight bearing. *Injury.* 2008 Jul;39(7):725–727.
17. **Koval KJ, Sala DA, Kummer FJ, et al.** Postoperative weight-bearing after a fracture of the femoral neck or an intertrochanteric fracture. *J Bone Joint Surg Am.* 1998 Mar;80(3):352–356.
18. **Kershaw CJ, Cunningham JL, Kenwright J.** Tibial external fixation, weight bearing, and fracture movement. *Clin Orthop Relat Res.* 1993 Aug(293):28–36.
19. **Joslin CC, Eastaugh-Waring SJ, Hardy JR, et al.** Weight bearing after tibial fracture as a guide to healing. *Clin Biomech (Bristol, Avon).* 2008 Mar;23(3):329–333.
20. **Gray FB, Gray C, McClanahan JW.** Assessing the accuracy of partial weight-bearing instruction. *Am J Orthop (Belle Mead NJ).* 1998 Aug;27(8):558–560.
21. **Kazemi N, Archdeacon MT.** Immediate full weightbearing after percutaneous fixation of anterior column acetabulum fractures. *J Orthop Trauma.* 2012 Feb;26(2):73–79.
22. **Segal D, Mallik AR, Wetzler MJ, et al.** Early weight bearing of lateral tibial plateau fractures. *Clin Orthop Relat Res.* 1993 Sep(294):232–237.
23. **Haak KT, Palm H, Holck K, et al.** Immediate weight-bearing after osteosynthesis of proximal tibial fractures may be allowed. *Dan Med J.* 2012 Oct;59(10):A4515.
24. **Solomon LB, Callary SA, Stevenson AW, et al.** Weight-bearing-induced displacement and migration over time of fracture fragments following split depression fractures of the lateral tibial plateau: a case series with radiostereometric analysis. *J Bone Joint Surg Br.* 2011 Jun;93(6):817–823.
25. **Smith TO, Sexton D, Mann C, et al.** Sutures versus staples for skin closure in orthopaedic surgery: meta-analysis. *BMJ.* 2010 Mar 16;340:c1199.
26. **Hemming K, Pinkney T, Futaba K, et al.** A systematic review of systematic reviews and panoramic meta-analysis: staples versus sutures for surgical procedures. *PLoS One.* 2013;8(10):e75132.
27. **Koval KJ, Egol KA, Polatsch DB, et al.** Tape blisters following hip surgery. A prospective, randomized study of two types of tape. *J Bone Joint Surg Am.* 2003 Oct;85-a(10):1884–1887.
28. **Polatsch DB, Baskies MA, Hommen JP, et al.** Tape blisters that develop after hip fracture surgery: a retrospective series and a review of the literature. *Am J Orthop (Belle Mead NJ).* 2004 Sep;33(9):452–456.
29. **Koval KJ, Egol KA, Hiebert R, et al.** Tape blisters after hip surgery: can they be eliminated completely? *Am J Orthop (Belle Mead NJ).* 2007 May;36(5):261–265.

30. **Pierannunzii L, Fossali A, De Lucia O, et al.** Suture-related pseudoinfection after total hip arthroplasty. *J Orthop Traumatol.* 2015 Mar;16(1):59–65.
31. **Willett KM, Simmons CD, Bentley G.** The effect of suction drains after total hip replacement. *J Bone Joint Surg Br.* 1988 Aug;70(4):607–610.
32. **Varley GW, Milner SA.** Wound drains in proximal femoral fracture surgery: a randomized prospective trial of 177 patients. *J R Coll Surg Edinb.* 1995 Dec;40(6):416–418.
33. **Tjeenk RM, Peeters MP, van den Ende E, et al.** Wound drainage versus non-drainage for proximal femoral fractures. A prospective randomised study. *Injury.* 2005 Jan;36(1):100–104.
34. **Akinyoola AL, Odunsi A, Yusu MB.** Use of wound drains following open reduction and internal fixation of femoral shaft fractures. *J Wound Care.* 2012 Jun;21(6):279–280, 282–284.
35. **Parker MJ, Livingstone V, Clifton R, et al.** Closed suction surgical wound drainage after orthopaedic surgery. *Cochrane Database Syst Rev.* 2007 Jul 18(3):CD001825.
36. **Brotman DJ, Jaffer AK.** Prevention of venous thromboembolism in the geriatric patient. *Cardiol Clin.* 2008 May;26(2):221–234, vi.
37. **Robert-Ebadi H, Le Gal G, Righini M.** Use of anticoagulants in elderly patients: practical recommendations. *Clin Interv Aging.* 2009;4:165–177.
38. **Sardar P, Chatterjee S, Chaudhari S, et al.** New oral anticoagulants in elderly adults: evidence from a meta-analysis of randomized trials. *J Am Geriatr Soc.* 2014 May;62(5):857–864.
39. **Stein PD, Hull RD, Kayali F, et al.** Venous thromboembolism according to age: the impact of an aging population. *Arch Intern Med.* 2004 Nov 08;164(20):2260–2265.
40. **Geerts WH, Bergqvist D, Pineo GF, et al.** Prevention of venous thromboembolism: American College of Chest Physicians Evidence-Based Clinical Practice Guidelines (8th Edition). *Chest.* 2008 Jun;133(6 Suppl):381S–453S.
41. **Amaragiri SV, Lees TA.** Elastic compression stockings for prevention of deep vein thrombosis. *Cochrane Database Syst Rev.* 2000 (3):CD001484.
42. **Kahn SR, Shapiro S, Wells PS, et al.** Compression stockings to prevent post-thrombotic syndrome: a randomised placebo-controlled trial. *Lancet.* 2014 Mar 08;383(9920):880–888.
43. **Guzelkucuk U, Skempes D, Kumnerddee W.** Common peroneal nerve palsy caused by compression stockings after surgery. *Am J Phys Med Rehabil.* 2014 Jul;93(7):609–611.
44. **AOTrauma Orthogeriatrics App (Orthogers).** Version 2.0. Dübendorf: AO or AO Technology AG; 2015 [Mobile application software].
45. **Bounameaux H, Perneger T.** Fondaparinux: a new synthetic pentasaccharide for thrombosis prevention. *Lancet.* 2002 May 18;359(9319):1710–1711.
46. **Garcia DA, Baglin TP, Weitz JI, et al.** Parenteral anticoagulants: Antithrombotic Therapy and Prevention of Thrombosis, 9th ed: American College of Chest Physicians Evidence-Based Clinical Practice Guidelines. *Chest.* 2012 Feb;141(2 Suppl):e24S–e43S.
47. **Lamont CT, Sampson S, Matthias R, et al.** The outcome of hospitalization for acute illness in the elderly. *J Am Geriatr Soc.* 1983 May;31(5):282–288.
48. **Tobu S, Noguchi M, Hashikawa T, et al.** Risk factors of postoperative urinary retention after hip surgery for femoral neck fracture in elderly women. *Geriatr Gerontol Int.* 2014 Jul;14(3):636–639.
49. **Tenke P, Koves B, Johansen TE.** An update on prevention and treatment of catheter-associated urinary tract infections. *Curr Opin Infect Dis.* 2014 Feb;27(1):102–107.
50. **Lahmann N, Dassen T, Kottner J.** Die Häufigkeit von Dekubitus in deutschen Krankenhäusern [Frequency of pressure ulcers in German hospitals]. *Gesundheitswesen.* 2012 Dec;74(12):793–797. German.
51. **Jaul E.** Assessment and management of pressure ulcers in the elderly: current strategies. *Drugs Aging.* 2010 Apr 01;27(4):311–325.
52. **Hofman A, Geelkerken RH, Wille J, et al.** Pressure sores and pressure-decreasing mattresses: controlled clinical trial. *Lancet.* 1994 Mar 05;343(8897):568–571.
53. **Lindgren M, Unosson M, Fredrikson M, et al.** Immobility—a major risk factor for development of pressure ulcers among adult hospitalized patients: a prospective study. *Scand J Caring Sci.* 2004 Mar;18(1):57–64.
54. **Grey JE, Harding KG, Enoch S.** Pressure ulcers. *BMJ.* 2006 Feb 25;332(7539):472–475.
55. **National Pressure Ulcer Advisory Panel.** NPUAP Pressure Injury Stages. Available at: www.npuap.org/resources/educational-and-clinical-resources/npuap-pressure-injury-stages/ between the 4 stages and the picture. Accessed March 2017.
56. **Moore ZE, Cowman S.** Wound cleansing for pressure ulcers. *Cochrane Database Syst Rev.* 2013 Mar 28(3):CD004983.

# 1.9 Postacute care

Bernardo Reyes, Nemer Dabage, Darby Sider

## 1 Introduction

For most hip fracture patients, the goal of postacute rehabilitation is the restoration of preinjury function and, when possible, functional independence. Postacute care includes not only physical rehabilitation but patient-specific multidisciplinary treatment of medical, social, nutritional and psychological contributors to disability, and typically produces significant benefits for most patients [1, 2]. Evidence on the comparative effectiveness of specific postacute rehabilitation settings is limited, but most successful programs involve more intensive exercise and multidisciplinary care than is available in many acute care hospital and outpatient settings. While rehabilitation following hip and other fragility fractures begins in the perioperative period, it is predominantly delivered in postacute care settings like skilled nursing facilities (SNFs), inpatient rehabilitation facilities (IRFs), rehabilitation with home health services, and outpatient settings [3, 4].

## 2 Postacute care settings

Depending on the structure and financing of the local healthcare system, postfracture rehabilitation can occur in the same acute care facility where the fracture was treated, in distinct postacute care facilities, or at home. Most studies have demonstrated that the outcomes after rehabilitation are similar regardless of the care setting.

Decisions regarding the setting where postacute care will be delivered often depend on factors including the patient's ability to participate in physical rehabilitation activities, insurance coverage and regulations, and local resources. Irrespective of these issues, a patient-specific rehabilitation plan is the best tool to promote optimal recovery, with a focus on high frequency rehabilitation; attendance of more than five physical therapy and occupational therapy sessions per week has been associated with better health outcomes [2].

### 2.1 Facility-based rehabilitation

Facility-based rehabilitation is common, effective and typically resource intensive. Most healthcare systems attempt to balance costs and benefits, so it is essential to assess the functional ability of the patient to determine if clinically appropriate care can be delivered in a lower intensity setting. The most common facility settings for rehabilitation are described below:

- When patients receive rehabilitation in inpatient geriatric wards, ie, in the same facility where the acute care was provided, placement in a geriatric care-based unit for the entire hospitalization appears to be superior to a 2-step model of postoperative transfer from an orthopedic surgical ward to a geriatric rehabilitation ward. This ward model can be more expensive but minimizes the risk of institutional transitions of care [5, 6]. Inpatient ward based rehabilitation is more common in European healthcare systems.
- Inpatient rehabilitation facilities can be located within a hospital or exist as standalone facilities. Patients that are managed in these facilities can typically tolerate intensive rehabilitation, ie, more than 3 hours per day, while still receiving access to comprehensive nursing care. These settings are appropriate if the intensity, frequency, and duration of therapeutic activities make it impractical to obtain the services in a less intensive setting. While younger and more robust patients may get superior outcomes from IRF-based rehabilitation, many fragility fracture patients (FFPs) cannot tolerate this intensity of services.
- A skilled nursing facility or postacute care setting is a setting of care where staff manages, observes and evaluates care including routine medication administration, postsurgical care, and rehabilitation. This is the most common FFP rehabilitation setting in North American healthcare systems, with multidisciplinary staff including nurses, physical and occupational therapists, social service workers, nutritionists and recreational therapists. Medical providers are not onsite at all times, and acute onsite medical evaluation is not always possible.

As suggested above, patients admitted to geriatric wards and IRFs should be generally able to participate in, and be likely to benefit from, at least 3 hours of rehabilitation activities per day, five times per week. In many of these settings a physician specialized in rehabilitation sees the patient at least three times per week.

Patients admitted to IRFs usually have shorter lengths of stay than those admitted to SNFs. In addition, IRF patients typically receive more physical and occupational therapy than patients admitted to SNFs. Some reports suggest that this comes at a higher cost without a significant change in functional outcomes [2, 7].

Patients can be transitioned to a less resource-intensive level of care from IRFs when all functional rehabilitation goals have been achieved or when therapy services are no longer required to meet rehabilitation goals. Patients should also be considered for transfer if further progress toward rehabilitation goals is not expected or can be achieved at a less resource-intensive level of care [8].

Most organized healthcare systems offer a predetermined number of covered rehabilitation days per eligibility period for patients to use when needed. Hip fracture patients admitted to SNFs can typically receive rehabilitation services at least five times per week. As the literature suggests, hip fracture patients admitted to SNFs have similar levels of recovery as those admitted to inpatient rehabilitation hospitals and at a lower cost.

The main difference between an acute rehabilitation hospital and an SNF is the level of staffing, the frequency of physician evaluation, and the intensity of the rehabilitation services. In the US, most insurers authorize payment for rehabilitation of FFPs in SNFs due to their lower operational cost.

### 2.2 Home and outpatient-based rehabilitation programs

Among patients who have completed standard rehabilitation after hip fracture, the use of a home-based functionally focused exercise program can provide some added improvement to mobility. Using home-based services as the only mode of rehabilitation after a hip fracture should be reserved for those with very high functional status in the immediate postfracture period or those that have a support system that allows them to receive adequate services in this setting [9, 10].

## 3 Postacute care assessments and evaluations

The primary assessment method during the postacute care phase is called the comprehensive geriatric assessment (CGA). The CGA is a structured survey and evaluation process commonly used to assess for medical, functional and socio-psychological issues that impact health and function. The components of the CGA vary depending on the specific setting and clinician preference, but typically cover the major areas above, as well as patient-specific goals of care and advance directives. The CGA requires time to complete and its results can be temporarily altered by acute illness. During the acute hospitalization, the results of the CGA can be influenced by many factors including pain, medications, and electrolyte abnormalities. Despite all this, using the CGA in these settings has been associated with improved outcomes [11].

During postacute recovery many of the complicating acute medical circumstances have resolved, allowing for a more appropriate assessment of patient factors to plan for optimal rehabilitation and restoration of health. Moreover, as the length of stay is longer in this setting, there is a greater ability to make and evaluate changes in long-term medications, promote recovery of lost function, and improve social factors.

This CGA can help identify medical, functional, environmental, and social contributors to the original injury, and it can identify issues that might affect the ability of the patient to thrive in their home setting. Environmental and other nonmedical issues like lack of bathroom bars and rails, inappropriate height of a bed, environmental clutter, limited access to groceries, and inappropriately complex drug regimens can negatively impact outcomes as much as any specific medical condition. In addition, the CGA helps identify social issues, including inadequate support systems to assist with activities of daily living (ADLs), or respond to an acute illness [12].

### 3.1 Multidisciplinary rehabilitation team

Once a comprehensive evaluation of the patient's needs has been completed, an individualized plan of care should be designed for each patient with the input of a multidisciplinary team. Team members often include physical and occupational therapists, medical providers, nurses, nutritionists and social workers. As mobility is the best overall predictor of a successful outcome, physical therapists play a central role in the rehabilitation process. Occupational therapists assist in specific ADL achievement, overall functioning, and reducing fall risk. If cognitive impairment is affecting communication or swallowing, a speech therapist can be helpful. The optimal degree of direct involvement of certified therapists has yet to be determined. When local resources permit, physicians with experience in geriatrics and rehabilitation typically manage the ongoing medical comorbidities and rehabilitation program.

Nursing care typically focuses on symptom assessment, pain control, managing medications and preventing pressure ulcers. Nurses involved in the care of FFPs should be familiar with common geriatric syndromes (eg, delirium, dementia, falls, and incontinence).

Nutritional enhancement in those who are malnourished or undernourished can improve outcomes [13]. Nutritionists are best suited to evaluate and recommend dietary regimens.

Social workers play an essential role in assisting with social or financial issues affecting long-term care needs. Moreover, the spouse, family, or caregivers play a significant role in providing psychological support and motivation to the patient. The medical and orthopedic providers are responsible for supervising the medical plan of care, monitoring clinical progress, and striving to avoid medical complications [14].

## 4 Disposition after postacute care

Most hip fracture patients experience some degree of disability even after postacute rehabilitation. Many studies indicate that a significant number of patients are still in need of further assistance with ADLs following their completion of a formal rehabilitation program. These needs, along with the patient's existing support system, determine the disposition of a patient after a postacute admission [15]. Even for those who do not require assistive devices for ambulation at the time of postacute discharge, there is often persistent need for assistance with some ADLs like putting on socks and shoes. Up to 25% of hip fracture patients will require long-term care placement in a nursing facility or transition to hospice after postacute rehabilitation. For the remaining 75%, key functional items including cognition, balance and gait may take up to 1 year to fully recover, and the degree of assistance with ADLs will determine the extent of home-based services they require [16].

In some parts of Europe, the first phase of the rehabilitation process occurs in acute care facilities. The implementation of a geriatric multiprofessional home rehabilitation program focused on supported discharge and independence in daily activities results in an improvement in balance confidence, independence and physical activity in previously community-dwelling older adults [17, 18].

In the US, where most of the rehabilitation occurs in postacute facilities, a basic array of follow-up home services is arranged. Such services include home physical therapy, home nursing for ongoing medical monitoring and wound care, and home aides to assist with specific ADLs. When in need, a social worker can assist with social issues such as transportation, assistance with meals, and advanced care planning.

## 5 Communication, transitions, and quality of care

Frail geriatric patients experience several potentially dangerous transitions of care between their home, the hospital and rehabilitation settings. Coordinating continuity of care and effective handoffs across these transitions is critical in order to optimize patient outcomes.

Handoffs should be structured and standardized to include all essential medical, functional and social information necessary for the next care setting. Accurate information about the patient's medical conditions and comorbidities, vision, hearing, language, and their prefracture functional status and limitations determine the approaches that the rehabilitation team will take [19].

Significant and valuable information that helps in clinical decision making includes the mechanism of injury, type of surgical intervention, functional restrictions, and the recommended weight-bearing status. It is important to provide essential information in a structured written and verbal format during care handoff [20]. The ability for the rehabilitation team to access the acute electronic healthcare record improves the efficiency greatly [21].

Including families in the handoff and plan of care, and face-to-face or verbal "warm hand-off communication" is anecdotally more successful. Providing a written plan of care to the family members may yield better outcomes as well as higher satisfaction for patients and family members.

More recently healthcare systems have invested in developing clinical care pathways that protocol acute and postacute needs and account for common barriers to recovery including pain, delirium, and cardiorespiratory status. Older adults have less predictable responses to standard therapy, and the care team needs to individualize treatment plans according to each patient's prognosis, goals of care and particular vulnerabilities [22].

## 6 Common clinical issues in the rehabilitation setting

Given the high morbidity and mortality associated with hip fractures, there should be intense focus on limiting postoperative complications, preventing readmissions, future falls and fractures, and regaining prefracture level of physical and cognitive functioning [23].

The best predictor of overall achievement in walking ability after early surgical repair is how quickly rehabilitation is initiated postoperatively. Weight bearing within hours after surgery is a positive prognostic indicator of future outcome for walking ability. Negative predictors in regaining mobility include low preinjury functional ability, cognitive deficit, postoperative delirium, age, male gender, and the presence of pressure ulcers [24, 25].

### 6.1 Delirium

Acute confusion or delirium is seen in 30% of hospitalized older patients. Delirium symptoms may last for weeks or months in some patients and can interfere with the ability to maximally participate in rehabilitation [26]. The prevalence of delirium in older patients is approximately 23% in postacute care facilities. Half of the patients that develop delirium during postacute care remain delirious a week later, and only 14% have complete resolution of symptoms. Patients with worsened delirium have more difficulty with their ADLs. Since delirium can persist in some instances up to 6 months, and there is variability in how patients recover, delirium does not mean that patients need to be hospitalized; the management is best individualized [26]. See chapter 1.14 Delirium for more details on the diagnosis and management of delirium.

### 6.2 Postoperative pain

Poorly controlled postoperative hip pain can affect functional outcomes significantly. Patients with uncontrolled pain in the postacute setting are less likely to participate in physical therapy and ambulate. Good pain control reduces the risk of delirium as well [27]. The level of pain can be affected by the type of fracture and surgical repair [28]. Bimodal pain regimens that include scheduled doses of acetaminophen and doses of opioids as needed have been used in several settings with acceptable results [29]. See chapter 1.12 Pain management for more on pain management.

### 6.3 Hypotension

Orthostatic hypotension often reflects degenerative impairments of the neuro-cardiovascular reflexes and can result in significant transient periods of hypotension. Hypotension is an important predictor of adverse outcomes in hip fracture patients and can be poorly recognized by patients and caregivers, as vital signs are often checked in the supine position. Orthostasis increases risk of falls and refracture and can also contribute to delirium among selected subpopulations. In the postacute setting, patients with dementia and a recent fall are more likely to suffer orthostatic hypotension [30].

In the immediate postoperative period, blood pressure is often attenuated by new anemia and opioids, and most patients will not require their prefracture antihypertensive medications. In the postacute setting blood pressure goals should be revised depending on age and function. Current evidence [30] favors a systolic blood pressure < 150 mm Hg among those who are 80 years or older and evaluation for orthostasis before and after administration of medications. If necessary, home blood pressure medications can be resumed at lower doses and slowly titrated to standing blood pressure targets.

### 6.4 Constipation

Constipation is frequently unrecognized by patients and caregivers alike and can contribute to anorexia, urinary retention, hospital readmission and poor outcomes. For those patients that report constipation in the first postoperative day, more than half will report the same problem 30 days later [31]. Many common medications, such as opioids, calcium supplements, and some antihypertensives, can contribute to constipation [32, 33]. Bowel regimens should be started in acute settings and continued during the postacute phase. For most patients a scheduled laxative should be part of the bowel regimen [34]. Moreover, the use of simple strategies such as stool charts for all patients and local dissemination of audits usually result in a significant reduction of constipation in the postacute setting [35].

### 6.5 Malnutrition

In the US, malnutrition occurs in approximately 20% of hospitalized older patients and in almost 40% of nursing home residents [36]. Malnutrition is associated with an impaired functional status and higher morbidity and mortality. In FFPs, proper nutrition is essential for recovery [37]. In the malnourished patient with dementia, smaller and more frequent meals sometimes result in better calorie intake [38].

Nutritional interventions with fortified food do not provide a significant benefit on nutritional and functional status in nursing home residents at risk of malnutrition, as standard nursing home food usually provides sufficient energy intake. Nonetheless, such interventions might result in fewer days with delirium and decreased risk of pressure ulcers [39, 40].

## 6.6 Depression

Depression has a significantly negative impact on rehabilitation during and after a postacute admission and is associated with worse adverse outcomes at 1 year [41].

Regarding the effectiveness of treatment, the involvement of a specialist such as a psychiatrist or a psychologist has not been shown to clearly improve outcomes of hip fracture patients suffering from depression [42].

Although oral antidepressants appear to be effective in the treatment of depression in community-dwelling older adults, their effect seems to be limited to SNF residents with advanced dementia [30]. Moreover, there is an increased risk of falls and fractures among geriatric patients using these medications [43]. Note that such increased risk appears to be dose-dependent, suggesting that pharmacological treatment of depression should be initiated with the lowest effective dose in patients that are most likely to benefit [44].

## 7 References


1. **Kramer AM, Steiner JF, Schlenker RE, et al.** Outcomes and costs after hip fracture and stroke. A comparison of rehabilitation settings. *JAMA.* 1997 Feb 5;277(5):396–404.
2. **Hoenig H, Rubenstein LV, Sloane R, et al.** What is the role of timing in the surgical and rehabilitative care of community-dwelling older persons with acute hip fracture? *Arch Intern Med.* 1997 Mar 10;157(5):513–520.
3. **Handoll HH, Sherrington C, Mak JC.** Interventions for improving mobility after hip fracture surgery in adults. *Cochrane Database Syst Rev.* 2011 Mar 16(3):CD001704.
4. **Handoll HH, Cameron ID, Mak JC, et al.** Multidisciplinary rehabilitation for older people with hip fractures. *Cochrane Database Syst Rev.* 2009 Oct 07(4):CD007125.
5. **Adunsky A, Lusky A, Arad M, et al.** A comparative study of rehabilitation outcomes of elderly hip fracture patients: the advantage of a comprehensive orthogeriatric approach. *J Gerontol A Biol Sci Med Sci.* 2003 Jun;58(6):542–547.
6. **Huusko TM, Karppi P, Avikainen V, et al.** Intensive geriatric rehabilitation of hip fracture patients: a randomized, controlled trial. *Acta Orthop Scand.* 2002 Aug;73(4):425–431.
7. **Dobson A, DaVanzo JE, El-Gamil A, et al.** Clinically Appropriate and Cost-Effective Placement (CACEP): Improving Health Care Quality and Efficiency. Final Report, 2012. Available at: http://ahhqi.org/images/pdf/cacep-report.pdf. Accessed 2015.
8. **Premera Blue Cross.** Criteria for Acute Inpatient Rehabilitation Care: Guideline for Admission and Transition of Care. Available at: https://www.premera.com/medicalpolicies/11.01.522.pdf. Accessed December 21, 2017.
9. **Latham NK, Harris BA, Bean JF, et al.** Effect of a home-based exercise program on functional recovery following rehabilitation after hip fracture: a randomized clinical trial. *JAMA.* 2014 Feb 19;311(7):700–708.
10. **Yu-Yahiro JA, Resnick B, Orwig D, et al.** Design and implementation of a home-based exercise program post-hip fracture: the Baltimore hip studies experience. *PM R.* 2009 Apr;1(4):308–318.
11. **Sletvold O, Helbostad JL, Thingstad P, et al.** Effect of in-hospital comprehensive geriatric assessment (CGA) in older people with hip fracture. The protocol of the Trondheim Hip Fracture trial. *BMC Geriatr.* 2011 Apr 21;11:18.
12. **Caplan GA, Williams AJ, Daly B, et al.** A randomized, controlled trial of comprehensive geriatric assessment and multidisciplinary intervention after discharge of elderly from the emergency department—the DEED II study. *J Am Geriatr Soc.* 2004 Sep;52(9):1417–1423.
13. **Gunnarsson AK, Lonn K, Gunningberg L.** Does nutritional intervention for patients with hip fractures reduce postoperative complications and improve rehabilitation? *J Clin Nurs.* 2009 May;18(9):1325–1333.
14. **NHS Choices.** Hip Fracture—Recovery. Recovering from a hip fracture. Available at: http://www.nhs.uk/Conditions/hip-fracture/Pages/recovery.aspx. Updated July 18, 2014. Accessed March 15, 2015.
15. **Magaziner J, Hawkes W, Hebel JR, et al.** Recovery from hip fracture in eight areas of function. *J Gerontol A Biol Sci Med Sci.* 2000 Sep;55(9):M498–M507.
16. **Ceder L, Thorngren KG, Wallden B.** Prognostic indicators and early home rehabilitation in elderly patients with hip fractures. *Clin Orthop Relat Res.* 1980 Oct(152):173–184.
17. **Ziden L, Frandin K, Kreuter M.** Home rehabilitation after hip fracture. A randomized controlled study on balance confidence, physical function and everyday activities. *Clin Rehabil.* 2008 Dec;22(12):1019–1033.
18. **Ziden L, Kreuter M, Frandin K.** Long-term effects of home rehabilitation after hip fracture—1-year follow-up of functioning, balance confidence, and health-related quality of life in elderly people. *Disabil Rehabil.* 2010;32(1):18–32.
19. **Packel L, Sood M, Gormley M, et al.** A pilot study exploring the role of physical therapists and transition in care of pediatric patients with cystic fibrosis to the adult setting. *Cardiopulm Phys Ther J.* 2013 Mar;24(1):24–30.
20. **Marks R.** Hip fracture epidemiological trends, outcomes, and risk factors, 1970-2009. *Int J Gen Med.* 2010 Apr 08;3:1–17.

21. **Bukata SV, Digiovanni BF, Friedman SM, et al.** A guide to improving the care of patients with fragility fractures. *Geriatr Orthop Surg Rehabil.* 2011 Jan;2(1):5–37.
22. **Lau TW, Fang C, Leung F.** The effectiveness of a geriatric hip fracture clinical pathway in reducing hospital and rehabilitation length of stay and improving short-term mortality rates. *Geriatr Orthop Surg Rehabil.* 2013 Mar;4(1):3–9.
23. **Marks R.** Physical activity and hip fracture disability: a review. *J Aging Res.* 2011 Apr 26;2011:741918.
24. **Duke RG, Keating JL.** An investigation of factors predictive of independence in transfers and ambulation after hip fracture. *Arch Phys Med Rehabil.* 2002 Feb;83(2):158–164.
25. **Vergara I, Vrotsou K, Orive M, et al.** Factors related to functional prognosis in elderly patients after accidental hip fractures: a prospective cohort study. *BMC Geriatr.* 2014 Nov 26;14:124.
26. **Lee HB, Mears SC, Rosenberg PB, et al.** Predisposing factors for postoperative delirium after hip fracture repair in individuals with and without dementia. *J Am Geriatr Soc.* 2011 Dec;59(12):2306–2313.
27. **Morrison RS, Magaziner J, McLaughlin MA, et al.** The impact of post-operative pain on outcomes following hip fracture. *Pain.* 2003 Jun;103(3):303–311.
28. **Singelyn FJ, Deyaert M, Joris D, et al.** Effects of intravenous patient-controlled analgesia with morphine, continuous epidural analgesia, and continuous three-in-one block on postoperative pain and knee rehabilitation after unilateral total knee arthroplasty. *Anesth Analg.* 1998 Jul;87(1):88–92.
29. **Aubrun F, Marmion F.** The elderly patient and postoperative pain treatment. *Best Pract Res Clin Anaesthesiol.* 2007 Mar;21(1):109–127.
30. **Messinger-Rapport BJ, Gammack JK, Thomas DR, et al.** Clinical update on nursing home medicine: 2013. *J Am Med Dir Assoc.* 2013 Dec;14(12):860–876.
31. **Trads M, Pedersen PU.** Constipation and defecation pattern the first 30 days after hip fracture. *Int J Nurs Pract.* 2015 Oct;21(5):598–604.
32. **Callard G, Schlinger B, Pasmanik M.** Nonmammalian vertebrate models in studies of brain-steroid interactions. *J Exp Zool Suppl.* 1990;4:6–16.
33. **Prince RL, Devine A, Dhaliwal SS, et al.** Effects of calcium supplementation on clinical fracture and bone structure: results of a 5-year, double-blind, placebo-controlled trial in elderly women. *Arch Intern Med.* 2006 Apr 24;166(8):869–875.
34. **Pappagallo M.** Incidence, prevalence, and management of opioid bowel dysfunction. *Am J Surg.* 2001 Nov;182(5A Suppl):11S–18S.
35. **Neighbour C, Weerasuriya N, McCulloch R.** Evaluating the Effect of Orthogeriatric Intervention on Bowel Care and Analgesia Following Hip Fracture. *Age Ageing.* 2014 Jun 1;43(suppl 1):i2.
36. **Guigoz Y, Lauque S, Vellas BJ.** Identifying the elderly at risk for malnutrition. The Mini Nutritional Assessment. *Clin Geriatr Med.* 2002 Nov;18(4):737–757.
37. **Bukata SV, Digiovanni BF, Friedman SM, et al.** A guide to improving the care of patients with fragility fractures. *Geriatr Orthop Surg Rehabil.* 2011 Jan;2(1):5–37.
38. **Alzheimer's Society.** Eating and drinking. Available at: http://www.alzheimers.org.uk/site/scripts/documents_info.php?documentID=149. Updated July 18, 2014. Accessed March 15, 2015.
39. **Smoliner C, Norman K, Scheufele R, et al.** Effects of food fortification on nutritional and functional status in frail elderly nursing home residents at risk of malnutrition. *Nutrition.* 2008 Nov–Dec;24(11–12):1139–1144.
40. **Olofsson B, Stenvall M, Lundstrom M, et al.** Malnutrition in hip fracture patients: an intervention study. *J Clin Nurs.* 2007 Nov;16(11):2027–2038.
41. **Morghen S, Bellelli G, Manuele S, et al.** Moderate to severe depressive symptoms and rehabilitation outcome in older adults with hip fracture. *Int J Geriatr Psychiatry.* 2011 Nov;26(11):1136–1143.
42. **Burns A, Banerjee S, Morris J, et al.** Treatment and prevention of depression after surgery for hip fracture in older people: randomized, controlled trials. *J Am Geriatr Soc.* 2007 Jan;55(1):75–80.
43. **Iaboni A, Seitz DP, Fischer HD, et al.** Initiation of Antidepressant Medication After Hip Fracture in Community-Dwelling Older Adults. *Am J Geriatr Psychiatry.* 2015 Oct;23(10):1007–1015.
44. **Bakken MS, Engeland A, Engesaeter LB, et al.** Increased risk of hip fracture among older people using antidepressant drugs: data from the Norwegian Prescription Database and the Norwegian Hip Fracture Registry. *Age Ageing.* 2013 Jul;42(4):514–520.

# 1.10 Osteoporosis

Rashmi Khadilkar, Krupa Shah

## 1 Introduction

Osteoporosis is the most common bone disease of older adults and is a major public health problem worldwide. Osteoporosis is characterized by low bone mass, deterioration of bone microstructure, and compromised bone strength resulting in an increased risk of fracture. Typically, patients with osteoporosis experience no symptoms until they sustain a fracture, making diagnosis and primary fracture prevention challenging.

## 2 Epidemiology and economic impact

The World Health Organization (WHO) defines osteoporosis as a bone mineral density (BMD) at the spine or hip of ≤ 2.5 standard deviations (SDs) below the mean BMD of a young woman, as measured by dual-energy x-ray absorptiometry (DEXA) (**Table 1.10-1**). A BMD between 2.5 and 1 SDs below the mean represents osteopenia.

A T-score of -1.0 represents a BMD 1 SD below the mean BMD for a young adult reference population.

The presence of a fragility fracture is diagnostic of osteoporosis even in the absence of a measurable decrease in BMD.

In the US, 10.2 million adults over 50 years of age are estimated to have osteoporosis and 43.4 million to have osteopenia [1]. These numbers will rise in the coming decades as the population ages, with 14 million older adults projected to have osteoporosis and 47 million to have osteopenia by 2020 [2].

The presence of osteoporosis or osteopenia increases the risk of fragility fractures which are defined as fractures secondary to a fall from standing or lower height and at a site associated with decreased BMD, including the hip, spine, and wrist. Such fractures increase in incidence after the age of 50 years [3].

There is a strong correlation between BMD and fragility fracture risk. In a 1993 study, each decrease of 1 SD in bone density at the femoral neck increased the risk of hip fracture by a factor of 2.5, and women in the lowest quartile of BMD had an 8.5-fold greater risk of hip fracture compared to women in the highest quartile [4]. However, more fragility fractures occur in patients with osteopenia than in those with osteoporosis because of the greater prevalence of osteopenia.

At the age of 50 years, the lifetime risk of sustaining any fragility fracture is estimated at 40% for women and 13% for men in the US; 46% and 22%, respectively, in Sweden, and 42% overall in Australia [3]. The risk of hip fracture for a 50-year-old Caucasian American woman is 17% [5]; the corresponding risk is 23% in Sweden and 17% in Australia [3].

This risk increases with aging. For each decade after age 50, the risk of hip fracture doubles, and a 90-year-old woman has approximately a 30% chance of sustaining a hip fracture in her remaining lifetime [6]. As the population ages, the worldwide incidence of hip fracture is projected to increase from 1.7 million in 1990 to 6.3 million in 2050 [7], with the largest increase expected in Asia and Latin America. Currently, age- and gender-adjusted 10-year rates of hip fracture are highest in Scandinavia [8]. The shifting demographics of aging will decrease the worldwide proportion of hip fractures that occur in North America and Europe from 50% in 2005 to 25% by 2050 [3].

| Diagnosis | Criteria |
|---|---|
| Normal | T-score at the spine of hip of -1.0 and above |
| Osteopenia (low bone mass) | T-score between -1.0 and -2.5 |
| Osteoporosis | T-score -2.5 and below |
| Severe osteoporosis | T-score -2.5 and below with one of more fractures |

**Table 1.10-1** World Health Organization's definitions of osteoporosis based on dual-energy x-ray absorptiometry criteria.

Hip fractures comprise only about 14% of fragility fractures, and vertebral and wrist fractures also have significant sequelae. At age 50, a Caucasian American woman has a 32% risk of sustaining a clinical or radiographic vertebral fracture and a 15% chance of sustaining a wrist fracture during her lifetime. A Swedish woman's risk is 15% and 21%, respectively; an Australian woman's risk is 10% and 13%, respectively [3]. As with hip fractures, the incidence of vertebral and wrist fractures increase with age.

Fragility fractures result in significant healthcare expenditures. In the US, osteoporosis contributes to 2 million fractures per year, resulting in about 430,000 hospital admissions, 2.5 million office visits, and 180,000 nursing home admissions and incurring costs of USD 18 billion per year. Despite comprising a minority of fragility fractures, hip fractures make up 72% of fracture cost; in 2002, a single hip fracture was estimated to cost USD 34,000–43,000 according to 2005 US governmental data [9]. By 2025, the annual cost of fracture care in the US is projected to be USD 25.3 billion [9]. Worldwide, the cost of hip fractures alone is estimated to rise to USD 131.5 billion by 2050 [10].

## 3 Clinical impact

Osteoporosis and fragility fractures carry significant morbidity and mortality:

- At 1 year more than 50% of patients with hip fractures continue to have significant functional limitations, with more than half of previously independent patients unable to walk one block, climb five stairs, get in and out of the shower, sit on the toilet, or rise from an armless seated position unassisted [11].
- About 30% of hip fracture sufferers require long-term nursing home care [12], and only 40% fully regain their prior level of functioning [2].
- Vertebral fractures can cause chronic pain; difficulty bending and reaching overhead; kyphosis and subsequent decreases in pulmonary function; and alterations in abdominal anatomy with resulting constipation, early satiety, and decreased oral intake.
- All fractures increase the risk of depression and cognitive impairment.
- A patient who sustains any type of fragility fracture is 50–100% more likely to sustain another, and fracture patients often develop a fear of falling, which in itself increases fracture risk.
- Fractures are also associated with increased mortality.
- Hip fracture surgery carries an overall mortality of 4%. Twenty percent of hip fracture patients die within 1 year of the fracture event; hip fractures confer a five- to eightfold increase in all-cause mortality in the first 3 months following the event, and this risk is higher for men. Vertebral fractures have been shown to have similar mortality to hip fractures [5]. This mortality risk is likely both a cause and a consequence of the fragility fracture. Functionally failing patients are likely to have fragility fracture as part of their terminal decline.

## 4 Practical considerations for the perioperative period

### 4.1 Diagnostic testing

Because the presence of a fragility fracture indicates osteoporosis even in the absence of a measurable decrease in BMD, DEXA is not warranted during the inpatient evaluation of the acute fracture patient. For patients without a prior study, DEXA at 6–12 weeks postfracture is reasonable to establish a baseline from which to monitor disease progression and efficacy of treatment. Diagnostic measures in the inpatient setting, particularly in men, should focus on the identification of modifiable risk factors and secondary causes of osteoporosis. Laboratory testing should include serum calcium (corrected for albumin), alkaline phosphatase, complete blood count, renal function, 25-hydroxyvitamin D, thyroid-stimulating hormone, serum protein electrophoresis (for patients with vertebral fractures and suspicion for multiple myeloma), and testosterone (for men). There is no role for measurement of markers of bone resorption in the inpatient setting.

### 4.2 Treatment of osteoporosis and secondary fracture prevention

Following fragility fracture, all patients should receive careful medication review, counseling on risk factor modification and fall prevention, and calcium and vitamin D supplementation.

In the absence of contraindications, patients with fragility fractures and a life expectancy greater than 1 year should be considered for bisphosphonate therapy [13]. In addition to improving BMD and reducing bone turnover markers, both intravenous and oral bisphosphonates are associated with reduced risk for subsequent fractures and mortality following hip fracture [14, 15]. However, no consensus exists regarding the optimal timing of bisphosphonate therapy for secondary prevention. On the one hand, the majority of patients who have sustained fragility fractures fail to receive adequate osteoporosis treatment as late as 2 years following the fracture. Early initiation of medication may reduce lapses in prescribing that can occur during transitions of care, underscore the importance of therapy, and maximize therapeutic benefit. On the other hand, the mechanism of action of bisphosphonates has raised concerns about whether these agents may delay fracture healing. Recent meta-analyses [16, 17] suggest that bisphosphonate administration within 3 months of fracture does not appear to clinically or radiographically impair fracture healing. Most osteoporosis experts support initiation of bisphosphonates between 6 and 12 weeks after fracture. It is reasonable to begin with weekly dosing of oral bisphosphonates (eg, alendronate 70 mg weekly). Intravenous bisphosphonates, eg, zolendronic acid and ibandronate) may offer advantages in compliance or inpatients who have gastrointestinal contraindications to oral agents. For patients with contraindications to bisphosphonate therapy, other therapies such as teriparatide and denosumab can be considered in consultation with an osteoporosis expert.

### 4.3 Ongoing management

Postoperative management of osteoporosis lies within the scope of quality primary care and does not routinely involve specialist referral. For patients with contraindications to oral therapy or disease refractory to oral therapy, subspecialist consultation may be warranted.

## 5 Basics of bone metabolism and pathophysiology of age-associated bone loss

Bone remodeling is the normal homeostatic process by which old bone is resorbed and replaced by new bone in order to maintain a healthy skeleton. This process occurs in several stages:

- Activation—osteoclast precursors arrive at the surface of formed bone.
- Resorption—osteoclast precursors convert to active osteoclasts and create an acidic environment, thus dissolving the mineral content of bone.
- Reversal—osteoclasts undergo apoptosis and are replaced by osteoblast precursors.
- Bone formation—osteoblast precursors undergo activation to osteoblasts and deposit collagen.
- Mineralization—osteocytes embedded within the collagen matrix contribute to its mineralization and hardening into new bone.

Bone remodeling occurs under the control of various hormones and cytokines, including estrogens and androgens, vitamin D, parathyroid hormone (PTH), osteoprotegerin, and receptor activator of nuclear factor-κB (RANK) and its ligand (RANK-L). Many of these factors have provided targets for the pharmacological treatment of osteoporosis. A schematic of the bone remodeling process is shown in **Fig 1.10-1**.

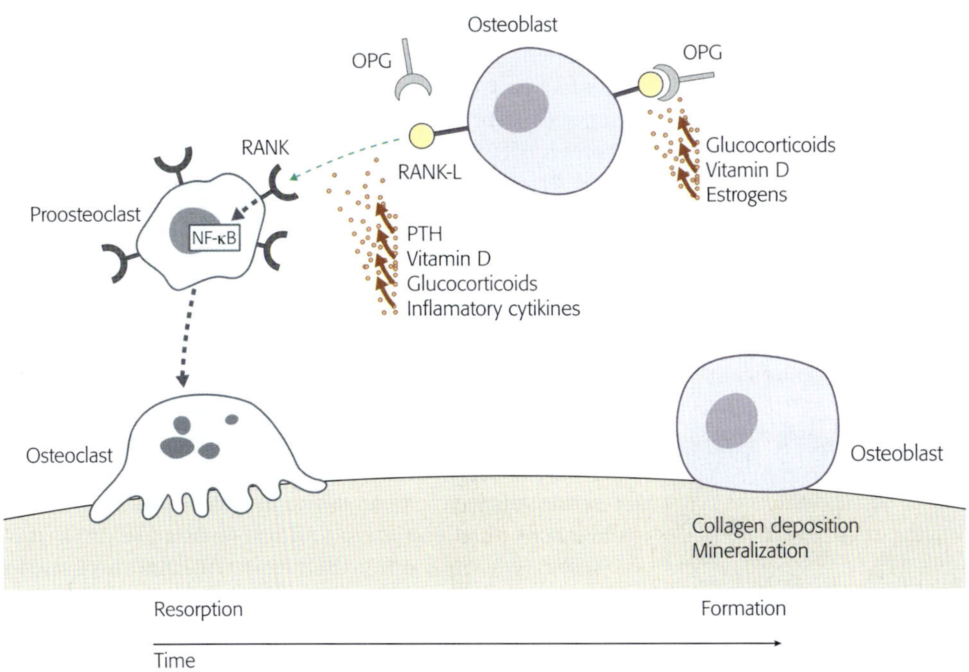


**Fig 1.10-1** Schematic of the key players in the bone modeling process. Abbreviations: OPG, osteoprotegerin; PTH, parathyroid hormone.

The remodeling process favors new bone formation until the 20s, when an individual's bone mass peaks. African Americans achieve the highest peak bone mass with Caucasians reaching lower peaks and Asians the lowest. A trend toward bone loss begins immediately after peak bone mass is reached. In women, bone loss accelerates after menopause, when lower estrogen levels allow increased bone resorption by osteoclasts without a corresponding increase in bone deposition by osteoclasts. In the seventh decade of life, age-related decreases in calcium absorption lead to a secondary hyperparathyroidism, which also increases bone resorption. Finally, in the very old, renal vitamin D production decreases while resistance to endogenous vitamin D increases, resulting in a further net increase in bone resorption. As she ages, a woman's bone mass may decrease by 30–40% from peak level.

Osteoporosis represents a pathological imbalance between bone resorption and bone formation, with the former predominating. In addition to decreased bone mass, osteoporosis is characterized by disruptions in the microarchitecture of bone, with fewer, more fragile bone trabeculae, as well as decreased viability of the osteocytes that maintain bone mineralization. **Figure 1.10-2** depicts the microscopic structure of normal and osteoporotic bone.

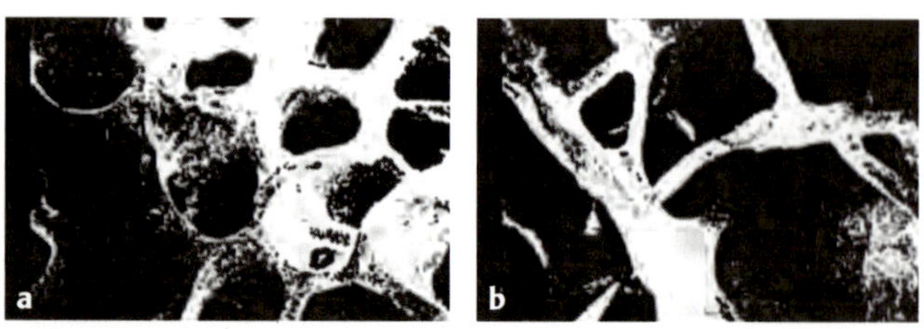


**Fig 1.10-2a–b** Normal (**a**) and osteoporotic bone (**b**)

## 6 Osteoporosis risk assessment, diagnosis, and evaluation

Any fracture at a major skeletal site, particularly at the hip or spine, in an adult 50 years or older should be considered osteoporosis-related unless clinical circumstances point to another clear etiology for the fracture, and the patient should be evaluated accordingly.

In addition, the National Osteoporosis Foundation (NOF) suggests assessment of osteoporosis and fall risk in all postmenopausal women and all men older than 50 years. Common risk factors for low BMD are listed in the following:

- Increasing age
- Early menopause
- Caucasian or Asian race
- Personal or family history of fragility fracture
- Inadequate calcium and vitamin D intake
- Excessive alcohol or tobacco use
- Low level of physical activity
- Medications:
  - Glucocorticoids
  - Anticonvulsants
  - Heparin
  - Excessive thyroid hormone
  - Proton pump inhibitors

Patients deemed to be at high risk for osteoporosis or falls should undergo BMD determination. The contribution of falls to fracture risk is discussed separately in chapter 1.11 Sarcopenia, malnutrition, frailty, and falls. Regardless of risk factors and fall and fracture history, the US Preventive Services Task Force recommends screening DEXA in all women 65 years and older; the NOF suggests screening in men 70 years and older as well.

Central DEXA as measured at the total hip, femoral neck, or spine is the most common method of BMD determination. A given patient's BMD, expressed in units of grams of mineral per square centimeter scanned ($g/cm^2$), is compared to two databases, one comprising an age-, gender-, and ethnicity-matched population and another comprising a young adult, gender-matched population. The SDs of the patient's BMD from these two database norms yield Z- and T-scores, respectively. As shown in **Table 1.10-1**, DEXA-based diagnoses of osteoporosis and osteopenia are defined by T-scores. Methods other than central DEXA also exist for the determination of BMD, but these have limitations. Quantitative computed tomography, for example, involves increased radiation exposure and cost compared to central

DEXA. Heel ultrasonography and peripheral DEXA, which measures BMD at the forearm, heel, and fingers, are portable but do not correlate as well with fracture risk as do central DEXA measurements.

Vertebral fractures define osteoporosis even in the absence of a DEXA diagnosis. These fractures often produce no symptoms and may go undiagnosed for months or years, but their presence is an indication for pharmacological treatment of osteoporosis. Therefore, some groups recommend yearly measurement of height in older patients. In addition, vertebral imaging should be considered in:

- Women older than 70 and men older than 80 years with DEXA-defined osteopenia
- Women from 65–69 years and men from 70–79 years with T-scores of less than -1.5
- Postmenopausal women and men older than 50 years with low-trauma fracture during adulthood, height loss of 4 cm or more or long-term treatment with glucocorticoids [18]

The majority of postmenopausal women with osteoporosis have no identifiable secondary cause. However, 50% of men and premenopausal women may have an underlying treatable condition, as the list of selected causes of secondary osteoporosis shows:

- Medications, eg, glucocorticoids, anticonvulsants, lithium, proton pump inhibitors, and others
- Rheumatic disease, eg, rheumatoid arthritis, systemic lupus erythematosus, and ankylosing spondylitis
- Endocrinopathies, eg, cushing syndrome, hyperthyroidism, hyperparathyroidism, hypogonadism, type 2 diabetes, and others
- Other medical conditions, ie, cystic fibrosis, chronic obstructive pulmonary disease, human immunodeficiency virus infection, renal insufficiency, and liver disease
- Nutritional factors, eg, excessive alcohol intake, anorexia, celiac disease, and vitamin D deficiency

While no formal guidelines exist for further evaluation, a careful clinical evaluation followed by laboratory testing may be warranted in patients suspected of having a secondary etiology of osteoporosis.

## 7 Osteoporosis in men

Although osteoporosis is more common in women than in men, a significant number of men are affected—in the US, 1.5 million older than 65 years, with another 3.5 million at risk [19]. One in eight American men sustains an osteoporotic fracture in his lifetime. Men are twice as likely as women to die as a result of their fractures but less than half as likely to be evaluated for osteoporosis and less than one-fifth as likely to be treated for osteoporosis following a fracture [20]. Despite the unclear validity of T-scores in men, DEXA remains the diagnostic method of choice. Approximately half of men with osteoporosis have a secondary cause or contributing factor, most commonly alcohol abuse, and most men diagnosed with osteoporosis should therefore undergo further evaluation. The treatment of osteoporosis in men follows principles similar to those in women.

## 8 Nonpharmacological treatment of osteoporosis

The treatment of osteoporosis involves a multimodal approach including education, fall prevention strategies, exercise, calcium and vitamin D supplementation, and pharmacological therapy. Unfortunately, despite the increased prevalence of osteoporosis, osteopenia, and fragility fractures, evidence suggests that many at-risk patients fail to receive education and treatment for decreased BMD. Time constraints often limit the amount of education that can be done during a routine office visit or hospitalization, and in one study of about 2,800 women with fragility fractures, only 4.6% were started on pharmacological treatment of osteoporosis immediately after the fracture, only 8.4% had BMD testing and only 42.4% received treatment in the 2 years following the fracture [21]. Fortunately, guidelines do exist for the therapy of patients with or at risk for osteoporosis or osteopenia. Please see chapter 2.8 Fracture liaison service and improving treatment rates for osteoporosis.

All postmenopausal women, men older than 50 years, and other patients at risk for accelerated bone loss should be counseled on risk factor modification, such as smoking cessation and moderation of alcohol consumption. Patients should also receive education on fall prevention strategies, including adequate lighting, grab bars, proper footwear, and removal of fall hazards such as throw rugs. Home safety evaluations can prove invaluable in reducing fall risk (for more information on falls and surgical management after the operation, see chapters 1.11 Sarcopenia, malnutrition, frailty, and falls and 1.8 Postoperative surgical management). Providers should minimize the use of medications that contribute to confusion, dizziness, hypotension, or fatigue, and they should also assess for visual impairments. Physical and occupational therapists can play critical roles in addressing existing balance and gait abnormalities and cognitive impairments, as well as in instructing patients in regular weight-bearing and muscle-strengthening exercises. While hip protectors, which provide padding around the hips to minimize the impact from a fall, were in common use in recent decades, a metaanalysis in 2006 showed that their efficacy is limited in the community and uncertain in institutional settings; moreover, poor fit and skin irritation led to poor compliance by many patients [22].

Patients with or at risk for accelerated bone loss should be educated on the importance of adequate calcium and vitamin D intake. In addition to its many other physiological functions, calcium is required for adequate bone mineralization. In older adults, serum calcium decreases, intestinal absorption of calcium decreases, and urinary calcium excretion increases. Vitamin D increases serum calcium by increasing intestinal absorption and renal reabsorption of calcium as well as resorption of calcium from bone. In older adults, the production of inactive vitamin D in the skin decreases, as does renal conversion of vitamin D to its active form, thereby leading to secondary hyperparathyroidism and subsequent hypocalcemia and bone resorption.

Studies have shown that calcium carbonate 600 mg twice daily reduces the incidence of clinical fracture as compared to placebo in patients who are at least 80% compliant; but despite minimal adverse effects, compliance can be as low as 43% [23]. Vitamin D supplementation alone has not been shown to be effective in decreasing fracture rates, although it can yield improvements in BMD [24]. However, the combination of calcium and vitamin D3 daily does appear both to reduce bone loss and to decrease the risk of both hip and other nonvertebral fractures among older women as compared to placebo [25, 26].

Based on these findings, it is recommended that patients at risk for bone loss consume 1,200 mg of calcium daily, along with vitamin D 800-1,000 international units (IUs) daily. Calcium supplements may be suggested for patients who cannot get enough calcium from dietary sources. Available calcium formulations include calcium carbonate and calcium citrate. The former is less expensive and must be taken with meals, while the latter is more expensive but may be taken at any time. Both formulations cause constipation and abdominal upset. For optimal absorption, a single dose of supplemental calcium should not exceed 500 mg elemental calcium, and calcium should not be given within several hours of levothyroxine, fluoroquinolones, phenytoin, angiotensin-converting enzyme inhibitors, and bisphosphonates, which can interfere with its absorption. Vitamin D is available as ergocalciferol (D2), which is commonly given at a dosage of 50,000 IU orally weekly for 8 weeks, followed by 50,000 IU every 2–4 weeks. Alternatively, patients can take cholecalciferol (D3) 1,000-2,000 IU orally once daily. The goal of vitamin D supplementation is a serum 25-hydroxyvitamin D level at or above 29.6 ng/mL (74 nmol/L).

## 9 Pharmacological treatment of osteoporosis

Varying recommendations exist about which patients should receive pharmacological treatment for decreased BMD. According to the NOF, postmenopausal women and men aged 50 years and older should be treated if:

- They have a clinical or radiographic hip or vertebral fracture, regardless of DEXA findings.
- They have a T-score equal to or less than -2.5 at the hip, femoral neck or lumbar spine.
- They have a T-score between -1.0 and -2.5 and a 10-year probability of hip fracture of at least 3% or a 10-year probability of a major fragility fracture of at least 20% as assessed by the WHO Fracture Risk Assessment (FRAX) tool [27].

Life expectancy is likely necessary to accrue enough pharmacological effect from osteoporosis therapy to make the benefits worth the risks. Canadian endorsed guidelines suggest a minimum life expectancy of 1 year to consider pharmacological treatment [13].

Developed after analysis of population-based cohorts from North America, Europe, Asia, and Australia, FRAX considers factors including age, gender, race, height and weight, fracture history, certain comorbidities, and medication and substance use, along with femoral neck BMD, to calculate the 10-year risk of hip or major fragility fractures. FRAX does not use spine BMD as this value can be falsely elevated in the presence of spinal osteoarthritis. The tool is validated only for postmenopausal women and men 50 years of age and older. It also lacks validity in patients already taking antiresorptive therapy and therefore cannot be used to determine the need for ongoing treatment.

Some experts suggest initiating antiresorptive therapy in any patients, particularly women, taking or anticipated to take glucocorticoids for longer than 3 months at doses exceeding the equivalent of prednisolone 7.5 mg daily given the strong negative effect of these agents on bone quality. In addition, some clinicians start therapy in patients with borderline bone mass and elevated markers of bone resorption, but the utility of these markers is not well established. Multiple pharmacological classes have been approved by the US Food and Drug Administration (FDA) for the treatment of osteoporosis and are summarized in **Table 1.10-2**.

## 9.1 Bisphosphonates

Bisphosphonates are the mainstay of treatment for osteoporosis and osteopenia. They are potent antiresorptive agents that bind to calcium hydroxyapatite in the bone mineral matrix and inhibit the activity of osteoclasts, thereby decreasing bone remodeling. Bisphosphonates actually incorporate themselves into the bone matrix, and their effects therefore persist for years. Salient characteristics of the various bisphosphonates are summarized in **Table 1.10-3**.

| Class | Example(s) |
|---|---|
| Bisphosphonates | • Alendronate<br>• Risedronate<br>• Ibandronate<br>• Zoledronic acid |
| Anabolic agent | Teriparatide (recombinant human parathyroid hormone) |
| Monoclonal antibody | Denosumab (human monoclonal antibody against RANK-L) |
| Hormone-based treatments | Estrogens, selective estrogen receptor modulators (SERMs) |
| Miscellaneous | Calcitonin |

**Table 1.10-2** Pharmacotherapeutical classes approved for the treatment of osteoporosis.

Oral bisphosphonates are associated with both poor gastrointestinal absorption and upper gastrointestinal side effects, including dysphagia, esophageal reflux, and esophageal inflammation. These medications must be taken on an empty stomach with a full glass of water; in addition, patients must wait 30–60 minutes before reclining or consuming other beverages, medications, and food. Not surprisingly, adherence to these agents is poor and can limit their efficacy. Intravenous bisphosphonates are better tolerated, though zoledronic acid can be associated with an infusion reaction characterized by fever, headache, and arthralgia and myalgia. Adequate hydration and premedication with acetaminophen reduce the risk of an infusion reaction, and the reaction is less likely to occur with subsequent infusions. Bisphosphonates are contraindicated in patients with significant renal impairment (typically defined as creatinine clearance < 30 mL/min); this can be a limiting factor for many frail older adults.

There have been reports in the literature of bisphosphonate-associated osteonecrosis of the jaw (ONJ), thought to result from the long-term suppression of bone remodeling and accumulation of microscopic damage to bone. Risk factors for this rare condition include the type and cumulative dose of bisphosphonate; most cases occur in patients with multiple myeloma and other malignancies involving lytic bone lesions who are receiving higher and more frequent doses of bisphosphonates than are used for the treatment of osteoporosis. Dental trauma and infection also seem to predispose patients to ONJ, and it is therefore suggested that patients receive ongoing routine dental care and undergo

| Drug name | Dosing | Efficacy | Indications |
|---|---|---|---|
| Alendronate | 70 mg orally weekly | Reduces hip and vertebral fracture risk | Prevention and treatment of:<br>• Postmenopausal osteoporosis<br>• Osteoporosis in men<br>• Glucocorticoid-induced osteoporosis |
| Risedronate | 35 mg orally weekly | Reduces hip and vertebral fracture risk | Prevention and treatment of:<br>• Postmenopausal osteoporosis<br>• Osteoporosis in men<br>• Glucocorticoid-induced osteoporosis |
| Risendronate | 150 mg orally monthly | As above | |
| Ibandronate | 150 mg orally monthly | Reduces vertebral fracture risk | Prevention and treatment of postmenopausal osteoporosis |
| Ibandronate | 3 mg intravenously every 3 months | Increases BMD, but no effect on fracture risk | Treatment of postmenopausal osteoporosis |
| Zoledronic acid | 5 mg intravenously yearly | Reduces hip and vertebral fracture risk | Prevention (when given every 2 years) and treatment of:<br>• Postmenopausal osteoporosis<br>• Osteoporosis in men<br>• Glucocorticoid-induced osteoporosis<br><br>Prevention of new clinical fractures in men and women with recent fragility hip fracture |

**Table 1.10-3** Bisphosphonate characteristics.

any necessary dental surgery or treatment of oral infections prior to initiation of a bisphosphonate, if at all possible. Treatment of ONJ involves pain management, infection control, debridement of necrotic tissue, and frequent cessation of bisphosphonate therapy. Because ONJ is a complication rarely seen in patients taking bisphosphonates for osteoporosis, concern over its occurrence should not preclude the initiation of these agents if otherwise indicated. Significantly higher rates of ONJ are reported in patients receiving frequent bisphosphonate dosing for malignancies [28].

Bisphosphonates have also been associated with atypical femoral fractures, defined as low-trauma fractures of the midfemoral diaphysis leading to a prodrome of vague thigh discomfort and weakness (see chapter 3.18 Atypical fractures). Again, oversuppression of bone remodeling may allow the accumulation of microscopic cracks in bone that eventually coalesce into clinically apparent injury. Studies have shown that while the relative risk of atypical femoral fractures does increase in patients taking bisphosphonates, the absolute risk remains very small [29–31]. Nevertheless, in patients found to have this type of fracture, bisphosphonate therapy should be discontinued.

The risk of both ONJ and atypical femoral fracture, though small in both cases, appears to increase with the duration of bisphosphonate use. This observation, coupled with the long half-life of bisphosphonates, has introduced uncertainty about the optimal duration of bisphosphonate therapy. In a 2006 study, women who took alendronate for 5 years, then were randomized to the drug for another 5 years, had higher BMD and a lower risk of vertebral fractures than women randomized to placebo for the second 5 years. There was no difference in the incidence of nonvertebral fractures [32]. Other studies have also shown inconsistent results with regards to BMD and fracture prevention benefits after 5 years of therapy. Various groups have therefore suggested a risk-stratified approach to ongoing treatment with bisphosphonates: patients at low risk for fracture could consider a "drug holiday" after 3–5 years, while higher risk patients should continue therapy for a longer duration with a shorter holiday, perhaps with use of an alternative agent during the holiday. In either case, patients should be reassessed within 1–3 years of cessation of therapy and a bisphosphonate resumed if BMD decreases or if fracture occurs. Currently, few data exist on the specific utility of markers of bone turnover for optimizing treatment duration.

### 9.2 Teriparatide and Abaloparatide

Parathyroid hormone has a net resorptive effect on bone when given continuously and a net anabolic effect when given intermittently. Teriparatide is a recombinant human PTH that, when dosed at 20 µg subcutaneously daily, is an agent approved for the treatment of osteoporosis that stimulates bone formation rather than limiting bone resorption. The mechanism of action of teriparatide involves the induction of cytokines including insulin growth factor 1, transforming growth factor B, and RANK-L, as well as the inhibition of sclerostin, resulting in the activation of bone-building osteoblasts. The anabolic effect of teriparatide begins within 1 month of initiation and peaks at 6–9 months. The agent increases vertebral, femoral, and total body BMD and decreases the risk of both vertebral and nonvertebral fractures [33]. It is approved for postmenopausal women and men with osteoporosis and high fracture risk and for patients intolerant of bisphosphonates. Teriparatide is generally well tolerated, with potential adverse effects including orthostatic hypotension, transient hypercalcemia, nausea, and leg cramps. In animal models, teriparatide was shown to increase the risk of osteosarcoma. Therefore, although there have been no reports of malignancy in humans who receive lower effective doses than the laboratory animals did, the agent is labeled as being contraindicated in patients with Paget's disease, a history of skeletal radiation, and unexplained elevations in serum alkaline phosphatase. Teriparatide is administered for 2 years, after which, one study suggests, patients should transition to bisphosphonate therapy in order to maintain the achieved gains in BMD [34]. Abaloparatide is a newer injectable analogue of PTH-related peptide. It is a daily subcutaneous administered drug with a pre-metered pen. Early data suggest similar performance in early study [35].

### 9.3 Denosumab

Denosumab is a fully human monoclonal antibody directed against RANK-L. This cytokine mediates the formation, function, and survival of osteoclasts (**Fig 1.10-1**); blockage of the interaction between RANK and RANK-L inhibits osteoclast-mediated bone resorption. Denosumab has been shown to increase BMD at the spine and to decrease the risk of both radiographic vertebral fractures and clinical hip and nonvertebral fractures [36]. Administered as a 60 mg subcutaneous injections every 6 months, it is approved for the treatment of osteoporosis in postmenopausal women and men at high risk of fracture, as well as for the treatment of bone loss in women and men receiving hormonal therapies for breast and prostate cancer, respectively. The most common adverse effects include hypocalcemia, rash, cellulitis, and flatulence. As with bisphosphonates, denosumab has been rarely associated with ONJ and atypical femoral fractures. The long-term efficacy and safety of denosumab are unknown.

## 9.4 Hormone-associated therapies

Endogenous estrogens limit bone resorption through stimulation of the cytokine osteoprotegerin (**Fig 1.10-1**). Osteoprotegerin, a natural antagonist of RANK-L, blocks the interaction of RANK with RANK-L, decreasing osteoclast activation and thus bone resorption. As endogenous estrogen levels sharply decline at menopause, osteoclast activation increases and leads to the accelerated bone loss seen in postmenopausal women. The administration of exogenous estrogens, with or without progesterone, has been shown to slightly reduce the risk of hip and vertebral fractures. However, estrogens confer an increased risk of stroke, thromboembolic disease, coronary artery disease, and breast cancer; and these risks outweigh the bone benefits. The FDA therefore recommends limiting the use of exogenous estrogen therapy for osteoporosis to women with moderate to severe vasomotor symptoms, and only for short periods of time.

Historically, selective estrogen receptor modulators (SERMs) provided another option for the treatment of osteoporosis in postmenopausal women, but may be falling out of favor. These agents act as estrogen agonists in bone tissue, where they have an antiresorptive effect, and as estrogen antagonists in breast and uterine tissue, where they decrease the risk of invasive breast cancer. They do not decrease the risk of coronary artery disease and actually increase the risk of thromboembolic disease and vasomotor symptoms. The most commonly prescribed SERM, raloxifene, has been shown to decrease the risk of vertebral fractures, but not hip fractures. Some organizations are beginning to remove raloxifene from their guidelines, due to the poor risk/benefit ratio for most patients [37]. Lasofoxifene is a third-generation SERM currently under investigation for the treatment of osteoporosis. Studies have shown that this drug decreases the risk of vertebral and nonvertebral fracture but not of hip fracture; and it also decreases the risk of breast cancer, stroke, and cardiovascular disease. However, there is a slight increase in overall mortality in patients taking lower-dose lasofoxifene rather than higher-dose lasofoxifene or placebo, and this finding is under further review.

Other hormone-associated therapies include combination conjugated estrogen-SERM products. Conjugated estrogens/bazedoxifene increases spine and hip BMD and reduces the risk of both vertebral and hip fractures with a neutral effect on breast and endometrial cancer risk. The combination agents, like others containing estrogen, should be used for the shortest possible duration and only after consideration of estrogen-free alternatives.

## 9.5 Calcitonin

Endogenous calcitonin, secreted by the thyroid gland, plays a role in normal calcium homeostasis, guarding against hypercalcemia by acting directly on osteoclasts to inhibit bone resorption. An intranasal salmon calcitonin formulation, sprayed into alternating nostrils daily at a dose of 200 IU, has been shown to decrease the incidence of vertebral fractures. It has also been found to have a small analgesic effect on vertebral compression fractures. It does not affect the risk of hip or other nonvertebral fracture. Intranasal calcitonin has few immediate side effects other than rhinitis, but studies have suggested an increased risk of unspecified malignancy with this agent. Calcitonin is a third-line agent for the treatment of osteoporosis given the availability of other medications with greater efficacy.

## 9.6 Other therapies

Strontium ranelate is used in some European countries for the treatment of osteoporosis. It has been shown to reduce the risk of vertebral and nonvertebral fractures in postmenopausal women and, in a high-risk subgroup, to reduce the risk of hip fracture as well. Its mechanism is unclear, but it is theorized to incorporate into the crystalline structure of bone and enhance matrix mineralization. Strontium has been associated with nausea, diarrhea, rash, and headache; and there have been reports of the drug reaction with eosinophilia and systemic symptoms syndrome, which is potentially fatal.

Our increased understanding of the pathways involved in bone metabolism and the pathophysiology of osteoporosis has led to the emergence of new targets for osteoporosis treatment. Two targeted agents currently under study include romosozumab and odanacatib. Romosozumab is a monoclonal antibody directed against sclerostin, an osteocyte-derived protein that downregulates the bone-formative effects of osteoblasts. A recent phase II study demonstrated that romosozumab improves BMD by enhancing bone formation and decreasing bone resorption [38]. Odanacatib inhibits cathepsin K, an osteoclast-derived protease involved in collagen degradation. Early trials have indicated that odanacatib increases spine and hip BMD [39]. Trials of fracture risk reduction for both romosozumab and odanacatib are in process [40]. Several other new agents are currently in preclinical trials.

## 10 Rescreening, treatment monitoring, and follow-up

Although screening for osteoporosis is recommended for women 65 years of age or older, there are few data to guide decisions about rescreening. In order to help clinicians determine optimal testing intervals, a recent study investigated the rates of transition to osteoporosis for older women with normal BMD or osteopenia at initial assessment. The investigators found that with rescreening intervals of 15 years for women with normal bone density or mild osteopenia, 5 years for women with moderate osteopenia, and 1 year for women with advanced osteopenia, less than 10% of the patients would develop osteoporosis [41].

In patients receiving treatment for osteoporosis, the need for ongoing therapy should be periodically reassessed to optimize the balance between treatment benefits and burdens. Some measures may be undertaken during routine office visits. Modifiable risk factors for bone loss, such as tobacco and alcohol consumption and calcium and vitamin D intake should be addressed, as should factors involving the risk of falls. Patients should receive ongoing education about the nature and sequelae of bone loss, fall prevention strategies, diet, and exercise. Patients should be asked about adverse effects and difficulties in adhering to the prescribed treatment regimen. They should have yearly height determination as an inexpensive screen for occult vertebral fractures, with follow-up imaging as indicated.

Many clinicians repeat BMD testing 2 years after the initiation of therapy, sooner in patients with risk factors for ongoing bone loss, such as long-term glucocorticoid therapy. If at all possible, a follow-up DEXA should be performed on the same DEXA scanner used to perform the initial screen, as variations between scanners can cloud test results. While an increase in BMD is the desired finding, particularly in patients taking anabolic therapies, a stable BMD may also indicate the efficacy of therapy in the face of a tendency towards ongoing bone loss. A decrease in BMD should prompt concerns about inadequate calcium and/or vitamin D intake, treatment nonadherence or failure, or a secondary cause of bone loss, and appropriate investigation should be undertaken. Some clinicians follow markers of bone resorption: defined decreases in urine N-telopeptide and serum C-telopeptide at 6 months as compared to baseline indicate treatment efficacy and compliance. However, these markers should not be the sole factor in decisions regarding continuation, modification, or cessation of treatment.

## 11 References

1. **Wright NC, Looker AC, Saag KG, et al.** The recent prevalence of osteoporosis and low bone mass in the United States based on bone mineral density at the femoral neck or lumbar spine. *J Bone Miner Res.* 2014 Nov;29(11):2520–2526.
2. **Office of the Surgeon General.** Reports of the Surgeon General. Bone Health and Osteoporosis: A Report of the Surgeon General. Rockville, MD: Office of the Surgeon General (US); 2004. Available at: www.surgeongeneral.gov/library/reports/index. Accessed February 12, 2015.
3. **Johnell O, Kanis J.** Epidemiology of osteoporotic fractures. *Osteoporos Int.* 2005 Mar;16 Suppl 2:S3–S7.
4. **Cummings SR, Black DM, Nevitt MC, et al.** Bone density at various sites for prediction of hip fractures. The Study of Osteoporotic Fractures Research Group. *Lancet.* 1993 Jan 9;341(8837):72–75.
5. **Friedman SM, Mendelson DA.** Epidemiology of fragility fractures. *Clin Geriatr Med.* 2014 May;30(2):175–181.
6. **Gallagher JC, Melton LJ, Riggs BL, et al.** Epidemiology of fractures of the proximal femur in Rochester, Minnesota. *Clin Orthop Relat Res.* 1980 Jul-Aug(150):163–171.
7. **Cooper C, Campion G, Melton LJ 3rd.** Hip fractures in the elderly: a world-wide projection. *Osteoporos Int.* 1992 Nov;2(6):285–289.
8. **Kanis JA, Johnell O, De Laet C, et al.** International variations in hip fracture probabilities: implications for risk assessment. *J Bone Miner Res.* 2002 Jul;17(7):1237–1244.
9. **Burge R, Dawson-Hughes B, Solomon DH, et al.** Incidence and economic burden of osteoporosis-related fractures in the United States, 2005–2025. *J Bone Miner Res.* 2007 Mar;22(3):465–475.
10. **Johnell O.** The socioeconomic burden of fractures: today and in the 21st century. *Am J Med.* 1997 Aug 18;103(2a):20S–25S; discussion 25S–26S.
11. **Magaziner J, Hawkes W, Hebel JR, et al.** Recovery from hip fracture in eight areas of function. *J Gerontol A Biol Sci Med Sci.* 2000 Sep;55(9):M498–M507.
12. **Magaziner J, Simonsick EM, Kashner TM, et al.** Predictors of functional recovery one year following hospital discharge for hip fracture: a prospective study. *J Gerontol.* 1990 May;45(3):M101–M107.
13. **Papaioannou A, Santesso N, Morin SN, et al.** Recommendations for preventing fracture in long-term care. *CMAJ.* 2015 Oct 20;187(15):1135–1144.
14. **Lyles KW, Colon-Emeric CS, Magaziner JS, et al.** Zoledronic acid and clinical fractures and mortality after hip fracture. *N Engl J Med.* 2007 Nov 1;357(18):1799–1809.
15. **Beaupre LA, Morrish DW, Hanley DA, et al.** Oral bisphosphonates are associated with reduced mortality after hip fracture. *Osteoporos Int.* 2011 Mar;22(3):983–991.
16. **Xue D, Li F, Chen G, et al.** Do bisphosphonates affect bone healing? A meta-analysis of randomized controlled trials. *J Orthop Surg Res.* 2014;9:45.

17. **Li YT, Cai HF, Zhang ZL.** Timing of the initiation of bisphosphonates after surgery for fracture healing: a systematic review and meta-analysis of randomized controlled trials. *Osteoporos Int.* 2015 Feb;26(2):431–441.
18. **Cosman F, de Beur SJ, LeBoff MS, et al.** Clinician's Guide to Prevention and Treatment of Osteoporosis. *Osteoporos Int.* 2014 Oct;25(10):2359–2381.
19. **Siddiqui NA, Shetty KR, Duthie EH Jr.** Osteoporosis in older men: discovering when and how to treat it. *Geriatrics.* 1999 Sep;54(9):20–22, 27–28, 30.
20. **Kiebzak GM, Beinart GA, Perser K, et al.** Undertreatment of osteoporosis in men with hip fracture. *Arch Intern Med.* 2002 Oct 28;162(19):2217–2222.
21. **Feldstein A, Elmer PJ, Orwoll E, et al.** Bone mineral density measurement and treatment for osteoporosis in older individuals with fractures: a gap in evidence-based practice guideline implementation. *Arch Intern Med.* 2003 Oct 13;163(18):2165–2172.
22. **Parker MJ, Gillespie WJ, Gillespie LD.** Effectiveness of hip protectors for preventing hip fractures in elderly people: systematic review. *BMJ.* 2006 Mar 11;332(7541):571–574.
23. **Prince RL, Devine A, Dhaliwal SS, et al.** Effects of calcium supplementation on clinical fracture and bone structure: results of a 5-year, double-blind, placebo-controlled trial in elderly women. *Arch Intern Med.* 2006 Apr 24;166(8):869–875.
24. **Lips P, Graafmans WC, Ooms ME, et al.** Vitamin D supplementation and fracture incidence in elderly persons. A randomized, placebo-controlled clinical trial. *Ann Intern Med.* 1996 Feb 15;124(4):400–406.
25. **Dawson-Hughes B, Harris SS, Krall EA, et al.** Effect of calcium and vitamin D supplementation on bone density in men and women 65 years of age or older. *N Engl J Med.* 1997 Sep 4;337(10):670–676.
26. **Chapuy MC, Arlot ME, Duboeuf F, et al.** Vitamin D3 and calcium to prevent hip fractures in the elderly women. *N Engl J Med.* 1992 Dec 3;327(23):1637–1642.
27. **Kanis JA.** Fracture Risk Assessment Tool (FRAX). Centre for Metabolic Bone Diseases. University of Sheffield, UK. Available at: www.shef.ac.uk/FRAX. Accessed 2016.
28. **Bamias A, Kastritis E, Bamia C, et al.** Osteonecrosis of the jaw in cancer after treatment with bisphosphonates: incidence and risk factors. *J Clin Oncol.* 2005 Dec 1;23(34):8580–8587.
29. **Black DM, Kelly MP, Genant HK, et al.** Bisphosphonates and fractures of the subtrochanteric or diaphyseal femur. *N Engl J Med.* 2010 May 13;362(19):1761–1771.
30. **Schilcher J, Michaelsson K, Aspenberg P.** Bisphosphonate use and atypical fractures of the femoral shaft. *N Engl J Med.* 2011 May 5;364(18):1728–1737.
31. **Schilcher J, Koeppen V, Aspenberg P, et al.** Risk of atypical femoral fracture during and after bisphosphonate use. *Acta Orthop.* 2015 Feb;86(1):100–107.
32. **Black DM, Schwartz AV, Ensrud KE, et al.** Effects of continuing or stopping alendronate after 5 years of treatment: the Fracture Intervention Trial Long-term Extension (FLEX): a randomized trial. *JAMA.* 2006 Dec 27;296(24):2927–2938.
33. **Neer RM, Arnaud CD, Zanchetta JR, et al.** Effect of parathyroid hormone (1–34) on fractures and bone mineral density in postmenopausal women with osteoporosis. *N Engl J Med.* 2001 May 10;344(19):1434–1441.
34. **Black DM, Bilezikian JP, Ensrud KE, et al.** One year of alendronate after one year of parathyroid hormone (1-84) for osteoporosis. *N Engl J Med.* 2005 Aug 11;353(6):555–565.
35. **Miller PD, Hattersley G, Riis BJ, et al.** Effect of abaloparatide vs placebo on new vertebral fractures in postmenopausal women with osteoporosis: a randomized clinical trial. *JAMA.* 2016 Aug 16;316(7):722–733.
36. **Cummings SR, San Martin J, McClung MR, et al.** Denosumab for prevention of fractures in postmenopausal women with osteoporosis. *N Engl J Med.* 2009 Aug 20;361(8):756–765.
37. **Qaseem A, Forciea MA, McLean RM, et al.** Treatment of low bone density or osteoporosis to prevent fractures in men and women: a clinical practice guideline update from the American College of Physicians. *Ann Intern Med.* 2017 Jun 6;166(11):818–839.
38. **McClung MR, Grauer A, Boonen S, et al.** Romosozumab in postmenopausal women with low bone mineral density. *N Engl J Med.* 2014 Jan 30;370(5):412–420.
39. **Bone HG, McClung MR, Roux C, et al.** Odanacatib, a cathepsin-K inhibitor for osteoporosis: a two-year study in postmenopausal women with low bone density. *J Bone Miner Res.* 2010 May;25(5):937–947.
40. **Bone HG, Dempster DW, Eisman JA, et al.** Odanacatib for the treatment of postmenopausal osteoporosis: development history and design and participant characteristics of LOFT, the Long-Term Odanacatib Fracture Trial. *Osteoporos Int.* 2015 Feb;26(2):699–712.
41. **Gourlay ML, Fine JP, Preisser JS, et al.** Bone-density testing interval and transition to osteoporosis in older women. *N Engl J Med.* 2012 Jan 19;366(3):225–233.

# 1.11 Sarcopenia, malnutrition, frailty, and falls

Claudia M Gonzalez Suarez

## 1 Introduction

Falls are common in older adults, occurring annually in more than 30% of community-dwelling adults aged 65 years and older, and half of those aged 85 years and older. Of those falls, 50% are recurrent. Of the 10–40% of falls that result in injury, 20% will require medical attention, and 10% will result in serious harm, including hip or other fracture, head injury or serious soft-tissue injury. Inability to rise without help, experienced by 50% of older persons after at least one fall, may result in dehydration, pressure ulcers, and rhabdomyolysis. Falls are associated with restricted mobility, reduced ability to carry out daily activities, and an increased risk of long-term institutional care. In addition to their physical toll, falls have psychosocial implications, including anxiety, depression, and social isolation [1].

Few falls have a single etiology; the majority of falls are a product of patient and environmental risk factors. Intrinsic physical and cognitive changes related to aging decrease functional reserve and predispose older patients to falling. Sarcopenia, frailty and malnutrition are three interrelated conditions to help identify and intervene in patients at risk for falls and fragility fractures [1]. Sarcopenia refers to the age-related loss of muscle mass and function. Frailty refers to the inherent vulnerability of older or comorbid persons to physiological stress [2]. Malnutrition is common and potentially treatable in many older adults [3]. This chapter gives an overview of these conditions, as well as strategies to evaluate fall risk and to prevent falls.

## 2 Falls

### 2.1 Risk factors and evaluation

With advancing age, the normal adult gait changes to a hesitant, broad-based, small stepped gait, often with a stooped posture, diminished arm swing and en bloc turns [4]. Disturbances of gait not only indicate the risk of falls but may herald or reflect serious underlying ill health [5]. The pattern of shortened step length and slowing of gait is particularly noticeable in individuals who have fallen repeatedly and is sometimes called the "post-fall syndrome", which is related to fear of further falling [6].

Since falls in older adults are usually the result of multiple conditions and circumstances, falls are classified as a geriatric syndrome rather than a discrete disease. The ability to transfer and walk safely depends on coordination among sensory (eg, vision, vestibular, proprioception), central and peripheral nervous, cardiopulmonary, musculoskeletal, and other systems. Falls that occur during usual daily activities generally result from impairments in one or more systems, such as occurs in frailty [7].

Common risk factors for falls include previous falls, age > 75 years, cognitive and visual impairment, arthritis, depression, and the use of four or more medications (ie, polypharmacy), particularly antihypertensive and psychiatric medications. The risk increases with increasing number of factors, from 8% with no risk factors to 78% among those with four or more risk factors [8].

A more comprehensive list of risk factors can be found in **Table 1.11-1**.

All patients should be asked about a history of falls, the specific circumstances of the falls, and any associated injury. Focused questions regarding dizziness, lightheadedness, weight loss, symptoms of neuropathy, gait instability and medication changes are necessary for adequate assessment for previous and future falls. Checking vision, postural blood pressure and a general neurological exam are appropriate for most patients who report falls [10].

Osteoporosis is an important consideration when assessing someone at risk for falls and fractures. This population is at greater risk of serious injuries related to falls; diagnostic tools like the Fracture Risk Assessment (FRAX) of the World Health Organization, as well as radiographic tools like bone densitometry using dual-energy x-ray absorptiometry or calcaneal quantitative ultrasound are useful methods to assess osteoporosis and fracture risk. If osteoporosis is diagnosed, management should be instituted including pharmacological and nonpharmacological interventions. Osteoporosis is further described in chapter 1.10 Osteoporosis.

### 2.2 Balance and gait evaluation

There are simple office-based assessments that can help evaluate gait and predict falls. The Timed Up and Go (TUG) test is the most frequently recommended screening test for mobility and entails having the patient get up from a chair, walk 3 meters (about 10 feet), turn and return to the chair, and sit down [11]. Any abnormality in movement suggests balance or gait impairment and increased risk of falling, requiring further assessment and suggest a likely need for treatment. Clear TUG completion times that indicate increased fall risk have not been definitively established, although cut points at 12 and 13.5 seconds have been suggested [12, 13].

| Domain | Factors |
|---|---|
| History | • History of falls<br>• Visual impairment<br>• Reported balance impairment or gait difficulties<br>• Cognitive impairment<br>• Age |
| Medications | • Number of medications, ie, use of more than four medications<br>• Medications by class:<br>– Sedatives and hypnotics<br>– Neuroleptics and antipsychotics<br>– Nonsteroidal antiinflammatory drugs<br>– Antidepressants<br>– Benzodiazepines |
| Functional status | • Impairments in ADLs and IADLs |
| Physical examination | • Gait and balance impairment<br>• Orthostatic hypotension<br>• Poor vision |
| Home hazards | • Lack of bathroom grab bars<br>• Dim lighting<br>• Slippery or uneven services<br>• Improper use of mobility aids |

**Table 1.11-1** Risk factors for falls in older adults [9].
Abbreviations: ADLs, activities of daily living; IADLs, instrumental activities of daily living.

The more detailed performance-oriented mobility assessment (POMA) involves assessing the quality of transfer, balance, and gait maneuvers used during daily activities and takes about 5–10 minutes to complete [14]. The POMA is not appropriate for highly functional patients or patients with a single disabling condition. It includes observing transfer and balance maneuvers such as getting up from a chair, performing side-by-side 1-leg and tandem stands (5–10 seconds each), turning in circle, and sitting down. In addition to the evaluation of gait during a 3-meter walk, gait initiation, heel-toe sequencing, step length, height, symmetry, path deviation, walk stance, steadiness on turning, arm swing, as well as neck, trunk, hip, and knee flexion are also assessed. These results can not only assess the risk of falling but also determine if there are balance and gait impairments that need intervention as well as assess the presence of neurological, musculoskeletal or other relevant disorders.

### 2.3 Prevention strategies

Trials of fall prevention strategies have shown that approximately 30% of falls can be prevented. Of those, several healthcare-based strategies have been shown to reduce the rate of falling; however, their implementation may be problematic, as clinicians tend to be more experienced at managing discrete diseases than at managing multifactorial conditions [15, 16].

Key domains of fall prevention typically include physical strengthening, medical evaluation and treatment, medication adjustment, environmental modification and education [10]. Key strategies for most patients include the following:

- Review and modify risk factors related to the patient's falls. Modifiable risk factors include correcting vision, reducing environmental hazards and obstacles, and education about using walking aids correctly.
- All patients should undergo a medication review to identify any medication-induced contributors to falls, including cardiovascular medications that may lead to orthostatic hypotension, and neuropsychiatric medications that may alter balance, awareness, or cognition.
- Vitamin D assessment for all patients and replacement for deficient patients.
- A history of one fall and no other balance or gait disturbances should be followed by participation in an exercise program that includes balance and strength training. Examples of these programs can include physical therapy, tai chi, or other programs.
- Two or more falls, and/or balance or gait difficulties should be followed by a detailed assessment and specialized physiotherapy.

Formal fall prevention programs can be divided into three main categories:

- Single programs including one intervention component, ie, supervised exercises
- Multicomponent programs including two or more intervention components, ie, exercises and environmental modifications
- Multifactorial programs including two or more customized interventions for each participant targeted at patient-specific risk factors

A recent metaanalysis found that single interventions failed to show a beneficial effect on fall-related outcomes in the nursing home population, since they are most often physically frail and the fall is frequently of a multifactorial nature [17]. Single programs targeted at more functionally intact older adults may be more successful.

Interventions, particularly those with strength and balance training, can successfully increase muscle strength and functional abilities. Avoiding iatrogenic harm related to excessive hospitalization, testing and polypharmacy is important when frailty is recognized [18–20].

Vitamin D levels fall with aging and low levels are associated with sarcopenia, falls, hip fracture, disability, and mortality. When levels are low, vitamin D replacement can reverse some functional deterioration, providing support for modest daily vitamin D supplementation [21]. A meta-analysis found positive effects of vitamin D supplementation on muscle strength, gait and balance suggesting that vitamin D supplementation of 800–1,000 international units (IUs) daily was associated with improvements of muscle strength and balance [22]. Vitamin D reduces the number of falls in those who are deficient, and the combination of calcium and vitamin D for older patients in long-term care can reduce fractures.

Other than vitamin D, few pharmacological agents have been investigated to improve muscle strength, balance and falls, including angiotensin-converting enzyme inhibitors, testosterone, and insulin-like growth factors (IGFs); none of these has emerged as safe and effective for fall prevention at this time.

## 3 Sarcopenia

Sarcopenia is defined as the loss of muscle mass, function, and efficiency. Aging is associated with sarcopenia and increased body fat, resulting from intrinsic metabolic changes and reduction in physical activity. Weight loss is a poorly sensitive indicator of sarcopenia, as increasing fat deposition can mask concurrent muscle loss [3].

At a microscopic level, sarcopenic muscle is characterized by a reduction in type II motor units and an associated loss of alpha motor neurons from the spinal cord. The contractile and mitochondrial protein synthesis rates of muscle are reduced with advancing age, resulting in loss of muscle mass and strength. As muscle mass decreases, there is also a lessened capacity for the mobilization of amino acids from muscle proteolysis for protein synthesis in vital organs and for immune processes. Physical inactivity leads to accelerated rates of muscle loss and can produce a cycle of falls, ie, increased fear of falling, reduced activity, muscle loss and increased falls [3, 23, 24].

### 3.1 Evaluation

Sarcopenia is identified by the presence of two of the following criteria: low muscle mass, low muscle strength, and low physical performance [25]. While low muscle mass and strength can be evaluated in the research setting using various imaging techniques and dynamic strength testing, most practical testing focuses on physical performance. The most commonly used office tests include usual gait speed and the short physical performance battery (SPPB). Slow gait speed is currently the simplest screen for sarcopenia, with a cutoff point of 0.8 m/s over a 4–6-m course as the threshold for poor performance [25]. The SPPB is a more time-intensive assessment, involving repeated chair stands, balance testing and gait speed measurements [26]. Sarcopenia is only typically quantified in research settings, using handgrip strength (so-called handgrip dynamometer) or knee extension strength (so-called isokinetic dynamometer).

### 3.2 Pathophysiology

Inactivity is one of the most prominent contributors to sarcopenia. Muscle contraction during exercise causes the release of muscle growth factors (IGF and mechano growth factor [MGF]) activating satellite cells, protein synthesis and muscle regeneration among other processes, all of which are decreased with aging. Nutritional deficiencies or insufficiencies also play a major role in the development of sarcopenia, as it is postulated that to maintain muscle mass an older adult requires at least 1.2 g of protein per kilogram of body weight per day.

Hormonal mediators such as testosterone also decline and contribute to the decline in muscle mass and to a lesser extent the decline in strength. This decline is more pronounced in females. Sarcopenia is also associated with elevated proinflammatory cytokines that also negatively impact muscle mass and function.

The major contributors to sarcopenia are delineated in **Table 1.11-2**.

### 3.3 Treatment

There are no standard or clearly safe drug treatments for sarcopenia. Current standard of care is focused on exercise and nutrition. Exercise can promote muscle anabolism, and this effect can become more pronounced with detailed training [1]. Even in very old individuals, resistance exercise has been reported to increase muscle mass and strength [24].

Testosterone and other anabolic steroids such as nandrolone have been shown to increase muscle mass and in higher doses muscle strength but can produce significant increase in cardiovascular risk [27].

Enobosarm is a potent oral selective androgen receptor molecule with tissue selectivity, still undergoing active study for both sarcopenia and osteoporosis treatment [28]. As such, it has been shown to improve lean body mass and measurements of physical function and power.

Other therapies such as myostatin antibodies have been developed and are still undergoing research, since they have shown to have no significant effect on muscle gain [29].

## 4 Frailty

Frailty refers to the general vulnerability of older or highly comorbid adults to physiological stress. It is related to the diminution of several interrelated physiological systems, beyond the expected gradual decrease in reserve that is seen with aging. This process results in the subsequent depletion of homeostatic reserve and vulnerability to disproportionate health complications after minor stressors [2].

Although frailty is not a specific disease, the frailty phenotype can be defined, measured and serves as one of the strongest and most useful factors in identifying fragility fracture patients at risk for surgical complications, perioperative morbidity and mortality, and poor functional prognosis [30-33].

Frailty is often clinically defined by the presence of three or more of the following: unintentional weight loss, self-reported exhaustion, weakness, slow walking speed, and low physical activity. See **Table 1.11-3** for formal criteria extracted from the Cardiovascular Health Study [34].

Simpler criteria (**Table1.11-4**) have been validated for falls and osteoporotic fractures as well, and are very easy to integrate into clinical physician or nursing practice. Frailty is increasingly predictive of falls, mortality and poor surgical outcomes [30, 31, 36].

| Domain | Contributor |
|---|---|
| Environmental | Malnutrition<br>Decreased physical activity |
| Vascular | Decreased capillary blood flow<br>Peripheral vascular disease |
| Endocrine | Insulin resistance<br>Decrease of hormones with anabolic properties (ie, testosterone, dehydroepiandrosterone, IGF 1, growth hormone) |
| Immunologic | Increased proinflammatory cytokines (ie, IL-6, TNF-α) |
| Genetic | Mitocondrial abnormalities |
| Neurogenic | Motor end plate degeneration<br>Peripheral neuropathy |

**Table 1.11-2** Major contributors to sarcopenia.
Abbreviations: IGF, insulin-like growth factor; IL, interleukin.

| Characteristic | Measure |
|---|---|
| Weight loss | Self-reported loss of more than 4.5 kg in prior year<br>Recorded loss of >5% of body weight in prior year |
| Exhaustion | 3–4 days per week or most of the time |
| Low-energy expenditure | Lowest quintile for gender<br>Men < 383 kcal/week<br>Women < 270 kcal/week |
| Slow gait speed | Lowest quintile for time to walk 4.57 m, adjusted for gender and height |
| Weak grip strength | Lowest quintile for grip strength, stratified by gender and body mass index |

**Table 1.11-3** Frailty phenotype—Fried criteria derive from the Cardiovascular Health Study [34].

Clinically important aspects of frailty include [2]:

- High prevalence in older adults, where 10–25% of persons aged 65 years and 30–45% of those aged 85 years and older are estimated to be frail [37]
- Highly associated with sarcopenia, exercise intolerance, frequent falls, immobility, and incontinence
- Poor response to standard medical and functional therapies
- Increased risk of functional decline and mortality

Although frailty is generally irreversible, exercise, protein-calorie supplementation, vitamin D, and reduction of polypharmacy may be able to slow its progression or delay complications [38, 39]. As noted previously, it is highly valuable in identifying patients with short life expectancies, poor prognosis for recovery, and poor responses to many traditional therapies.

### 4.1 Pathophysiology

Aging can be explained by the lifelong accumulation of molecular and cellular damage that is usually regulated by complex maintenance and repair network. There seem to be multiple organ systems that are closely interrelated in the development of frailty: the central nervous system, endocrine system, immune system, and skeletal muscle, mediated by intrinsic and extrinsic factors, such as nutritional status. Frailty results from and contributes to impairments in all of these areas. In 2009, Fried et al [34] used twelve measures to assess for cumulative dysfunction in aging women, reporting a nonlinear relation between the number of abnormal systems and frailty, independent of age and comorbidity. Abnormal results in three or more systems were a strong predictor of frailty, supporting the idea that there is an aggregate crucial level beyond which frailty becomes evident.

| Criteria | Points* |
|---|---|
| 5% weight loss over 1 year | 1 |
| Inability to do five chair stands without using arms | 1 |
| Feeling low energy | 1 |

**Table 1.11-4** Simple frailty screening tool, adapted from Ensrud et al [35].
*Points: 2–3 = frail
1 = prefrail
0 = robust

## 5 Malnutrition

Inadequate nutritional intake and malabsorption are common findings in hip fracture patients and associated with delirium, susceptibility to infection, poor recovery and mortality [40–42]. Alterations in taste, smell, mental status, depression, physical incapacity, dysphagia, medication side effects, chronic disease, and relative financial poverty are all contributors to the development of malnutrition [43].

Monitoring for weight loss in the community and particularly in the long-term care setting is the most common measure of quickly identifying those who may be at risk for nutritional insufficiency. There are several validated screening tools, including the simplified nutritional appetite questionnaire, the geriatric nutritional risk index, the Mini-Nutritional Assessment (MNA), or its 6-item version MNA-Short Form which can distinguish malnutrition from nutritional risk and normal nutritional status. Nutritional and swallowing assessments should be part of all fragility fracture programs.

### 5.1 Nutritional strategies

There is no high-quality evidence of improved outcomes to support specific nutritional supplementation strategies in hip fracture populations [44]. Current practice is to provide high protein, nutrient dense oral nutrition when able [45, 46], as well as to provide adequate calcium and vitamin D supplementation. Oral nutrition supplements seem to be of some value in preventing pressure ulcers in patients after hip fracture in the hospital and postacute care settings [47]. However, these studies are small and further investigation is required. Routine iron administration for the treatment of anemia has not been shown to be beneficial [48] and can be complicated by side effects, eg, dyspepsia, constipation.

Postoperative identification of oropharyngeal dysphagia is common; many patients likely have preexisting swallowing dysfunction and even small amounts of functional decline and precipitate inability to manage adequate swallowing from nutritional and respiratory standpoints. Invasive forms of nutritional supplementation, ie, nasogastric tube feeding, are not recommended, as they place older adults at risk for delirium as well as infectious complications, ie, aspiration pneumonia. Parenteral nutrition carries risk and expense as well.

Nutritional support and supplementation is an important component of functional optimization in older adults in the postacute setting. Therapeutic diets (eg, low fat or calorie restricted) should generally be avoided in the long-term care population [15]. In a 2009 systematic review, Milne and his colleagues [16] found 62 trials with more than 10,000 older adults at risk of malnutrition, who demonstrated a significant increase in weight of 2.2% with oral nutrition supplements (ONSs); however, the study failed to find mortality benefit or functional improvement in the treatment group. In another study of community-dwelling women [49], the combination of supplemental protein and exercise improved muscle mass and strength, and walking speed.

The American Geriatrics Society advocates for clinicians to avoid using prescription appetite stimulants or high-calorie ONS for treatment of anorexia or cachexia in older adults, and it encourages healthcare providers to instead optimize social supports, provide feeding assistance and clarify patient goals and expectations, particularly in patients with dementia [50, 51]. Oral nutrition supplements may be of limited benefit in specific subgroups, such as those with specific nutrient deficiencies, recently hospitalized patients, and patients recovering from fracture.

## 6 References

1. **Kinney JM.** Nutritional frailty, sarcopenia and falls in the elderly. *Curr Opin Clin Nutr Metab Care.* 2004 Jan;7(1):15–20.
2. **Fried LP, Waltson JD, Ferrucci L.** Frailty. In: Halter, JB, ed. *Hazzard's Geriatric Medicine and Gerontology.* 6th ed. New York: McGraw-Hill; 2009:631–645.
3. **Hebuterne X, Bermon S, Schneider SM.** Ageing and muscle: the effects of malnutrition, re-nutrition, and physical exercise. *Curr Opin Clin Nutr Metab Care.* 2001 Jul;4(4):295–300.
4. **Sudarsky L.** Geriatrics: gait disorders in the elderly. *N Engl J Med.* 1990 May 17;322(20):1441–1446.
5. **Toots A, Rosendahl E, Lundin-Olsson L, et al.** Usual gait speed independently predicts mortality in very old people: a population-based study. *J Am Med Dir Assoc.* 2013 Jul;14(7):529.e1–529.e6.
6. **Martin FC, Hart D, Spector T, et al.** Fear of falling limiting activity in young-old women is associated with reduced functional mobility rather than psychological factors. *Age Ageing.* 2005 May;34(3):281–287.
7. **Nowak A, Hubbard RE.** Falls and frailty: lessons from complex systems. *J R Soc Med.* 2009 Mar;102(3):98–102.
8. **Dionyssiotis Y.** Analyzing the problem of falls among older people. *Int J Gen Med.* 2012;5:805–813.
9. **Fuller GF.** Falls in the elderly. *Am Fam Physician.* 2000 Apr 01;61(7):2159–2168, 2173–2154.
10. **Panel on Prevention of Falls in Older Persons.** Summary of the Updated American Geriatrics Society/British Geriatrics Society clinical practice guideline for prevention of falls in older persons. *J Am Geriatr Soc.* 2011 Jan;59(1):148–157.
11. **Podsiadlo D, Richardson S.** The timed "Up & Go": a test of basic functional mobility for frail elderly persons. *J Am Geriatr Soc.* 1991 Feb;39(2):142–148.
12. **Close JC, Lord SR.** Fall assessment in older people. *BMJ.* 2011 Sep 14;343:d5153.
13. **Barry E, Galvin R, Keogh C, et al.** Is the Timed Up and Go test a useful predictor of risk of falls in community dwelling older adults: a systematic review and meta-analysis. *BMC Geriatr.* 2014 Feb 01;14:14.
14. **Tinetti ME.** Performance-oriented assessment of mobility problems in elderly patients. *J Am Geriatr Soc.* 1986 Feb;34(2):119–126.
15. **Messinger-Rapport BJ, Gammack JK, Little MO, et al.** Clinical update on nursing home medicine: 2014. *J Am Med Dir Assoc.* 2014;15(11):786–801.
16. **Milne AC, Potter J, Vivanti A, et al.** Protein and energy supplementation in elderly people at risk from malnutrition. *Cochrane Database Syst Rev.* 2009 Apr 15(2):CD003288.
17. **Vlaeyen E, Coussement J, Leysens G, et al.** Characteristics and effectiveness of fall prevention programs in nursing homes: a systematic review and meta-analysis of randomized controlled trials. *J Am Geriatr Soc.* 2015 Feb;63(2):211–221.
18. **Fiatarone MA, O'Neill EF, Ryan ND, et al.** Exercise training and nutritional supplementation for physical frailty in very elderly people. *N Engl J Med.* 1994 Jun 23;330(25):1769–1775.
19. **Laosa O, Alonso C, Castro M, et al.** Pharmaceutical interventions for frailty and sarcopenia. *Curr Pharm Des.* 2014;20(18):3068–3082.
20. **Vina J, Borras C, Sanchis-Gomar F, et al.** Pharmacological properties of physical exercise in the elderly. *Curr Pharm Des.* 2014;20(18):3019–3029.
21. **Rondanelli M, Faliva M, Monteferrario F, et al.** Novel insights on nutrient management of sarcopenia in elderly. *Biomed Res Int.* 2015;2015:524948.
22. **Muir SW, Montero-Odasso M.** Effect of vitamin D supplementation on muscle strength, gait and balance in older adults: a systematic review and meta-analysis. *J Am Geriatr Soc.* 2011 Dec;59(12):2291–2300.
23. **Janssen I.** The epidemiology of sarcopenia. *Clin Geriatr Med.* 2011 Aug;27(3):355–363.
24. **Fiatarone MA, O'Neill EF, Ryan ND, et al.** Exercise training and nutritional supplementation for physical frailty in very elderly people. *N Engl J Med.* 1994 Jun 23;330(25):1769–1775.
25. **Cruz-Jentoft AJ, Baeyens JP, Bauer JM, et al.** Sarcopenia: European consensus on definition and diagnosis: Report of the European Working Group on Sarcopenia in Older People. *Age Ageing.* 2010 Jul;39(4):412–423.
26. **Perera S, Mody SH, Woodman RC, et al.** Meaningful change and responsiveness in common physical performance measures in older adults. *J Am Geriatr Soc.* 2006 May;54(5):743–749.
27. **Morley JE.** Sarcopenia in the elderly. *Fam Pract.* 2012 Apr;29(Suppl 1):i44–i48.
28. **Girgis CM, Mokbel N, Digirolamo DJ.** Therapies for musculoskeletal disease: can we treat two birds with one stone? *Curr Osteoporos Rep.* 2014 Jun;12(2):142–153.
29. **Morley JE, von Haehling S, Anker SD.** Are we closer to having drugs to treat muscle wasting disease? *J Cachexia Sarcopenia Muscle.* 2014 Jun;5(2):83–87.
30. **Krishnan M, Beck S, Havelock W, et al.** Predicting outcome after hip fracture: using a frailty index to integrate comprehensive geriatric assessment results. *Age Ageing.* 2014 Jan;43(1):122–126.
31. **Kistler EA, Nicholas JA, Kates SL, et al.** Frailty and Short-Term Outcomes in Patients With Hip Fracture. *Geriatr Orthop Surg Rehabil.* 2015 Sep;6(3):209–214.

32. **Rolland Y, Abellan van Kan G, Benetos A, et al.** Frailty, osteoporosis and hip fracture: causes, consequences and therapeutic perspectives. *J Nutr Health Aging.* 2008 May;12(5):335–346.
33. **Kua J, Ramason R, Rajamoney G, et al.** Which frailty measure is a good predictor of early post-operative complications in elderly hip fracture patients? *Arch Orthop Trauma Surg.* 2016 May;136(5):639–647.
34. **Fried LP, Tangen CM, Walston J, et al.** Frailty in older adults: evidence for a phenotype. *J Gerontol A Biol Sci Med Sci.* 2001 Mar;56(3):M146–M156.
35. **Ensrud KE, Ewing SK, Taylor BC, et al.** Comparison of 2 frailty indexes for prediction of falls, disability, fractures, and death in older women. *Arch Intern Med.* 2008 Feb 25;168(4):382–389.
36. **Makary MA, Segev DL, Pronovost PJ, et al.** Frailty as a predictor of surgical outcomes in older patients. *J Am Coll Surg.* 2010 Jun;210(6):901–908.
37. **Ferrucci L, Guralnik JM, Studenski S, et al.** Designing randomized, controlled trials aimed at preventing or delaying functional decline and disability in frail, older persons: a consensus report. *J Am Geriatr Soc.* 2004 Apr;52(4):625–634.
38. **Regional Health Council.** Frailty in elderly people. Florence (Italy): Regione Toscana, Consiglio Sanitario Regionale; 2013. Available at: www.guideline.gov/summaries/summary/47484. Accessed December 2017.
39. **Turner G, Clegg A.** Best practice guidelines for the management of frailty: a British Geriatrics Society, Age UK and Royal College of General Practitioners report. *Age Ageing.* 2014 Nov;43(6):744–747.
40. **Koren-Hakim T, Weiss A, Hershkovitz A, et al.** The relationship between nutritional status of hip fracture operated elderly patients and their functioning, comorbidity and outcome. *Clin Nutr.* 2012 Dec;31(6):917–921.
41. **Bell JJ, Bauer JD, Capra S, et al.** Multidisciplinary, multi-modal nutritional care in acute hip fracture inpatients—results of a pragmatic intervention. *Clin Nutr.* 2014 Dec;33(6):1101–1107.
42. **Juliebo V, Bjoro K, Krogseth M, et al.** Risk factors for preoperative and postoperative delirium in elderly patients with hip fracture. *J Am Geriatr Soc.* 2009 Aug;57(8):1354–1361.
43. **Bell CL, Tamura BK, Masaki KH, et al.** Prevalence and measures of nutritional compromise among nursing home patients: weight loss, low body mass index, malnutrition, and feeding dependency, a systematic review of the literature. *J Am Med Dir Assoc.* 2013 Feb;14(2):94–100.
44. **Avenell A, Smith TO, Curtain JP, et al.** Nutritional supplementation for hip fracture aftercare in older people. *Cochrane Database Syst Rev.* 2016 Nov 30(11):CD001880.
45. **Roberts KC, Brox WT, Jevsevar DS, et al.** Management of hip fractures in the elderly. *J Am Acad Orthop Surg.* 2015 Feb;23(2):131–137.
46. **Eneroth M, Olsson UB, Thorngren KG.** Nutritional supplementation decreases hip fracture-related complications. *Clin Orthop Relat Res.* 2006 Oct;451:212–217.
47. **Houwing RH, Rozendaal M, Wouters-Wesseling W, et al.** A randomised, double-blind assessment of the effect of nutritional supplementation on the prevention of pressure ulcers in hip-fracture patients. *Clin Nutr.* 2003 Aug;22(4):401–405.
48. **Parker MJ.** Iron supplementation for anemia after hip fracture surgery: a randomized trial of 300 patients. *J Bone Joint Surg Am.* 2010 Feb;92(2):265–269.
49. **Kim HK, Suzuki T, Saito K, et al.** Effects of exercise and amino acid supplementation on body composition and physical function in community-dwelling elderly Japanese sarcopenic women: a randomized controlled trial. *J Am Geriatr Soc.* 2012 Jan;60(1):16–23.
50. **Hanson LC, Ersek M, Gilliam R, et al.** Oral feeding options for people with dementia: a systematic review. *J Am Geriatr Soc.* 2011 Mar;59(3):463–472.
51. **American Geriatrics Society.** Ten Things Clinicians and Patients Should Question. Available at: www.choosingwisely.org/wp-content/uploads/2015/02/AGS-Choosing-Wisely-List.pdf Accessed January 22, 2017.

# 1.12 Pain management

Timothy Holahan, Daniel A Mendelson

## 1 Introduction

Uncontrolled pain is a common contributor to poor outcomes in both medical and surgical settings. Treatment of acute, chronic and perioperative pain in older adults with hip fractures has been recognized as inadequate [1–3]. Pain management is particularly complicated in older adults due to the significant physiological and cognitive vulnerabilities of this population. In light of the many factors necessary to achieve safe and adequate pain control, a thoughtful and thorough approach is required to appropriately treat pain in the perioperative period [3–5].

### 1.1 Prevalence of preexisting pain

Estimates of chronic pain range from 20% to 46% in community-dwelling older adults and from 28% to 73% in older adults living in residential care facilities or nursing homes [6]. The prevalence of daily pain tends to increase with age with as many as 75% of adults older than 75 years reporting pain [6, 9]. The prevalence appears to be higher in women [6].

### 1.2 Recognition

Older adults with cognitive impairment are a specific high-risk group for poor pain control, due both to inadequate recognition and a tendency to undertreatment [6]. Identification of pain is particularly challenging in the perioperative and postoperative period when delirium and medical instability complicate the clinical assessment.

Reasons for underrecognition and undertreatment of pain in older adults include difficulties in assessment, particularly in patients with dementia, fear of side effects and overdose, and general provider uncertainty regarding the response to opioids in a highly complex and comorbid population.

A reluctance to use standing orders for analgesics in hip fracture patients after surgery illustrates this issue [10].

### 1.3 Negative effects of poor pain control

Regardless of the underlying cause, uncontrolled pain has negative effects on the physiology and clinical outcomes in older adults, especially in the inpatient setting. Pain is a contributor to tachycardia and myocardial oxygen consumption [3]. Poor pain control in hip fracture patients has been shown to lead to increased rates of postoperative delirium, increased length of stay and poor participation in therapy [3]. Uncontrolled pain delays postoperative ambulation and time to recovery. Decreased rates of delirium and early ambulation have been shown to reduce length of stay and postoperative complications including pneumonia [11]. While there is a paucity of evidence about the impact of specific pain regimens on hip fracture outcomes [12], improved pain control is suspected to lead to less morbidity in hip fracture patients postoperatively [10].

### 1.4 Unique pain pathophysiology in older adults

The neurophysiological mechanism of pain in older adults has been shown to be substantially altered when compared to the pathways in younger adults. Neurochemical and electrophysiological aspects of nociceptive pain pathways change as a person ages [4]. There is a known age-related loss in several relevant neurotransmitters including serotonin, gamma-aminobutyric acid as well as in opioid receptors, and a decrease in the function of the descending inhibitory pain pathway. A slight increase in pain threshold, or a reduced sensitivity to mild pain, has been demonstrated in older adults, particularly to thermal stimuli [13].

From a treatment perspective, frail older adults typically have reduced capacities for drug absorption, distribution and metabolism, and a higher risk for drug toxicity [14]. There is also evidence to suggest that the physiological response to pain may be blunted in older adults with dementia [15].

**Table 1.12-1** [16] summarizes the many physiological and pharmacokinetic changes that are common in older adults. These factors are the basis for the unique issues with pain assessment, management, and expected response to therapy in older adults [15].

### 1.5 Types of pain

While the specific nature and intensity of pain is subjective, clinically meaningful categories exist. Pain can be usefully characterized as acute or chronic, and further divided into different pathophysiological subtypes [17]:

- Acute pain is characterized by an abrupt onset, linked to a specific insult and only lasts for a relatively short period of time.
- Chronic pain persists for more than 3–6 months and is characterized by the ongoing pain in the absence of specifically identified stimuli. Lower socioeconomic status, inactivity, chronic illness, and lack of social support are some of the factors that have been associated with the development of chronic pain in older adults [17].

There are three different pathophysiological subtypes of pain: nociceptive, neuropathic and mixed [4]:

- Nociceptive pain is due to the activation of sensory receptors by noxious stimuli, and can be further divided into either somatic or visceral pain. Somatic pain tends to originate in the skin, muscle or bone and is often easily localized. Pain related to an acute hip fracture is typically a nociceptive, somatic type of pain. Visceral pain is a referred pain originating from an internal organ such as the heart, lungs or gastrointestinal (GI) tract. Usually visceral pain is relatively difficult to localize and is described as aching, dull or vague.
- Neuropathic pain is caused by irritation or inflammation of nerve fibers and/or neurons, and is usually described as burning, tingling or numbness. It is usually localized easily but may have a radiating component that follows the path of the nerve itself. This can also be seen in hip fracture patients postoperatively if nerve fibers were disturbed during the fracture or the procedure or by postoperative edema and inflammation. Neuropathic pain may have a variable or inadequate response to typical pain medications, including antiinflammatory analgesics or opioids. Nontraditional pain medications like anticonvulsants and antidepressants may be more effective for neuropathic pain.
- The third subtype of pain is a mixed type with features of both nociceptive and neuropathic pain; this typically requires multiple different modalities to treat adequately. One example of this mixed type is a vertebral fracture with nerve impingement resulting in both somatic and neuropathic components [4, 16, 18].

## 2 Pain assessment

While pain assessment can be difficult in any patient population, it can be particularly challenging in the fragility fracture patient due to the high prevalence of cognitive and communication impairments. The most common and valid methods for pain assessment include patient self-report, visual rating scales, and behavioral pain assessment tools for patients unable to effectively communicate.

| | Changes in older adults | Clinical effect |
|---|---|---|
| Gastrointestinal absorption | Decrease in GI transit time<br>Bowel more sensitive to opioid dysmotility<br>Altered gastric pH (usually from other medications) | More prolonged effect of sustained release pain medications<br>Increased risk of side effects such as constipation<br>Variable absorption of medications |
| Drug distribution | Decrease in lean body mass and increase in lipid distribution | Could lead to longer drug half-life and increased risk of drug side effects |
| Drug metabolism | Decreased oxidation of medications in the liver | Increased drug half-life and increased risk of drug side effects |
| Drug excretion | Glomerular filtration rate decreases with age | Decreased rate of excretion of drug<br>Increased risk of accumulation of toxic metabolites |

**Table 1.12-1** Pharmacological changes in older adults. Adapted from: American Geriatrics Society Panel on Pharmacological Management of Persistent Pain in Older Persons [16].
Abbreviation: GI, gastrointestinal.

Pain is one of the major obstacles to good surgical and functional outcomes, and is typically present in all but the most minor of orthopedic trauma. Accurate assessment requires a thoughtful and methodical approach based on staff observation, physical exam, and the use of validated pain assessment tools. Improved perioperative pain control is a cornerstone of delirium prevention, preservation of function and avoidance of complications [3, 10, 11].

## 2.1 Self-report

Self-report is the primary method in pain assessment for older adults. This should be attempted first; if the patient is unable to respond appropriately, then other clinical indicators of pain should be sought. Autonomic symptoms such as diaphoresis, hypertension and tachycardia can sometimes suggest a high likelihood of pain. The following scales are commonly used for pain assessment:

- The numerical rating scale (NRS) is a verbally obtained numerical pain scale ranging from 0 to 10 (0 is considered no pain and 10 is considered the most severe pain imaginable); patients are asked to ascribe a number to their pain from this continuum. The NRS is the most common and most valid pain scale in older adults capable of self-report [19].
- The Visual Analog Scale is a related tool that prompts a patient to indicate a pain rating on a printed line between two extremes of no pain (0) and excruciating pain (10). This has been shown to be less effective in older adults and has a higher error rate [20].
- The Verbal Descriptor Scale (VDS) has also been validated in older adults and consists of verbal indicators (eg, mild, moderate, severe) to quantify the intensity of a patient's pain. The VDS is preferred by older adults and has been demonstrated to be effective in moderate and severe dementia [19].
- Other self-report options include the Faces Pain Scale, commonly used in children but has also been validated in older adults [21]. It requires the patient to identify the facial expression which best indicates the pain they are experiencing. This can be helpful in older adults who are nonverbal.

All of these tools have limitations including inability to describe pain location, problems with identifying dynamic pain with activity, and inaccuracies with monitoring the response to the treatment of chronic pain.

## 2.2 Cognitively impaired patients

The assessment of pain in a nonverbal or severely cognitively impaired patient can present a dilemma for clinicians and nurses. In order to obtain an accurate assessment, clinician and staff observation of nonverbal indicators is necessary. The American Geriatrics Society (AGS) recommends the evaluation of six behavioral domains including facial expressions, verbalizations/vocalizations, body movements, changes in interpersonal interactions, changes in activity patterns, and changes in mental status [16].

A number of behavioral pain assessment tools have been validated for use in older adults with severe cognitive impairment [20]. These include the Pain Assessment in Advanced Dementia scale [8], which consists of five items that aid in the interpretation of nonverbal pain as seen in **Table 1.12-2**.

Other validated scales include the Abbey pain scale and the pain assessment checklist for seniors with limited ability to communicate [20, 21]. All of these can be used to assess and track acute pain as well as measure the effectiveness of the treatment.

| | 0 | 1 | 2 |
|---|---|---|---|
| Breathing (independent of vocalization) | Normal | Occasional labored breathing | Noisy labored breathing<br>Long period of hyperventilation |
| Negative vocalization | None | Occasional moan or groan | Loud moaning or groaning<br>Crying |
| Facial expression | Smiling<br>No expression | Sad<br>Frightened<br>Frowning | Facial grimacing |
| Body language | Relaxed | Tense<br>Distressed pacing<br>Fidgety | Rigid<br>Fists clenched<br>Knees pulled up<br>Pulling or pushing away |
| Consolability | No need to console | Distracted<br>Reassured by voice or touch | Unable to console, distract or reassure |

**Table 1.12-2** Pain assessment in advanced dementia (adapted from the Pain Assessment in Advanced Dementia scale).
A possible interpretation of the scores is:
1–3 = mild pain; 4–6 = moderate pain; > 6 = severe pain

## 3 Treatment

As previously described, there are physiological changes that occur in older adults that can affect the efficacy and tolerance of pain medications and limit the effectiveness of nonstandardized pain management strategies in older adults. Using a standardized and predictable approach can significantly reduce adverse effects while improving pain control [4, 6, 15, 16]. This is especially true in postoperative patients when blood loss, dehydration, and changes in mental status can lead to uncertainty regarding appropriate pharmacological and nonpharmacological treatment.

### 3.1 General principles

The first principle is "start low and go slow" as recommended by the AGS. This refers to using the lowest dose possible when starting a medication in an older adult and titrating up slowly until the desired effect is achieved. In light of the reduced metabolic capabilities of older adults, this principle is useful when starting any medication, and similarly important to the development of standardized treatment.

A second principle is to maximize the use of nonpharmacological modalities to treat pain. The third one is to be attentive for common adverse effects of (and other) medications, allowing for early recognition and adjustment to prevent further morbidity [14, 15].

### 3.2 Nonpharmacological interventions

Nonpharmacological interventions, eg, early surgery, early mobilization, positioning, and ice have an excellent benefit to risk ratio, and should be a consistent part of pain control strategies in both the pre- and postoperative setting:

- Early mobilization and physical therapy are likely to contribute to adequate pain control and lead to reductions in overall mortality, reduced length of stay, and physical disability [22]. A delay in ambulation postoperatively promotes postoperative delirium and pneumonia as well as prolonged pain [11].
- Ice applied before and after physical therapy can reduce inflammation and lead to reductions in pain. Care should be taken not to injure the skin by overexposure.
- Other therapies such as massage therapy, acupuncture/acupressure, and use of transcutaneous electrical nerve stimulation (TENS) units have also helped in the management of postoperative pain in selected hip fracture patients. Limited data suggests TENS units can accelerate recovery in range of movement and lead to a reduction in pain after hip surgery [23]. Acupressure has also been shown to reduce pain in hip fracture patients preoperatively [24]. These interventions are safe and can complement the pharmacological management of pain and lead to lower medication dosing and reduced adverse effects.
- Traction is not typically used in high-performing fracture centers due to risks of skin injury and delirium in this population [25].

Nonpharmacological interventions are recommended by the American Academy of Orthopaedic Surgeons [5] to treat perioperative and postoperative pain after hip fracture in older adults, supporting the multidisciplinary and multimodal approach necessary to treat pain in some older adults effectively.

### 3.3 Pharmacological interventions

Pharmacological agents, including opioids and acetaminophen, are necessary for pain control in virtually all hip fracture patients during both the preoperative and postoperative phases:

- For patients without liver disease or other contraindications, most current protocols utilize immediate use of scheduled dose acetaminophen and scheduled doses of opioids or as needed (eg, morphine, oxycodone, hydromorphone).
- Nonsteroidal antiinflammatory medications (eg, ibuprofen, naproxen sodium, ketorolac) are avoided in the perioperative phase due to cardiovascular, renal, and cognitive effects.
- Combination medications (eg, acetaminophen plus opioid) typically fail to allow appropriate dosing of the individual components.

| | **Usual starting doses*** |
|---|---|
| Morphine immediate release (low potency) | 2.5–5 mg by mouth every 3–4 hours as needed<br>2–4 mg intravenously every 3–4 hours as needed |
| Oxycodone immediate release (moderate potency) | 2.5–5 mg by mouth every 3–4 hours as needed<br>No intravenous formulation available |
| Hydromorphone (high potency) | 1–2 mg by mouth every 3–4 hours as needed<br>0.25–0.5 mg intravenously every 2–3 hours as needed |

**Table 1.12-3** Usual starting doses for acute pain in opioid naïve older adults.
* Please note that the initial starting does recommended for older adults (> 65 years old) are approximately half the starting dose for younger opioid naïve adults. Intravenous preparations are more potent compared to a similar dose in an oral preparation.

- Specific dosing and monitoring recommendations can be found through the AOTrauma Orthogeriatrics Pain smartphone app [25], as well as the American College of Surgeons' National Surgical Quality Improvement Program/AGS best practice guidelines for preoperative assessment of the geriatric surgical patient [26].

### 3.3.1 Opioids

Opioid preparations are often necessary to provide optimal pain relief in the perioperative setting for geriatric patients, and can be used safely. Medical and surgical clinicians should acquire familiarity with common issues related to adequate dosing, side effects and toxicities of specific opioid preparations:

#### Opioid preparation, dose, and route considerations

Oral opioid administration offers a longer duration of action, but also a longer time to onset (up to 1 hour). Using parenteral medications in older adults requires clinician attention to avoid excessive sedation, nausea, or delirium. Different opioids have different potencies and careful selection is important (Table 1.12-3). Sustained release formulations are usually not necessary in older adults for whom the half-life of short-acting opioids is typically prolonged. For younger patients with normal renal function, sustained release preparations may be helpful to meet more significant opioid requirements, and reduce the need for frequent additional doses. Transdermal fentanyl is generally not appropriate in the acute setting due to prolonged onset/peak (12–24 hours) and offset (12–24 hours), and it can be difficult to calculate rescue/breakthrough doses. Parenteral fentanyl may be useful but because of short duration and potency, it is often limited to monitored settings such as operating room, post-anesthesia care unit, and intensive care unit.

#### Long-term opioid therapy

Patients on long-term opioid therapy are likely to require modestly increased opioid dosing for perioperative pain control. Acute reductions in routine home doses may precipitate opioid withdrawal. One option for patients with significant opioid tolerance due to long-term therapy includes continuing the long-acting home regimen, and ordering 10–30% of this total dose as a short-acting equivalent every 2–3 hours as needed for breakthrough pain. Patients may need a 25–50% increase in baseline long-term regimen in the perioperative period. We recommend titrating doses based on pain assessment and side effect monitoring. Medical or pain specialist consultation for the pain management of patients on long-term opioid therapy may be appropriate [27].

#### Opioid side effects

Opioids have multiple side effects that need to be identified, treated, and prevented when possible (**Table 1.12-4**) [7, 28].

One of the most common and serious side effects of opioid medications is constipation, mostly through a direct effect on gut motility, with contributions from decreased oral intake, hydration and immobility. Since constipation is already a common issue in the older adult population, a constipation protocol for all patients is typically warranted. Scheduled doses of bowel stimulants (eg, sennosides) and an osmotic laxative (eg, polyethylene glycol or lactulose), in addition to early ambulation and physical therapy, can limit constipation. Once a bowel movement is achieved, the regimen can be reduced if needed. For patients who develop severe opioid-induced constipation resistant to multiple therapies, a μ-opioid-receptor antagonist such as methylnaltrexone may be indicated but should only be used in consultation with a geriatrician or GI specialist.

Nausea and vomiting can be a side effect of opioid therapy although this is not commonly seen with low-dose regimens and typically resolves after the first few days of therapy. Managing constipation, lowering doses, switching opioids or treatment with antiemetics is usually effective [29].

Respiratory depression is perhaps the most feared side effect of opioid therapy. It is typically seen with high doses and/or rapid dose titration. The risk may also be increased in older adults with previous respiratory pathology or who are taking concurrent sedating medications. Sedation almost always occurs prior to clinically significant respiratory depression so careful monitoring can help identify at-risk patients.

| Opioid side effect | Treatment |
|---|---|
| Mild to moderate constipation | Early ambulation<br>Scheduled sennoside and polyethylene glycol or lactulose |
| Severe constipation (no bowel movement in > 4 days) | Bisacodyl suppository<br>Enema<br>Methyl naltrexone (as last resort and in consultation with geriatrician) |
| Nausea and vomiting | Treat constipation<br>Antiemetics<br>Lower opioid dose<br>Opioid rotation |
| Delirium | Ensure adequate treatment of pain<br>Consider opioid rotation |

**Table 1.12-4** Opioid side effects and treatment strategies.

Naloxone is an opioid antagonist used to reverse respiratory depression. However, it can precipitate a pain crisis and lead to worsening delirium in a postoperative patient. Naloxone should only be used if significant respiratory depression (< 6 breaths per minute) or worsening hypoxia is present. Usually, appropriate dose reduction is sufficient to prevent any life-threatening respiratory depression and the use of an opioid antagonist should rarely be needed. Naloxone also has a significant side effect profile particularly in the older adult [30].

Concerns for opioid-induced delirium or cognitive impairment can be confused with delirium caused by poorly controlled pain [10]. In general, it can be assumed that almost all hip fracture patients will require opioids for adequate pain control, even if they are unable to communicate this need. Uncontrolled pain is likely to precipitate delirium, and appropriate pain treatment has been demonstrated to reduce the incidence of delirium in hip fracture cohorts [10]. Trials of small doses of opioids are often necessary to distinguish these causes. Synthetic opioids (eg, oxycodone, hydromorphone) may lead to less delirium than morphine [31, 32].

### 3.3.2 Preoperative pain control

In the preoperative period, modest doses of intravenous (IV) opioids (eg, morphine sulfate 2–4 mg every 1–2 hours as needed) are typically necessary to achieve rapid and effective pain relief.

Using protocols and order sets facilitates safe initial dosing and can promote more clinician familiarity with medication effectiveness and toxicities. See chapter 2.7 Protocol and order set development for more information on protocols and order set development.

Acute femoral nerve blockade is another excellent option to improve pain control and to achieve a reduction in opioid needs; this has been best studied in the emergency department setting [33, 34]. Nerve blocks are most appropriate in the preoperative setting, as postoperative nerve blocks can limit mobility. Nerve blockade has been shown to reduce the risk of delirium, presumably through improved pain control and reduced opioid use [12]. Peripheral nerve blocks include fascia iliaca blockade and femoral nerve blockade with local anesthetic. Fascia iliaca blockade may be performed by nonanesthesia personnel; femoral nerve blockade typically involves consulting an anesthesiologist and the use of ultrasound-guided technology. Preoperative femoral nerve block can also provide some degree of postoperative pain control. All of these techniques complement the use of systemic pain medications and can provide some opioid-sparing benefits in the short term. See chapter 1.3 Principles of orthogeriatric anesthesia for more details.

### 3.3.3 Postoperative pain control

After surgical fixation, IV opioids are usually not required, and the risks of continued administration like excessive sedation and short duration can outweigh the benefits. Routine acetaminophen and low-dose oral opioids are generally safe and effective, along with nonpharmacological methods including extremity positioning, ice and mobilization (**Table 1.12-5**).

Acetaminophen (650–1,000 mg three times per day) is typically the first line oral agent chosen due to its low incidence of side effects.

Combination medications of acetaminophen with an opioid increase the hazard of inadvertent acetaminophen overdose, and otherwise limit the ability to titrate opioid doses. There are no GI or renal side effects described with the use of acetaminophen in older adults. In addition to routine acetaminophen, a low-dose, moderate potency opioid should be available for moderate to severe pain (ie, oxycodone 2.5–5 mg every 3 hours as needed). If this dosing is inadequate, then a dose increase of 25–50% is usually appropriate while monitoring for any new adverse effects.

Cognitively impaired persons frequently have difficulty with pain assessment and inability to request pain medications.

| Clinical setting | Dosing and strategies |
|---|---|
| Preoperative dosing:<br>Frail older adult<br>Chronic kidney disease | Acetaminophen:<br>650–1,000 mg orally three times per day<br>Routinely scheduled<br>Morphine sulfate:<br>2–4 mg intravenously every 2 hours as needed<br>OR<br>Hydromorphone:<br>0.25–0.5 mg intravenously every 2 hours as needed |
| Postoperative dosing:<br>Frail older adult<br>Chronic kidney disease | Acetaminophen:<br>650–1,000 mg orally three times per day, routinely scheduled<br>Oxycodone:<br>2.5–5 mg orally every 3 hours as needed<br>OR<br>Hydromorphone:<br>1–2 mg orally every 3 hours as needed |
| Other situations | More robust patients may need higher dosing to achieve adequate pain control<br>For patients unable to report pain adequately, schedule doses of opiates may be necessary |

**Table 1.12-5** Pain medication dosing guidelines.

Scheduled analgesic medications, with instructions to hold for excessive sedation, are necessary in these situations where inadequately controlled pain is suspected. It is also appropriate to schedule analgesic medications prior to situational pain episodes such as a dressing changing or prior to physical therapy, and may improve participation in therapy-reduced pain afterwards.

### 3.3.4 Problematic medications

- Nonsteroidal antiinflammatory drugs (NSAIDs) are contraindicated in patients with known chronic kidney disease, cerebrovascular disease, bleeding disorders, congestive heart failure, or heart disease, and carry significantly increased risk of adverse effects including GI bleeding, myocardial ischemia, heart failure and delirium. Nonsteroidal antiinflammatory drugs are also listed on the AGS Beers Criteria for medications to avoid in older adults [35].
- Cyclooxygenase 2 (COX-2) inhibitors such as celecoxib purport to have less GI effects, but have the same renal toxicities and are usually avoided in the dynamic postoperative period. Some COX-2 inhibitors have been withdrawn from the market due to associated cardiovascular events.
- Proton pump inhibitors (PPIs) can be prescribed concomitantly with NSAIDs to provide a GI protective effect, but PPIs have their own risks (eg, *Clostridium dificile* infection, osteoporosis, pneumonia) and do not mitigate the renal and cardiovascular toxicities of NSAIDs or COX-2 inhibitors.
- Tramadol is a combined opioid agonist and serotonin/norepinephrine reuptake inhibitor with a significant side effect profile including delirium, nausea, headaches, sweating and tremors. It is not tolerated by up to one-third of patients due to these adverse effects [27]. One study implicated its use as a risk factor for new hip fracture [36].
- Meperidine use has largely fallen out of favor due to severe delirium, especially in older adults, and numerous other toxic effects [10].
- Muscle relaxants (eg, cyclobenzaprine, benzodiazepines) have a poor side effect profile in older adults.
- Gabapentin, pregabalin, and duloxetine all have significant risks for delirium and medication interactions during the dynamic perioperative period. In general, they should not be initiated for standard hip fracture pain.

### 3.3.5 Patient controlled analgesia

Patient-controlled analgesia (PCA) is problematic for cognitively impaired patients, and carries the disadvantage of restricting mobility. It is typically not appropriate for use in most older FFPs. It is important to consider consultation with geriatrics and/or a pain management specialist when using a PCA in an older patient, since intense monitoring of side effects and attenuated dosing may be needed.

## 4 References


1. **Markey, G, Rabbani, W, and Kelly, P.** Association of dementia with delayed ED analgesia in patients over 70 with acute musculoskeletal injury. *Emerg Med J.* 2013;30(10):875.
2. **McDermott JH, Nichols DR, Lovell ME.** A case-control study examining inconsistencies in pain management following fractured neck of femur: an inferior analgesia for the cognitively impaired. *Emerg Med J.* 2014 Oct;31(e1):e2–e8.
3. **Morrison RS, Magaziner J, McLaughlin MA, et al.** The impact of post-operative pain on outcomes following hip fracture. *Pain.* 2003 Jun;103(3):303–311.
4. **Bruckenthal P.** Pain in the Older Adult. In: Fillit HM, Rockwood K, Woodhouse K, eds. *Brocklehurst's textbook of geriatric medicine and gerontology.* 7th ed. Philadelphia: Saunders/Elsevier Health Sciences; 2010:965–972.
5. **American Academy of Orthopaedic Surgeons (AAOS).** Management of Hip Fractures in the Elderly: Evidence Based Clinical Practice Guideline. Adopted by the American Academy of Orthopaedic Surgeons Board of Directors, September 5, 2014. Available at: http://www.aaos.org/research/guidelines/HipFxGuideline_rev.pdf. Accessed 2014.
6. **Abdulla A, Adams N, Bone M, et al.** Guidance on the management of pain in older people. *Age Ageing.* 2013 Mar;42 Suppl 1:i1–57.
7. **Achterberg WP, Pieper MJ, van Dalen-Kok AH, et al.** Pain management in patients with dementia. *Clin Interv Aging.* 2013;8:1471–1482.
8. **Warden V, Hurley AC, Volicer L.** Development and psychometric evaluation of the Pain Assessment in Advanced Dementia (PAINAD) scale. *J Am Med Dir Assoc.* 2003 Jan–Feb;4(1):9–15.
9. **Brattberg G, Thorslund M, Wikman A.** The prevalence of pain in a general population. The results of a postal survey in a county of Sweden. *Pain.* 1989 May;37(2):215–222.
10. **Morrison RS, Magaziner J, Gilbert M, et al.** Relationship between pain and opioid analgesics on the development of delirium following hip fracture. *J Gerontol A Biol Sci Med Sci.* 2003 Jan;58(1):76–81.

11. **Kamel HK, Iqbal MA, Mogallapu R, et al.** Time to ambulation after hip fracture surgery: relation to hospitalization outcomes. *J Gerontol A Biol Sci Med Sci.* 2003 Nov;58(11):1042–1045.
12. **Abou-Setta AM, Beaupre LA, Rashiq S, et al.** Comparative effectiveness of pain management interventions for hip fracture: a systematic review. *Ann Intern Med.* 2011 Aug 16;155(4):234–245.
13. **Gibson SJ, Farrell M.** A review of age differences in the neurophysiology of nociception and the perceptual experience of pain. *Clin J Pain.* 2004 Jul-Aug;20(4):227–239.
14. **McLachlan AJ, Bath S, Naganathan V, et al.** Clinical pharmacology of analgesic medicines in older people: impact of frailty and cognitive impairment. *Br J Clin Pharmacol.* 2011 Mar;71(3):351–364.
15. **Kunz M, Mylius V, Schepelmann K, et al.** Effects of age and mild cognitive impairment on the pain response system. *Gerontology.* 2009;55(6):674–682.
16. **American Geriatrics Society Panel on Pharmacological Management of Persistent Pain in Older Persons.** Pharmacological management of persistent pain in older persons. *J Am Geriatr Soc.* 2009 Aug;57(8):1331–1346.
17. **Periyakoil VS.** Persistent Pain. In: Durso SC, Sullivan GM, eds. *Geriatrics Review Syllabus: A Core Curriculum in Geriatric Medicine.* 8th edition. New York American Geriatrics Society 2013:128–139.
18. **Tosounidis TH, Sheikh H, Stone MH, et al.** Pain relief management following proximal femoral fractures: Options, issues and controversies. *Injury.* 2015 Nov;46 Suppl 5:S52–58.
19. **Lukas A, Niederecker T, Gunther I, et al.** Self- and proxy report for the assessment of pain in patients with and without cognitive impairment: experiences gained in a geriatric hospital. *Z Gerontol Geriatr.* 2013 Apr;46(3):214–221.
20. **Hadjistavropoulos T, Herr K, Prkachin KM, et al.** Pain assessment in elderly adults with dementia. *Lancet Neurol.* 2014 Dec;13(12):1216–1227.
21. **Corbett A, Husebo B, Malcangio M, et al.** Assessment and treatment of pain in people with dementia. *Nat Rev Neurol.* 2012 Apr 10;8(5):264–274.
22. **Siu AL, Penrod JD, Boockvar KS, et al.** Early ambulation after hip fracture: effects on function and mortality. *Arch Intern Med.* 2006 Apr 10;166(7):766–771.
23. **Gorodetskyi IG, Gorodnichenko AI, Tursin PS, et al.** Non-invasive interactive neurostimulation in the post-operative recovery of patients with a trochanteric fracture of the femur. A randomised, controlled trial. *J Bone Joint Surg Br.* 2007 Nov;89(11):1488–1494.
24. **Barker R, Kober A, Hoerauf K, et al.** Out-of-hospital auricular acupressure in elder patients with hip fracture: a randomized double-blinded trial. *Acad Emerg Med.* 2006 Jan;13(1):19–23.
25. **American Academy of Orthopaedic Surgeons (AAOS).** Management of Hip Fractures in the Elderly: Summary. Available at: http://www.aaos.org/Research/guidelines/HipFxSummaryofRecommendations.pdf. Accessed September 2014.
26. **ACS NSQIP/AGS.** Best Practice Guidelines: Optimal Preoperative Assessment of the Geriatric Surgical Patient. Available at: www.facs.org/~/media/files/quality%20programs/nsqip/acsnsqipagsgeriatric2012guidelines.ashx. Accessed 2012.
27. **Schofield PA.** The assessment and management of peri-operative pain in older adults. *Anaesthesia.* 2014 Jan;69(Suppl 1):54–60.
28. **O'Neil CK, Hanlon JT, Marcum ZA.** Adverse effects of analgesics commonly used by older adults with osteoarthritis: focus on non-opioid and opioid analgesics. *Am J Geriatr Pharmacother.* 2012 Dec;10(6):331–342.
29. **Webster LR.** Opioid-Induced Constipation. *Pain Med.* 2015 Oct;16(Suppl 1):S16–21.
30. **Clarke SF, Dargan PI, Jones AL.** Naloxone in opioid poisoning: walking the tightrope. *Emerg Med J.* 2005 Sep;22(9):612–616.
31. **Maddocks I, Somogyi A, Abbott F, et al.** Attenuation of morphine-induced delirium in palliative care by substitution with infusion of oxycodone. *J Pain Symptom Manage.* 1996 Sep;12(3):182–189.
32. **Hallingbye T, Martin J, Viscomi C.** Acute postoperative pain management in the older patient. *Aging Health.* 2011;7(6):813–828.
33. **Foss NB, Kristensen MT, Kristensen BB, et al.** Effect of postoperative epidural analgesia on rehabilitation and pain after hip fracture surgery: a randomized, double-blind, placebo-controlled trial. *Anesthesiology.* 2005 Jun;102(6):1197–1204.
34. **Foss NB, Kristensen BB, Bundgaard M, et al.** Fascia iliaca compartment blockade for acute pain control in hip fracture patients: a randomized, placebo-controlled trial. *Anesthesiology.* 2007 Apr;106(4):773–778.
35. **American Geriatrics Society.** 2015 Updated Beers Criteria for Potentially Inappropriate Medication Use in Older Adults. *J Am Geriatr Soc.* 2015 Nov;63(11):2227–2246.
36. **Hirst A, Knight C, Hirst M, et al.** Tramadol and the risk of fracture in an elderly female population: a cost utility assessment with comparison to transdermal buprenorphine. *Eur J Health Econ.* 2016 Mar;17(2):217–227.

# 1.13 Polypharmacy

Bernardo Reyes, Justinder Malhotra

## 1 Introduction

Long medication lists are a typical feature of fragility fracture patients (FFPs) for many reasons. The presence of multiple comorbidities, advances in disease-specific drug treatment, increased diagnostic testing and changing thresholds for treatment have contributed to significant increases in the number of medications prescribed for older adults. The majority of older adults take more than five prescribed medications [1] and 40% of nursing home residents use nine or more medications each day [2]. The potential benefits of these medications are often offset by risks related to interactions and toxicities in frail older patients. Adverse drug reactions due to common medications (ie, anticoagulants, antithrombotics, antidiabetic medications, and digoxin) account for a significant number of emergency hospitalizations [3], and benzodiazepenes, antihistamines, and opioids are often implicated in delirium [4].

Common postoperative complications related to polypharmacy include:

- Hypotension due to the combination of blood loss, opiates and home antihypertensive agents
- Acute renal failure related to diuretics and angiotensin-converting enzyme inhibitors
- Sedation and delirium due to interactions between postoperative pain medications and home medications (eg, antidepressants, muscle relaxants, and psychiatric medications)
- Urinary retention and constipation due to opioids and anticholinergic agents

Addressing polypharmacy is fundamental to optimal short- and long-term outcomes for orthogeriatric fracture patients. Standardized medication reconciliation by appropriate orthogeriatric team members at each transition of care is the primary tool to reduce unnecessary and harmful medications during hospitalization and at the time of discharge.

## 2 Unique prescribing issues for older adults

There are a number of issues that make current disease specific prescribing guidelines problematic for older adults:

- Lack of valid clinical trials:
  The vast majority of clinical trials of pharmacological interventions are not validated in older or highly comorbid populations, making risks and benefits uncertain, even for many standard medications.
- Lower dose thresholds for toxicity:
  Age- and disease-related changes in drug absorption, distribution, metabolism and excretion can result in lower thresholds for drug toxicity in older adults.
- Limited lifespan:
  Older adults may not have sufficient remaining lifespan to realize the benefit of many standard chronic disease-directed drug therapies, making potential benefits unlikely.

Common drug side effects like delirium, constipation, anorexia and hypotension often complicate the perioperative and postsurgical course of orthogeriatric patients and have a big impact on recovery and outcomes. These factors should result in a general reluctance to routinely prescribe many medications found in standard disease-specific guidelines, and support the geriatric maxim to "start low, go slow" whenever choosing medications and doses in this population.

## 3 Definitions and challenges

Polypharmacy can be defined in many ways:

- Five or more medications [5]. This is the most common definition but other studies use cut-offs as low as two and as high as eleven.
- The use of one or more medications, herbal remedies, or supplements with potential interactions.

- Inappropriate use of any specific medication in an older adult. Each medication should have a clear indication and be prescribed at the minimum effective dose. Short life expectancy, side effects, and goals of care can all impact the appropriateness of specific medications for individual patients.

The risk of drug-related adverse events is higher as the number of medications increases, with nearly 20% of patients on eight or more medications likely to experience an adverse drug event [6].

Obtaining an accurate admission medication list for all orthogeriatric patients is essential, but not the only step in managing medications in the hospital setting. Regardless of the criteria, polypharmacy occurs as a result of a lack of appropriate and thoughtful review of the patients' medication regimen [7–9]. Many home medications may need to be stopped or the dose reduced during the perioperative period.

It can be challenging to correctly identify polypharmacy, as most patients take medications consistent with disease-specific clinical guidelines. Despite having appropriate indications, individual patients can have side effects or toxicities that make the risks of a particular medication or medication dose excessive. The cumulative effect of medications can produce symptoms that sometimes are mistakenly attributed to other etiologies or new medical problems. Acutely compromised orthogeriatric patients can become vulnerable to previously well-tolerated medications. For any significant sign or symptoms, the clinician should always evaluate the patient's current medication regimen as a potential contributor.

## 4 Strategies to safely reduce medications

Despite the need to stop or reduce the dose of some long-term medications in the perioperative setting, specific approaches to achieve this are not well studied or specified [10]. Moreover, the few available studies are limited by being observational and short term.

We offer the following 3-step approach to evaluating and modifying the medication regimen for FFP (**Table 1.13-1**).

1. Stop medications that are likely to delay surgical repair or are expected to produce clinically significant side effects in the perioperative period. Each prescribed medication should be reviewed to ensure that it is clinically necessary at the time of surgery, and it is being prescribed at the most appropriate dose. Moreover, clinicians should verify that there are no other treatment alternatives with significantly less side effects.
2. Stop medications that are likely to interfere with postoperative recovery and rehabilitation, especially those that produce excessive sedation, hypotension, or delirium.
3. Stop medications that have no obvious clinical indication, might produce significant side effects, or lead to complications.

With each of these steps, the clinician needs to consider the risk for medication withdrawal, especially for those medications for which there are known withdrawal syndromes, eg, benzodiazepines, opiates, some antidepressants, clonidine, and beta-blockers. Rapid discontinuation of some of these medications—most likely drugs with cardiovascular and neurological indications—can cause adverse events [11].

Medication management needs to be coordinated by team members with experience in perioperative and geriatric medicine. Some common issues are summarized in **Table 1.13-2**.

The STOPP/START criteria are the best studied single point of care intervention aimed at modifying drug regimens [12]. These criteria use a structured and detailed approach to evaluating patient and disease factors that should prompt appropriate prescribing. The benefits of applying these criteria have been demonstrated up to 6 months after hospitalization.

In addition, the STOPP/START criteria make appropriate suggestions for dosage selection, particular for older adults with reduced renal function [12]. Patients with high degrees of inappropriate prescribing as measured by STOPP/START criteria appear to be at higher risk for mortality after hip fracture [11]. These criteria are generally too cumbersome to use in a busy clinical setting but do support the rationale for more limited prescribing.

| Strategy | Example |
|---|---|
| Stop/reduce dose of medications causing immediate harm or likely to delay surgery | Anticoagulants during the preoperative period<br>Antihypertensive medications in hypotensive patients |
| Stop/reduce dose of medications likely to interfere with postoperative recovery | Diabetes medications in patients with poor intake<br>Anticholinergic medications<br>(eg, diphenhydramine, bladder antispasmodics)<br>Sedatives |
| Stop medications without clear indications | Proton pump inhibitors in patients without recent gastrointestinal bleeding |

**Table 1.13-1** Stepwise approach to reducing polypharmacy in the perioperative period.

## 5 Medication reconciliation

Medication reconciliation is the process used to verify and intentionally adjust medications during transitions of care either between settings (ie, inpatient admission or discharge) or providers (ie, from a specialist office to the primary care physician).

The majority of admission order errors in the inpatient setting are associated with poor medication reconciliation [13]. The process of medication reconciliation is usually limited by clinician time, availability of medical records, and the literacy level of the patient and family members. Based on previous studies, almost half of the patients have unintended medication discrepancies in their discharge medication list [11].

Patients at the highest risk for errors during medication reconciliation include older adults with multiple comorbidities, multiple medications, and cognitive impairment.

| Medication class/examples | Common complications | Strategies/special issues |
|---|---|---|
| Antihypertensives | Excessive hypotension in the setting of blood loss, anesthesia, and opioids | Stop/reduce dose of medications until the patient demonstrates hypertension<br>Beta-blocker and clonidine withdrawal can occur, may need to continue at reduced doses<br>Some antihypertensives also used for arrhythmia control, may need to continue drug |
| Diabetes medications | Hypoglycemia due to reduced oral intake | Hold oral agents; reduce long-acting insulins until patient demonstrates significant hyperglycemia |
| Anticoagulants | Excessive bleeding | Hold until hemostasis is achieved (see chapter 1.6 Anticoagulation in the perioperative setting) |
| Chronic opiates | Sedation<br>Constipation | Dose reduction may precipitate opiate withdrawal<br>Often need to use increased doses for pain control in the perioperative period<br>May need to limit other sedating medications and aggressively treat constipation |
| Anticholinergic medications | Delirium<br>Constipation | Avoid the use of highly anticholinergic medications (eg, diphenhydramine, antispasmodics for urinary incontinence) |
| Diuretics | Hypotension<br>Volume depletion | Hold medications until hemodynamically stable<br>Urine output may be limited until these are resumed |

**Table 1.13-2** Common perioperative prescribing issues in the orthogeriatric patient.

Keys to success:

- Standardizing the reconciliation process. It is helpful to clearly define the team member responsible for medication list verification. Setting the requirement that all providers update the medication list may create opportunities for error if there is inadequate time, training, or information for the provider to accomplish this task.
- Respecting medical record system capabilities from the accepting and referring facilities to ensure that accurate medication lists are received and processed between settings.

Although most facilities in different settings of care use electronic medical records, the systems may not be compatible. Communication via paper forms is often still necessary. Efforts should be made to improve the format of discharge documents in order to have a clear, readable medication list that includes correct dosing, frequency and duration, particularly for time-limited medications like antibiotics and some anticoagulants. In addition, specific attention must be directed to identifying active medications not on the current electronic medication lists and confirming the actual frequency of use by the patient, especially for "as needed" medications. Any medication started during the surgical admission should be highlighted and appropriate monitoring should be specified if indicated. Medications with an "as needed" indication should be ordered only for clearly anticipated needs, placing emphasis on those to treat pain, nausea, constipation, and dyspepsia.

Additional communication points to consider include:

- For patients on thromboembolic prophylaxis, a clear stop date should be specified in the discharge documents.
- Reconciling the dose of each medication is also important, particularly if patients are not taking the exact doses that were prescribed, or if doses have been reduced during the postoperative period.
- The final list of medications should be shared with all the providers that are going to care for the patient during the postacute rehabilitation phase and also upon discharge back to the community. This typically includes the rehabilitation facility or ward, the primary care and subspecialty physicians, and any involved nursing or home care agencies. Being on a shared medical record has the potential to have the same medication list display in all appropriate settings.
- Patients and their families must receive appropriate and sufficient counseling and education about the medications throughout the continuum of care. They should participate

in the maintenance of the medication list and should be empowered to provide feedback to providers regarding any changes in the dose or frequency of the medications as well as side effects [14].

## 6 Pharmacist-based evaluation

The addition of a pharmacist to the care team may contribute to reductions in polypharmacy and improving the self-rated health of older adults. Some research has found that patients who have their medications reviewed by a pharmacist have a lower hospitalization rate and shorter length of stay.

Even when using ordering systems with decision-support alerts that fire to the prescriber, there is likely an additional benefit of pharmacist medication review [15]. When electronic flagging is used by a pharmacist to identify potentially inappropriate medications pharmacists are able to rapidly screen for inappropriate prescribing and deliver timely point-of-care interventions [16].

There is conflicting evidence of how long-term outcomes are influenced by such single point of care interventions [17, 18, 19]. In the postacute setting, the involvement of a clinical pharmacist to evaluate patients for polypharmacy shows similar reductions in the overall number of medications. The cost effectiveness and long-term benefits of these interventions are still to be determined [19, 20].

## 7 References

1. **Tinetti ME, Bogardus ST Jr, Agostini JV.** Potential pitfalls of disease-specific guidelines for patients with multiple conditions. *N Engl J Med.* 2004 Dec 30;351(27):2870–2874.
2. **Dwyer LL, Han B, Woodwell DA, et al.** Polypharmacy in nursing home residents in the United States: results of the 2004 National Nursing Home Survey. *Am J Geriatr Pharmacother.* 2010 Feb;8(1):63–72.
3. **Budnitz DS, Lovegrove MC, Shehab N, et al.** Emergency hospitalizations for adverse drug events in older Americans. *N Engl J Med.* 2011 Nov 24;365(21):2002–2012.
4. **Clegg A, Young JB.** Which medications to avoid in people at risk of delirium: a systematic review. *Age Ageing.* 2011 Jan;40(1):23–29.
5. **Wallace J, Paauw DS.** Appropriate prescribing and important drug interactions in older adults. *Med Clin North Am.* 2015 Mar;99(2):295–310.
6. **Onder G, Petrovic M, Tangiisuran B, et al.** Development and validation of a score to assess risk of adverse drug reactions among in-hospital patients 65 years or older: the GerontoNet ADR risk score. *Arch Intern Med.* 2010 Jul 12;170(13):1142–1148.
7. **Lee RD.** Polypharmacy: a case report and new protocol for management. *J Am Board Fam Pract.* 1998 Mar–Apr;11(2):140–144.
8. **Viktil KK, Blix HS, Moger TA, et al.** Polypharmacy as commonly defined is an indicator of limited value in the assessment of drug-related problems. *Br J Clin Pharmacol.* 2007 Feb;63(2):187–195.
9. **Gleason KM, McDaniel MR, Feinglass J, et al.** Results of the Medications at Transitions and Clinical Handoffs (MATCH) study: an analysis of medication reconciliation errors and risk factors at hospital admission. *J Gen Intern Med.* 2010 May;25(5):441–447.
10. **Schuling J, Gebben H, Veehof LJ, et al.** Deprescribing medication in very elderly patients with multimorbidity: the view of Dutch GPs. A qualitative study. *BMC Fam Pract.* 2012 Jul 09;13:56.
11. **Gosch M, Wortz M, Nicholas JA, et al.** Inappropriate prescribing as a predictor for long-term mortality after hip fracture. *Gerontology.* 2014;60(2):114–122.
12. **Gallagher PF, O'Connor MN, O'Mahony D.** Prevention of potentially inappropriate prescribing for elderly patients: a randomized controlled trial using STOPP/START criteria. *Clin Pharmacol Ther.* 2011 Jun;89(6):845–854.
13. **Wong JD, Bajcar JM, Wong GG, et al.** Medication reconciliation at hospital discharge: evaluating discrepancies. *Ann Pharmacother.* 2008 Oct;42(10):1373–1379.
14. **Commonwealth of Massachusetts, Board of Registration in Medicine. Quality and Patient Safety Division.** Advisory Medication Reconciliation, January 2015. Available at: http://c.ymcdn.com/sites/www.mashp.org/resource/resmgr/medication-reconciliation-ja.pdf. Accessed March 5, 2015.
15. **Zaal RJ, Jansen MM, Duisenberg-van Essenberg M, et al.** Identification of drug-related problems by a clinical pharmacist in addition to computerized alerts. *Int J Clin Pharm.* 2013 Oct;35(5):753–762.
16. **O'Sullivan D, O'Mahony D, O'Connor MN, et al.** The impact of a structured pharmacist intervention on the appropriateness of prescribing in older hospitalized patients. *Drugs Aging.* 2014 Jun;31(6):471–481.
17. **Crotty M, Rowett D, Spurling L, et al.** Does the addition of a pharmacist transition coordinator improve evidence-based medication management and health outcomes in older adults moving from the hospital to a long-term care facility? Results of a randomized, controlled trial. *Am J Geriatr Pharmacother.* 2004 Dec;2(4):257–264.
18. **Chisholm-Burns MA, Kim Lee J, Spivey CA, et al.** US pharmacists' effect as team members on patient care: systematic review and meta-analyses. *Med Care.* 2010 Oct;48(10):923–933.
19. **Hughes CM, Lapane KL.** Pharmacy interventions on prescribing in nursing homes: from evidence to practice. *Ther Adv Drug Saf.* 2011 Jun;2(3):103–112.
20. **Mueller SK, Sponsler KC, Kripalani S, et al.** Hospital-based medication reconciliation practices: a systematic review. *Arch Intern Med.* 2012 Jul 23;172(14):1057–1069.

# 1.14 Delirium

Markus Gosch, Katrin Singler

## 1 Introduction

The two most important cognitive issues affecting hospitalized older adults are delirium and dementia, impacting areas such as memory, awareness, perception, reasoning, and judgment.

While these two disturbances in cognition have overlapping causes, clinical findings and management, they should be understood as distinct conditions that warrant unique approaches to evaluation and treatment. The history, time course, and progression of these deficits allow clinicians to distinguish between delirium and dementia. Delirium is an acute medical condition that develops quickly, waxes and wanes, and has the potential to resolve. Dementia is a progressive and irreversible loss of cognition. This chapter focuses on summarizing the impact of delirium on patient outcomes and identifying optimal prevention, diagnostic and treatment strategies.

## 2 Prevalence in older adults

There is a high prevalence of delirium and dementia in older adults, particularly during hospitalization:

- Among older adults in healthcare settings, delirium is common, occurring in 10–34% of those living in long-term care facilities, 30% of those in emergency departments, and 10–42% during a hospital stay [1, 2, 3].
- Delirium complicates 17–61% of major surgical procedures and occurs in 25–83% of patients at the end of life [1, 4]. This huge range reported in the literature may be explained by historical difficulties in accurately diagnosing delirium as well as by the use of other descriptive terms, eg, acute brain failure, acute confusional state, acute organic brain syndrome, cerebral insufficiency, encephalopathy, postoperative psychosis, or toxic psychosis.
- As with delirium, dementia also strongly correlates with age. Starting at age 65 years, the risk of developing dementia doubles every 5 years. By age 85 years and older, between 25% and 50% of persons will exhibit signs of Alzheimer's disease, the most common type of dementia. Dementia is a particularly strong risk factor for delirium.
- Globally, 24 million people have dementia today and this prevalence is likely to double every 20 years to 42 million by 2020, and 81 million by 2040.
- Of those with dementia, 60% live in developing countries, with the number expected to rise to 71% by 2040 [5].
- The increasing prevalence of dementia is mainly due to increased life expectancy and the increasing proportion of older adults in modern society.

## 3 Definitions

### 3.1 Delirium

Delirium is an acute and fluctuating disturbance in cognition characterized by inattention.

In the Diagnostic and Statistical Manual of Mental Disorders (DSM-V) [6], delirium is defined by the following criteria:

A A disturbance in attention (ie, reduced ability to direct, focus, sustain, and shift attention) and awareness (ie, reduced orientation to the environment)

B The disturbance develops over a short period of time (usually hours to a few days), represents a change from baseline attention and awareness, and tends to fluctuate in severity during the course of a day

C An additional disturbance in a second cognitive domain (eg, memory deficit, disorientation, language, visuospatial ability, or perception)

The disturbances in criteria A and C are not better explained by another preexisting, established, or evolving neurocognitive disorder. There is evidence from the history, physical examination, or laboratory findings that the disturbance is a direct physiological consequence of another environmental or medical condition, substance intoxication or withdrawal (ie, due to drug abuse or to medication).

Delirium can be clinically subclassified as hyperactive (ie, marked by agitation), hypoactive (ie, marked by lethargy and sedation), or mixed [7].

### 3.2 Dementia

Unlike delirium, dementia represents a progressive and irreversible loss in cognitive function. Current DSM criteria include memory impairment, but also emphasize deterioration in other cognitive domains like speech or language ability. Dementia, also called major neurocognitive disorder, is defined by the following [6]:

- Evidence of substantial decline in one or more cognitive domains (ie, attention, awareness, memory, language, visuospatial ability, and perception), and a decline in neurocognitive performance (ie, two or more standard deviations below appropriate norms on formal testing or equivalent clinical evaluation)
- The cognitive deficits are sufficient to interfere with independence
- The cognitive deficits do not occur exclusively in the context of delirium
- The cognitive deficits are not primarily attributable to another mental disorder (eg, major depressive disorder, and schizophrenia)

According to the DSM-V criteria, individuals with major neurocognitive disorder exhibit cognitive deficits that interfere with independence. Persons with mild neurocognitive disorder may retain the ability to be independent.

Typical assessment tools for dementia are of limited use in the acutely hospitalized fragility fracture patient (FFP), as these assessments are only valid when patients are at their baseline cognitive function. Abnormalities in dementia testing like the Mini-Mental Status Exam, Montreal Cognitive Assessment, or clock drawing tests can also be found in delirious patients. Information gained from patient history, such as the progressive inability to manage home medications or finances, may be of more use in identifying patients with previously undiagnosed dementia [8].

## 4 Delirium

Delirium during hospitalization of FFPs has an enormous impact on the patient outcomes and is an independent risk factor for many complications including:

- Increased length of hospitalization
- Increase in functional impairment
- Complications including urinary incontinence, falls and pressure ulcers
- Increase in admission to nursing homes [1, 9]
- Increased mortality (as much as fivefold) [9]
- Significant cognitive impairment in > 50%, and impairment may persist for more than one year [9]

Only one third of hospitalized older adults fully recover from delirium [1]. Delirium is likely a marker of overall frailty, an indicator of clinical instability, and a contributor to poor long-term function. Delirium is always a medical emergency, and requires a prompt diagnostic process and initiation of therapy.

### 4.1 Pathogenesis

Delirium is typically due to multiple causal mechanisms. Several interacting biological factors result in disruption of the neuronal networks of the brain, leading to acute cognitive dysfunction. Current evidence suggests that neuroinflammatory processes, changes in balances of neurotransmitters, physiological stressors, metabolic derangements as well as electrolyte disorders and genetic factors contribute to the development of delirium [9].

Many neurotransmitters are implicated, but cholinergic deficiency and/or dopaminergic excess are of special importance. These systems are often influenced by drugs known to interfere with synaptic transmission and cause delirium. Cytokines, such as interleukin-1 (IL-1), IL-2, IL-6, tumor necrosis factor-α (TNF-α) and interferon, influence the permeability of the blood-brain barrier and disturb the process of neurotransmission. In addition, systemic inflammatory processes including trauma, hypoxia and surgery result in an increase of cytokine levels, causing activation of the microglia and increasing the risk for delirium [9].

### 4.2 Risk factors

Delirium typically results from acute stressors in a vulnerable patient. Identifying high-risk patients and common triggers are an essential workflow for optimal care of orthogeriatric patients. A standardized workup for the diagnosis and management of delirium should be integrated in an orthogeriatric comanagement model.

Patients with dementia are at particularly high risk for the development of delirium. This group should be identified as soon as possible and receive all available nonpharmacological prevention measures for delirium.

Common patient-related risk factors for delirium:

- Preexisting dementia
- Previous delirium
- Older age
- Severe comorbidities and polypharmacy
- Visual and/or hearing impairment
- Major fractures, eg, hip fracture

Because of the high prevalence of risk factors and the high incidence of delirium [4], all older patients should be managed as high-risk patients. One proposed risk assessment tool is described in **Table 1.14-1**.

## 4.3 Common etiologies

Many common hospital treatments and minor complications are triggers for the development of delirium. These are essential to recognize and manage, and include:

- Poorly controlled pain
- Medication effects, eg, toxicity, withdrawal, and anesthesia
- Infections
- Metabolic derangements, eg, hypogylcemia, hyponatremia, hypoxia, fever
- Systemic organ failure, eg, heart failure, renal failure
- Urinary obstruction and constipation
- Physical restraints and tethers, eg, telemetry, intravenous lines, and urinary catheters
- Impaired perception of the environment, eg, missing glasses and hearing aids
- Withdrawal of benzodiazepines or alcohol

| Predisposing risk factors for delirium | Points |
|---|---|
| Delirium during previous hospitalization | 5 |
| Dementia | 5 |
| Clock drawing (displaying 10 past 11): | |
| • Small mistakes | 1 |
| • Big mistakes, unrecognizable or no attempt | 2 |
| Age: | |
| • 70–85 years | 1 |
| • > 85 years | 1 |
| Impaired hearing, ie, patient is not able to hear speech | 1 |
| Impaired vision, ie, vision less than 40% | 1 |
| Problems in activities of daily living: | |
| • Domestic help or help with meal preparation | 0.5 |
| • Help with physical care | 0.5 |
| Use of heroin, methadone or morphine | 2 |
| Daily consumption of four or more units of alcohol | 2 |
| Total score | |

**Table 1.14-1** Risk model for delirium according to Vochteloo et al [10]. Patients with a score of 5 or more are considered high-risk patients.

## 4.4 Diagnosis

Delirium may be the first sign of critical medical decompensation in older patients. Since drug treatment of delirium is potentially harmful, it is very important to detect and reverse underlying medical causes as soon as possible.

### 4.4.1 Clinical presentation

Up to 70% of delirium is unrecognized by clinicians [9], in part due to the variability of clinical manifestations of a delirium.

Patients with a hyperactive state of delirium are often easily recognized, as these patients show increased psychomotor activity, agitation, aggression, mood lability, and, in some cases, hallucinations and delusions.

On the other hand, it can be difficult to detect a patient in hypoactive delirium. This form is characterized by decreased psychomotor activity, with the presence of lethargy and drowsiness, apathy, and confusion.

Conversation with the patient may elicit memory difficulties, disorientation, or speech that is tangential, disorganized, or incoherent. The clinician should be aware of superficially appropriate conversation that follows social norms but is poor in content. It is important that the clinicians are sensitive to the patient's flow of thoughts and do not attribute tangential or disorganized speech to age, dementia, or fatigue.

A focused clinical examination, targeted laboratory tests, and occasionally intracranial imaging are necessary for all patients with new symptoms of delirium. If no easily reversible causes are identified and nonpharmacological methods of control are insufficient, pharmacological symptom control may be necessary to prevent harm or to allow evaluation and treatment. There are limited data to guide treatment. Delirium is still managed empirically and there is no evidence in the literature to support change to current practice at this time.

### 4.4.2 Confusion Assessment Method

Standardized tools help to accurately diagnose delirium. They can be easily and quickly administered. The Confusion Assessment Method (CAM) is a widely used delirium screening instrument based on DSM-III-R criteria [11]. A diagnosis of delirium requires according to the CAM the presence of item 1 and 2 plus either 3a or 3b:

1. Acute onset and fluctuating course (required)
   - Is there evidence of an acute change in mental status from the patient's baseline?
   - Did the abnormal behavior fluctuate during the day?
2. Inattention (required)
   - Did the patient have difficulty focusing attention, being easily distractible or having difficulty keeping track of what was being said?

3a. Disorganized thinking
   - Was the patient's thinking disorganized or incoherent, such as rambling or irrelevant conversation, unclear or illogical flow of ideas, or unpredictable switching from subject to subject?

3b. Altered level of consciousness?
   - Any condition other than alert, eg, vigilant, lethargic, drowsy, comatose.

### 4.4.3 Delirium Observation Screening Scale

The Delirium Observation Screening Scale (DOSS) (**Table 1.14-2**) is a validated surveillance tool that can be performed by the nursing staff throughout the day [12]. In addition to identifying delirium, the DOSS is also useful to describe the course of a delirium over time. In clinical practice it can be used like a pain score. The DOSS includes 13 items and the final score is calculated from the three scores per day and divided by 3. If the final score is 3 or higher, delirium is likely present.

## 4.5 Delirium prevention

It is important to maximize nonpharmacological attempts to prevent or minimize delirium by all healthcare providers, since treatment strategies are less effective and more harmful than preventive measures.

Prevention is based upon four principles:

- Avoid triggers and worsening factors
- Identify and treat possible causes
- Start mobilization and rehabilitation early in a supportive environment to avoid further physical and cognitive decline
- Prevent/control potentially injurious behavior

Early surgery and proactive geriatric management are crucial. The following preventive measures can be taken in clinical practice:

- Early volume and electrolyte repletion
- Adequate pain therapy
- Medication review:
  - Avoidance of anticholinergic (eg, diphenhydramine) and sedative medications, particularly new introduction of benzodiazepines
  - Avoidance of acute medication or substance withdrawal, eg, continuation of long-term opiate or benzodiazepine therapy, management of alcohol withdrawal
- Early mobilization
- Avoidance of physical restraints and/or tethers
- Routine evaluation for urinary retention and constipation
- Environmental modification and nonpharmacological sleeping aids for patient with insomnia
- Orientation protocol and cognitive stimulation for patients with cognitive impairment
- Monitoring high-risk patients with validated scoring tools, like the DOSS or CAM

| DOSS criteria | Never | Sometimes |
|---|---|---|
| Dozes off during conversation or activities | 0 | 1 |
| Is easily distracted by stimuli from the environment | 0 | 1 |
| Maintains attention to conversation or action | 1 | 0 |
| Does not finish question or answer | 0 | 1 |
| Gives answer that do not fit the question | 0 | 1 |
| Reacts slowly to instructions | 0 | 1 |
| Thinks they are somewhere else | 0 | 1 |
| Knows which part of the day it is | 1 | 0 |
| Remembers recent events | 1 | 0 |
| Is picking, disorderly, restless | 0 | 1 |
| Pulls intravenous tubing, feeding tubes, catheters etc | 0 | 1 |
| Is easily or suddenly emotional | 0 | 1 |
| Sees/hears things which are not there | 0 | 1 |

**Table 1.14-2** Delirium Observation Screening Scale [12]. Patients with a score of 5 or more are considered high-risk patients. Abbreviation: DOSS, Delirium Observation Screening Scale.

For most FFPs, pharmacological prevention using haloperdidol, atypical neuroleptics or rivastigmine is not recommended, with only one study suggesting that the use of low dose haloperidol or atypical neuroleptics preoperatively may reduce the length and severity of delirium.

Specific pharmacological prevention for some individual high-risk patients can be considered, after risks and benefits have been carefully considered [13].

### 4.6 Delirium treatment

There are no large placebo-controlled randomized trials that recommend the use of antipsychotics to treat hyperactive delirium. If nonpharmacological measures fail to keep the agitated patient and the treating staff safe, both the American Geriatrics Society [14] and the National Institute for Health and Care Excellence guidelines [15] state that the prescription of a low dose of any antipsychotic drug for a short period may be considered (**Table 1.14-3**).

No adequately controlled trials support the use of benzodiazepines in the treatment of most cases of delirium, with exceptions for delirium clearly linked to alcohol withdrawal or benzodiazepine withdrawal. Many older adults have paradoxical reactions to benzodiazepines, including worsening confusion, and this class of medication should generally be avoided.

After initiation of therapy, pharmacological delirium treatment should be reviewed for discontinuation as soon as possible. Improvement can be suggested by repeat clinical examinations and use of the validated tools noted earlier, eg, DOSS. Consultation with geriatric or psychiatric teams may be necessary for complicated or high-risk cases.

| Medication | Dosage | Comment |
|---|---|---|
| Haloperidol | 0.25–0.5 mg oral or intramuscular every 6 hours as needed | • Increase in side effects > 3 mg/d<br>• Avoid in patients with Parkinson's disease<br>• Toxicity: QTc prolongation, sedation, extrapyramidal side effects |
| Risperidone | 0.25–1 mg repeated every 12 hours as needed | • Toxicity: QTc prolongation, sedation, extrapyramidal side effects |
| Quetiapine | 12.5–25 mg every 8 hours as needed | • Can be used in Parkinson's disease<br>• Toxicity: QTc prolongation, sedation, extrapyramidal side effects |
| Olanzapine | 2.5 mg to 5 mg every 12 hours as needed | • Toxicity: QTc prolongation, sedation, extrapyramidal side effects |

**Table 1.14-3** Pharmacological treatment for delirium [16].

## 5 References


1. **Inouye SK.** Delirium in older persons. *N Engl J Med.* 2006 Mar 16;354(11):1157–1165.
2. **de Lange E, Verhaak PF, van der Meer K.** Prevalence, presentation and prognosis of delirium in older people in the population, at home and in long term care: a review. *Int J Geriatr Psychiatry.* 2013 Feb;28(2):127–134.
3. **Siddiqi N, House AO, Holmes JD.** Occurrence and outcome of delirium in medical in-patients: a systematic literature review. *Age Ageing.* 2006 Jul;35(4):350–364.
4. **Marcantonio ER.** Postoperative delirium: a 76-year-old woman with delirium following surgery. *JAMA.* 2012 Jul 4;308(1):73–81.
5. **Ferri CP, Prince M, Brayne C, et al.** Global prevalence of dementia: a Delphi consensus study. *Lancet.* 2005 Dec 17;366(9503):2112–2117.
6. **American Psychiatric Association, ed.** *Diagnostic and statistical manual of mental disorders.* 5th ed. Arlington: American Psychiatric Association; 2013.
7. **Fong TG, Tulebaev SR, Inouye SK.** Delirium in elderly adults: diagnosis, prevention and treatment. *Nat Rev Neurol.* 2009 Apr;5(4):210–220.
8. **Cromwell DA, Eagar K, Poulos RG.** The performance of instrumental activities of daily living scale in screening for cognitive impairment in elderly community residents. *J Clin Epidemiol.* 2003 Feb;56(2):131–137.
9. **Inouye SK, Westendorp RG, Saczynski JS.** Delirium in elderly people. *Lancet.* 2014 Mar 8;383(9920):911–922.
10. **Vochteloo AJ, Moerman S, van der Burg BL, et al.** Delirium risk screening and haloperidol prophylaxis program in hip fracture patients is a helpful tool in identifying high-risk patients, but does not reduce the incidence of delirium. *BMC Geriatr.* 2011 Aug 11;11:39.
11. **Wei LA, Fearing MA, Sternberg EJ, et al.** The Confusion Assessment Method: a systematic review of current usage. *J Am Geriatr Soc.* 2008 May;56(5):823–830.
12. **Schuurmans MJ, Shortridge-Baggett LM, Duursma SA.** The Delirium Observation Screening Scale: a screening instrument for delirium. *Res Theory Nurs Pract.* 2003 Spring;17(1):31–50.
13. **Gosch M, Nicholas JA.** Pharmacologic prevention of postoperative delirium. *Z Gerontol Geriatr.* 2014 Feb;47(2):105–109.
14. **American Geriatrics Society Expert Panel on Postoperative Delirium in Older Adults.** Postoperative delirium in older adults: best practice statement from the American Geriatrics Society. *J Am Coll Surg.* 2015 Feb;220(2):136–148.e1.
15. **Young J, Murthy L, Westby M, et al.** Diagnosis, prevention, and management of delirium: summary of NICE guidance. *BMJ.* 2010 Jul 28;341:c3704.
16. **Fruhwald T, Weissenberger-Leduc M, Jagsch C, et al.** Delir: eine interdisziplinäre Herausforderung [Delirium: an interdisciplinary challenge]. *Z Gerontol Geriatr.* 2014 Jul;47(5):425–438; quiz 439–440. German.

# Section 2
# Improving the system of care

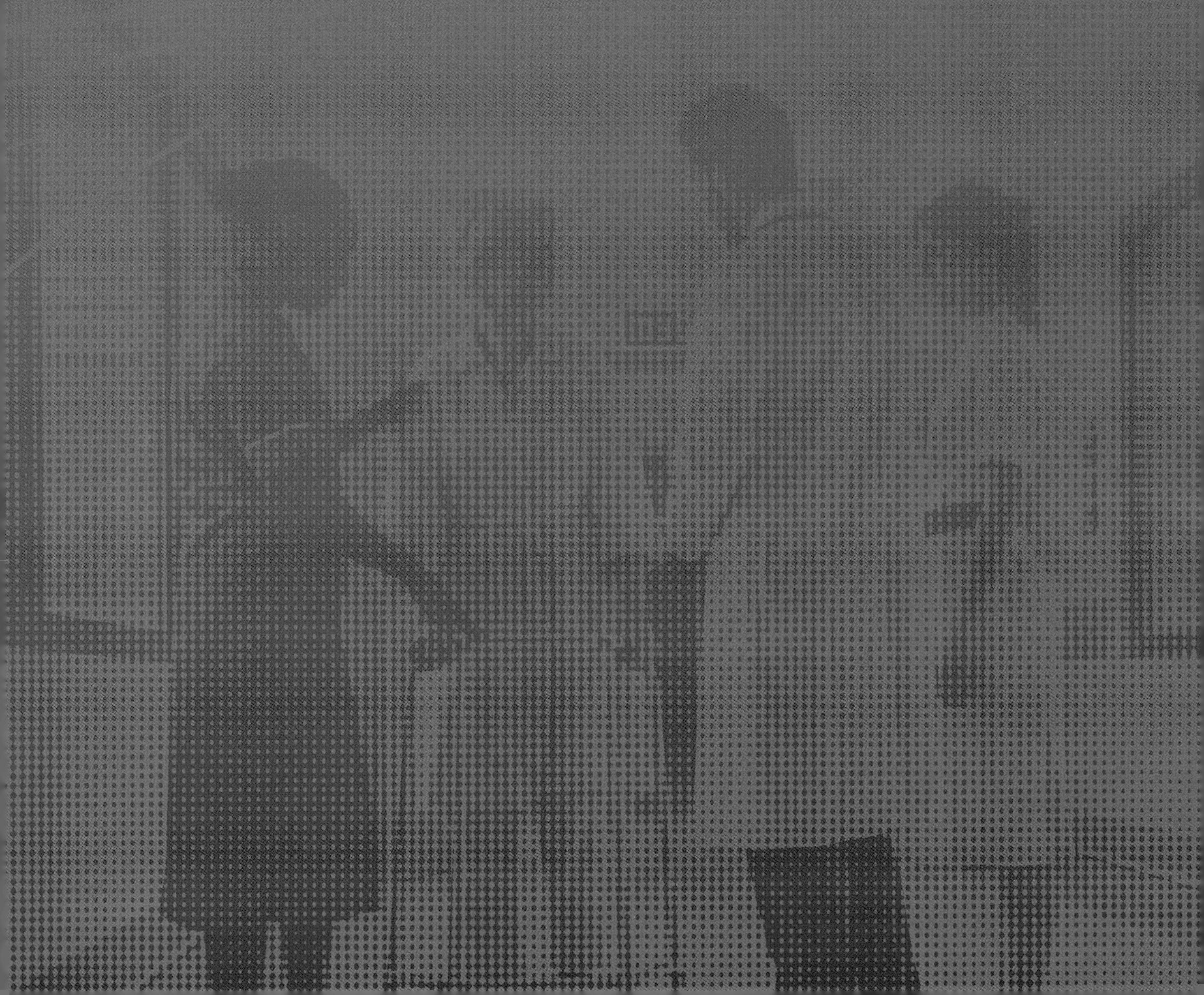

# Section 2
## Improving the system of care

# 2.1 Models of orthogeriatric care

Andrea Giusti, Giulio Pioli

## 1 Introduction

The growing awareness of the consequences of hip and other fragility fractures, the expected rise in the total number of osteoporotic fractures worldwide, and improvements in surgical techniques have led to the development and implementation of alternative models of care for the acute and postacute management of older adults with fractures [1–5].

These services seek to achieve the following major goals:

- Improve functional and clinical outcomes
- Minimize in-hospital complications
- Streamline hospital care
- Promote early discharge
- Reduce direct and indirect healthcare costs

The main features that distinguish these innovative models of care from the traditional ones are:

- A multidisciplinary and interprofessional team of healthcare professionals that share responsibilities for the patient
- The organization of an orthogeriatric service unit [4, 5]

It is not possible to define the single best model of care for fragility fracture patients (FFPs) based on evidence. However, randomized controlled trials (RCTs) and before-after observational studies have demonstrated superior outcomes for organized, sophisticated multidisciplinary programs when compared to the traditional models [4–8].

A number of reviews and two metaanalyses support these conclusions, demonstrating a trend toward better short-term and long-term outcomes with the more recent models based on geriatric orthopedic comanagement [4–9]. In particular, the results of two metaanalyses demonstrate that most models are able to reduce length of hospital stay (LOS), time to surgery, and, in some but not all studies, mortality [6, 7]. On the other hand, these metaanalyses emphasize the limitations of available studies and the need for well-designed RCTs with standardized end points, complete reporting, and inclusion of functional outcomes [6, 7].

This chapter provides a brief description of the models implemented in the last 20 years, describes their potential benefits on short-term and long-term outcomes, defines the strengths and limitations of these models, highlights the areas of uncertainty, and considers the future of orthogeriatric care.

## 2 Variables involved in the implementation of orthogeriatric care models

### 2.1 Which patients should be targeted?

Theoretically, all older adults presenting with hip or other disabling fragility fractures (eg, ankle) should be managed within an orthogeriatric service unit. Randomized controlled trials and before-after observational studies include primarily hip fracture patients older than 65 or 70 years [4, 5]. In some cases, it has been proposed to include subjects older than 70 years presenting with relevant comorbidities and any patients older than 80 years. Indeed, the characteristics of the patients eligible for an orthogeriatric service unit should be based also on the available resources, since the setting of a given criterion may significantly influence the volume of patients.

There are no established criteria from the available literature, and, due to the small number of RCTs, cost-effectiveness analyses are lacking. Moreover, the baseline characteristics of hip fracture patients are of limited benefit in identifying subjects at greatest risk of adverse outcomes, given the high degree of frailty in almost all FFPs. Therefore, we believe that orthogeriatric services should make an effort to include all older adults with hip or other disabling fractures by optimizing the resources available.

## 2.2 Responsibility and leadership—who is in charge?

The multidisciplinary approach is now the gold standard in the care of older adults presenting with hip or other osteoporotic fractures. The basic multidisciplinary team of these orthogeriatric models includes an orthopedic surgeon, a geriatrician or internist, an anesthesiologist during the perioperative phase, and other healthcare providers, such as a physiotherapist, clinical nurse, nutritionist, and a social worker, during the acute and postacute phases [4]. Direct communication, scheduled meetings, and written orders are the usual way to share information and communicate between team members, even if, in some cases, a skilled care manager takes on the role of coordinating the pathway of care and fostering communications between professionals [4, 10].

The main difference between the variety of orthogeriatric models concerns which professional discipline retains the primary responsibility for the management of the patients throughout the care pathway (**Fig 2.1-1**) [4, 5]:

- In both the traditional model (**Fig 2.1-1a**) and the routine geriatric consultation model (**Fig 2.1-1b**), the primary responsibility for oversight and coordination lies with the orthopedic surgical staff.
- The comanaged care model is characterized by the comanagement of the fracture patient by the geriatrician and the orthopedic surgeon, with shared responsibility and leadership from admission to discharge (**Fig 2.1-1c**).
- Finally, geriatrician leadership distinguishes the third model, usually referred to as the geriatric-led model (**Fig 2.1-1d–e**).

## 2.3 Time to surgery

Recent data and metaanalyses support the beneficial effect of early surgery in the management of older adults presenting with hip fractures [4, 5, 11]. Indeed, there is no clear definition of early surgery, since, in the various studies, it has been defined as "within 24 hours", "within 48 hours" or even "as soon as medical conditions are stable" [4, 5, 11]. Although the meaning of "early surgery" is debatable, guidelines suggest that medically stable patients should undergo surgery as soon as possible, while unstable ones should be quickly optimized to avoid detrimental delays [5, 11].

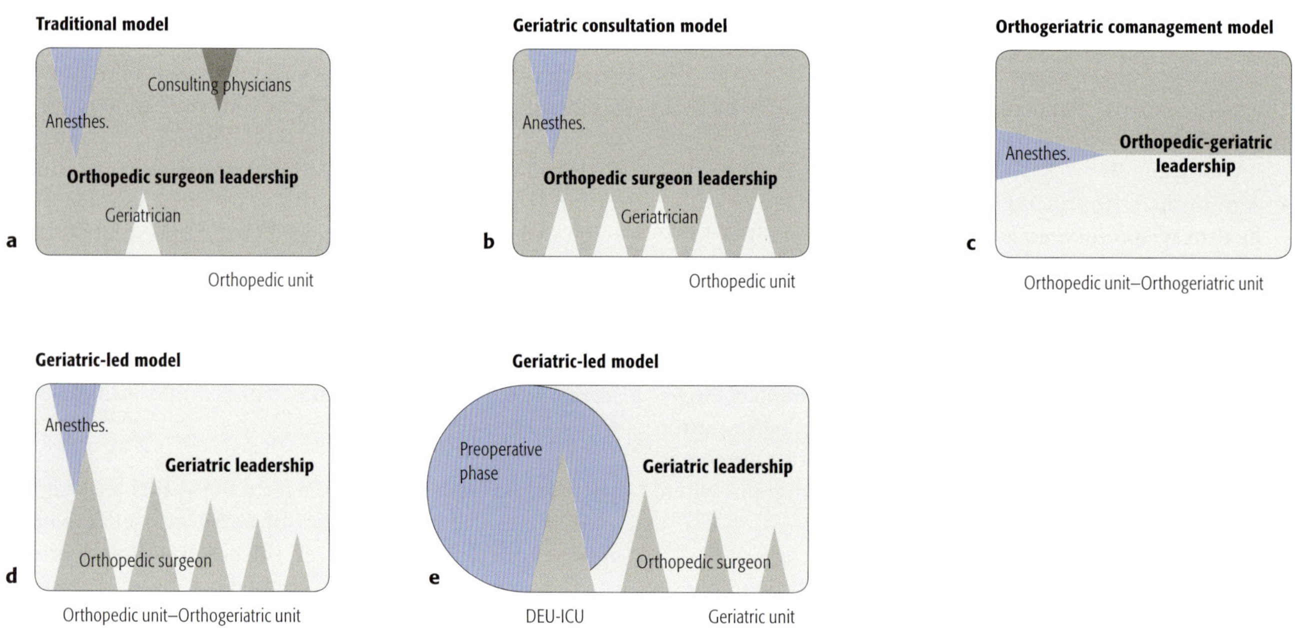


**Fig 2.1-1a–e** Models of orthogeriatric care for the management of the older adults presenting with hip fracture. The models distinguish themselves by the team of different healthcare professionals that retain the responsibility for managing the patients throughout the care pathway. The setting of the care is described at the bottom of each figure.
Abbreviations: Anesthes, anesthesiologist; DEU-ICU, Department of Emergency Unit-Intensive Care Unit.

The recognition of hip fracture as an urgent scenario requiring early surgery has significantly impacted the organization and implementation of the orthogeriatric models. In an ideal model, the patient may be transferred directly to the operating room from the emergency department and admitted to a hospital ward only after surgical repair. The feasibility of this approach has been tested in a study undertaken at the Pitié-Salpêtrière Hospital in Paris, where the FFPs, following a fast-track procedure, are quickly repaired and are postoperatively admitted to a dedicated geriatric unit within 1–2 days from their arrival in the emergency department (**Fig 2.1-1e**) [12]. Although at least in part still theoretical, it is highly probable that this approach will significantly affect the development of orthogeriatric models in the near future.

In conclusion, early surgery appears to produce potential advantages in the management of older adults with hip fractures, without significant risks for the patients, and it is the most ethical and humane approach to deal with FFPs. Therefore, all orthogeriatric models should clearly support this goal, addressing underlying problems and identifying solutions through intensive teamwork involving physicians and hospital management staff.

## 2.4 Length of hospital stay, early and late rehabilitation

In many countries, orthogeriatric models of care have also been influenced by the need to reduce acute hospital stay and promote early discharge, and by the availability of rehabilitation facilities in the community. Even when strategies to reduce the LOS are implemented, LOS is largely dependent on the features of the local healthcare system and often related to local organizational factors [4].

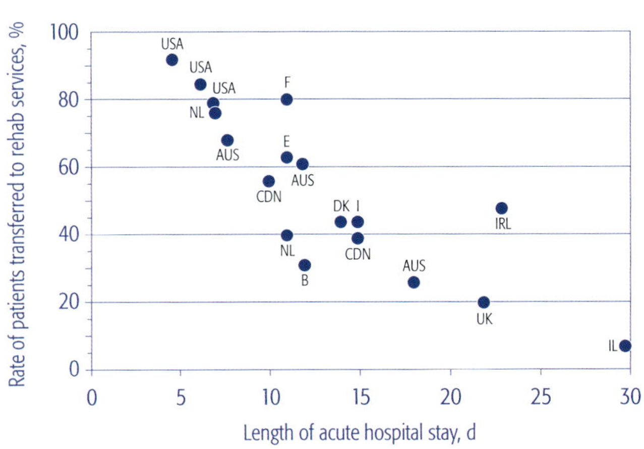


In general, there is an inverse relationship between LOS and rate of transfer to rehabilitation services in the community (**Fig 2.1-2**):

- Models characterized by short LOS require the support of postdischarge rehabilitation services, with the ability to take care of the patients undergoing early discharge, and community rehabilitation. In the US, where the LOS for hip fracture has decreased dramatically over the last 20 years to a national average of 6.3 days [13, 14], patients are usually discharged on the third postoperative day if they are clinically stable and able to transfer from bed to a chair with assistance. In these circumstances, more than 70% of hip fracture patients should be transferred to inpatient rehabilitation or community skilled nursing facilities (SNFs) to continue rehabilitation. A similar picture has been observed in other countries where the LOS is less than 1 week [12, 15, 16].
- The opposite scenario is typically represented by the UK system, where patients complete functional recovery during the hospital stay [17–20]. Although decreasing in recent years, the mean LOS in the UK remains more than 20 days, as less than 30% of hip fracture patients are discharged to rehabilitation facilities [18, 19].
- In between these two scenarios are most European (and some other) countries with LOS between 10 and 15 days [21–31]. In the European models, the rehabilitation is usually broken down into two phases, ie, early rehabilitation that occurs during hospital stay and late rehabilitation that takes place after discharge.

The rehabilitation program and discharge planning should be the result of a comprehensive evaluation involving the different members of the orthogeriatric team. To optimize use of resources, the orthogeriatric team should also decide which patients are most likely to benefit from using rehabilitation.

**Fig 2.1-2** Inverse relationship between length of hospital stay and rate of transfer to rehabilitation services in the community examined by different published studies.
Abbreviations: d, days; rehab, rehabilitation;
AUS, Australia [16, 27, 28]; B, Belgium [23]; CDN, Canada [25, 26]; DK, Denmark [31]; E, Spain [21]; F, France [12]; I, Italy [29, 30]; IL, Israel [20]; IRL, Ireland [22]; NL, the Netherlands [15, 24]; UK, United Kingdom [18, 19]; USA, United States of America [13, 14].

## 2.5 Case volumes

A positive relationship between case volume and improved outcomes has been shown for a wide range of surgical procedures across a variety of specialties [4]. In particular, higher surgeon and hospital procedure volumes have been associated with lower mortality rates, fewer complications, and shorter LOS [4]. A minimum of 100 cases per year has been suggested to develop sufficient expertise in managing FFPs and to adopt an efficient orthogeriatric model of care [4, 32]. There are no studies to clearly define a precise minimum caseload.

In the case of hip fractures, current literature [4, 32–34] offers conflicting results about the optimum number of cases required to implement a successful fragility fracture program. Some additional considerations include:

- Even if a precise minimum number of cases needed to implement a service for the management of FFPs cannot be defined, low-volume hospitals are at risk for suboptimal outcomes.
- Both the acute care ward volume and the rehabilitation unit volume may be relevant.
- The concentration of orthogeriatric services in high-volume hospitals may have significant implications in the (re)distribution of resources, (re)organization of healthcare, and costs in developed countries.

# 3 Models of orthogeriatric care

## 3.1 General considerations

Innovative models of care for the management of FFPs have been developed and implemented over the past 30 years, with the first RCT comparing a traditional model with an orthopedic geriatric inpatient service published by Gilchrist et al in 1988 [35].

High-level evidence establishing superiority of any specific model is still limited. Ideally, several features of these innovative models of care would be compared and clarified by head-to-head RCTs. One example where this approach would be helpful concerns the creation of an emergency department "fast track" for FFPs. While the evaluation and optimization of patients within the emergency department by the emergency staff or multispecialty team can reduce time to surgery, and, theoretically, improve in-hospital outcomes, this has not been demonstrated. Without clear evidence of benefit, it can be difficult to justify the costs of staff reorganization and changes in workload and workflow.

## 3.2 Traditional model

In the traditional model, the key elements are:

- The patient is managed on a general orthopedic ward.
- The orthopedic service holds primary responsibility for inpatient plan of care while nonsurgical concerns and complications are dealt with by consultative medical services upon request (**Fig 2.1-1a**) [4, 5, 8].
- The medical physician is only involved when requested by the orthopedic service.
- Early rehabilitation typically takes place on the orthopedic ward.
- The patient is discharged directly home, to an SNF, or to a rehabilitation facility, without strong emphasis on continuity of care and careful handoffs.

While several lines of evidence have demonstrated that this approach is appropriate for younger adults presenting with a simple traumatic fracture, it is not adequate for the management of the complex needs of FFPs [1–5]. As a result, several care models involving collaboration between orthopedic surgeon and geriatrician have been developed [4, 5]. The first models introduced were simple variations of the traditional model. They were characterized by routine input from a specific consultant team of different professionals, with the overall responsibility of the care remaining with the orthopedic surgical staff.

Over the years these models evolved and were replaced by multidisciplinary and coordinated approaches that have been demonstrated to be more effective to meet patients' complex needs. These experiences have been designated with different names, such as orthogeriatric units (OGUs), comanaged geriatric fracture centers, or geriatric hip fracture clinical pathways, which in most cases distinguish unique models in terms of setting and organization. The common goals of most of these models were to define a multidisciplinary team dedicated to the surgical and medical care of FFPs, to promote rapid management of the comorbid medical conditions, early surgical repair, mobilization and rehabilitation, coordinated discharge planning, and continuity of care [4].

Although a variety of experiences have been described, nontraditional services can be summarized by the following models (**Fig 2.1-1b–e**).

### 3.3 Geriatric consultant in the orthopedic ward

The geriatric consultant in the orthopedic ward model is the simplest model [4, 5, 8].

The key elements are:

- The patient is managed on the orthopedic ward.
- The overall responsibility of the care is under the orthopedic surgical staff.
- A geriatric consultant is involved either preoperatively or postoperatively.
- A multidisciplinary team holds regular rounds to develop and monitor treatment plans of all FFPs on the ward. Although many relevant clinical services may participate, these are typically not coordinated or integrated, and do not clearly impact the overall plan of care.
- Prevention and management of common problems and complications are based on the individual choices of the surgeon or geriatric consultant.

This model and closely related variations have been investigated with the largest amount of studies including RCTs. Interpretation of the results of these trials is limited by the huge heterogeneity in design and outcomes, the small sample sizes, and the absence of long-term follow-up [4–7].

Significantly improved outcomes compared to usual care could not be demonstrated when the consultant team's contribution started postoperatively [4]. Slightly better results were reported with involvement of the geriatric consultant team at the time of admission and in models with daily medical visits [4]. This approach reduced the LOS and the number of medical complications.

The implementation of a geriatric consultant team on the orthopedic ward seems to add some benefits to the traditional model of care, but only when the consultant team is involved early in the process of care. These benefits are probably related to an earlier identification of common issues and complications compared to the traditional model [8]. However, the absence of an active, integrated, and coordinated interdisciplinary care can increase the risk of delays or errors, produce a detrimental fragmentation of care, and compromise an early and adequate discharge [4, 8].

### 3.4 Orthogeriatric comanaged care

This is probably the most sophisticated and complex model implemented for the management of older adults with fractures. The geriatric fracture center developed at the University of Rochester (New York) is the reference model of the orthogeriatric comanaged care [14, 32], and it has been adopted by many other hospitals, mainly in North America and Europe [3, 15, 17, 22, 24, 31, 36–42]. This model has evolved over the last 10–15 years with gradual improvements over time.

Its key elements are:

- The patient is managed on the orthopedic ward or orthogeriatric unit.
- Co-ownership—the orthogeriatric team shares responsibility and leadership from admission to discharge [4, 8].
- An interdisciplinary team including several healthcare professionals skilled in the care of FFPs supports this codirection, working in close and integrated collaboration.
- Standardized patient-centered, protocol-driven treatments and pathways are implemented.
- Geriatrician and surgeon visit the patient daily, write their own orders, and communicate frequently, sharing their opinions and choices with the other members of the interdisciplinary team. This approach reduces the risk of delays, inappropriate variations in care, and iatrogenic errors, and it promotes clinical coordination. Even traditionally surgical issues like evaluation of surgical fitness, timing of procedure, and preoperative planning are usually shared and discussed between both the medical and surgical service to optimize the management of the patients.

The beneficial effects on short-term and long-term functional and clinical outcomes of this innovative model have been illustrated in a number of well-designed before-after observational studies and RCTs, in their reviews, and meta-analyses [4–7, 43]. **Table 2.1-1** and **Table 2.1-2** describe most relevant studies published in the last 15 years. Trials are heterogeneous in terms of design, duration of follow-up, and outcomes considered.

In most of the studies, the implementation of a comanaged care model for FFPs demonstrates a clinically significant reduction in both short-term and long-term adverse events. Compared to the traditional model, the comanaged care model has been shown to improve many short-term outcomes, including length of stay, time to surgery, in-hospital complications, and in-hospital mortality. Specifically, three of five studies demonstrated a significant decrease in the incidence of in-hospital complications [14, 37, 41], and four well-designed trials reported a significant reduction of in-hospital mortality [3, 15, 40, 41].

Few long-term trials have been published (**Table 2.1-2**), with inconsistent and sometimes skewed results. In these studies, this model has been shown to increase long-term survival, and possibly improve functional recovery compared to the traditional model. For example, in three studies (ie, one RCT and two before-after trials), the 1-year survival rates were about 10% higher in the orthogeriatric comanaged care group than in the controls [3, 22, 41]. Vidan et al [41] also reported, after adjustment for confounding variables, a 45% lower probability of death or major complications, and a significantly greater functional recovery at 3 months.

In conclusion, the orthogeriatric comanaged care service represents a valuable and more effective alternative to the traditional approach to inpatient management of FFPs. Unfortunately, there are no published head-to-head RCTs comparing this model with the geriatric consultant in the orthopedic ward service. The fully implemented model requires considerable effort, consistent administrative support, strong physician leadership, and a commitment to continuous quality improvement. Given the relevant resources needed to implement an orthogeriatric comanaged care model, additional studies are warranted for a better understanding of its impact on long-term functional outcomes, to evaluate its cost-effectiveness, and whether this service is translatable and applicable to any hospital organization and framework [4].

### 3.5 Geriatric-led fracture service with orthopedic consultant

The key elements of this model are:

- The geriatric ward is under the leadership of the geriatrician [4, 5, 43]. Usually, the FFP is admitted directly from the emergency department, evaluated and prepared for surgery in the geriatric ward, transferred to the operating room, and then returned to the geriatric ward.

| | | Khan et al [36] | Khasraghi et al [37] | Friedman et al [14] | Gonzalez-Montalvo et al [38] | Folbert et al [24] | Biber et al [39] | Zeltzer et al [40] | Bhattacharyya et al [17] | Flikweert et al [15] |
|---|---|---|---|---|---|---|---|---|---|---|
| **Study design** | | **Before-after prospective** | **Before-after prospective** | **Retrospective cohorts** | **Randomized-controlled** | **Before-after prospective** | **Before-after retrospective** | **Retrospective multicenter** | **Before-after prospective** | **Before-after prospective** |
| Country | | United Kingdom | United States | United States | Spain | Netherlands | Germany | Australia | United Kingdom | Netherlands |
| Number of patients | Intervention | 208 | 273 | 193 | 101 | 140 | 114 | 4,575 | 249 | 256 |
| | Control | 537 | 237 | 121 | 123 | 90 | 169 | 5,026 | 274 | 145 |
| Mean age, y | Intervention | 82 | 80 | 85* | 85 | 81 | 82 | 84 | 83 | 78 |
| | Control | 81 | 80 | 82 | 87 | 82 | 82 | 84 | 83 | 80 |
| In-hospital mortality, % | Intervention | 11.1 | NA | 1.6 | 5.9 | 5.0 | 4.4 | 6.5* | 8.4 | 2.0* |
| | Control | 10.4 | NA | 2.5 | 6.5 | 8.9 | 5.9 | 8.1 | 12.4 | 5.5 |
| Length of stay [mean days (SD or IQR)] | Intervention | 27 (23) | 6 (NR)* | 5 (3)* | 12 (4)* | 11 (7–18) | 14 (7)* | 30 (23)* | 20 (NR) | 7 (6–10)* |
| | Control | 26 (26) | 8 (NR) | 8 (6) | 18 (8) | 12 (6–20) | 17 (10) | 29 (30) | 25 (NR) | 11 (7–16) |
| Time to surgery [mean days (SD or IQR)] | Intervention | NA | 1.1 (NR)* | 1.0 (0.7)* | 5 (3–6)* | NR | 2.1 (1.8)* | 1.8 (2.7) | NR | NR |
| | Control | NA | 1.9 (NR) | 1.6 (2.7) | 6 (5–9) | NR | 3.1 (4.6) | 1.7 (13.2) | NR | NR |
| In-hospital complications, % | Intervention | NA | 36* | 31* | NA | NR | NA | NA | NA | 51 |
| | Control | NA | 51 | 46 | NA | NR | NA | NA | NA | 49 |

**Table 2.1-1** Studies evaluating the in-hospital beneficial effects of a comanaged care service in the management of hip fractures in older adults. Abbreviations: IQR, interquartile range; NA, not assessed; NR, data assessed but not reported; SD, standard deviation.
* Significant difference between intervention and control.

- The geriatrician, as the primary attending physician for all patients from hospital admission to discharge, plays a central role. He/she evaluates the patient on admission and during the in-hospital stay, coordinates the timing of surgery, procedures, diagnostics, treatments, and transition/discharge planning.
- The geriatrician, orthopedic surgeon, and anesthesiologist manage the patients together in the perioperative phase. In the postoperative phase, the orthopedic surgeon is a consulting physician who follows the patients until complete wound healing.
- An interdisciplinary team, including different healthcare professionals, is integrated in the service and participates in the care of the patients.
- Standardized orders and protocols are implemented.

On the basis of the clinical/rehabilitative pathway following these preoperative and perioperative phases, different experiences have been described [4].

The first geriatric-led fracture service with an orthopedic consultant dedicated to older adults presenting with hip fractures was implemented at the Sheba Hospital in Tel Aviv in 1999 [20, 44, 45]. This experience was unique since the patient was cared for throughout the acute and postacute rehabilitative phases in the same setting, with an overall high LOS. In the most recent experiences, the geriatric-led fracture service was restricted to the acute phase, followed by an early transfer to a community SNF for further rehabilitation, with the attention focused on reducing the time to surgery and LOS [12, 46–48].

Actually, the relevant difference in the organization of the postacute phase seems to be attributable to the organization of the healthcare system in the country where the program is adopted, to the resources available, and to the main objectives of the program. For example, in the Sheba model all the care takes place in the same setting with the same intensity of care [20, 44, 45]. This is a strong point, producing

| | | Vidan et al [41] | Barone et al [3] | Cogan† et al [22] | Gregersen et al [31] | Watne et al [42] |
|---|---|---|---|---|---|---|
| **Study design** | | **Randomized controlled** | **Before-after prospective** | **Before-after retrospective** | **Before-after retrospective** | **Randomized controlled** |
| Country | | Spain | Italy | Ireland | Denmark | Norway |
| Number of patients | Intervention | 155 | 272 | 98 | 233 | 163 |
| | Control | 164 | 252 | 103 | 262 | 166 |
| Mean age, y | Intervention | 81 | 84 | 82* | 83 | 84 |
| | Control | 83 | 84 | 75 | 82 | 85 |
| In-hospital mortality, % | Intervention | 0.6* | 4.8* | 8.2 | 7.7 | 3.7 |
| | Control | 5.5 | 9.9 | 20.4 | 6.1 | 1.8 |
| 3- or 4-month mortality, % | Intervention | NR | NR | NR | 16.3 | 17.2 |
| | Control | NR | NR | NR | 14.9 | 14.5 |
| 12-month mortality, % | Intervention | 18.9 | 25.0* | 33.7 | NA | 28.2 |
| | Control | 25.6 | 35.3 | 44.6 | NA | 25.9 |
| 3- or 4-month readmission, % | Intervention | NA | NA | NA | 12.9 | 17.4 |
| | Control | NA | NA | NA | 12.2 | 17.4 |
| Length of stay [mean days (SD or IQR)] | Intervention | 16 (5) | 21 (11) | 30 (NR) | 13 (NR)* | 11 (8–15)* |
| | Control | 18 (8) | 21 (13) | 23 (NR) | 15 (NR) | 8 (5–11) |
| Time to surgery [mean days (SD or IQR)] | Intervention | 3.2 (1.8) | NA | 1.9 (0.9) | 0.9 (0.8)* | 1.1 (0.7–1.8) |
| | Control | 3.3 (2.2) | NA | 1.9 (1.9) | 0.7 (1.0) | 1.0 (0.7–1.6) |
| In-hospital complications, % | Intervention | 45* | NA | NA | NA | 44 |
| | Control | 62 | NA | NA | NA | 46 |
| Functional status recovery 3 month, % | Intervention | 57* | NA | NA | NA | NA |
| | Control | 44 | NA | NA | NA | NA |

**Table 2.1-2** Studies evaluating the short- and long-term beneficial effects of a comanaged care service in the management of hip fractures in older adults.
Abbreviations: IQR, interquartile range; NA, not assessed; NR, data assessed but not reported; SD, standard deviation.
* Significant difference between intervention and control.
† The authors did not report the statistical significance in the between-groups comparisons.

continuous geriatric supervision for the prevention of common geriatric syndromes, and reducing the detrimental effects of fragmentation of care. On the other hand, it seems that this model design may be not acceptable (in terms of costs and resources) for the healthcare systems of most European countries or in the US, where the trend in the last 10 years has been to separate the settings of the acute and intermediate care to appropriately use available resources and reduce costs.

**Table 2.1-3** depicts relevant studies designed to evaluate the geriatric-led fracture service [12, 45–49]. In contrast to the wealth of data published for the other models described, information regarding the efficacy of the geriatric-led fracture service is relatively limited. The model originally proposed by Adunsky et al [44] has been shown in one study to improve long-term functional outcomes and in other studies to reduce time to surgery and hospital stay compared to the traditional orthopedic-centered approach [12, 45–49].

However, none of the trials published to date report a significant beneficial effect on short- and long-term mortality. Interestingly, Miura et al [46] demonstrated a significant reduction in the direct and indirect costs when the geriatric leadership was implemented only for the acute phase and followed by early discharge.

In conclusion, on the basis of the few papers published, a geriatric-led fracture service with orthopedic consultant approach seems feasible, applicable, and efficacious in terms of functional outcomes when the overall care takes place in the same setting with the same intensity of care. The beneficial effects of models in which the geriatric leadership is limited to the acute phase still need to be established, in light of the common separation of acute and postacute care in many health systems.

| | | Stenvall et al [49] | Miura et al [46] | Adunsky et al [45] | Della Rocca et al [47] | Boddaert et al [12] | Gupta [48] |
|---|---|---|---|---|---|---|---|
| **Study design** | | **Randomized controlled** | **Before-after† prospective** | **Retrospective cohort** | **Before-after retrospective** | **Prospective cohorts** | **Before-after† prospective** |
| Country | | Sweden | United States | Israel | United States | France | United Kingdom |
| Number of patients | Intervention | 102 | 91 | 847 | 115 | 203 | 259 |
| | Control | 97 | 72 | 2,267 | 31 | 131 | 235 |
| Mean age, y | Intervention | 82 | 80 | 82* | 82 | 86 | 81 |
| | Control | 82 | 81 | 81 | 82 | 85 | 82 |
| In-hospital mortality, % | Intervention | 5.9 | NA | 1.9 | 4.3 | 3.0 | NA |
| | Control | 7.2 | NA | 3.0 | 9.7 | 7.6 | NA |
| Long-term mortality, % | Intervention | 15.7 | NA | 14.8 | 31.3 | 14.3 | NA |
| | Control | 18.6 | NA | 17.3 | 45.2 | 23.7 | NA |
| Length of stay [mean days (SD or IQR)] | Intervention | 30 (18)* | 5 (1)* | 32 (20)* | 7 (NR)* | 11 (8–16)* | 15 (NR)* |
| | Control | 40 (41) | 6 (2) | 25 (31) | 10 (NR) | 13 (10–20) | 19 (NR) |
| Time to surgery [mean days (SD or IQR)] | Intervention | 1.0 (0.7) | NA | 3.0 (2.9)* | 1.2 (NR) | 0.9 (0.5–1.4) | NA |
| | Control | 1.0 (0.6) | NA | 2.9 (6.5) | 1.5 (NR) | 1.0 (0.6–1.7) | NA |
| Discharge to preadmission place of residence, % | Intervention | 84 | NA | NA | NA | NR | NA |
| | Control | 76 | NA | NA | NA | NR | NA |
| In-hospital complications, % | Intervention | NA | NA | NA | NA | NR | NA |
| | Control | NA | NA | NA | NA | NR | NA |
| Functional status (ADLs) recovery 12 months , % | Intervention | 58* | NA | NA | NA | NA | NA |
| | Control | 36 | NA | NA | NA | NA | NA |

**Table 2.1-3** Studies assessing the beneficial effects of a geriatric-led model with orthopedic consultant in the management of hip fractures in older adults.
Abbreviations: ADLs, activities of daily living; IQR, interquartile range; NA, not assessed; NR, data assessed but not reported; SD, standard deviation.
* Significant difference between intervention and control.
† Control: retrospective chart review.

## 4 Early supported discharge and postacute care

### 4.1 General considerations

The concept of using forms of skilled and dedicated postacute care like a geriatric orthopedic rehabilitation unit and early home-based care for FFPs was originally introduced in the United States and more recently also adopted in the United Kingdom and other European countries [4, 18]. These strategies were implemented primarily to improve functional recovery by offering dedicated services skilled in the rehabilitation of older adults presenting with hip fractures, in contradistinction to traditional inpatient rehabilitation [2, 4, 5, 50]. They also offered the opportunity to reduce acute hospital stay and promote early discharge in FFPs while maintaining an acceptable quality of care and short-term and long-term outcomes. Geriatric orthopedic rehabilitation units and home-based supported discharge represent the more consistently implemented approaches to achieve these goals [2, 4, 50–54].

Since they focus on only a part of the overall care, these innovative rehabilitation schemes should be considered as possible postacute transitions that could be used in tandem with any of the aforementioned models, rather than as a standalone and comprehensive model of care [4]. Indeed, the implementation of these services without including a specific orthogeriatric acute model may not produce the expected outcomes.

### 4.2 Geriatric orthopedic rehabilitation units

The geriatric orthopedic rehabilitation unit (GORU) is a variation of the traditional geriatric rehabilitation unit, fully dedicated to the care and rehabilitation of older adults presenting with a fracture. In general, the transition to a GORU may follow the admission to one of the services previously described. Once the orthopedic surgeon, the geriatrician, or the orthogeriatric team judges that the patient is fit to be moved to a rehabilitation ward, he/she is rapidly transferred to a GORU [4].

The presence of an interdisciplinary team skilled in the care of older adults distinguishes this service from other rehabilitation programs. The orthopedic specialist is not routinely present but advises the team on demand. The healthcare providers of the interdisciplinary team hold weekly or more frequent meetings to evaluate progress and problems arising during the rehabilitation. The specific contents, frequency, duration, and intensity of the training or rehabilitative program vary from one program to another.

Since their implementation, these units have produced better short-term and long-term outcomes than those from traditional rehabilitation units [49, 53–57]. A number of well-designed trials have demonstrated significant reduction in LOS in the rehabilitation setting, greater recovery of functional status, lower risk of institutionalization, and higher rates of survival compared to those treated in the traditional rehabilitation ward. Finally, it should be emphasized that this rehabilitation approach was also demonstrated to be successful in patients with moderate to severe dementia [56].

### 4.3 Home-based rehabilitation

Early discharge and home-based rehabilitation (HBR) approaches after hip fracture have been developed since 1986 in Europe, Australia, and North America [4]. The implementation of this alternative to traditional inpatient rehabilitation requires adequate community resources and the presence of home rehabilitation and community nursing services in the patient's healthcare district [4].

Patients potentially suitable for early discharge to home are usually those living at home with relatives or with other types of social support and are medically fit enough to be discharged to an outpatient setting, ie, clinically stable without relevant acute illness [2, 4]. Patient and relatives should be assessed on admission for suitability, informed about the service, and agreeable to this discharge plan. In some experiences, a trained geriatric nurse, a physiotherapist, or an occupational therapist visits the patient's home before discharge to evaluate the home for suitability and identify any necessary equipment. Then, soon after surgery, the patient is transferred directly home for rehabilitation. An interdisciplinary team, including a geriatrician and a geriatric nurse, is usually involved in the care of the older adult in collaboration with the general practitioner.

A number of RCTs and prospective observational studies have evaluated the potential benefits of HBR [2, 4, 50, 52, 57–61]. Published studies demonstrate that HBR services in older adults after hip fracture are feasible, safe, and effective producing comparable results in terms of functional outcomes and reduced LOS to traditional rehabilitation programs. These results were also confirmed in patients with prefracture cognitive decline or disability [2, 50].

## 5 References


1. **Pioli G, Barone A, Giusti A, et al.** Predictors of mortality after hip fracture: results from 1-year follow-up. *Aging Clin Exp Res.* 2006 Oct;18(5):381–387.
2. **Giusti A, Barone A, Oliveri M, et al.** An analysis of the feasibility of home rehabilitation among elderly people with proximal femoral fractures. *Arch Phys Med Rehabil.* 2006 Jun;87(6):826–831.
3. **Barone A, Giusti A, Pizzonia M, et al.** A comprehensive geriatric intervention reduces short- and long-term mortality in older people with hip fracture. *J Am Geriatr Soc.* 2006 Apr;54(4):711–712.
4. **Giusti A, Barone A, Razzano M, et al.** Optimal setting and care organization in the management of older adults with hip fracture. *Eur J Phys Rehabil Med.* 2011 Jun;47(2):281–296.
5. **Pioli G, Giusti A, Barone A.** Orthogeriatric care for the elderly with hip fractures: where are we? *Aging Clin Exp Res.* 2008 Apr;20(2):113–122.
6. **Grigoryan KV, Javedan H, Rudolph JL.** Orthogeriatric care models and outcomes in hip fracture patients: a systematic review and meta-analysis. *J Orthop Trauma.* 2014 Mar;28(3):e49–e55.
7. **Buecking B, Timmesfeld N, Riem S, et al.** Early orthogeriatric treatment of trauma in the elderly: a systematic review and metaanalysis. *Dtsch Arztebl Int.* 2013 Apr;110(15):255–262.
8. **Mendelson DA, Friedman SM.** Principles of comanagement and the geriatric fracture center. *Clin Geriatr Med.* 2014 May;30(2):183–189.
9. **Prestmo A, Hagen G, Sletvold O, et al.** Comprehensive geriatric care for patients with hip fractures: a prospective, randomised, controlled trial. *Lancet.* 2015 Apr 25;385(9978):1623–1633.
10. **Doshi HK, Ramason R, Azellarasi J, et al.** Orthogeriatric model for hip fracture patients in Singapore: our early experience and initial outcomes. *Arch Orthop Trauma Surg.* 2014 Mar;134(3):351–357.
11. **Moja L, Piatti A, Pecoraro V, et al.** Timing matters in hip fracture surgery: patients operated within 48 hours have better outcomes. A meta-analysis and meta-regression of over 190,000 patients. *PLoS One.* 2012;7(10):e46175.
12. **Boddaert J, Cohen-Bittan J, Khiami F, et al.** Postoperative admission to a dedicated geriatric unit decreases mortality in elderly patients with hip fracture. *PLoS One.* 2014;9(1):e83795.
13. **Gehlbach SH, Avrunin JS, Puleo E.** Trends in hospital care for hip fractures. *Osteoporos Int.* 2007 May;18(5):585–591.
14. **Friedman SM, Mendelson DA, Bingham KW, et al.** Impact of a comanaged Geriatric Fracture Center on short-term hip fracture outcomes. *Arch Intern Med.* 2009 Oct 12;169(18):1712–1717.
15. **Flikweert ER, Izaks GJ, Knobben BA, et al.** The development of a comprehensive multidisciplinary care pathway for patients with a hip fracture: design and results of a clinical trial. *BMC Musculoskelet Disord.* 2014 May 30;15:188.
16. **Chia PH, Gualano L, Seevanayagam S, et al.** Outcomes following fractured neck of femur in an Australian metropolitan teaching hospital. *Bone Joint Res.* 2013;2(8):162–168.
17. **Bhattacharyya R, Agrawal Y, Elphick H, et al.** A unique orthogeriatric model: a step forward in improving the quality of care for hip fracture patients. *Int J Surg.* 2013;11(10):1083–1086.
18. **Jarman B, Aylin P, Bottle A.** Discharge destination and length of stay: differences between US and English hospitals for people aged 65 and over. *BMJ.* 2004 Mar 13;328(7440):605.
19. **The National Hip Fracture Database.** National Report 2012. Available at: www.nhfd.co.uk/20/hipfractureR.nsf/vwcontent/2012ReportDownload/$File/NHFD+National+Report+2012.pdf?openelement. Accessed October 1, 2014.
20. **Adunsky A, Arad M, Levi R, et al.** Five-year experience with the 'Sheba' model of comprehensive orthogeriatric care for elderly hip fracture patients. *Disabil Rehabil.* 2005 Sep 30-Oct 15;27(18-19):1123–1127.
21. **Alvarez-Nebreda M, Vidan M, Serra J.** Hip fracture management and outcomes in Spain. *Eur Geriatr Med.* 2010;1(2):108–111.
22. **Cogan L, Martin AJ, Kelly LA, et al.** An audit of hip fracture services in the Mater Hospital Dublin 2001 compared with 2006. *Ir J Med Sci.* 2010 Mar;179(1):51–55.
23. **Deschodt M, Braes T, Broos P, et al.** Effect of an inpatient geriatric consultation team on functional outcome, mortality, institutionalization, and readmission rate in older adults with hip fracture: a controlled trial. *J Am Geriatr Soc.* 2011 Jul;59(7):1299–1308.
24. **Folbert EC, Smit RS, van der Velde D, et al.** Geriatric fracture center: a multidisciplinary treatment approach for older patients with a hip fracture improved quality of clinical care and short-term treatment outcomes. *Geriatr Orthop Surg Rehabil.* 2012 Jun;3(2):59–67.
25. **Auais M, Morin S, Nadeau L, et al.** Changes in frailty-related characteristics of the hip fracture population and their implications for healthcare services: evidence from Quebec, Canada. *Osteoporos Int.* 2013 Oct;24(10):2713–2724.
26. **Beaupre LA, Cinats JG, Senthilselvan A, et al.** Reduced morbidity for elderly patients with a hip fracture after implementation of a perioperative evidence-based clinical pathway. *Qual Saf Health Care.* 2006 Oct;15(5):375–379.
27. **Chong C, Christou J, Fitzpatrick K, et al.** Description of an orthopedic-geriatric model of care in Australia with 3 years data. *Geriatr Gerontol Int.* 2008 Jun;8(2):86–92.
28. **Sivakumar BS, McDermott LM, Bell JJ, et al.** Dedicated hip fracture service: implementing a novel model of care. *ANZ J Surg.* 2013 Jul;83(7-8):559–563.
29. **Pioli G, Frondini C, Lauretani F, et al.** Time to surgery and rehabilitation resources affect outcomes in orthogeriatric units. *Arch Gerontol Geriatr.* 2012 Sep-Oct;55(2):316–322.
30. **Pioli G, Lauretani F, Davoli ML, et al.** Older people with hip fracture and IADL disability require earlier surgery. *J Gerontol A Biol Sci Med Sci.* 2012 Nov;67(11):1272–1277.
31. **Gregersen M, Morch MM, Hougaard K, et al.** Geriatric intervention in elderly patients with hip fracture in an orthopedic ward. *J Inj Violence Res.* 2012 Jul;4(2):45–51.
32. **Kates SL, Mendelson DA, Friedman SM.** Co-managed care for fragility hip fractures (Rochester model). *Osteoporos Int.* 2010 Dec;21(Suppl 4):S621–S625.
33. **Sund R.** Modeling the volume-effectiveness relationship in the case of hip fracture treatment in Finland. *BMC Health Serv Res.* 2010 Aug 13;10:238.
34. **Forte ML, Virnig BA, Swiontkowski MF, et al.** Ninety-day mortality after intertrochanteric hip fracture: does provider volume matter? *J Bone Joint Surg Am.* 2010 Apr;92(4):799–806.
35. **Gilchrist WJ, Newman RJ, Hamblen DL, et al.** Prospective randomised study of an orthopaedic geriatric inpatient service. *BMJ.* 1988 Oct 29;297(6656):1116–1118.

36. **Khan R, Fernandez C, Kashifl F, et al.** Combined orthogeriatric care in the management of hip fractures: a prospective study. *Ann R Coll Surg Engl.* 2002 Mar;84(2):122–124.
37. **Khasraghi FA, Christmas C, Lee EJ, et al.** Effectiveness of a multidisciplinary team approach to hip fracture management. *J Surg Orthop Adv.* 2005 Spring;14(1):27–31.
38. **Gonzalez-Montalvo JI, Alarcon T, Mauleon JL, et al.** The orthogeriatric unit for acute patients: a new model of care that improves efficiency in the management of patients with hip fracture. *Hip Int.* 2010 Apr–Jun;20(2):229–235.
39. **Biber R, Singler K, Curschmann-Horter M, et al.** Implementation of a co-managed Geriatric Fracture Center reduces hospital stay and time-to-operation in elderly femoral neck fracture patients. *Arch Orthop Trauma Surg.* 2013 Nov;133(11):1527–1531.
40. **Zeltzer J, Mitchell RJ, Toson B, et al.** Orthogeriatric services associated with lower 30-day mortality for older patients who undergo surgery for hip fracture. *Med J Aust.* 2014 Oct 06;201(7):409–411.
41. **Vidan M, Serra JA, Moreno C, et al.** Efficacy of a comprehensive geriatric intervention in older patients hospitalized for hip fracture: a randomized, controlled trial. *J Am Geriatr Soc.* 2005 Sep;53(9):1476–1482.
42. **Watne LO, Torbergsen AC, Conroy S, et al.** The effect of a pre- and postoperative orthogeriatric service on cognitive function in patients with hip fracture: randomized controlled trial (Oslo Orthogeriatric Trial). *BMC Med.* 2014 Apr 15;12:63.
43. **Kammerlander C, Roth T, Friedman SM, et al.** Ortho-geriatric service—a literature review comparing different models. *Osteoporos Int.* 2010 Dec;21(Suppl 4):S637–S646.
44. **Adunsky A, Lusky A, Arad M, et al.** A comparative study of rehabilitation outcomes of elderly hip fracture patients: the advantage of a comprehensive orthogeriatric approach. *J Gerontol A Biol Sci Med Sci.* 2003 Jun;58(6):542–547.
45. **Adunsky A, Lerner-Geva L, Blumstein T, et al.** Improved survival of hip fracture patients treated within a comprehensive geriatric hip fracture unit, compared with standard of care treatment. *J Am Med Dir Assoc.* 2011 Jul;12(6):439–444.
46. **Miura LN, DiPiero AR, Homer LD.** Effects of a geriatrician-led hip fracture program: improvements in clinical and economic outcomes. *J Am Geriatr Soc.* 2009 Jan;57(1):159–167.
47. **Della Rocca GJ, Moylan KC, Crist BD, et al.** Comanagement of geriatric patients with hip fractures: a retrospective, controlled, cohort study. *Geriatr Orthop Surg Rehabil.* 2013 Mar;4(1):10–15.
48. **Gupta A.** The effectiveness of geriatrician-led comprehensive hip fracture collaborative care in a new acute hip unit based in a general hospital setting in the UK. *J R Coll Physicians Edinb.* 2014;44(1):20–26.
49. **Stenvall M, Olofsson B, Nyberg L, et al.** Improved performance in activities of daily living and mobility after a multidisciplinary postoperative rehabilitation in older people with femoral neck fracture: a randomized controlled trial with 1-year follow-up. *J Rehabil Med.* 2007 Apr;39(3):232–238.
50. **Giusti A, Barone A, Pioli G.** Rehabilitation after hip fracture in patients with dementia. *J Am Geriatr Soc.* 2007 Aug;55(8):1309–1310.
51. **Parker MJ, Pryor GA, Myles J.** 11-year results in 2,846 patients of the Peterborough Hip Fracture Project: reduced morbidity, mortality and hospital stay. *Acta Orthop Scand.* 2000 Feb;71(1):34–38.
52. **Hollingworth W, Todd C, Parker M, et al.** Cost analysis of early discharge after hip fracture. *BMJ.* 1993 Oct 09;307(6909):903–906.
53. **Reid J, Kennie DC.** Geriatric rehabilitative care after fractures of the proximal femur: one year follow up of a randomised clinical trial. *BMJ.* 1989 Jul 01;299(6690):25–26.
54. **Kennie DC, Reid J, Richardson IR, et al.** Effectiveness of geriatric rehabilitative care after fractures of the proximal femur in elderly women: a randomised clinical trial. *BMJ.* 1988 Oct 29;297(6656):1083–1086.
55. **Huusko TM, Karppi P, Avikainen V, et al.** Intensive geriatric rehabilitation of hip fracture patients: a randomized, controlled trial. *Acta Orthop Scand.* 2002 Aug;73(4):425–431.
56. **Huusko TM, Karppi P, Avikainen V, et al.** Randomised, clinically controlled trial of intensive geriatric rehabilitation in patients with hip fracture: subgroup analysis of patients with dementia. *BMJ.* 2000 Nov 04;321(7269):1107–1111.
57. **Chudyk AM, Jutai JW, Petrella RJ, et al.** Systematic review of hip fracture rehabilitation practices in the elderly. *Arch Phys Med Rehabil.* 2009 Feb;90(2):246–262.
58. **Crotty M, Whitehead CH, Gray S, et al.** Early discharge and home rehabilitation after hip fracture achieves functional improvements: a randomized controlled trial. *Clin Rehabil.* 2002 Jun;16(4):406–413.
59. **Crotty M, Whitehead C, Miller M, et al.** Patient and caregiver outcomes 12 months after home-based therapy for hip fracture: a randomized controlled trial. *Arch Phys Med Rehabil.* 2003 Aug;84(8):1237–1239.
60. **Kuisma R.** A randomized, controlled comparison of home versus institutional rehabilitation of patients with hip fracture. *Clin Rehabil.* 2002 Aug;16(5):553–561.
61. **Tinetti ME, Baker DI, Gottschalk M, et al.** Home-based multicomponent rehabilitation program for older persons after hip fracture: a randomized trial. *Arch Phys Med Rehabil.* 1999 Aug;80(8):916–922.

# 2.2 Overcoming barriers to implementation of a care model

Stephen L Kates

## 1 Introduction

Over the past several years, a great deal of literature has been published about the benefits of starting and using an enhanced care model for fragility fracture patients (FFPs). Many care models have been described in the literature [1, 2], four of which are presented in chapter 2.1 Models of orthogeriatric care. The benefits of such models include improved quality of patient care, shorter length of hospital stay (LOS), fewer adverse events during and after the hospital stay, improved collegiality among healthcare providers, and reduced costs of care [3–7].

Despite these reported benefits, most hospitals have not yet adopted a comanaged care model. Many possible reasons exist for not implementing such a program. This chapter covers some of these barriers to the implementation of an organized geriatric fracture program.

## 2 If an organized program is better, why doesn't everyone want one?

In some centers, physicians and institutional team members may be of the opinion that their usual care model is acceptable and performing adequately. Although there has been a universal emphasis on the reduction of LOS, few hospitals have made the direct association between a standardized geriatric fracture care program, reduced LOS, and improved quality of care. Additionally, there are a number of surgeons and physicians who believe no one else needs to tell them how to take better care of their FFPs. Some perceive the model as too hard to implement [8]. Other centers suffer from a lack of physician leadership, resulting in failure to implement such a model of care [8]. In some centers, there are major institutional barriers to implementing a program [8]. Additionally, many other issues have been described that interfere with the implementation of an organized, standardized, and comanaged geriatric fracture program (**Table 2.2-1**). In such cases, the patients suffer from a lack of organized care and experience more adverse events and longer LOSs as a result.

## 3 Institutional barriers

There are certainly many potential barriers that exist from an institutional standpoint.

### 3.1 Other priorities

One of the more common barriers includes capacity of the hospital or institutional leadership team because of the range of tasks allocated to the team members. In this situation, there are often more pressing matters that present themselves to the institutional leadership [8]. These include regulatory and payment changes, local, state, and national dictums, space concerns, recruitment of physician concerns, and potential penalties, or punitive measures facing the hospital externally.

### 3.2 Other clinical service lines

Additionally, there are numerous other diagnoses and programs competing for the attention of hospital leadership, many of which are perceived as more commercially attractive. Fragility fractures do not usually make it to that level of significant attention from hospital administration. It is the job of the physician leaders to elevate the importance of the FFP to the hospital leadership to get it into the queue of projects needing to be accomplished.

### 3.3 Overcrowded emergency department

Other common barriers to implementation include overcrowded emergency departments which often hinder the FFP from being treated efficiently. More pressing matters, such as acute high-energy or penetrating-trauma patients, take on higher priority for the emergency department staff [9]. Also, patients using the emergency department for common, often nonurgent medical problems clog up the emergency department, preventing the FFP from being seen promptly and receiving the appropriate attention [9].

### 3.4 Overcrowded floors

Once seen in the emergency department, bed capacity of the hospital becomes a major issue. Oftentimes, hospitals are full to capacity, preventing the FFP from being admitted in a timely manner. In which case, the patient may be boarded in the emergency department for a prolonged period, in some cases with a LOS measured in days.

### 3.5 Lack of operating room capacity

Operating room capacity also represents a significant issue for the FFP [8]. If the operating room is full to capacity, more pressing acute cases will be treated first, relegating the FFP to the end of the queue. Here again, appropriate medical and surgical leadership are required to help the administrative team understand the importance of early surgery for this patient group. The hospital without any operating room capacity remaining will often decline to institute an organized fragility fracture program because they will be fearful of success.

### 3.6 Minimum caseload

Another institutional problem relates to the number of patients seen. There have been a few published estimates of patient volumes needed to implement a successful fragility fracture program. These range from 49 to 159 patients [10]. Published work suggests the average number of patients seen yearly should be 100 or greater for an organized program to be worthwhile [5].

| Barrier | Countermeasure | Personnel needed for implementation |
|---|---|---|
| Program leadership | • Select committed:<br>– Surgeon<br>– Medical leaders | • Can be selected by:<br>– Department<br>– Chairman<br>– Peers<br>– Hospital<br>– Administration |
| Hospital administration | • Engage, educate, and persuade, with an emphasis on expected improvements in:<br>– Patient satisfaction<br>– Cost reduction<br>– Hospital prestige | • Program champions with departmental support |
| Skeptical surgeons | • Education to explain the problem<br>• Review data<br>• Emphasize physician benefits including improved patient outcomes and ease of care | • Surgeon champion |
| Regulatory | • Education<br>• Collaboration with other centers<br>• Business planning that documents outcomes/costs | • Program champions |
| Technical implementation | • Read published literature<br>• Visit a successful center<br>• Attend a course and/or webinars<br>• Engage a consultant if needed | • Program leaders<br>• Hospital administration |
| Bed capacity | • Collect data on LOS<br>• Examine ways to shorten LOS and recognition that a 50% reduction in LOS doubles the bed capacity of the unit | • Program leaders with hospital administrators |
| Operating room capacity | • Look for designated time for geriatric fracture cases<br>• Emphasize need for early surgery to improve outcomes and reduce LOS<br>• Sometimes requires negotiation and helping the operating room personnel to learn how to shorten turnaround times | • Surgeon leader |
| Anesthesia buy-in | • Select an anesthesia champion to educate and lead colleagues to a collaborative and collegial approach to caring for geriatric fracture patients | • Program leaders<br>• Hospital administration |
| Cardiac clearance | • This is a problem of tradition and lack of education. It can be ameliorated with education and trust-building of the medical and anesthesia colleagues<br>• Published literature clearly documents when an echocardiogram is required and when to consult a cardiologist | • Medical, anesthesia, and surgical champions |
| Need a case manager | • A case manager can be a nurse, physician's assistant, or nurse practitioner<br>• This is an important position for a busy program<br>• Designating an experienced, respected individual already employed by the hospital is a good strategy<br>• The hospital administration will need to accept the cost in return for cost savings realized by the program with time | • Administration with program leader input |

**Table 2.2-1** Barriers to the implementation of an organized, standardized, and comanaged geriatric fracture program, as well as countermeasures to overcome them [8].
Abbreviation: LOS, length of hospital stay.

### 3.7 Costs and effectiveness

An additional institutional concern is based on the cost of running such a program, particularly if the savings are not realized until future years. Support costs can run from minimal to significantly more than USD 150,000 depending on whether or not a consulting firm is used to implement the program or if new employees are hired. If a program requires employees to be hired, costs will obviously be ongoing and higher than if existing employees can be used. Likewise, if existing space and other resources can be used, costs will be considerably lower for both implementation and the ongoing operation of an organized standardized fragility fracture program.

Finally, institutional administration leadership expects such a program to be both cost-effective and the outcomes to be measurable. Both cost-effectiveness and outcomes are measurable, but this requires work and ongoing attention to these metrics. Creation of a monthly scorecard to be reviewed by the hospital administration officials is one good method for management of cost and outcomes.

## 4 Provider barriers

Published literature has identified a number of provider barriers to implementing a standardized fragility fracture program [8]. These include lack of surgeon or medical champions, lack of a case manager, anesthesia department problems, and difficulty obtaining cardiology clearance in a timely manner [8].

### 4.1 Surgical and medical leadership

Surgical and medical leadership of the program represents an essential element for success of any organized standardized orthogeriatric fracture program [5]. The leaders should agree to work together and have a collegial relationship with one another. It is also important to engage the anesthesiologists by finding a suitable committed leader to help with implementation and ongoing operation of the program. Regular and ongoing communication between the individual physician leaders is essential to proactively identify new problems and to ensure the representation and support of the care team members. Communication forums can include regular team meetings, routine review of processes and outcomes, and reinforcement of best-practice efforts. In addition, as members of the extended care team change over time, basic educational efforts about orthogeriatric care are always needed. The leaders should have departmental support, administration support, and be respected by the care team. It is a long-term commitment that must be considered carefully when choosing leaders.

Individual medical and surgical physicians may not agree with the program and may in fact strongly wish to continue their traditional approach to care (ie, usual care). A combination of education and persuasion with good communication is required here. The program leaders should recognize that about 70% of the physicians and surgeons must agree to participate in the program and comply with policies to get it successfully started. Once running, the outcome data are frequently persuasive to stubborn providers to show them the new program is better. For undermining or recalcitrant providers, replacement may be necessary if all else fails.

## 5 Regulatory barriers

In most locales, some forms of regulatory barriers exist to implementing a fragility fracture program. These may be relatively simple or more complex.

### 5.1 Hospital board approval

Hospital board approval is commonly required and can be a barrier if the program is not presented to them in the proper manner. The program should be presented by the surgeon champion to the board emphasizing the quality, safety, and economic benefits of the program and include an abbreviated business plan overview. This presentation should last 7–10 minutes in most cases and will likely be successful if presented well.

### 5.2 Regional and/or provincial barriers

In some systems, changing the care model will require regional and/or provincial approval. Again, a focus on the quality and safety aspects of the program along with potential cost savings should be emphasized. The regional system data should be included in such a presentation to demonstrate the economic aspects of the program to the regional authorities. It may also need to include consensus from other regional centers or a plan to scale the program regionally in order to be successful. The Canadian province of Ontario has successfully implemented an improved care system in this manner.

### 5.3 National approval barriers

National approval barriers are considerably greater. Few nations have successfully changed the hip fracture care model. The UK is an excellent example of consensus building, governmental lobbying, and outstanding leadership from surgeons, physicians, and thought leaders to successfully implement the Best Practice Tariff nationally in the National Health Service. The program has shown reduced mortality rates at 30 days along with a high level of compliance by hospitals. This program required a committed group of champions from across the nation to achieve this success that now serves as a model for other diagnoses in the UK. There are analogous efforts in the US to reward systems with organized fracture programs [11, 12].

## 6 Cultural barriers

Cultural barriers are many and are difficult to change. As with the regulatory barriers, cultural ones come in many forms.

### 6.1 Traditions and attitudes

Local cultural barriers consist of traditions and attitudes toward care held by the care provider team. There is a common issue of tradition, ie, "we have always done it this way and it works." Likewise, the care team may not understand that providing the care in an organized manner is actually better. Education of the team is an effective countermeasure. Education can include reading literature, attending lectures and programs by visiting professors, site visits to successful programs, and attending face-to-face educational events such as a regional AO orthogeriatric course. It is essential here to show that a better quality of care is actually easier once the model has been implemented.

### 6.2 Patient-related cultural barriers

It is important to educate patients and families about a new system and emphasize the safety and quality benefits. Consistent messaging from a committed care team is essential here. Because care is delivered locally, local education efforts should extend into the local community to educate primary care physicians, nursing home staff, and groups of senior citizens about the new care model to achieve buy-in and understanding of the program goals.

## 7 References

1. **Giusti A, Barone A, Razzano M, et al.** Optimal setting and care organization in the management of older adults with hip fracture. *Eur J Phys Rehabil Med.* 2011 Jun;47(2):281–296.
2. **Grigoryan KV, Javedan H, Rudolph JL.** Orthogeriatric care models and outcomes in hip fracture patients: a systematic review and meta-analysis. *J Orthop Trauma.* 2014 Mar;28(3):e49–e55.
3. **Friedman SM, Mendelson DA, Bingham KW, et al.** Impact of a comanaged Geriatric Fracture Center on short-term hip fracture outcomes. *Arch Intern Med.* 2009 Oct 12;169(18):1712–1717.
4. **Friedman SM, Mendelson DA, Kates SL, et al.** Geriatric co-management of proximal femur fractures: total quality management and protocol-driven care result in better outcomes for a frail patient population. *J Am Geriatr Soc.* 2008 Jul;56(7):1349–1356.
5. **Kates SL, Mendelson DA, Friedman SM.** Co-managed care for fragility hip fractures (Rochester model). *Osteoporos Int.* 2010 Dec;21(Suppl 4):S621–S625.
6. **Della Rocca GJ, Moylan KC, Crist BD, et al.** Comanagement of geriatric patients with hip fractures: a retrospective, controlled, cohort study. *Geriatr Orthop Surg Rehabil.* 2013 Mar;4(1):10–15.
7. **Kates SL, Mendelson DA, Friedman SM.** The value of an organized fracture program for the elderly: early results. *J Orthop Trauma.* 2011 Apr;25(4):233–237.
8. **Kates SL, O'Malley N, Friedman SM, et al.** Barriers to implementation of an organized geriatric fracture program. *Geriatr Orthop Surg Rehabil.* 2012 Mar;3(1):8–16.
9. **Rashid A, Brooks TR, Bessman E, et al.** Factors associated with emergency department length of stay for patients with hip fracture. *Geriatr Orthop Surg Rehabil.* 2013 Sep;4(3):78–83.
10. **Clement RC, Ahn J, Mehta S, et al.** Economic viability of geriatric hip fracture centers. *Orthopedics.* 2013 Dec;36(12):e1509–e1514.
11. **Neuburger J, Currie C, Wakeman R, et al.** The impact of a national clinician-led audit initiative on care and mortality after hip fracture in England: an external evaluation using time trends in non-audit data. *Med Care.* 2015 Aug;53(8):686–691.
12. **Johansen A, Boulton C, Hertz K, et al.** The National Hip Fracture Database (NHFD)—using a national clinical audit to raise standards of nursing care. *Int J Orthop Trauma Nurs.* 2017 Aug;26:3–6.

# 2.3 Clinical practice guidelines

Stephen L Kates, Michael Blauth

## 1 Introduction

Clinical practice guidelines (CPGs) are designed to inform practice, and offer guidance and direction on clinical care. Clinical practice guidelines are typically evidence-based and constructed by a workgroup of interested physicians. Most CPGs are supported by governments or medical societies with endorsement from other stakeholders. A CPG helps to set care standards that physicians and surgeons can use to guide their patient care practices. Typically, CPGs on orthogeriatric comanagement will cover the time period from hospital admission to completion of healing including secondary fracture prevention.

Clinical practice guidelines are not designed to specifically dictate care but serve as a framework for care. Individual physicians should consider the recommendations and the strength of these recommendations when providing care to specific patients. Clinical practice guidelines, when done well, can highlight evidence-based best practices and also point out gaps in knowledge that will require future study to answer. They also serve as a convenient reference for evidence on specific aspects of care for medical and surgical providers.

## 2 Commonality of national clinical practice guidelines

Many national guidelines exist for the care of hip fractures but not as many exist for osteoporotic fractures in general. Among these national CPGs, several will be discussed in this chapter, including the American Academy of Orthopaedic Surgeons (AAOS) CPG, the National Institute for Health and Care Excellence (NICE) guidelines, and the Australian and New Zealand Hip Fracture Registry (ANZHFR) guidelines [1–3]. These three sets of CPGs are among the finest created and often serve as templates for future efforts in other countries and regions.

Since all these guidelines are evidence-based, they contain a significant amount of commonality and the recommendations made are similar. Specific topics covered include use of advanced diagnostic imaging, timing of surgery, postoperative weight-bearing status, medical comanagement, management of femoral neck and trochanteric fractures, and postfracture osteoporosis management. For a more comprehensive list, see **Table 2.3-1**. Review of this table shows considerable commonality exists in topics covered and similar recommendations as well [1–3]. The reassuring aspect of comparing CPGs from

| Recommendation | AAOS | NICE | ANZHFR |
|---|---|---|---|
| MRI for undisplaced fracture | ✔ | ✔ | ✔ |
| Pain management | ✔ | ✔ | ✔ |
| Early assessment | | ✔ | ✔ |
| Early surgery | ✔ | ✔ | ✔ |
| Early weight bearing | | ✔ | ✔ |
| Multidisciplinary care model | ✔ | ✔ | ✔ |
| Presurgical optimization | | ✔ | ✔ |
| Anesthetic choice | ✔ | ✔ | ✔ |
| Surgical team composition | | ✔ | ✔ |
| Displaced femoral neck fracture | ✔ | ✔ | ✔ |
| Physical therapy | ✔ | ✔ | ✔ |
| Delirium avoidance | | ✔ | ✔ |
| Falls assessment | | ✔ | |
| Early discharge | | ✔ | ✔ |
| Nursing home involvement | | ✔ | ✔ |
| Nondisplaced femoral neck fracture | ✔ | ✔ | |
| Implant for trochanteric fracture | ✔ | ✔ | ✔ |
| Anticoagulation postsurgery | ✔ | No clear advice | No clear advice |
| Transfusion threshold | ✔ | | |
| Nutrition | ✔ | ✔ | ✔ |
| Osteoporosis assessment | ✔ | ✔ | |
| Osteoporosis treatment | ✔ | ✔ | |

**Table 2.3-1** Commonality of recommendations of clinical practice guidelines for hip fracture care.
Abbreviations: AAOS, American Academy of Orthopaedic Surgeons; ANZHFR, Australian and New Zealand Hip Fracture Registry; MRI, magnetic resonance imaging; NICE, National Institute for Health and Care Excellence.

different regions is the general agreement on evidence-based best practices that are most useful for hip fracture patients. This international agreement is based on existing literature, which covers the most important aspects of care for the hip fracture patient. There are no guidelines offered for osteoporosis-related fractures or fragility fractures in general; all the existing guidelines are concerned specifically with hip fractures. However, there are two well-written monographs on fragility fractures that offer guidance, the BOA/BGS Blue Book [4, 5] and the *A Guide to Improving the Care of Fragility Fractures* by Mears et al [6]. The national guidelines have clearly focused on hip fracture due to its prevalence and high societal costs combined with frequent suboptimal outcomes.

## 3 Local adaptation and implementation

Once CPGs have been published by a national organization or society, the stepwise adaptation and implementation of these guidelines to the local or hospital setting becomes important. In some cases, hospitals will adopt the national CPGs to be their local guidelines and set these as a standard of care.

Creating consensus, and publishing and communicating local guidelines with all stakeholders in the process is the most important step in implementing optimal orthogeriatric fracture care. Often, national guidelines are not detailed. Local guidelines can be explicit including the choice and dosage of drugs in specific situations.

In large institutions, typically university departments, core team members like orthopedic trauma surgeons, geriatricians, anesthetists, and staff nurses can be complemented by local specialists like a cardiologist, microbiologist, and specialist for anticoagulation and thrombosis prophylaxis. These specialists can give input on specific topics, strengthen the significance and power of the local guidelines and help to avoid disagreement during implementation. The treatment team in smaller institutions may simply adopt the recommendations of those local guidelines.

Consensus guidelines are a strong tool to implement best practices standard in hospitals with many different "players". Since CPGs are typically based on best available evidence, their adoption is expected to benefit the majority of patients [1–3].

The following steps have proven to be key success factors in the local adoption of CPGs:

1. Creating awareness: The first step is making clinicians and care providers aware of the publication of the guidelines and the evidence basis used to create these documents. It should not be assumed that all clinicians are aware of the guidelines or of their content, and it may require repeated efforts on the hospital level to make clinicians aware of their publication and content. Communication with care providers is an essential element for local implementation. Repeated communication and repeated review of new guidelines should be strongly considered by hospital and physician leadership to inform clinicians of their content.
2. Meetings: Well-organized meetings with team members help to convey information, build trust, and enhance mutual understanding. The meetings should result in written and agreed upon local guidelines that address all steps in the treatment of fragility fracture patients (FFPs).
3. Internal communication systems: Guidelines should be made readily available, for example via the hospital or department intranet. Local guidelines should be studied and their important messages and recommendations should be incorporated into order sets, care plans, and surgical tactics and approaches (**Table 2.3-2**).
4. Monitoring and supervision: Adherence to the guidelines must be monitored, especially after implementation. A practical way to do so is the discussion of cases while doing rounds or in morbidity and mortality meetings. Particularly, when adverse events occur in the care of a FFP, the specific deviations in practice should be identi-

| CPG recommendation | Standard order |
|---|---|
| Osteoporosis assessment | • Admission order<br>• Vitamin D level<br>• Intact parathyroid hormone level<br>• Thyroid-stimulating hormone level<br>• Ionized calcium level |
| Blood transfusion | • Do not transfuse patient unless the hemoglobin level is < 8 grams |
| Anticoagulation | • Enoxaparin 40 mg SQ daily |
| Nutrition | • High-calorie, low-bulk dental soft diet |
| Delirium avoidance | • Be certain the patient retains and uses glasses and hearing aids<br>• Do not restrain patient<br>• Avoid use of diphenhydramine, meperidine, and H2 blockers |
| Osteoporosis treatment | • Vitamin D3, 2,000 international units daily |

**Table 2.3-2** Examples of order sets matching CPGs.
Abbreviations: CPG, clinical practice guidelines; SQ, subcutaneous.

fied and it should be determined if these are also deviations from national guidelines, and if this variation was appropriate. Educational efforts for the care team should focus on adherence to these guidelines in most cases unless there is a strong clinical reason not to. In such cases, the physician should be encouraged to carefully document reasons for not adhering to the local guidelines.

5. Outcome measurement: Measurement of guideline adherence linked to outcomes is a reasonable approach to determining if guidelines are actually being used by treating physicians. One helpful approach is to provide a "dot plot" of adherence and identify and inform specific physician outliers. This will help the physician understand their actual adherence to the guidelines in relation to their peers. Because physicians are typically competitive individuals, the underperforming physician will have a strong incentive to improve their performance. Such underperforming individuals should have education and counseling offered to them by departmental leaders on how they can improve results. The collection of a small amount of key data to monitor the outcome of FFPs is an appropriate quality control in countries without national hip fracture registry. If done regularly, trends and patterns can identify issues related to outcomes.

## 4 Nationwide initiatives

Some nations with CPGs are developing process measures for guideline adherence and the impact of guideline deviation. These so-called process measures are often obtained from claims data or from national hip fracture registry data. A powerful approach to change physician behavior is to modify reimbursement according to the level of adherence to guidelines and participation in registries for benchmarking.

### 4.1 The Best Practice Tariff

The British Best Practice Tariff was developed for osteoporotic hip fractures to encourage two key clinical characteristics of best practice: prompt surgery and appropriate involvement of geriatric medicine [7, 8]. The key clinical characteristics of best practice were chosen by a group of clinicians and service managers chaired by the National Clinical Director for trauma care. The following best practices focused on FFPs aged 60 years and older:

- Time to surgery within 36 hours from arrival in an emergency department, or time of diagnosis if an inpatient, to the start of anesthesia
- Admission under the joint care of a consultant geriatrician and a consultant orthopedic surgeon
- Application of a standard assessment protocol agreed upon by geriatric medicine, orthopedic surgery and anesthesia
- Assessment by a geriatrician in the preoperative period, within 72 hours of admission
- Postoperative geriatrician-directed multiprofessional rehabilitation team
- Fracture prevention assessments (falls and bone health)

### 4.2 Certification

In Germany, so-called centers for fragility fractures can be certified by the Academy of the German Trauma Association [9]. The requirements aim to foster an orthogeriatric interdisciplinary approach and to improve the quality of care and results documented in the national hip fracture registry. In order to become certified, a long list of items that are in concordance with national and international guidelines need to be audited. This process creates positive competition between providers. Reimbursement can be significantly increased if the ambitious requirements for a diagnosis-related group dedicated to orthogeriatric management are fulfilled.

### 4.3 Indicators used by the government

In the Netherlands, evidence-based guidelines, made by practicing professionals serve as a basis for indicators used by the government [10]. This set of parameters must be recorded by each hospital yearly and includes a pain score, time to surgery within 24 hours, reoperation rate within 60 days, pressure ulcers, nutritional status, and delirium. The parameters change over time.

The healthcare inspectorate may visit places with suboptimal performance, come up with a list of corrective actions, and may even initiate legal action if required.

The National Hip Fracture Database in the UK is designed by professionals. It is a web-based audit of hip fracture treatment and prevention. Similar to the British Best Practice Tariff, departments get a bonus if the patient is operated within 36 hours, care is taken by trauma and geriatric professionals, if there is an agreement on protocols of standard care by surgeon, geriatrician and anesthetist, if there is pre- and perioperative assessment by geriatricians, if the geriatricians take the lead in multidisciplinary revalidation, and if secondary fracture and falls prevention is addressed [8].

## 5 Periodic reassessment and revision of guidelines

Because CPGs are based on the best available evidence on a specific topic, best practices can be expected to change with time as new or better evidence becomes available. It is probably wise to revisit CPGs every 3–5 years to be sure that they are still consistent with best available evidence on the topic [3]. The task of reevaluating and revising CPGs should be undertaken by an expert group of physicians and surgeons assembled by the national group sponsoring the guidelines [1]. In some cases, this group will be governmental, whereas in other cases the group will be the medical or surgical specialty society. Because tremendous effort and rigid methodology is used to prepare CPGs, practicing physicians and surgeons should closely study CPG recommendations and try to adopt them in their clinical practice.

## 6 References

1. **American Academy of Orthopaedic Surgeons (AAOS).** Management of hip fractures in the elderly. Available at: www.aaos.org/Research/guidelines/HipFxSummaryofRecommendations.pdf. Published 2014. Accessed 2017.
2. **Australian and New Zealand Hip Fracture Registry (ANZHFR).** Australian and New Zealand Guideline for Hip Fracture Care: Improving Outcomes in Hip Fracture Management of Adults. Available at: www.anzhfr.org/guidelines-and-standards. Published 2014. Accessed 2017.
3. **National Institue for Health and Care Excellence (NICE).** Hip fracture: the management of hip fracture in adults. Clinical guideline [CG124]. Available at: https://www.nice.org.uk/guidance/cg124. Published 2014. Accessed 2017.
4. **British Orthopaedic Association and British Geriatrics Society.** The care of patients with fragility fracture. Available at: www.nhfd.co.uk. Published 2007. Accessed 2018.
5. **Marsh D, Curry C, Brown P, et al.** The Care of Patients with Fragility Fracture: British Orthopaedic Society Available at: www.bgs.org.uk. Published 2007. Accessed 2017.
6. **Mears SC, Kates SL.** A guide to improving the care of patients with fragility fractures, edition 2. *Geriatr Orthop Surg Rehabil.* 2015 Jun;6(2):58–120.
7. **Khan SK, Shirley MD, Glennie C, et al.** Achieving best practice tariff may not reflect improved survival after hip fracture treatment. *Clin Interv Aging.* 2014;9:2097–2102.
8. **Khan SK, Weusten A, Bonczek S, et al.** The Best Practice Tariff helps improve management of neck of femur fractures: a completed audit loop. *Br J Hosp Med (Lond).* 2013 Nov;74(11):644–647.
9. **Krause U, Jung K.** Geriatric Fracture Centre (German Trauma Society): guidelines and certification to improve geriatric trauma care. *Innovative Surg Sci.* 2016;1(2):79–85.
10. **Zielinski SM, Meeuwis MA, Heetveld MJ, et al.** Adherence to a femoral neck fracture treatment guideline. *Int Orthop.* 2013 Jul;37(7):1327–1334.

# 2.4 Elements of an orthogeriatric comanaged program

Carl Neuerburg, Christian Kammerlander

## 1 Introduction

In light of the historically poor perioperative outcomes in fragility fracture patients (FFPs) [1–3], unique interdisciplinary team approaches in the treatment of these patients have been implemented to reduce peri- and postoperative complications. Orthogeriatric models of care were developed in England in the late 1950s and are now widely accepted [4]. Geriatricians are specialized in addressing comorbidities, ensuring optimal medical management for older multimorbid individuals, and can help to improve the outcomes of older patients with fragility fractures [3]. These interdisciplinary approaches have been described in various terms including orthogeriatric management, comprehensive geriatric care, or comanagement [5, 6]. The implementation of a successful orthogeriatric comanagement model of care varies from one hospital to another, but some key elements have to be considered.

Key elements of the comanaged care model, adapted from Lisk and Yeong [7], are:

- Prompt admission to orthopedic care
- Rapid and comprehensive medical, surgical, and anesthesiologic assessment
- Minimal delay to surgery
- Accurate and well-performed surgery (single-shot surgery)
- Prompt mobilization and rehabilitation
- Early supported discharge and ongoing community rehabilitation
- Secondary prevention, addressing bone protection and falls assessment

In order to ensure these elements, certain principles must be applied:

- Interdisciplinary teamwork and co-ownership: Patients should be treated in a coordinated manner and without conflicts among orthopedic, geriatric, and anesthesiological teams.
- Interdisciplinary communication including team meetings.
- Goal setting: Based on protocols and guidelines, patient-specific short-term and medium-term treatment goals must be set and revised according to the dynamic status and functional potential of each patient. Diagnostic and therapeutic interventions must be aligned with those goals. Consented goal setting is an excellent technique to get all clinicians and family members on the same page and to ease interprofessional and interdisciplinary communication.

These elements require a lot of additional resources, thus the importance of the individual elements have to be further discussed.

## 2 Key elements of comanaged care

### 2.1 Rapid comprehensive medical, surgical, and anesthesiologic assessment

Up to a quarter of patients with hip fractures have a preexisting cardiovascular disease, and some patients already have subclinical infections prior to their fracture [8, 9]. The postoperative course is often marked by an increased incidence of chest infections due to the combination of pain, immobility and reduced ability to cough [7].

The following correctable comorbidities should be identified and addressed immediately in order not to delay surgery [10] (see chapter 1.4 Preoperative risk assessment and preparation):

- Anemia
- Anticoagulation
- Volume depletion
- Electrolyte imbalance
- Uncontrolled diabetes
- Uncontrolled heart failure
- Correctable cardiac arrhythmia or ischemia
- Acute chest infection
- Exacerbation of chronic chest conditions

Data on the power of rapid comprehensive assessment still remain weak. It is recommended that an interdisciplinary prioritization of orthogeriatric trauma patients should start in the emergency department and the postoperative care unit should be informed as soon as possible to allocate capacities.

### 2.2 Minimal delay to surgery

There is growing emphasis on the benefits of minimizing surgical delay for orthogeriatric hip fracture patients [11]. It has been shown that a prolonged time to surgery is a risk factor for delirium, whereas delirium was found to be associated with a poor functional outcome and increased mortality [12, 13].

However, there are still authors querying the necessity of early surgery. Lizaur-Utrilla et al [14] stated recently that delaying surgery up to 4 days was not associated with higher morbidity or mortality rates. The authors recommended concentrating more on preoperative optimization with sufficient medical treatment rather than being bound by a universal timing of surgery [14].

The majority of studies consistently show that early surgery has a strong impact on reducing patient's mortality (**Fig 2.4-1**).

### 2.3 Single-shot surgery

Adapted surgical techniques respecting the low bone quality, bleeding issues, and reduced reserves in the soft tissues are required (see chapter 1.2 Principles of orthogeriatric surgical care). Revision surgeries must be avoided because they usually lead to significant deterioration.

### 2.4 Prompt mobilization

Immobilization of FFPs can be associated with various medical complications such as pressure ulcers, venous thromboembolism, wound and systemic infections, loss of muscle mass and muscle strength, or demineralization of bone that deteriorates during postoperative recovery. Postoperative mortality is known to be associated with the extent of postoperative mobilization. This was shown for patients suffering from femoral periprosthetic fractures (**Fig 2.4-2**) [16].

The importance of targeting the vulnerability of these patients at an early stage to prevent functional decline in the long run was also illustrated in the Trondheim Hip Fracture Trial [17]. Geriatric trauma patients were investigated in a randomized controlled trial comparing comprehensive geriatric care (CGC) to conventional orthopedic care. In this study, participants who received CGC had significantly higher gait speed, less asymmetry, better gait control, and more efficient gait patterns. Furthermore, the CGC participants were more often able to walk and reported better mobility at 4 and 12 months.

In conclusion, prompt mobilization remains an essential element for the treatment of orthogeriatric patients (see chapter 1.8 Postoperative surgical management).

### 2.5 Early multidisciplinary rehabilitation

In orthogeriatric patients, it is of particular importance to start rehabilitation immediately after surgery to prevent a loss of self-care and independence. Especially in patients with high degrees of comorbidity, frailty and polypharmacy, a multidisciplinary rehabilitation process is an important factor leading to optimal outcomes and a successful surgical procedure [18]. To determine the most appropriate rehabilitation program, the individual's baseline health status should be assessed. The assessment of prefracture mobility, cognition, depression, fall risk, nutritional status, incontinence, and visual function are of importance to plan the optimal rehabilitation program [19]. Interdisciplinary rehabilitation programs are known to have the best outcomes in terms of quality of life, reduced readmission rates, depression and fall prevention, highlighting the importance of early multidisciplinary rehabilitation [20].

| Timeframe and study | Early surgery, n | Delayed surgery, n | RR (95% CI) |
|---|---|---|---|
| **Short-term** | | | |
| Davie et al | 105 | 95 | 0.66 (0.28–1.56) |
| Harries et al | 40 | 40 | 1.00 (0.21–4.71) |
| Parker et al* | 290 | 178 | 0.68 (0.28–1.65) |
| Smektala et al | 139 | 22 | 0.79 (0.19–3.33) |
| Moran et al* | 982 | 1,372 | 0.98 (0.75–1.28) |
| Rae et al* | 137 | 85 | 0.62 (0.24–1.59) |
| Overall | 1,693 | 1,792 | 0.90 (0.71–1.13) |
| **Medium-term** | | | |
| Davis et al* | 45 | 185 | 0.80 (0.43–1.50) |
| Mullen et al† | 8 | 52 | 2.17 (1.42–3.31) |
| Dorotka et al | 158 | 24 | 0.42 (0.21–0.84) |
| Orosz et al | 398 | 780 | 0.70 (0.50–0.97) |
| Overall | 609 | 1,041 | 0.87 (0.44–1.72) |
| **Long-term** | | | |
| Zuckerman et al‡ | 267 | 100 | 0.58 (0.35–0.99) |
| Beringer et al | 133 | 70 | 0.54 (0.39–0.75) |
| Elliott et al | 169 | 1,611 | 0.35 (0.21–0.59) |
| Doruk et al§ | 38 | 27 | 0.36 (0.14–0.92) |
| Siegmeth et al* | 3,454 | 174 | 0.50 (0.34–0.74) |
| Smektala et al | 609 | 1,629 | 0.90 (0.71–1.15) |
| Overall | 4,670 | 3,673 | 0.55 (0.40–0.75) |

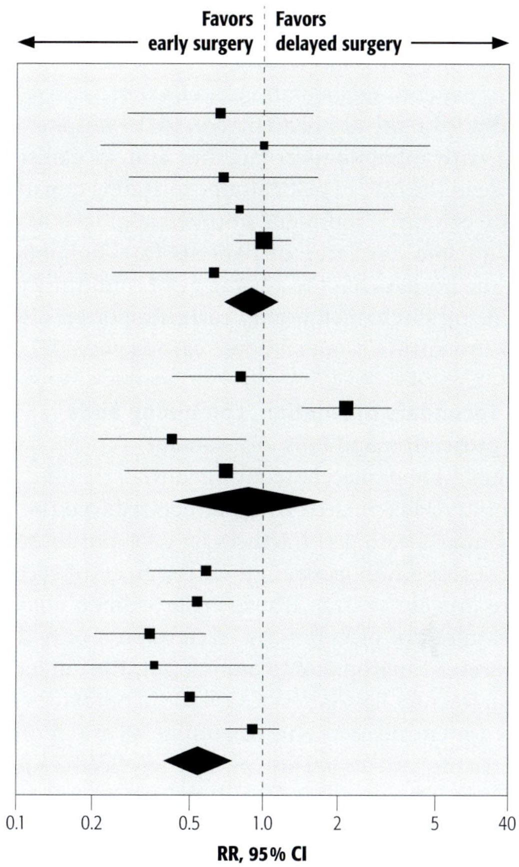


**Fig 2.4-1** Stratified analysis by time of death adapted from Simunovic et al [15]. Forrest plot of unadjusted relative risks for the effect of early compared with delayed surgery for hip fractures on all-cause mortality assessed in hospital or at 30 days (short-term), at 3–6 months (medium-term) or at 1 year (long-term) (random-effects model based on inverse variance method). Studies used a cut-off for delay of 24 hours, except as indicated otherwise.
Abbreviations: CI, confidence interval; n, number of patients included in the study group analyzed by the authors; RR, relative risk.
*Study used a cut-off of 48 hours for delay.
†Data based on patients who had medical illness in combination with hip fracture.
‡Study used a cut-off of 72 hours for delay.
§Study used a cut-off of 5 days for delay.

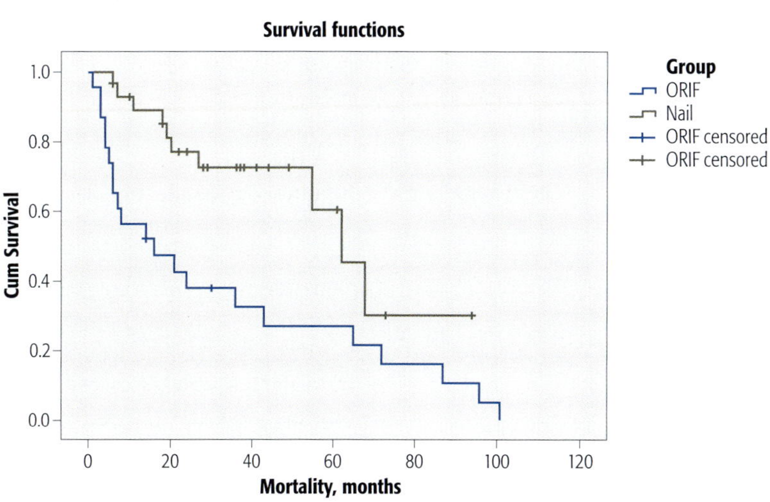


**Fig 2.4-2** Kaplan-Meier survival analysis for total mortality adapted from Langenhan et al [16] in patients being treated with either open reduction and internal fixation (ORIF) or a modular prosthesis nail. Patients in the ORIF group underwent a prolonged period of partial or non-weight bearing.

### 2.6 Early supported discharge and ongoing community rehabilitation

Planning patients' rehabilitation should start as early as possible, ideally on the day of admission to the hospital. Cooperation with rehabilitation facilities and specialists with expertise in the care of older adults, including departments for acute geriatrics, represent a proven approach to ensure early and safe discharge of patients [21]. Rehabilitation within the hospital has the advantage of continuity of care. When being discharged home, early supported discharge should also ensure as much home care as possible.

### 2.7 Secondary prevention, combining bone protection and falls assessment

In a double-blind, placebo-controlled trial, treatment with zoledronic acid compared with placebo reduced the risk of morphometric vertebral fractures by 70% during a 3-year period. These findings strengthen the need of secondary fracture prevention [22]. However, in women eligible for the treatment of osteoporosis in Germany, only 23% of them received appropriate treatment [23]. The implementation of a fracture liaison service (FLS) that provides a standardized identification and treatment of osteoporosis to orthogeriatric patients has proven to be an effective approach for secondary fracture prevention (see also chapter 2.8 Fracture liaison service and improving treatment rates for osteoporosis). In one trial, the FLS produced a 30% reduction for any fracture and a 40% reduction for major refractures compared to a standard approach hospital, whereas only 20 patients needed to be treated to prevent one new fracture over 3 years [24]. The impact of comprehensive geriatric care on the patients' mobility and subsequent fall prevention is also important for secondary fracture prevention.

## 3 Cost of care

At first glance, the comprehensive orthogeriatric model appears to require a lot of additional resources. Cost-utility analyses integrating epidemiological and economic aspects for hip fracture patients treated within a comprehensive orthogeriatric model of care, as compared with the standard of care model, are of interest. In hip fracture patients it has been shown that a comprehensive orthogeriatric care modality is more cost-effective, as it provides additional quality-adjusted life years (QALYs) while using fewer resources compared with standard care [25].

Another prospective randomized controlled trial compared the effectiveness of comprehensive geriatric care in a dedicated geriatric ward with usual orthopedic care and supported the above findings (**Table 2.4-1**). The staffing ratios of medical professionals used in this study is listed in **Table 2.4-2**.

| | Comprehensive geriatric care (n = 198) | Orthopedic care (n = 198) | Difference | |
|---|---|---|---|---|
| | Mean (SD) | Mean (SD) | Estimate (95% CI) | *P* value |
| Index stay* | 11,868 (4,185) | 9,537 (4,393) | 2,331 (1,483 to 3,178) | < .0001 |
| Hospital costs after discharge* | 7,745 (15,006) | 11,022 (20,119) | -3,277 (-6,784 to 230) | .07 |
| Rehabilitation stay* | 8,105 (9,076) | 9,633 (11,125) | -1,529 (-3,535 to 477) | .14 |
| Nursing home stay* | 14,874 (30,153) | 18,798 (32,959) | -3,923 (-10,164 to 2,318) | .22 |
| Other primary health and care services* | 11,741 (15,128) | 10,496 (14,498) | 1,246 (-1,683 to 4,173) | .40 |
| Total cost* | 54,332 (38,048) | 59,486 (44,301) | -5,154 (-13,311 to 3,007) | .22 |

**Table 2.4-1** Overall costs per patient in a comprehensive geriatric care model compared to conventional orthopedic care. Adapted from Prestmo et al [26].
Abbreviations: CI, confidence interval; SD, standard deviation.
* Costs are in euros for 2010.

| | Comprehensive geriatric care | Orthopedic care |
|---|---|---|
| Department | • Department of Geriatrics<br>• Clinic of Internal Medicine | • Department of Orthopedic Surgery<br>• Clinic of Orthopedics and Rheumatology |
| Facilities* | • Geriatric ward:<br>– Five 1-bed rooms organized in a group together reserved for patients with hip fractures within a 15-bed ward | • Orthopedic trauma ward:<br>– 1-, 2-, or 4-bed rooms in a 19-bed ward before, or single rooms in a 24-bed ward after relocation<br>– Mixed orthopedic trauma patient population |
| Team members, number per bed †: | | |
| • Geriatricians | 0.13 | No geriatrician in this setting |
| • Registered nurses, licensed practical nurses | 1.67 | 1.48 |
| • Physiotherapists | 0.13 | 0.09 (0.07 after relocation) |
| • Occupational therapists | 0.13 | None |
| • Orthopedic surgeons | No geriatrician in this setting | 0.11 (0.08 after relocation) |
| Treatment | • Structured, systematic interdisciplinary comprehensive geriatric assessment and care focusing on:<br>– Somatic health (comorbidity management, review of drug regimens, pain, nutrition, elimination, hydration, osteoporosis, and prevention of falls)<br>– Mental health (depression, delirium)<br>– Function (mobility, PADL, and IADL)<br>– Social situation<br>• Early discharge planning<br>• Early mobilization and initiation of rehabilitation | Following routines of Department of Orthopedic Surgery |

**Table 2.4-2** Supply of medical professionals and management in the comprehensive geriatric assessment and care and the orthopedic care groups. Adapted from Prestmo et al [26].
Abbreviations: IADL, instrumental activity of daily living; PADL, personal activity of daily living.
*Orthopedic care was relocated to a new hospital building after 219 of 397 patients were recruited.
†Separate teams with no collaboration.

## 4 Standard care pathways, protocols, and order sets

The implementation of standard treatment approaches is a crucial part of the treatment of FFPs to ensure routine use of best practice in the areas of osteoporotic fracture repair, anticoagulant management, treatment of comorbidities, and early mobilization (see chapter 2.3 Clinical practice guidelines). In the National Institute for Health and Care Excellence guideline, a standardized pathway for the treatment of hip fractures in orthogeriatric patients has been proposed (**Fig 2.4-3**).

In a prospective study of orthogeriatric patients that suffered from a hip fracture, Ogilvie-Harris et al [27] observed significantly improved outcomes for those patients treated with standardized medical and nursing protocols. See chapter 2.7 Protocol and order set development for concepts and issues regarding standardizing care.

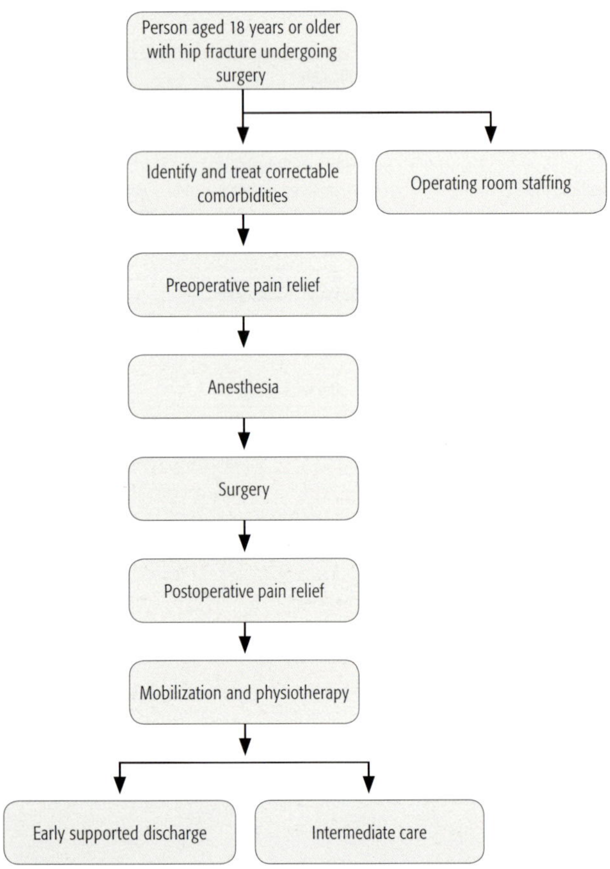


**Fig 2.4-3** Pathway proposed in the National Institute for Health and Care Excellence guideline for the treatment of hip fractures in fragility fracture patients.

## 5 Data collection

There are a variety of outcome parameters to assess the effectiveness of an orthogeriatric service. Specific parameters including the time to surgery, length of hospitalization, and 1-year mortality are easily comparable measures to monitor a system's effectiveness (**Table 2.4-3**) As stated above, in patients with a hip fracture, longer preoperative waiting times increase the risk of medical complications due to immobility [3]. Thus, patients should undergo surgery as soon as possible. Similarly, the length of hospitalization is an important parameter, as it can be associated with development of complications and there is a direct correlation with costs [28].

Ideally, the goal of optimal fracture care is the restoration of the patients' function, with the lowest mortality possible. To measure these parameters, appropriate geriatric assessment scores can be useful. Functional outcome and activities of daily living (ADLs) can be assessed with the Barthel Index that is used to measure performance in basic ADLs by scaling the presence or absence of fecal or urinary incontinence, the help needed with grooming, toilet use, feeding, transfers (eg, from chair to bed), walking, dressing, climbing stairs, and bathing. For each question there are two to four ordinal responses with a fixed count that are summed up. The maximum of 100 points implies that the patient is independent in his basic ADLs. This score was found to be a reliable outcome parameter for FFPs [29, 30].

Another frequently used index to assess ADLs is the Katz score. It analyzes the patient's performance in six functions using yes or no questions to evaluate their performance while bathing, dressing, toileting, transferring, feeding, and being continent. A score of 6 indicates full function, 4 moderate impairment, and 2 or less describes a relevant impairment of the patient's ADLs. The Functional Independence Measure uses similar items to evaluate motor and cognitive performance and is frequently used to describe the ADLs of the patient at discharge. Another simple tool to evaluate mobility is the Parker Mobility Score. The Timed Up and Go test is another commonly used mobility score known to be a valid and reliable tool to assess patient mobility [31]. Assessment of geriatric function is addressed in greater detail in chapters 1.4 Preoperative risk assessment and preparation and 1.11 Sarcopenia, malnutrition, frailty, and falls.

Furthermore, perioperative and postoperative complications must be evaluated. Common complications of patients having suffered fragility fracture are cardiac, cerebral, thromboembolic, and pulmonary complications such as renal failure, urinary tract infection, delirium, pressure ulcers, gastrointestinal complications, adverse drug reactions, and subsequent fractures. The main surgical problems are surgical site infection and other surgical complications such as catastrophic failures [28].

Further parameters to assess quality are the readmission rate, analysis of the quality of life, pain (see chapter 1.12 Pain management), and patient satisfaction.

Given the high financial burden of osteoporosis-related fractures with estimated annual costs of EUR 31.7 billion (about USD 33.6 billion in 2017) in Europe [32], cost-effectiveness remains another tool to evaluate a program's effectiveness.

| Outcome parameter | Assessment tool | Admission* | Discharge† | 30 days | 90 days | 1 year |
|---|---|---|---|---|---|---|
| Mortality | Mortality rate (%) | | | X | | X |
| Length of stay | Midnight census method | | X | | | |
| Time to surgery | Time from admission until arrival in operating room (h) | | X | | | |
| Complications: | Complication rate (%) using the complication list | | | | | |
| • Medical | | | X | X | | |
| • Surgical | | | X | X | | X |
| Readmission: | Readmission rate (%) using the complication list | | | | | |
| • Medical | | | | X | X | |
| • Surgical | | | | X | X | X |
| Mobility | • Parker Mobility Score | X | | | X | X |
| | • Timed Up and Go test | | | | X | X |
| Quality of life | EQ-5D | X | | | X | X |
| Pain | Verbal rating scale | X‡ | | | X | X |
| Satisfaction | No appropriate tool available | | | | | |
| ADLs | Barthel Index | X | X | | X | X |
| Falls | No appropriate tool available | | | | | |
| Medication use: | | | | | | |
| • Inappropirate | • Adverse drug reaction with complications | | X | X | | |
| • Osteoporosis | • Medication list | X | X | | X | X |
| Place of residence | Living situation list | X | | | X | X |
| Costs | Percentage of expected national costs | | X | | | |

**Table 2.4-3** Overview of the relevant outcome parameters, assessment tools, and their follow-up to monitor system's effectiveness [28].
Abbreviations: ADLs, activities of daily living; EQ-5D, EuroQoL-5 dimension (questionnaire to assess quality of life); h, hour.
* Assessment of prefracture status.
†Discharge from the acute hospital.
‡Two days postoperative.

## 6 References

1. **Friedman SM, Mendelson DA, Bingham KW, et al.** Impact of a comanaged Geriatric Fracture Center on short-term hip fracture outcomes. *Arch Intern Med.* 2009 Oct 12;169(18):1712–1717.
2. **Kammerlander C, Gosch M, Kammerlander-Knauer U, et al.** Long-term functional outcome in geriatric hip fracture patients. *Arch Orthop Trauma Surg.* 2011 Oct;131(10):1435–1444.
3. **Kammerlander C, Roth T, Friedman SM, et al.** Ortho-geriatric service—a literature review comparing different models. *Osteoporos Int.* 2010 Dec;21(Suppl 4):S637–S646.
4. **Hempsall VJ, Robertson DR, Campbell MJ, et al.** Orthopaedic geriatric care—is it effective? A prospective population-based comparison of outcome in fractured neck of femur. *J R Coll Physicians Lond.* 1990 Jan;24(1):47–50.
5. **Kammerlander C, Gosch M, Blauth M, et al.** The Tyrolean Geriatric Fracture Center: an orthogeriatric co-management model. *Z Gerontol Geriatr.* 2011 Dec;44(6):363–367.
6. **Prestmo A, Saltvedt I, Helbostad JL, et al.** Who benefits from orthogeriatric treatment? Results from the Trondheim hip-fracture trial. *BMC Geriatr.* 2016 Feb 19;16:49.
7. **Lisk R, Yeong K.** Reducing mortality from hip fractures: a systematic quality improvement programme. *BMJ Qual Improv Rep.* 2014;3(1).
8. **Cameron ID, Chen JS, March LM, et al.** Hip fracture causes excess mortality owing to cardiovascular and infectious disease in institutionalized older people: a prospective 5-year study. *J Bone Miner Res.* 2010 Apr;25(4):866–872.
9. **Roche JJ, Wenn RT, Sahota O, et al.** Effect of comorbidities and postoperative complications on mortality after hip fracture in elderly people: prospective observational cohort study. *BMJ.* 2005 Dec 10;331(7529):1374.
10. **National Clinical Guideline Centre.** The Management of Hip Fracture in Adults. Available at: www.ncbi.nlm.nih.gov/books/NBK83014. Accessed 2018.
11. **Khan SK, Jameson SS, Avery PJ, et al.** Does the timing of presentation of neck of femur fractures affect the outcome of surgical intervention. *Eur J Emerg Med.* 2013 Jun;20(3):178–181.
12. **Juliebo V, Bjoro K, Krogseth M, et al.** Risk factors for preoperative and postoperative delirium in elderly patients with hip fracture. *J Am Geriatr Soc.* 2009 Aug;57(8):1354–1361.
13. **Lee KH, Ha YC, Lee YK, et al.** Frequency, risk factors, and prognosis of prolonged delirium in elderly patients after hip fracture surgery. *Clin Orthop Relat Res.* 2011 Sep;469(9):2612–2620.
14. **Lizaur-Utrilla A, Martinez-Mendez D, Collados-Maestre I, et al.** Early surgery within 2 days for hip fracture is not reliable as healthcare quality indicator. *Injury.* 2016 Jul;47(7):1530–1535.
15. **Simunovic N, Devereaux PJ, Sprague S, et al.** Effect of early surgery after hip fracture on mortality and complications: systematic review and meta-analysis. *CMAJ.* 2010 Oct 19;182(15):1609–1616.
16. **Langenhan R, Trobisch P, Ricart P, et al.** Aggressive surgical treatment of periprosthetic femur fractures can reduce mortality: comparison of open reduction and internal fixation versus a modular prosthesis nail. *J Orthop Trauma.* 2012 Feb;26(2):80–85.
17. **Thingstad P, Taraldsen K, Saltvedt I, et al.** The long-term effect of comprehensive geriatric care on gait after hip fracture: the Trondheim Hip Fracture Trial—a randomised controlled trial. *Osteoporos Int.* 2016 Mar;27(3):933–942.
18. **Pils K, Muller W, Likar R, et al.** Rehabilitation nach Hüftfraktur [Rehabilitation after hip fracture]. *Wien Med Wochenschr.* 2013 Oct;163(19–20):462–467. German.
19. **Givens JL, Sanft TB, Marcantonio ER.** Functional recovery after hip fracture: the combined effects of depressive symptoms, cognitive impairment, and delirium. *J Am Geriatr Soc.* 2008 Jun;56(6):1075–1079.
20. **Huusko TM, Karppi P, Avikainen V, et al.** Intensive geriatric rehabilitation of hip fracture patients: a randomized, controlled trial. *Acta Orthop Scand.* 2002 Aug;73(4):425–431.
21. **Friedman SM, Mendelson DA, Kates SL, et al.** Geriatric co-management of proximal femur fractures: total quality management and protocol-driven care result in better outcomes for a frail patient population. *J Am Geriatr Soc.* 2008 Jul;56(7):1349–1356.
22. **Black DM, Delmas PD, Eastell R, et al.** Once-yearly zoledronic acid for treatment of postmenopausal osteoporosis. *N Engl J Med.* 2007 May 03;356(18):1809–1822.
23. **Kanis JA, McCloskey E, Branco J, et al.** Goal-directed treatment of osteoporosis in Europe. *Osteoporos Int.* 2014 Nov;25(11):2533–2543.
24. **Nakayama A, Major G, Holliday E, et al.** Evidence of effectiveness of a fracture liaison service to reduce the re-fracture rate. *Osteoporos Int.* 2016 Mar;27(3):873–879.
25. **Ginsberg G, Adunsky A, Rasooly I.** A cost-utility analysis of a comprehensive orthogeriatric care for hip fracture patients, compared with standard of care treatment. *Hip Int.* 2013 Nov–Dec;23(6):570–575.
26. **Prestmo A, Hagen G, Sletvold O, et al.** Comprehensive geriatric care for patients with hip fractures: a prospective, randomised, controlled trial. *Lancet.* 2015 Apr 25;385(9978):1623–1633.
27. **Ogilvie-Harris DJ, Botsford DJ, Hawker RW.** Elderly patients with hip fractures: improved outcome with the use of care maps with high-quality medical and nursing protocols. *J Orthop Trauma.* 1993;7(5):428–437.
28. **Liem IS, Kammerlander C, Suhm N, et al.** Identifying a standard set of outcome parameters for the evaluation of orthogeriatric co-management for hip fractures. *Injury.* 2013 Nov;44(11):1403–1412.
29. **Bryant DM, Sanders DW, Coles CP, et al.** Selection of outcome measures for patients with hip fracture. *J Orthop Trauma.* 2009 Jul;23(6):434–441.
30. **Kammerlander C, Riedmuller P, Gosch M, et al.** Functional outcome and mortality in geriatric distal femoral fractures. *Injury.* 2012 Jul;43(7):1096–1101.
31. **Hutchings L, Fox R, Chesser T.** Proximal femoral fractures in the elderly: how are we measuring outcome? *Injury.* 2011 Nov;42(11):1205–1213.
32. **Kanis JA, Johnell O.** Requirements for DXA for the management of osteoporosis in Europe. *Osteoporos Int.* 2005 Mar;16(3):229–238.

# 2.5 Adapting facilities to fragility fracture patients

Edgar Mayr

## 1 Introduction

With future demographic changes, an increasingly large number of geriatric fracture patients are expected. As an example, the total number of 80- to 100-year old patients with a proximal femoral fracture will more than double by 2050 [1]. Notably, these injuries carry a 1-year mortality rate of up to 30%. Furthermore, many of these patients are threatened by the loss of their independence and about 50% require nursing care or general support within the first year [2].

Specialized centers for geriatric fracture care nicely address some of the problems associated with the treatment of fragility fracture patients (FFPs). Two approaches can be differentiated:

- The "ward round model" or "network model" has the patients being treated on a standard trauma ward with additional regularly scheduled ward rounds by a geriatrician to address the specific geriatric problems.
- The "ward model" or "comanaged program" on the other hand has FFPs treated on a specialized ward, whereby the specialization also concerns its construction. Ward rounds are made by a trauma surgeon as well as a geriatrician resulting in comanaged care [3].

## 2 Rationale for adaptation

Older patients often have an altered cognitive status as well as physical condition. Their health and well-being are at risk as an inpatient and therefore require special caution:

- The healing process is complicated for older adults [4, 5]. Patients on a geriatric fracture ward should therefore be protected from harm. The patient's unsteady gait must be considered [6].
- Facilities should be designed to avoid the development of delirium; nursing interventions to enhance patients' activity and early mobilization are helpful in this regard [7]. It is necessary to provide the appropriate patient rooms, therapy rooms, and bathroom facilities. These must be accessible without obstacles and offer enough space and safety, ie, handrails to help the patients with their personal hygiene.
- A therapy room located on the ward helps to avoid patient transportation, which is both time-consuming, costly in terms of manpower, and provocative for the onset of a delirium by changing the familiar environment.

## 3 General measures

As with children, older adults have unique needs and requirements, which need to be met by specialized facilities. The creation of a completely new special geriatric fracture ward will in many cases not be feasible, but is also not mandatory. Many existing structural factors can be modified to meet these special requirements at an economically justifiable cost and effort.

Typical examples are:

- Wards
- Walls and colors
- Common rooms
- Patient rooms and beds
- Common areas
- Washrooms and bathroom facilities
- Therapy rooms

On a specialized geriatric trauma ward, these measures will prove extremely valuable and may be indispensable.

### 3.1 Inpatient ward

Suitable wards are essential (**Fig 2.5-1**, **Fig 2.5-2**):

- Usually a hospital's hallways are sufficiently wide but are often used for the storage of carts with bandaging materials, food, wheelchairs, material for ward rounds, etc. This creates a lot of obstacles that hinder the mobilization of the patient. Such hallway clutter should be avoided.
- The hallways of a geriatric fracture ward should not only allow for patient transport, but also for gait training and exercise. For these reasons, the halls need to be free of barriers and obstacles, steps, thresholds, or tripping hazards. Furthermore they should offer solid handrails and benches to sit down and recover from strenuous practice. Seating for intermittent recovery breaks enhances mobility.
- Good lighting is also important to prevent tripping and assist with reduced visual acuity. Contrasting colors on the walls, such as pictures, can aid patient's orientation and motivation by, for instance, defining an area to be covered in mobilization. A visible scaling along the floor can also be helpful.
- Floors that reduce tripping have proper visual characteristics for aging eyes and reduction of doorway thresholds.
- Mobile telemetry units can be retrofitted to nearly any ward without difficulty.

### 3.2 Walls and colors

Suitable wall equipment and colors are important (**Fig 2.5-3**):

- The color scheme of the ward can also be designed to meet the needs of older adults. Smooth, pastel shades are both calming and mood-lifting. Sufficient contrast between walls, floors, and doors allow good orientation even with impaired eyesight. Differing colors of doors and walls can be used to illustrate the covered distance.
- For the patient's optimal mobilization, the hallways should be equipped with a sufficient amount of handlebars or handrails. Fold-out seating offers possibilities for breaks, and they do not obstruct when in a hinged position. Both increase the ability of older adults to ambulate.

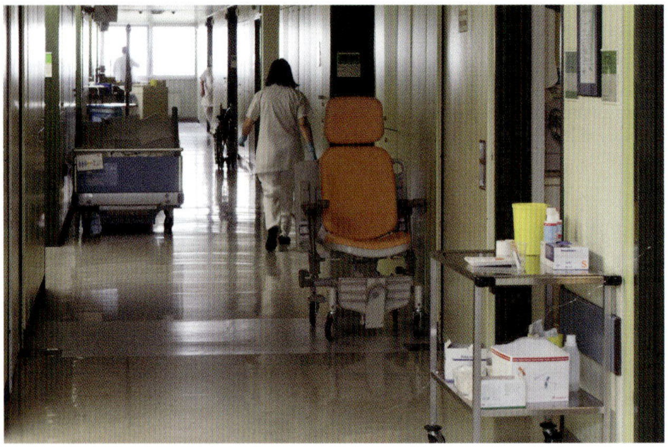

**Fig 2.5-1** The hallway on a regular ward is dark, monotonous, and full of obstacles.

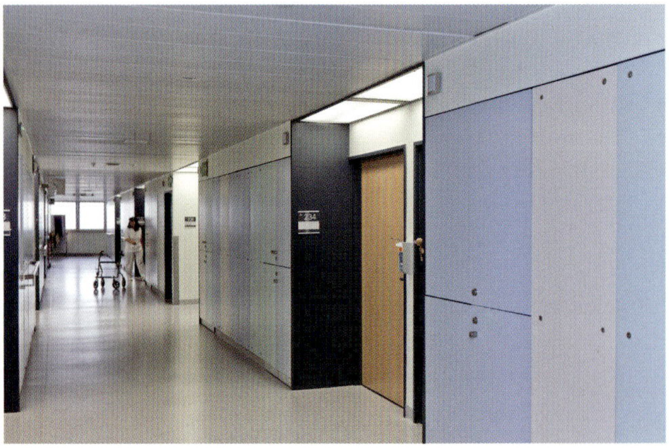

**Fig 2.5-2** The hallway on a geriatric trauma ward has abundant light, contrasting colors and is free of obstacles to assure good mobilization of patients.

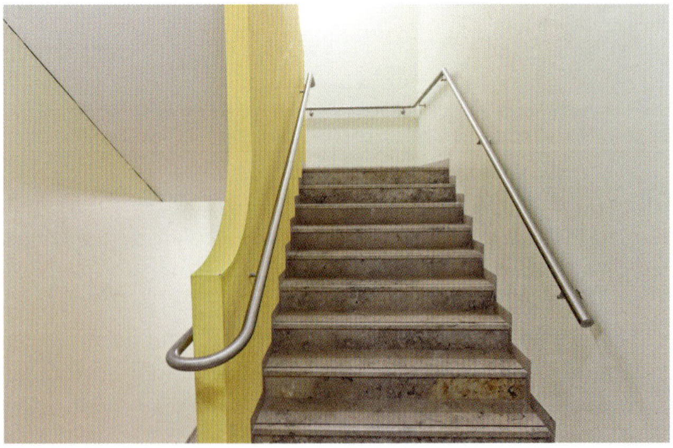

**Fig 2.5-3** Staircase with handrails on both sides to assure secure mobilization of the patient.

## 3.3 Patient room

- A large clock and calendar help to maintain orientation. Adequate lighting and a night light are necessary. Large windows provide daylight, which is mood lifting and maintains a circadian rhythm.
- The patient should be allowed to personalize his or her room by, for example, putting up pictures of his or her family and relatives. This helps to maintain family recognition and links positive memories and associations to the room.
- Room changes throughout the stay should be avoided. A patient room needs to be spacious and functional enough on the one hand, but designed to make it resemble a hospital as little as possible on the other (**Fig 2.5-4**). It should offer the patient a comforting atmosphere in a familiar environment.
- As a rule we find 2-bed rooms to be a reasonable size, as it offers needed space and a conversational partner, but still does not create a noisy or disturbing environment.
- Certain patients, such as those that are difficult to mobilize, or are delirious, will benefit from single patient rooms. In these few cases, the extra space is needed to provide the required nursing care including aids, ie, for mobilization (**Fig 2.5-5**).
- As an aid to avoid falls, especially with delirious patients, low-to-floor beds with adjustable height have proved to be very valuable (**Fig 2.5-6**). The low height level reduces risk of falls without having to restrain the patient to the bed. Evidence shows that this sort of bed should be available for about 30% of the patients [8].
- Other equipment should include a bedside locker of proper height and a mobile bed, since the patient may need to be transferred to another bed or a wheelchair for transport within the hospital.

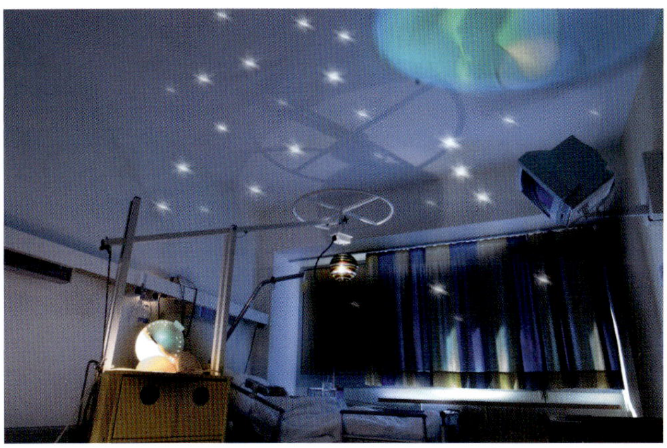

**Fig 2.5-4** Patient room with mobile mirror ball unit providing visual, acoustic, and olfactory stimulus.

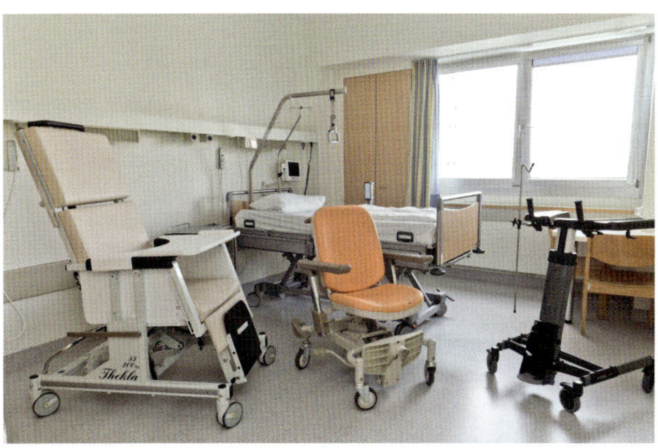

**Fig 2.5-5** Patient room with required auxiliary material and assistive devices for patients with difficult mobilization. Almost the entire room is occupied.

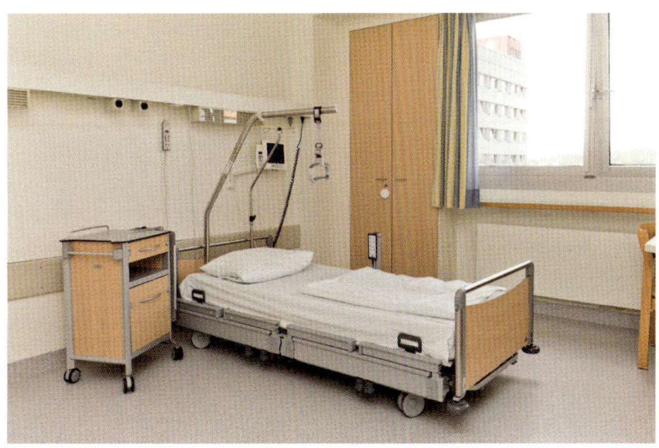

**Fig 2.5-6** Patient room with height-adjustable low-floor bed.

### 3.4 Common areas

A room for common activities is another important element (**Fig 2.5-7**):

- A common room suitable to the patients of a geriatric trauma ward can be simply designed. When put to proper use, this space can be used not just as a meeting place, but also as an extensive therapy concept.
- Simple measures can help to address many issues for an older patient. Repeated transfers every day from the patient room to the common space, for instance, offer mobility of the patient.
- Dining in the company of other patients and sitting at a table rather than dining in bed may increase the patient's appetite and counter malnourishment.
- The predetermined day's structure can be a prophylactic measure against the development of delirium.
- Shared parlor games and activities not only provide amusement but are also helpful with cognitive activation.
- Overall, the patient is engaged in a normal day structure and their independence is strengthened [3].
- The furnishing of such a common room includes suitable tables and diverse seating opportunities ranging from a couch to a specialized chair for mobilization, a sufficiently large TV set, possibly equipped with headphones, an overall ambience with recognizable objects, ie, bus stop sign to prevent patients from leaving the ward, old piano, old posters, toys. With help from volunteers an alternating program with parlor games, singalongs, or pottery can be offered.
- A common room has the additional advantage that patients with delirium can be taken care of much more easily and with fewer staff, as they are together in a group instead of their own rooms.

### 3.5 Washrooms and bathrooms

Bathrooms should be appropriately equipped (**Fig 2.5-8, Fig 2.5-9**):

- Easy access without obstacles is essential for older adults.
- Seating in the shower is also important.
- Handlebars, which should always be installed on both sides since one side of the patient may be impaired due to his or her injury, are also needed in the shower.

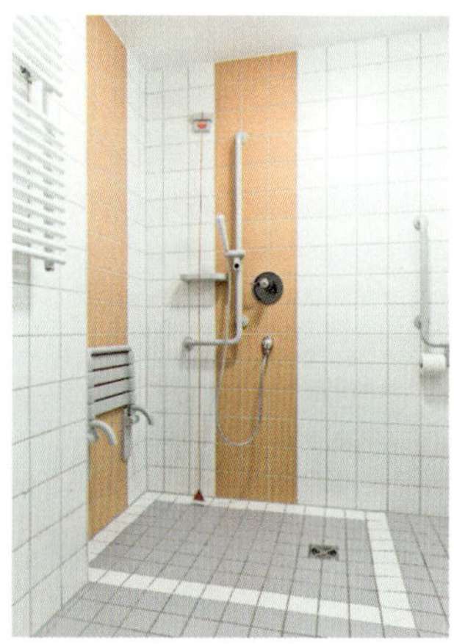

**Fig 2.5-8** Patient bathroom with barrier-free access to the shower and handlebars with fold-out seating.

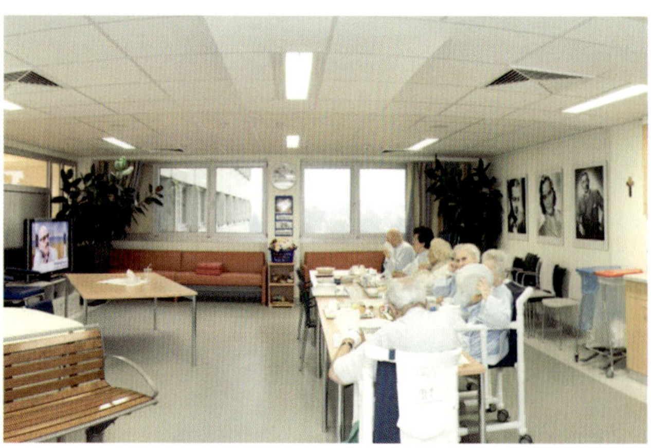

**Fig 2.5-7** Common room with patients having lunch together. The open and friendly design with old movie posters offers great recognition value. A calendar and clock offer temporal orientation.

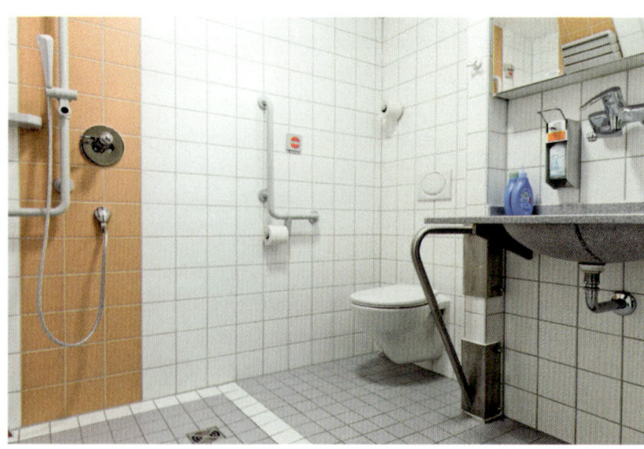

**Fig 2.5-9** Patient bathroom free of obstacles, equipped with plenty of handlebars and enough room for the patient, a nurse, and an occupational therapist, along with auxiliary material.

- Enough space for the patient plus an additional nurse and occupational therapist with assistive equipment should be available to allow autonomous personal hygiene with corresponding practice.

### 3.6 Therapy room

A spacious therapy room is an essential element:

- All necessary equipment is available (**Fig 2.5-10**).
- It offers sufficient open space to permit group therapy sessions (**Fig 2.5-11**).

## 4 Delirium prevention

Prevention of delirium is a multimodal exercise. Many non-pharmacological concepts are important [9]. In this context environmental factors in wards play a major role and should not be underestimated. They can promote but also counteract delirium as follows:

- A friendly and colorful but soothing wall design can have a prophylactic effect.
- Large windows and good lighting promote the maintenance of a circadian rhythm.
- The same applies to patient activation, meals, games, or music, and watching TV during daytime in a common room [6]. This room should, just like the patient rooms, be designed in a considerate way concerning the patient's age by creating points with recognition value, such as old movie posters or an old piano (**Fig 2.5-7**).
- The patient rooms should, if possible, be personalized during and throughout the stay by, for example, decorating them with family pictures. Switching rooms during one stay on the ward must be avoided.
- Frequent changes of environment can also be reduced with a therapy room on the ward by reducing the number of required transports and changes of location, thereby reducing the likelihood of delirium.

See chapter 1.14 Delirium for a more thorough discussion.

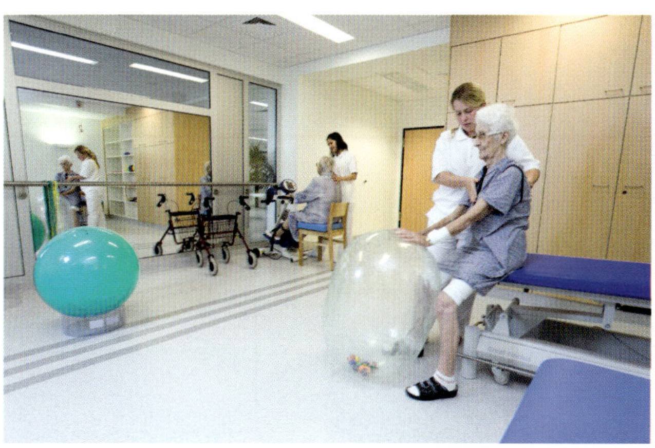

**Fig 2.5-10** Therapy room on the ward with necessary auxiliary material and training devices.

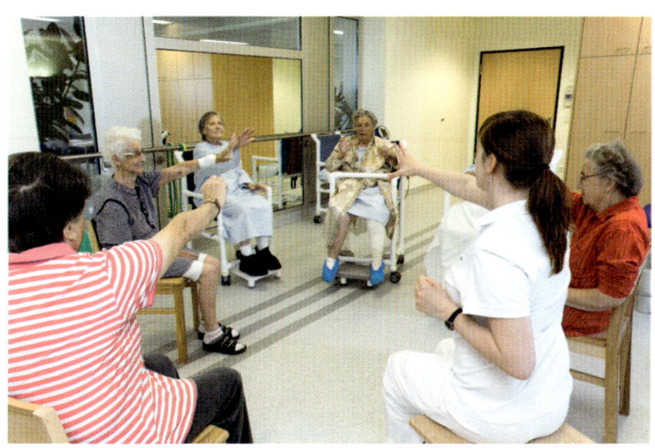

**Fig 2.5-11** Therapy room on the ward with enough space for group sessions.

## 5 References

1. **Lohmann R, Haid K, Stockle U, et al.** Epidemiologie und Perspektiven der Alterstraumatologie [Epidemiology and perspectives in traumatology of the elderly]. *Unfallchirurg.* 2007 Jun;110(6):553–560; quiz 561–552. German.
2. **Muller-Mai CM, Schulze Raestrup US, Kostuj T, et al.** Einjahresverläufe nch proximalen Femurfracturen. Poststationäre Analyse von Letalität und Pflegestufen durch Kassendaten. [One-year outcomes for proximal femoral fractures: Posthospital analysis of mortality and care levels based on health insurance data]. *Unfallchirurg.* 2015 Sep;118(9):780–794. German.
3. **Werther SFJ, Mayr E.** Interdisziplinäres Management im Zentrum für geriatrische Traumatologie. [Interdisciplinary management at the center for geriatric traumatology]. *Orthopäd Unfallchirur.* 2014;9(05):387–406. German.
4. **Bellelli G, Mazzola P, Morandi A, et al.** Duration of postoperative delirium is an independent predictor of 6-month mortality in older adults after hip fracture. *J Am Geriatr Soc.* 2014 Jul;62(7):1335–1340.
5. **Marcantonio ER, Flacker JM, Michaels M, et al.** Delirium is independently associated with poor functional recovery after hip fracture. *J Am Geriatr Soc.* 2000 Jun;48(6):618–624.
6. **Gillespie LD, Robertson MC, Gillespie WJ, et al.** Interventions for preventing falls in older people living in the community. *Cochrane Database Syst Rev.* 2012 Sep 12(9):CD007146.
7. **Holroyd-Leduc JM, Khandwala F, Sink KM.** How can delirium best be prevented and managed in older patients in hospital? *Can med Assoc J.* 2010 Mar 23;182(5):465–470.
8. **Tzeng HM, Yin CY, Anderson A, et al.** Nursing staff's awareness of keeping beds in the lowest position to prevent falls and fall injuries in an adult acute surgical inpatient care setting. *Medsurg Nurs.* 2012 Sep-Oct;21(5):271–274.
9. **Tabet N, Howard R.** Non-pharmacological interventions in the prevention of delirium. *Age Ageing.* 2009 Jul;38(4):374–379.

# 2.6 Orthogeriatric team—principles, roles, and responsibilities

Markus Gosch, Michael Blauth

## 1 Introduction

Fragility fracture patients (FFPs) are medically complex and typically present with more than a single medical problem. While some of these problems are apparent, others may remain unrecognized and lead to complications and adverse outcomes. Because of this typical complexity, systematic efforts are necessary to routinely obtain detailed patient-specific clinical information and to set patient-specific goals. This approach requires a coordinated team of health professionals, each of whom is focused on specific aspects of care (**Fig 2.6-1**).

A systematic approach helps to manage this information and to detect underlying cognitive, functional, medical, and social problems that are likely to impact outcomes and effect prognosis. For the team to work effectively, it is essential to clearly define the orthogeriatric team and the roles of each member. This chapter is written based on the academic and clinical experience of a mature orthogeriatric team using the principles of orthogeriatric comanagement (see chapters 2.1 Models of orthogeriatric care and 2.4 Elements of an orthogeriatric comanaged program) [1].

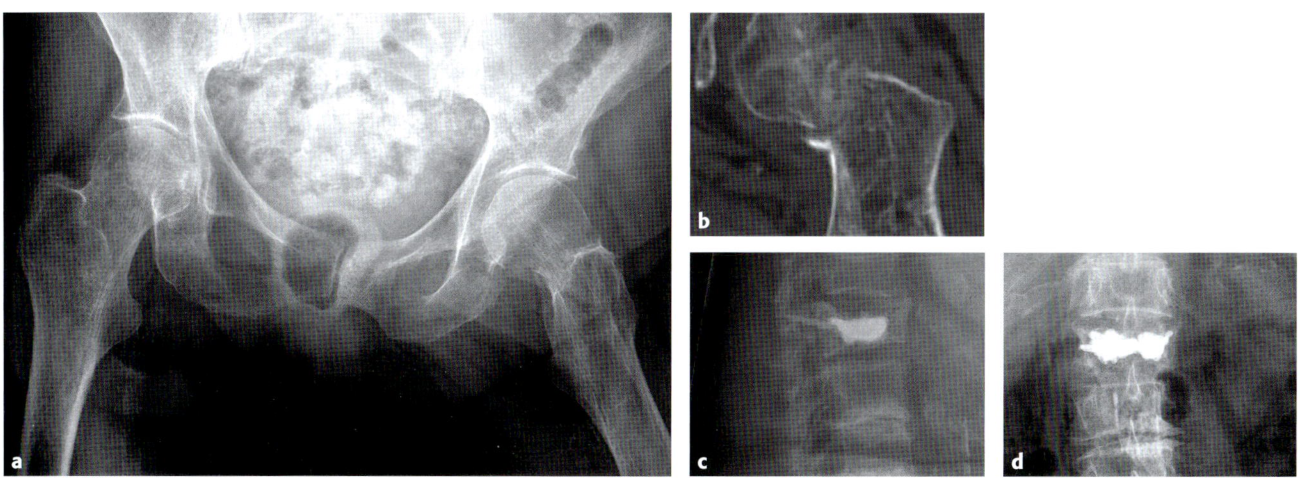


**Fig 2.6-1a–d** An 88-year-old woman was admitted to the emergency department following a fall on the way to the bathroom. The x-rays of her left hip showed a femoral neck fracture (**a–b**). Her body weight was 46 kg. Nine months before, a kyphoplasty was performed after a fracture of the first lumbar vertebra (**c–d**). She had many comorbidities, including osteoporosis, heart failure, hypertension, depression, mild cognitive impairment, and urinary incontinence, and was taking 10 different drugs daily. Additionally, she had difficulty swallowing her medication and sometimes her food. To that point, she had been living alone and independently and had received help from her neighbors. She had to climb the stairs to enter her second-floor apartment. Her son worked in another town and was not able to come to the hospital.

## 2 The comorbidity construct

The comorbidity construct (**Fig 2.6-2**) is a useful tool to get a better overview of the complexity that needs to be addressed for most FFPs [2]. This approach should help illustrate the necessary components and goals of the orthogeriatric team.

Usually, the index disease (ie, fragility fracture) leads to hospital admission. In order to prioritize the treatment goals, it is worthwhile to identify and define additional important conditions:

- Comorbidities are medical conditions that are strongly interrelated with the index disease and the outcomes of interest. When treating the index disease, you have to include the comorbidities in the treatment plan for an optimal outcome.
- Multimorbidity refers to the total burden of other diseases in a patient. These may play a general role in outcomes, but may not be modifiable, or need to be specifically addressed during the hospitalization.
- Interestingly, the impact of the chronological age is not as significant. The biological age of patients and the estimated life expectancy are more relevant for the outcome.
- Fragility fractures are mainly a result of a low-energy trauma, eg, a fall from standing height. In older patients, intrinsic factors are a major contributor in terms of falls. Besides comorbidities, health-related individual attributes must be taken into consideration. Health-related attributes are existing or developing functional disabilities and geriatric syndromes (eg, frailty, gait instability, cognitive impairment, urinary incontinence). They all contribute to the overall morbidity burden.
- Finally, the complexity of patients' conditions result from their nonhealth-related individual attributes (eg, personality, social supports, and financial supports).

By using this systematic framework in the rather simple example described in **Fig 2.6-1**, the team is more likely to identify the relevant medical and social problems and better address those conditions that are likely to impact recovery from fracture repair and attainment of the highest level of function (**Fig 2.6-3**). When applying the comorbidity construct to this specific example, it becomes clear that:

- The index disease for hospital admission is the hip fracture.
- A contributing comorbidity is osteoporosis. There is a strong relationship between the fracture and osteoporosis. When treating FFPs, you should initiate osteoporosis care. Otherwise, you will miss an opportunity; probably the most important in terms of secondary fracture prevention, and your case management will be at risk to fail.
- Other potentially important comorbidities are heart failure, hypertension, and depression. Their impact on short-term recovery is not entirely clear and may be influenced by the severity of each disease and other individual factors. The team must evaluate which medical conditions might have an impact on the outcome of the patient and need to be included in the team's treatment plans.
- Gender aspects should also be considered. Usually, male patients have worse outcomes than female patients. Social environments are not comparable.
- The correlation of increased age and mortality is mainly the result of the higher prevalence of disease and functional disabilities with increasing age. For highly functional and healthy adults, the correlation between age and mortality is not strong [3].

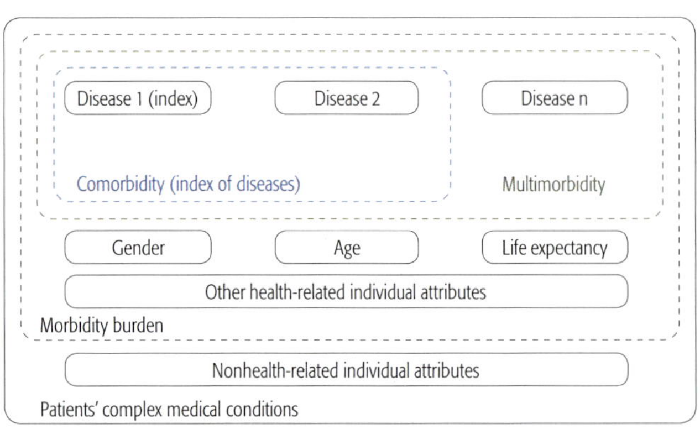


**Fig 2.6-2** Comorbidity construct according to Valderas et al [2].

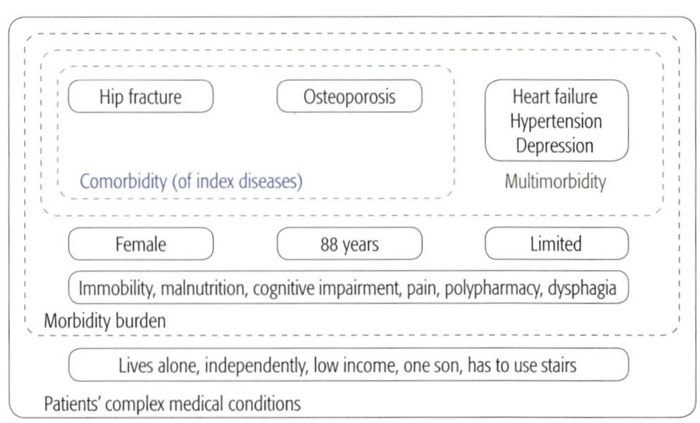


**Fig 2.6-3** Comorbidity construct applied to **Fig 2.6-1**.

- In terms of goal setting, life expectancy should be estimated. Functional and robust older adults may still have a remarkably long life expectancy. In the example case, the life expectancy was limited, but not so much as to preclude fracture repair and an attempt at rehabilitation (see chapter 1.5 Prognosis and goals of care).
- Different functional disabilities such as immobility, malnutrition, cognitive impairment, pain, polypharmacy, and dysphagia may be present. These health-related individual attributes can have more impact on the outcome than the index diagnosis and should be specifically and systematically addressed by the team.
- Finally, morbidity burden not only reflects the diagnosis but also the functional disabilities of a patient.
- Based on a holistic approach, the orthogeriatric team also has to assess for nonhealth-related individual attributes including the social environment. The social network is not only extremely important for discharge planning but also for reduction of readmissions and secondary fracture prevention.

## 3 Goal setting

After having collected all information by using the comorbidity construct, the process of goal setting starts. This process should be based on the following principles:

- Ensure the goal you set is specific, clear, and attainable.
- The goal should be measurable, ie, if you cannot measure it, you cannot manage it.
- A goal needs to be attractive and acceptable to the patient, family, and team.
- The timeline should be considered by setting short-term as well as long-term goals. Usually, the long-term goal is the expected outcome in several weeks, ie, "to live independently" or "to walk without using a walking aid". In order to achieve the long-term goal, it is necessary to meet different short-term goals for each problem, like walking with a roller after the first week or removing the urine catheter within 2 or 3 days after surgery. The goals may be changed due to medical complications or if patients were to become unwilling or unable to continue or if they progress more slowly or quickly than expected.

Goal setting should be integrated into the regular team meetings.

## 4 Team members and roles

For FFPs, a team approach is essential to attain success. A frequently asked question concerns leadership. The comanagement paradigm is based on shared leadership from all core team members (ie, surgeons, anesthesiologists, and geriatricians) and decisions are made collaboratively [4]. Leadership is not regulated by hierarchical structure but by medical qualification. Based on the knowledge and the expertise in the involved disciplines, leadership changes depend on the clinical situation. In addition to providing leadership, each team member has a specific role within the team.

All team members play their role at different phases of the treatment and even in different facilities. Depending on local resources and practices, they may have different roles and responsibilities to those suggested below. But they all must agree on the basic principles of treatment according to the guidelines, and they all must feel responsible with a sense of co-ownership of the patient. This obviously requires regular communication and meetings around specific patient issues as well as system concerns.

### 4.1 Orthopedic trauma surgeon

The orthopedic trauma surgeon has specific roles and tasks when seeing an FFP. He/she:

- Is often the first member of the core team to evaluate the patient.
- Obtains the history of the patient including the mechanism of injury. In some settings, the surgeon decides if an older patient requires admission to a geriatric-based unit, based on age, comorbidities, and fracture details.
- Starts the interdisciplinary process by contacting the geriatrician and anesthesiologist if a surgery is planned.
- Initiates the diagnostic workup regarding injuries, makes diagnoses, and classifies fracture(s).
- Activates standard preoperative order sets and protocols.
- Takes part in the process of goal setting in cooperation with the geriatrician and anesthesiologist.
- Plans and performs surgery, typically determining the optimal technique to promote full weight bearing during the immediate postoperative period.
- Cares for anticoagulation management preoperatively and postoperatively in cooperation with the geriatrician and the anesthesiologist. Especially among patients receiving chronic anticoagulation, these team members should weigh risks and benefits for each patient.
- Initiates and reviews pain management, starting on evaluation and including local anesthesia, enteral and parenteral drug treatment, and nonpharmacological measures.

- Plans perioperative antibiotic management.
- Supervises wound healing and the control of wound infections [5].

### 4.2 Geriatrician or medical leader

The geriatrician or medical leader takes part in the interdisciplinary ward rounds and team meetings, evaluates treatment progress, and adjusts treatments and goals together with the other team members. She/he:

- Should be involved as soon as possible, ideally in the emergency department.
- Performs a physical examination, particularly focused on the cardiopulmonary and neurological status. Collects medical history, especially comorbidities and medication. Basic assessment tools, like prefracture functional scores (eg, Parker Mobility Score) or cognitive assessments (eg, Confusion Assessment Method or Mini-Cog tests) should be part of the clinical examinations. Standard orders and protocols should have already been initiated, but the medical team is responsible for any nonstandard tests or consultations.
- Has, if surgery is required, the most important task to exclude conditions (eg, uncontrolled heart failure) that could result in surgical delay. In these rare cases the core team has to set a clear goal for the optimization and a time line.
- Optimizes the patient for surgical repair, focused on preoperative fluid support, hemodynamic stability, and acute pain management.
- Identifies patient-specific goals of care, and surrogate decision makers and advanced directives in the event of cardiac arrest or need for cardiopulmonary resuscitation.
- Is in charge of medical treatment postoperatively, particularly of the comorbidities, and supervises prevention and treatment of complications (eg, delirium, pneumonia, heart failure, and renal insufficiency).
- Is primarily responsible for medication management and avoidance of polypharmacy. Usually, FFPs are medically complex patients in an unstable situation. Many chronic medications can be dangerous during this dynamic situation, and a high level of prescribing expertise is needed. Potentially inappropriate medications should be avoided. Some medications issues, like anticoagulants, antibiotics, or pain medications, should be discussed by the interdisciplinary team.
- Is primarily responsible for initiating secondary fracture prevention. Osteoporosis and fall assessment have to be completed. Geriatricians should evaluate for metabolic bone disease, ensure adequate calcium intake and vitamin D supplementation, and consider specific osteoporosis drug treatment for every patient. Geriatricians must look for fall risk factors and work out a specific treatment plan to reduce the risk of subsequent falls and fractures.

### 4.3 Anesthesiologist

The anesthesiologist is an essential team member that is closely involved in the decision to operate and the management of fracture pain. He/she:

- Should be involved as soon as possible.
- Is often responsible for the procedure to achieve acute pain relief in the emergency department, eg, local anesthetic nerve blocks.
- Evaluates patient fitness for surgery together with medical and surgical teams. Identifies additional optimization strategies for each patient.
- Helps to determine the timing of surgery.
- Determines the perioperative anesthesia plan and anticipates postanesthesia recovery needs (eg, postanesthesia care unit [PACU] or intensive care unit [ICU] recovery).
- Is responsible for the immediate postoperative care of the patient, eg, PACU or ICU.
- Benefits from cooperation between surgeons and geriatricians.

### 4.4 Orthopedic staff nurse

The orthopedic nurse spends a great deal of time and effort taking care of the FFP and communicating with the family. She/he:

- Spends the most time with the patients. Therefore, the nursing staff play a major role in the interprofessional team and in the treatment process.
- Provides essential care such as pain assessment, medication administration, vital sign tracking, wound care, and communication of patient status with medical and surgical teams.
- Focuses on prevention of falls, pressure ulcers, malnutrition, delirium, and infections.
- Assesses and encourages nutritional intake and any factors that may impair optimal oral nutrition (eg, dysphagia, nausea, consistency, and taste).
- Ensures that sensory aides (eg, glasses and hearing aids) are present and working.
- Implements specific tools to assess pain, delirium, and fluid and nutrition management.
- Manages incontinence and catheters. Urinary retention should be excluded using ultrasound. If urinary incontinence occurs, it has to be documented and included in the treatment process.
- Encourages patients in activities of daily living (ADLs).

- As a specialized orthopedic nurse, they are involved in secondary fracture prevention. They choose the appropriate walking aid, and counsel their patients and relatives about osteoporosis and fall risk factors [6].
- Is involved in discharge management together with social workers.

### 4.5 Physiotherapist

The physiotherapist is closely involved with the FFP and their rehabilitation and physical function assessment. He/she:

- Implements and adjusts a physiotherapy plan for FFPs.
- Prepares patients for transfer to the next setting (ie, rehabilitation facility, nursing home, or home).
- Obtains details regarding home setting and home resources to assist with ADLs.
- Helps to encourage development and facilitates recovery, adjusting for common geriatric issues like gait instability, orthostatic hypotension, dyspnea, and delirium.
- Identifies obstacles to mobility (eg, pain with activity and room clutter) and is extremely important for mobilization and specific exercises as well as for checking further functional problems.
- Trains patients and family in the proper use of walking aids.
- Trains patients how to use stairs safely.
- Provides feedback to the team regarding functional limits, pain, or other obstacles to recovery.

### 4.6 Occupational therapist

The occupational therapist is focused on the patient's return to independence with ADLs. She/he:

- Addresses the needs of rehabilitation, disability, and participation.
- Practices activities like eating, bathing, or toileting. Activities of daily living are very important for independence.
- Assists the team in determining a safe discharge plan.
- Teaches ADLs, the use of walking aids, and special devices.
- Should also be involved in the treatment of delirium. Occupational therapy is charged with evaluating patient cognition, as it relates to home safety and ability to be independent. They have different options to work with confused patients and to help them to recover earlier from delirium. Environmental stimuli may help to reduce the risk of delirium.

### 4.7 Speech therapist

The speech pathologist has an essential and unique role in care of the FFP. He/she:

- Provides treatment, support, and care for older adults that have difficulties with eating, drinking, and swallowing. Pneumonia is a frequent complication after surgery with aspiration being a common cause. Postoperative swallowing disturbances are frequent in older adults. In confused patients, sedation during or after anesthesia aggravates the risk for aspiration.
- Helps to confirm the risk of aspiration and is able to treat them successfully. An assessment of swallowing should be integrated in the treatment process.

### 4.8 Medical social worker

The involvement of the medical social worker should ideally begin at hospital admission [4]. She/he:

- Stays in contact with the relatives, nursing homes, and rehabilitation centers.
- Evaluates home environment and social support of the patients.
- Is extremely important in terms of goal setting and discharge planning.

### 4.9 Dietitian or nutritionist

Many older adults suffer from poor nutrition. As a result, the involvement of a dietician or nutritionist is important. Malnutrition is common among older FFPs for many reasons. Supplementation of protein improves the outcome of these patients and is able to prevent sarcopenia. See chapter 1.11 Sarcopenia, malnutrition, frailty, and falls for more discussion on malnutrition. The dietitian:

- Assesses patients for presence of malnutrition.
- Creates a dietary plan that maximizes nutritional intake of protein, calories, water, and micronutrients.
- If food intake is insufficient, the dietitian can develop a special food plan.
- Can be helpful in the management of swallowing disturbances.

### 4.10 Care coordinator or case manager

A care coordinator or case manager can help to manage an optimal treatment process, organize team meetings, and stays in contact with general practitioners, nursing homes, and rehabilitation centers. This role is often filled by a nonclinical nurse or a social worker dedicated to overall unit efficiency.

### 4.11 Pharmacist

Polypharmacy is a widespread problem among older FFPs [7]. Drug-drug interactions and adverse drug reactions are strongly associated with the number of drugs. A pharmacist:

- Or pharmacy assistant can verify the accuracy of home medication lists, identify appropriate drug dosing for frail older adults, and assist with the education of patients around specific medication issues (eg, anticoagulant teaching).
- Can be involved as a part of ward rounds or in team meetings.
- Advises the geriatrician, trauma surgeon, and nursing staff on prescribing and administration, with a focus on avoiding adverse drug reactions.
- Can ensure that the discharge medication list is accurate.

### 4.12 Psychiatrist

Delirium is the most frequent complication. Usually, a well-trained orthogeriatric team is able to care for patients suffering from delirium. However, in severe cases of delirium, a psychiatrist may need to be involved.

Depression and fear of falling are other frequent symptoms. Older FFPs frequently fear losing their autonomy. The hospital stay is a source of psychological stress for these patients.

The indication for antidepressants should be evaluated by the psychiatrist. Particularly regarding secondary fracture prevention, antidepressants have a negative effect on risk of falls and bone quality. Therefore, the risks and benefits of treatment should be considered.

### 4.13 Emergency physicians and emergency team

The role of the emergency physicians and the emergency team depends on the local situation and structure of the hospital. Based on their expertise, they can assume some responsibilities from trauma surgeons, anesthesiologists, and geriatricians.

The treatment process starts at the location of accident, especially pain treatment and delirium prevention. The emergency team collects all available information including medications, medical reports, and patient's advanced directives. The team typically focuses on initiating standard protocols and order sets focused on diagnostic workup, restoration of intravascular volume, and acute pain control.

### 4.14 Cardiologist or other specialists

The majority of FFPs can be managed without further subspecialty consultation, and consultation does carry the risk of inappropriate surgical delay or delay in initiation of rehabilitation [8]. Occasionally, patients will require consultation for new medical complications or complex chronic disease. The primary team should incorporate subspecialty advice along with other goals to limit polypharmacy and adapt medical treatment to life expectancy and goals of care.

## 5 References

1. **Gosch M, Hoffmann-Weltin Y, Roth T, et al.** Orthogeriatric co-management improves the outcome of long-term care residents with fragility fractures. *Arch Orthop Trauma Surg.* 2016 Oct;136(10):1403–1409.
2. **Valderas JM, Starfield B, Sibbald B, et al.** Defining comorbidity: implications for understanding health and health services. *Ann Fam Med.* 2009 Jul–Aug;7(4):357–363.
3. **Keeler E, Guralnik JM, Tian H, et al.** The impact of functional status on life expectancy in older persons. *J Gerontol A Biol Sci Med Sci.* 2010 Jul;65(7):727–733.
4. **Friedman SM, Mendelson DA, Kates SL, et al.** Geriatric co-management of proximal femur fractures: total quality management and protocol-driven care result in better outcomes for a frail patient population. *J Am Geriatr Soc.* 2008 Jul;56(7):1349–1356.
5. **Mears SC, Kates SL.** A guide to improving the care of patients with fragility fractures, edition 2. *Geriatr Orthop Surg Rehabil.* 2015 Jun;6(2):58–120.
6. **Bunta AD, Edwards BJ, Macaulay WB Jr, et al.** Own the bone, a system-based intervention, improves osteoporosis care after fragility fractures. *J Bone Joint Surg Am.* 2016 Dec 21;98(24):e109.
7. **Harstedt M, Rogmark C, Sutton R, et al.** Polypharmacy and adverse outcomes after hip fracture surgery. *J Orthop Surg Res.* 2016 Nov 24;11(1):151.
8. **Kates SL, Mendelson DA, Friedman SM.** Co-managed care for fragility hip fractures (Rochester model). *Osteoporos Int.* 2010 Dec;21(Suppl 4):S621–S625.

# 2.7 Protocol and order set development

Stephen L Kates, Joseph A Nicholas

## 1 Introduction

High-performing geriatric fracture centers report the institution of protocols and order sets as one of the major tools to improve outcomes. These attempts at standardization of care are often focused on many different members of the care team, including providers, nursing, ancillary services, and administrative staff responsible for arranging safe and timely surgery.

Standardization of care is an essential part of providing optimal care for fragility fracture patients (FFPs). Order sets, protocols, and care plans are tools that can help organize safe and efficient care, and avoid errors due to inappropriate variation. These tools are the centerpiece of fracture programs that yield significant gains in safety and reductions in harm.

This chapter will discuss the rationale for increased standardization of care, as well as issues to consider in the development, adoption, and maintenance of these tools.

## 2 Why are standard protocols and order sets needed?

The primary concept is to create a standard work flow for a specific diagnosis. The concept of standard work is ubiquitous in industry dating back to the early 20th century in the automotive industry [1]. Standard order sets offer a lot of benefits, as the following list and **Table 2.7-1** show:

- They may help to reduce unnecessary variations [2–6]. This avoids what is referred to as "inappropriate creativity" by the physician when writing orders and devising treatment plans.
- They ensure that patient care follows a predetermined pathway that has been shown to be effective and hopefully is based on evidence-based best practices [7].
- When all patients are managed using standard protocols and order sets, outcomes can be better assessed and compared. When an order or pathway is changed, it is considerably easier to assess the effects of the change.
- An unspoken benefit of standard protocols and order sets is that all members of the care team come to accept them as being the norm, and recognize potentially harmful deviations. When there is a variation from the norm, the team members will question why, often avoiding harm or an adverse event. Use of standard order sets offers the opportunity for significant cost savings by reducing the use of "physician preference" medications and other variations. This results in measurable cost savings and offers the opportunity to avoid medication errors.

## 3 Development of a standard care pathway

The essential steps in developing a standard pathway are:

- To reach a clinical and administrative consensus that the pathway and order sets are needed to improve patient care. The benefits of standardizing pathways should be carefully explained to members of the care team. One benefit of the implementation of electronic health records is that it becomes much simpler to have standard order sets. Once an order set is created for a specific diagnosis, it becomes the easier path for physicians to follow.
- To obtain buy-in from all team members affected by the protocols and order sets. This is best accomplished by meeting as a team and requesting the assistance of a representative from each discipline involved in care of the patients with the diagnosis.
- Use of an older order set or an order set from a successful program is a good starting place. Each order should be examined in detail and discussed with the entire team to improve it. It should be understood that such order sets will need to be revisited and upgraded over time to improve outcomes and to adapt them to the availability of new medical evidence.

| Area | Benefit | Example | Team members |
|---|---|---|---|
| Emergency department order sets | • Rapid admission<br>• Avoid unnecessary tests and x-rays | • Emergency department order set | • Surgeon<br>• Medical doctor<br>• Nurses<br>• Pharmacist<br>• Emergency physician |
| Admission orders | • Optimize patient<br>• Appropriate tests<br>• Avoid bad medications | • Admission order set for hip fractures | • Surgeon<br>• Geriatrician<br>• Nurses<br>• Pharmacist<br>• Social worker<br>• Therapists<br>• Mid-level providers |
| Postoperative orders | • Streamlined postoperative care<br>• Appropriate medications ordered<br>• Avoid unnecessary tests<br>• Early discharge<br>• Avoid delirium | • Postoperative hip fracture order set | • Surgeon<br>• Geriatrician<br>• Nurses<br>• Pharmacist<br>• Social worker<br>• Therapists<br>• Mid-level providers |
| Consultation form | • Standard assessment for preoperative patient<br>• Risk stratification<br>• Avoid unnecessary consultations | • Preoperative geriatric fracture consultation form | • Geriatrician<br>• Surgeon<br>• Anesthesiologist |
| Surgical choices | • Develop decision tree based on radiographic pattern for evidence-based correct hip fracture fixation<br>• Goal is stable fixation that allows immediate weight bearing | • Hip fracture poster to hang in surgical area | • Surgeon champion |
| Metabolic bone workup | • Standardized assessment for osteoporosis, primary or secondary | • Set of orders, including vitamin D level, PTH level, TSH level, calcium | • Surgeon and medical physicians<br>• Mid-level providers |
| Transfer protocol | • Standard method for streamlined acceptance of transfers from other facilities | • Transfer protocol and poster | • Surgeon<br>• Medical physician<br>• Mid-level providers<br>• Hospital administration |
| Direct admission | • Standard method for streamlined acceptance of direct admission to the orthopedic floor from other facilities | • Direct admission protocol | • Surgeon<br>• Medical physician<br>• Mid-level providers<br>• Hospital administration |
| Nursing care | • Plan that follows each step of the standard order sets<br>• Everyone is on the same page | • Nursing care map | • Surgeon<br>• Medical physician<br>• Nursing leaders |
| Discharge process | • Early hospital discharge | • Standardized social work assessment done prior to surgery after admission | • Social worker<br>• Surgeon and medical champion |
| Consent forms | • Preprinted procedure-specific consent forms | • Expedite consent process with legible complete form<br>• Avoid liability issues | • Surgeon champion |
| Outcomes report | • Collect standard outcome measures for hip fracture patients | • Monitor program performance | • Surgeon and medical champions<br>• Hospital administration |
| Comorbidity scoring | • Score patients with a standard score that predicts outcomes | • Helps to risk-stratify patients<br>• For outcomes, and understand patient comorbidity severity | • Surgeon and medical champion<br>• Hospital quality department and information technology personnel |

**Table 2.7-1**: Areas to address in a standardized program.
Abbreviations: PTH, parathyroid hormone; TSH, thyroid-stimulating hormone.

- For team members to compromise on some of the specific aspects (eg, specific medications and dosages) selected for the order set in order to produce a straightforward, concise, and safe pathway.

## 4 Creation or adaptation of standard order sets for fragility fracture patient care

Order sets should:

- Help the physician to follow clinical practice guidelines when caring for their patients, as these are becoming more prevalent for FFPs. Two examples would be use of prophylactic anticoagulation in the perioperative period and obtaining a mini-metabolic bone workup as part of the admission order set. The physician has only to sign the order if this order has been defaulted in the order set.
- Default to the best available evidence and serve as a template for individual patient care plans; they should also offer an opportunity for variation if clinically indicated.
- Be patient centered, meaning that they can be adapted to the individual patient's needs. For example, most patients with a hip fracture typically should not be managed with a knee brace following surgery. However, in certain instances, it may be necessary to utilize a knee brace and therefore an unchecked box would be placed in the order set for knee brace.
- Indicate that a particular medication or treatment is known to be harmful and should not be used in a patient group to which it is specifically harmful. That may include use of medications such as meperidine, diphenhydramine, or H2 receptor blockers for older adults [8]. These are all known to be problematic in older FFPs and should be avoided in essentially all cases.
- Encourage specific treatment or protocols that are known to be helpful, such as the retention of eye glasses and hearing aids throughout the hospital stay [6, 9]. This helps to avoid the complication of delirium yet these aids are often taken away from the older patient upon hospital admission.
- Reach a practical compromise when there is a question on a specific area and lack of agreement.
- Be based on a comprehensive literature search or consultation with experts in the field as indicated if there is considerable uncertainty on a specific area. There are many unanswered questions remaining in the field of osteoporotic fracture management.
- Not be too long or cumbersome to effectively use. A complicated or exhaustive order set may not result in standardized and efficient care for most patients. The final electronic or paper product should be piloted with the team members who will use these tools; this can help identify content or formatting issues that may impair safety and efficiency.
- Be periodically revisited by the team, especially if a problem is identified upon review of quality management data.
- Offer the opportunity to help physicians comply with hospital, local, and governmental regulations for care provision. Such regulatory mandates should be built into an order set. For example, it may be required to document the patient's preferences for resuscitation in the event of respiratory or cardiac arrest. The standard order set can include a mandatory order where the physician documents the resuscitation status.

Once an order set has been created and agreed to by the team, it should be reviewed and approved by the hospitals order set committee to be certain it is in full compliance with all hospital policies and procedures as well as national requirements. At that point, the order set will be given to the electronic medical record team to create a usable electronic document. For centers still using paper medical records, at this stage it would be sent to the printer to be printed.

After creation of the new order set, it is essential to make sure that the nursing care map matches the order sets step by step. Typically, the medical and surgical program leaders meet with nursing leaders caring for the patients to be certain that the nursing care map matches the order sets.

## 5 Standardized protocols for accepting patients transferred from another facility

An organized orthogeriatric program will tend to attract medically complex patients from smaller or less experienced hospitals for transfer. This, in fact, is a service to the patient and the transferring center and should be considered as such. It is important for the receiving orthogeriatric fracture program to have a standardized and organized method for accepting such transfers that include the following steps:

- It is helpful if the transferring center can transfer the patient with one telephone call explaining the need for the transfer and other particular important medical and social information.
- Electronic transfer of x-rays and other data may help with the assessment of the patient in question from the receiving center.

- When the patient is transferred, it is helpful to use a transfer envelope in which to place all pertinent medical information. On the front of the transfer envelope, there should be a checklist that helps the transferring team provide all necessary information to facilitate care at the receiving center.
- Development of a written protocol is extremely helpful. All members of the team need to know about the receiving protocol. Patients should be accepted if at all possible, and their care should be streamlined and facilitated at the receiving center. Transfers are best received during daylight hours when the team is present to assess the patient in a timely manner after admission. Use of a transfer protocol and transfer envelope is recommended for both the transferring center and the receiving center. Examples can be found in **Fig 2.7-1** and **Fig 2.7-2**.

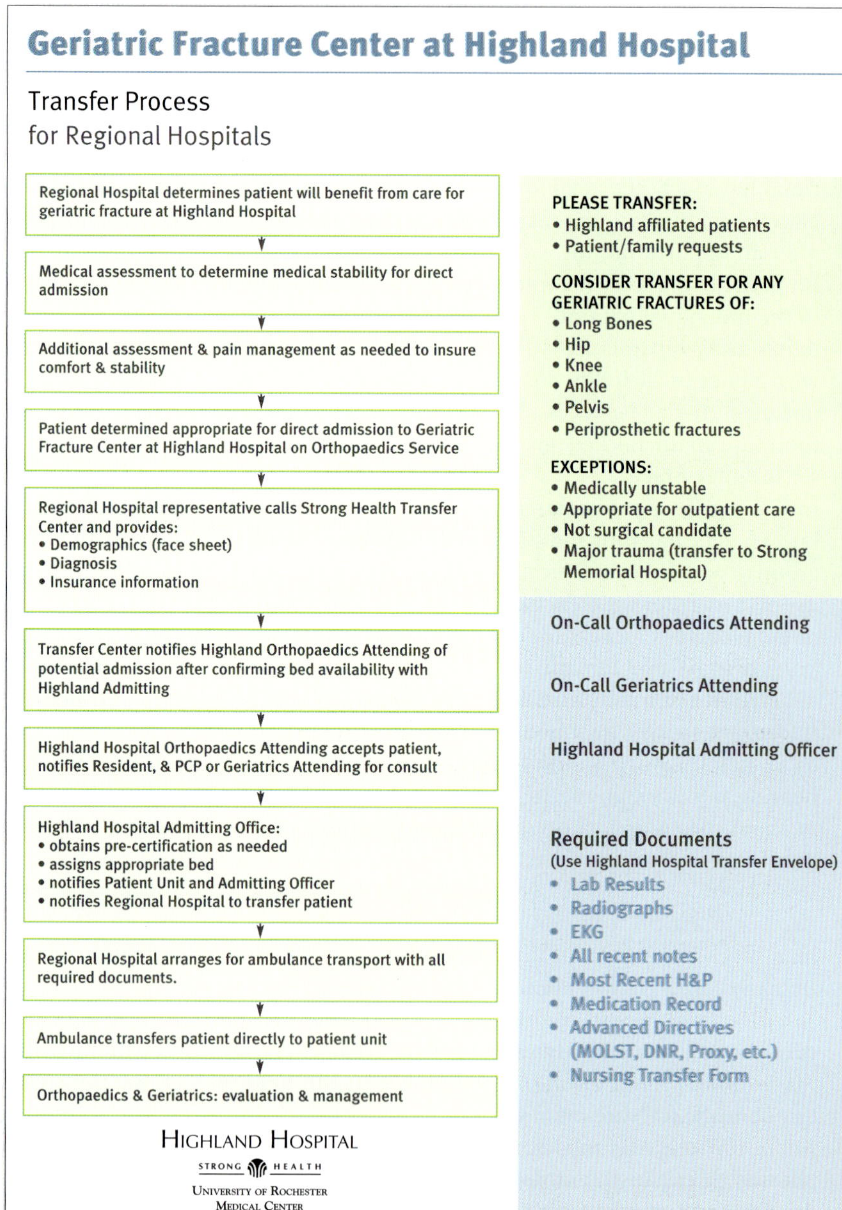


**Fig 2.7-1** Example of a transfer protocol.

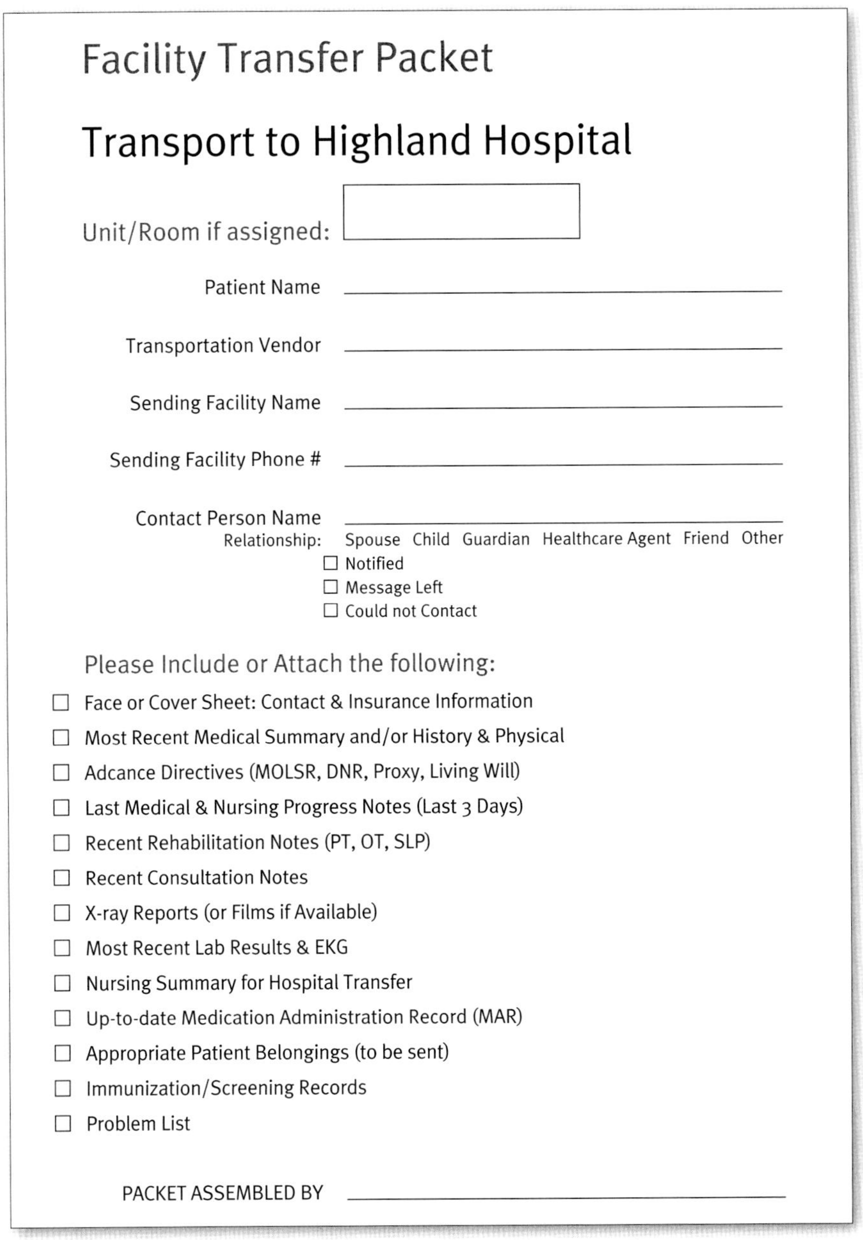

Facility Transfer Packet

Transport to Highland Hospital

Unit/Room if assigned: ______

Patient Name ______

Transportation Vendor ______

Sending Facility Name ______

Sending Facility Phone # ______

Contact Person Name ______

Relationship: Spouse Child Guardian Healthcare Agent Friend Other

☐ Notified

☐ Message Left

☐ Could not Contact

Please Include or Attach the following:

☐ Face or Cover Sheet: Contact & Insurance Information

☐ Most Recent Medical Summary and/or History & Physical

☐ Adcance Directives (MOLSR, DNR, Proxy, Living Will)

☐ Last Medical & Nursing Progress Notes (Last 3 Days)

☐ Recent Rehabilitation Notes (PT, OT, SLP)

☐ Recent Consultation Notes

☐ X-ray Reports (or Films if Available)

☐ Most Recent Lab Results & EKG

☐ Nursing Summary for Hospital Transfer

☐ Up-to-date Medication Administration Record (MAR)

☐ Appropriate Patient Belongings (to be sent)

☐ Immunization/Screening Records

☐ Problem List

PACKET ASSEMBLED BY ______

**Fig 2.7-2** Example of a transfer envelope. The checklist on the front of the envelope enables the transferring team to assemble all the needed data to facilitate the transfer. This helps avoid wasting time and errors.

## 6 Standard consultation form to document and prevent case cancellation

The standard consultation form in the medical record helps the medical consultant accurately document the results of the patient's history and physical examination. The forms should be designed to fit the physician's workflow in documenting their findings and assessment. Using a standardized consultation form as a template, documentation is improved and is readily searchable by members of the care team. This avoids a loss of sometimes difficult to gather but important information specifically in demented patients.

Standardized consultation forms ease and speed up the treatment progress. They may be used in the emergency department and for daily ward rounds. If possible they should be integrated in the electronic chart of the patient to be readily available for all team members.

Early surgery for the optimized patient has shown to be beneficial in the care of geriatric fracture patients [10, 11]. The frequent concern of surgeons is that the patient's surgery will be canceled for reasons that they deem inappropriate. Case cancellation is often the result of poor communication or poor documentation in the preoperative notes by the surgeon and medical physician. When an anesthesiologist reviews the medical record, they look for a legible and comprehensive medical assessment of the patient. A short note stating "cleared for surgery" is meaningless and not helpful to the anesthesiologist. What is beneficial is a comprehensive history and physical review of the past medical history, medications, allergies, family history, social history, preoperative functional status, and response to prior surgery. Additionally, the patient needs to be medically optimized, fluid resuscitated, and truly ready for surgery. This status should be clearly documented in the preoperative medical assessment.

Other areas that standardized consultation forms can promote include attention to goals of care, such as resuscitation status and also patient decision regarding resuscitation during surgery, healthcare proxy designation, and advanced directives in the event of a poor outcome. These consultation forms can also display standardized care plan recommendations for predictable issues like venous thromboembolism prophylaxis, delirium prevention, disposition needs, and suggest wording indicating to other providers that a high-risk procedure is still appropriate for highly comorbid or frail patients. The standard consultation form should not recommend the type of anesthetic to be used, nor should it specify intraoperative management by the anesthesiologist unless there is a critical piece of information that needs to be shared, for instance, a critical aortic stenosis.

Another benefit of a standard consultation form is appropriate hospital and team documentation of the patient's preoperative status. Very few to no liability cases will result from outstanding documentation. Care needs to be taken to avoid excessive amounts of imported or highly detailed documentation; key clinical communication should be consolidated in a consistent and easy to find section of the notes, ie, the beginning or the end.

## 7 Development of standard protocols for assessment and risk stratification

It is frequently beneficial that the patient is risk-stratified into a category of low risk, intermediate risk, high risk, or extremely high risk [3]. This risk assessment helps the anesthesiologist and the team members to understand the patient's true surgical risk. It also helps the medical consultant to appropriately document whether the patient is optimized for surgery and their level of risk [2, 6]. Some perioperative risk assessment tools (eg, Revised Cardiac Risk Index) can help anchor risk estimates to those from the literature, but all team members should recognize that risk estimation is less accurate in frail older adults (see chapter 1.4 Preoperative risk assessment and preparation for further discussion of these issues).

Typically in the perioperative period, the anesthesiologist will assign an American Society of Anesthesiologists (ASA) score to the patient. The ASA score has been shown to accurately correlate with patient outcomes [12]. Recently, a mini-frailty index has been developed, which also helps to predict short-term adverse events that can occur in the perioperative period [13]. Risk stratification supports the orthopedic surgeon in the determination of surgical or nonsurgical treatment for fractures without a clearly superior standard of care, typically after fractures of the upper extremity.

## 8 Standardization of discharge processes

Geriatric fractures, especially hip fracture, create the highest risk for hospital readmission at 30 and 90 days among orthopedic patients [14]. Although there are multiple causes of readmission and no obvious way to avoid all of them [15], appropriate discharge documentation including all needed information to appropriately care for the patient should be provided to the receiving facility (eg, nursing home) at the time of hospital discharge.

Standardizing the discharge process is a way to improve the packaging of the patient at the time of discharge to reduce errors and complications. A thoughtful and well-documented handoff to the receiving providers will help to reduce medical errors and readmissions. It is important to recognize that many patients will be discharged to a facility that has no prior medical knowledge of the patient; discharge documentation that contains a clear summary of the patient's prefracture medical history, medications, functional status and goals of care are essential to minimizing readmissions for lapses in care.

Placement of appropriate documentation in a large envelope with a checklist on the front is one useful strategy to nicely package the patient for discharge (**Fig 2.7-2**). Included in this package should be:

- The most recent medication list
- The most recent history, physical examination, and discharge summary
- Necessary orders
- Name and contact information for care providers at the hospital
- Date of next recommended follow-up visit
- Any specifics such as laboratory workup or wound care

Careful documentation and creation of an appropriate package upon discharge reduces errors and improves the quality of the patient handoff. It is well-known that most errors occur at the time of a handoff to another provider [16].

## 9 Periodic reassessment and revision of standard protocols in order sets

Orthogeriatric programs should typically collect data and look at the results over time [6]. Graphing the results over time will visually demonstrate variation in some of the measured parameters. If there is a negative progression in outcomes or metrics or a serious adverse event occurs, the reasons for this should be sought and corrected. This may require reassessment of the treatment protocol or order sets. Sometimes the change in the order sets reflects a change in what is best practice. Other times, changes in the order set will be needed to meet hospital or regulatory requirements. As time progresses, it is certain that all order sets will need to be revisited and appropriately amended to benefit the patient and the system. When such changes are needed, it is extremely important to include care team members at the table when decisions are made. That way each representative of the discipline can report their recent changes to their coworkers and help them understand the need to make changes. In this manner, care can improve with time.

Order set improvements will be needed more commonly soon after implementation and, as time passes, the changes required will become less frequent. Nonetheless, as science and medical evidence improves, changes will be needed to benefit the patients.

## 10 References

1. **Womack JP, Jones DT, Roos D.** *The Machine That Changed the World.* New York: Simon&Schuster; 1990.
2. **Kates SL, Mendelson DA, Friedman SM.** Co-managed care for fragility hip fractures (Rochester model). *Osteoporos Int.* 2010 Dec;21(Suppl 4):S621–S625.
3. **Friedman SM, Mendelson DA, Kates SL, et al.** Geriatric co-management of proximal femur fractures: total quality management and protocol-driven care result in better outcomes for a frail patient population. *J Am Geriatr Soc.* 2008 Jul;56(7):1349–1356.
4. **Friedman SM, Mendelson DA, Bingham KW, et al.** Impact of a comanaged Geriatric Fracture Center on short-term hip fracture outcomes. *Arch Intern Med.* 2009 Oct 12;169(18):1712–1717.
5. **Kates SL.** Lean business model and implementation of a geriatric fracture center. *Clin Geriatr Med.* 2014 May;30(2):191–205.
6. **Mears SC, Kates SL.** A guide to improving the care of patients with fragility fractures, edition 2. *Geriatr Orthop Surg Rehabil.* 2015 Jun;6(2):58–120.
7. **Neuman MD, Archan S, Karlawish JH, et al.** The relationship between short-term mortality and quality of care for hip fracture: a meta-analysis of clinical pathways for hip fracture. *J Am Geriatr Soc.* 2009 Nov;57(11):2046–2054.
8. **Fick DM, Semla TP.** 2012 American Geriatrics Society Beers Criteria: new year, new criteria, new perspective. *J Am Geriatr Soc.* 2012 Apr;60(4):614–615.
9. **Inouye SK.** Delirium after hip fracture: to be or not to be? *J Am Geriatr Soc.* 2001 May;49(5):678–679.
10. **Bottle A, Aylin P.** Mortality associated with delay in operation after hip fracture: observational study. *BMJ.* 2006 Apr 22;332(7547):947–951.
11. **Moran CG, Wenn RT, Sikand M, et al.** Early mortality after hip fracture: is delay before surgery important? *J Bone Joint Surg Am.* 2005 Mar;87(3):483–489.
12. **Michel JP, Klopfenstein C, Hoffmeyer P, et al.** Hip fracture surgery: is the pre-operative American Society of Anesthesiologists (ASA) score a predictor of functional outcome? *Aging Clin Exp Res.* 2002 Oct;14(5):389–394.
13. **Kistler EA, Nicholas JA, Kates SL, et al.** Frailty and short-term outcomes in patients with hip fracture. *Geriatr Orthop Surg Rehabil.* 2015 Sep;6(3):209–214.
14. **Goodman DC, Fisher ES, Chang C-H, et al.** *After Hospitalization: a Dartmouth Atlas Report on Post-Acute Care for Medicare Beneficiaries.* Hanover, NH: The Dartmouth Institute for Health Policy and Clinical Practice. 2011;28.
15. **Kates SL, Behrend C, Mendelson DA, et al.** Hospital readmission after hip fracture. *Arch Orthop Trauma Surg.* 2015 Mar;135(3):329–337.
16. **Starmer AJ, Spector ND, Srivastava R, et al.** Changes in medical errors after implementation of a handoff program. *N Engl J Med.* 2014 Nov 06;371(19):1803–1812.

# 2.8 Fracture liaison service and improving treatment rates for osteoporosis

**Paul J Mitchell**

## 1 What is a fracture liaison service?

The fracture liaison service (FLS) was developed in response to a pervasive and persistent postfracture care gap evident among fragility fracture patients (FFPs) throughout the world [1]. The majority of people aged 50 years and older who present with a fragility fracture do not receive the osteoporosis assessment and management as advocated in clinical guidelines [2–7]. Furthermore, interventions intended to identify and mitigate risk factors for falls are often not a standard component of postfracture care. The secondary fracture prevention care gap and the role that FLS can play to reduce it have been highlighted by international and national campaigns, including:

- International Osteoporosis Foundation's (IOF) Capture the Fracture Campaign [1, 7, 8]
- Osteoporosis Canada's Make the FIRST break the LAST with Fracture Liaison Services [9]
- Osteoporosis New Zealand's Bone Care 2020 [10]
- Falls and Fractures Alliance in England [11]
- National Bone Health Alliance in the United States [12–14]

The rationale for prioritizing secondary fracture prevention stems from epidemiological observations that about half of all hip fracture patients break another bone before they fracture their hip [15–18]. Among postmenopausal women, estimates suggest that one-sixth will have suffered a fragility fracture at any relevant skeletal site (ie, generally excluding fractures of the skull, fingers, and toes) [5]. Taken together, among women aged 50 years and older, these data suggest that half of all future cases of hip fracture will emanate from the one-sixth of the population who have suffered a prior fragility fracture. Older men account for 30% of the world's hip fractures. Information on the prevalence of prior fracture history is not broadly available. However, several studies suggest that 30–59% of men who have suffered a hip fracture had previously broken another bone [15, 16, 18]. The IOF [8, 19], the Endocrine Society [20], and other organizations [6, 9, 21, 22] endorse secondary fracture prevention as a requirement for men too.

A broad array of pharmacological interventions has been demonstrated to reduce future fracture risk for individuals who have suffered a fragility fracture [23]. Given that these treatments have been available for 20 years, why are they not routinely being targeted to individuals at high risk of suffering further fractures? This question has been considered by investigators from several countries [2, 3]. A study that evaluated the practice of orthopedic surgeons and general practitioners (GPs) in the UK provided an insight into why this apparent breakdown in chronic disease management is occurring [24]. Surgeons and GPs were asked about their routine clinical practice when confronted with three clinical scenarios:

- A 55-year-old woman with a low-trauma Colles wrist fracture
- A 60-year-old women with a vertebral wedge fracture
- A 70-year-old woman with a low-trauma femoral neck fracture

Both groups agreed in principle that FFPs should be investigated for osteoporosis, ie, 81% of surgeons and 96% of GPs. However, as indicated in **Fig 2.8-1**, in most scenarios both surgeons and GPs would not take direct responsibility to do so themselves. This study mirrors the findings of systematic reviews that considered barriers to secondary fracture prevention in clinical practice. There is a tendency for orthopedic surgeons and primary care providers to rely upon one another to implement secondary fracture prevention, resulting in its omission for the majority of FFPs. The fracture liaison service was developed to overcome the lack of clarity regarding clinical ownership of secondary prevention efforts, and to eliminate the care gap.

The fracture liaison service is a program designed to ensure that all FFPs above a specific age receive secondary preventive care. This program includes both osteoporosis assessment and treatment, and where appropriate, an intervention to reduce the risk of falls. A critical component of an FLS is personnel dedicated to identifying, investigating, and initiating secondary preventive care for fracture patients. While this FLS coordinator is often a nurse practitioner or registered nurse, some FLS have employed physicians in training or allied healthcare professionals to fulfil this role. An FLS will adhere to protocols of care agreed with all relevant local hospital specialists, primary care providers, and health system administrators.

The scope of an FLS may vary, depending on the case mix of fracture patients presenting to the particular hospital or health system. The FLS may manage all FFPs, just those admitted as inpatients to a hospital, or just those managed in the outpatient setting. The operational structure of an FLS will be influenced by local orthopedic service configurations, particularly the presence or absence of orthopedic-geriatric comanagement services for FFPs also known as geriatric fracture centers or orthogeriatrics services [25, 26].

The place of an FLS in a systematic approach to hip fracture care and prevention is illustrated in **Fig 2.8-2**, which describes the approach being taken in New Zealand [10]. This approach was based on previous experience from the UK [27], which has also been adopted in Australia [28], Canada [9], and the United States [14], and internationally by IOF [1]. The FLS can be configured to provide secondary preventive care for all FFPs. In institutions with established orthopedic-geriatric comanagement services, which usually manage osteoporosis and fall risks for hip fracture patients, the FLS can serve the nonhip FFPs, which usually represents 80–85% of the fragility fracture case load [25, 26].

The process of planning for an FLS, considerations during implementation, and results achieved from well-established, high-performing FLS will be discussed in the next topics of this chapter.

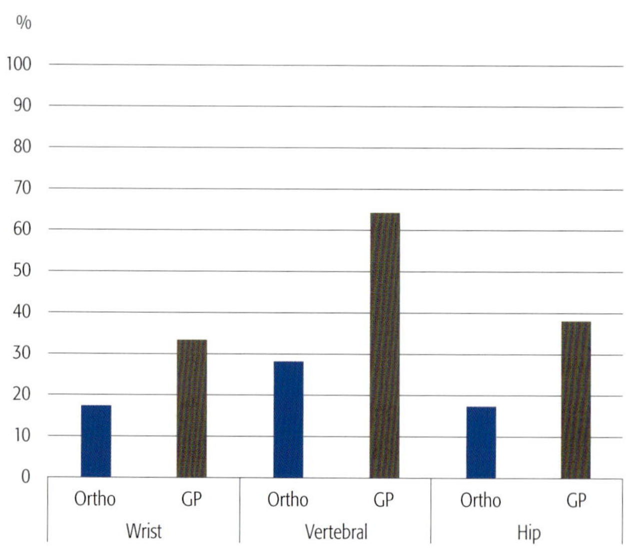


**Fig 2.8-1** The proportion of orthopedic surgeons and general practitioners who would routinely assess the fracture patient and/or initiate osteoporosis treatment, or would refer the fracture patient to a local osteoporosis clinic [24].
Abbreviations: GP, general practitioner; Ortho, orthopedic surgeon.

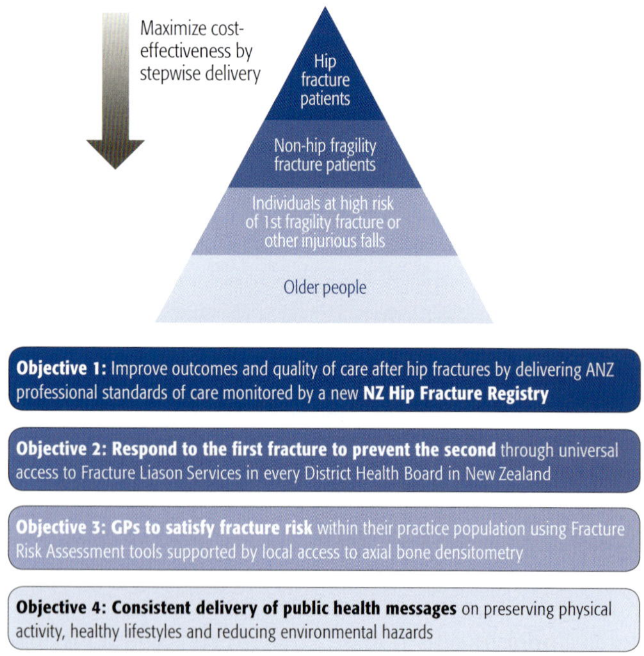


**Fig 2.8-2** Fracture liaison service in the context of a systematic approach to hip fracture care and prevention for New Zealand (reproduced with kind permission of Osteoporosis New Zealand) [10].
Abbreviations: ANZ, Australian and New Zealand; GP, general practitioner.

## 2 Planning

All successful FLS programs have required an individual to champion the case for FLS implementation within their institution or health system. This person is often formally or informally designated as the "lead clinician for osteoporosis" in his/her place of work. In the hospital setting, the FLS champion may be an endocrinologist, rheumatologist, geriatrician, or orthopedic surgeon. Some FLS programs have been established in primary care, where the FLS champion is a GP (ie, a family physician) with a special interest in osteoporosis or musculoskeletal disease [29]. A selection of useful resources to support champions embarking upon their FLS development efforts is available in topic 5 of this chapter. The key steps in planning for an FLS that a physician champion should consider are illustrated in **Fig 2.8-3**.

### 2.1 Stakeholders

The care of FFPs involves a broad group of health professionals and administrative staff. The champion's first task is to identify which individuals should become members of a multidisciplinary stakeholder group that will guide and enable development of the FLS. This group is likely to include:

- The FLS champion
- Orthopedic surgeons with an interest in hip or fragility fracture surgery
- Geriatricians, orthogeriatricians, hospitalists, or internists working in orthopedic-geriatric comanagement services
- A radiologist and/or nuclear medicine specialist
- Relevant specialist nurses, physiotherapists, and other allied healthcare professionals
- Information technology (IT) professionals responsible for development and/or installation of an FLS database
- Hospital and primary care pharmacy or medicines management representatives
- Hospital administration and/or business planning group representatives
- Local primary care-based service commissioning group representatives
- Local primary care practice representatives
- Local public health authority representatives

### 2.2 Needs assessment

Numerous published audits of secondary fracture prevention have reported, in the absence of a systematic approach, that most FFPs do not receive guideline-based care [7]. To illustrate that a need exists for development of a new FLS, an audit is likely necessary to quantify the local care gap. Analysis of the following key performance indicators over a 1–3-month period would provide an adequate overview of postfracture care at baseline:

- How many women and men aged 50 years and older presented to the hospital or health system with a fragility fracture, which resulted from a fall from standing height or less, and who were managed either as inpatients or outpatients?
- Of these, what percentage received an osteoporosis assessment? This question needs to be answered for two groups, ie, those that were assessed with bone mineral density (BMD) measurement by axial dual-energy x-ray absorptiometry (DEXA) scan and those assessed without a DEXA scan.

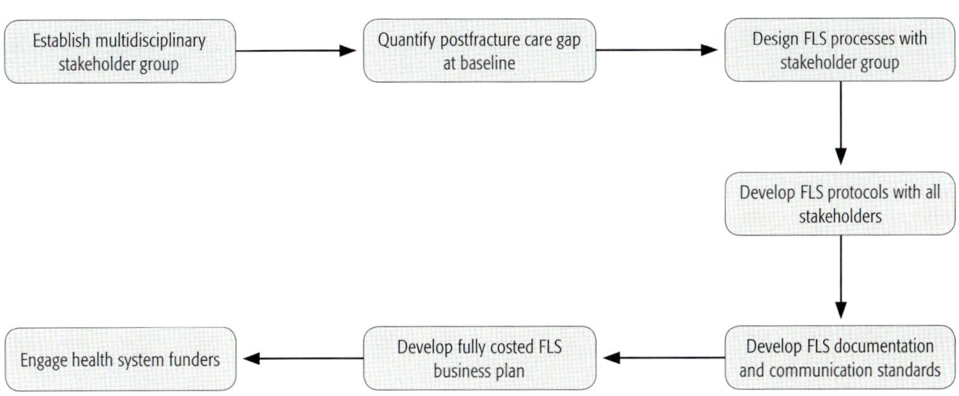


**Fig 2.8-3** Key steps in planning for a fracture liaison service. Abbreviation: FLS, fracture liaison service.

- What percentage received an assessment of fall risk factors, either delivered by an appropriately skilled clinician within an FLS or by referral to a local falls service, or equivalent, operating independently of an FLS?
- Of these, what percentage received lifestyle advice relating to osteoporosis, including diet and activity? What percentage received specific medication for osteoporosis, and what percentage received advice and/or intervention to mitigate fall risk for identified risk factors?

The processes for identification, investigation, and initiation of secondary preventive care need to be designed by the stakeholder group. It can be more efficient to establish a subgroup to define draft processes, documentation, and communication mechanisms that can be reviewed and amended by the entire stakeholder group membership. Key considerations will include:

- Defining the initial scope of the FLS, eg, inpatients and/or outpatients, patients aged 50 years and older or 65 years and older
- Determining how existing IT systems can aid identification of fracture patients, and facilitate ordering of investigations and communication with local primary care providers
- Considering the impact of FLS on capacity of local bone densitometry services

## 2.3 Business plan

Development of a formal business plan for the new FLS is a critical step in the development of a service. Fracture liaison service business plan templates are available in Canada [9], New Zealand [30], and the United States [14] (see topic 5 in this chapter). As the costs related to FLS implementation will vary between and within countries, the following list provides an illustration of the sources of costs that will generally apply:

- Fracture liaison service coordinator salary
- Fracture liaison service lead clinician offering one session per week
- Administrative support
- Bone density scans
- Drug treatment
- Fracture liaison service database and IT costs
- Patient literature
- Printing of reports and questionnaires
- Postage
- Office costs

The potential sources of savings that will be relevant to the funder(s) of the FLS business plan will depend upon the reimbursement system for healthcare in the particular country. In a health and social care system with unified budgets, reductions in direct costs for acute fracture care and hospital admissions, reductions in postdischarge fracture-related visits to primary care providers, and avoidance of admissions to centrally funded nursing homes will all contribute to offset the cost of implementing the FLS. In a different environment, the United States for example, reimbursement for providers of healthcare can be higher for those organizations that achieve higher quality ratings for postfracture care (eg, Medicare Advantage's Five-Star Quality Rating System). The business plan must clearly articulate why implementation of FLS is in the funder's interest. Early engagement with representatives of the hospital, the health system administration, and/or the business planning group, by inviting a representative to join the multidisciplinary stakeholder group, should ensure that the preparatory work and comprehensive business plan is presented in a fashion most likely to meet with success.

In 2013, the IOF published a best practice framework (BPF), which provides globally endorsed standards of care for FLS [8]. Given the variation in structure of healthcare systems throughout the world, the IOF consulted with leading experts from many countries who had established FLS in their localities and undertaken beta testing to ensure that the standards were internationally relevant and fit for purpose. The BPF sets an international benchmark for FLS, which defines essential and aspirational elements of service delivery. For those in the early stages of FLS development, the BPF clearly shows what a high-performing FLS would actually deliver. To expedite sharing of best practice between centers, the IOF developed a process for best practice recognition, which can result in FLS featuring on the "map of best practice" [7]. The map provides an opportunity for those undertaking FLS development to learn from the experience of colleagues elsewhere who have successfully established a service.

## 3 Implementation

Once funding has been identified to establish an FLS, staff recruited, and the service has been launched to the local medical community, ongoing evaluation of FLS performance is required. The key steps in such a process are illustrated in **Fig 2.8-4**.

Plan-Do-Study-Act methodology has been successfully applied to support continuous improvement of FLS performance [31]. Aspects of service delivery that will benefit from close monitoring include:

- Patient identification—knowledge of the proportion of all FFPs presenting to the hospital or health system that are receiving care from the FLS is essential. This data may be available from hospital IT systems for patients admitted as inpatients. However, robust mechanisms must be in place to ensure a basic level of information is also known about patients managed only in the outpatient setting.
- Communication with patients—ongoing assessment should be undertaken of the effectiveness of information relating to lifestyle advice and treatment recommendations.
- Communications with primary care—in systems where primary care providers take responsibility for management of chronic diseases, the effectiveness of all aspects of FLS-initiated communications with primary care should be scrutinized.
- Interaction with hospital specialists—FLS care must be delivered in a patient-centered manner, keeping in mind that patients may find interactions with multiple healthcare professionals bewildering. The FLS must work seamlessly with orthopedic doctors and nursing staff and, for patients admitted to hospital, with colleagues in geriatric medicine.

## 4 Result and impact of fracture liaison services

A growing number of FLS programs have published articles describing aspects of the development of their service and process of care outcomes, while a comparatively small number of publications have described impacts on secondary fracture rates and health economic aspects.

### 4.1 Process of care outcomes

To date, there has been a lack of standardized reporting of outcomes from FLS. In an attempt to determine how the organization of an FLS impacts on process of care outcomes, Ganda et al [32] undertook a systematic review and metaanalysis. This study established a classification system for FLS, relating to the intensity of service provision, based on the premise that FLS can identify, investigate, and initiate (hence 3i) interventions for FFPs:

- Type A models undertake identification, investigation, and initiation (ie, 3i model).
- Type B models undertake identification and investigation, but leave initiation to the primary care provider (ie, 2i model).
- Type C models undertake just identification, whereby the primary care provider is alerted that the fracture has occurred and further assessment should be conducted (ie, 1i model).
- Type D models only provide education on osteoporosis to the patient and do not alert the primary care provider or recommend investigation (ie, zero i model).

The findings of the metaanalysis in relation to the process outcomes of BMD testing and initiation of osteoporosis treatment are shown in **Fig 2.8-5**. Clearly, type A (3i) and type B (2i) models outperform the less intensive type C (1i) and type D (zero i) models.

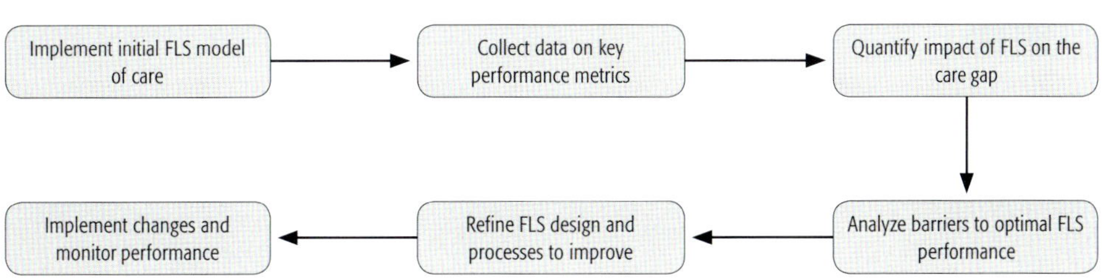


**Fig 2.8-4** Key steps in fracture liaison service implementation. Abbreviation: FLS, fracture liaison service.

### 4.2 Impact on secondary fractures

Studies to evaluate the impact of FLS on secondary fracture rates can be challenging to undertake. The presence of national clinical guidelines that recommend or mandate that FFPs should undergo osteoporosis assessment, and be initiated on treatment where appropriate, can eliminate the appropriateness of a control group that are denied access to care by the FLS. Two approaches have been taken to establish contemporaneous control groups to enable evaluation of the impact of FLS on fracture rates.

Dutch investigators evaluated subsequent nonvertebral fracture experience and mortality for patients managed by their own hospital-based FLS as compared to the experience of patients managed at another hospital that lacked an FLS [33]. The risk for subsequent nonvertebral fractures and mortality were analyzed and adjusted for age, gender, and baseline fracture location. Over 2 years of follow-up, patients managed at the FLS hospital had a 56% reduction in nonvertebral fracture incidence and 35% lower mortality compared to those managed at the hospital without an FLS.

In Australia, two groups of investigators based in New South Wales compared the fracture experience of patients managed by their own FLS with that of patients who chose not be managed by their FLS [34, 35]. Over 4 years the FLS based in Sydney observed an 80% ($P < .01$) difference between nonvertebral fracture rates between the FLS group (4.1%) and the control group (19.7%). Over 2 years the FLS based in Newcastle observed similar differences in fracture incidence between the FLS group (5.1%) and the control group (16.4%) [35].

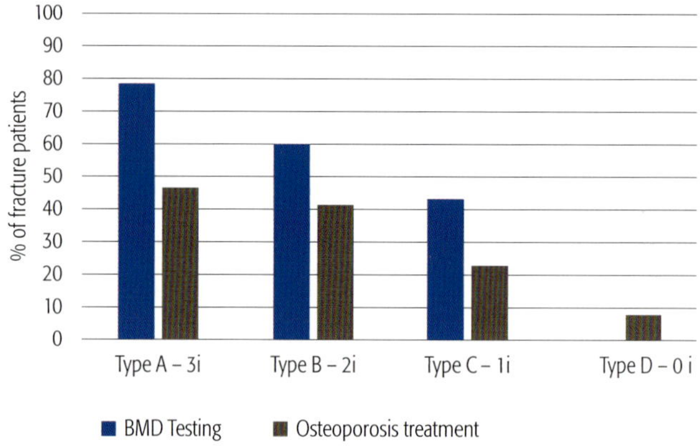


**Fig 2.8-5** Intensity of fracture liaison service model and process of care outcomes [32].
Abbreviation: BMD, bone mineral density.

In Germany, Niedhart et al [36] described a significant reduction of osteoporosis fracture-related hospitalization rate due to an intensified, multimodal treatment in the integrated healthcare network Osteoporosis North Rhine. A retrospective cross-sectional analysis was performed using routine data from the regional public health insurer for the years 2007–2010. Patients were included if they were 50–89 years old, had a diagnosis of osteoporosis, and at least three prescriptions of osteoporosis-specific medication. Data were analyzed separately for integrated and regular healthcare. Of the 22,040 patients identified, 3,173 were participants in the integrated healthcare group (IV). The hospitalization rate for hip fractures was significantly lower in the IV group, ie, 5.93 per 1,000 patient-years versus 22.96 per 1,000 patient-years (-74%, $P < .05$). Also the hospitalization rate of all other osteoporosis-related fractures was reduced by 73% to 46.92 per 1,000 patient-years versus 172.88 per 1,000 patient-years ($P < .05$).

### 4.3 Cost-effectiveness evaluations

A number of formal cost-effectiveness analyses of FLS have been published from several countries.

#### 4.3.1 Australia

A Markov model [37] was developed, which incorporated fracture probabilities and resource utilization data obtained directly from study of the FLS in Sydney mentioned in topic 4.2 of this chapter [34]. Findings included that:

- A mean improvement in discounted quality-adjusted life expectancy per patient of 0.089 quality-adjusted life years (QALYs) was gained.
- There was a partial offset of the higher costs of the FLS by a decrease in subsequent fractures, which lead to an overall discounted cost increase of AUD 1,486 per patient over the 10-year simulation period.
- The incremental costs per QALY gained (ie, incremental cost-effectiveness ratio) were AUD 17,291, which is well below the Australian accepted maximum of AUD 50,000 to pay for one QALY gained.

#### 4.3.2 Canada

A 1-year decision-analysis model was developed to evaluate the FLS at St Michael's Hospital in Toronto [38]. Findings included the following:

- A hospital that hired an FLS coordinator managing 500 patients with fragility fractures annually could reduce the number of subsequent hip fractures by 9% in the first year.

- A net hospital cost saving of CND 48,950 would be realized (Canadian dollars in year 2004 values).
- Hiring an FLS coordinator would be a cost-saving measure even when the coordinator manages as few as 350 patients annually.

### 4.3.3 Germany

Osteoporosis-related medication costs were doubled in the integrated healthcare group (IV), while total medication costs were lower in the IV group (EUR 1,438 versus EUR 1,702).

### 4.3.4 United Kingdom

A Markov model was developed, utilizing detailed audit data collected by the West Glasgow FLS [39]. The model compared costs and outcomes for a hypothetical cohort of 1,000 FFPs, of whom 740 required treatment, managed by the FLS with usual care in the UK according to data from a comprehensive national audit program. Considerably more patients (n = 686) managed by the FLS received treatment as compared to those who received usual care (n = 193). Findings included:

- Assessments and osteoporosis treatments cost an additional £ 83,598 and £ 206,544, respectively, in the FLS.
- The FLS prevented 18 fractures (including 11 hip fractures), with an overall saving of £ 21,000.
- Setup costs for widespread adoption of FLS across the UK were estimated at £ 9.7 million.

### 4.3.5 United States of America

A Markov model was developed to evaluate an FLS that provided postfracture osteoporosis care specifically for hip fracture patients [40]. The model considered remaining lifetime fracture incidence (mean 8.6 years) and associated costs for 10,000 men and women who had experienced an index hip fracture. Treatment delivered by a universal FLS for this population was compared to usual care. Implementation of the FLS was predicted to result in the following:

- There would be 153 fewer fractures, ie, 109 hip, 5 wrist, 21 spine, and 17 other fractures.
- Patients would gain 37.4 more QALYs.
- The healthcare system would save USD 66,879 compared with usual care.

## 5 Useful resources

The following online resources may prove useful to FLS champions and multidisciplinary teams at the outset of FLS development:

- IOF Capture the Fracture Campaign website www.capture-the-fracture.org [7]
- Osteoporosis Canada's Make the FIRST break the LAST with Fracture Liaison Services www.osteoporosis.ca/fracture-liaison-service [9]
- NBHA Fracture Prevention CENTRAL website www.FracturePreventionCENTRAL.org [14]

## 6 References


1. **Åkesson K, Mitchell PJ.** Capture the fracture: a global campaign to break the fragility fracture cycle. Nyon: International Osteoporosis Foundation; 2012. Available at: http://share.iofbonehealth.org/WOD/2012/report/WOD12-Report.pdf. Accessed 2017.
2. **Elliot-Gibson V, Bogoch ER, Jamal SA, et al.** Practice patterns in the diagnosis and treatment of osteoporosis after a fragility fracture: a systematic review. *Osteoporos Int.* 2004 Oct;15(10):767–778.
3. **Giangregorio L, Papaioannou A, Cranney A, et al.** Fragility fractures and the osteoporosis care gap: an international phenomenon. *Semin Arthritis Rheum.* 2006 Apr;35(5):293–305.
4. **Cooper C, Mitchell P, Kanis JA.** Breaking the fragility fracture cycle. *Osteoporos Int.* 2011 Jul;22(7):2049–2050.
5. **Marsh D, Akesson K, Beaton DE, et al.** Coordinator-based systems for secondary prevention in fragility fracture patients. *Osteoporos Int.* 2011 Jul;22(7):2051–2065.
6. **Eisman JA, Bogoch ER, Dell R, et al.** Making the first fracture the last fracture: ASBMR task force report on secondary fracture prevention. *J Bone Miner Res.* 2012 Oct;27(10):2039–2046.
7. **International Osteoporosis Foundation.** Capture the fracture: break the worldwide fragility fracture cycle 2014. Available at: www.capturethefracture.org. Accessed: 2017.
8. **Akesson K, Marsh D, Mitchell PJ, et al.** Capture the Fracture: a Best Practice Framework and global campaign to break the fragility fracture cycle. *Osteoporos Int.* 2013 Aug;24(8):2135–2152.
9. **Osteoporosis Canada.** Make the FIRST break the LAST with Fracture Liaison Services. Available at: www.osteoporosis.ca/wp-content/uploads/FLS-TOOLKIT.pdf. Accessed 2017.
10. **Osteoporosis New Zealand.** Bone Care 2020: a systematic approach to hip fracture care and prevention for New Zealand. Available at: https://osteoporosis.org.nz/wp-content/uploads/2013/10/Bone-Care-2020.pdf. Published 2012. Accessed 2017.

11. **National Osteoporosis Society.** The Falls and Fractures Alliance 2014. Available at: nos.org.uk/about-nos/public-affairs/falls-and-fractures-alliance. Accessed 2017.
12. **National Bone Health Alliance.** Secondary Fracture Prevention Initiative. Available at: www.nbha.org/projects/secondary-fracture-prevention-initiative. Published 2012, Accessed 2017.
13. **Lee DB, Lowden MR, Patmintra V, et al.** National Bone Health Alliance: an innovative public-private partnership improving America's bone health. *Curr Osteoporos Rep.* 2013 Dec;11(4):348–353.
14. **National Bone Health Alliance.** Fracture Prevention CENTRAL. Available at: www.nbha.org/fpc. Published 2014. Accessed 2017.
15. **Gallagher JC, Melton LJ, Riggs BL, et al.** Epidemiology of fractures of the proximal femur in Rochester, Minnesota. *Clin Orthop Relat Res.* 1980 Jul-Aug(150):163–171.
16. **Port L, Center J, Briffa NK, et al.** Osteoporotic fracture: missed opportunity for intervention. *Osteoporos Int.* 2003 Sep;14(9):780–784.
17. **McLellan A, Reid D, Forbes K, et al.** *Effectiveness of Strategies for the Secondary Prevention of Osteoporotic Fractures in Scotland (CEPS 99/03).* Scotland: NHS Quality Improvement; 2004.
18. **Edwards BJ, Bunta AD, Simonelli C, et al.** Prior fractures are common in patients with subsequent hip fractures. *Clin Orthop Relat Res.* 2007 Aug;461:226–230.
19. **Ebeling P.** Osteoporosis in men: Why change needs to happen. Nyon: International Osteoporosis Foundation, 2014. Available at: share.iofbonehealth.org/WOD/2014/thematic-report/WOD14-Report.pdf. Accessed 2017.
20. **Watts NB, Adler RA, Bilezikian JP, et al.** Osteoporosis in men: an Endocrine Society clinical practice guideline. *J Clin Endocrinol Metab.* 2012 Jun;97(6):1802–1822.
21. **Papaioannou A, Morin S, Cheung AM, et al.** 2010 clinical practice guidelines for the diagnosis and management of osteoporosis in Canada: summary. *CMAJ.* 2010 Nov 23;182(17):1864–1873.
22. **National Osteoporosis Foundation.** Clinician's guide to prevention and treatment of osteoporosis. Washington: 2013. Available at: emri.tums.ac.ir/upfiles/158936855.pdf. Accessed 2017.
23. **Kanis JA, McCloskey EV, Johansson H, et al.** European guidance for the diagnosis and management of osteoporosis in postmenopausal women. *Osteoporos Int.* 2013 Jan;24(1):23–57.
24. **Chami G, Jeys L, Freudmann M, et al.** Are osteoporotic fractures being adequately investigated? A questionnaire of GP & orthopaedic surgeons. *BMC Fam Pract.* 2006 Feb 07;7:7.
25. **Mendelson DA, Friedman SM.** Principles of comanagement and the geriatric fracture center. *Clin Geriatr Med.* 2014 May;30(2):183–189.
26. **New South Wales Agency for Clinical Innovation.** The orthogeriatric model of care: summary of evidence. North Ryde: NSW Agency for Clinical Innovation, 2010. Available at: www.aci.health.nsw.gov.au/__data/assets/pdf_file/0013/153400/aci_orthogeriatrics_clinical_practice_guide.pdf. Accessed 2017.
27. **Department of Health.** Falls and fractures: effective interventions in health and social care. Available at: http://www.laterlifetraining.co.uk/wp-content/uploads/2011/12/FF_Effective-Interventions-in-health-and-social-care.pdf. Published 2009. Accessed 2017.
28. **Agency for Clinical Innovation.** *Musculoskeletal Network: NSW Model of Care for Osteoporotic Refracture Prevention.* Chatswood: Agency for Clinical Innovation; 2011.
29. **Brankin E, Mitchell C, Munro R.** Closing the osteoporosis management gap in primary care: a secondary prevention of fracture programme. *Curr Med Res Opin.* 2005 Apr;21(4):475–482.
30. **Osteoporosis New Zealand.** Fracture Liaison Service Resource Pack. Available at: https://osteoporosis.org.nz/news/fracture-liaison-service-resource-pack-published-today. Published 2014. Accessed 2017.
31. **Harrington JT, Barash HL, Day S, et al.** Redesigning the care of fragility fracture patients to improve osteoporosis management: a health care improvement project. *Arthritis Rheum.* 2005 Apr 15;53(2):198–204.
32. **Ganda K, Puech M, Chen JS, et al.** Models of care for the secondary prevention of osteoporotic fractures: a systematic review and meta-analysis. *Osteoporos Int.* 2013 Feb;24(2):393–406.
33. **Huntjens KM, van Geel TA, van den Bergh JP, et al.** Fracture liaison service: impact on subsequent nonvertebral fracture incidence and mortality. *J Bone Joint Surg Am.* 2014 Feb 19;96(4):e29.
34. **Lih A, Nandapalan H, Kim M, et al.** Targeted intervention reduces refracture rates in patients with incident non-vertebral osteoporotic fractures: a 4-year prospective controlled study. *Osteoporos Int.* 2011 Mar;22(3):849–858.
35. **Van der Kallen J, Giles M, Cooper K, et al.** A fracture prevention service reduces further fractures two years after incident minimal trauma fracture. *Int J Rheum Dis.* 2014 Feb;17(2):195–203.
36. **Niedhart C, Preising A, Eichhorn C.** Signifikante Reduktion von Krankenhauseinweisungen aufgrund osteoporoseassoziierter Frakturen durch intensivierte multimodale Therapie–Ergebnisse der Integrierten Versorgung Osteoporose Nordrhein [Significant reduction of osteoporosis fracture-related hospitalisation rate due to intensified, mulitmodal treatment—results from the integrated healthcare network osteoporosis North Rhine]. *Zeitschrift für Orthopädie und Unfallchirurgie.* 2013;151(01):20–24. German.
37. **Cooper MS, Palmer AJ, Seibel MJ.** Cost-effectiveness of the Concord Minimal Trauma Fracture Liaison service, a prospective, controlled fracture prevention study. *Osteoporos Int.* 2012 Jan;23(1):97–107.
38. **Sander B, Elliot-Gibson V, Beaton DE, et al.** A coordinator program in post-fracture osteoporosis management improves outcomes and saves costs. *J Bone Joint Surg Am.* 2008 Jun;90(6):1197–1205.
39. **McLellan AR, Wolowacz SE, Zimovetz EA, et al.** Fracture liaison services for the evaluation and management of patients with osteoporotic fracture: a cost-effectiveness evaluation based on data collected over 8 years of service provision. *Osteoporos Int.* 2011 Jul;22(7):2083–2098.
40. **Solomon DH, Patrick AR, Schousboe J, et al.** The potential economic benefits of improved postfracture care: a cost-effectiveness analysis of a fracture liaison service in the US health-care system. *J Bone Miner Res.* 2014 Jul;29(7):1667–1674.

# 2.9 Use of registry data to improve care

Colin Currie

## 1 Introduction

This chapter discusses the importance and utility of registry data to improve the care of fragility fracture patients. It focuses upon hip fracture because, as the most common serious fracture, it is the tracer condition for the current pandemic of osteoporotic fractures, and because the evidence base for care is good and hip fracture registries are now well established. The chapter aims to help the reader understand the importance of registry participation and the use of registry data at the hospital, national, and international levels to drive improvements in the quality, effectiveness, and cost-effectiveness of care.

## 2 Overview of registries for osteoporotic fracture care and their current and future impact

Hip fracture is the most common serious osteoporotic fracture. It is well defined anatomically. Its presentation is acute and normally results in hospital admission. Hip fracture care costs are high, and care quality and patient outcomes vary greatly. Hip fracture care is therefore an ideal subject for clinical audit and has been implemented at local, national, and international levels since the mid-1980s. Over time, an audit has often helped to raise the quality of care [1].

In contrast, nonhip osteoporotic fractures are less well defined, more variable in their presentation, and may, as in the case of vertebral fractures, be clinically silent. The evidence base for the care of such fractures is generally less robust than that for hip fracture. For these reasons, a large-scale audit of nonhip osteoporotic fractures is challenging, and no such audits could be identified in a recent literature search. For the purposes of this brief chapter, the focus is on hip fracture registries and hip fracture care; the terms audit, register, and registry are regarded as interchangeable.

Hip fracture is increasingly acknowledged as the tracer condition for the rapidly growing challenge of osteoporotic fracture care. As more orthopedic trauma units are able to deliver high-quality hip fracture care as a result of audit participation, they now deploy the skills, expertise, and systems that can meet the care and rehabilitation needs of frail older adults with the full range of nonhip osteoporotic fractures. This "halo effect" is a beneficial and welcome result of rising standards in hip fracture care.

Large-scale hip fracture audits began with the Swedish Rikshoft register [2], launched in 1989. Generously supported by Rikshoft expertise and technology, both the Scottish Hip Fracture Audit [3] and the multinational Standardized Audit of Hip Fracture in Europe (SAHFE) project [4] followed in the 1990s. A third national audit, the UK National Hip Fracture Database (NHFD) [1], drew on Swedish and Scottish experience and was developed from 2004 as a collaboration between the British Orthopaedic Association (BOA) and the British Geriatrics Society (BGS). The NHFD incorporated continuously reported feedback technology derived from a National Health Service (NHS) cardiac audit. This proved to be a considerable advance on the annual reports of the two national audits cited above. The NHFD was launched in 2007 alongside *The Care of Patients with Fragility Fracture* (ie, the Blue Book), also a BOA/BGS collaboration, with the NHFD monitoring compliance with the six consensus-derived clinical standards for hip fracture care set out in the Blue Book [5]. The following list shows the six standards monitored by NHFD. All patients:

1. With hip fractures should be admitted to an acute orthopedic ward within 4 hours of presentation.
2. With hip fractures that are medically fit should have surgery within 48 hours of admission, during normal working hours.
3. With hip fractures should be assessed and cared for with a view to minimizing the risk of developing a pressure ulcer.

4. Presenting with fragility fractures should be managed on an orthopedic ward with routine access to orthogeriatric medical support from the time of admission.
5. Presenting with fragility fractures should be assessed to determine their need for antiresorptive therapy to prevent future osteoporotic fractures.
6. Presenting with fragility fractures following a fall should be offered multidisciplinary assessment and intervention to prevent future falls.

Since then, national hip fracture audits have been established successively in Norway [6], Denmark [7], Ireland [8], and Australia and New Zealand [9]—all essentially Rikshoft-derived, and incorporating datasets and clinical standards similar to those used in the NHFD. In Germany, an extensive national fragility fracture registry [10] includes key elements of hip fracture audit data compatible with NHFD standards 1–6 [11].

The rise of such large-scale hip fracture audits, and of similar local initiatives, can be seen as a rational response to the aging of populations and the consequent pressures on orthopedic services and healthcare delivery systems. In parallel, commendable surgical and industry interest in an injury once regarded as burdensome has led to the development of more reliable fixation methods and has also resulted in the rise of collaborative care, with geriatricians and other physicians becoming involved in nonsurgical aspects of the care of frail older adults [12, 13]. Importantly, major recent developments in information technology and internet communication have made data collection, transfer, and analysis all faster and cheaper, so that international collaboration has become easier and more cost-effective. Large-scale audits with high data quality and audit-based research with large prospective observational series and case-mix-adjusted outcomes, for example in anesthetic care, [14] are now possible.

Another major factor in the rise of effective hip fracture audits has been the increasing availability of guidelines. These have taken various forms. An early example is *United They Stand: Coordinating care for elderly patients with hip fracture* from 1995 [15]. The more formally evidence-based Scottish Intercollegiate Guideline Network guideline [16] *Prevention and Management of hip fracture in older people* followed in 2002 and was updated in 2009. More recently, the UK National Institute for Health and Care Excellence followed with *Hip fracture: management (CG124)* [17]. In the US, *A Guide to Improving the Care of Patients with Fragility Fractures* [18] covers both hip and nonhip fractures. Another recent US guideline adopted by the American Academy of Orthopaedic Surgeons *Management of Hip Fractures in the Elderly* focuses only on hip fracture care [19].

Clearly the nature of the gathered data greatly influences the effectiveness of a hip fracture audit. In general, the data must be sufficient in scope, volume, and quality to influence behavior and improve care. In most audits, the data need not, and will not, be of research quality, but it will serve its main purpose of quantifying and improving clinical care. The work of gathering, recording, and uploading audit data are a serious responsibility. Experience has shown that it is risky to rely on its casual delegation to voluntary or conscripted nursing staff or junior medical colleagues employed for other duties. Recruiting, training, and supporting competent and committed audit staff is essential.

A supportive approach pays dividends, and advancing technology, eg, offering drop-down definitions of data items, can contribute much. Regional data quality workshops, bringing together audit staff from a number of hospitals, have proved to be popular and effective in the case of the NHFD. Working alone or in pairs in participating units can be isolating, and for such staff peer support, exchanging views and troubles, and learning and lunching together serves to promote and maintain enthusiasm and to help people wanting to do a good job to do it better. The involvement of such staff, alongside clinicians, managers, and central audit staff, in the larger regional meetings described in the following topics serve to recognize their essential contribution to the wider effort.

Where nursing professionals are involved in data collection, professional standards apply inasmuch as to willfully enter false and misleading information about a patient could lead to a disciplinary process. Awareness of this might in itself deter such practice. In a few instances in the work of the NHFD, suspiciously low 30-day death rates prompted suspicions of the possible omission of poor prognosis patients, and these were checked by the use of nonaudit routine NHS data, ie, the Hospital Episode Statistics data, which records hospital admissions for hip fracture. Current NHFD advice on data quality assurance recommends that service lead clinicians check random monthly samples of records against data uploaded. Where sites have joint lead clinicians (eg, a surgeon and a geriatrician), data quality and performance standards are higher.

Issues arise in some jurisdictions where individual patient consent for inclusion in an audit is mandatory, and data completeness suffers accordingly. When it is accepted that a clinical audit is an integral part of good care, there are fewer problems. The cost of gathering specific data for audit at around GBP 80 per case, a negligible sum when compared to the price of care ("if you think information is expensive, try ignorance"), when routinely collected hospital data might suffice, has been raised as an objection to free-standing audits, although there is a broad counterview that the latter form of data are not fit for audit purposes. These and other questions have been helpfully addressed by Martyn Parker [20] in a guest editorial. In broader terms, and on the basis of experience, single-payer healthcare systems offer a more favorable environment for hip fracture audits than those that are less developed, or developed but commercially fragmented. If demographic and societal needs in coming decades dictate the development of hip fracture audits, the difficulties encountered in these varying environments must eventually be addressed.

Hip fracture audits are therefore now a mature web-based technology and an effective change agent, and also a platform for both quality improvement [1], research collaboration [14], and for the development of patient-reported outcome measures [21]. Given the current predictions for the worldwide rise in osteoporotic fractures, the status of hip fracture as its tracer condition, and the halo effect of audit-driven improvements in hip fracture for other fragility fracture cases, the potential international influence of hip fracture audits in developed and less well-developed healthcare economies is considerable. Over the next few decades standards of fragility fracture care could rise substantially, and audit-based research collaborations could drive forward evidence-based care in a range of national and international settings.

## 3 Using audits and feedback to improve patient care and outcomes

The purpose of hip fracture audits is to change behavior in ways that improve patient care and outcomes. Individual audits vary greatly in scope, methods, and impact. Access to the detailed information on hip fracture audits also varies greatly, and clearly a great many local audit initiatives fail to surface in the literature. Audits may range from single-hospital efforts that are transient or more enduring and largely unreported to established national audits, currently few in number, though with other national initiatives emerging in Japan, the Netherlands, and Spain. Such audits can document thousands of cases annually, deliver measurable improvements in care, and are now making substantial contributions to the hip fracture literature.

What matters most for any hip fracture audit is its impact on care teams, which is best addressed in terms of hearts and minds. So it is worth considering audit characteristics likely to achieve this. Reporting methods matter. Annual reports of multicenter audits seem to have relatively little impact on meaningful individual program improvement. Units in the top percentiles may enjoy temporary satisfaction while those at the bottom of the league table may temper remorse with a vague intention, or a hope, that things might improve in time for the next report.

Conversely, regular feedback, ideally continuous, confers on clinical teams the benefits of what production engineers call statistical process control. At regular meetings clinical teams can look at their data and ask, for instance, what happened the previous month that resulted in longer preoperative delay: more cases, lack of operating room time, poor management of operating room time, an unenthusiastic anesthetist, or unnecessary preoperative investigations? In this way local teams can use data to address local problems and find local solutions. In effect they are empowered by information, which produces a mindset different from that of an annual league-table.

A successful audit is likely to be supportive not only via regular feedback, but by making available examples of good practice, providing practical online support with a regularly updated "key papers" literature library, model business cases for funding, and even job descriptions for various audit and clinical roles. A regular web-based newsletter featuring relevant meetings and news from teams and from the audit's leadership will supplement the above measures in creating a hip fracture audit community with the real sense of itself and its purpose.

Meetings matter. Within a large national audit, regional meetings bring people together. Such meetings with 100 or more clinicians, audit staff, managers, and a program of presentations, lunch, and coffee breaks can promote and maintain enthusiasm. And they may have a competitive edge too, and successive local presentations often reflect this, adding to the enjoyment and effectiveness of the meetings. Of course there are other approaches quite different from the above, such as an audit as a top-down bureaucratic exercise, departmentally controlled, and lacking in central clinical leadership, judgmental rather than supportive, and communicating only via annual reports. However, they are less likely to create "a critical mass of enthusiasm and expertise in hip fracture care" with a demonstrable and sustained impact achieved by overall quality improvement and resulting in improved survival [1].

An early and interesting example of a regional audit was carried out in East Anglia, England, in 1992 and repeated in 1997 [22]. The 1992 findings showed no significant differences in case-mix across the eight participating hospitals, meaning that differences in outcome were likely to be attributable to variance in care. There were significant differences in 90-day mortality. Results showed that only around half of the survivors regained their prefracture physical function, with a marked decrease in physical function (for 31%) being associated with postoperative complications. Key measures for improvement identified for scrutiny in the 1997 audit were processes likely to reduce postoperative complications and improve outcomes at 90 days.

The 1997 findings showed reduced pneumonia, wound and hip joint infections, pressure sores, and fatal pulmonary embolism. Two relevant interventions were more widely applied, leading to a rise in thromboembolic prophylaxis from 45% to 81% and early mobilization from 56% to 70%. However, 90-day functional outcomes and mortality were unchanged. The 1997 population sample was older, but again there were no significant differences across the hospitals. In 1992, one hospital had impressively low mortality, but by 1997 this hospital "had lost its ... preeminence, perhaps partly because of the improvement of some other hospitals, but primarily because of failure to maintain and improve its overall package of care ... We therefore recommend that hospitals continue to audit the care of patients with hip fractures." [22].

National hip fracture audits remain few in number, and where they exist, their relationships with their respective health departments will vary by context. Some audits may have developed with independent funding and subsequently been recognized as innovative and effective and therefore meriting funding from national sources, as was the case with the UK NHFD. Others may have had to negotiate the complexities of a federal system, together with predetermined national processes and conditions for audit development, as was the case in Australia. In smaller nations, such as Scotland, Ireland, and New Zealand, tighter networks may make things easier. But once established, effective nationwide clinically-led audits may find themselves in a position to influence policy. In this respect the UK NHFD was fortunate, with various NHFD activists working within the Whitehall village where the profiles of hip fracture care and fragility fractures generally rose quite markedly [23]. The political element of hip fracture audit work should be openly recognized, and is essential if the goal of influencing policy is to be achieved.

## 4 Hospital-level use of audits—the impact of good practice on care quality and outcomes

Together, audits, standards, and regular or continuous feedback offer clinical teams actionable data to address barriers to good practice. When solving emergent problems requires management support and/or additional resources, discussion with management is more likely to be rational, objective, and productive than it would be in the absence of audit data. Perhaps the most productive use of audit data are in prompting and monitoring changes in clinical care and/or service structure.

The NHFD issues annual reports [24] aimed at a broad readership that includes Department of Health officials, NHS regional and local management, national press and media, and participating hospitals. These reports include a section called *Using Audit to Improve Care: Good Practice Examples*, from which the following have been extracted:

- Northumbria Healthcare NHS Foundation Trust: Wansbeck General Hospital and North Tyneside General Hospital:
  A quality improvement program for hip fracture care began in October 2009. A multidisciplinary steering group worked to improve care from admission to discharge. Pain control improved, with 79% of patients receiving a nerve block on admission. A total of 90% of patients now undergo surgery within 36 hours. Of medically fit patients, 25% are mobilized on the day of surgery and 100% by the following day. With the help of newly appointed nutrition assistants, 81% received additional feeding. An information booklet on hip fracture is now provided for patients and caregivers. Feedback on care from patients and families is high, with monthly average scores consistently above 9.3 of 10.
- Salisbury NHS Foundation Trust: Salisbury District Hospital:
  In 2010, with no orthogeriatrician, a noncollaborative approach, and long preoperative delays, Salisbury ranked 98th out of 100 NHS England trusts in Best Practice Tariff (BPT) achievement (see topic 5 in this chapter). A change program introduced orthogeriatric and nurse practitioner staffing, additional operating room capacity, and active leadership shared by an orthopedic surgeon, the lead anesthetist, and the consultant orthogeriatrician. By 2012, 80% of patients reached orthopedic care within 4 hours, 95% had a preoperative othogeriatric assessment, 92% had surgery within 48 hours and 84% within 36 hours; pressure ulcer incidence fell from 5.4% to 1.2%. Mortality fell from 10.1% to 8.4% and acute length of stay from 27.6 days to 19.8 days. Best Practice Tariff

attainment rose from 1.5% to 84.4%, with BPT income of GBP 187,790 and efficiency savings of GBP 391,000 (calculated as 1,955 bed-days at GBP 200 per day). Importantly, feedback from patients, relatives, and clinical staff was positive.
- St Peter's Hospitals NHS Foundation Trust: St Peter's Hospital, Chertsey:
  In 2010, the trust invested in a 4-day efficiency, quality, improvement, and productivity initiative on the hip fracture pathway. Analysis of NHFD data showed that the longest delays occurred during or just after the weekend. To address this, an all-day Saturday operating room list was split into two half-day lists. As a result, 60% of patients underwent surgery within 24 hours and 80% within 36 hours. Time to trauma ward admission was reduced by the introduction of a priority hip fracture pager. Weekend physiotherapy and a hip fracture exercise class improved mobilization rates within 24 hours of surgery. Length of stay dropped from 25 days to 22 days, with considerable efficiency savings. Importantly, discharge to original residence improved to 60% within 25 days compared with 44% within 30 days 2 years previously.

These initiatives have been described in some detail because they illustrate a wide range of clinical and service improvements that were locally driven, informed by baseline data, monitored by continuing feedback, and went beyond simple compliance with the six clinical standards embodied in the NHFD audit. Patient-centered measures promoting improved pain control, weekend rehabilitation, and improved nutrition are good in themselves but also contribute to overall efficiency through quicker recovery, sometimes with substantial savings. Patient and caregiver involvement, in the form of leaflets and surveys, is unusual but admirable. Many teams might hesitate but more should attempt it. And since acute length of stay is less important for patients than getting home as soon as possible, St Peter's Hospital's achievement in discharging more patients straight home earlier is patient-centered and probably cost-effective too, since rehabilitation costs can rise rapidly as a result of the unnecessary use of postacute hospital care.

Together, and importantly, the three local reports just mentioned show that, in general, quality and cost are not in conflict. "Looking after hip fracture patients well is cheaper than looking after them badly" [5] is a simple message that makes sense to clinicians, managers, health departments, and politicians, and might itself be the best short argument for the wider implementation of effective hip fracture audits.

## 5 Incentives for hospitals to improve care like the Best Practice Tariff

In 1988, a US community hospital retrospective study [25] assessed the impact on the care of hip fracture patients admitted from home of a prospective payment system (PPS) introduced in 1983. Some 330 eligible cases were identified, 149 before the implementation of PPS, 189 thereafter. Mean hospital stay fell from 21.9 days to 12.6 days following implementation. Other main findings gave serious cause for concern. Maximum walking distance prior to discharge fell from 27 meters to 11 meters. The proportion of patients discharged to nursing homes rose from 38% to 60%, and the proportion remaining in nursing homes a year later rose from 9% to 33% ($P < .0001$ for all values quoted). While the aim of the PPS may have been to contain acute sector costs, its overall impact on the quality and cost effectiveness of subsequent patient care appeared adverse. Rehabilitation and return home were seriously affected, and the human and economic costs of one-third of the patients still in nursing home care at 1 year are truly alarming, and illustrate the problems raised by a focus purely on acute care.

A 2009 Israeli report [26] on a retrospective analysis of two samples of patients (ie, total number of 10,620 patients from 1999–2006 and from seven hospitals participating in a trauma registry) was carried out to assess the impact of a change in 2004 that reduced significantly the diagnosis-related group (DRG) tariff for patients undergoing surgery more than 48 hours after admission. This data showed a 35% increase in the number of patients having surgery within 48 hours and a 30% reduction in inpatient mortality for all operated patients.

A 2013 report from Lazio, Italy, [27] retrospectively analyzed data on 12,433 hip fracture admissions from a variety of local, teaching, religious, and private hospitals in the region. A 2009 change in DRG payment led to full reimbursement only for patients having surgery within 48 hours, with further reductions proportionate to longer preoperative delay. A comparison of the years preceding and following this change showed that the proportion of patients having surgery within 48 hours rose from 11.7% to 22%. Some improvement was seen in all types of hospitals, with the greatest improvement in the private sector.

These two studies have limitations, the former for its duration, over which many non-DRG factors may have contributed to mortality reduction, the latter in its relatively modest impact on serious baseline preoperative delay.

The UK NHFD, which has documented more than half a million cases since its launch in 2007 and now captures over 95% of eligible hip fractures, made hip fracture care an obvious topic for the BPT when it was introduced by the English Department of Health in 2010. The standards set reflected those of the NHFD, with the early surgery target tightened from 48 hours to 36 hours. The incentive was an incremental payment of GBP 445 ("differential") over the base tariff. The BPT base tariff remained constant, but the differential increased relative to the base tariff from the original GBP 445 to GBP 890 for 2011–2012 and further still thereafter. At the same time the base tariff was cut by a similar amount to put a "carrot and stick" incentive on participants to improve. As intended, an increase in BPT achievement occurred [15].

## 6 Progress, challenges, and opportunities in hip fracture audits

In the year 2000, 1.6 million hip fractures occurred globally. Numbers will rise dramatically as a result of mass aging of the baby boomer generation in some populations, and more dramatically in others such as Brazil, China, and India where a first mass aging cohort will dominate the demography for the coming decades [28]. Progress in hip fracture audit and improvements in hip fracture care since 2000 should give grounds for cautious optimism, not least that over the next few decades, comparable further progress and improvements are still to come.

The rise of collaborative care, with orthopedic surgeons and orthogeriatricians working together, has greatly improved the care and outcomes for hip fracture patients, who are often the frailest and most vulnerable presenting to the acute healthcare sector. The care of their multiple comorbidities, including cognitive impairment, has been transformed and their outcomes much improved [13]. A recent NHFD-based study [29] showed that increased orthogeriatrician hours per patient were associated with higher rates of prompt surgery, but were independently associated with lower 30-day mortality. Such access to orthogeriatric care, however, is available in few healthcare systems. In the UK, geriatricians and orthopedic surgeons constitute the largest medical and surgical specialties respectively, and the absence of fee-for-service in trauma care makes collaborative care simple and cost-effective. In other contexts, where geriatricians are few or absent, other contributors who can offer geriatric medical expertise, such as hospitalists, physician assistants, and nurse specialists, might be identified and trained. These clinicians may benefit greatly from modular training programs focusing on key topics, such as the International Geriatric Fracture Society CORE Certification initiative [30].

Other more recent progress includes successful large-scale prospective observational audit-based research studies such as the one by White et al [14] which observed 5-day and 30-day case mix-adjusted mortality in 11,085 patients and highlighted statistically significant increased mortality associated with intraoperative hypotension. This study now transcends the vast majority of previous hip fracture anesthesia reports that were small and/or selective, eg, in excluding patients with mental impairment, generally around one-third of the hip fracture population.

In addition, one serious criticism of hip fracture audits, namely that of the moral hazard arising from the fact that they are self-reporting, has been addressed and its value as a quality improvement initiative established [1]. This study used national nonaudit data and examined trends in early surgery and mortality at 30 and 90 days and 1-year in a series of 471,590 patients admitted from 2003–2011, ie, spanning 4 years before and following the NHFD's launch in 2007. The 30-day mortality fell from 10.9% to 8.5% over the second 4-year period compared with a small reduction from 11.5% to 10.9% over the first. The 2007–2011 decrease in 90-day mortality was greater in absolute terms than the decrease in 30-day mortality and similar in magnitude to the decrease in 1-year mortality. This suggests that better acute hip fracture care reduces mortality by minimizing the collateral damage of poor care, and that this reduction is maintained at 1 year. This is consistent with the evidence that between 17% and 32% of deaths after hip fracture are potentially avoidable [31].

Unfortunately, acute care dominance is embedded in the developed healthcare economies. This is reflected in the hip fracture care with its focus on the first few weeks of care and its failure to engage seriously with postacute care and rehabilitation. There is no more costly and undesirable outcome of hip fracture care than avoidable permanent institutionalization, which can be a personal tragedy and often an unjustifiable cost, however that cost is met [25].

Postacute care varies greatly and generally reflects service structure and provision rather than the individual patient's needs and potential. Complexities around costs and responsibilities, divisions between health and social care, and commercial interests present vast challenges to researchers. And, in contrast to technical advances in acute care such as those in surgery and anesthetics, the findings from such research are, for similar reasons, not easily generalizable.

Ideally, the development of community services that offer social services, nursing, and rehabilitation, and are capable of dealing confidently and well with patients discharged directly home from acute care following early in-hospital rehabilitation, would deliver on the mantra that "looking after hip fracture patients well is cheaper than looking after them badly" [5], but such services are currently the exception. Sadly, care that is both bad and expensive is accepted as the norm. There are no simple one-size-fits-all remedies, but the combination of spiraling costs and patient discontent, much more likely as the baby boomer generation ages, may serve to focus attention and lead to local or national initiatives, such as the much-discussed merger of health and social care services in the UK context, which would make sense in both economic and human terms. Addressing these challenges requires a political response, ideally that of building a common agenda, with government and the professions working on better and cheaper care, and better patient and caregiver satisfaction.

In less developed healthcare economies, even greater challenges exist. The nations with the greatest challenges are also those least equipped to address them. But again, progress will depend on a broadly based political medium to long-term clinical and political responses, most probably with the establishment of pioneer initiatives in academic settings and an outward diffusion of improving practice compatible with the national context.

Such progress is a central goal of the Fragility Fracture Network (FFN), an international nonprofit organization that brings together a broad international membership of activists, including orthopedic surgeons, geriatricians, nurses, and other clinical disciplines, together with scientists with relevant interest. It seeks to promote the dissemination globally of the best multidisciplinary practice in preventing and managing fragility fractures, the promotion of research aimed at better treatment, and the generation of political priority for fragility fracture care in all countries. With the status of hip fracture as the tracer condition of the wider fragility fracture epidemic, an FFN consensus strategic document *The Future of Hip Fracture Audit* was developed over 2013–2015 [32].

The Hip Fracture Audit Database Implementation Group in the FFN worked, via an international expert group meeting on Skype, to use a consensus approach to develop a concise and practical minimum common dataset (MCD) capturing key elements of case-mix, care and outcomes in hip fracture care [11]. This work was based on the much more extensive and largely Rikshoft-based datasets already in use in established national audits, and was therefore compatible with them for comparison purposes, but sufficiently user-friendly for the purposes of start-up audits, and cost-effective where resources were limited. Subsequently, a small-scale pilot phase using the MCD has established the feasibility of international web-based hip fracture audit in collaboration between five European centers (Barcelona, Spain; Celje, Slovenia; Lübeck, Germany; Msida, Malta; Stuttgart, Germany) from which valuable lessons have been learned [11]. The pilot phase also allowed the MCD-based international comparison of data on case-mix, care, and early outcomes from established audits, most recently those in Sweden, the UK, Ireland, Australia and New Zealand.

In summary, hip fracture audits are already a mature technology that have established their effectiveness in improving care and outcomes at a national level. Now, given the status of hip fracture as the tracer condition for the looming pandemic of fragility fractures worldwide, the implementation of effective hip fracture audits has the potential to play an important part in responding to the clinical and organizational challenges posed by that pandemic.

One recent publication [33] has expressed support for the concept of international progress in extending the implementation of effective hip fracture audits, with dataset comparability offering a practical basis for collaboration in mutual learning, and also bringing opportunities for collaborative research, in the form of prospective observational studies or even RCTs. The challenge of the coming decades is great, but there are now at least some grounds for cautious optimism, and the outlines of a strategy for delivering on that optimism are now emerging.

## 7 References

1. **Neuburger J, Currie C, Wakeman R, et al.** The impact of a national clinician-led audit initiative on care and mortality after hip fracture in England: an external evaluation using time trends in non-audit data. *Med Care.* 2015 Aug;53(8):686–691.
2. **Rikshöft.** Swedish National Registry of hip fracture patient care. Available at: rikshoft.se/about-rikshoft. Published 2013. Accessed 2017.
3. **Currie CT, Hutchison JD.** Audit, guidelines and standards: clinical governance for hip fracture care in Scotland. *Disabil Rehabil.* 2005 Sep 30–Oct 15;27(18-19):1099–1105.
4. **Parker M, Currie C, Mountain J, et al.** Standardised audit of hip fracture in Europe (SAHFE). *Hip International.* 1998;8:11–18.
5. **British Orthopaedic Association and British Geriatrics Society.** The care of patients with fragility fracture. Available at: www.nhfd.co.uk. Published 2007. Accessed 2018.
6. **Gjertsen JE, Engesaeter LB, Furnes O, et al.** The Norwegian Hip Fracture Register: experiences after the first 2 years and 15,576 reported operations. *Acta Orthop.* 2008 Oct;79(5):583–593.
7. **DrHoftebrud.** Dansk Tværfagligt Register for Hoftenære Lårbensbrud. National årsrapport 2016. Available at: https://www.sundhed.dk/content/cms/62/4662_hofte-fraktur_årsrapport-2016.pdf. Published 2016. Accessed 2017. Danish.
8. **National Office of Clinical Audit (NOCA).** Irish Hip Fracture Database National Report 2015. Available at: https://www.noca.ie/irish-hip-fracture-database. Published 2016. Accessed 2017.
9. **Australian and New Zealand Hip Fracture Registry (ANZHFR).** Annual Report 2016. Available at: www.anzhfr.org/reports. Published 2016. Accessed 2017.
10. **AUC Geschäftsstelle Register und Forschungskoordination.** AltersTraumaRegister DGU. Available at: www.alterstraumazentrum-dgu.de/de/qualitaet_sicherheit/alterstraumaregister_dgur.html. Published 2016. Accessed 2017. German.
11. **Hip Fracture Audit Database (HFAD).** Minimum Core Dataset for hip fracture audit. Available at: http://web1.crownaudit.org/ffn/info.nsf. Accessed 2017.
12. **Wakeman R, Sheard PD, Jenner GH.** Ortho-geriatric liaison—the missing link? *J Bone Joint Surg Br.* 2004 Jul;86(5):636–638.
13. **Johansen A.** The future of orthogeriatrics. *Age Ageing.* 2010 Nov;39(6):664–665.
14. **White SM, Moppett IK, Griffiths R, et al.** Secondary analysis of outcomes after 11,085 hip fracture operations from the prospective UK Anaesthesia Sprint Audit of Practice (ASAP-2). *Anaesthesia.* 2016 May;71(5):506–514.
15. **United Kingdom National Audit Commission.** *United They Stand: Coordinating Care for Elderly Patients With Hip Fractures.* London: HMSO; 1995.
16. **Scottish Intercollegiate Guidelines Network (SIGN).** Prevention and Management of hip fracture in older people. A national clinical guideline (Guideline 56). Edinburgh: SIGN Executive; 2002. Available at: www.sif-fisioterapia.it/wp-content/uploads/2014/12/Hip-Fracture-Management-Prevention-Scotland-2002.pdf. Accessed 2017.
17. **National Institute for Health and Care Excellence (NICE).** Hip fracture: management. Clinical guideline [CG124]. Available at: www.nice.org.uk/guidance/cg124. Published 2011. Accessed 2017.
18. **Bukata SV, Digiovanni BF, Friedman SM, et al.** A guide to improving the care of patients with fragility fractures. *Geriatr Orthop Surg Rehabil.* 2011 Jan;2(1):5–37.
19. **American Academy of Orthopaedic Surgeons (AAOS).** Management of hip fractures in the elderly. Available at: http://www.aaos.org/Research/guidelines/HipFxSummaryofRecommendations.pdf. Published 2014. Accessed 2017.
20. **Parker MJ.** Databases for hip fracture audit. *Acta Orthop.* 2008 Oct;79(5):577–579.
21. **Griffin XL, Parsons N, Achten J, et al.** Recovery of health-related quality of life in a United Kingdom hip fracture population. The Warwick Hip Trauma Evaluation—a prospective cohort study. *Bone Joint J.* 2015 Mar;97-B(3):372–382.
22. **Freeman C, Todd C, Camilleri-Ferrante C, et al.** Quality improvement for patients with hip fracture: experience from a multi-site audit. *Qual Saf Health Care.* 2002 Sep;11(3):239–245.
23. **Oliver D.** Development of services for older patients with falls and fractures in England: successes, failures, lessons and controversies. *Arch Gerontol Geriatr.* 2009 Dec;49 Suppl 2:S7–S12.
24. **Royal College of Physicians.** The National Hip Fracture Database. Part of the Falls and Fragility Fracture Audit Programme. Available at: www.nhfd.co.uk/docs/reports. Accessed November 29, 2017.
25. **Fitzgerald JF, Moore PS, Dittus RS.** The care of elderly patients with hip fracture. Changes since implementation of the prospective payment system. *N Engl J Med.* 1988 Nov 24;319(21):1392–1397.
26. **Peleg K, Savitsky B, Yitzhak B, et al.** Different reimbursement influences surviving of hip fracture in elderly patients. *Injury.* 2011 Feb;42(2):128–132.
27. **Colais P, Pinnarelli L, Fusco D, et al.** The impact of a pay-for-performance system on timing to hip fracture surgery: experience from the Lazio Region (Italy). *BMC Health Serv Res.* 2013 Oct 7;13:393.
28. **Cooper C, Campion G, Melton LJ 3rd.** Hip fractures in the elderly: a world-wide projection. *Osteoporos Int.* 1992 Nov;2(6):285–289.
29. **Neuburger J, Currie C, Wakeman R, et al.** Increased orthogeriatrician involvement in hip fracture care and its impact on mortality in England. *Age Ageing.* 2017 Mar 01;46(2):187–192.
30. **Mears SC, Suk M, Cobbe F, et al.** International Geriatric Fracture Society CORE Certification: turning knowledge into action. *Geriatr Orthop Surg Rehabil.* 2014 Sep;5(3):91–92.
31. **Kanis JA, Oden A, Johnell O, et al.** The components of excess mortality after hip fracture. *Bone.* 2003 May;32(5):468–473.
32. **Currie C, Mitchell P.** The Future of Hip Fracture Audit. A Draft Consensus Statement. Available at: http://fragilityfracturenetwork.org/files/future_of_hip_fracture_audit_-_a_consensus_statement.pdf. Published 2015. Accessed 2017.
33. **Saez-Lopez P, Branas F, Sanchez-Hernandez N, et al.** Hip fracture registries: utility, description, and comparison. *Osteoporos Int.* 2017 Apr;28(4):1157–1166.

# 2.10 Lean business principles

Stephen L Kates, Andrew J Pugely

## 1 Introduction

There are multiple clinical and health system models of care pertaining to orthogeriatric care. Guisti et al [1] described five distinct organizational models in their landmark paper (see chapter 2.1 Models of orthogeriatric care for a summary and discussion of these models). However, from a business model standpoint, there are only three models to discuss. These include "craft production", semiorganized care using "mass production" principles, and highly organized care using "lean business principles". These three business models derive from the automotive industry and can be applied within a medical care context.

With the use of lean business methods, considerable improvement in program outcomes can be achieved. The dual goals of quality improvement and cost saving are achievable and more cost-effective care can be delivered [2]. Lean business methods are a win for the institution, patients, and healthcare teams. This chapter is designed to discuss the use of business modeling and its role in care improvement.

## 2 Models from the automotive industry

### 2.1 Craft production

Before 1911, all manufacturing of cars and other goods and services used craft production principles. Craft production was dependent on the skills of the individual craftsman. Supplies were purchased in a disorganized manner and were variable. The manufacturing process was done one at a time, and there were no standards applied to each car. There was no standard quality management program and each product was different. The results were thus variable even for skilled craftsmen.

### 2.2 Mass production

Mass production began in 1911 with Henry Ford's introduction of interchangeable parts. In 1914, Ford introduced the moving assembly line and focused routinely on reducing waste in the manufacturing process by prescribing standard work and the use of recycled defective steel parts. Ford standardized the size of the boards composing the wooden shipping crates including where the drill holes were made. When emptied, the crates were disassembled at the factory and became the floorboards of the Model T car. He actually reduced the price of the vehicle every year, passing on the realized savings to the customers.

However, about 25% of the cars would not start and run properly at the end of the assembly line and required reworking from the "craftsmen" he employed to correct the defects. Mass production quality control efforts often failed to determine the true root cause of an error, thus the error was repeated over and over again. Despite its shortcomings, mass production was a tremendous success and mass production principles greatly increased output of all factories employing the principles.

### 2.3 Lean production

Lean production began in postwar Japan with the Toyoda family, their engineer Taiichi Ohno, and Dr W Edwards Deming who was serving in MacArthur's army of occupation. In 1950, no cars were produced in Japan, but the Toyoda family and Ohno, with the help of Deming, developed new manufacturing principles now known as lean production [3].

In lean production, the space used for manufacturing was less, changeover times were relentlessly reduced, the quality of the parts and cars dramatically improved, and the costs of production fell as a result. Concepts such as just-in-time delivery of parts and poka-yoke, ie, error-proofing, were introduced.

The supply chain was managed by an inventory-control system (kanban), involving signaling cards to indicate the need to replenish parts as they were used, which was combined with just-in-time delivery of the parts to the assembly line. The assembly line was "production leveled" (heijunka) by sequencing the models of car built by their complexity and components. At the end of the line, all of the cars started and ran, and could be immediately transported to the freighter for shipping to their intended destination. Quality was improved continuously using the Deming cycles of plan-do-check-act (PDCA) and use of frequent "improvements" (kaizens) to solve problems encountered in the manufacturing process. By the late 1990s, Toyota became the number one manufacturer of cars in the world.

## 3 Where are we now and what is value in healthcare?

Based on the business models described above, orthogeriatric care is usually delivered in a craft production mode with some mass production features such as a quality management system, a supply chain, and a large volume of cases managed in some centers. Typical care produces variable results including many readily avoidable adverse events such as medication errors, and poor sequencing of surgeries and consults, resulting in long delays, depletion of necessary supplies, avoidable infections, the ordering of unnecessary tests such as head CT scans and echocardiograms, and the list goes on.

If the reader is still not convinced, ask yourself the following question: If I needed urgent surgery on my fracture, would I like to choose my surgeon and care team? Most readers would answer "yes, definitely". Because traditional fracture care is highly variable and unorganized, you surely want to choose your craftsman wisely. Of course this is highly inefficient and rarely possible in the urgent setting. As cost pressures mount on health systems around the world, there is an increasing need to improve quality of care at lower cost. Fortunately, there is often an inverse relationship between the costs of care and quality of care, ie, high-value care typically costs less. Health systems and patients are demanding better value care be delivered [4]. The value equation is [5]:

$$\frac{\text{Outcomes}}{\text{Costs}} = \text{Value}$$

In most cases we know the costs. Typically, only outcomes as defined by "process measures" like length of stay, mortality rate, and infection rate are known but not the truly important patient-reported outcomes. Patient-reported outcomes are important to show if the care provided actually improved the patient's health status. It is hard to have a true measure of value, but with time this issue will surely be corrected.

## 4 Implementation of lean business methods

Each episode of care for a fragility fracture can be broken down into a series of steps or processes. These processes, strung together, will encompass the flow of the patient through the health system during their care. Using lean business methods, these processes can be studied and improved repeatedly to improve the patient flow through the system, reduce errors, and improve patient satisfaction. This is called a value stream map [6]. To embark on such a journey, prerequisites such as the following are needed:

- Support of hospital administration is essential.
- Solid leadership from surgeon champion and medical champion [2] is required.
- The care team should be involved and empowered so that any changes made will "stick".
- There must be an element of commitment among the care providers to understand that there are better ways to care for their patients.
- Excellent communication around the lean practices is also essential with an emphasis that the idea is to improve patient care and provider satisfaction rather than to eliminate jobs.

Some programs will employ a team of consultants to assist them with the process of creating a value stream map; others employ a facilitator to help oversee the process. In all cases, employees must participate actively in lean processes to ensure a successful outcome. When starting to implement lean processes in a department, choosing a discrete diagnosis such as hip fracture is important so that the care team member can focus their efforts clearly.

## 5 Examples of wastes and ways to mitigate them

A primary focus of lean business methods is to eliminate waste from the process [7]. In healthcare, an estimated 30–47% of delivered services are estimated to be "waste" [8]. Waste is something that adds no value to the process of care and is often harmful. Failure of care coordination is an example of harmful waste. Processes that add value in healthcare include a necessary test, time spent with the doctor or nurse, and a needed surgery.

Waste comes in many varieties and these are listed below as the classic seven wastes [2, 3] with relevant examples:

1. Transportation—transporting a patient too many times to radiology when once was enough
2. Inventory—too much or too little inventory
3. Motion—a staff member running around to find a needed item
4. Waiting—waiting for surgery, waiting to see the physician, etc; waiting is aggravating and disrupts the flow of care
5. Overprocessing and overtreatment—ordering too many tests and/or an unnecessary echocardiogram
6. Overproduction—repeatedly performing the same test when the answer was acceptable to begin with
7. Defects—avoidable errors resulting in rework, readmission, and reoperation; this is the worst waste

An added eighth waste is not seeking employees' opinions, thus wasting their good ideas.

As lean processes are implemented, elimination of wastes is a focal point of the methodology [6]. Some wastes are readily eliminated with the use of standardized order sets, by prescribing only generic medications (with geriatric doses) and by standardizing the timing and type of laboratory tests needed for each day of the hospital stay. This helps to eliminate unnecessary medication costs, duplication of laboratory tests, and allows for more predictable staffing for phlebotomy.

In surgery, use of a prominently displayed care algorithm poster to determine the appropriate implant for specific fracture types based upon patient age and functional status enables both good care and tremendous cost savings. It avoids use of costly implants to treat patients with a minimal functional status. This is referred to as "demand matching" the implant to the patient's specific needs and is truly patient-centered care. [9]

## 6 Kaizen—and how is it useful

### 6.1 Lean Six Sigma

Once a decision is reached to embark on the process improvement journey and adopt a lean approach, the goals must be set to allow the leaders to choose the correct methodology to employ it. For a single focused problem, like operating room changeover time, a Lean Six Sigma approach is likely best. Lean Six Sigma is focused on detail and employs a specific methodology to improve the processes and reduce the process variation greatly.

### 6.2 Lean business flow model

For the overall care process of a fracture patient, use of a lean business flow model is preferred. This methodology examines the flow of the patient through the system from emergency department admission to hospital discharge. The process begins at "gemba", ie, the place where the work is done. The team leaders and process facilitator walk the flow of the patient through the system, asking questions, taking notes, and developing an understanding of the complexity of care received. Ideas for improvement are generated but not yet shared or acted upon.

### 6.3 Kaizen

The next step is to plan a "kaizen". Kaizen is a Japanese word that means to take apart (kai), and to make new (zen). To be successful, a kaizen must be carefully planned in advance. A kaizen is a short burst of activity usually lasting 1–5 days. During this time all participating employees are relieved of their usual job responsibilities and required to attend the entire event:

- The specific goal of the kaizen is set by hospital administration.
- The facilitator may be an employee or a specialist hired to facilitate the kaizen.
- Employees are carefully chosen from the usual care team including physicians, nurses, clerical staff, nursing assistants, and even housekeepers if that is appropriate.
- Employees selected should be interested in improvement, engaged, and not naysayers or disruptive individuals.
- A complainer is acceptable to include as long as they are seeking improvement in the system of care.
- The goal of the process improvements is to make them revenue neutral or cost saving.

The event begins with the kaizen leader providing a short presentation, typically 30–45 minutes, explaining the problem and the background, and charging the group with their responsibilities. If the team assembled is not familiar with the process of a kaizen, there is an introductory explanation of the process. A kaizen is biased toward action rather than analysis and is focused on identifying all relevant processes and problems.

After the introduction of the problem and background, the next step is to create a process map or value stream map for the care process being studied. One useful way to do this is to put large white sheets of paper on the wall, side to side, as a first step. The process steps are next mapped out with smaller uniform color sticky notes. Each individual step is mapped in order of occurrence. If there is more than one pathway, parallel paths are made. When all of the steps from beginning to end have been mapped out, the team looks at each step individually and assigns problems that are associated with that step (**Fig 2.10-1**).

The next step is to identify the problems that impact each process step. Each individual problem is written on a sticky note of a different color to the process steps. These are placed vertically above or below the process step. There are typically many more problems per step then there are steps in the process.

When the value stream map is completed, the team usually takes a break to eat. It is important that even for meals, the team remains together. Therefore, the sponsoring organization, typically the hospital, should provide good food for the kaizen. Next, the team collects all the problems by process division. These are studied briefly by the team which is now split into 2–3 groups. The problems are broken into four groups based on problem impact and difficulty, using the grid shown in **Fig 2.10-2**.

After all the problems have been assigned to one of the four squares, problems in squares 3 and 4 are discarded. Problems in square 1 (ie, high impact/low difficulty) are assigned equally amongst the groups. The team is asked to come up with innovative solutions to the problems they have been assigned. Problems in square number 2 (ie, high impact/high difficulty) are placed in a "parking lot" for later assessment. The difficulty level of these is typically too high and may require its own kaizen or may need to be dealt with over time.

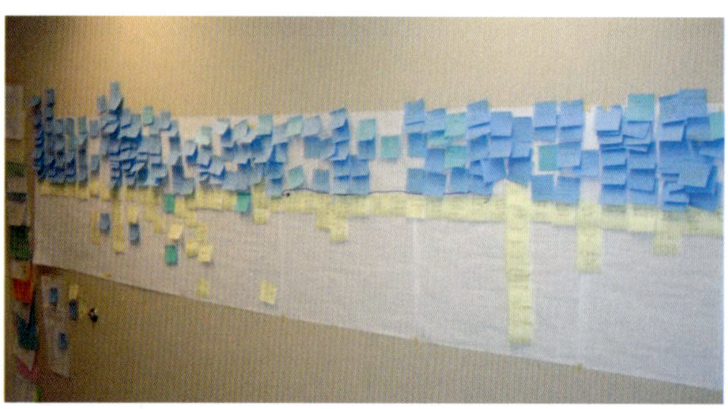

**Fig 2.10-1** Process map used at a kaizen session to solve problems and improve processes.

As the kaizen prepares to close, a summary presentation is created by the groups listing the problems, what step they are at in the care process, and the proposed solutions. When each group has come up with solutions to the problems, they are asked to pilot these solutions in the workplace. Sometimes this can be tried right away, and sometimes it will require a planned pilot phase with a small subgroup of the overall organization. Pilot studies may require calling in employees from the particular area performing the process to ask if the proposed solution will work. In no instance is a detailed analysis done, the kaizen is biased toward action.

The final hour of the kaizen is spent presenting the summary audiovisual presentation to the institutional leadership. During this presentation, no questions are permitted. The solutions are listed, and the team expects that the institutional leadership will support trying these solutions to solve the problems. This is an essential aspect of the kaizen. It requires true support from the institutional leadership. If support is not there, process improvements will not succeed. After time has passed, another kaizen may be required for the same topic as new problems arise or when some of the solutions have failed to solve the original problem. Problems assigned to square 2 (ie, high impact/high difficulty) may often need their own kaizen.

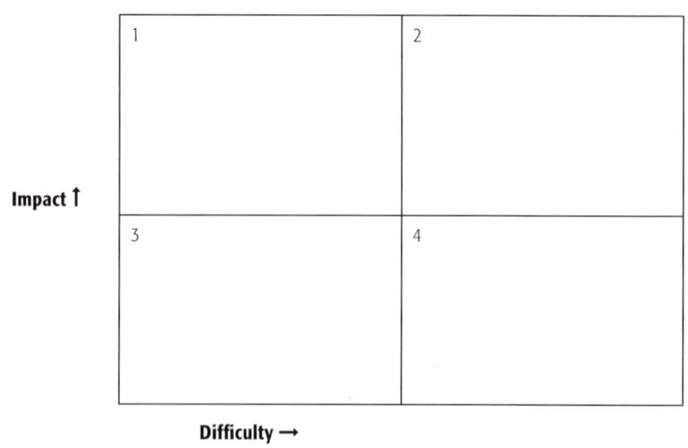


**Fig 2.10-2** Difficulty-opportunity analysis grid helps divide problems into four groups based on problem impact and difficulty (ie, high impact/low difficulty, high impact/high difficulty, low impact/low difficulty, and low impact/high difficulty).

## 6.4 Implementation

Implementing process improvements in the clinical setting is next. This is an ongoing effort. A spreadsheet is devised with the problem, individuals responsible are assigned, and the colors of red (ie, halted, needs attention), green (ie, going well) and blue (ie, completed) are assigned to indicate the progress (**Fig 2.10-3**).

A timeline is often assigned as well. Weekly short team meetings are held and only processes coded red are reviewed. The meetings continue until the process improvements have been completed. Obviously, support from the hospital leadership is required for this to be a success.

Initially, employees may be wary of change. This is particularly true for employees in leadership roles of an area where they feel they "own the processes" already in use. This is why it is essential for the members on the kaizen team to take ownership of the process improvements and sell the new concepts to their coworkers. When a team takes ownership of process improvements, this greatly reduces backsliding to the old ways. When processes are implemented in a top-down manner (ie, traditional for medical centers), employee resistance and backsliding are common. The team should be praised and supported by leadership during process changes.

## 6.5 Results

Assessment of the results of process improvements is critical. Lean business methods are data-driven, so the collection of before and after outcomes is essential. Periodic review of the progress is important as is asking for employee and patient feedback, which typically requires data collection. For financial data, the hospital finance department will need to be involved; they should be aware of the specific data points requested in advance, and these should be compared to historical data for reference. Many other process measures will be already collected by the hospital such as length of stay, complication rates, and operating room measures. Some metrics, like time to surgery, can require extra effort to collect and should have an employee assigned to report these metrics regularly to monitor progress. For outpatient measures, additional effort is required to collect data and an employee will likely need to be tasked with this responsibility.

## 6.6 Program monitoring

A scorecard or dashboard should be assembled with program data and monitored monthly. Outcomes should be available to team members to help them understand their performance improvements. Consider creating graphical dashboards for employees to view. Visual dashboards are an important example of lean business controls (**Fig 2.10-3**). Regular review of outcomes, progress, and backsliding is essential. With use of lean business methods, considerable improvement in program outcomes can be achieved. The dual goals of quality improvement and cost saving are achievable and more cost-effective care will be delivered [6]. Lean business methods are a win for the institution, patients, and healthcare teams.

| Deliverable | Benefit | Owner | Team | Time to complete | Due date | Status | Comments |
|---|---|---|---|---|---|---|---|
| **Registration and checkout** | | | | | | | |
| Ask for photo ID and scan | Once patient is in the system, no longer have to ask for ID (saves time and improves customer satisfaction). | | | 2 weeks | 03-Mar | Complete | |
| Update and relocate provider board to vestibule | Reduce patient walking, improves communications and customer satisfaction. | | | | 01-May | G | Getting info on adding department names to front window. |
| Ban sales reps from area who do not have appointments | Less distractions. | | | | 12-Mar | Complete | New signs posted. No sales reps can enter clinic area without appt. |
| Call for patient transportation when patients are roomed | Current process is to call for patient transport (if required) at end of appointment. This causes long patient wait times and requires staff to make multiple (4–5) calls to check on transport status (improve customer satisfaction and staff efficiency). | | | | 15-Feb | Complete | Send out policy to providers and have it posted in clinic area. |
| Notify patients of their wait times at all stages | Improve patient satisfaction by setting expectations. Try to give a range of times. | | | | 19-Feb | Complete | Send out email. |
| Have new patient registration forms arrive directly to CCO | Direct ships, saves on labels (need to estimate annual savings in USD). This will also ensure that correct info is on labels. | | | | 19-Mar | G | |
| Communicate and distribute minors policy. State during appointment scheduling, with physician liaison and signage | Reduces loss of revenue, saves patient time, and increases customer satisfaction. | | | | 15-Feb | Complete | |
| Standardize to one general patient form with specialty areas/one adult and one pediatric form. | Reduce the need to fill out multiple forms with the same info. Saves time and increases customer satisfaction. | | | 2 weeks | 01-Apr | G | Draft completed on Feb 15. Need space for stickers on each page. Revising form. |
| Order two new high capacity fax machines | Saves time, higher quality faxes, lower supply costs. | | | 1 week | | R | On order. |
| **X-rays and visits** | | | | | | | |
| Post x-ray requirements in modules | Improves communication with x-ray team/ efficiency in radiology. Results in quicker patient visit (customer satisfaction) This will eliminate the 5–10% of x-rays which are repeated today due to lack of communication. | | | | 15-Mar | Complete | |
| Gowns no longer required for most x-rays | Eliminates tying up room to hold patient valuables, huge customer satisfaction issue, reduces cycle time and room utilization. Patient is uncomfortable and inattentive in gown. Saves in buying and cleaning gowns. | | | | 05-Mar | Complete | |
| Mandatory for gowned patients to wear slippers or shoes | Hygiene improvement. | | | 2 Days | 26-Feb | Complete | Signs are posted in each room and slippers are now located next to gowns. |

**Fig 2.10-3** Example of a kaizen dashboard.
Abbreviations: appt, appointment; CCO, Clinton Crossings Office; reps, representatives.

| Deliverable | Benefit | Owner | Team | Time to complete | Due date | Status | Comments |
|---|---|---|---|---|---|---|---|
| **Internal** | | | | | | | |
| Appointment will remind patients to wear lose-fitting clothing | Helps eliminate the need to change into gown. | | | | 17-Feb | Complete | Appts informed and are informing patients. |
| When two or more patients are waiting in checkout line, staff will approach line and ask who needs a follow-up appointment. If no follow up is required, take encounter form, give back yellow copy, tell patient they will be billed or their copay if they have one. | Eliminates patient from standing in line and waiting when they can leave! Increase customer satisfaction. | | | | 16-Feb | Complete | |
| Perform 5S–pick a pilot area and set the standards | This will ensure that all forms are stored in the same place and called by the same name. | | | | 15-Mar | G | Once pilot is complete, the entire building will perform 5S. Peg will call. Bill to schedule audit for mid-April. |
| Perform 5S–pick a pilot area and set the standards (Dr's Bay area) | This will ensure that all forms are stored in the same place and called by the same name. | | | | 15-Mar | G | |
| Need for additional magazines | Improve customer satisfaction | | | 08-Mar | 08-Mar | Complete | Additional magazine order went out with renewals. |
| Team huddle–tech and provider, at start of day and throughout day | Improve patient flow, tech and provider satisfaction | | | | TBD | G | |
| Future potential kaizen | | | | | | | |
| We documented many proposals during the kaizen. We need to add them to this document. | | | | | | | |
| Billing issues | Insurance not entered correctly | | | | | | |
| Allow for copay for x-ray | | | | | | | |
| | | | | | KEY | G | Action is on target |
| | | | | | | Complete | Action closed, fully implemented |
| | | | | | | R | Behind schedule, or having issues |

**Fig 2.10-3 (cont)** Example of a kaizen dashboard.

## 7 References


1. **Giusti A, Barone A, Razzano M, et al.** Optimal setting and care organization in the management of older adults with hip fracture. *Eur J Phys Rehabil Med.* 2011 Jun;47(2):281–296.
2. **Kates SL.** Lean business model and implementation of a geriatric fracture center. *Clin Geriatr Med.* 2014 May;30(2):191–205.
3. **Ohno T.** *Toyota Production System: Beyond Large-Scale Production.* Cambridge: Productivity Press; 1988.
4. **Morden NE, Colla CH, Sequist TD, et al.** Choosing wisely—the politics and economics of labeling low-value services. *N Engl J Med.* 2014 Feb 13;370(7):589–592.
5. **Porter ME.** What is value in health care? *N Engl J Med.* 2010 Dec 23;363(26):2477–2481.
6. **Wormack JP, Jones DT.** *Lean Thinking: Banish Waste and Create Wealth in Your Corporation.* 2nd ed. New York: Free Press; 2003.
7. **Womack JP, Jones DT, Roos D.** *The Machine That Changed the World.* New York: Simon & Schuster; 1990.
8. **Berwick DM, Hackbarth AD.** Eliminating waste in US health care. *JAMA.* 2012 Apr 11;307(14):1513–1516.
9. **Swart E, Makhni EC, Macaulay W, et al.** Cost-effectiveness analysis of fixation options for intertrochanteric hip fractures. *J Bone Joint Surg Am.* 2014 Oct 01;96(19):1612–1620.

# Section 3
# Fracture management

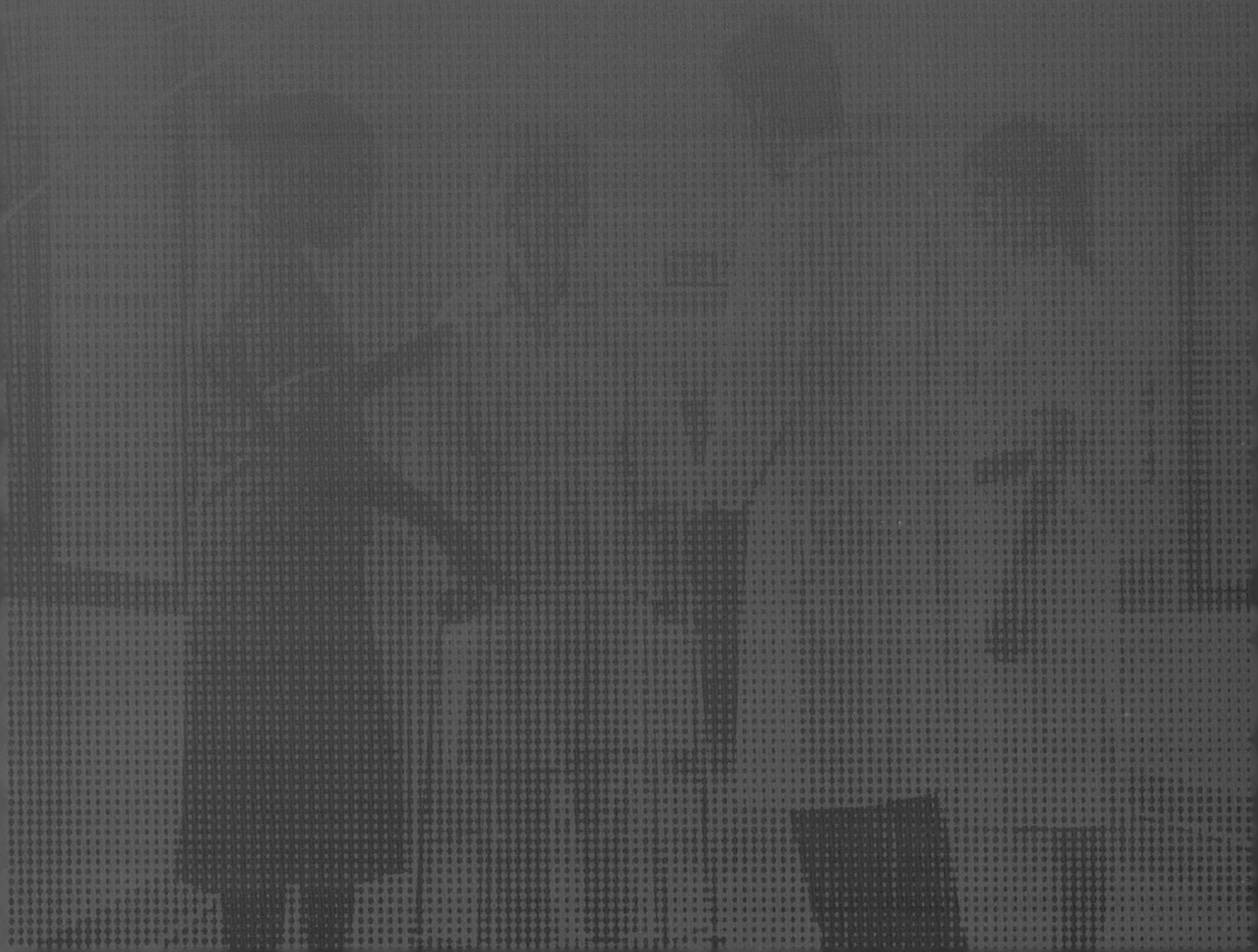

# Section 3
## Fracture management

# 3.1 Proximal humerus

Franz Kralinger, Michael Blauth

## 1 Introduction

The treatment of proximal humeral fractures (PHFs) is controversial for a number of reasons:

- There is an ongoing debate about the benefits of operative versus nonoperative treatment even of displaced, unstable fractures.
- The rate of "mechanical" complications after surgical treatment is 30–35% in prospective studies with surgical revision rates from 20–30% [1–3]. Nevertheless, up to 74% of PHFs actually received surgical treatment [4].
- Multiple available operative options from pinning to arthroplasty with varying selection criteria are mainly based on bone and fracture characteristics without considering the patient's functional status.
- There is a lack of randomized studies investigating distinct fracture entities and treatment modalities.
- Unspecific outcome measures. While using the Constant and Disabilities of the Arm, Shoulder, and Hand (DASH) scores, ceiling effects may make it difficult to detect substantial advantages of surgical fixation over nonoperative management [5]. If the scores or patient-reported outcome measures (PROMs) used were more precise, differences between different procedures might be detected more easily. A ceiling effect of a score describes the fact that a score at its upper end of values loses the ability to detect changes in a patient's health status in a sufficient manner. Therefore ceiling effects can lead to artefactual data, eg, showing no effect of an intervention when in reality there is one.
- More traditional ways to evaluate treatment results like range of motion (ROM), muscle strength, fracture reduction, and bone healing may not apply to the proximal humerus where objective parameters often do not match subjective appraisals [6].

Since there is no single clear-cut approach to a PHF, treatment recommendations depend largely on surgeon experience, skills, and preference. An improvement of this situation can only be achieved with larger and higher level clinical studies and specifically designed PROMs to address the geriatric population. This chapter summarizes the current situation from a practical approach to guide proper patient- and treatment-specific decision making. This seems to be the most important factor in achieving a good outcome as well as for the most appropriate treatment selection and avoidance of complications.

### 1.1 Epidemiology

Proximal humeral fractures:

- Are the third most common fractures in adults older than 60 years.
- Affect 70–80% of women with a history of osteoporosis who have fallen from a standing height [1].
- Have been increasing by up to 15% in the past decades [7, 8]. There are major differences between ethnicities and the rate of fractures are significantly lower in countries like Japan [9] compared to Europe or America.

Interestingly, the clear rise in the rate of low-trauma PHFs in older Finnish women from the early 1970s until the mid-1990s has stabilized at a high level. The reasons for this are largely unknown, but a cohort effect toward a healthier aging population with improved functional ability and reduced risk of injurious falls cannot be ruled out [10]. In Austria, on the other hand, this levelling off effect could not be confirmed and absolute numbers of PHFs are still rising due to increased life expectancy [11].

## 1.2 Etiology

- Proximal humeral fractures occur mostly after low-energy falls [12].
- Comorbidities increase the risk for PHFs. Factors like decreased neuromuscular response, delayed reaction time, cognitive impairment, impaired balance, intoxication as well as early menopause are all associated with PHFs [13].
- Middle-aged patients who sustain PHFs are physiologically older than their numerical age indicates and have a higher incidence of medical comorbidities often related to alcohol, tobacco, and drug usage (**Case 1: Fig 3.1-1**) [14].

CASE 1

### Young woman suffering from alcoholism and severe osteoporosis, multiple fractures including bilateral proximal humeral fractures with special solution on one side

#### Patient

A 48-year-old woman with no obvious signs of dementia or confusion; she was cooperative. She was living with her husband and wanted to remain independent. Over the years, she sustained continuously major fractures of the distal radius, lumbar spine, and proximal tibia.

#### Comorbidities

- Alcohol addiction
- Nicotine abuse
- Chronic obstructive pulmonary disease
- Osteoporosis
- Grand mal seizures
- Multiple other comorbidities

#### Treatment and outcome

In 2005 the female patient sustained a subcapital fracture of the left humerus (**Fig 3.1-1a–c**). The fracture was treated nonoperatively leading to healing in malalignment. The bone was clearly osteoporotic, but no action was taken with regard to this.

In 2008 she presented with a fracture of the right proximal humerus (**Fig 3.1-1d–f**). The fracture was first treated nonoperatively, which resulted in a painful and debilitating condition. Since fracture healing was not to be expected, the decision to perform surgery was made.

After the fracture was aligned (**Fig 3.1-1g**), an almost normal anatomical condition could be reestablished with a massive central allograft (**Fig 3.1-1h**). Then the plate was preliminarily fixed (**Fig 3.1-1i**).

The intraoperative (**Fig 3.1-1j–k**), 3-month (**Fig 3.1-1l**), and 1-year (**Fig 3.1-1m**) follow-up x-rays showed an uneventful clinical course. Range of motion was 120° of abduction/flexion and 60° of external rotation.

#### Treatment options

- Nonanatomical fixation in valgus of the humeral head and massive shortening may result in an impaired functional outcome due to a shorter lever arm of the rotator cuff muscles.
- Nailing: Head fragment is too short for stable anchorage of the fifth anchor point.
- Hemiarthroplasty: Overtreatment when stable reconstruction is possible. Midterm function of the shoulder is questionable.
- Reverse total shoulder arthroplasty is not indicated with intact rotator cuff and well-centered shoulder joint.

#### Key points

- Central voids can be successfully filled with massive allografts to prevent early varus failure and subsidence of the head fragment with cut-through of the screws, even in patients with severe osteoporosis [15].
- In a retrospective case series, this procedure leads to bony union in a noncompliant or high-risk patient population [16].
- Treatment of the underlying osteoporosis may be challenging in noncompliant patients.

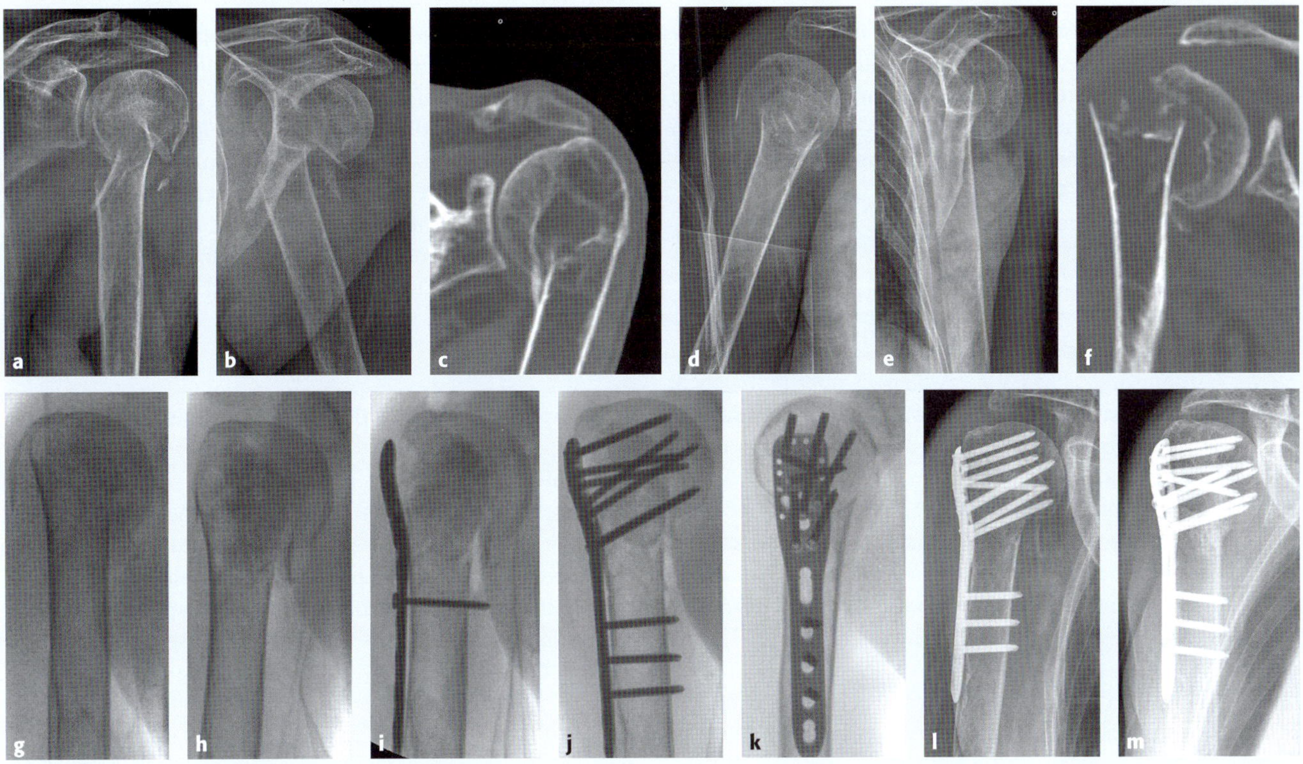


**Fig 3.1-1a–m** A 48-year-old woman with multiple fractures.
**a–c** X-rays showing a subcapital fracture of the left humerus.
**d–f** X-rays showing a fracture of the right proximal humerus.
**g–i** X-rays showing aligned fracture (**g**), an almost normal anatomical condition achieved with a massive central allograft (**h**) and preliminary plate fixation (**i**).
**j–m** Intraoperative result (**j–k**), follow-up after 3 months (**l**), and 1 year (**m**). Note the different projection in the last picture which can be read from the PHILOS plate.

## 2 Diagnostics and classification

In order to give a viable therapeutic recommendation, the preoperative workup must go beyond fracture analysis, although there seems to be a high degree of uncertainty as how to measure and implement clinical information into the decision-making process.

In a recent study 238 surgeons rated 40 x-rays of patients with PHFs. Participants were randomly selected to receive information about the patient and mechanism of the injury. Patient information, particularly older age, was associated with a higher likelihood of nonoperative treatment recommendation rather than x-rays alone. Clinical information did not improve agreement with the actual treatment or the generally poor interobserver agreement on treatment recommendations [17].

### 2.1 Clinical evaluation

History and physical examination include:

- Mechanism of injury
- Vascular and neurological status, especially distal circulation and the axillary nerve function
- Soft-tissue injuries, including the skin
- Muscle status, specifically the muscles of the rotator cuff (**Diagnostics 1: Fig 3.1-2, Fig 3.1-3, Fig 3.1-4**)
- Preinjury level of function
- Occupation
- Hand dominance
- History of malignancy
- History of previous fragility fractures
- Rehabilitation potential
- Presence of concomitant injuries
- Geriatric workup including comorbidities, functional and mental status

Evidence of how the mental status may influence the outcome is poor. In most studies, patients with significant mental impairment are excluded or this factor is not considered at all. Advanced age and higher degrees of dementia with increased risk of postoperative delirium usually lead to nonoperative treatment (**Case 2: Fig 3.1-5**).

Other patient factors like level of independence, housing situation, or the need to use walking aids also potentially affect outcomes after both operative and nonoperative management and should therefore be evaluated very carefully. Complications such as infection, nonunion, osteonecrosis, fixation failure, and compliance with rehabilitation can all be related to medical comorbidities [13]. Alcohol abuse particularly increases a patient's risk of noncompliance and nonunion, and tobacco use increases the risk of nonunion [18].

DIAGNOSTICS 1

## Evaluation of rotator cuff muscles status with standardized 2-D computed tomographic reconstructions

### Patients

An 85-year-old woman with chronic rotator cuff deficiency and complete atrophy of the supra- and infraspinatus muscles (**Fig 3.1-2**).

A 78-year-old woman with posterior and superior cuff deficiency (**Fig 3.1-3**).

An 87-year-old man with no muscle atrophy or fatty degeneration of the rotator cuff muscles (**Fig 3.1-4**).

### Discussion

A fracture reconstruction in a patient like the one in **Fig 3.1-3** does not seem to be indicated. Even if the pretrauma status of the computed tomographic angiography was compensated, the risk of decompensation after the reconstruction with the need of revision surgery is high; the authors recommend reverse shoulder arthroplasty in these cases.

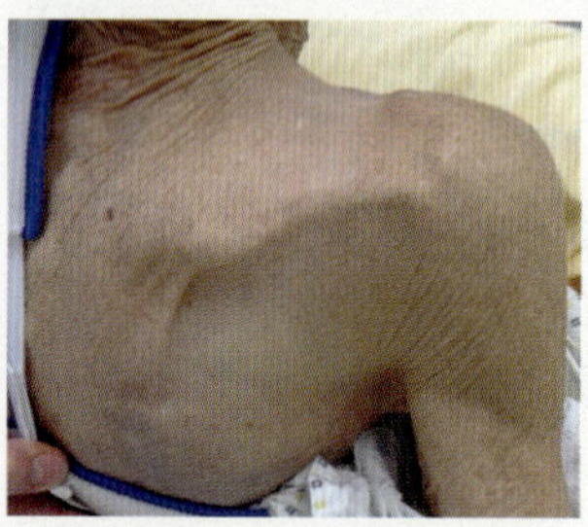

**Fig 3.1-2** Clinical picture of an 85-year-old woman with chronic rotator cuff deficiency and complete atrophy of the supraspinatus muscle and infraspinatus muscles. The diagnosis can be easily made by visual inspection.

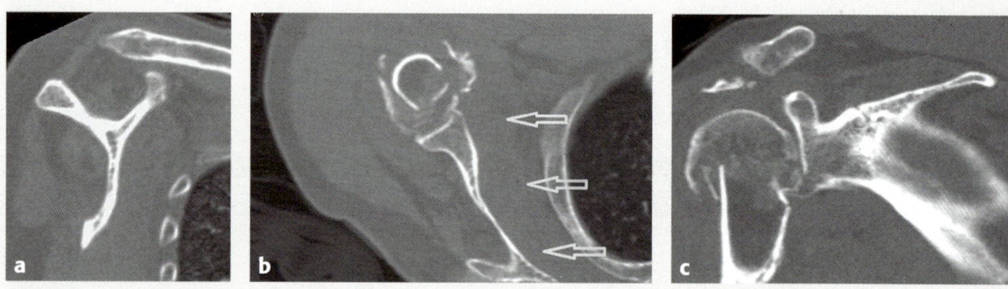

**Fig 3.1-3a–c** Parasagittal 2-D reconstruction of a 78-year-old woman with posterior and superior cuff deficiency. Inhomogeneous presentation of the supraspinatus muscle and infraspinatus muscle because of atrophy and fatty degeneration (**a, c**). The subscapularis (SSC) is still in good shape in the caudal aspects (**b**).

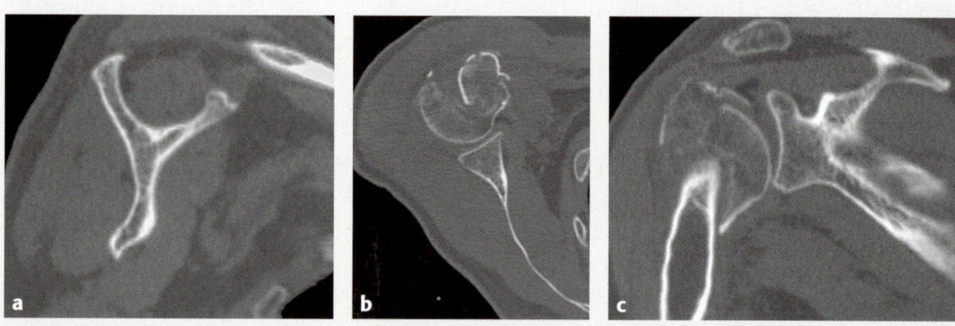

**Fig 3.1-4a–c** In contrast, parasagittal 2-D reconstruction of an 87-year-old man shows no muscle atrophy or fatty degeneration of the rotator cuff muscles. Note the muscle belly of the supraspinatus muscle (**a, c**). The head fragment is internally rotated due to the pull of the subscapularis tendon, and the corresponding muscle is without atrophy (**b**). The full cuff without significant atrophy or fatty infiltration is visible in the parasagittal plane at the coracoid and base of the spinal junction [19].

## Evaluation of mental status and comorbidities

### Patient

A 90-year-old slow-go, ie, unfit, female patient, was living in a nursing home and required a walker to assist with ambulation.

### Comorbidities

- Dementia
- Coronary heart disease
- Hypertension
- Multiple falls
- A pertrochanteric fracture 2 years ago, treated with a cephalomedullary nail with an augemented head neck element or so-called proximal femoral nail antirotation plus augmentation
- Osteoporosis

### Treatment and outcome

The female patient had a displaced 2-part proximal humeral fracture (**Fig 3.1-5a–b**) and an undisplaced superior and inferior anterior pelvic ring fracture (**Fig 3.1-5c**). Her therapy comprised shoulder sling, pain medication, and pain-adapted mobilization. She was hospitalized for 16 days, mobilized to sit in a wheelchair, and transferred to a nursing home (**Fig 3.1-5d**).

The follow-up x-rays at 6 weeks showed a rapid ongoing healing process in varus malalignment (**Fig 3.1-5e–g**). She had only little pain and could reach her head with her hand. She did not walk any more but was satisfied with her situation and refused further follow-ups. Her situation was still the same 2 years later.

### Discussion

- From a geriatric standpoint, everything should be done to get the patient out of bed: adapt pain medication, keep motivating her and help her to walk again. Bed rest with loss of muscle mass, staring at the ceiling all the time and eating in bed has to be avoided. Nutritional aspects should also be considered.
- To answer the question if surgical treatment under a nerve block would improve the patient's prognosis, her prefracture status needs to be carefully evaluated (ie, "What was she really able to do?") as well as her mental status, ability to cooperate, and motivation. This may take a few days. Finally her risk for surgery must be estimated.
- In this case, despite a low risk for surgery, nonoperative treatment was recommended, because the patient had poor cognitive function and did not require high functional demands. In her case bone healing took place quickly despite her severe osteoporosis. Surgical stabilization would most probably not have caused any change in the rehabilitation process.
- From a surgical standpoint, if a nailing procedure would have been chosen, a low risk for failure would have been expected.

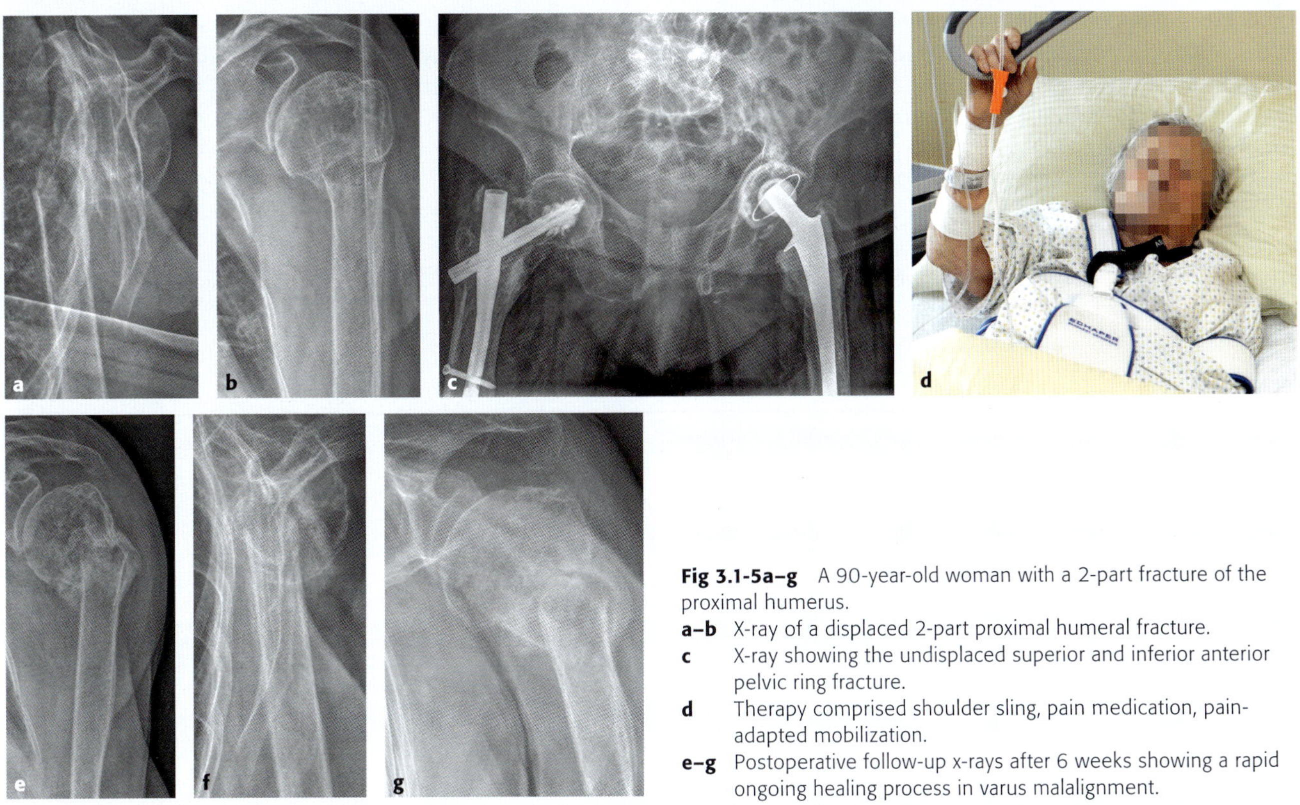


**Fig 3.1-5a–g** A 90-year-old woman with a 2-part fracture of the proximal humerus.
**a–b** X-ray of a displaced 2-part proximal humeral fracture.
**c** X-ray showing the undisplaced superior and inferior anterior pelvic ring fracture.
**d** Therapy comprised shoulder sling, pain medication, pain-adapted mobilization.
**e–g** Postoperative follow-up x-rays after 6 weeks showing a rapid ongoing healing process in varus malalignment.

To describe the functional status of the patient, a simple distinction between go-go, slow-go and no-go patients (**Table 3.1-1**, see topic 3.1 in this chapter) is useful. The Parker Mobility Score and the WHO performance status (**Table 3.1-2**, see topic 3.3 in this chapter) may also be helpful.

## 2.2 Imaging

### 2.2.1 Plain x-rays

Surgeons can only make clear and unambiguous statements if the fracture is clearly visualized by x-ray(s). If criteria are defined to classify and treat PHFs, the proximal humerus must be displayed in a manner that those criteria can be reliably evaluated.

The trauma series consists of a true AP view, an axial view, and an outlet view. The first two x-rays are most important to check the displacement of fragments and the instability of the fracture. Acute pain should be treated before images are taken.

Analyzing the projection of the proximal humerus in published serial x-ray studies suggests that the position of the patient's arm often varies within one case. Recommendations about the "standard position" also vary widely. According to geometrical studies by Hengg et al [20], especially different degrees of internal rotation (IR) distort the measurement of the head-shaft angle on the AP view substantially: 30°, 45°, and 60° of IR result in a projection of the head-shaft angle of 144°, 150°, and 159°. Standardized and above all comparable visualizations of the proximal humerus are therefore crucial to make decisions and to collate results (**Diagnostics 2: Fig 3.1-6**).

The true AP view (**Diagnostics 3: Fig 3.1-7, Fig 3.1-8**) shows:

- Varus and valgus deformity and amount of displacement
- Medial displacement of the shaft consistently produced by the pectoralis major muscle
- Posterosuperior displacement of the greater tuberosity (GT)

Rotational displacement of the head fragment is due to the pull of the subscapularis (SSC) in 3-part GT fractures. This pathology needs to be derotated in percutaneous procedures. When placing the arm in a sling or holding it in a relieving posture, this type of view cannot be achieved.

The axial view (**Diagnostics 4: Fig 3.1-9, Fig 3.1-10**):

- Is paramount to assess anterior or posterior displacement of the humeral head in relation to the glenoid
- Determines anteversion and retroversion
- Displays displacement and fragmentation of the GT (**Diagnostics 5: Fig 3.1-11**) and the overlap of the head by the minor tuberosity
- Shows posterior dislocation of the humeral head associated with PHF, which is often missed without an appropriate axillary lateral view. Alternatively, a dynamic investigation under image intensifier may be performed

The Velpeau view is an alternative to the axial view and can be obtained with the arm in a sling.

The lateral view (= lateral scapula, = Y view, = outlet view) (**Diagnostics 6: Fig 3.1-12, Fig 3.1-13**) is easy to shoot in the trauma situation but often very difficult to interpret because of poor quality and superimposed structures. It is definitely the third most important view of the trauma series. If only two views are done, they should be the true AP and axial views.

The lateral view shows:

- Greater tuberosity posterior displacement due to the pull of the infraspinatus (ISP) and supraspinatus (SSP) muscles.
- The relation of the head fragment to the glenoid.

## Comparable projections are of utmost importance

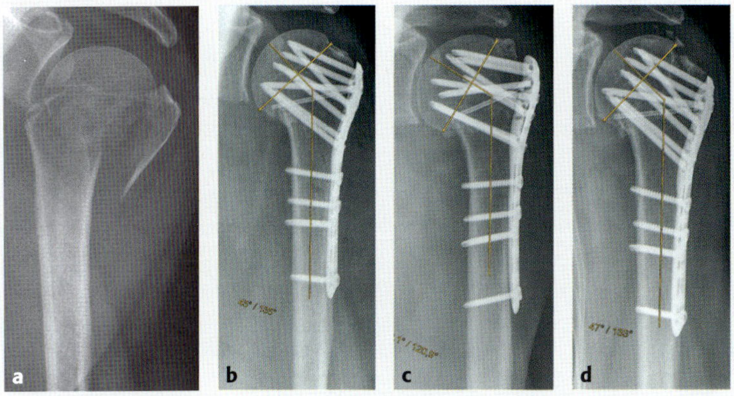

**Fig 3.1-6a–d** X-ray series after a displaced 3-part fracture in a 58-year-old woman (**a**). In a true AP view taken postoperatively the head-shaft angle (HSA) amounts to 135°, which is equivalent to an anatomical reduction (**b**). The 8-week follow-up displays varus malalignment of 120.9° which is due to only another arm rotation and also an x-ray beam projection. This can be easily detected by comparing the projection of the standard locking plate in both views (**c**). The 1-year follow-up shows again the initial situation with a HSA of 133° and no relevant loss of reduction (**d**). This example clearly demonstrates the great importance of comparable standardized projections.



## True AP view

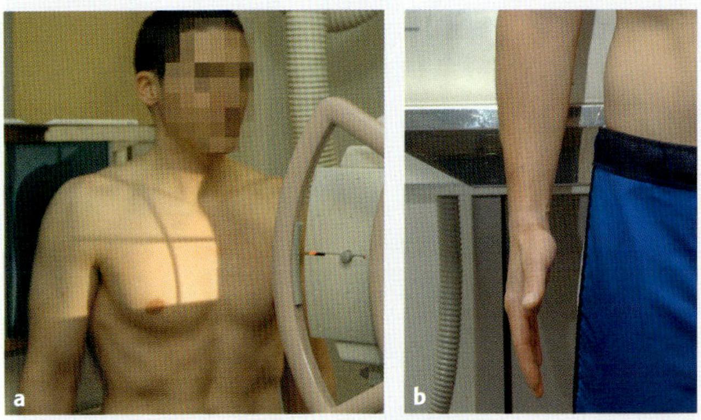

**Fig 3.1-7a–b** The patient's affected shoulder should be placed against the x-ray plate with his trunk tilted approximately 40° toward the beam. The scapula of the affected shoulder should be parallel to the cassette (**a**). The patient's arm is in neutral rotation, ie, with the thumb bent forward; this position is reproducible and complies with the geometrical reflections of a true AP view (**b**). The central beam is orientated 20–25° caudally.

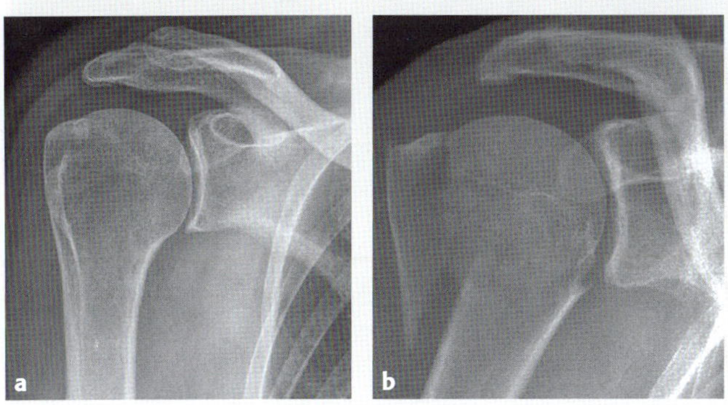

**Fig 3.1-8a–b** Orthograde and tangential projection of the glenoid, and free projection of the humeral head with the greater tuberosity (GT) marginalized and the subacromial space visible. Examples of an uninjured shoulder of a 32-year-old man without pathology (**a**) and a 3-part GT valgus-impacted proximal humeral fracture in a 42-year-old woman (**b**), both in correct AP view.

DIAGNOSTICS 4

## Axial view

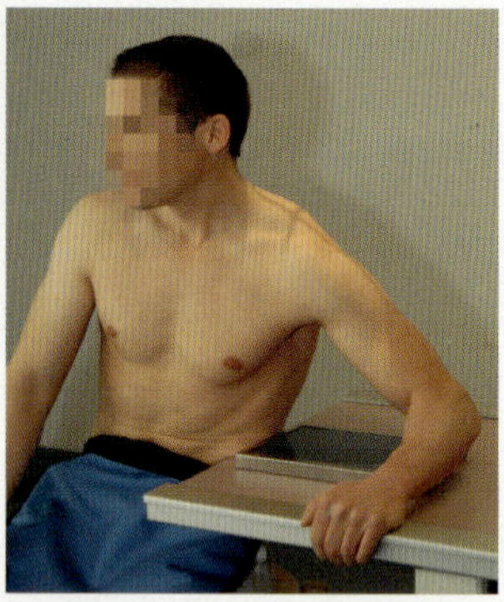

**Fig 3.1-9** Axial view in 30–40° of abduction and the forearm parallel to the table. This can be achieved in most acute cases after administering some pain medication.

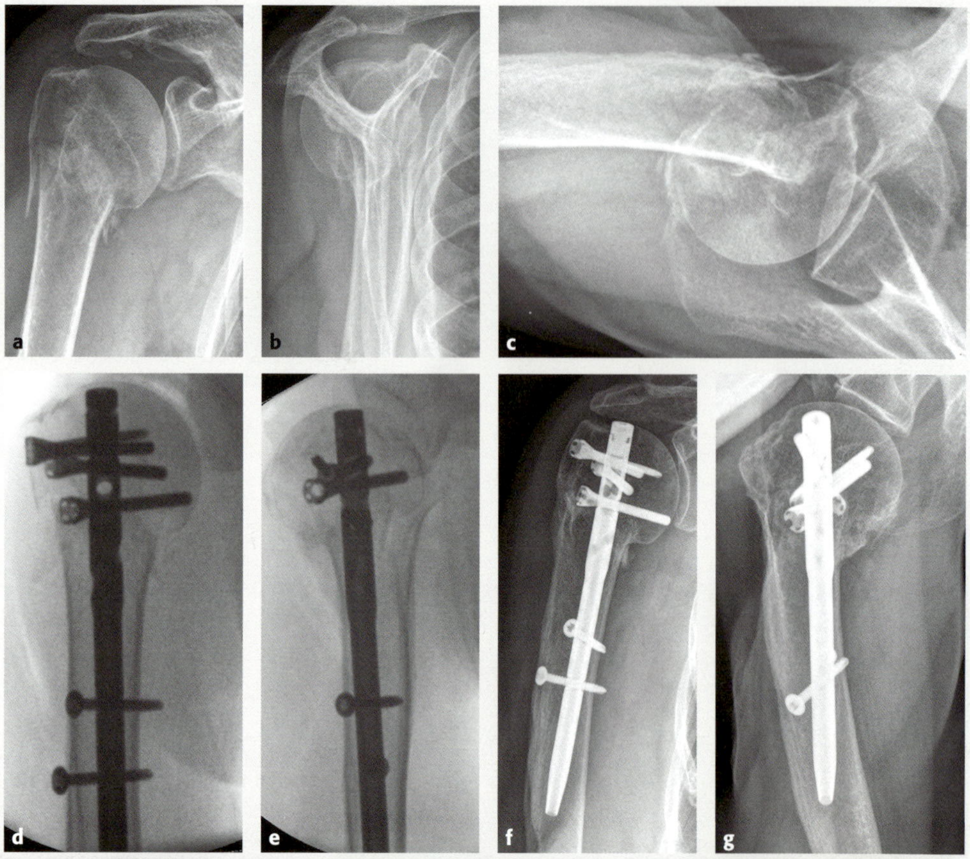

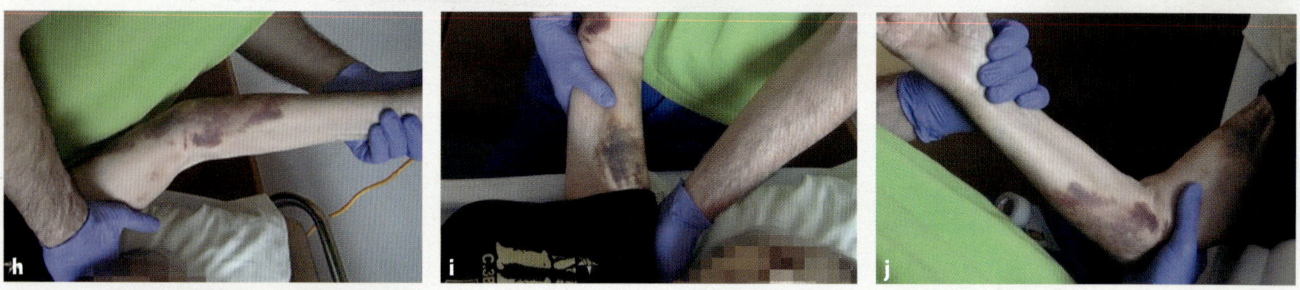

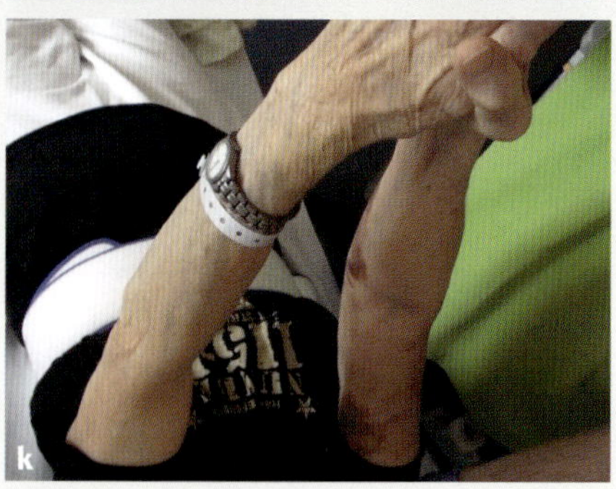

**Fig 3.1-10a–k** A 72-year-old woman with a 2-part fracture.

**a–c** True AP, outlet, and axial views of a displaced 2-part fracture in a go-go, ie, fit, 72-year-old female patient. Displacement and instability is best demonstrated in the axial view.

**d–e** Fracture fixation with an intramedullary nail.

**f–g** Result after 6 months. Note that the projection is different from the postoperative views.

**h–k** Functional rehabilitation 8 days after surgery.

DIAGNOSTICS 5

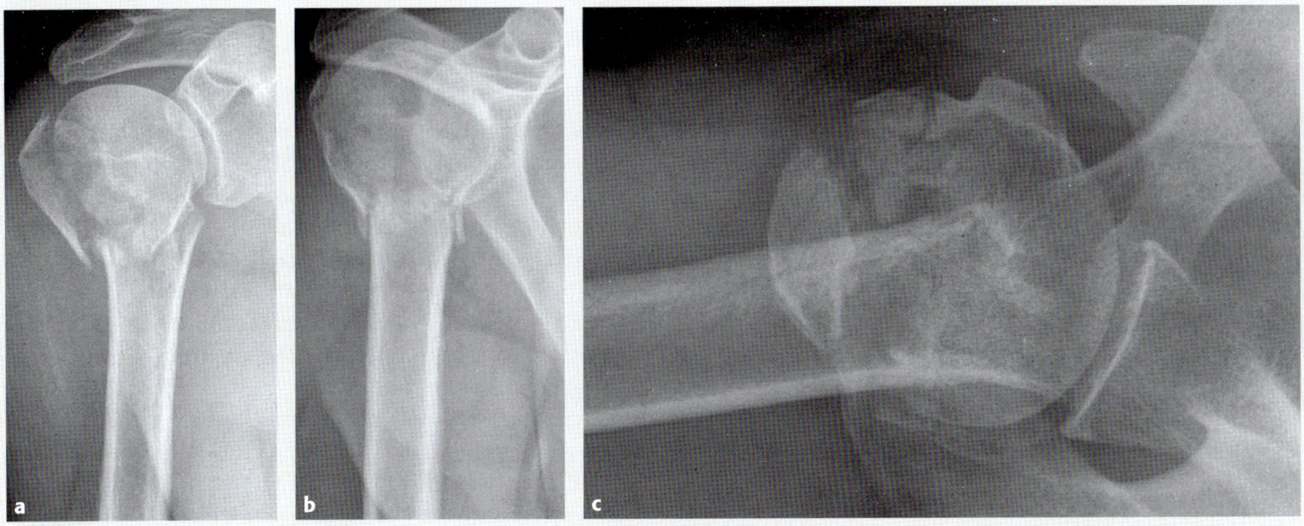

**Fig 3.1-11a–c** The AP and outlet views (**a–b**) provide sufficient information about the greater tuberosity (GT), shaft and head fragment. The axial view (**c**) displays all missing information to classify the HL-G-S fracture. Note the comminution and dorsal displacement of the GT.

DIAGNOSTICS 6

## Lateral view

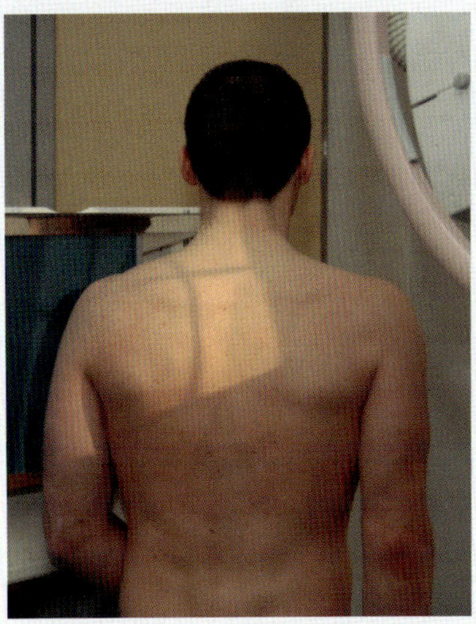

**Fig 3.1-12** For the lateral view, the anterior shoulder is placed on the x-ray plate with the unaffected shoulder tilted forward 40°. The beam is placed posteriorly and directed along the scapular spine.

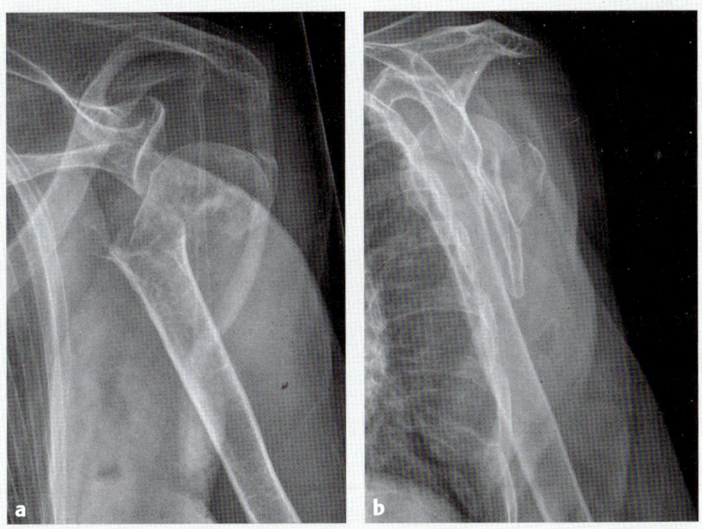

**Fig 3.1-13a–b** The AP view (**a**) of an 80-year-old patient shows a fracture involving the greater tuberosity, the shaft, and the head fragment. The lateral view (**b**) does not add much information. Especially the lesser tuberosity (LT) cannot be visualized well, be it in the AP view or in the lateral view. The axial view generates this critical information, and if unavailable, a computed tomographic scan is necessary to show the involvement of the LT.

### 2.2.2 Computed tomographic scan

In most hospitals, a CT scan is part of the standard workup of PHFs. Certainly, if surgical treatment is an option, a CT scan with 3-D reconstructions adds important information in fracture dislocations, humeral head-split fractures, and comminuted fractures. Three-dimensional CT scan reconstructions have been shown to provide the highest interobserver agreement with regard to classification and treatment recommendations among upper-extremity specialists [21].

CT scans:

- Help to precisely determine fracture lines and pieces, ie, fracture characteristics needed for surgical planning.
- Provide enhanced understanding of fracture comminution, impaction, humeral head involvement and its size and remaining thickness, and additional glenoid articular surface injury (**Case 3: Fig 3.1-14**).
- Allow for manual 2-D reconstructions along the axes of the humerus to show the exact angulation and displacement of fragments as well as the length of the metaphyseal fracture extension.
- Facilitate soft-tissue imaging specifically rotator cuff muscles. In case of a rotator cuff arthropathy with limited preoperative function and an indication for surgery, an inverse prosthesis instead of fracture fixation is indicated.

CASE 3

## Importance of a detailed computed tomographic analysis

#### Patient

An 80-year-old woman sustained a low-energy proximal humeral fracture and a distal radial fracture of the left upper extremity.

#### Comorbidities

- No relevant comorbidities besides osteoporosis—already treated

#### Treatment and outcome

The AP and lateral views showed a 2-part fracture of the surgical neck (HGL-S) and the medial calcar seemed comminuted (**Fig 3.1-14a–b**). Both fractures were initially treated nonoperatively. After 10 days, progressive tilting of the head fragment with pronounced displacement was visible in the lateral view (**Fig 3.1-14c–d**). In addition, the patient was unable to participate in rehabilitation because of pain. The surgeon and patient decided on plating. The 2-D computed tomographic scans showed the narrow head fragment (**Fig 3.1-14e–f**). Only very few thread pitches of the locked screws could be anchored.

Intraoperative x-rays demonstrated a residual varus position of the head fragment and a lack of medial support due to "wrong impaction" (**Fig 3.1-14g–h**).

Insufficient medial support and residual varus together with the small osteoporotic head fragment led to a mechanical varus failure. After 4 weeks (**Fig 3.1-14i**) and 6 months (**Fig 3.1-14j–k**) the fracture was malunited with a severe varus deformity; since the screws did not perforate, the patient was not revised.

#### Discussion

In cases such as shown in **Fig 3.1-14**, a sustainable medial bone contact can only be achieved by reducing the head fragment into a slight valgus position. Because the length of the proximal humerus is then reduced, the plate must be placed in a nonanatomical position, ie, with a gap between lateral cortex and the plate.

An impaction with valgus position and with additional cement augmentation of the screws might have helped, but if in doubt a structural allograft could definitely provide the mechanical stability for a functional rehabilitation as desired in orthogeriatrics.

In a surgical neck 2-part fracture we would not consider arthroplasty.

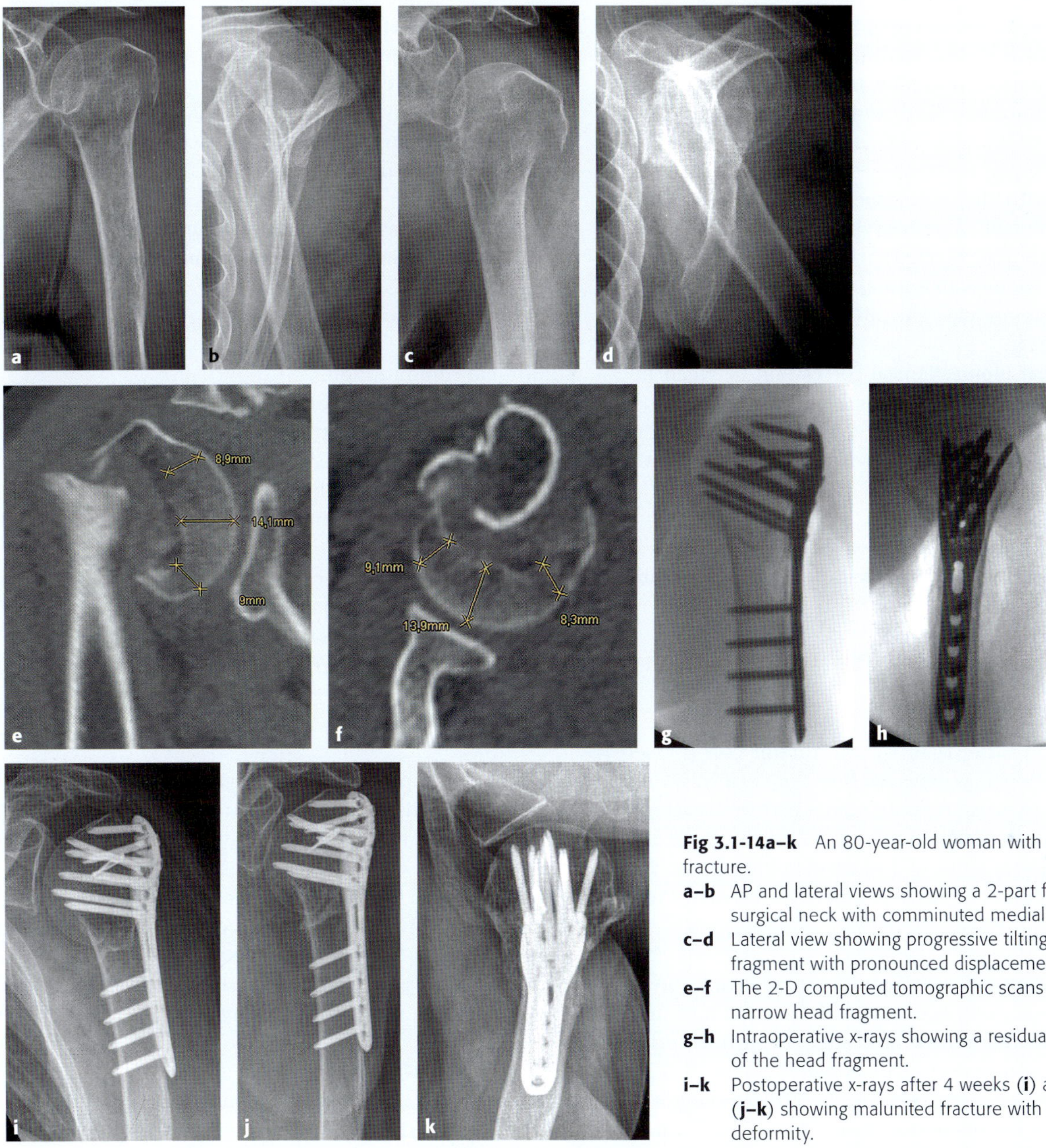


**Fig 3.1-14a–k** An 80-year-old woman with a surgical neck fracture.

**a–b** AP and lateral views showing a 2-part fracture of the surgical neck with comminuted medial calcar.
**c–d** Lateral view showing progressive tilting of the head fragment with pronounced displacement.
**e–f** The 2-D computed tomographic scans showing the narrow head fragment.
**g–h** Intraoperative x-rays showing a residual varus position of the head fragment.
**i–k** Postoperative x-rays after 4 weeks (**i**) and 6 months (**j–k**) showing malunited fracture with severe varus deformity.

### 2.2.3 Magnetic resonance imaging

Magnetic resonance imaging (MRI) adds little to the initial evaluation of PHFs [22].

### 2.2.4 Local bone quality

- Promising attempts have been made to experimentally measure the local bone quality (LBQ) with a torque measurement tool (DensiProbe) which was adapted to a standard locking plate. The mechanical peak torque correlates with the local bone mineral density (BMD) and screw failure load in anatomical specimens [23].
- With modern picture archiving and communication systems, the local bone density (LBD) can be measured in standardized regions of interest given in Hounsfield units [24] and converted into BMD values. The aforementioned measurement gives an estimate of the LBQ.

The significance of local osteoporosis for the outcome of the treatment is unclear. In a multicenter trial, patients with mechanical complications after plate fixation of unstable PHFs had the same low BMD as patients with uneventful healing [1].

Experiments with anatomical specimens have shown that periimplant polymethylmethacrylate (PMMA) cement augmentation cannot be injected through a cannulated screw into cancellous bone with normal density [25, 26]. If implant augmentation is intended, the LBQ needs to be determined.

There is a linear biomechanical correlation between LBQ and cycles to failure [27, 28]. Common sense dictates that osteoporosis is clinically associated with increased rates of comminution and defects due to impaction, loss of fixation and reduction after surgical management.

Recent clinical trial results suggest that LBQ constitutes at most one contributing factor to fixation failures after plating [1, 28].

For the typical patient with PHF, LBQ must be expected [1].

### 2.3 Soft-tissue injuries

With fractures of the GT or LT, the rotator cuff is essentially nonfunctional, as expected [13]. Conversely, we may presume that a 4-part PHF only occurs with an intact rotator cuff. Without a functioning rotator cuff, displaced avulsion fractures are rare due to the lack of pulling forces. With a preexisting cuff arthropathy, 2-part fractures are more likely.

A complete rotator cuff examination cannot usually be performed in an acute setting due to pain and swelling, but the rotator cuff function should be monitored throughout the typical clinical course to ensure adequate function [22]. Due to the age of most patients who sustain PHFs previous rotator cuff injuries are likely, and a new rotator cuff tear can certainly occur in conjunction with PHFs [29]. As an indirect measurement, the status of the rotator cuff muscle can be determined with the CT scan (**Diagnostics 1: Fig 3.1-2, Fig 3.1-3, Fig 3.1-4**).

### 2.4 Instability and displacement

Instability and displacement are often used as criteria for determining the treatment strategy. Imaging usually only shows a momentary situation of unstable fractures. Whether or not fracture fragments are displaced may depend on the position of the arm while x-rays or CT scans were taken.

If in doubt, perform repeat x-rays examinations to help rule out misinterpretation or secondary displacement.

Signs for stability are [21, 30]:

- Minimal comminution
- Three or fewer fragments
- Absence of significant tuberosity displacement
- Cortical contact
- Relative impaction of the shaft into the head
- No history of dislocation

If the fracture is stable, gentle and careful movements of the affected arm can be performed with no or very little pain during a physical examination. This should only be done after imaging, though.

Signs of instability are:

- Significant displacement with segments angulated more than 45° or displaced more than 0.5–1 cm from their normal anatomical position, best detected on the axial view [31].
- A difference in fragment angulation between plain x-rays and CT scans with 2-D reconstruction along the axes of the humerus.
- Extraordinary pain which does not subside with adequate pain medication within a few days.

### 2.5 Classification

Codman's 4-part model laid the foundations of modern understanding of PHFs. All of the following classifications were based on the four parts, ie, the shaft, GT, LT, and the head fragment. The most common classifications used over the last decades were the Neer and the AO/OTA classifications. Both systems are characterized by a poor interobserver reliability [32, 33] which improves with advanced imaging like 3-D CT scans [34], education and experience [35].

### 2.5.1 Neer's classification

Neer focused on the patterns of displacement rather than the location of fracture lines. In his retrospective study he attempted to identify fractures that would benefit from open reduction. Similar to Hertel, he also wanted to predict the risk of avascular necrosis (AVN) which again would have an impact on decision making (see topic 2.5.2 in this chapter). Neer's system remains the most commonly used today, because it is easy to apply and yet has a prognostic value. Four-part fractures generally have worse outcomes than 2- and 3-part fractures regardless of the treatment.

Neer randomly defined the borderline between displaced and nondisplaced at a displacement of 1 cm and an angulation of 45°. A fracture that is below this threshold is called 1-part fracture irrespective of the number of fragments.

These criteria have evolved to make a displacement of 5 mm or more an acceptable indication for fixation provided the direction of displacement creates a functional limitation. A good example is the superior displacement of the GT, which has the potential of restricting abduction.

### 2.5.2 Hertel's classification

Hertel [36] fundamentally changed the approach by using a binary system based on Lego bricks. He proposed fracture planes instead of fracture fragments. To classify a fracture, possible fracture planes between head and GT, GT and shaft, head and LT, LT and shaft, and finally between GT and LT need to be identified.

This results in six options for 2-part fractures, five for 3-part fractures and obviously just one 4-part fracture. In contrast to Neer, Hertel rated any cortical discontinuity as a fracture irrespective of the amount of displacement or angulation. Particular attention has to be paid to seven other parameters, such as the length of the posteromedial metaphyseal head extension, the integrity of the medial hinge with displacement of the shaft in respect to the head, the displacement of the tuberosities, the amount of angular displacement of the head, the occurrence of glenohumeral dislocation, a head impression fracture, a head-split component and the mechanical quality of the bone.

### 2.5.3 Hertel's modified classification

Sukthankar et al [37] modified Hertel's system by replacing numbers with a comprehensive nomenclature. H(ead), G(reater) and L(esser tuberosity) and S(haft) identify possible fracture parts, a fracture plane is represented by a hyphen (-) and represents a cortical disruption between the parts, regardless of displacement and angulation. H-G-L-S therefore indicates the classic 4-part fracture. The letter "d"(dislocation) as a prefix to "H" and "c" followed by the length of the intact calcar fragment in millimeters as postfix in brackets can be added as well as "a" for the head-neck angulation. The simplicity and intuitive nature of this nomenclature may be the reason for a higher reliability compared to the original Hertel, AO/OTA, and Neer systems.

Prediction of head necrosis does not play an important role in decision making in geriatric patients. Fracture pattern interpretation mainly serves to differentiate stable from unstable fractures and to forecast the likelihood of achieving a stable fixation.

## 2.6 Summary

Clinical evaluation:

- In addition to fracture pattern analysis, the patient's functional and cognitive status must be considered to determine the best approach.
- Nonfracture-related geriatric parameters play an important role in choosing the adequate therapeutic approach for each individual patient.

Imaging:

- The main purpose of imaging PHF is to determine instability and fragment displacement.
- Standardized views are paramount to determine angulation, displacement, and detection of any changes postoperatively.
- The axial view displays instability and displacement between shaft and head and should be part of the standard trauma x-ray series.
- CT scans should be used for precise fracture analysis and measurement of local bone density. Two- and three-dimensional reconstructions are essential for precise classification and surgical planning.

Classification:

- Codman's 4-part model and Neer's classification (1970) are still the basis for understanding PHFs [31].
- Hertel's system and the HGLS classification are recommended for more detailed description of the fracture situation.
- Other factors like the degree of shaft displacement and angulation/rotation of the head fragment should also be described.

## 3 Decision making

Since little high-level evidence exists, there is still much uncertainty about which patients will benefit from nonoperative treatment, plate fixation, nailing, or arthroplasty [38, 39]. Overall, conflicting results between studies favoring operative intervention and others failing to show much benefit for more displaced and unstable fractures have been described. This demands careful consideration of the patient-specific benefits and risks of operative and nonoperative therapy [22].

Older patients tend to have worse functional outcomes [30]. This trend has been attributed to factors such as fragility, cognitive deficits, rotator cuff injuries, osteoporosis, and poor rehabilitation potential [40].

The indication for surgery in PHFs is usually a relative one. Therefore comorbidities play an important role in deciding whether or not to perform surgery. In cases where deterioration of comorbid medical conditions like renal insufficiency is likely to happen, it is usually better to refrain from surgery even if the fracture type would justify it.

General remarks and thoughts:

- The severity of comminution in displaced fractures may have a more significant effect on functional outcomes than the choice of treatment; there is also a clear difference in prognosis between 3- and 4-part fractures, but not between 2- and 3-part fractures [5]. In many studies 4-part fractures yielded worse outcomes compared to 2- or 3-part fractures regardless of the treatment chosen [41].
- The functional outcome is difficult to assess, as many variables contribute to a successful patient outcome. Fortunately, functional expectations for older individuals are lower than for younger patients—a less than satisfactory result for a young patient can therefore be completely acceptable for an older person. Even with decreased outcome scores, older patients' perception of outcome and quality of life can be acceptable [30].
- As evidence supporting routine operative treatment is limited and complication rates are high, decision making should include individual factors such as living situations, comorbidities, and the patient's attitude towards surgery. With surgeons' increasing knowledge about appropriate patient selection and limits of specific procedures, results become more predictable. That means, however, that more than one operative method is necessary to address different situations.
- If we think about operative fixation, it seems expedient to ask what kind of difference the patient will experience after surgery. There must be some tangible benefit in terms of an increased functional result. This also holds true if an older patient's functional status benefits from immediate use of the injured extremity by using a cane, for instance (**Case 4: Fig 3.1-15**).
- It is helpful to discuss all relevant aspects among the interdisciplinary team members in addition to the patient and relatives. If the patient seems motivated to make use of an expedited rehabilitation process after surgery and has no contraindications, the patient may receive the same treatment as a younger adult (**Case 5: Fig 3.1-16**).
- With enhanced techniques like the use of fibular strut grafting or allograft bone blocks, better and more reliable results can be achieved both in younger and in geriatric patients (**Case 6: Fig 3.1-17**) [16, 42].
- As in other areas, outcomes may also be correlated with the level of surgeon experience, the time of surgery and the soft-tissue handling. These potentially important factors are hardly ever reported or investigated in studies and neither is the precise amount of displacement with a standardized CT scan measurement.

## Potential benefit of operative fixation in geriatric patients

### Patient

A 90-year-old woman sustained a left pertrochanteric fracture after a fall from standing height and was treated with a proximal femoral nail antirotation (PFNA) plus augmentation. She was living alone and mostly self-reliant with some help from her daughter who lived close by. No signs of dementia and she was cooperative and go-go, ie, fit. Osteoporosis treatment was initiated and the patient has been using a walking cane ever since.

### Comorbidities

- Hypertension
- Chronic renal deficiency
- Heart failure
- Osteoporosis (T-score: spine = -3.6, hip = -3.6).

### Treatment and outcome

Five months later the patient presented with a 2-part surgical neck fracture (HGL-S) after a low-energy trauma at home with medial comminution and varus displacement (**Fig 3.1-15a–e**). After careful and extensive consultation with the team, the patient and her daughter decided on operative treatment. Stable fixation was achieved with PHILOS augmentation (**Fig 3.1-15f–g**). Nonanatomical plate position was chosen to maintain the medial support, which was achieved by slight shortening and impaction of the shaft into the head, as well as a slight valgus position of the head fragment. Peri-implant augmentation with 0.5 cc of polymethylmethacrylate cement per cannulated screw was used. With this measure, additional fixation was added. Five days after surgery, pain restricted the patient's mobilization and usage of the affected arm (**Fig 3.1-15h**); this made it impossible for her to return home as early as possible and to limit care dependency to a minimum. After 12 days the patient was transferred to the internal medicine and rehabilitation department.

Six weeks postoperatively a comparison with previous x-rays was not possible, as they were blurred by different projections. Active flexion and abduction was 140°, active rotation in 90°, and abduction 80°. She used a cane to support the right side; she was pain free (**i–l**) and back home.

### Other treatment options

- Nonoperative treatment: The patient would be unable to use crutches at least for some time because of pain and she would depend on care. It is likely that the fracture would displace more and could lead to a more restricted functional outcome.
- Proximal nailing would be a good alternative, as the reduction in valgus and shortening would be beneficial.
- Hemiarthroplasty and reverse arthroplasty are not an option for this type of fracture (overtreatment).

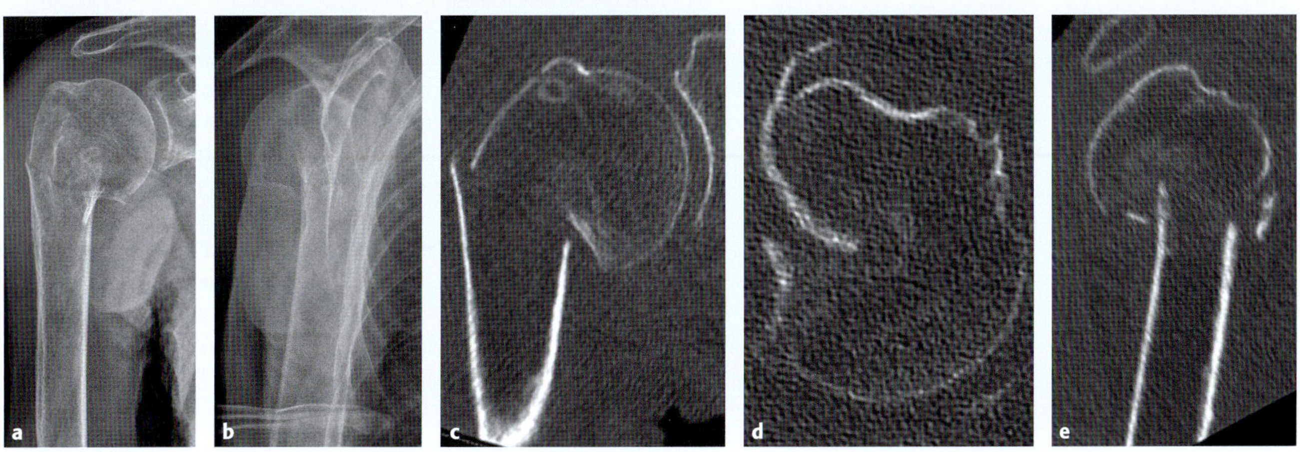


**Fig 3.1-15a–l** A 90-year-old woman after a low-energy trauma.
**a–e** X-rays showing a 2-part surgical neck fracture with medial comminution and varus displacement. Note the poor bone quality and the shallow head fragment in the computed tomographic scan reconstructions (**a–d**).

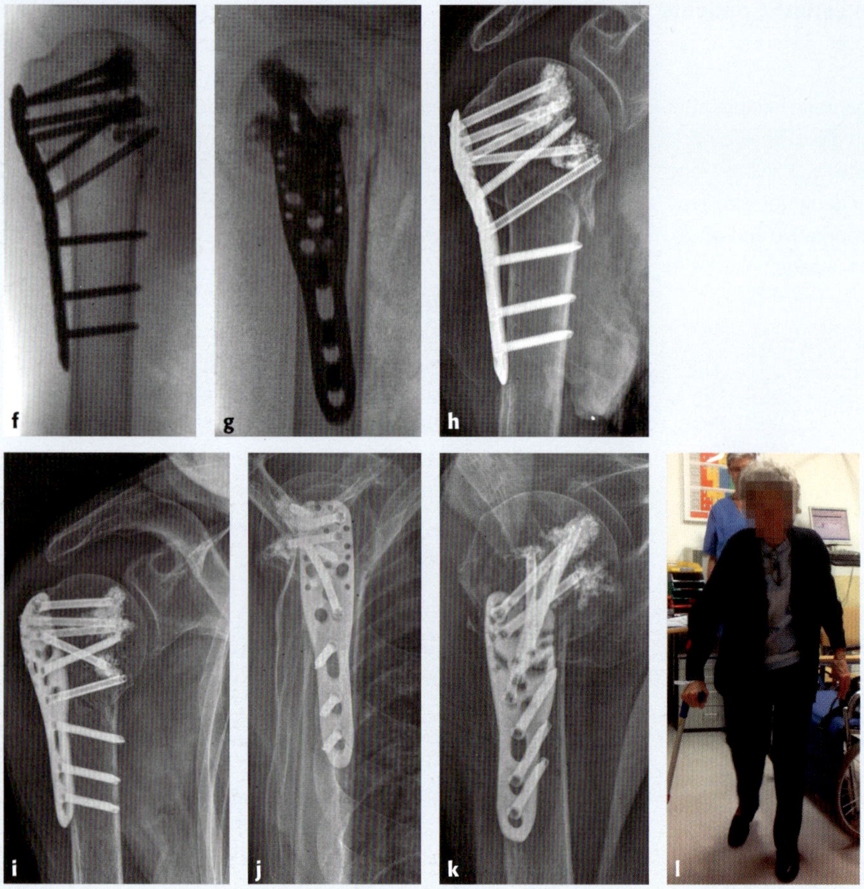


**Fig 3.1-15a–l (cont)** A 90-year-old woman after a low-energy trauma.
**f–g** Stable fixation was achieved with PHILOS augmentation. The medial support is maintained by nonanatomical plate position.
**h** X-ray at 5 days postoperative.
**i–l** Six-week postoperative x-rays and clincal image of pain-free patient.

CASE 5

## Operative fixation for rapid rehabilitation

### Patient

A 71-year-old woman was living an active social life. She was motivated, cooperative and go-go, ie, fit. The patient sustained a valgus-impacted 4-part fracture (H(c0)-G-L-S) (**Fig 3.1-16a–c**). The medial head extension was 0 mm, which indicated a high risk of avascular necrosis (**Fig 3.1-16d–f**).

### Comorbidities

- Arterial hypertension
- Varicosis
- Polyarthritis
- Osteoporosis

### Treatment and outcome

The patient opted for surgery. Due to the osteoporotic bone, an anatomomical reduction and stable osteosynthesis with PHILOS augmentation was accomplished (**Fig 3.1-16g–i**). Immediate active rehabilitation without sling and without relevant postoperative pain led to an excellent active range of motion (ROM) after 3 weeks (**Fig 3.1-16j**).

One year later the fracture healed uneventfully without secondary displacement (**Fig 3.1-16k–l**). The patient achieved full ROM without pain (**Fig 3.1-16m–o**).

### Other treatment options

- According to the current authors' treatment algorithm, displaced 4-part fractures in go-go, ie, fit, patients should be treated operatively.
- Nonoperative treatment may lead to consecutive cranial and/or posterior greater tuberosity (GT) displacement with functional impairment in abduction and rotation.
- Osteotomies after malunions of the GT usually fail to heal in proper position. With a varus malunion, an anatomical prosthetic solution is also no longer possible.
- According to the current authors' opinion antegrade nailing is not the first choice in 4-part fractures.
- Arthroplasty was not an option because a stable and anatomical reconstruction was to be expected.

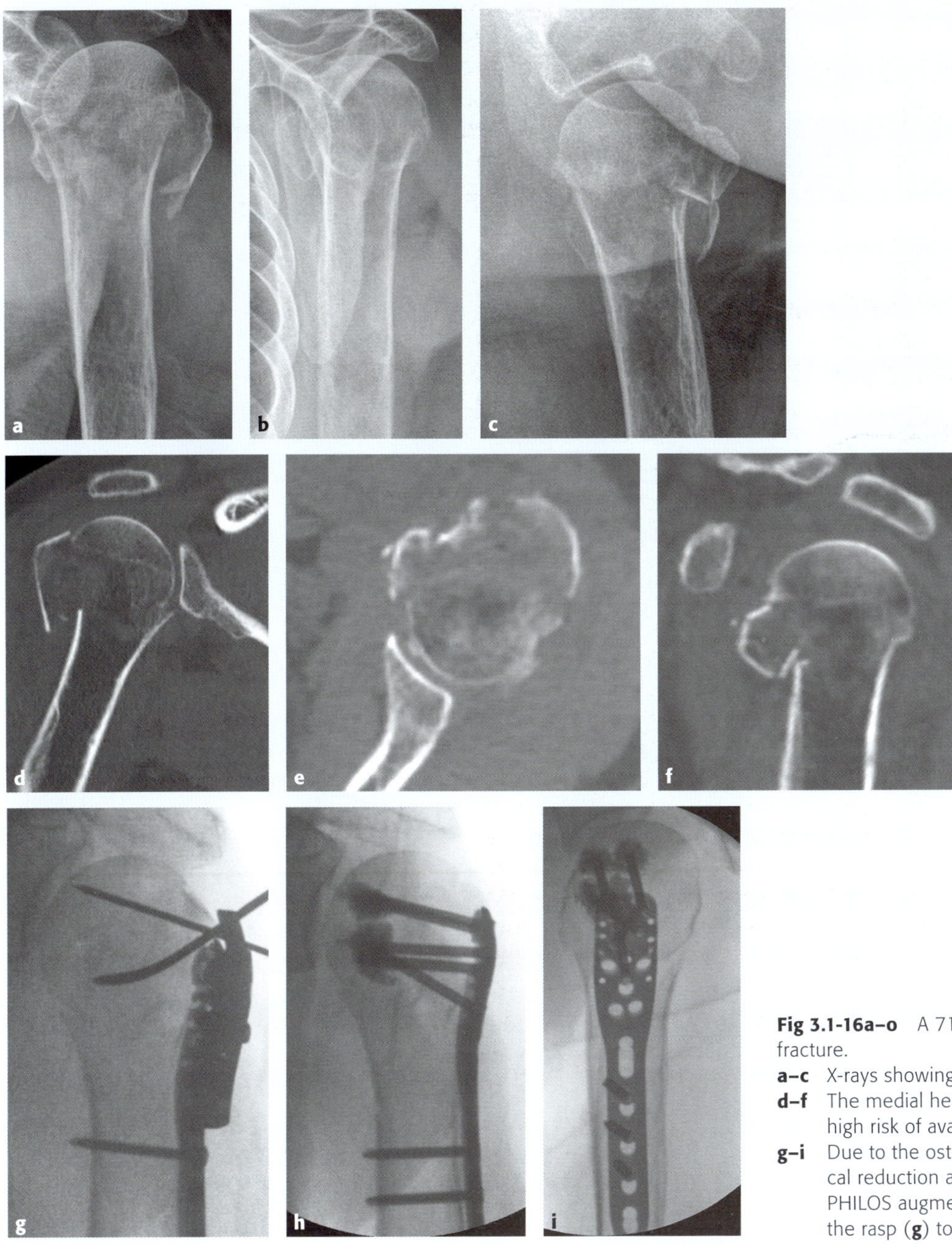

**Fig 3.1-16a–o** A 71-year-old woman with a 4-part fracture.
**a–c** X-rays showing valgus-impacted 4-part fracture.
**d–f** The medial head extension of 0 mm indicates a high risk of avascular necrosis.
**g–i** Due to the osteoporotic bone, an anatomomical reduction and stable osteosynthesis with PHILOS augmentation was accomplished. Note the rasp (**g**) to elevate the head fragment.

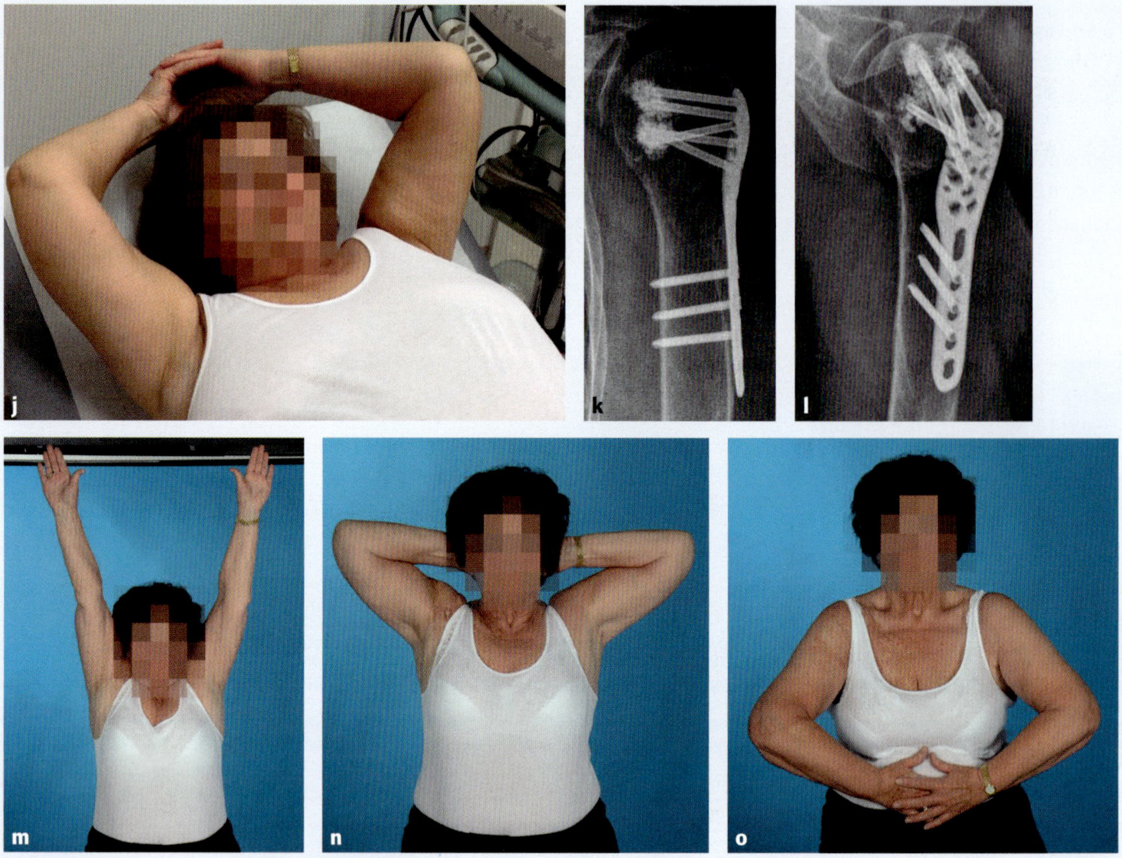

**Fig 3.1-16a–o (cont)** A 71-year-old woman with a 4-part fracture.
**j** Clinical photograph showing excellent active range of motion (ROM) after 3 weeks due to immediate active rehabilitation without sling and without relevant postoperative pain.
**k–l** One year later the fracture healed uneventfully without secondary displacement.
**m–o** The patient achieved full ROM without pain.

CASE 6

## Massive central allograft to ease reduction and prevent secondary displacement of fracture fragments

### Patient

A 65-year-old female patient sustained a low-energy trauma resulting in a 4-part fracture (H-G-L-S). The patient suffered from chronic alcoholism. Although she was not cognitively impaired, her compliance was uncertain.

### Comorbidities

- Osteoporosis with a wide proximal shaft and rarefied cancellous bone

### Treatment and outcome

The head was in varus, the greater tuberosity severely comminuted and ultrashort, ie, without lateral extension that could be fixed directly with the plate. The patient also suffered from osteoporosis with a wide proximal shaft and rarefied cancellous bone, as the computed tomographic scan of the opposite proximal humerus showed (**Fig 3.1-17a–c**). The head fragment was damaged by the shaft and the patient complained about pain (**Fig 3.1-17d**). This led the authors to decide on reconstruction with allograft. The allograft resembling a champagne cork (**Fig 3.1-17e**) locked itself in the shaft and the head fragment and the tuberosities sat on the graft (**Fig 3.1-17f–g**). The ultrashort greater tuberosity was fixed transosseously to the graft without additional hardware (**Fig 3.1-17h**). The intraoperative C-arm follow-ups (**Fig 3.1-17i–j**) demonstrated the huge allograft supporting the reconstruction (**Fig 3.1-17i**). Follow-up x-rays were taken after 1 week (**Fig 3.1-17k–m**).

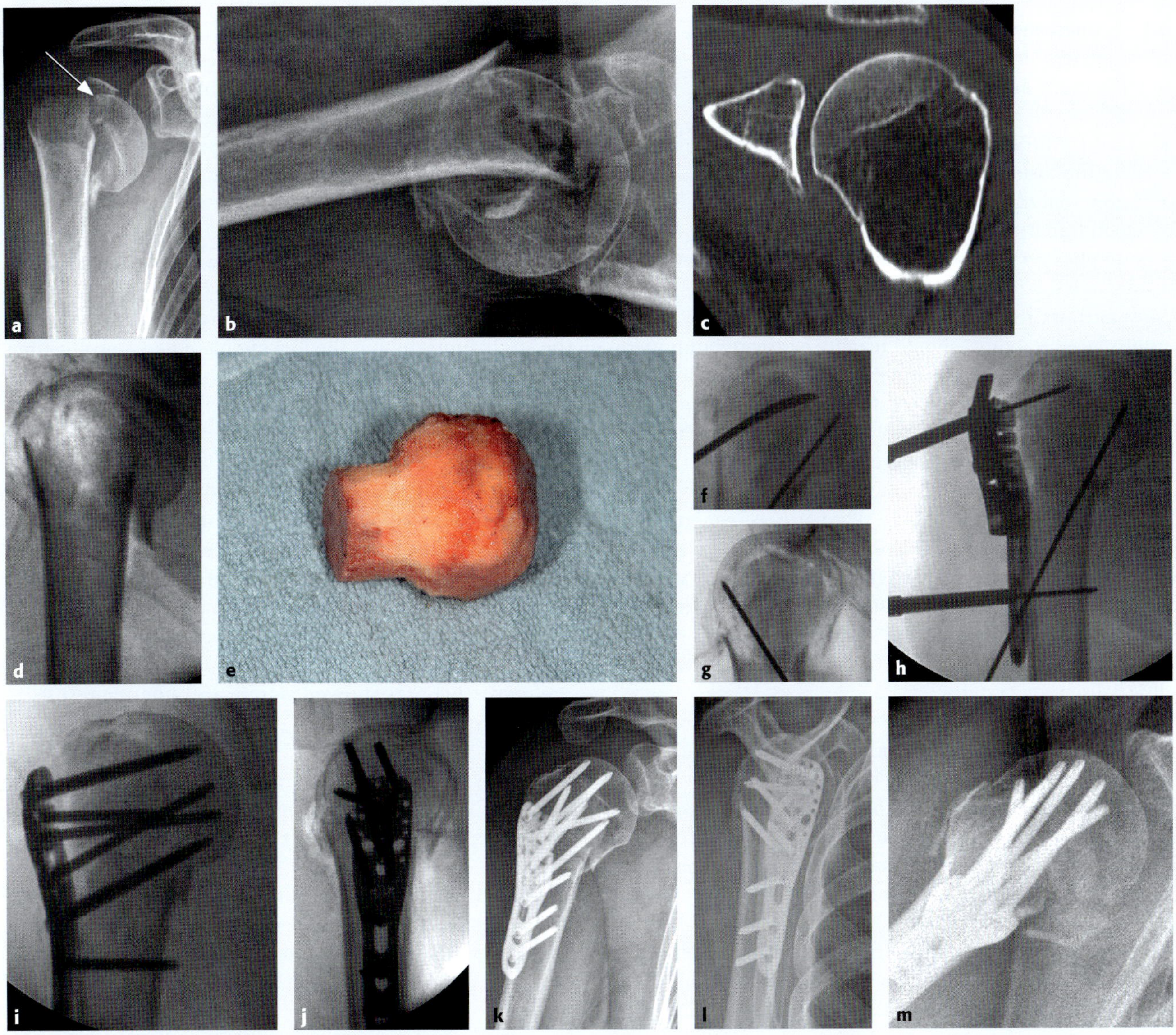

**Fig 3.1-17a–m** A 65-year-old woman with a 4-part fracture after a low-energy trauma.

**a–c** X-rays (**a–b**) showing the head in varus, the greater tuberosity severely comminuted and ultrashort, ie, without lateral extension that could be fixed directly with the plate. Osteoporosis with a wide proximal shaft and rarefied cancellous bone is visible on the computed tomographic scan of the opposite proximal humerus (**c**).

**d–h** X-ray showing the head fragment damaged by the shaft (**d**). Reconstruction performed with allograft that resembles a champagne cork (**e**) and locked itself in the shaft and the head fragment and the tuberosities sitting on the graft (**f–g**). The ultrashort greater tuberosity was fixed transosseously to the graft without additional hardware (**h**).

**i–j** Intraoperative C-arm follow-ups showing the huge allograft supporting the reconstruction (**i**).

**k–m** Follow-up x-rays at 1 week.

## 3.1 Operative or nonoperative?

More or less undisputed indications for surgery even in older patients are:

- Head-split fracture
- Fracture dislocation
- Segmental fracture
- Open fracture
- Complicated fracture with additional vascular injury

Most authors also agree that according to the Neer criteria, undisplaced fractures should usually be treated nonoperatively, irrespective of the number of fragments. Moreover, a lack of consistently successful surgical techniques and common complications has resulted in a preference for nonoperative treatment over surgery [6, 43].

Clinical experience has shown that patients regularly benefit from operative fixation even if it is only for the first few weeks after the trauma. The effect of a pain-free extremity on patients, especially on older ones, may be strikingly positive. As mentioned in the introduction of this chapter, it may be difficult to measure this kind of success with traditional scoring systems.

Careful decision making and safe procedures, ie, with a limited risk and performed to the best of the surgeon's knowledge, are required, as everything must be done to avoid complications. The worst outcomes usually result from poor open surgery and soft-tissue handling during surgery leading to unstable fracture fixation.

It is often observed that the functional status deteriorates after sustaining a PHF. Patients immediately become dependent on help and in many instances require full-time nursing care, at least temporarily. If this could be prevented by operative fixation, which has been demonstrated only by anecdotal evidence, operative fixation would be a good option for some patients. The patient's living condition also has an impact on making a therapeutic decision.

In **Table 3.1-1** different aspects and parameters are discussed.

### 3.1.1 Outcome

At 1-year follow-up of a randomized controlled trial (RCT), Fjalestad et al [44] found no evident difference in functional outcome between operative treatment and nonoperative treatment of displaced PHFs in older patients. Only radiographic scores turned out to be better after operative interventions.

Only one RCT exists comparing 3-part PHFs treated nonoperatively versus with a locking plate. Olerud et al [2] investigated 60 patients aged 74 years on average. The results of the study indicate that the locking plate had a positive impact on the functional outcome and health-related quality of life (HRQoL), but at the cost of additional surgery in 30% of the patients.

In another RCT, fracture arthroplasty and nonoperative treatment were compared. 55 patients, aged 77 years, ie, 58–92 years, on average, with displaced 4-part fractures were randomly allocated to the two treatment options and monitored for 2 years. The Constant score, ROM, DASH score and pain (visual or verbal analogue scale) did not differ significantly among the patients. The quality of life assessment (EQ-5D) showed significantly better results in favor of surgery [45].

Metaanalyses of 3- and 4-part fractures revealed that patients treated nonoperatively had more pain and a worse ROM than those treated with either fixation or arthroplasty [46].

Van den Broek et al [47] compared antegrade nailing (n = 27) with nonoperative treatment (n = 16). The Constant score was 67.1 in the nailing group and 81.4 in the nonsurgical group.

Krettek et al [6] compared two PHF studies dealing with patients after nonoperative and operative treatments respectively, supported by the AO Clinical Investigation and Documentation (AOCID) team. They found more complications (34% versus 28.8%), more revision surgeries (19% versus 7.2%) and a 10% lower Constant score in the surgical group.

The extent to which PHFs impact functionality of geriatric patients has not yet been thoroughly investigated. Einsiedel et al [4] described a significant deterioration of walking ability, leading to two or more new falls in 24% of patients with distal radial fractures (DRFs) and 28% of PHF patients in a prospective study of 104 patients.

| | Nonoperative treatment | Grey zone | Operative treatment |
|---|---|---|---|
| **Findings in favor of pain** | | | • Patient cannot be managed with ambulatory care because of fracture-related pain<br>• Crepitation as a sign for instability |
| **Displacement of the GT** | • Nondisplaced<br>• No displacement during follow-up | • Short GT fragment with lateral comminution and impaction: difficult to address operatively<br>• "Functional 2-part fracture" (with multiple fracture lines of the GT fragment, yet undisplaced), good medial support of the head fragment | • Posterosuperior displacement of GT of > 0.5 cm: GT overlaps the posterior articular surface with loss of external rotation and early glenoidal impingement<br>• Cranialization of GT into the subacromial space<br>• Large GT fragment with high success rate after fixation |
| **Displacement shaft** | • Nondisplaced and stable<br>• Impacted | | • > 50% displacement<br>• Unstable medial hinge |
| **Angulation head vs shaft** | • < 45° varus/valgus<br>• < 45° anteversion/retroversion | • Stable operative fixation is questionable because of medial comminution, allograft is an alternative | • > 45° varus/valgus<br>• > 45° anteversion/retroversion |
| **Calcar** | | • Stable surgical fixation is questionable because of medial comminution<br>• Impaction must result in medial stability, otherwise bone grafting | • Calcar can be perfectly reduced |
| **Use of walking aids** | • Has to use walking aids | • If the patient cannot be mobilized within the first week, augmented fixation may be considered | |
| **Surgical skills and feasability** | • Doubts that the surgeon will be able to accomplish it<br>• The worst case is a failed surgery | | • The surgeon is able to do it right because of the size of the fragments, a long cortical extension of the GT fragment and other fracture characteristics like the feasibility of creating intraoperatively intrinsic stability |
| **Concomitant injuries or disabilities** | • With cuff arthropathy, nonoperative treatment may be preferred<br>• In case of problems, a reversed arthoplasty is indicated | • Compensated cuff arthropathy with good function may be a good nailing indication | • Multilevel injuries |
| **Low bone quality** | • May have an impact on the choice of operative treatment but not on the question of whether operative treatment is indicated | | |
| **Age, comorbidities, functional status** | • No-go or frail patients. They are mostly ≥ 85 years, suffer from three or more comorbidities and geriatric syndromes, and are constantly limited in their daily activities | • Slow-go, intermediate or vulnerable patients may be dependent in one or more IADLs but not ADLs, and suffer from one to two comorbidities but no geriatric syndromes | • Go-go or fit patients are functionally independent in terms of ADLs and IADLs and without serious comorbidities or geriatric syndromes |
| **Compliance, mental status, abuse** | • Dementia<br>• In patients with polytoxicomania there is only risk and barely any benefit | • Demanding and cooperative | • Normal or slightly impaired<br>• Highly motivated |
| **Risk of surgery** | • High | • Moderate | • Low |
| **Rehabilitation potential** | • Mostly sitting only, needs constant care | | • High |
| **Functional expectations** | • Low | | • High |
| **Financial aspects** | No significant difference between operative and nonoperative treatment [44] | | |

**Table 3.1-1** Nonoperative versus operative treatment. Factors that may influence decision making in proximal humeral fractures. Items where either direction is possible are in the "grey zone".
Abbreviations: ADLs, activities of daily living; GT, greater tuberosity; IADLs, instrumental activities of daily living.

## 3.2 Fixation or arthroplasty?

The question whether stable fixation will be possible is much more important in terms of the predicted outcome than the presumed extent of AVN. Therefore, if stable fixation is possible, there is no need to be concerned about future osteonecrosis.

Whether stable fixation is possible may be questionable mainly in 4-part fractures. In critical cases, ie, cases with a low probability of achieving stable fixation, surgeons should be prepared to perform joint replacement. In cases where stable fixation turns out to be impossible and the surgeon does not feel comfortable performing arthroplasty, it may be advisable to get the help of an experienced team to preliminarily fix the fracture with K-wires and perform an early secondary arthroplasty procedure.

## 3.3 Treatment algorithm

In the authors' own practices, approximately 30% of all fractures with pronounced comminution and/or dislocation are treated operatively. The majority of all PHFs are minimally or nondisplaced and can therefore be successfully treated without surgery. It should also be taken into consideration that many studies are older and retrospective and focus mainly on objective parameters like ROM or x-rays. Patients are getting older nowadays and attitudes and demands may change.

Fragile patients have limited reserves of physical strength and even short-term functional decline may be difficult to compensate. Some patients may therefore benefit from operative fixation to restore functionality earlier.

Obviously, one type of treatment does not fit all pathologies and patient profiles. Most surgical methods can be applied to a variety of fracture types, but they each have strengths and weaknesses. Avoiding complications is one of the main goals, so surgeons should be able to choose between modalities servicing their actual need, which also includes arthroplasty.

The following questions need to be answered in daily practice:

- Are the fracture fragments displaced enough to require surgery?
- Is the patient a good candidate for surgery ie, mentally fit and demanding?
- Is the surgical risk within the normal range?
- Is it unlikely to produce a surgical complication?

The type of treatment will be decided based on the criteria listed in **Table 3.1-2**.

## 3.4 Summary

Decision making:

- Though improving, evidence is not yet sufficient to allow for robust treatment recommendations. Surgeons' skills and preferences play an important role. Most current treatment recommendations are based on expert opinion and low-powered studies.
- Treatment with locked plates and antegrade nails has failed to demonstrate better results than nonoperative treatment and is fraught with a complication rate of ~ 30%.
- Selection of patients suitable for a particular treatment seems to be of paramount importance. Criteria for a successful outcome have not yet been fully identified.
- In patients older than 60 years, nonoperative and operative protocols, including arthroplasty, yield similar functional results despite better x-rays after operative fixation. Operative indications must therefore be well justified individually.
- Obvious operative indications are fracture dislocations, head-split fractures, open fractures, pathological fractures, and segmental fractures.
- For patients unfit for surgery or with important risk factors indicating deterioration after operative, surgical procedures should only be suggested with great caution and in accordance with the whole orthogeriatric team.
- Nonoperative treatment is indicated in simple and nondisplaced PHFs. The same approach may apply in selected cases of more complex injuries and if patients are unfit for surgery.
- Arthroplasty should only be chosen if all other options will presumably fail.

| Grade | Explanation of activity |
|---|---|
| 0 | Fully active, able to carry on all predisease performance without restriction |
| 1 | Restricted in physically strenuous activity but ambulatory and able to carry out work of a light or sedentary nature, eg, light house work, office work |
| 2 | Ambulatory and capable of all self-care but unable to carry out any work activities. Up and about more than 50% of waking hours |
| 3 | Capable of only limited self-care, confined to bed or chair more than 50% of waking hours |
| 4 | Completely disabled. Cannot carry on any self-care. Totally confined to bed or chair |
| 5 | Dead |

**Table 3.1-2** World Health Organization performance status.

## 4 Therapeutic options

Apart from nonoperative treatment, several operative options are at the surgeon's disposal, but there are no evidence-based recommendations to specifically guide selection.

General remarks and thoughts:

- Soft-tissue handling is critical for a successful outcome, but it has not been studied in detail. It is the factor often not considered in any study and may not be comparable even if the type of fracture, approach, and implant are the same.
- Open fixation must result in a stable construct which allows for immediate postoperative physiotherapy. If this is not achievable, a prosthetic replacement should be used. Sometimes it is necessary to switch strategies during an operation.
- Angular stable implants alone do not solve the problem. Anatomical reduction with either cortical contact or void filling must also be provided in order to prevent secondary displacement of parts with subsequent cut-through or cut-out of screws.
- It seems important to mention again that nonoperative treatment is more desirable than a poorly performed operative procedure regardless of the method of fixation [13]. The surgeon must know the chosen method very well.
- At the moment, discussion about anatomical hemiarthroplasty and reverse arthroplasty is open; there are no clear guidelines for the orthopedic trauma surgeon to treat these disabling fractures in geriatric patients.

### 4.1 Nonoperative treatment

The vast majority of PHF are successfully treated nonoperatively. The rotator cuff, remnants of periosteum and capsular tissue (so-called ligamentotaxis effect) often provide enough intrinsic stability to resist further displacement of fracture fragments. Minimal tuberosity displacement combined with controlled shaft impaction reduces the risk of nonunion.

#### 4.1.1 Pain treatment

Initial pain control after the injury includes a combination of oral medications, topical modalities, and sling immobilization. Providing adequate pain control over the first couple of days after injury is of paramount importance for functional recovery.

Regional nerve blocks like the interscalene block, ie, Winnie block, the supraclavicular perivascular (subclavian perivascular) block or the suprascapular nerve block should be considered.

Exercises should never be painful, otherwise a complex regional pain syndrome may result.

#### 4.1.2 Fracture reduction

Attempts to reduce a PHF have little, if any, effect on rates of malalignment or functional outcomes. Given the potential risk for soft-tissue and plexus injuries caused by manipulation, surgeons should critically reconsider the indication for fracture reduction (**Case 7: Fig 3.1-18**) [48]. Moreover, the typical varus malalignment may develop after several weeks (**Case 8: Fig 3.1-19**) and is not predictive of the outcome [49].

CASE 7

## Spontaneous realignment with nonoperative treatment

### Patient

Nonoperative treatment of a proximal humeral fracture (PHF) in an 87-year-old woman.

### Treatment and outcome

Five years before PHF the patient sustained a displaced, intraarticular right distal radial fracture (**Fig 3.1-18a**) that healed after nonoperative management with acceptable malalignment (**Fig 3.1-18b–c**). Initially, the 2-part PHF was minimally displaced (**Fig 3.1-18d–e**).

The patient was treated with a sling. After 1 week pronounced displacement could be seen in a true AP view (**Fig 3.1-18f**). The fracture was still markedly displaced 2 and 4 weeks later (**Fig 3.1-18g–h**). After 6 weeks the situation improved (**Fig 3.1-18i**) and after 10 weeks the fracture progressed to healing in a good position (**Fig 3.1-18j–k**).

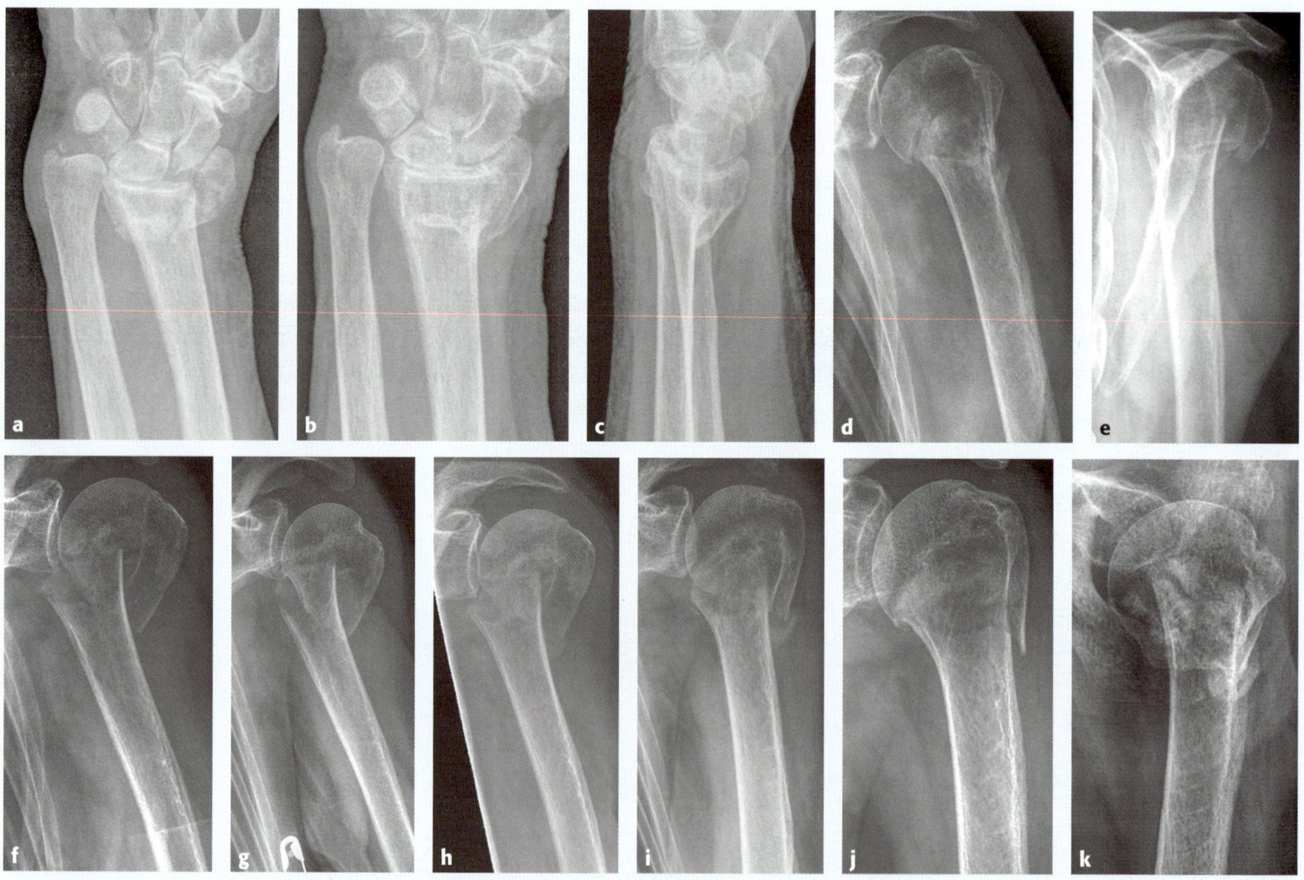


**Fig 3.1-18a–k** An 81-year-old woman with a 2-part fracture.
**a–e** X-rays showing a displaced, intraarticular right distal radial fracture (**a**) that healed with acceptable malalignment after nonoperative treatment (**b–c**). Initial displacement of the 2-part proximal humeral fracture occurred (**d–e**).
**f–k** True AP view (**f**) at 1 week showing pronounced displacement. X-rays showing the still markedly displaced fracture at 2 and 4 weeks (**g–h**) but improved situation at 6 weeks (**i**) and fracture progressing to healing in good position at 10 weeks (**j–k**).

## Typical course of nonoperative treatment

### Patient

An 81-year-old woman in excellent condition sustained a 2-part fracture.

### Comorbidities

- No relevant comorbidities but obvious radiological signs of severe osteoporosis.

### Treatment and outcome

The 2-part fracture (**Fig 3.1-19a–b**) showed obvious radiological signs of osteoporosis (25-hydroxyvitamin D3: 11.2 ng/mL [28 nmol/L]; PTH: 56 μg/L; T-score: lumbar spine = -2.0; proximal femur = -2.2). The patient was administered 3 mg IV of ibandronate every 3 months, 1,000 mg of calcium, 400 IU of vitamin D. Otherwise, the patient was in excellent condition without relevant comorbidities.

Nonoperative treatment was chosen. The patient's arm was put in a sling, adequate pain treatment was administered (**Fig 3.1-19c–d**), and the arm was mobilized as soon as possible. After 4 weeks the alignment was good and the patient had little pain (**Fig 3.1-19e**). After 9 weeks the fracture was well aligned and the function improved (**Fig 3.1-19f–g**). Five months after the injury the typical varus malalignment by continuous pull of the supraspinatus muscle occurred (**Fig 3.1-19h–i**).

The function was excellent and the patient was satisfied with the outcome (**Fig 3.1-19j–m**).

At the 5-year follow-up, the patient broke her right proximal femur which was treated with a proximal femoral nail antirotation augmentation (**Fig 3.1-19n–o**). The T-score of the opposite hip was -3.4 and of the lumbar spine was -2.3. A computed tomographic scan of her right shoulder revealed a stable nonunion of the proximal humeral fracture without any complaints and near to normal function (**Fig 3.1-19p–q**).

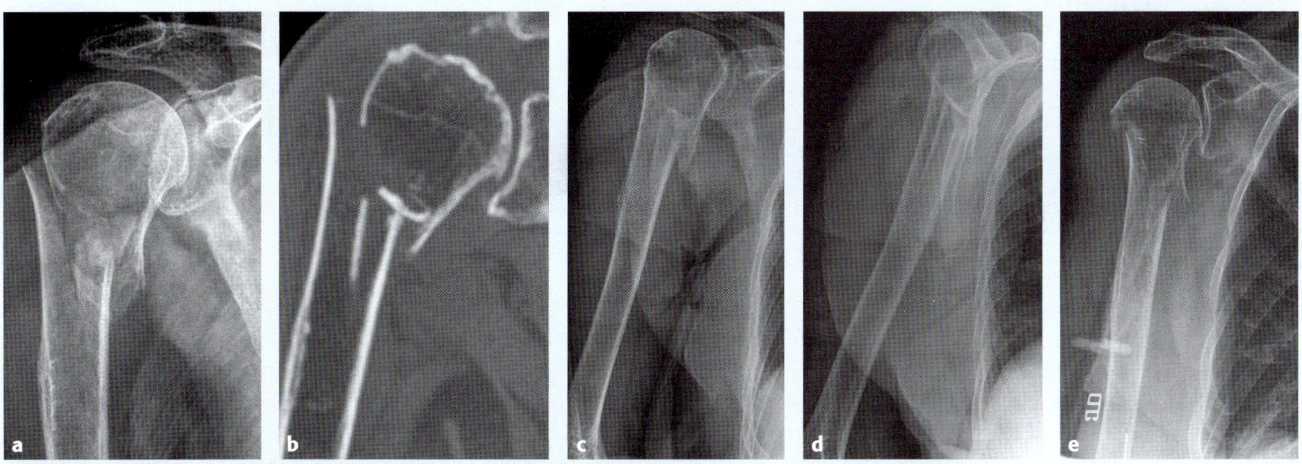


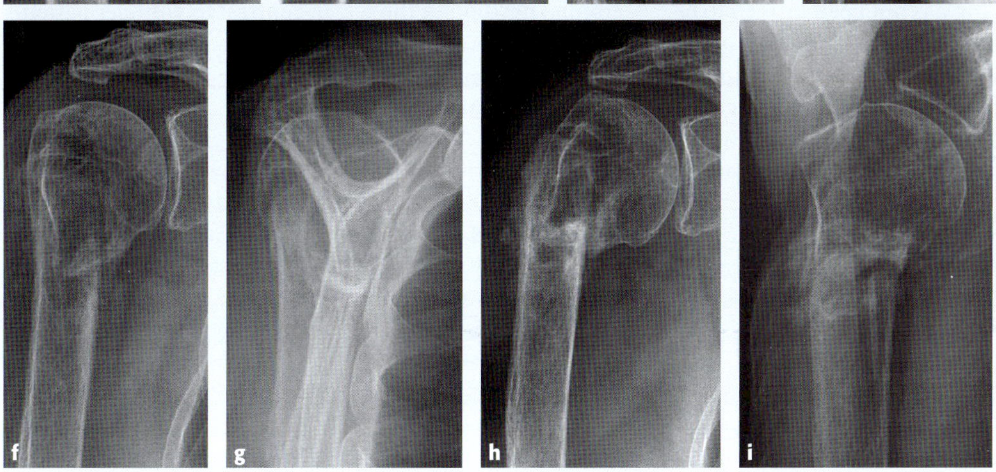


**Fig 3.1-19a–q** An 81-year-old woman with a 2-part fracture.
**a–b** X-rays showing a 2-part fracture with obvious radiological signs of osteoporosis.
**c–e** X-rays after nonoperative treatment, ie, arm in sling (**c–d**), showing good alignment (**e**).
**f–g** Well-aligned fracture after 9 weeks.
**h–i** X-rays 5 months post-injury showing typical varus malalignment.

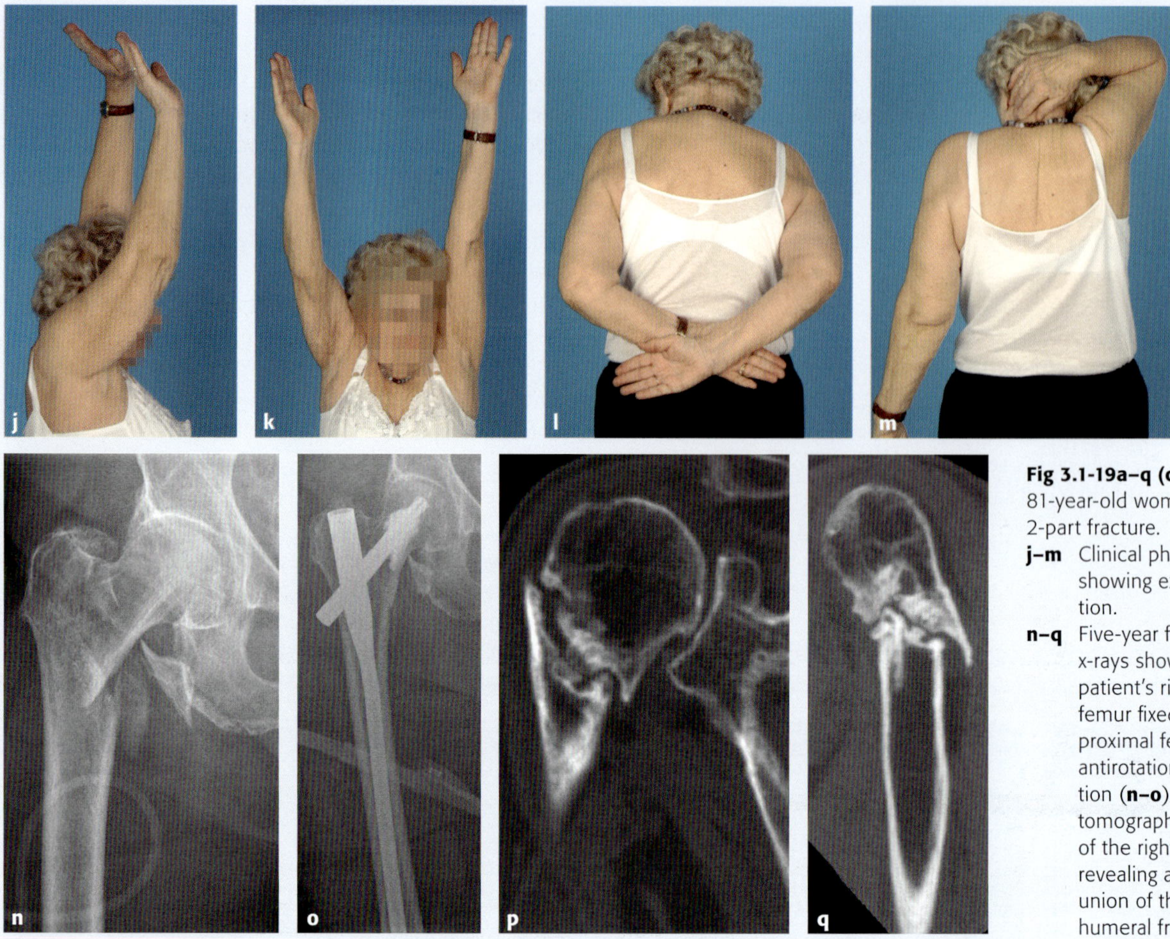


**Fig 3.1-19a–q (cont)** An 81-year-old woman with a 2-part fracture.
**j–m** Clinical photographs showing excellent function.
**n–q** Five-year follow-up x-rays showing the patient's right proximal femur fixed with a proximal femoral nail antirotation augmentation (**n–o**). Computed tomographic scans of the right shoulder revealing a stable nonunion of the proximal humeral fracture (**p–q**).

### 4.1.3 Immobilization

Generally, the treatment strategy should be as functional as possible, allowing patients to use their injured shoulder as much as pain allows (**Table 3.1-1**). Prolonged immobilization with a Gilchrist type of sling has not been proven to be effective. The authors encourage patients to use their upper extremity as much as possible while performing daily activities. With clinical and x-ray follow-ups, those fractures that are more unstable than initially anticipated can be identified. If necessary, the treatment strategy may be changed eventually (**Case 9: Fig 3.1-20**).

A slab splint from the forearm to the shoulder or Desault's bandage may cause iatrogenic problems like skin abrasions, swelling, or stiffness.

The predicted risk of delayed and/or nonunion is 7% with nonoperative management. The risk for nonunion in smokers is 5.5 times higher than in nonsmokers.

### 4.1.4 Outcome

Radiologically, nonoperative treatment usually results in some malalignment. In 2-part fractures this typically leads to a varus position of the proximal fragment with a subacromial position of the GT. In contrast to younger patients and to patients after operative treatment, this does not interfere with a reasonable or even good function of the shoulder in older patients [49].

Retrospective studies have shown a near functional normality in 80% of geriatric patients with only minor restrictions in strength and ROM to vigorous activities especially if the fracture is only minimally displaced [50, 51]. Most patients should be able to perform activities of daily living (ADLs) (**Case 10: Fig 3.1-21**). There is robust evidence that nonoperative management of PHFs is safe and effective, mainly in AO/OTA type A and B fractures [5].

## Secondary displacement with change of treatment modality

### Patient

An 83-year-old woman with severe osteoporosis and a 2-part fracture after a fall at home. She was go-go, ie, fit, had no relevant comorbid conditions, and took only one medication for bradyarrhythmia.

### Treatment and outcome

There existed a trauma series of the fracture including an axial view without relevant displacement. The patient expressly said that she did not want operative treatment so ambulatory nonoperative treatment was started (**Fig 3.1-20a–c**).

The 1-week follow-up showed complete dislocation and the patient had distinct pain despite oral pain medication (**Fig 3.1-20d–f**). Operative fixation was therefore recommended.

One day later, operative fixation with 9.5 mm/160 mm intramedullary nail, statically locked, 3 head screws, one screw in screw (**Fig 3.1-20g–h**).

Three months later there was no change in position, bone healing, and excellent function (**Fig 3.1-20i–k**). Two years later she presented again in the emergency department with a knee distortion after lifting a clothes basket.

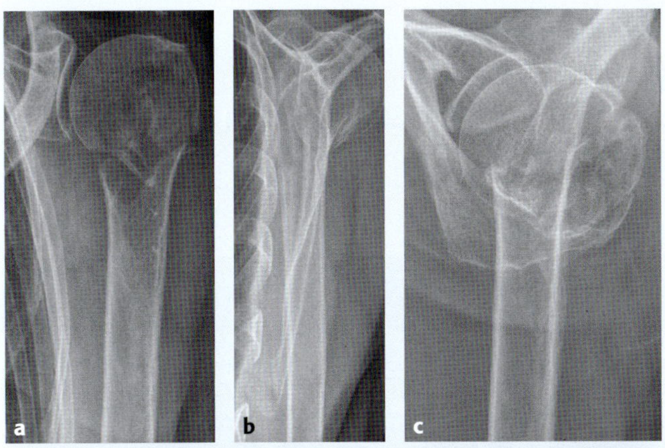


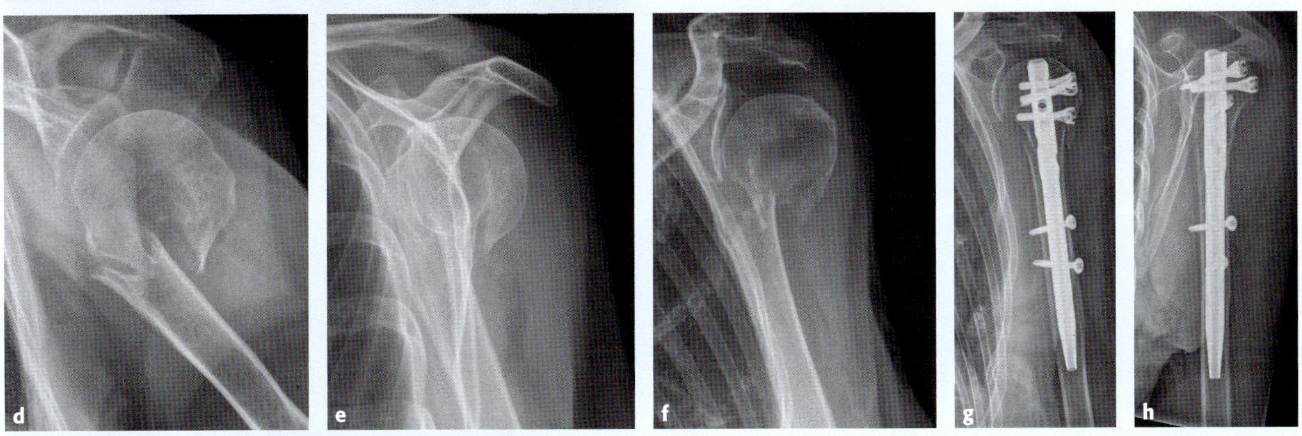


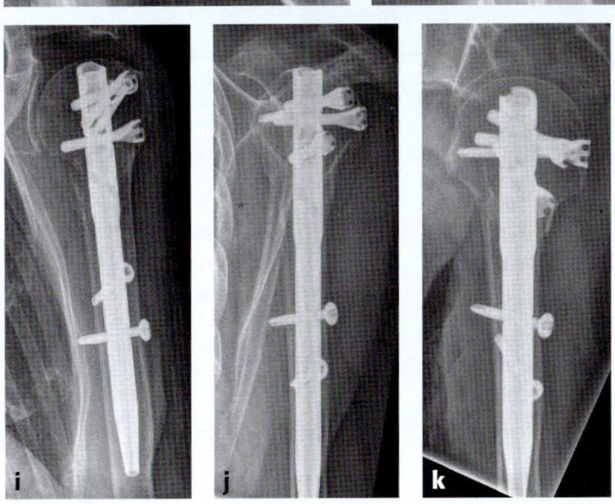


**Fig 3.1-20a–k** An 83-year-old woman after a fall at home.
**a–c** A trauma series of the 2-part fracture including an axial view without relevant displacement.
**d–f** Follow-up after 1 week showing complete dislocation.
**g–h** X-rays showing fracture treated operatively with 9.5 mm/160 mm intramedullary (IM) nail, three locked screws in proximal end of IM nail and standard distal interlocking screws.
**i–k** X-rays after 3 months showing no change in position, bone healing, and excellent function.

CASE 10

## Adequate functional result despite massive malalignment in a very old patient

### Patient

A 96-year-old female patient with a 3-part proximal humeral fracture (HL-G-S) after a fall at home.

### Treatment and outcome

Nonoperative treatment was chosen because of the patient's age. The greater tuberosity (GT) was pulled posteriorly and superiorly (**Fig 3.1-21a–e**).

Six months later the head fragment was displaced more into varus and anteversion (**Fig 3.1-21f–h**). Some anterior part of the GT was still attached to the head fragment which allowed some supraspinatus muscle functions. Posterosuperior displacement of the GT occurred. The pain was tolerable and the patient could flex the arm 150°, reach her mouth and the back of her head; she could also reach her buttocks.

### Discussion

Progression into varus malalignment within the first 6–8 weeks is frequent in patients treated nonoperatively. Large series show little functional impairment in 2-part surgical neck fracture. In contrast, posttraumatic malunion of the GT is problematic to treat. Reverse arthroplasty is the preferred choice in this age group, yet the amount of external rotation depends on the displacement of the GT limiting range of motion in the "hinged door" mechanism of the reversed polarity.

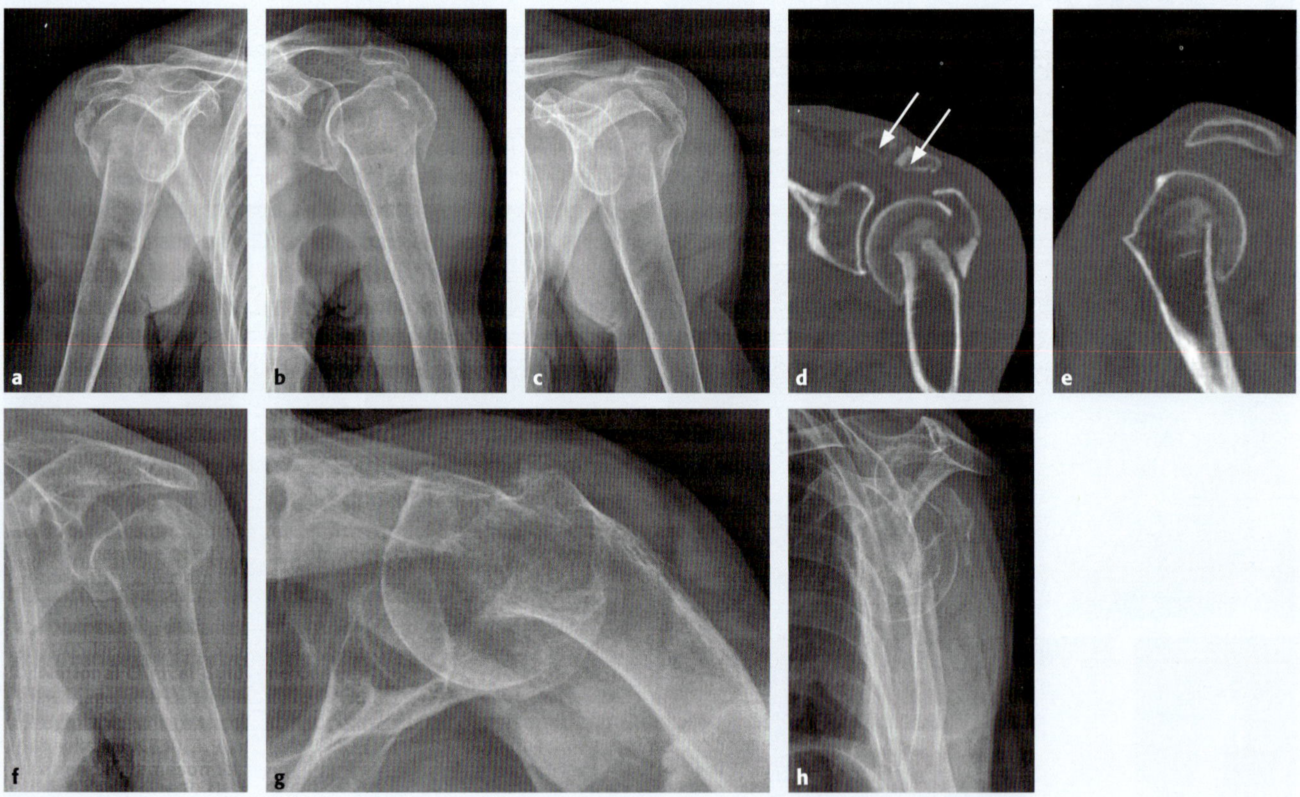


**Fig 3.1-21a–h** A 96-year-old woman after a fall.
**a–e** X-rays showing the greater tuberosity (GT) pulled to posterior and superior—note the intact supraspinatus muscle (SSP) (arrows).
**f–h** Six months later the head fragment was displaced more into varus and anteversion. Some anterior part of the GT was still attached to the head fragment which allowed some SSP functions. Posterosuperior displacement of the GT.

## 4.2 Locking plate

After the introduction of the locking plate concept in the early 1990s, it rapidly became the most frequently used technique for fixation of PHFs. This still holds true today despite an unacceptably high rate of reported complications. Many patients, however, achieve good to excellent results. Factors predicting failure are understood better nowadays and can be avoided more easily.

Regardless of the approach, soft-tissue management seems to be at least as important as biomechanical issues. No data exists on the impact of soft-tissue handling on the outcome, since it is very difficult to control this in studies.

Topic 4.2 focuses on lessons that have been learned over the past years. For a systematic description of the technique, see Acklin et al [52] and Plecko et al [53].

### 4.2.1 Approaches

Deltoid-split approach for minimally invasive plate osteosynthesis (MIPO):

- The use of this minimally invasive approach should not result in malreduction, specifically of the varus and valgus positions of the head fragment.
- The surgeon should be familiar with MIPO techniques such as indirect reduction and the use of joysticks as the fracture zone cannot be visualized directly.
- It offers complete access to the entire GT, especially when parts of it are posteriorly displaced, and to the plating area.
- On the other hand, there is an increased risk of limited access to the head fragment, and the axillary nerve is in danger. Options to extend the approach are limited.
- In a comparative study with the deltopectoral approach, the use of the deltoid-split approach resulted in a lower Constant score due to poorer ROM. According to a retrospective study there is no difference between the two approaches including electrophysiological investigations [54, 55].

Deltopectoral approach (**Approach 1: Fig 3.1-22**):

- Although the skin incision is longer in this approach than in the deltoid-split approach, the procedure should be as minimally invasive as possible, which can be achieved by preserving periosteal bridges, using sutures to manipulate the fracture fragments, and using the plate to indirectly reduce the fracture. For excellent exposure, no deeper structures need to be dissected.
- Manipulation of tuberosities should only be performed by sutures through the tendon of the rotator cuff. They should never be pulled directly to avoid further fragmentation and iatrogenic periosteal detachment.
- The affected arm should be positioned on a Mayo side stand in abduction. By internal rotation and abduction, the deltoid muscle can be retracted and the GT exposed.
- Rounded retractors are inserted underneath the deltoid muscle.
- A longitudinal split of the SSP tendon does not cause important damage and can be closed easily. The quality of the GT reduction can be clinically assessed with the SSP split and is also easy to extend.
- The so-called tendon-free rotator interval between SSC and SSP muscles should not be dissected. The whole complex together with smaller anterior fracture fragments act like a hood that can be pulled over the humeral head at the end of the surgery.
- This approach is used for revision surgery as well.

APPROACH 1

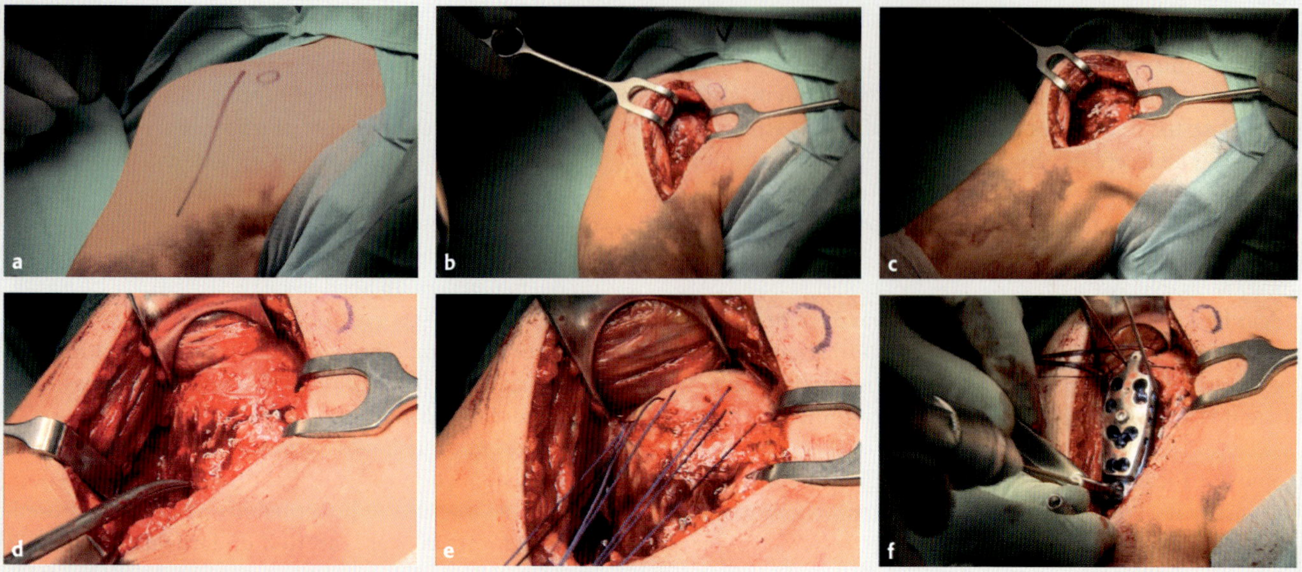


**Fig 3.1-22a–f** Deltopectoral approach.

- **a** The skin incision runs along the humerus, starting lateral to the palpable tip of the coracoid.
- **b–c** The cephalic vein is retracted laterally and the subdeldoital space is opened by exposing the clavipectoral fascia. The lateral tendon border of the conjoined tendon and the coracoacromial ligament are identified (not shown in the pictures). By simple abduction of the arm on a Mayo side stand the tension of the deltoid is relieved and the exposure can be nicely extended laterally (**c**).
- **d** No soft-tissue structures are dissected or stripped including those already injured.
- **e** Stay sutures through the cuff are placed from anterior to posterior. The anterior suture allows manipulation of the head to place the next one until the posterior cuff is reached. The tuberosities are never manipulated with sharp instruments.
- **f** The authors' preferred method is first to fix the plate to the shaft and then to manipulate and temporarily fix the fracture with pins without interfering with the plate position. Two pins, one just below the bony edge of the greater tuberosity and one just behind the bicipital groove, are used for guidance of the final plate position.

### 4.2.2 Biceps tendon

Sutures or cerclages crossing the bicipital groove with the tendon underneath act like a tenodesis (**Fig 3.1-23**, **Fig 3.1-24**, **Case 11: Fig 3.1-25**). Therefore, whenever this approach is necessary, surgeons are advised to tentomize the biceps tendon, perform a tenodesis by suturing the distal stump to the insertion of the pectoralis muscle and resect the proximal part of the tendon.

### 4.2.3 Typical complications

Screw cut-through is typically caused by subsidence of the head fragment over the locked screws. This is possible because of some comminution at the fracture zone and the big central void that characterizes the proximal humerus in the elderly. Subsidence may be combined with varus displacement of the head fragment and usually takes place in the first several weeks after the surgery; it should not be confused with AVN. Typically, the screw tips perforate the head fragment and damage the glenoid fossa. Changing the screws immediately may prevent serious damage to the joint (**Case 11: Fig 3.1-25a–j**).

Screw cut-out goes hand in hand with a loss of reduction. Driven by the pull of the rotator cuff, the humeral head "moves" into a varus position. Cut-through and cut-out often occur at the same time and may lead to irreversible destruction of the glenoid if action is taken belatedly. Revision is challenging and often ends with reverse arthroplasty as a last resort.

Boileau et al [56] described the "unhappy triad after locking plate" fixation as a combination of:

- Humeral head necrosis
- Loss of reduction with posterior migration of the GT and posterosuperior cuff insufficiency
- Glenoid erosion and destruction because of screw penetration

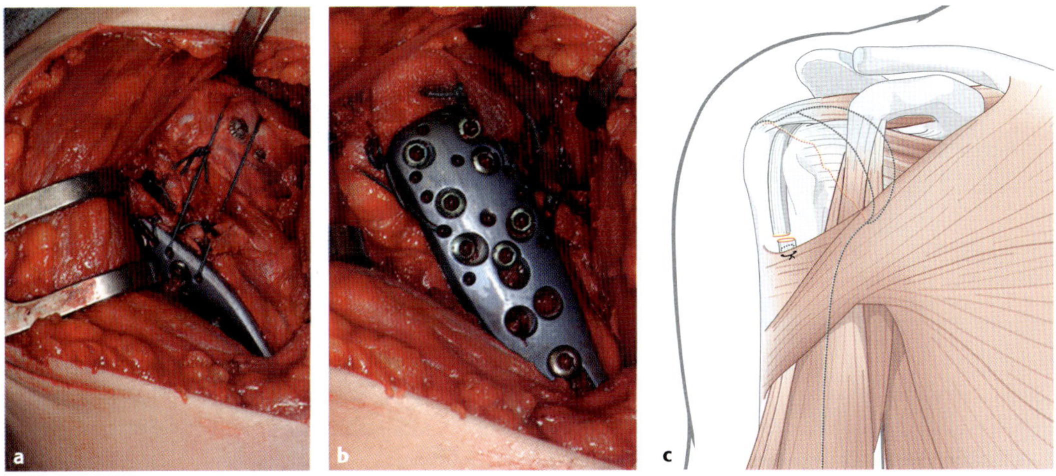

**Fig 3.1-23a–c**

**a–b** Whenever sutures cross the sulcus of the biceps, the physiological gliding of the biceps in the groove is made impossible. Adhesion between the interval tissue and the biceps tendon, which is no longer gliding, generates pain and loss of external rotation. Therefore, in these cases a tenodesis of the long head of the biceps (LHB) tendon is recommended. The authors' preferred technique is to suture the tendon to the upper edge of the pectoralis major tendon. The biceps tendon is then cut proximally and the intraarticular portion is harvested through the fracture plane between the tuberosities.

**c** Note the plane of the intertuberosity fracture, running 8–10 mm behind the sulcus, as the sulcus provides the best bone quality in this area. Frequently the supraspinatus muscle (SSP) tendon is already split minimally at the end of the fracture plane. If needed, eg, in the case of a head-split fracture, when resection of the intraarticular portion of the LHB is difficult, the split of the SSP tendon can be prolonged in line of the fibers and the whole posterior part of the cuff can be pushed back like a curtain providing excellent exposure to the head fragment.

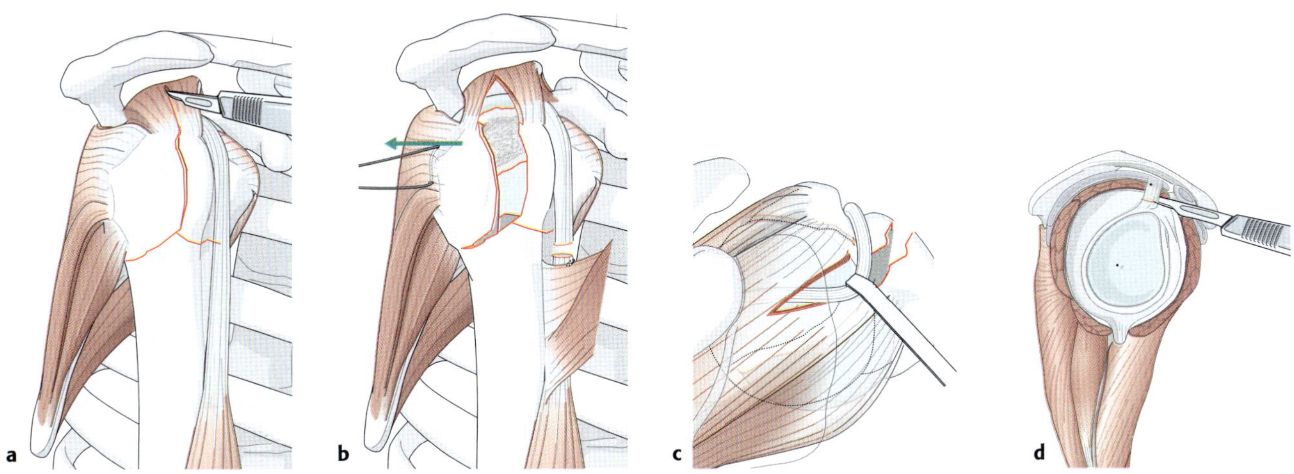

**Fig 3.1-24a–d** The long head of the biceps tendon is first sutured to the upper border of pectoralis major tendon and then cut above. The intraarticuar portion can be harvested without compromising the interval through the existing fracture between the tuberosities. If needed, the supraspinatus tendon can be split along the fibers to extend the needed exposure. Likewise, this method to extend the intraarticular exposure can be used in head-split reconstruction.

CASE 11

## Typical "mechanical" complication due to varisation and subsiding of the head fragment

### Patient

An 83-year-old patient, living in a nursing home, suffered a fall from standing height.

### Comorbidities

- Hypertension
- Aortic valve replacement
- Mitral valve insufficiency
- Atrial fibrillation
- Left bundle branch block
- Coronary heart disease after bypass surgery
- Multiple vertebral fractures
- Mastectomy after breast cancer 26 years ago

### Treatement and outcome

The patient sustained a 3-part fracture (HG-L-S) with sufficient alignment for nonoperative treatment (**Fig 3.1-25a–b**). The computed tomographic scan confirmed the diagnosis and classification (**Fig 3.1-25c–e**).

X-rays after 11 days showed severe displacement and the patient had great pain (**Fig 3.1-25f–g**). The geriatric evaluation rated the patient as slow-go, ie, unfit, and pain treatment was adapted. Mobilization and pain control deteriorated and after another 8 days of inpatient treatment the decision in favor of surgery was made. Intraoperative x-rays showed good alignment and plate fixation. Medial support reconstruction was questionable (**Fig 3.1-25h–j**).

Within 5 weeks the head fragment subsided and screw penetration occurred. Revision surgery with shorter screws was performed. Arthroscopy demonstrated erosion of the glenoid surface (**Fig 3.1-25k–l**).

Within 1 year the head collapsed (**Fig 3.1-25m–n**). The patient refused revision surgery, as she was pain free. The function was poor, though.

Within the same year she suffered a pertrochanteric fracture that was treated with a long proximal femoral nail antirotation (**Fig 3.1-25o–q**). Four years later she suffered a periimplant humeral shaft fracture that was treated with a long locking compression plate (**Fig 3.1-25r–s**).

### Discussion

Retrospectively, an important reason for failure was the lack of medial support, a lesson learned in the past. A well-fixed straight antegrade nail with impaction might have resulted in sufficient stability for healing. The further course was characterized by an overall poor result, but pain was still tolerable. Also in this age group, secondary fracture prophylaxis was required.

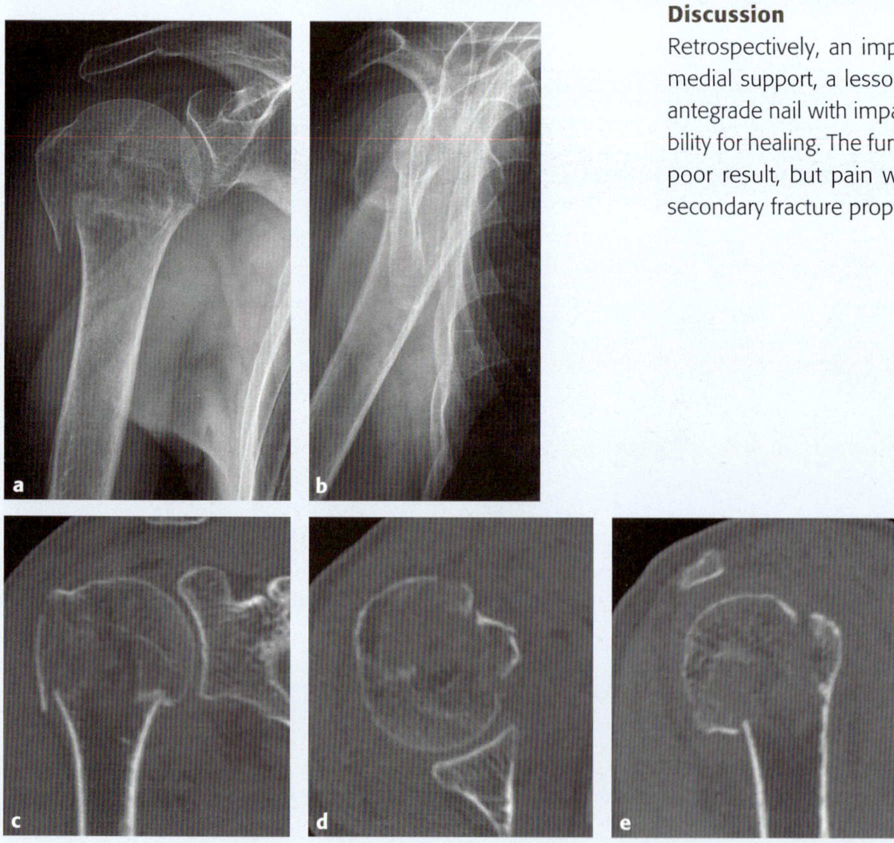


**Fig 3.1-25a–s** An 83-year-old patient after a fall from standing height.
**a–b** X-rays showing a 3-part fracture with sufficient alignment for nonoperative treatment.
**c–e** Computed tomographic scan of the fracture.

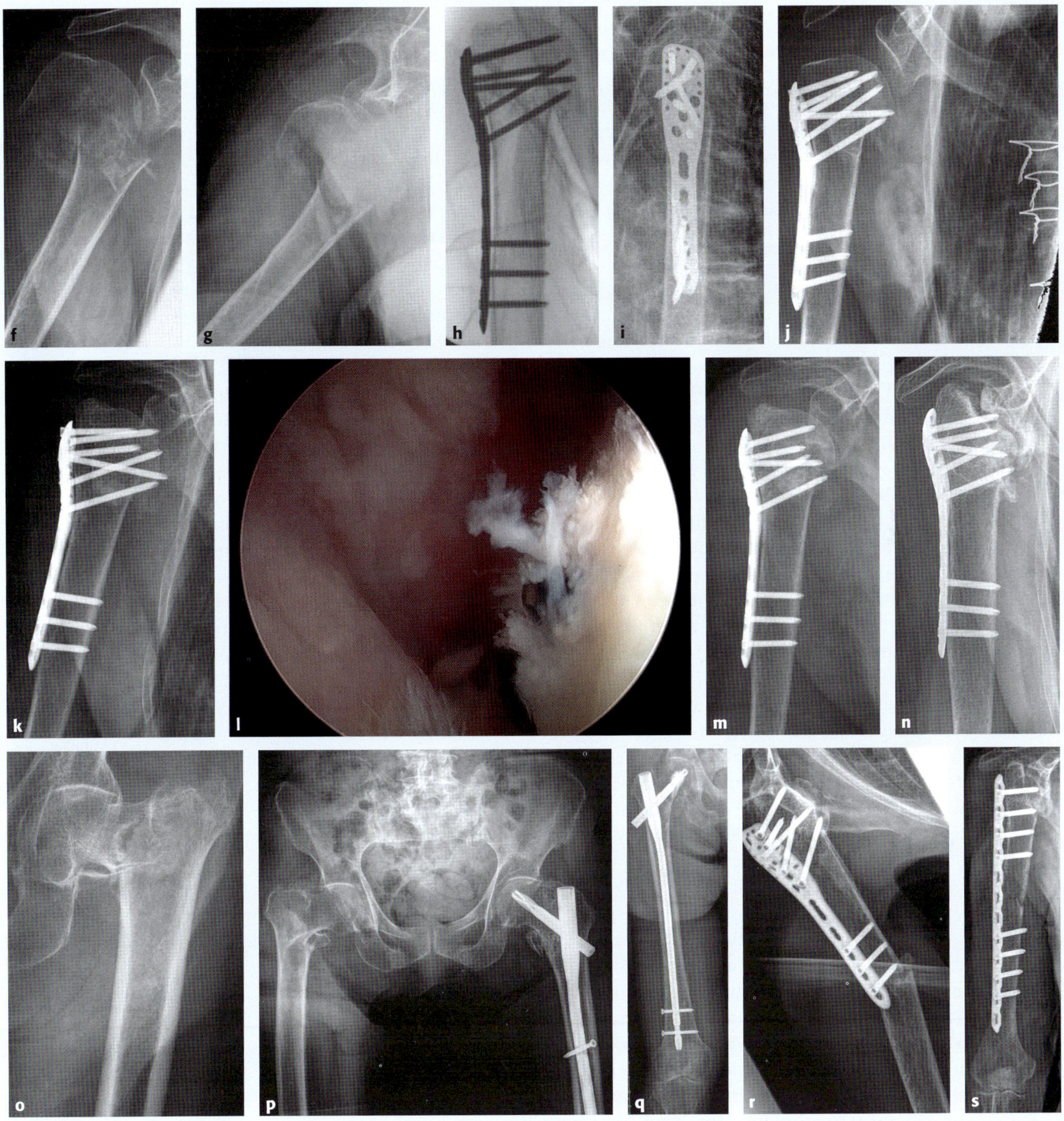

**Fig 3.1-25a–s (cont)** An 83-year-old patient after a fall from standing height.

**f–g** X-rays after 11 days showing severe displacement.

**h–j** Postoperative x-rays after surgery showing good alignment and plate fixation.

**k–l** Within 5 weeks the head fragment subsided and screw penetration occurred. Revision surgery with shorter screws was performed. Arthroscopy demonstrating erosion of the glenoid surface (**l**).

**m–n** Within 1 year the head collapsed.

**o–q** Pertrochanteric fracture treated with a long proximal femoral nail antirotation.

**r–s** Periimplant humeral shaft fracture treated with a long locking compression plate.

Boileau et al [56] also stated that a failure after a locking plate fixation cannot be reversed. A revision with hemiarthroplasty is not possible because of glenoid erosion and GT migration. An anatomical total shoulder arthroplasty cannot be performed for the same reasons, specifically because of the posterosuperior cuff insufficiency. Unfortunately, reverse shoulder arthroplasty (RSA) will yield poor functional results because of stiffness and absence of the external rotator muscles.

There are several ways to avoid these complications:

- Careful evaluation of the thickness of the head fragment in the preoperative CT scan. If it is below 8–10 mm, the risk increases and additional measures like augmentation should be considered, especially in osteoporotic bone (**Case 3: Fig 3.1-14**).
- Careful "percussion" drilling and measuring screw lengths without perforating the articular surface. Perforation of the subchondral bone increases the risk drastically. A blunt probe for length measurement should be used.
- Filling the void after reduction and supporting the humeral head are other options to prevent fragments from being displaced. Techniques that used allograft bone or fibular strut graft [57, 58] have turned out to be more successful even in unfavorable conditions [16, 42]. Ideally, massive bone blocks from femoral heads are available from a local bone bank (**Case 12: Fig 3.1-26**). This applies specifically to those cases with a shallow head fragment (which is particularly pronounced in osteoporotic cases), comminution zones, and/or a short or multifragmentary GT fragment that would not be able to take any screws but can only be fixed with sutures.
- Enhancing the anchorage of the screws in the reduced cancellous subchondral bone is another approach that is currently under evaluation. Injecting small amounts of PMMA cement through cannulated and perforated screws leads biomechanically to significantly more cycles to cut out. This only works in osteoporotic bone structure.
- Medial hinge (calcar) reconstruction either by meticulous reduction or in case of comminution by shortening to achieve mechanical stability. Indirect techniques like employing a bone rasp to reduce the head fragment through the fracture can be used. When the plate is already in situ, reduction can be secured by using a preliminary pin through the plate. The quality of medial calcar restoration should be carefully checked by image intensification.
- Controlled impaction of the head fragment onto the humeral shaft or vice versa in case of medial comminution and highly osteoporotic bone quality. Impaction may contribute to the overall stiffness and has to be done correctly, ie, no varus malalignment must result.
- Accepting a nonanatomical position of the PHILOS plate after shortening. When approximating the humeral shaft to the plate, the achieved medial support will be lost (**Case 13: Fig 3.1-27**). If the head is impacted, the plate cannot be applied in an anatomical position (**Case 13: Fig 3.1-27**). Frequently the shaft is shifted laterally by the first screw and pulled out of the medial support, which is to be avoided.
- Under no circumstances should a residual varus position of the head fragment be accepted. A slight overcorrection into valgus may be beneficial and is preferred.
- The GT functions as a capstone that completes the corpus and offers intrinsic stability at least in cases with reasonable bone quality. The implant must then only keep the position, as loads are transferred by the bone.
- To support the medial corner and to prevent varus malalignment, calcar screws have proven to be effective [59].
- In situations with lateral comminution of the GT and/or a short GT fragment that is fractured close to the tendon, insertion the standard plate position does not address the superior part of the GT any more. Additional suture fixation of the GT through the SSP tendon-bone-interface to the prepared holes in the plate may be particularly helpful. In cases with a big central void it is of paramount importance that enough bony substance underneath the GT and the head fragment is provided to restore mechanical stability and promote healing. A massive allograft works well in these cases.
- Isolated screws should not be used for fixation of the lesser tuberosity in this population. The screws often loosen and may cause problems culminating in revision surgery.

## Central massive allogenic bone block to prevent secondary loss of reduction

### Patient

An 89-year-old woman sustained a 2-part proximal humeral fracture (PHF) with additional metaphyseal fragments after a fall in her nursing home (**Fig 3.1-26a–b**). Her World Health Organization performance status was 4, Parker Mobility Score 3, and she used a cane; CAM 0, Lachs Score 10, local bone mineral density 70.9 mg/cm$^3$. She had sustained an L1 fracture many years ago (**Fig 3.1-26c**).

### Comorbidities

- Parkinson's disease
- Epilepsy

### Treatment and outcome

The fracture was operatively reconstructed with a massive allogenic bone block from the local bone bank (**Fig 3.1-26d–f**). Three months later the fracture healed uneventfully (**Fig 3.1-26g–i**).

A computed tomographic scan after 6 months showed integration of the graft without loss of reduction and also a reasonable function (**Fig 3.1-26j–l**).

### Discussion

Nonoperative management must be discussed in this case. If surgery is chosen, additional measures apart from fixation are necessary, as otherwise failure of any fixation is likely.

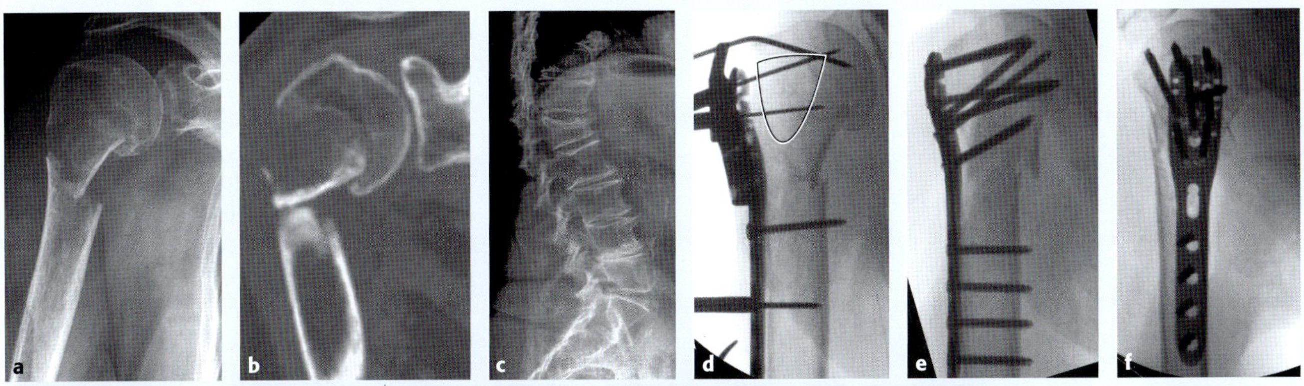

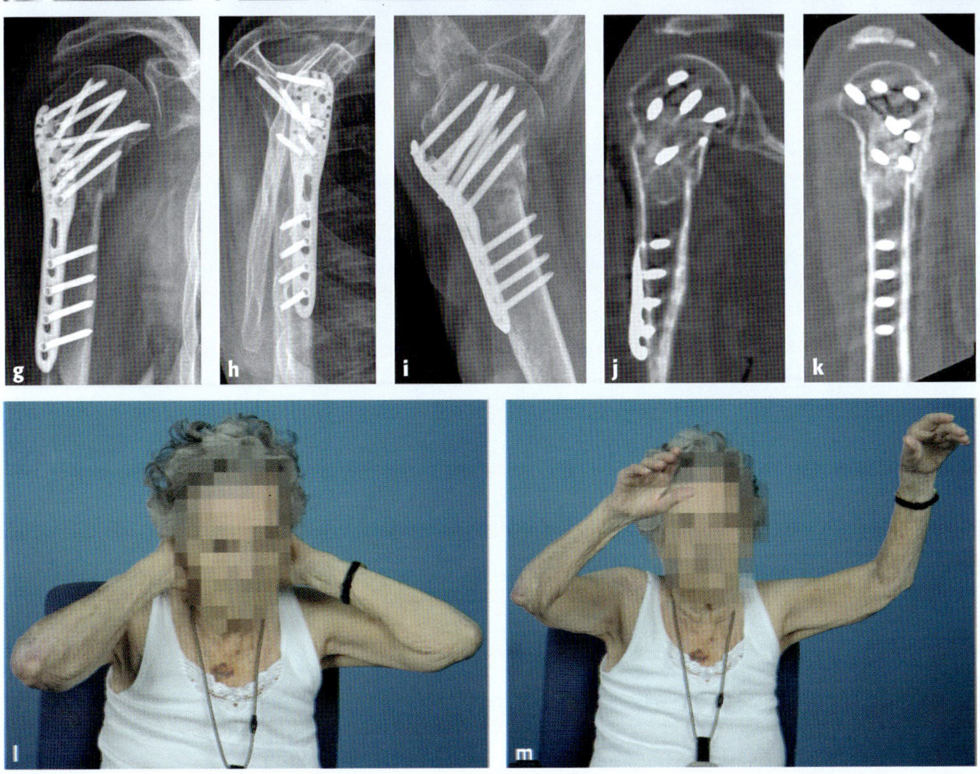

**Fig 3.1-26a–m** An 89-year-old woman after a fall.

**a–b** X-rays showing the 2-part proximal humeral fracture with additional metaphyseal fragments.

**c** X-ray of L1 fracture taken 2 years prior to the proximal humeral fracture.

**d–f** Operative reconstruction with massive allograft bone block from the local bone bank.

**g–i** X-rays after 3 months showing uneventful healing of the fracture.

**j–k** Computed tomographic scan at 6 months showing integration of the graft without loss of reduction.

**l–m** Follow-up range of motion examination.

CASE 13

## Importance of calcar reconstruction

### Patient

A 79-year-old female patient who experienced a fall at home. The patient sustained a displaced 3-part proximal humeral fracture with a head-split component (**Fig 3.1-27a–d**).

### Comorbidities

- Hypertension
- Hyperlipidemia
- Osteoporosis

### Treatment and outcome

The fracture was reduced and preliminarily fixed with K-wires (**Fig 3.1-27e–g**) and the calcar was reconstructed (**Fig 3.1-27h–l**). Moving the shaft to the plate would lead to uncontrolled impaction of the shaft into the head of the humerus with loss of reduction (**Fig 3.1-27h–i**). After 4 weeks (**Fig 3.1-27m–n**) and 1 year (**Fig 3.1-27 o–q**) there was no change in position. Constant score right/left was 78/77. Range of motion and power were almost equal on both sides.

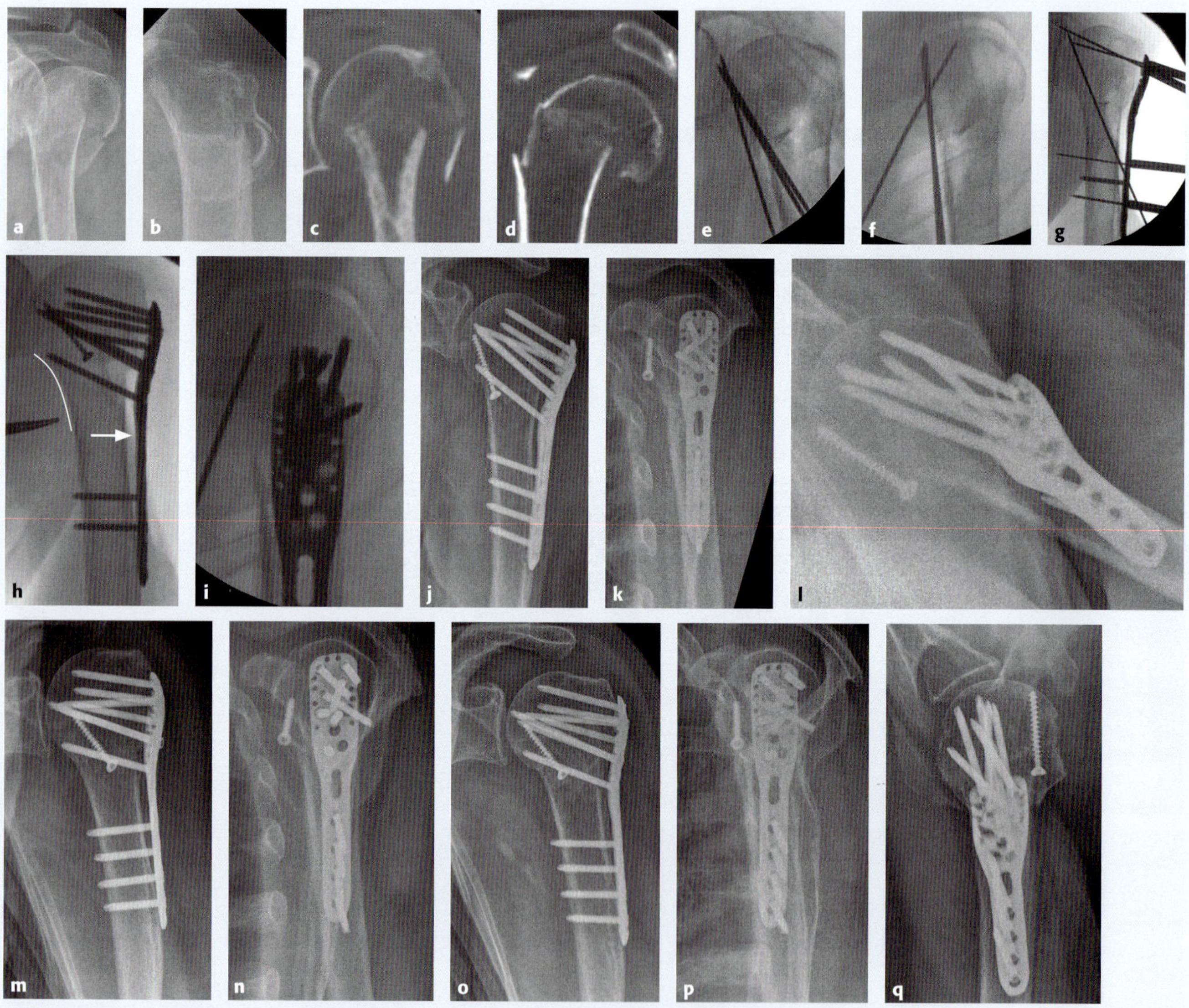

**Fig 3.1-27a–q** A 79-year-old woman after a fall.
**a–d** X-rays showing a displaced 3-part proximal humeral fracture with a head-split component.
**e–g** X-rays showing reduced fracture and preliminarily fixed with K-wires.
**h–l** X-rays showing reconstructed calcar. Note the distance of the plate from the humeral shaft (arrow). Moving the shaft to the plate would lead to uncontrolled impaction of the shaft into the head of the humerus with loss of reduction (**h–i**). Postoperative follow-up x-rays (**j–l**).
**m–q** No change in position after 4 weeks (**m–n**) and 1 year (**o–q**).

### 4.2.4 Aftercare

Postoperative physiotherapy and self-directed exercises play a crucial role in achieving a good outcome. The stability of the fixation should always allow for immediate and active treatment.

Patients should never experience pronounced pain, ie, a differentiated pain regimen including nerve blocks is vital. Passive mobilization is allowed from day 1, active motion as soon as pain subsides. Using a sling is not mandatory but many patients feel more comfortable with a sling at least in the first couple of days.

We encourage patients to stretch the elbow and use the hand of the affected arm as soon as possible for ADLs.

### 4.2.5 Outcome

Comparing results from different studies is challenging, because the amount of displacement and angulation is rarely quantified and the term unstable is not clearly defined and is difficult to measure preoperatively.

Complications are hardly ever monocausal. Krappinger et al [28] reported that age, local BMD, anatomical reduction, and restoration of the medial cortical support to be important predictors for failure. The probability of mechanical failure increased significantly when at least three of the following risk factors were present: higher age, lower local BMD, less than anatomical reduction, no medial cortical support.

A thorough and prospective analysis of 150 patients with unstable PHFs failed to show any of the suspected parameters to be significant including surgical characteristics, smoking, alcohol consumption, fracture type, medical comorbidities, and delay of surgery [1]. Loss of reduction and secondary screw loosening with perforation or both were the most frequent mechanical complications.

Spross et al [60] reported 294 patients, aged 72.9 years on average, with a complication rate of 28.2% and 24.5% required revision surgeries. Screw cut-out was the most frequent reason due to secondary displacement. Smokers with more than 20 pack years had significantly more complications.

Other studies reported similar rates [3, 61]. Clearly, patients with complications have worse functional outcomes [1, 62].

## 4.3 Antegrade nailing

Antegrade humeral nailing has gone through an evolution with regard to nail and screw designs. With improved options of the latest nails, this type of osteosynthesis has become an alternative to plate fixation.

A straight nail design seems to be superior to a curvilinear one for many reasons [63]. With a modular concept, implant configuration can be adapted to fracture morphology.

Nail insertion via a split of the SSP tendon is more widely accepted in older than in younger patients. Antegrade nailing is most often indicated in displaced 2-part PHFs.

### 4.3.1 Advantages

- It is a minimally invasive surgical procedure.
- Biomechanically, an IM nail comes closer to the calcar than a plate and may support this important structure more effectively (**Case 14: Fig 3.1-28**). This can be further enhanced by an ascending calcar screw and the so-called screw-in-screw concept to address the posteromedial area of the humeral head [64].
- Some nails offer a modular system with angular stable proximal and distal locking options.
- Ipsilateral segmental fractures of the proximal humerus and the humeral diaphysis can be stabilized by using a long version of the nail.

### 4.3.2 Disadvantages

- These demanding operative techniques require hands-on training so as to avoid errors and complications.
- Subacromial scarring may cause painful limited ROM.
- Despite improved locking options, loss of reduction and varus malalignment still occur (**Case 15: Fig 3.1-29**).

For a systematic description of the technique, see Hessmann et al [65].

CASE 14

## Straight intramedullary nail to address unstable 2-part fracture

### Patient

A 91-year-old female patient fell in her nursing home in the middle of the night. She suffered a massive hematoma, but her neurovascular status was intact.

### Comorbidities

- Urinary tract infection with *Escherichia coli*
- Atrial fibrillation after myocardial infarction 5 years ago
- Chronic obstructive pulmonary disease

### Treatment and outcome

The patient sustained a displaced 2-part proximal humeral fracture with metaphyseal comminution (**Fig 3.1-28a**). She was under general anesthesia when closed reduction and fixation with an 8 mm intramedullary (IM) nail was performed (**Fig 3.1-28b–e**). Postoperative AP and lateral x-rays showed good alignment (**Fig 3.1-28f–g**).

After 6 months the patient sustained two minor strokes. The fracture healed in anatomical position. She used a wheelchair, did not report any pain and had equal range of motion on both sides (**Fig 3.1-28h–i**).

### Discussion

This case shows the power of IM nailing. With IM nailing surgeons should strive for a medial support. In this case, it was decided not to open up the fracture and to take some risk in terms of stability.

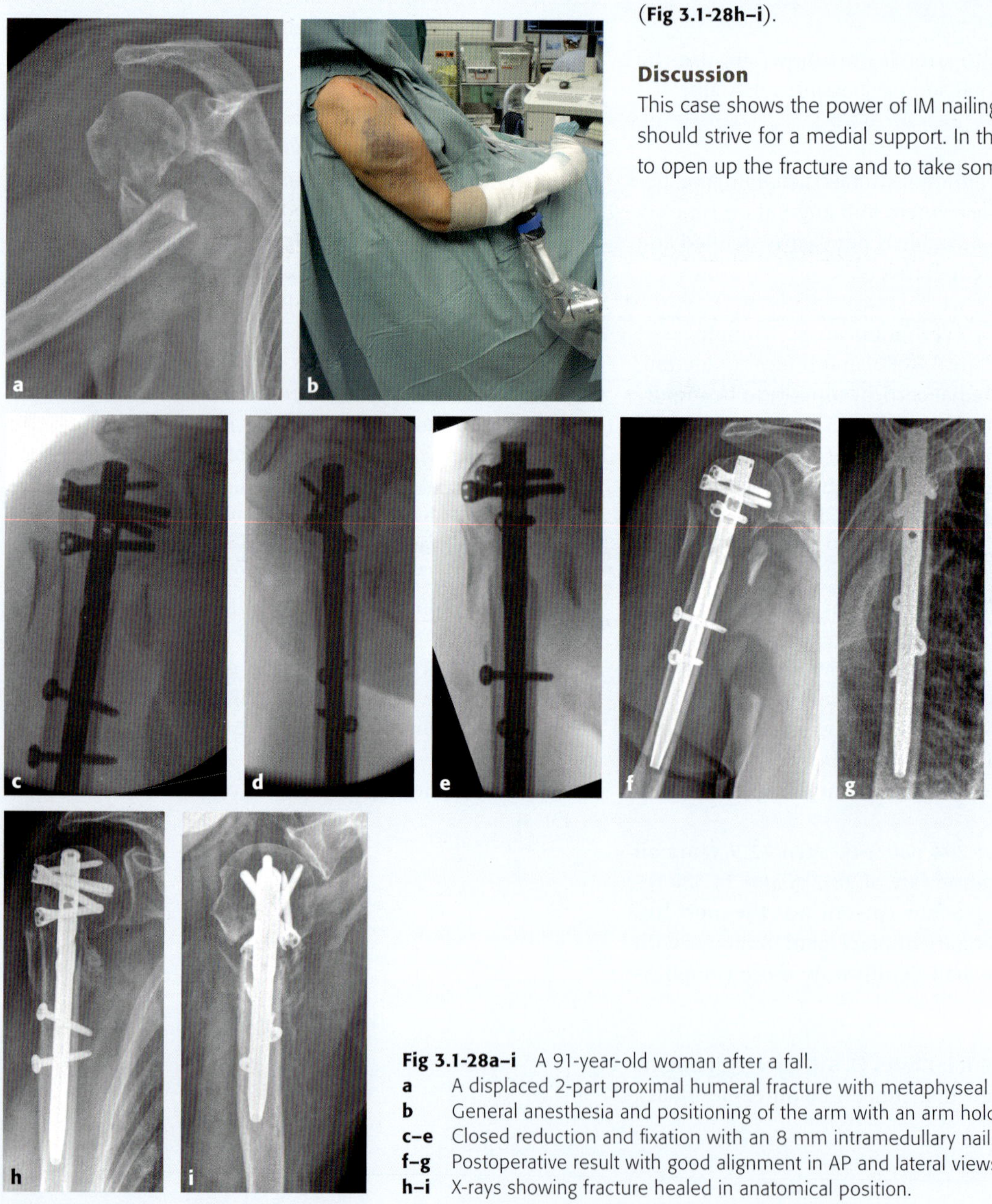

**Fig 3.1-28a–i** A 91-year-old woman after a fall.
**a** A displaced 2-part proximal humeral fracture with metaphyseal comminution.
**b** General anesthesia and positioning of the arm with an arm holder.
**c–e** Closed reduction and fixation with an 8 mm intramedullary nail.
**f–g** Postoperative result with good alignment in AP and lateral views.
**h–i** X-rays showing fracture healed in anatomical position.

## Typical course after intramedullary nailing of a 2-part proximal humeral fracture

### Patient

An 81-year-old, clearly go-go, ie, fit, male patient sustained a displaced 2-part proximal humeral fracture 4 days after a fall (**Fig 3.1-29a–b**). Two years previously, he had sustained a type A fracture of L1 with no treatment of the underlying osteoporosis (**Fig 3.1-29c**).

### Comorbidities

- Myocardial infaction
- Type 2 diabetes
- Chronic renal insufficiency

### Treatment and outcome

The fracture was anatomically reduced and fixed including a calcar screw (**Fig 3.1-29d–e**).

One week (**Fig 3.1-29f**), 3 weeks (**Fig 3.1-29g**), 6 weeks (**Fig 3.1-29h**), and 8 months (**Fig 3.1-29i–k**, **Fig 3.1-29j** in internal rotation) after surgery there was limited loss of reduction into varus and osseous healing. The patient experienced residual pain; flexion/abduction was 100°.

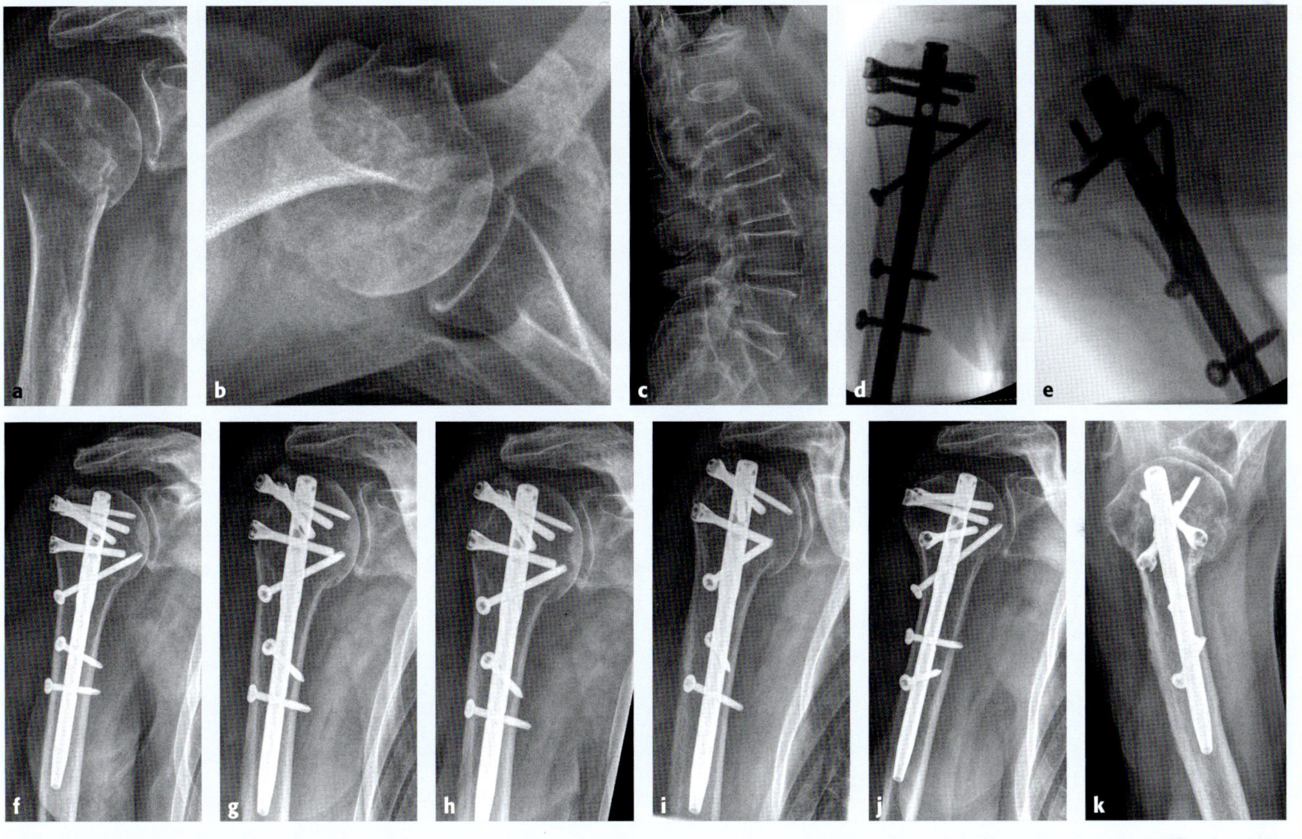

**Fig 3.1-29a–k** An 81-year-old man after a fall.
**a–c** X-rays showing a displaced 2-part proximal humeral fracture. Note the amount of displacement in the axial view.
**d–e** Anatomical reduction and fixation including a calcar screw.
**f–k** X-rays 1 week (**f**), 3 weeks (**g**), 6 weeks (**h**), and 8 months (**i–k**, **j** in internal rotation) after surgery showing limited loss of reduction into varus and osseous healing.

### 4.3.3 Typical complications

Iatrogenic rotator cuff injury:

- This is the main reason why many surgeons are reluctant to use IM antegrade fixation techniques in younger adults. Since the rotator cuff already shows some signs of degeneration, this concern is of less importance in older adult patients.
- Nails with a straight design are inserted through the muscular part of the SSP and the superior part of the humeral head, thus potentially avoiding the delicate tendinous part at the footprint of the tendon.
- Euler et al [16] analyzed CT scans of bilateral proximal humeri in 200 patients with an average age of 45.1 years (SD 19.6; 18–97) without humeral fractures. They defined the entry point of the nail and the region of interest, ie, the biggest entry hole that would not encroach on the insertion of the SSP tendon. This showed that 38.5% of the humeral heads had to be categorized as critical types due to morphology in which the predicted offset of the entry point would encroach on the insertion of the SSP tendon that might damage the tendon and reduce the stability of fixation. The authors recommended studying the preoperative x-rays accordingly and to choose another treatment option in critical cases (**Case 16: Fig 3.1-30**).

Subacromial impingement:

- A straight nail design helps to avoid this complication. Instrumentation should allow for precise determination of the nail's proximal end.
- Countersunk proximal screw head reduces the risk of subacromial mechanical impingement.

Nail toggling:

- With two sizes, the diameter of the nail can be adapted to the diameter of the medullary cavity.
- Angular stability, also distal if required, is possible with the angular stable locking system.

Suboptimal initial reduction:

- Preexisting osteoarthritis of the shoulder, shoulder stiffness, and inability to recline the arm may be serious obstacles to reaching the optimal entry portal.
- Manipulation of fragments may be difficult. Only minimally invasive techniques such as K-wires and sutures (eg, joystick, stay suture) should be applied.
- In addition to the correct entry point, the direction of the bony canal in the humeral head is extremely important; it must be parallel to the humeral shaft both horizontally and vertically and cannot be changed. The surgeon needs to get it right the first time, otherwise the head fragment may break (**Case 17: Fig 3.1-31**).

Loss of reduction:

- The central entry point offers an additional "fifth" anchor point in the humeral head. Prior to the operation the surgeon should check carefully if the bone quality around the entry portal is sufficient. A wrongly chosen entry portal cannot be changed. If fixation will not be stable, the surgeon must be able to switch to a plate or an arthroplasty.
- Locking screws in the humeral head should aim towards areas that are known to be denser even in the older patients, ie, the posteromedial part of the head.
- If anatomically possible, the calcar screw should be used.

## Importance of correct entry portal

### Patient

An 88-year-old woman had a fall from standing height. She was living alone and had good cognitive function at baseline. The patient sustained a 3-part greater tuberosity (GT) fracture (HL-G-S), yet the GT was not displaced (**Fig 3.1-30a–c**).

### Treatment and outcome

The contralateral side was a 2-D reconstruction along the shaft axis; the shape of a straight nail with 8.5 mm in diameter was superimposed (**Fig 3.1-30d–f**). Note the estimated insertion site at the lateral end of the head fragment, even involving part of the supraspinatus footprint. This situation is critical in the use of antegrade straight nails, as the so-called "fifth anchoring point" does not offer an advantage any longer. The authors' experience has shown that this can be compensated with a slight valgus reduction, or else a different operative procedure, eg, angular stable plate, has to be chosen. The reconstruction showed the entry point problem and consecutive loss of reduction as shown in **Fig 3.1-30d–f**. Since the insertion was lateral, the "fifth" anchoring point was not established (**Fig 3.1-30g–i**). Progressive displacement of the reconstruction proved the insufficiency of the implant (**Fig 3.1-30j–k**). When the implant becomes insufficient, the course of the fracture healing process cannot be predicted (**Fig 3.1-30l–m**). In this case the patient accepted limited range of motion (90° flexion, external rotation 10°, internal rotation to L1), as she could reach her head and pain was tolerable.

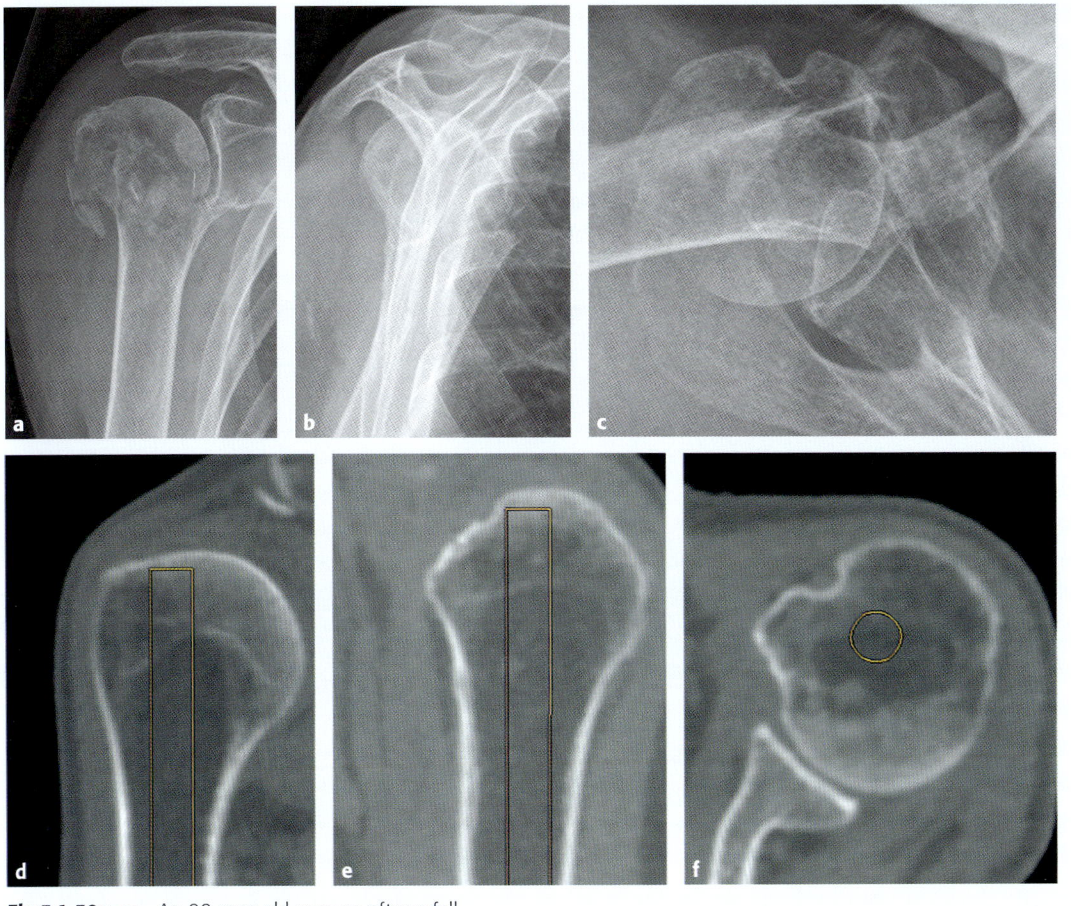


**Fig 3.1-30a–m** An 88-year-old woman after a fall.
**a–c** X-rays showing a 3-part greater tuberosity (GT) fracture without displaced GT. Note the lateral comminution creating a medium length GT fragment.
**d–f** The contralateral side is a 2-D reconstruction along the shaft axis; the shape of a straight nail with 8.5 mm in diameter is superimposed. Note the estimated insertion site at the lateral end of the head fragment, even involving part of the supraspinatus footprint.

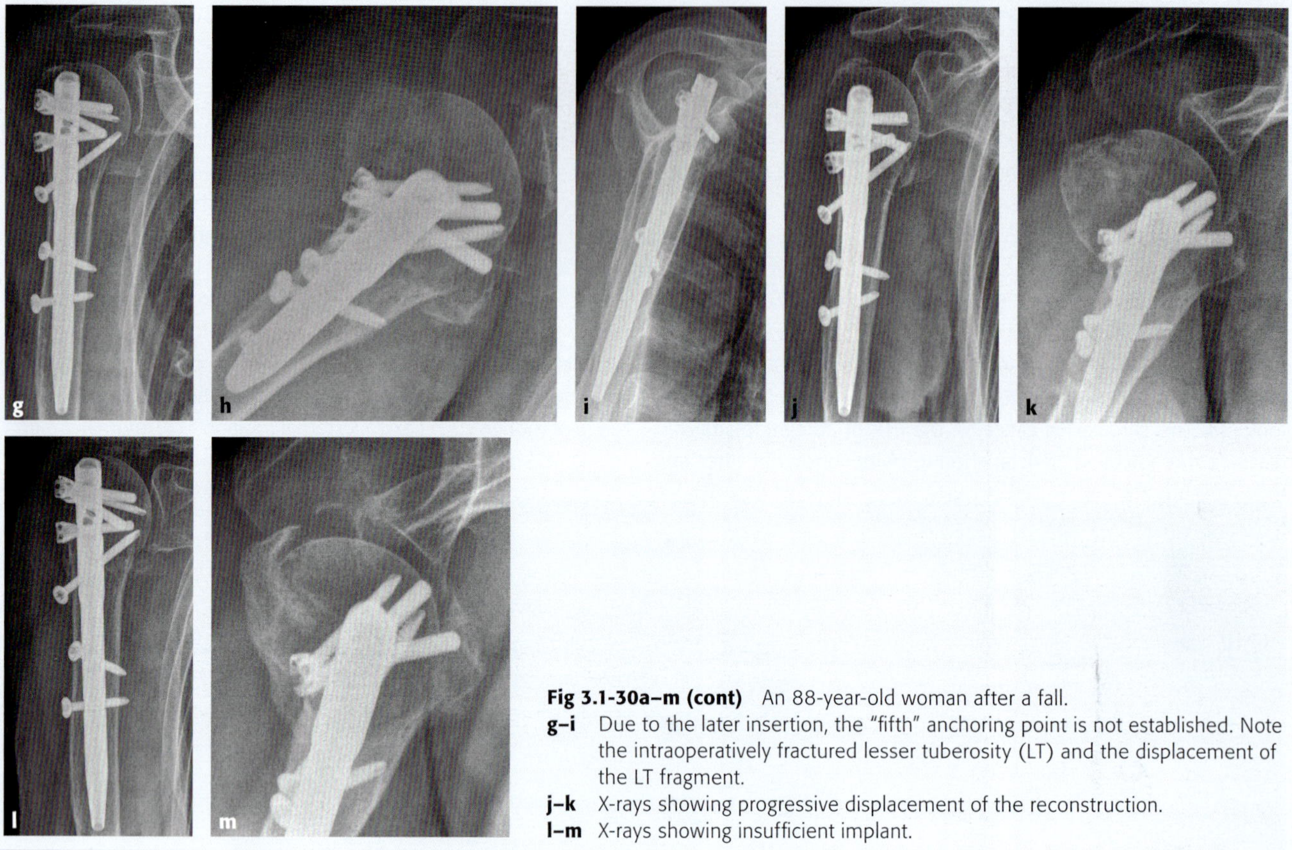


**Fig 3.1-30a–m (cont)** An 88-year-old woman after a fall.
**g–i** Due to the later insertion, the "fifth" anchoring point is not established. Note the intraoperatively fractured lesser tuberosity (LT) and the displacement of the LT fragment.
**j–k** X-rays showing progressive displacement of the reconstruction.
**l–m** X-rays showing insufficient implant.

CASE 17

## Wrong entry point leads to change of procedure

### Patient

A 72-year-old male patient presented with a low-energy proximal humeral fracture. The patient sustained an unstable, displaced 2-part surgical neck fracture (HGL-S).

### Comorbidities

- Type 2 diabetes
- Hypertension
- Chronic obstructive pulmonary disease
- Osteoporosis
- Hyperparathyroidism

### Treatment and outcome

The patient was scheduled for antegrade nailing after informed consent (**Fig 3.1-31–b**). The computed tomographic scans provided no additional information for the chosen treatment (**Fig 3.1-31c–e**).

The guide wire might have been placed too far anterior or lateral (**Fig 3.1-31f–h**). If this was the case, the direction of the guide wire was not checked properly. The hollow reamer was then driven in without aligning it with the humeral canal, resulting in severe malalignment when the straight nail was introduced (**Fig 3.1-31g**). In an effort to achieve better reduction by manipulating the nail, the head fragment cracked and the greater tuberosity split off from the head. Shoulder hemiarthroplasty was then the treatment option selected.

Postoperatively, the tuberosities were anatomically fixed (**Fig 3.1-31i–j**). In the following weeks, the tuberosities resorbed and the head was migrating cranially (**Fig 3.1-31k–l**). The patient had only little pain, but the overall result was poor with less than 40° of abduction and flexion, 0° of external rotation and internal rotation to the gluteal region.

### Conclusion

Prosthetic standby may be necessary even in relatively simple cases if severe complications are identified intraoperatively. Prolonged surgical time combined with increased iatrogenic trauma and comorbidities increase the risk of complications like infection, malunion of the tuberosities, or reabsorption.

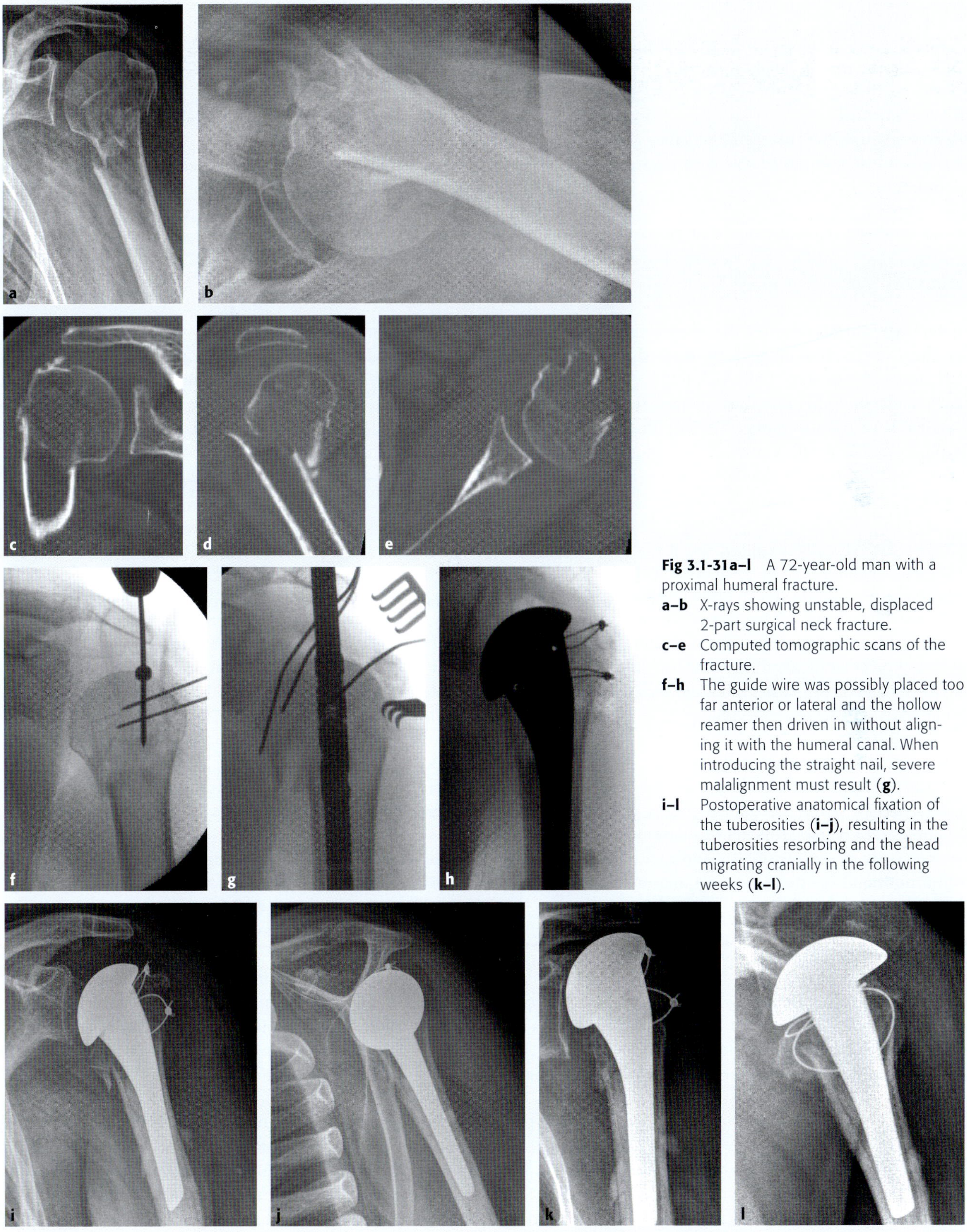

**Fig 3.1-31a–l** A 72-year-old man with a proximal humeral fracture.

**a–b** X-rays showing unstable, displaced 2-part surgical neck fracture.

**c–e** Computed tomographic scans of the fracture.

**f–h** The guide wire was possibly placed too far anterior or lateral and the hollow reamer then driven in without aligning it with the humeral canal. When introducing the straight nail, severe malalignment must result (**g**).

**i–l** Postoperative anatomical fixation of the tuberosities (**i–j**), resulting in the tuberosities resorbing and the head migrating cranially in the following weeks (**k–l**).

### 4.3.4 Aftercare
Physiotherapy programs following antegrade nailing are similar to the ones following plating.

### 4.3.5 Outcome
Reports about procedures with the latest generation of nails designs are sparse, especially with regard to the geriatric population.

Lopiz et al [63] observed that 9 of 26 patients had rotator cuff symptoms and 11.5% needed reoperations with the MultiLock nail.

Hatzidakis et al [66] reported that the fractures of 38 patients aged 65 years on average were treated with an angular stable locked antegrade nail. All fractures healed primarily. The mean follow-up Constant score (and standard deviation) was 71 ± 12 points (range: 37–88 points), with a mean age-adjusted Constant score of 97% (range: 58–119%). All fractures but one healed with a neck-shaft angle of ≥ 125°.

Despite improved locking options and anatomical initial reduction, a minor loss of reduction into varus but without any implant perforations can often be observed. The clinical significance has not yet been investigated sufficiently. Although this may be interpreted as an implant failure, cut-through or cut-out seem to occur less frequently than in plate fixation. Fracture healing improves the situation, but some malalignment is expected.

## 4.4 Shoulder hemiarthroplasty
Because of unpredictable results of shoulder hemiarthroplasty (SHA), surgeons tend to choose between fracture fixation and reverse arthroplasty (**Case 18: Fig 3.1-32**). If reconstruction is not possible possible, the tuberosities are often not good enough to expect anatomical healing and function with SHA.

### 4.4.1 Indications

- Shoulder hemiarthroplasty may be indicated in nonreconstructible 3- and 4-part PHFs, head-split injuries and fracture dislocations in older patients.
- Suspected AVN does not necessarily require joint replacement as long a stable anatomical reconstruction and fixation can be achieved.
- Stable and anatomical reconstruction as well as immediate postoperative physiotherapy are decisive factors in achieving a good result. The decision to go for SHA may be taken intraoperatively if attempts to fix the fracture with preservation of the humeral head fail.

An arthroplasty set should be readily available (**Case 17: Fig 3.1-31**). The best outcome after fracture arthroplasty results from surgery on day 6 according to the Swedish registry. Thus, fractures that are likely to require a joint replacement procedure should only be operated on if an optimal infrastructure is available.

### 4.4.2 Approach
The approach most widely used for the anatomical fracture arthroplasty is the deltopectoral approach which can be minimally invasive. When releasing the deltoid muscle close to the clavicle and all the way down to its humeral insertion, the muscle can be retracted far posteriorly in abduction giving full exposure to all aspects of the proximal humerus.

As mentioned earlier, performing a tenodesis of the long head of the biceps (LHB) tendon to prevent scarring of an insufficient LHB to the SSC-SSP-interval with subsequent pain and loss of ROM is strongly recommended. Technically, the interval between the SSC and SSP muscles should not be dissected. The LHB can be sutured to the upper pectoralis tendon and cut directly above. The proximal part of the tendon is resected intraarticularly, in case of fracture arthroplasty after the head fragment is removed.

### 4.4.3 Typical complications
Insufficient fixation, malpositioning and resorption of the tuberosities:

- Healing in anatomical position is essential for the result of hemiarthroplasty. "Embracing" fixation of the tuberosities offers superior fixation strength, even more so when applied with flexible cables.
- With most systems, the slim metaphyseal part of the stem needs cancellous bone graft underneath the tuberosities to create the bony socket needed for the fixation in the anatomical position. Without this support, the tuberosities are pulled to the metaphyseal stem with the embracing cerclage wires, which results in too low a position. Usually the whole cancellous part of the head fragment is interposed.
- Resorption of the tuberosities or consecutive cranialization of the SHA is the reason for inferior functional results comparable to cuff-deficient shoulders. In the worst case scenario an anterosuperior escape with a painful disabling upper extremity might be the result.

## Typical course of a shoulder hemiarthroplasty

### Patient

A 77-year-old male patient sustained a 4-part fracture (H-G-L-S) with severely displaced fragments after a fall from a ladder (**Fig 3.1-32a–b**).

### Comorbidities

- Prostate cancer diagnosed 5 years ago
- No relevant other comorbidities present

### Treatment and outcome

The fracture was considered unsuitable for stable anatomical reconstruction and treated with an anatomical head-shaft angle with embracing flexible cables (**Fig 3.1-32c–d**). The tuberosities were in a good position and the glenohumeral joint was centered in both planes. By that time a lower plexus lesion was diagnosed. Four months later, the proximal humerus was migrating upward indicating an insufficiency of more than two tendons of the rotator cuff (**Fig 3.1-32e–f**). Heterotopic bone formation was also present indicating the severe soft-tissue trauma. Eighteen months after the fall, the patient had pain; the range of motion of the shoulder was 30° of forward flexion, 0° of external rotation, and when internally rotating he could reach the outer gluteal region (**Fig 3.1-32g–i**). All parts of the deltoid muscle were working. Almost 3 years after the index trauma the revision to a cemented long stemmed reverse shoulder arthroplasty was carried out, as the patient had been operated in 2010 for a colon carcinoma (**Fig 3.1-32j–k**). The patient was pain free, function was limited to 80° of forward flexion, 0° of external rotation, and the patient could reach the buttocks.

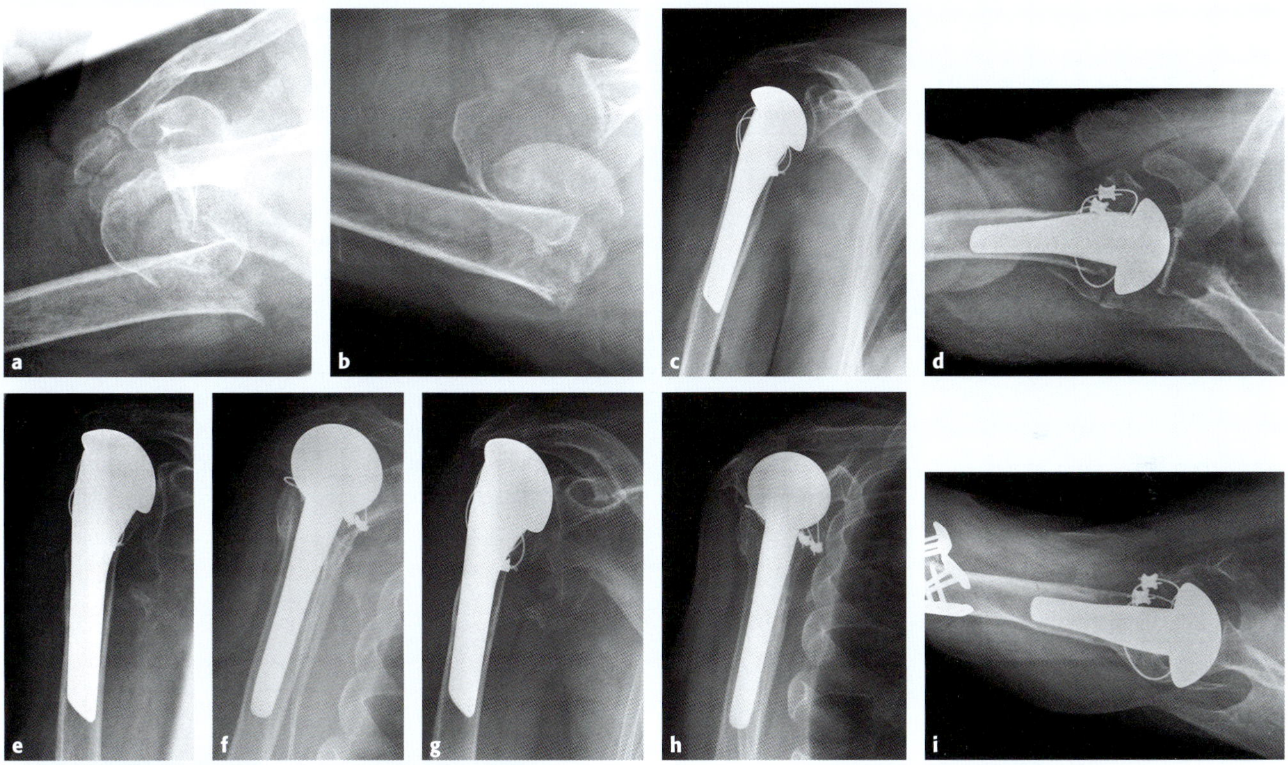


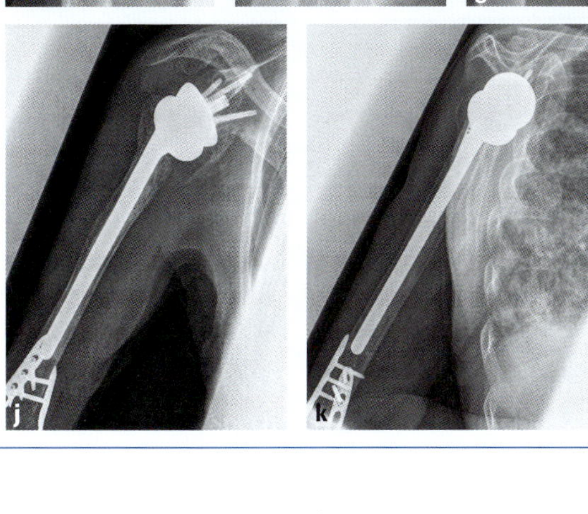


**Fig 3.1-32a–k** A 77-year-old man after a fall from a ladder.
**a–b** X-rays showing a 4-part fracture with severely displaced fragments.
**c–d** The tuberosities were in a good position and the glenohumeral joint centered in both planes.
**e–f** X-rays taken 4 months later: note the ongoing upward migration of the proximal humerus indicating an insufficiency of more than two tendons of the rotator cuff. Heterotopic bone formation is also present indicating the severe soft-tissue trauma.
**g–i** X-rays 18 months after the fall.
**j–k** Almost 3 years after the index trauma, the revision to a cemented long stemmed reverse shoulder arthroplasty was carried out.

Incorrect height and retroversion of the implant are other factors of major importance. The most accurate reference is the length of the medial head extension, which can be measured accurately. With the shaft dislocated for preparation and implantation of the shaft component, the head can be anatomically reduced and in many cases the anatomical retrotorsion of the given patient can be mimicked perfectly. Too much retrotorsion puts excessive strain on the GT fixation, as it has to be reattached more anteriorly, which potentially leads to more healing problems.

#### 4.4.4 Aftercare

Early passive ROM is essential to avoid stiffness. Immobilization has not been proven to increase the healing rate of the tuberosities but the problem of stiffness.

#### 4.4.5 Outcome

The outcome of an individual patient is difficult to predict. The results of managing pain are generally good, yet the functional results may vary extremely from very good to unsatisfactory. Anatomical healing of the tuberosities yields good results, outperforming those of RSA (**Case 19: Fig 3.1-33**). Unfortunately, in contrast to the latter, results of SHA are much less predictable. Radiographic healing can be expected in about 60% of patients and depends greatly on the selection of patients [67].

Cuff et al [67] followed up 47 patients, aged 74.4 years on average, with 3- and 4-part fractures prospectively for a minimum of 2 years. Three patients (13%) in the hemiarthroplasty group preferred revision to RSA because of failed tuberosity healing and resultant shoulder pseudoparesis. Reverse shoulder arthroplasty resulted in better clinical outcomes and a similar complication rate compared with hemiarthroplasty for the treatment of comminuted PHFs in older adults.

Ferrel et al [68] performed a systematic review to compare SHA and RSA; they found no significant clinical difference in either the American Shoulder and Elbow Surgeons Shoulder Score (RSA: 64.7, Hemi: 63.0) or the Constant score (RSA: 54.6, Hemi: 58.0). Reverse shoulder arthroplasty was associated with an increased rate of clinical complications (9.6%) and a lower revision rate (0.93%) at short-term to medium-term follow-ups compared with hemiarthroplasty. They concluded that "RSA offers an acceptable surgical option for patients after complex acute PHFs".

## Healing of tuberosities is unpredictable

### Patient

An 87-year-old man suffered a 3-part greater tuberosity head-split fracture (HL-G-S) resulting from low-energy trauma (**Fig 3.1-33a–b**).

### Comorbidities

- Condition after cerebral stroke with full recovery and good compliance
- Type 2 diabetes

### Treatment and outcome

The supraspinatus tendon insertion was intact, and the muscle belly was without any fatty degeneration or atrophy (**Fig 3.1-33c**). The reconstruction (**Fig 3.1-33d**) revealed that the lesser tuberosity was still attached to the head fragment, and due to the pull of the subscapularis (SSC) tendon the shallow head fragment was rotated internally. The muscle belly of the SSC was without atrophy and fatty infiltration.

The postoperative series showed good alignment of the tuberosities and a centered glenohumeral joint (**Fig 3.1-33e–f**).

At the 4-year follow-up, the healing of the tuberosities was successful (**Fig 3.1-33g–h**). The joint was centered, the patient was pain free and had an almost full range of motion. The absolute values of the Constant score were 74 points compared to 81 for the healthy uninvolved extremity.

### Discussion

Although the patient's result is exceptionally favorable, anatomical healing of the tuberosities is unpredictable. Nowadays, a combination of an 87-year-old man, diabetes mellitus and a nonreconstructable head-split fracture would be treated with a reverse shoulder arthroplasty giving a reasonable result independently of the healing of the tuberosities.

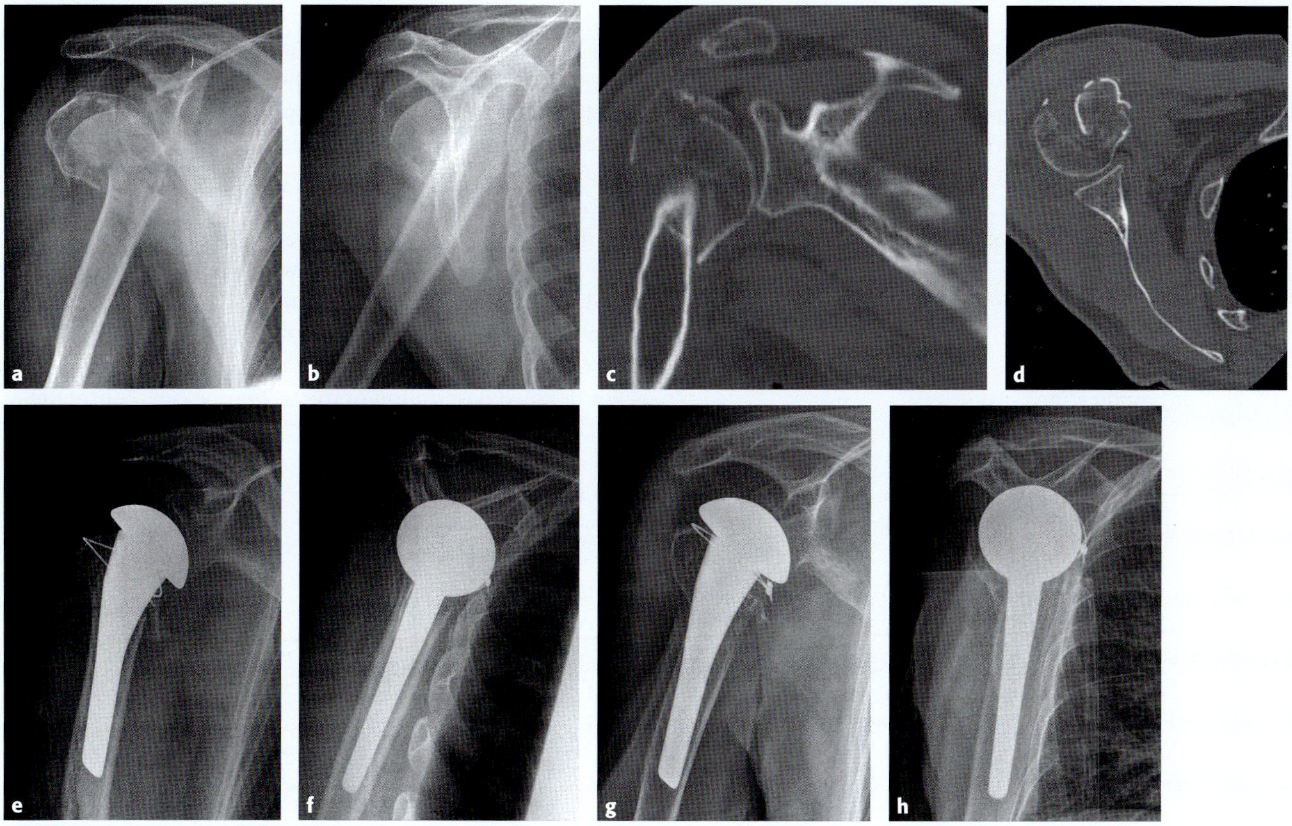


**Fig 3.1-33a–h** An 87-year-old man with a low-energy trauma.
**a–b** X-rays showing a 3-part greater tuberosity head-split fracture.
**c–d** Supraspinatus tendon insertion was intact, the muscle belly was without any fatty degeneration or atrophy (**c**). The reconstruction (**d**) revealed that the lesser tuberosity was still attached to the head fragment, and due to the pull of the subscapularis tendon, the shallow head fragment was rotated internally.
**e–f** The postoperative series showed good alignment of the tuberosities and a centered glenohumeral joint.
**g–h** The 4-year follow-up x-rays showed successful healing of the tuberosities with the joint centered.

## 4.5 Reverse shoulder arthroplasty

Due to the unpredictability of SHA results, RSA is used more often in orthogeriatric patients. Especially in patients older than 75 years, there seems to be consensus on the use of a primary RSA if a stable and anatomical reconstruction is not possible. Results are promising and unaffected by the status of the tuberosities healing. Therefore rehabilitation is less critical or even unnecessary.

Be aware that a functioning deltoid muscle is essential and in the fracture setting the testing might be difficult at times. Reverse shoulder arthroplasty results in better functional scores than SHA, especially in forward flexion, whereas the RSA result for external rotation is lower than that for SHA. The complication rate seems not considerably higher for patients undergoing RSA compared to SHA, and yet it accounts for lower revision rates.

### 4.5.1 Indications

- Complex 3- and 4-part fractures that are not suitable for a stable and anatomical reconstruction due to poor bone quality.
- Fractures that have "short" and comminuted tuberosities and a high risk of losing the tuberosities when treated with SHA.
- Head-split fractures are selected for SHA or RSA under the same criteria as already mentioned.
- Preexisting computed tomographic angiography (**Case 20: Fig 3.1-34**).

### 4.5.2 Contraindications

- Substantial glenoid bone loss or lack of glenoid bone stock might be a contraindication. Complex bony reconstruction and revision of metaglene fixation is not yet being discussed for acute fracture care.
- Axillary nerve deficiency or palsy. An intact deltoid muscle is vital for a functional RSA, therefore axillary nerve investigation is crucial in the acute fracture patient. Reverse shoulder arthroplasty is contraindicated in this situation as the increased risk for instability and the expected low functional result do not outweigh the risk of the intervention.

### 4.5.3 Approach

In the literature for primary cuff tear arthropathy, arthroplasty with RSA, deltopectoral or superior lateral approaches are described. The superior lateral approach is associated with a lower risk of instability and lower incidence of consecutive acromial and scapular spine fractures. In the acute fracture setting, instability seems to play an inferior role and perfect exposure of the bony glenoid seems essential to lower the risk of malpositioning of the metaglene and consecutive loosening or scapular notching. Therefore the deltopectoral approach remains the main approach in acute fracture care, as it leaves all options open, including complex revision if needed.

### 4.5.4 Implant selection

Currently, there are more than 20 different systems on the market. Medialized or lateralized RSA systems are available. As all systems promote their given designs, it is difficult to choose.

### 4.5.5 Fixation of the tuberosities

Rival concepts concerning repair of the tuberosities fuel an ongoing debate. Total resection of the tuberosities to full repair maintaining the full cuff (including SSP) are described. In order to gain more external rotation, some surgeons advocate cutting the SSC tendon or resecting the LT and peforming an isolated repair of the GT. The authors resect the SSP and the upper part of ISP with their bony attachment and fix the LT and the remaining GT with cerclage sutures to the prosthesis.

For detailed description of the technique, see Reuther et al [69].

### 4.5.6 Typical complications

- Scapular notching is the most common complication, responsible for polyethylene wear and consequent loosening.
- Acromial or scapular spine insufficiency fractures due to the high stress levels on the implant-bone-interface are reported.
- The risk of infection is supposed to be higher in RSA fracture arthroplasty compared to SHA; however this could not be proven in recent systematic reviews.
- Neuropathy and instability are other typical complications.

### 4.5.7 Outcome

Three recent systematic reviews and metaanalyses [68–71] compare RSA and SHA for acute fracture care. The results concerning complication rates, functional outcome, revision rates, and cost factors are conflicting.

According to Namdari et al [71] both systems have the potential to restore pain-free function. They believe that the higher complication rates and costs in RSA should be considered individually. Mata-Fink et al [70] saw better forward flexion and functional outcome of RSA, whereas in their study complication rates did not differ substantially. Ferrel et al [68] stated better forward flexion, lower external rotation, but no statistical differences according to the American Shoulder and Elbow Surgeons Shoulder Score (RSA: 64.7, Hemi: 63.0) or the Constant score (RSA: 54.6, Hemi: 58.0). Complication rates for RSA were higher, yet in contrast with this finding revision rates were lower compared with the SHA.



**Patient**

A 78-year-old woman fell from a standing height, sustaining a 2-part surgical neck fracture (HGL-S) (**Fig 3.1-34a–c**). One year prior to the fall the patient was treated with a proximal femoral nail antirotation for a pertrochanteric fracture. No relevant comorbidities are present and the patient is not cognitively impaired.

**Treatment and outcome**

The patient sustained a 2-part surgical neck fracture (HGL-S) (**Fig 3.1-34a–c**). She was known from the shoulder outpatient department (see **Fig 3.1-2**, **Fig 3.1-3**, **Fig 3.1-4**). Reconstruction in the presence of a preexisting computed tomographic angiography in a 78-year-old patient was not indicated (**Fig 3.1-34d–f**).

The fracture was addressed with a reverse shoulder arthroplasty and the tuberosities were reattached in an overlapping mode (tile technique) with embracing sutures. The supraspinatus muscle and upper part of infraspintus muscle inserted on top of the greater tuberosity was released (**Fig 3.1-34g–h**).

At the 2-year follow-up the patient herself was satisfied, as her range of motion was 140° of flexion, external rotation in 0° of abduction was -10°, and in internal rotation she could reach the lower lumbar spine. She continued to live independently and could even do some gardening (**Fig 3.1-34i–j**).

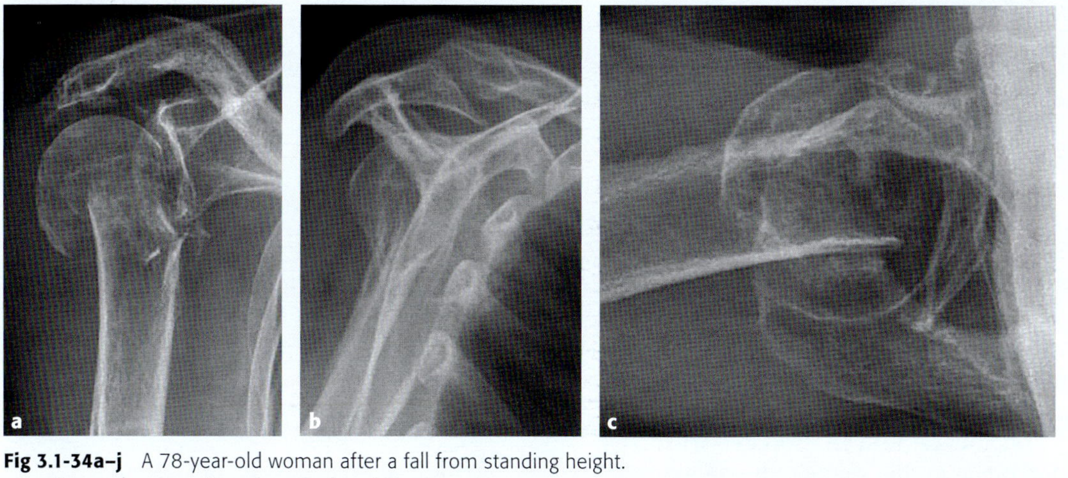


**Fig 3.1-34a–j** A 78-year-old woman after a fall from standing height.
**a–c** X-rays showing a 2-part surgical neck fracture.

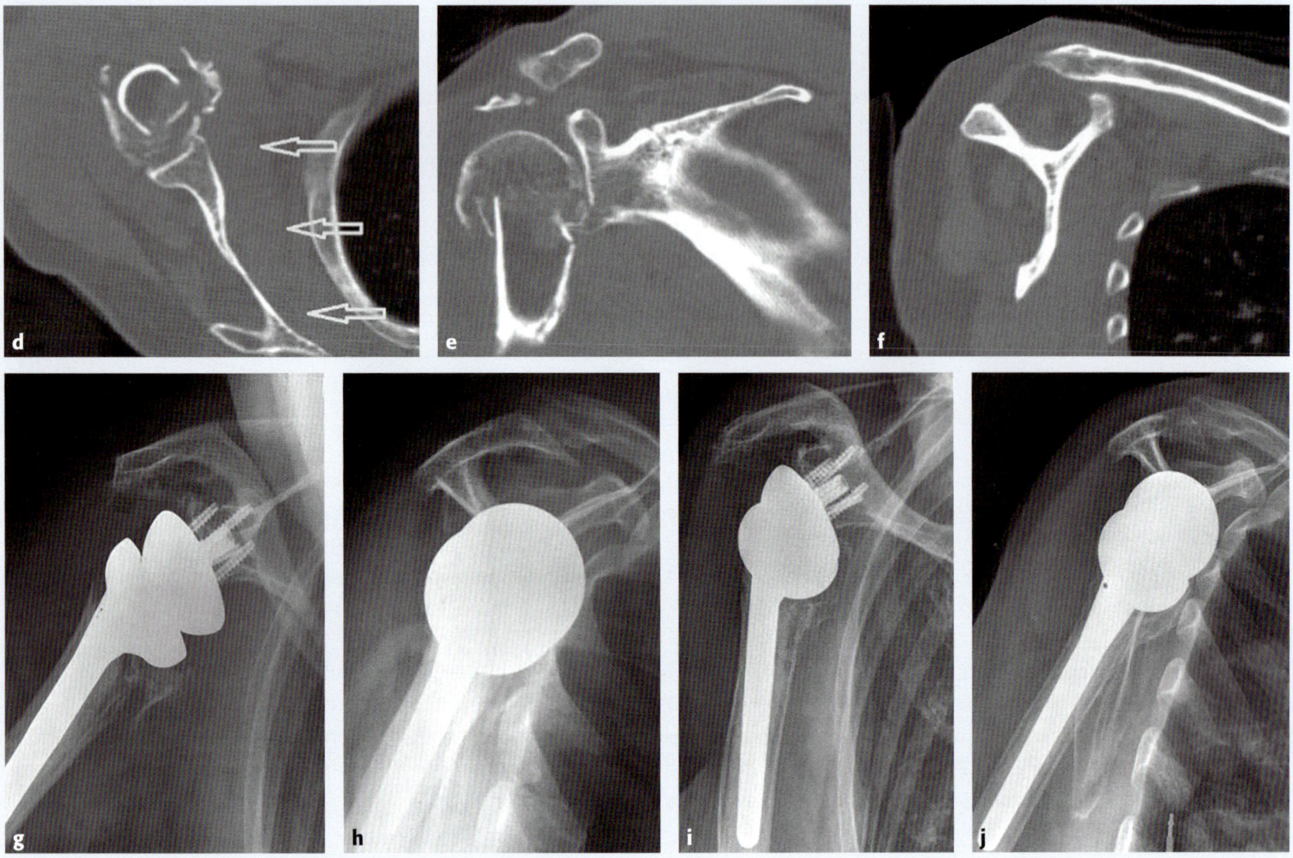


**Fig 3.1-34a–j (cont)** A 78-year-old woman after a fall from standing height.
**d–f** A preexisting computed tomographic angiography.
**g–h** Tuberosities reattached in an overlapping mode with embracing sutures. The supraspinatus muscle and upper part of infraspintus muscle inserted on top of the greater tuberosity is released.
**i–j** Two-year follow-up x-rays.

### 4.6 Summary

Reconstruction of complex orthogeriatric PHF remains challenging and high complication rates are reported. In selected patients and with stable and anatomical reconstruction good results can be achieved. Supportive techniques like allografts or implant augmentation with cement may improve the outcome. Anatomical SHA is associated with inconsistent results depending on the status of the tuberosities. In more recent studies with modern stem designs and adequate embracing fixation of the tuberosities, results are comparable with RSA, consistently better regarding external rotation. Reverse shoulder arthroplasty is increasing in use for primary fracture care. Many surgeons advocate the exclusive use of this type of joint replacement in patients aged 70 years and over, when treating complex 3- and 4-part fractures. Outcome data are conflicting and the need for prospective randomized studies is obvious.

## 5 References


1. **Kralinger F, Blauth M, Goldhahn J, et al.** The Influence of Local Bone Density on the Outcome of One Hundred and Fifty Proximal Humeral Fractures Treated with a Locking Plate. *J Bone Joint Surg Am.* 2014 Jun 18;96(12):1026–1032.
2. **Olerud P, Ahrengart L, Ponzer S, et al.** Internal fixation versus nonoperative treatment of displaced 3-part proximal humeral fractures in elderly patients: a randomized controlled trial. *J Shoulder Elbow Surg.* 2011 Jul;20(5):747–755.
3. **Sudkamp N, Bayer J, Hepp P, et al.** Open reduction and internal fixation of proximal humeral fractures with use of the locking proximal humerus plate. Results of a prospective, multicenter, observational study. *J Bone Joint Surg Am.* 2009 Jun;91(6):1320–1328.
4. **Einsiedel T, Becker C, Stengel D, et al.** Frakturen der oberen Extremität beim geriatrischen Patienten—Harmlose Monoverletzung oder Ende der Selbstständigkeit? Eine prospektive Studie zum Outcome nach distaler Radius- und proximaler Humerusfraktur bei über 65-jährigen [Do injuries of the upper extremity in geriatric patients end up in helplessness? A prospective study for the outcome of distal radius and proximal humerus fractures in individuals over 65]. *Z Gerontol Geriatr.* 2006 Dec;39(6):451–461. German.
5. **Hanson B, Neidenbach P, de Boer P, et al.** Functional outcomes after nonoperative management of fractures of the proximal humerus. *J Shoulder Elbow Surg.* 2009 Jul–Aug;18(4):612–621.
6. **Krettek C, Wiebking U.** Proximale Humerusfraktur. Ist die winkelstabile Plattenosteosynthese der konservativen Behandlung überlegen? [Proximal humerus fracture: is fixed-angle plate osteosynthesis superior to conservative treatment?]. *Unfallchirurg.* 2011 Dec;114(12):1059–1067. German.
7. **Palvanen M, Kannus P, Niemi S, et al.** Update in the epidemiology of proximal humeral fractures. *Clin Orthop Relat Res.* 2006 Jan;442:87–92.
8. **Roux A, Decroocq L, El Batti S, et al.** Epidemiology of proximal humerus fractures managed in a trauma center. *Orthop Traumatol Surg Res.* 2012 Oct;98(6):715–719.
9. **Hagino H, Yamamoto K, Ohshiro H, et al.** Changing incidence of hip, distal radius, and proximal humerus fractures in Tottori Prefecture, Japan. *Bone.* 1999 Mar;24(3):265–270.
10. **Kannus P, Palvanen M, Niemi S, et al.** Rate of proximal humeral fractures in older Finnish women between 1970 and 2007. *Bone.* 2009 Apr;44(4):656–659.
11. **Dimai HP, Svedbom A, Fahrleitner-Pammer A, et al.** Epidemiology of proximal humeral fractures in Austria between 1989 and 2008. *Osteoporos Int.* 2013 Sep;24(9):2413–2421.
12. **Lind T, Kroner K, Jensen J.** The epidemiology of fractures of the proximal humerus. *Arch Orthop Trauma Surg.* 1989;108(5):285–287.
13. **Robinson CM.** Proximal humerus fractures. In: Bucholz RW, Court-Brown CM, Heckman JD, et al, eds. *Fractures in Adults.* Philadelphia: Lippincott Williams & Wilkins; 2010:1039–1105.
14. **Nguyen TV, Center JR, Sambrook PN, et al.** Risk factors for proximal humerus, forearm, and wrist fractures in elderly men and women: the Dubbo Osteoporosis Epidemiology Study. *Am J Epidemiol.* 2001 Mar 15;153(6):587–595.
15. **Euler SA, Kralinger FS, Hengg C, et al.** Allograft augmentation in proximal humerus fractures. *Oper Orthop Traumatol.* 2016 Jun;28(3):153–163.
16. **Euler SA, Hengg C, Wambacher M, et al.** Allogenic bone grafting for augmentation in two-part proximal humeral fracture fixation in a high-risk patient population. *Arch Orthop Trauma Surg.* 2015 Jan;135(1):79–87.
17. **Hageman MG, Jayakumar P, King JD, et al.** The factors influencing the decision making of operative treatment for proximal humeral fractures. *J Shoulder Elbow Surg.* 2015 Jan;24(1):e21–e26.
18. **Volgas DA, Stannard JP, Alonso JE.** Nonunions of the humerus. *Clin Orthop Relat Res.* 2004 Feb(419):46–50.
19. **Goutallier D, Postel JM, Bernageau J, et al.** Fatty infiltration of disrupted rotator cuff muscles. *Rev Rhum Engl Ed.* 1995 Jun;62(6):415–422.
20. **Hengg C, Mayrhofer P, Euler S, et al.** The relevance of neutral arm positioning for true ap-view X-ray to provide true projection of the humeral head shaft angle. *Arch Orthop Trauma Surg.* 2016 Feb;136(2):213–221.
21. **Foroohar A, Tosti R, Richmond JM, et al.** Classification and treatment of proximal humerus fractures: inter-observer reliability and agreement across imaging modalities and experience. *J Orthop Surg Res.* 2011;6:38.
22. **Twiss T.** Nonoperative Treatment of Proximal Humerus Fractures. In: Crosby LN, R., eds. *Proximal Humerus Fractures: Evaluation and Management.* Cham: Springer; 2015:23–41.
23. **Scola A, Gebhard F, Weckbach S, et al.** Mechanical quantification of local bone quality in the humeral head: a feasibility study. *Open Orthop J.* 2013;7:172–176.
24. **Krappinger D, Roth T, Gschwentner M, et al.** Preoperative assessment of the cancellous bone mineral density of the proximal humerus using CT data. *Skeletal Radiol.* 2012 Mar;41(3):299–304.
25. **Roderer G, Scola A, Schmolz W, et al.** Biomechanical in vitro assessment of screw augmentation in locked plating of proximal humerus fractures. *Injury.* 2013 Oct;44(10):1327–1332.
26. **Unger S, Erhart S, Kralinger F, et al.** The effect of in situ augmentation on implant anchorage in proximal humeral head fractures. *Injury.* 2012 Oct;43(10):1759–1763.
27. **Gradl G, Knobe M, Stoffel M, et al.** Biomechanical evaluation of locking plate fixation of proximal humeral fractures augmented with calcium phosphate cement. *J Orthop Trauma.* 2013 Jul;27(7):399–404.
28. **Krappinger D, Bizzotto N, Riedmann S, et al.** Predicting failure after surgical fixation of proximal humerus fractures. *Injury.* 2011 Nov;42(11):1283–1288.
29. **Gallo RA, Sciulli R, Daffner RH, et al.** Defining the relationship between rotator cuff injury and proximal humerus fractures. *Clin Orthop Relat Res.* 2007 May;458:70–77.
30. **Court-Brown CM, Cattermole H, McQueen MM.** Impacted valgus fractures (B1.1) of the proximal humerus. The results of non-operative treatment. *J Bone Joint Surg Br.* 2002 May;84(4):504–508.
31. **Neer CS 2nd.** Displaced proximal humeral fractures. I. Classification and evaluation. *J Bone Joint Surg Am.* 1970 Sep;52(6):1077–1089.
32. **Majed A, Macleod I, Bull AM, et al.** Proximal humeral fracture classification systems revisited. *J Shoulder Elbow Surg.* 2011 Oct;20(7):1125–1132.
33. **Sjoden GO, Movin T, Guntner P, et al.** Poor reproducibility of classification of proximal humeral fractures. Additional CT of minor value. *Acta Orthop Scand.* 1997 Jun;68(3):239–242.
34. **Brunner A, Honigmann P, Treumann T, et al.** The impact of stereo-visualisation of three-dimensional CT datasets on the inter- and intraobserver reliability of the AO/OTA and Neer classifications in the assessment of fractures of the proximal humerus. *J Bone Joint Surg Br.* 2009 Jun;91(6):766–771.
35. **Sidor ML, Zuckerman JD, Lyon T, et al.** The Neer classification system for proximal humeral fractures. An assessment of interobserver reliability and intraobserver reproducibility. *J Bone Joint Surg Am.* 1993 Dec;75(12):1745–1750.

36. **Hertel R.** Fractures of the proximal humerus in osteoporotic bone. *Osteoporos Int.* 2005 Mar;16(Suppl 2):S65–S72.
37. **Sukthankar AV, Leonello DT, Hertel RW, et al.** A comprehensive classification of proximal humeral fractures: HGLS system. *J Shoulder Elbow Surg.* 2013 Jul;22(7):e1–e6.
38. **Bhandari M, Matthys G, McKee MD.** Four part fractures of the proximal humerus. *J Orthop Trauma.* 2004 Feb;18(2):126–127.
39. **Handoll HH, Gibson JN, Madhok R.** Interventions for treating proximal humeral fractures in adults. *Cochrane Database Syst Rev.* 2003 (4):CD000434.
40. **Olsson C, Nordqvist A, Petersson CJ.** Increased fragility in patients with fracture of the proximal humerus: a case control study. *Bone.* 2004 Jun;34(6):1072–1077.
41. **Torrens C, Corrales M, Vila G, et al.** Functional and quality-of-life results of displaced and nondisplaced proximal humeral fractures treated conservatively. *J Orthop Trauma.* 2011 Oct;25(10):581–587.
42. **Hinds RM, Garner MR, Tran WH, et al.** Geriatric proximal humeral fracture patients show similar clinical outcomes to non-geriatric patients after osteosynthesis with endosteal fibular strut allograft augmentation. *J Shoulder Elbow Surg.* 2015 Jun;24(6):889–896.
43. **Schmidt A.** Proximal humeral fractures and shoulder dislocations. In: Stannard JP, Schmidt AH, Kregor PJ, eds. *Surgical treatment of orthopaedic trauma.* New York: Thieme; 2007.
44. **Fjalestad T, Hole MO, Hovden IA, et al.** Surgical treatment with an angular stable plate for complex displaced proximal humeral fractures in elderly patients: a randomized controlled trial. *J Orthop Trauma.* 2012 Feb;26(2):98–106.
45. **Olerud P, Ahrengart L, Ponzer S, et al.** Hemiarthroplasty versus nonoperative treatment of displaced 4-part proximal humeral fractures in elderly patients: a randomized controlled trial. *J Shoulder Elbow Surg.* 2011 Oct;20(7):1025–1033.
46. **Misra A, Kapur R, Maffulli N.** Complex proximal humeral fractures in adults—a systematic review of management. *Injury.* 2001 Jun;32(5):363–372.
47. **van den Broek CM, van den Besselaar M, Coenen JM, et al.** Displaced proximal humeral fractures: intramedullary nailing versus conservative treatment. *Arch Orthop Trauma Surg.* 2007 Aug;127(6):459–463.
48. **Lill H, Bewer A, Korner J, et al.** Konservative Therapie dislozierter proximaler Humerusfrakturen [Conservative treatment of dislocated proximal humeral fractures]. *Zentralbl Chir.* 2001 Mar;126(3):205–210. German.
49. **Court-Brown CM, McQueen MM.** The impacted varus (A2.2) proximal humeral fracture: prediction of outcome and results of nonoperative treatment in 99 patients. *Acta Orthop Scand.* 2004 Dec;75(6):736–740.
50. **Gaebler C, McQueen MM, Court-Brown CM.** Minimally displaced proximal humeral fractures: epidemiology and outcome in 507 cases. *Acta Orthop Scand.* 2003 Oct;74(5):580–585.
51. **Koval KJ, Gallagher MA, Marsicano JG, et al.** Functional outcome after minimally displaced fractures of the proximal part of the humerus. *J Bone Joint Surg Am.* 1997 Feb;79(2):203–207.
52. **Acklin YP, Sommer C.** Plate fixation of proximal humerus fractures using the minimally invasive anterolateral delta split approach. *Oper Orthop Traumatol.* 2012 Feb;24(1):61–73.
53. **Plecko M, Kraus A.** Internal fixation of proximal humerus fractures using the locking proximal humerus plate. *Oper Orthop Traumatol.* 2005 Feb;17(1):25–50.
54. **Hepp P, Theopold J, Voigt C, et al.** The surgical approach for locking plate osteosynthesis of displaced proximal humeral fractures influences the functional outcome. *J Shoulder Elbow Surg.* 2008 Jan–Feb;17(1):21–28.
55. **Wu CH, Ma CH, Yeh JJ, et al.** Locked plating for proximal humeral fractures: differences between the deltopectoral and deltoid-splitting approaches. *J Trauma.* 2011 Nov;71(5):1364–1370.
56. **Boileau P, d'Ollone T, Hatzidakis AM, et al.** Intramedullary Locking Nail Fixation of Proximal Humerus Fractures: Rationale and Technique. In: Crosby LA, Neviaser RJ, eds. *Proximal Humerus Fractures: Evaluation and Management.* Cham: Springer International Publishing; 2015:73–98.
57. **Hettrich CM, Neviaser A, Beamer BS, et al.** Locked plating of the proximal humerus using an endosteal implant. *J Orthop Trauma.* 2012 Apr;26(4):212–215.
58. **Osterhoff G, Baumgartner D, Favre P, et al.** Medial support by fibula bone graft in angular stable plate fixation of proximal humeral fractures: an in vitro study with synthetic bone. *J Shoulder Elbow Surg.* 2011 Jul;20(5):740–746.
59. **Osterhoff G, Ossendorf C, Wanner GA, et al.** The calcar screw in angular stable plate fixation of proximal humeral fractures—a case study. *J Orthop Surg Res.* 2011;6:50.
60. **Spross C, Platz A, Rufibach K, et al.** The PHILOS plate for proximal humeral fractures—risk factors for complications at one year. *J Trauma Acute Care Surg.* 2012 Mar;72(3):783–792.
61. **Clavert P, Adam P, Bevort A, et al.** Pitfalls and complications with locking plate for proximal humerus fracture. *J Shoulder Elbow Surg.* 2010 Jun;19(4):489–494.
62. **Bahrs C, Kuhle L, Blumenstock G, et al.** Which parameters affect medium- to long-term results after angular stable plate fixation for proximal humeral fractures? *J Shoulder Elbow Surg.* 2015 May;24(5):727–732.
63. **Lopiz Y, Garcia-Coiradas J, Garcia-Fernandez C, et al.** Proximal humerus nailing: a randomized clinical trial between curvilinear and straight nails. *J Shoulder Elbow Surg.* 2014 Mar;23(3):369–376.
64. **Rothstock S, Plecko M, Kloub M, et al.** Biomechanical evaluation of two intramedullary nailing techniques with different locking options in a three-part fracture proximal humerus model. *Clin Biomech (Bristol, Avon).* 2012 Aug;27(7):686–691.
65. **Hessmann MH, Nijs S, Mittlmeier T, et al.** Internal fixation of fractures of the proximal humerus with the MultiLoc nail. *Oper Orthop Traumatol.* 2012 Sep;24(4–5):418–431.
66. **Hatzidakis AM, Shevlin MJ, Fenton DL, et al.** Angular-stable locked intramedullary nailing of two-part surgical neck fractures of the proximal part of the humerus. A multicenter retrospective observational study. *J Bone Joint Surg Am.* 2011 Dec 7;93(23):2172–2179.
67. **Cuff DJ, Pupello DR.** Comparison of hemiarthroplasty and reverse shoulder arthroplasty for the treatment of proximal humeral fractures in elderly patients. *J Bone Joint Surg Am.* 2013 Nov 20;95(22):2050–2055.
68. **Ferrel JR, Trinh TQ, Fischer RA.** Reverse total shoulder arthroplasty versus hemiarthroplasty for proximal humeral fractures: a systematic review. *J Orthop Trauma.* 2015 Jan;29(1):60–68.
69. **Reuther F, Kohut G, Nijs S.** [Newly developed modular reverse fracture endoprosthesis in non-reconstructable humeral head fracture in old people]. *Oper Orthop Traumatol.* 2014 Aug;26(4):369–382; quiz 382–384.
70. **Mata-Fink A, Meinke M, Jones C, et al.** Reverse shoulder arthroplasty for treatment of proximal humeral fractures in older adults: a systematic review. *J Shoulder Elbow Surg.* 2013 Dec;22(12):1737–1748.
71. **Namdari S, Horneff JG, Baldwin K.** Comparison of hemiarthroplasty and reverse arthroplasty for treatment of proximal humeral fractures: a systematic review. *J Bone Joint Surg Am.* 2013 Sep 18;95(18):1701–1708.

# 3.2 Humeral shaft

Clemens Hengg, Vajara Phiphobmongkol

## 1 Introduction

Humeral shaft fractures are common in geriatric patients with a clinically significant impact on upper extremity function, independence, gait, balance, and mobilization.

Historically, nonoperative treatment has been common. However, surgical fixation may restore patients' independence more rapidly and allow for safer mobilization. As with proximal humeral fractures, treatment recommendations depend in part on surgeon experience, skills, and preference.

## 2 Epidemiology and etiology

Humeral shaft fractures account for 1–3% of all fractures [1]. They are less frequent than fractures of the proximal humerus. In one series of 2011 humeral fractures 79% were proximal, 13% shaft, and 8% distal humeral fractures [2]. Fractures of the humeral shaft have a bimodal age distribution, with a minor peak in the third decade and a major peak in the eighth decade. In the younger population, most fractures occur in men and are predominantly due to high-energy trauma. In older adults, simple falls are the most common mechanism of injury and the overwhelming majority are in women [2].

## 3 Diagnostics and classification

Patients present with arm pain, swelling and hematoma. Depending on the amount of fracture displacement, axis and rotation of the arm may deviate. The arm may be shortened and may demonstrate crepitus with manipulation. A careful neurovascular evaluation of the extremity is essential.

Usually plain x-rays in AP and lateral including the adjacent joints are sufficient for diagnosis and classification.

Complex or combined fractures of the shaft and the proximal or distal end of the humerus should be assessed with computed tomographic (CT) scan.

The AO/OTA Fracture and Dislocation Classification is recommended and can be applied to older patients as well.

## 4 Decision making

### 4.1 Nonoperative treatment

Historically, nonoperative treatment has been widely used for these injuries [3]. The authors prefer conservative treatment especially in simple long spiral fractures. However, short oblique or transverse fractures are also suitable for nonoperative treatment [4, 5].

The risk of nonunion and impaired shoulder function after nonoperative treatment must not be underestimated (**Case 1: Fig 3.2-1**).

If nonoperative treatment is considered, bone fragments must align and approximate without suspicion of interposed muscle tissue.

It may be necessary to revise the decision for nonoperative treatment if bone healing appears unlikely and/or if the burden of nonoperative treatment mainly in terms of pain and functional restriction cannot be handled by the patient (**Case 2: Fig 3.2-2**) [6, 7].

CASE 1

## Patient

An 82-year-old man had an unobserved fall. He sustained a fracture of the right humerus (**Fig 3.2-1a–b**).

## Comorbidities

- Alcoholism
- Renal failure
- Failure to thrive

## Treatment and outcome

Decision making—Due to the fracture type, general state of the patient (eg, alcoholism and frailty), and concerns for noncompliance, nonoperative fracture treatment was chosen. The x-rays showed the initial position in a hanging cast (**Fig 3.2-1c–d**).

Course of treatment—After 3 weeks, the fracture was significantly displaced by the traction of the deltoid muscle with fracture angulation of 45°. Due to inability to comply with immobilization the fracture reduction could not be maintained with bracing (**Fig 3.2-1e–f**). The patient had little pain and no soft-tissue problems. After 5 weeks the situation was unchanged so the treatment decision was revised (**Fig 3.2-1g–h**).

Operative treatment—The nonunion was explored and reduced using an anterior approach by pushing the biceps muscle medially and performing a centric split of the upper portion of the brachialis muscle. Reduction was retained temporarily with a reduction clamp, while the antegrade nailing was performed (**Fig 3.2-1i–j**). The anterolateral approach was used for nailing and the anterior approach to the humeral shaft was used for addressing the nonunion (**Fig 3.1-2k**).

Postoperative—Anatomical fracture fixation was achieved with no soft-tissue complications and little pain (**Fig 3.2-1l–m**). At the 6-month follow-up, the fracture had healed with restoration of adequate function (**Fig 3.2-1n–r**).

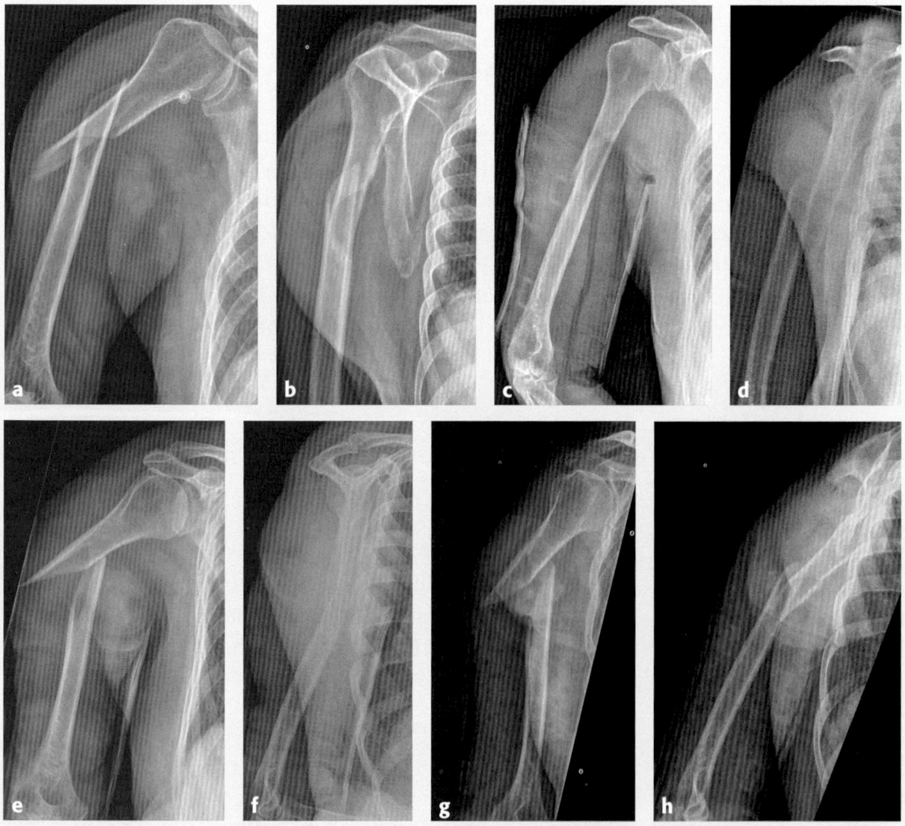


**Fig 3.2-1a–r** An 82-year-old man with a right humeral fracture.
**a–b** Closed spiral fracture of the proximal shaft of the right humerus (AO/OTA 12A1) without comminution.
**c–d** AP (**c**) and lateral (**d**) views showing almost full restoration of the anatomical position and acceptable displacement, respectively.
**e–f** X-rays showing significant fracture displacement as a result of noncompliance to immobilization.
**g–h** Postoperative x-rays at 5 weeks showing a still significantly displaced fracture.

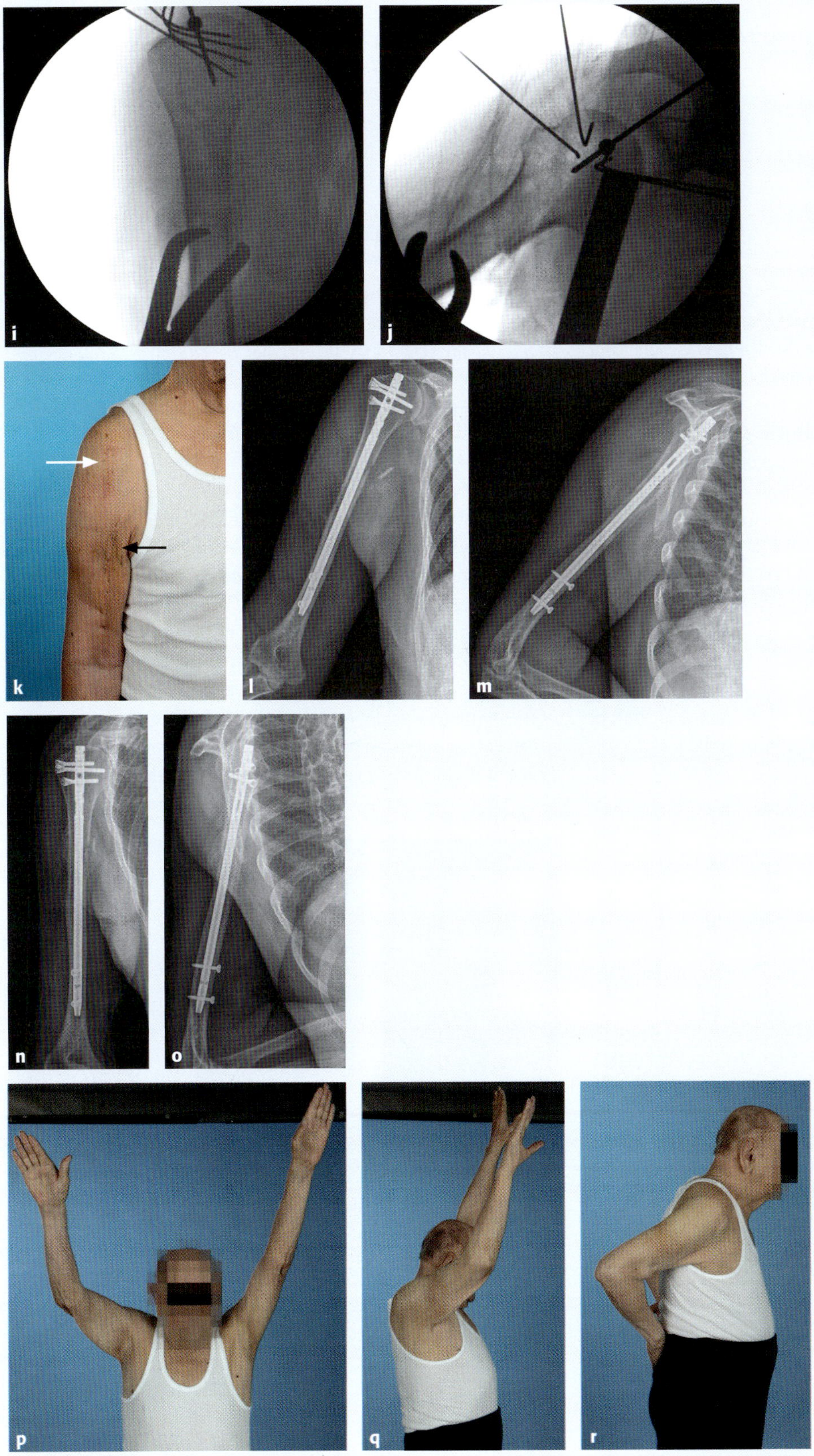


**Fig 3.2-1a–r (cont)** An 82-year-old man with a right humeral fracture.

**i–j** Temporary reduction with a clamp.

**k** Anterolateral approach (white arrow) for nailing and anterior approach (black arrow) to the humeral shaft for treating the nonunion.

**l–m** Postoperative x-rays.

**n–r** Postoperative x-rays (**n–o**) and clinical photographs (**p–r**) at 6 months showing a healed fracture with good function.

CASE 2

## Patient

A 92-year-old woman with left humeral shaft fracture related to low-energy trauma.

## Comorbidities

- Dementia
- Hypertension
- Diabetes mellitus
- Osteoporosis

## Treatment and outcome

History—The patient was initially treated with a sugar-tong splint and arm sling in another hospital (**Fig 3.2-2a–b**). There was significant displacement and angulation. At the 3-month follow-up (**Fig 3.2-2c**), the alignment was unacceptable and the skin was tenting with a bone spike. The patient still had pain and there was no sign of bone union. Despite this, this treatment plan was continued for 4 months.

Current situation—The treatment decision was revised to operative treatment. Soft-tissue irritation also was a cause of pain (**Fig 3.2-2d–f**).

Diagnosis and classification—The initial diagnosis was closed fracture of the proximal shaft of the left humerus (AO/OTA 12A1). The current diagnosis is nonunion.

Indication for surgery—A painful nonunion of the proximal shaft of the left humerus. Skin complication due to bony spike.

Treatment planning:

- Fixation: open reduction and internal fixation (ORIF) with a narrow locking compression plate and iliac bone grafting
- Positioning: supine on transparent x-ray table
- C-arm: located on the opposite side
- Preparation and draping: from shoulder to hand and free to move in any direction
- Surgical approach: anterolateral, direct reduction

Intraoperative technique—Soft tissues were removed at the fracture site and the bone ends were freshened (**Fig 3.2-2g**). The sharp spike of the proximal fragment (**Fig 3.2-2h**) and the V-shaped cortical fracture site of the distal fragment corresponding with the shape of the proximal end (behind the sharp spike in **Fig 3.2-2g**) could be seen. The incision was extended distally to identify and protect the radial nerve. The sharp spike of the proximal fragment was pushed into the intramedullary canal through a V-shaped opening of the distal fragment to create a stable bone construction before plating (**Fig 3.2-2i**). This provides significant stability of fixation in osteoporotic bone, which even with the use of many locking head screws may not be able to withstand the bending and rotational deforming forces. Through a proximal incision of the deltoid split, PHILOS was inserted submuscularly into position on the lateral aspect of the humerus. Correct positioning of the plate was confirmed through a true AP x-ray of the proximal humerus using image intensification, then temporarily fixed with a K-wire (**Fig 3.2-2j–k**). The sharp bony spike of the proximal fragment was pushed into the intramedullary canal of the distal fragment to create primary stability and the screws were fixed in compression holes close to the fracture site to add more stability (**Fig 3.2-2l–m**). An iliac bone graft was impacted in the fracture gap on the medial side after complete plate fixation (**Fig 3.2-2n–p**). Immediate postoperative x-rays showed good alignment and stable bone-implant construction (**Fig 3.2-2q–r**).

Postoperative care—Gentle active assistive exercise for range of motion (ROM) of the shoulder and elbow were started on the second day postoperatively. No pushing or pulling were allowed until bone union (**Fig 3.2-2s–t**). The patient could flex the shoulder forward (**Fig 3.2-2u–v**), though her ROM was limited due to her prolonged preoperative immobility and her dementia, both of which limited rehabilitation capabilities. She could perform adequate, pain-free flexion and extension of the elbow. Rotational movement of the humerus was done gently in light of risk of screw failure due to severe osteoporosis. The patient had no pain and had good ability to perform daily living activities (**Fig 3.2-2s–v**).

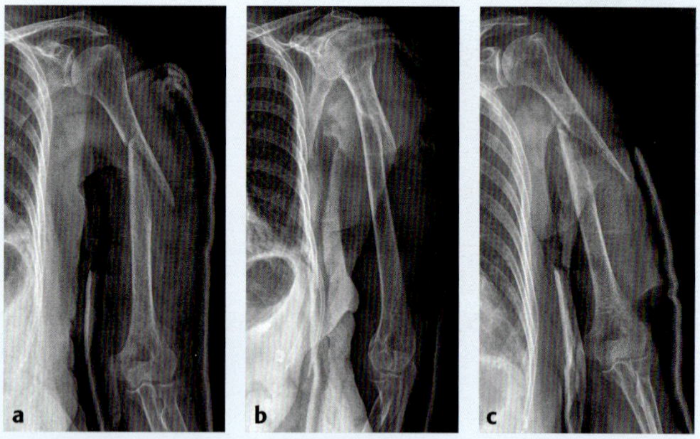


**Fig 3.2-2a–v** A 92-year-old woman with a fracture of the left humeral shaft after a low-energy trauma.
**a–c** Initial AP (**a**) and lateral (**b**) x-rays showing significant displacement and angulation. The 3-month follow-up (**c**) showing unacceptable alignment and no sign of bone union.

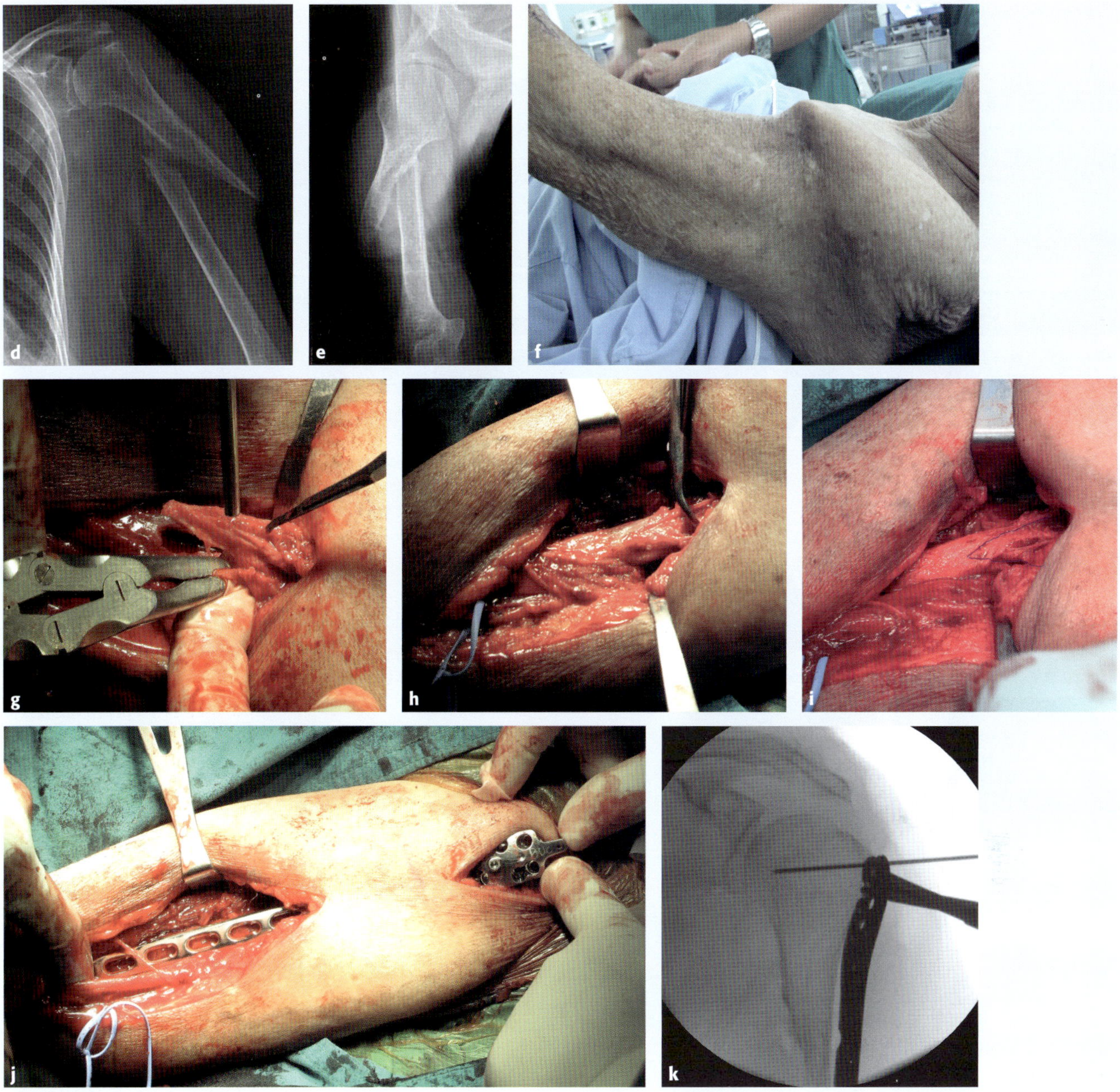

**Fig 3.2-2a–v (cont)** A 92-year-old woman with a fracture of the left humeral shaft after a low-energy trauma.

**d–f** Nonunion after 4 months.

**g–h** Removal of soft tissue at the fracture ends (**g**). Note the sharp spike of the proximal fragment (**h**) and the V-shaped cortical fracture site of the distal fragment.

**i** Clinical photograph showing the radial nerve (blue tape).

**j–k** Clinical photograph (**j**) showing proximal incision of the deltoid-split approach and AP x-ray (**k**) of the proximal humerus.

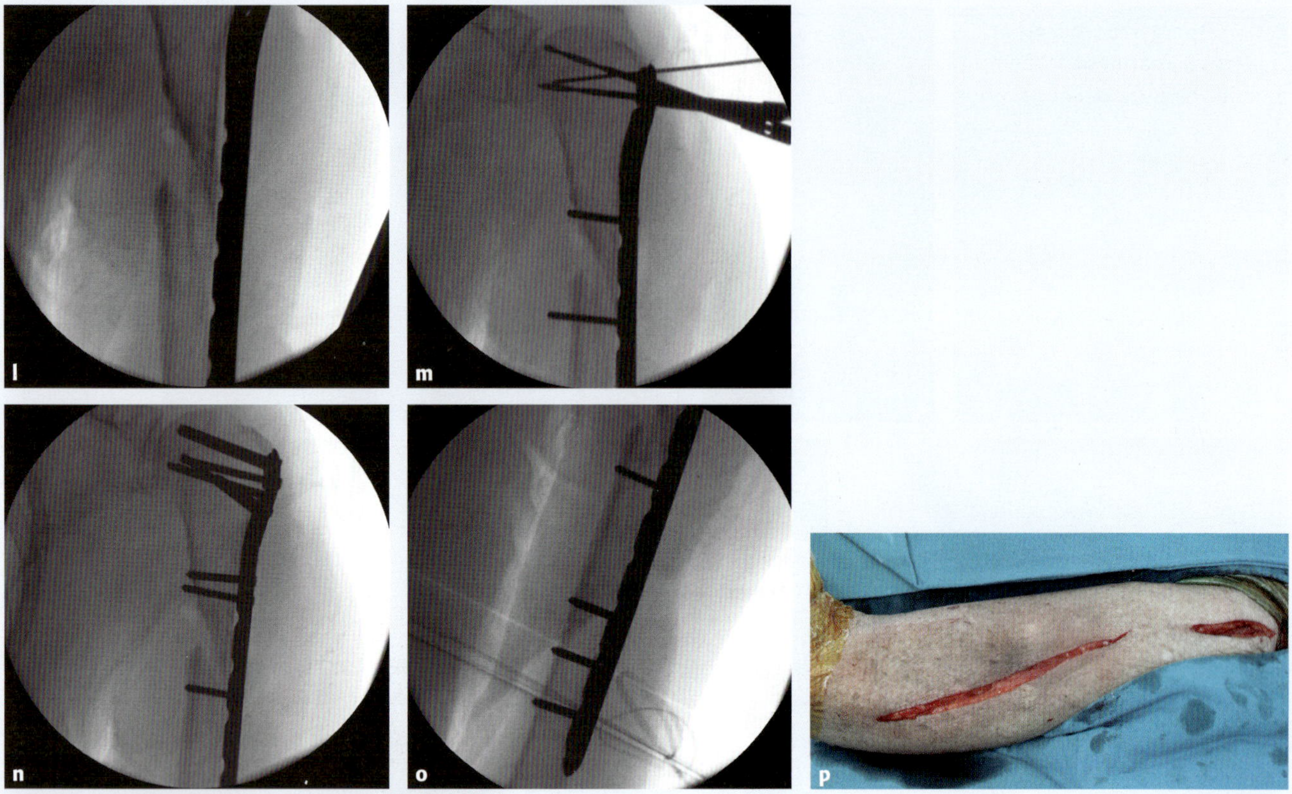

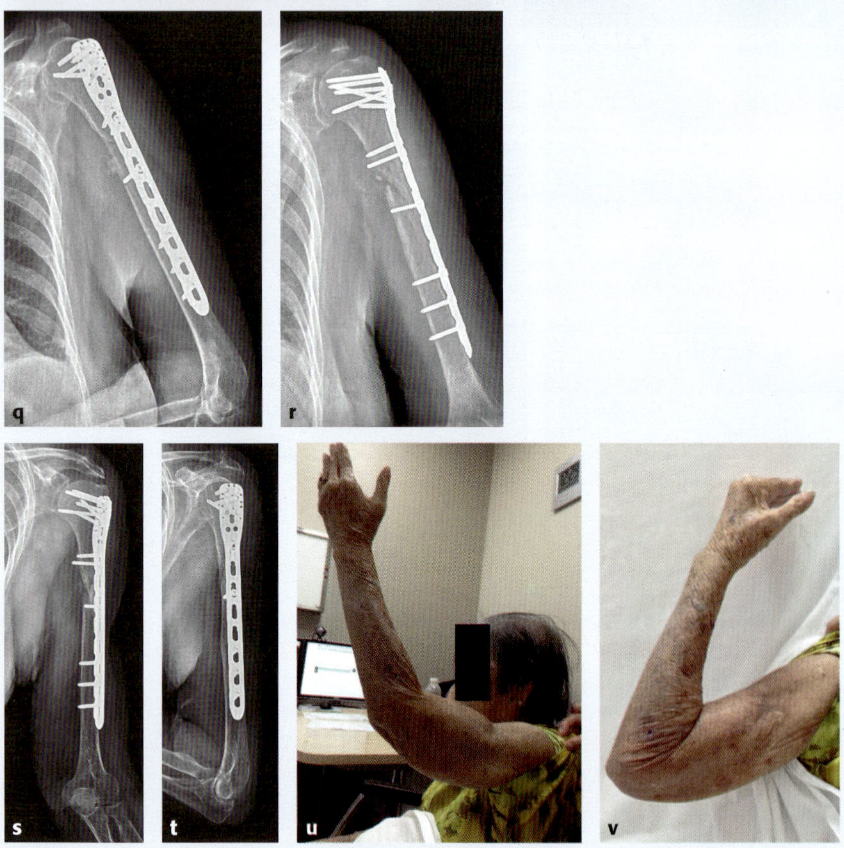

**Fig 3.2-2a–v (cont)** A 92-year-old woman with a fracture of the left humeral shaft after a low-energy trauma.

**l–m** X-rays showing the proximal fragment pushed into the distal fragment (**l**) and the screws in compression holes close to the fracture site (**m**).

**n–p** X-rays and clinical photograph showing the iliac bone graft impacted into the fracture gap on the medial side (**n–o**) and the separate skin incisions of anterolateral and deltoid split approaches (**p**), respectively.

**q–r** Immediate postoperative x-rays showing good alignment.

**s–v** Postoperative x-rays and clinical photographs at 16 months showing bone union (**s–t**) and adequate forward flexion of the shoulder and extension of the elbow (**u–v**).

(Courtesy of Dr Suthorn Bavonratanavech)

## 4.2 Operative treatment

Operative treatment of the humeral shaft should be considered in the following situations:

- Inability to maintain nonoperative fracture reduction. This depends on fracture patterns and the degree of displacement, comminution, whether short oblique or transverse fractures, as well as patient factors, such as obesity or ability to comply with activity and weight-bearing restrictions.
- Complicated mobilization because of concomitant fractures of the lower extremities
- Bilateral humeral fractures: fixation of at least one side to maximize the patient's independence with activity
- Ipsilateral fracture of the proximal or distal humerus, especially articular fracture extension
- Ipsilateral fracture of the elbow joint or forearm
- Open fractures
- Polytrauma
- Pathological fractures
- Fractures associated with a neurovascular injury

In addition, operative fixation may help to preserve patients' independence by earlier and safer mobilization.

Management of humeral shaft fractures associated with radial nerve palsy is controversial [8–11]. Radial nerve injury is a common complication of humeral shaft fractures, occurring in up to 18% of closed injuries [4, 12]; spontaneous recovery can be expected in 90% of cases at 4 months after injury.

If there are no objective clinical signs of radial nerve recovery at 6 weeks postinjury (ie, return of brachioradialis, extensor carpi radialis longus, and brevis muscle function), electromyography and nerve conduction studies should be performed. In the absence of recovery at 12 weeks, as indicated by clinical examination and neurophysiological testing, surgical exploration of the radial nerve is recommended [4].

If in doubt, ultrasonographic assessment of the integrity of the radial nerve may inform the treatment decision [13].

## 4.3 Plating versus nailing

Plating and nailing can achieve similar reduction. Antegrade nailing can potentially cause shoulder pain or restricted range of motion because the involvement of the rotator cuff. We are not aware of any study focussing on shoulder problems after antegrade nailing in older patients [14].

In their metaanalysis, Liu et al [15] found that intramedullary (IM) nailing appears comparable to plate fixation in terms of rates of nonunion, postoperative infection, and radial nerve palsy. The only minor difference they identified was a higher delayed healing rate in patients treated with a nail.

Kumar et al [16] came to a similar conclusion in their prospective study of 30 patients: finding that plating offered advantages in less time to union, better joint function, and reduced reoperation, whereas nailing offers a minimally invasive approach, less infection, less nerve injury, and less chance of implant failure.

Retrograde nailing became unpopular mainly because of the somehow unpredictable risk of creating iatrogenic distal humeral fractures while inserting the nail.

As the literature does not clearly support a superior procedure, the experience and preference of the surgeon must also be considered.

## 4.4 Minimally invasive plate osteosynthesis versus open reduction and internal fixation

Selecting minimally invasive plate osteosynthesis (MIPO) or open reduction and internal fixation (ORIF) depends on the fracture type: in case of type A fractures (simple fracture), ORIF is preferred to close the fracture, create adequate contact, and reduce the strain of the fracture site [17].

On the other hand, in case of type C (multifragmentary) fractures of the midshaft of the humerus, bridging plate with MIPO on the anterior surface is a good option, as the strain of the fracture sites is lower and the procedure preserves the blood supply of the fragments [18, 19].

The treatment decision in type B fractures is controversial: it depends on many details such as size, type of wedge, displacement, and quality of reduction, if indirect reduction leaves a significant gap and creates so-called high-strain condition, ORIF to reduce the fracture with adequate soft-tissue handling is required to preserve nutritional soft-tissue attachment to the fracture fragments.

## 5 Treatment

### 5.1 Nonoperative techniques

The fracture should be reduced to ensure length, axis, and rotation. Then it has to be immobilized (Desault plaster, hanging cast, U-plaster splint). The achieved reduction should be documented and monitored radiographically.

After 2–3 weeks of cast immobilization, the authors switch to functional bracing for 6–8 weeks until the fracture is healed.

Case 3: **Fig 3.2-3** [20, 21] shows nonoperative treatment of a midshaft humeral fracture.

CASE 3

**Patient**

A 68-year-old woman fell and had right arm pain and swelling.

**Comorbidities**

- Hypertension
- Diabetes mellitus
- Previous cerebrovascular accident
- Osteopenia

**Treatment and outcome**

Diagnosis—The diagnosis was a closed fracture of the right humeral shaft (AO/OTA 12A3). There was minimal displacement and no distraction (**Fig 3.2-3a**).

Treatment plan—Nonoperative treatment with a coaptation splint and arm sling. After closed manipulation and immobilization in a U-slab, AP and lateral x-rays of the right humerus showed adequate apposition (**Fig 3.2-3b–c**), the axial alignment was acceptable in both views. X-ray at the 2-week follow-up with coaptation splint showed that alignment was maintained (**Fig 3.2-3d**). At the 2-month follow-up, there were signs of callus formation at the fracture site (**Fig 3.2-3e–f**). The patient had minimal pain, good elbow flexion/extension (**Fig 3.2-3g–h**), and forward flexion of the shoulder (**Fig 3.2-3i**). At the 3-month follow-up, there was adequate callus formation. The patient was pain free, and the splint was removed (**Fig 3.2-3j–k**).

**Discussion**

Nonoperative treatment was possible in this case as there were many favorable factors including:

- Mild displacement with adequate apposition visible on the initial x-rays
- Axial alignment was adequate with acceptable angulation
- No distraction at the fracture site

These x-ray findings reflect the condition of the periosteum around the fracture which might be intact.

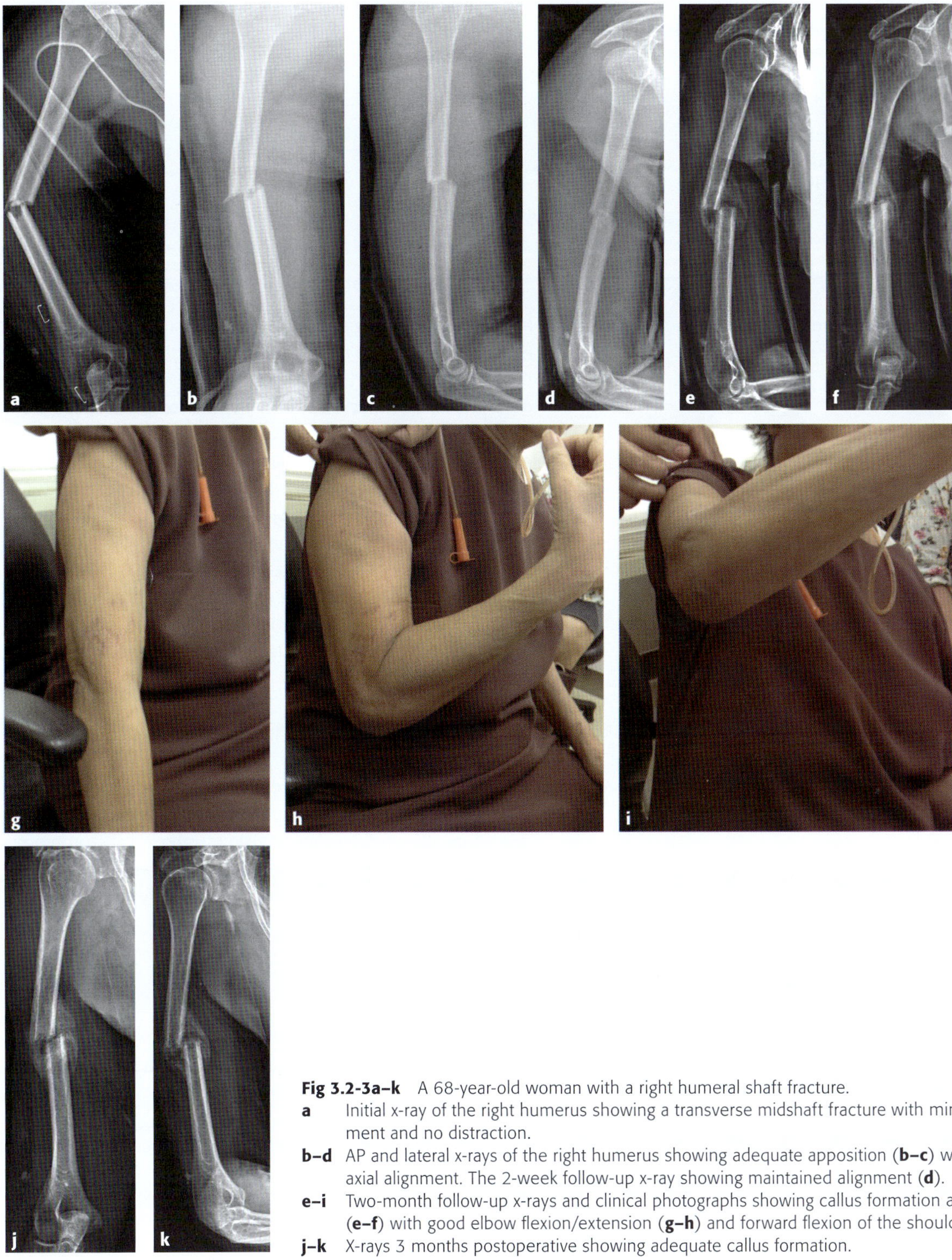

**Fig 3.2-3a–k** A 68-year-old woman with a right humeral shaft fracture.

**a** Initial x-ray of the right humerus showing a transverse midshaft fracture with minimal displacement and no distraction.

**b–d** AP and lateral x-rays of the right humerus showing adequate apposition (**b–c**) with acceptable axial alignment. The 2-week follow-up x-ray showing maintained alignment (**d**).

**e–i** Two-month follow-up x-rays and clinical photographs showing callus formation at the fracture site (**e–f**) with good elbow flexion/extension (**g–h**) and forward flexion of the shoulder (**i**).

**j–k** X-rays 3 months postoperative showing adequate callus formation.

## 5.2 Open reduction and plate fixation in proximal shaft fractures

Open reduction and plate fixation with PHILOS plate via the standard anterolateral approach is one treatment option for long spiral fractures of the proximal shaft; additional wiring helps achieve reduction, maintain alignment, and provide stability (**Case 4: Fig 3.2-4**) [22, 23].

CASE 4

### Patient

An 80-year-old woman with severe osteoporosis. She had a minor fall with pain and deformity of the right arm.

### Comorbidities

- Dementia
- Osteoporosis
- Hypertension
- Coronary heart disease
- Chronic kidney disease
- Thoracic and lumbar spine spondylosis with kyphoscoliosis. Multiple thoracic compression fractures (**Fig 3.2-4a–d**)
- Severe osteoporosis with multiple levels of collapsed vertebra. The patient had never been treated for osteoporosis.

### Treatment and outcome

Diagnosis and classification—Closed fracture of the proximal shaft of the right humerus (AO/OTA 12A1), spiral fracture without comminution. A long spiral fracture is a common finding in geriatric patients after low-energy trauma (**Fig 3.2-4e–f**).

Indications for surgery:

- Displaced fracture with severe pain
- Malalignment in the proximal shaft after nonoperative treatment
- Requirement for functional independence for acceptable quality of life

Treatment planning:

- Fixation: open reduction and internal fixation with PHILOS
- Positioning: supine on a radiolucent table, C-arm located on the opposite side
- Preparation and draping: from shoulder to hand and free to move in any direction
- Surgical approach: deltopectoral approach with extension to the anterolateral approach

Intraoperative technique—Direct reduction and wiring is simple and effective to reduce the fracture and maintain the alignment. Due to the fracture location, PHILOS was selected. Plate positioning is crucial and should be checked by image intensification. In true AP view, proximal and distal temporary K-wire fixation ensures the correct positioning (**Fig 3.2-4g–i**). As many locking head screws (LHSs) as possible were used proximally together with four distal screws in this osteoporotic bone (**Fig 3.2-4j–k**). Postoperative x-rays in AP and lateral views showed good alignment, implant positioning, and adequate fixation (**Fig 3.2-4l–m**). Leaving cerclage wires in place helps to maintain fracture stability in osteoporotic fractures. Lag screw fixation was not used because lag screw application in osteoporotic bone may not provide adequate stability and lead to iatrogenic fractures.

Postoperative care—The rehabilitation program was started early for the right shoulder and elbow. Early patient mobility and rehabilitation is often necessary to prevent common complications and loss in overall functional status. The postoperative x-rays at 2 months (**Fig 3.2-4n–o**) revealed a stable construct without change in implant position and the ones at 4 months (**Fig 3.2-4p–q**) showed good bone healing. The patient could return to her daily activities without pain.

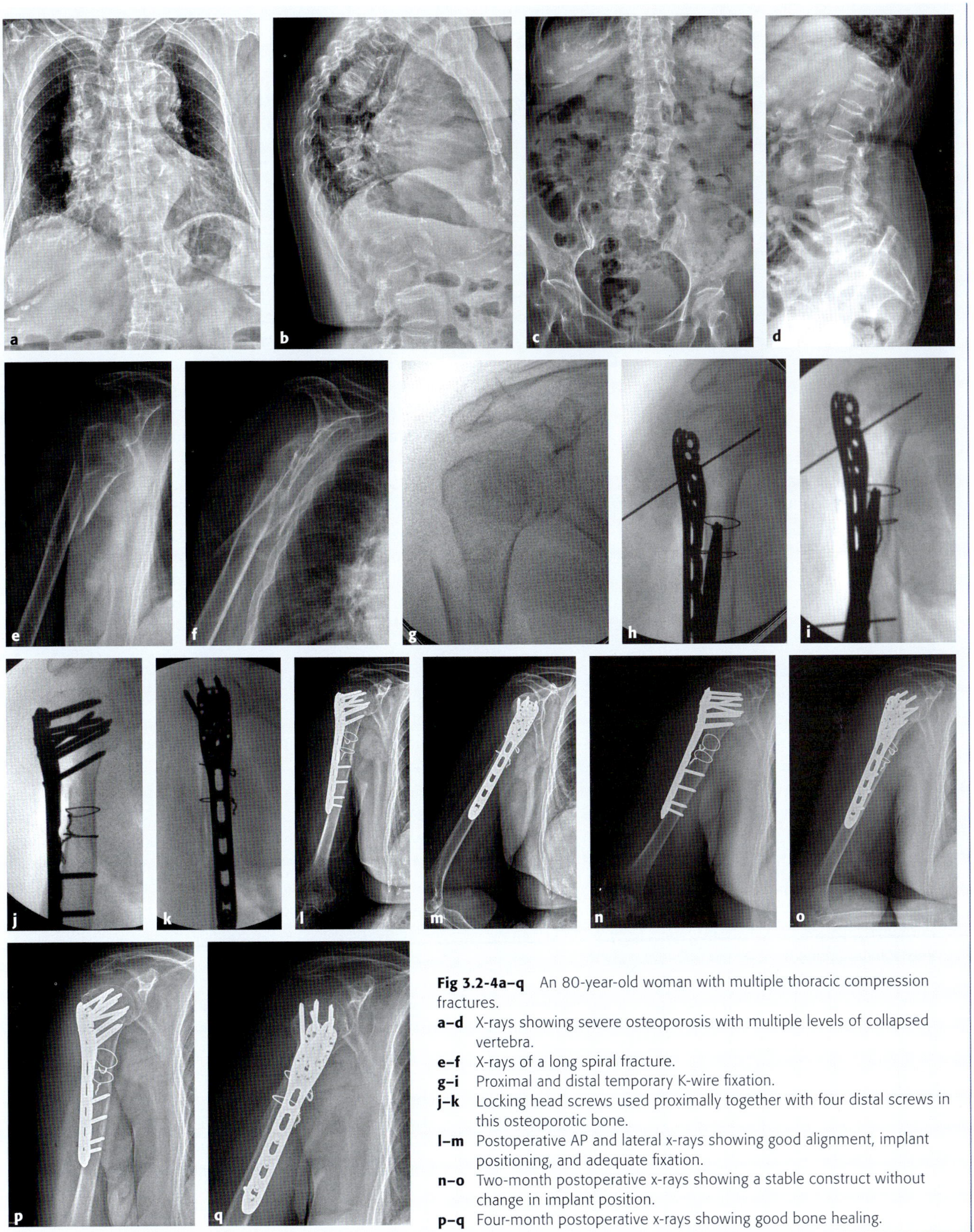


**Fig 3.2-4a–q** An 80-year-old woman with multiple thoracic compression fractures.

**a–d** X-rays showing severe osteoporosis with multiple levels of collapsed vertebra.

**e–f** X-rays of a long spiral fracture.

**g–i** Proximal and distal temporary K-wire fixation.

**j–k** Locking head screws used proximally together with four distal screws in this osteoporotic bone.

**l–m** Postoperative AP and lateral x-rays showing good alignment, implant positioning, and adequate fixation.

**n–o** Two-month postoperative x-rays showing a stable construct without change in implant position.

**p–q** Four-month postoperative x-rays showing good bone healing.

## 5.3 Open reduction and plate fixation in distal shaft fractures

Distal humeral fractures can be nicely approached and fixed by posterior approach and posterior plating (**Case 5: Fig 3.2-5**) [24, 25].

CASE 5

### Patient

A 70-year-old woman sustained a left humeral fracture in a previously hemiparetic arm from a minor fall in her house 5 weeks previously. She had persistent pain and deformity of the left arm and no new neurological deficit. X-rays showed malalignment, a large gap, and no sign of healing.

### Comorbidities

- Coronary artery disease
- Coronary artery bypass graft 3 years ago
- Cardiac arrhythmia
- Atrial fibrillation
- Old cerebrovascular accident with left hemiparesis
- Obesity
- Dementia
- Osteopenia on dual energy x-ray absorptiometry scan

### Treatment and outcome

Diagnosis and classification—Spiral fracture of the distal shaft of the left humerus (AO/OTA 12A1). The AP and lateral x-rays of the left humerus taken 5 weeks after nonoperative treatment showed malalignment, a large gap, and no sign of healing (**Fig 3.2-5a–b**).

Indication for surgery—Displaced fracture of the humeral shaft with failure of nonoperative treatment.

Treatment planning:

- Open reduction and internal fixation
- Positioning: prone, on x-ray transparent table with the elbow flexed and dropped down at the side of the table
- C-arm: located on same side
- Preparation and draping: from shoulder to hand and free to move in any direction
- Surgical approach: posterior approach, lateral paratriceps
- Implant: locking compression plate (LCP) extraarticular distal humerus plate

Intraoperative technique—In prone position, the elbow was flexed to facilitate exposure and fracture reduction as gravity helped balance the rotational force. Skin markings to identify all structures were important to clarify appropriate surgical orientation (**Fig 3.2-5c**), to clearly identify the humerus, fracture site, olecranon, and course of the radial nerve. **Figure 3.2-5d** shows the plane of dissection via a lateral paratriceps approach. The radial nerve was identified proximally and along the course distally.

The radial nerve was identified and protected during the entire operation (**Fig 3.2-5e–g**). The plate was long and needed to be fixed proximally to the area of the radial nerve crossing the posterior aspect of the midshaft of the humerus. The nerve was elevated and freed from the humeral shaft, and then the plate was inserted close to the cortex, under the nerve.

Postoperative care—Early gentle range of motion (ROM) of the elbow and shoulder. No pushing or pulling activity is allowed until the bone heals. The fracture is in good alignment, and the patient could perform pain-free active ROM exercises of the elbow from 10° to 120° (**Fig 3.2-5h–m**).

### Discussion

There were options in both surgical approach and implant selection:

- An anterior approach and straight LCP anteriorly would be possible but—due to short distal segment—may not result in adequate distal fixation. In addition, the distal tip of the plate and screws should not be placed in the coronoid fossa and obstruct elbow flexion.
- Anterolateral plating with contoured LCP on the anterolateral surface was also an option, but the plate must be contoured well in three dimensions and the radial nerve must also be identified and protected.
- Posterior plating with a well-designed anatomical plate for fixation along the lateral column of the distal humerus and the more proximal shaft provides good stability but the radial nerve must be identified, protected, and elevated. In this case, the plate was placed carefully and the patient had no radial nerve complications.

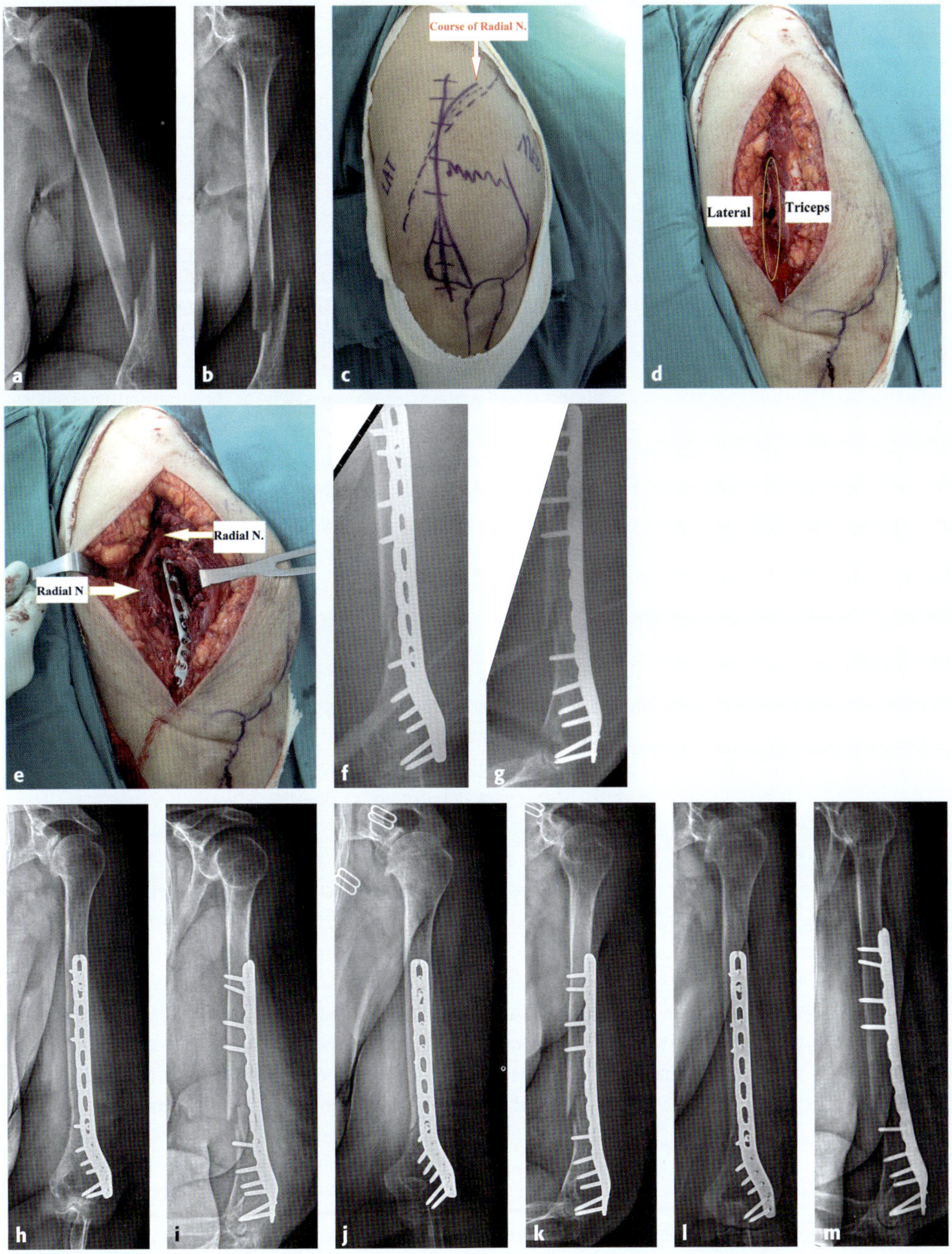


**Fig 3.2-5a–m** A 70-year-old woman with a fracture of the distal shaft of the left humerus.

**a–b** AP and lateral x-rays of the left humerus at 5 weeks after nonoperative treatment showing malalignment, a large gap, and no sign of healing.

**c–d** Skin markings to identify all structures and clarify appropriate surgical orientation (**c**). A lateral paratriceps approach used for the plane of dissection (**d**).

**e–g** The radial nerve was identified and protected during the operation (**e**). Immediate postoperative x-rays (**f–g**).

**h–m** X-rays showing 2 weeks (**h–i**), 5 weeks (**j–k**), and 10 weeks (**l–m)** postoperative follow-up.

## 5.4 Anterior minimally invasive plate osteosynthesis

**Case 6: Fig 3.2-6** [19, 26] shows minimally invasive plate osteosynthesis with anterior plating technique for humeral shaft fracture (straight locking compression plate).

CASE 6

### Patient

A 69-year-old man tripped and fell; he had pain and swelling in his right arm.

### Comorbidities

- Hypertension
- Osteoporosis

### Treatment and outcome

Diagnosis and classification—Long spiral intact wedge fracture of the midshaft of the right humerus (AO/OTA 12B2) (**Fig 3.2-6a–b**). After a primary treatment with a plaster splint, the alignment of the fracture was unacceptable and the patient consented to operative repair.

Indication for surgery—Painful, displaced fracture, and failure of nonoperative treatment.

Treatment planning:

- Minimally invasive plate osteosynthesis (MIPO) technique, anterior plating
- Positioning: supine on x-ray transparent table
- C-arm: located on the opposite side
- Preparation and draping: from shoulder to hand and free to move in any direction
- Surgical approach:
  - Proximal incision: anterior incision for the proximal humerus
  - Distal incision: anterior approach to the distal humeral shaft
- Implant: 12-hole narrow locking compression plate (LCP) (4.5/5 mm)

Intraoperative technique—After the proximal and distal incisions, a supraperiosteal tunnel was created anteriorly, the 12-hole narrow LCP was inserted from distal to proximal, passing the plate on the anterior surface of the humerus. The plate was positioned using image intensifier guidance. As this fracture had lateral angulation, reduction was performed by direct pressure outside the skin on the lateral aspect to correct the axis (**Fig 3.2-6c**). A thin bump of cloth can be used to support the humerus to correct sagittal plane alignment. This was followed by temporary K-wire fixation (**Fig 3.2-6d–e**).

After reduction was achieved and plate positioning was assured, cortical screw fixation of the proximal and distal fragments was initially preformed on each main fragment. This stabilized the fracture and guided the plate closer to the anterior cortex. Then, locking head screws were fixed on each side of the fragment to stabilize the whole shaft with relative stability. Three AP x-rays confirmed good alignment and screw fixation (**Fig 3.2-6f–h**). Further imaging showed the bridging plate with relative stability (**Fig 3.2-6j–k, Fig 3.2-6l–m**). Four screws on each side of the fragment should be adequate to stabilize the fracture in relative stability mode, suitable for this type C shaft fracture.

### Discussion

There are many techniques and implant options in this case:

- Long spiral wedge fractures can be addressed with open direct reduction with lag screw or wiring to maintain alignment and fixation with neutralization plate. However, soft-tissue damage is always a risk during an open technique. Preservation of the spiral wedge fragment blood supply is essential to prevent delayed union or nonunion.
- Closed reduction and bridge plating technique is technically demanding, especially for MIPO technique. These procedures require specific training in manipulation for closed reduction, plate placement and fixation, and prevention of radial nerve injury. Once MIPO is achieved with good alignment with bridge plating stabilization for relative stability, the postoperative rehabilitation can start early and good bone healing can be expected.
- Closed intramedullary nailing is also a good option, however, this is also technically demanding and carries risk of radial nerve injury and further displacement of the fragment.

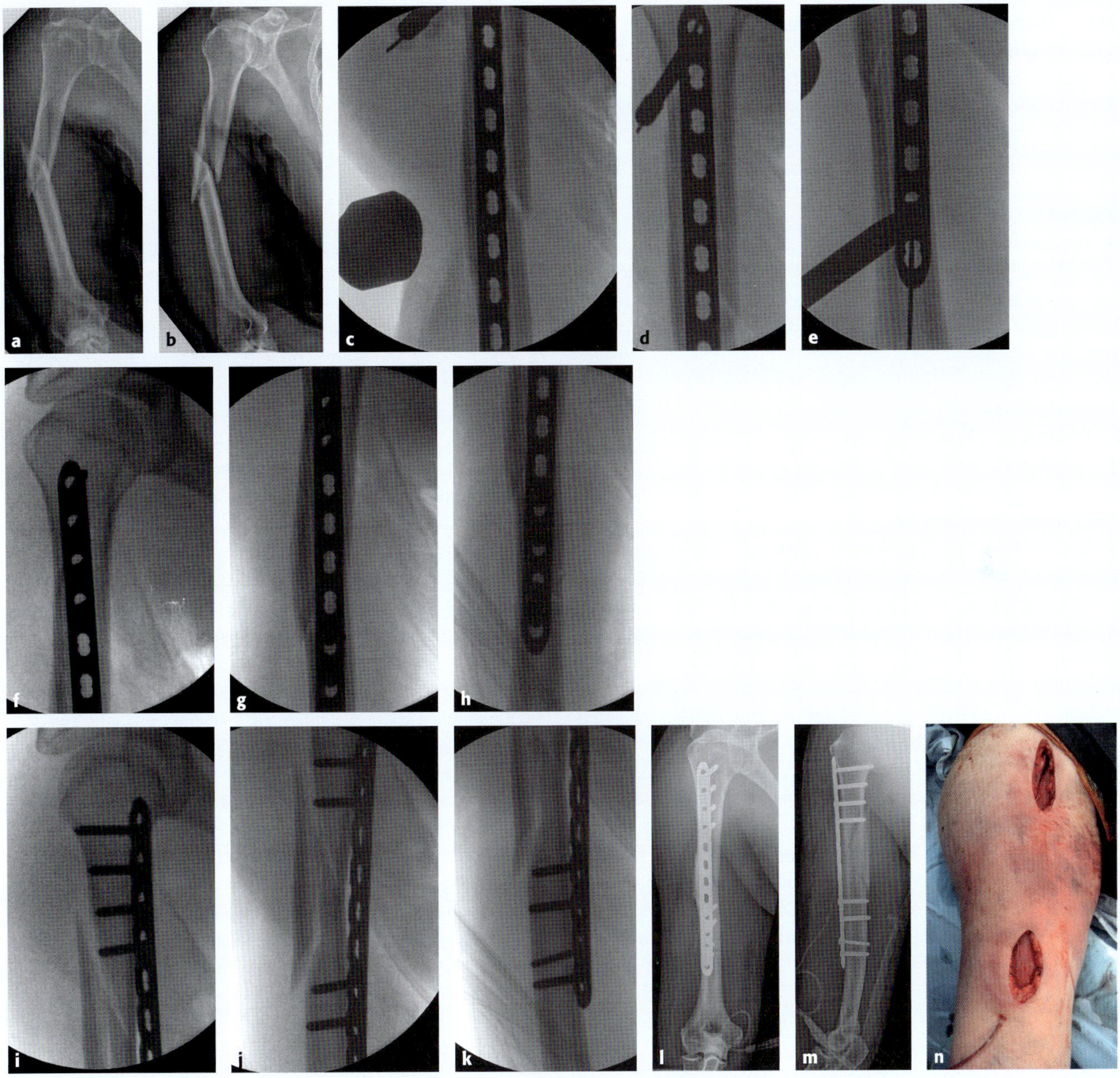


**Fig 3.2-6a–n** A 69-year-old man with a wedge fracture of the midshaft of the right humerus.
**a–b** Initial x-rays of the right humerus showing a long spiral wedge fracture at the midshaft.
**c–e** Direct pressure outside the skin was applied on the lateral aspect to correct the axis (**c**), followed by temporary K-wire fixation (**d–e**).
**f–h** AP x-rays confirming good alignment and screw fixation.
**i–k** Bridging plate with relative stability.
**l–n** X-rays of the anterior bridge-plating technique in AP and lateral views (**l–m**). Skin incisions of minimally invasive plate osteosynthesis technique is shown in (**n**).

### 5.5 Anterolateral minimally invasive plate osteosynthesis

Minimally invasive plate osteosynthesis can be safe and appropriate for osteoporotic fractures (**Case 7: Fig 3.2-7**) [27, 28].

CASE 7

#### Patient

A 57-year-old man with osteopenia suffered a low-energy injury while sitting in the back seat of a public taxi. The injury occurred during sudden braking while he was grasping a grab handle on the roof. He was taken directly to the hospital for evaluation of severe pain and deformity.

#### Comorbidities

- Diabetes
- Osteopenia

#### Treatment and outcome

Diagnosis and classification—Multifragmentary fractures involving the proximal one third to middle of the left humeral shaft (AO/OTA 12C3) (**Fig 3.2-7a**). After primary treatment with a splint from an emergency department, the x-rays were done. The alignment of the fracture was unacceptable.

Indication for surgery—A displaced fracture with malalignment after reduction and immobilization.

Treatment planning—Due to the configuration of the AO/OTA Fracture and Dislocation Classification type

C shaft fracture, minimally invasive plate osteosynthesis (MIPO) technique was the treatment of choice. Conventional plating would have damaged the blood supply of the middle fragments and likely resulted in delayed or nonunion.

- Positioning: supine on x-ray transparent table
- C-arm: located on the opposite side
- Preparation and draping: from shoulder to hand and free to move in any direction
- Surgical approach: proximal incision, deltoid split
- Distal incision: anterior approach to distal humeral shaft
- Implant: PHILOS (long)

PHILOS is appropriate to fix the proximal part with various locking screws. This well-designed low plate profile can be fixed suitably in this high-level fracture with short proximal main fragment (**Fig 3.2-7b**). Narrow locking compression plate can also be contoured and fixed on the anterior surface with MIPO technique but it is a relatively thick implant. This may interfere with the proximal anterior structures such as the long-head biceps tendon or the insertion of the deltoid. Furthermore, it provides fewer screw options for the proximal fragment than the PHILOS plate. An intramedullary nail with multiple locking screws in the proximal part is another option. This is technically demanding and there is no tolerance for error.

The deltoid-split incision is to prevent injury to the deltoid branch of the axillary nerve which lay just 1–2 cm from the distal part of this incision (**Fig 3.2-7c1**). **Figure 3.2-7c2** shows the longitudinal split of the deltoid fiber to identify the lateral part of the proximal humerus. A string-like structure, just distal to this point under the deltoid muscle, is the branch of the axillary nerve. Care must be taken not to stretch or cut this nerve. Use a periosteal elevator to separate the subdeltoid space and lateral surface of the proximal humerus to create a tunnel for plate insertion (**Fig 3.2-7c3**).

The length of the distal incision is 5–6 cm (**Fig 3.2-7d**). After opening the anterior fascia to identify the biceps muscle, the musculocutaneous nerve was identified under the biceps muscle (between the two retractors). The biceps and nerve were retracted and protected medially to expose the anterior surface of the brachialis muscle.

When splitting the brachialis muscle anteriorly in the middle, care must be taken not to use any bone retractor (eg, Hohmann retractor) to retract directly between the lateral cortex of the humerus and the muscles as the radial nerve is at risk of traction injury (**Fig 3.2-7e**).

In this case, only a simple soft-tissue retractor was used on the skin and subcutaneous tissue, and deeper on the brachialis muscle just enough to gently expose the anterior cortex for plate positioning and screw fixation. At this step, a periosteal elevator (or a tunneller, if available) was used to create a submuscular tunnel to connect to the previously created tunnel from the proximal surgical wound (**Fig 3.2-7f**).

To protect the axillary nerve branch during insertion, the plate was passed along the previously created submuscular plane, supraperiosteal tunnel by pointing anteriorly. This prevents slipping into the wrong tract and injuring the radial nerve at the distal lateral surface of the shaft (**Fig 3.2-7g**).

Reduction was done indirectly by manipulation with traction and rotational control followed with temporary K-wire fixation or unicortical drill bits for proximal and distal plate stabilization (**Fig 3.2-7h**). For MIPO with PHILOS, screw fixation was limited above the axillary nerve area leaving some screw holes empty (**Fig 3.2-7i**). There was initial distal fixation with a positioning screw (cortical screw) before performing the locking head screw fixation (**Fig 3.2-7j**, **Fig 3.2-7k**).

Immediate postoperative x-rays show proper alignment and good plate positioning as planned preoperatively (**Fig 3.2-7l**). This was a bridge plating with relative stability which is suitable for multifragmentary fractures.

Postoperative care—An arm sling was used to support and rest the muscle and soft tissue on the first day. The patient was allowed to start early active gentle range-of-motion exercise as tolerated (**Fig 3.2-7m**, **Fig 3.2-7n–o**).

## Discussion

Fixation in this case can be done by IM nailing or MIPO. Minimally invasive plate osteosynthesis with long PHILOS can be done with or without helical plate-like contouring. If the plate is not contoured to a helical type, the distal incision should be lateral and the radial nerve has to be identified.

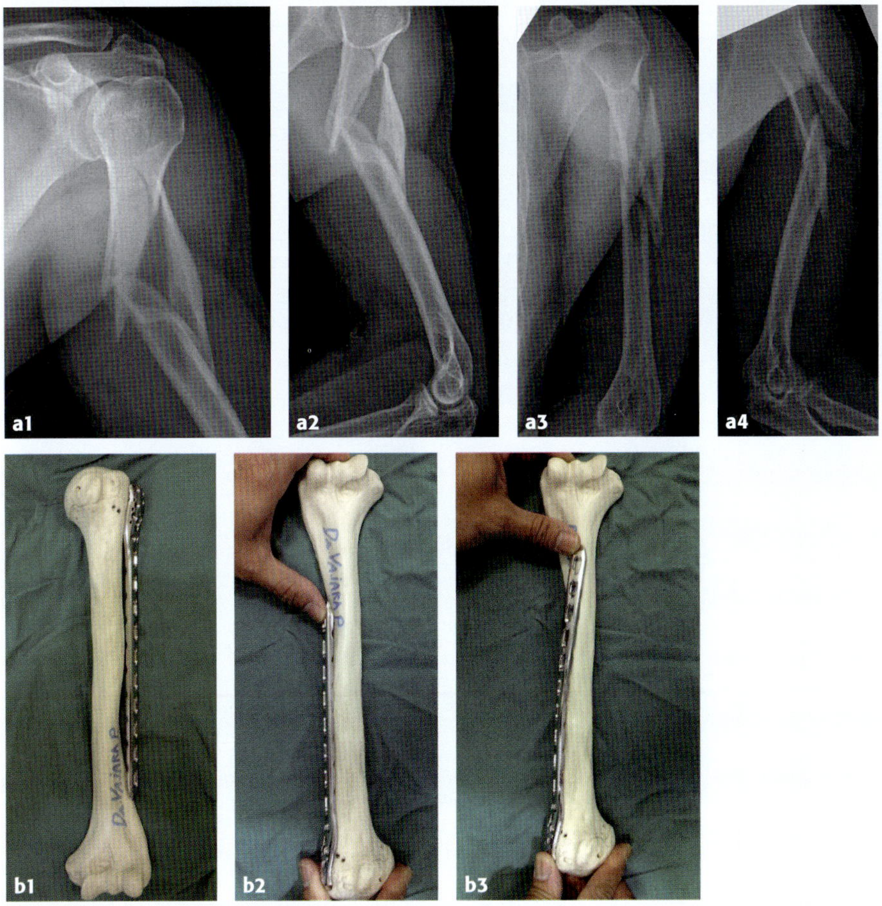


**Fig 3.2-7a–o** A 57-year-old man with multifragmentary fractures after a low-energy injury.

**a** X-rays showing multifragmentary fractures involving the proximal one third to middle of the left humeral shaft.

**b** A long PHILOS (**b1**) was prepared and contoured with a plan to fix it proximally to the normal lateral surface and distally to the anterior surface to avoid manipulation and retraction of the radial nerve on the lateral surface of the shaft (**b2–b3**). Plastic bone was used as a template to contour it like a helical plate.

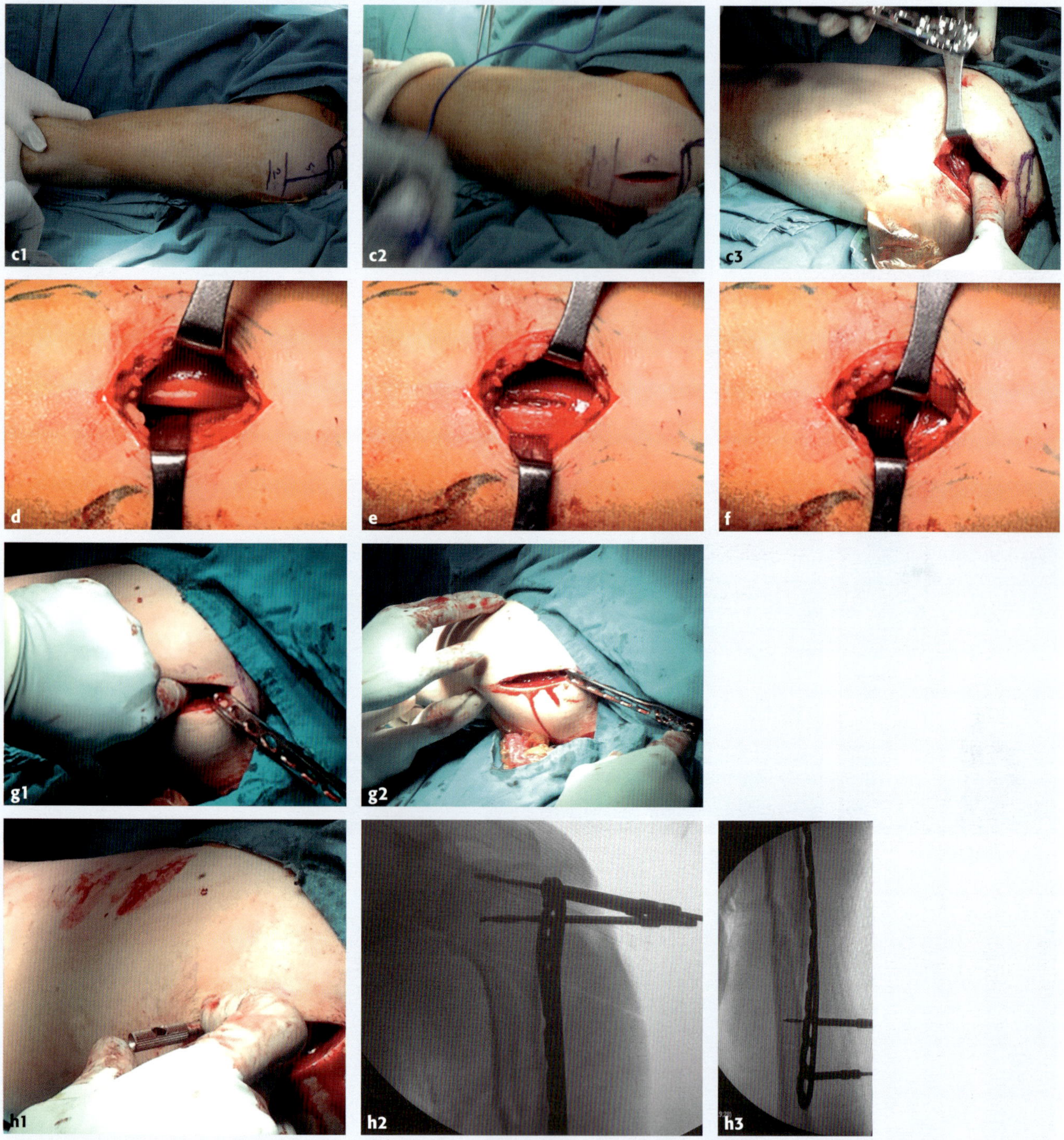


**Fig 3.2-7a–o (cont)** A 57-year-old man with multifragmentary fractures after a low-energy injury.

- **c** Acromion landmarks and a longitudinal deltoid-split incision were marked starting from the anterior one third of the length of the acromion and extend not more than 5 cm.
- **d** The distal incision on the anterior surface of the left arm.
- **e** Splitting of the brachialis muscle anteriorly in the middle fracture site and full range of motion (ROM) of the elbow and shoulder.
- **f** A periosteal elevator (or a tunneller, if available) was used to create a submuscular tunnel to connect to the previously created tunnel from the proximal surgical wound.
- **g** The plate was passed along the previously created submuscular plane, supraperiosteal tunnel by pointing anteriorly.
- **h** The plate was inserted and set for proper positioning by direct visualization and use of image intensification.

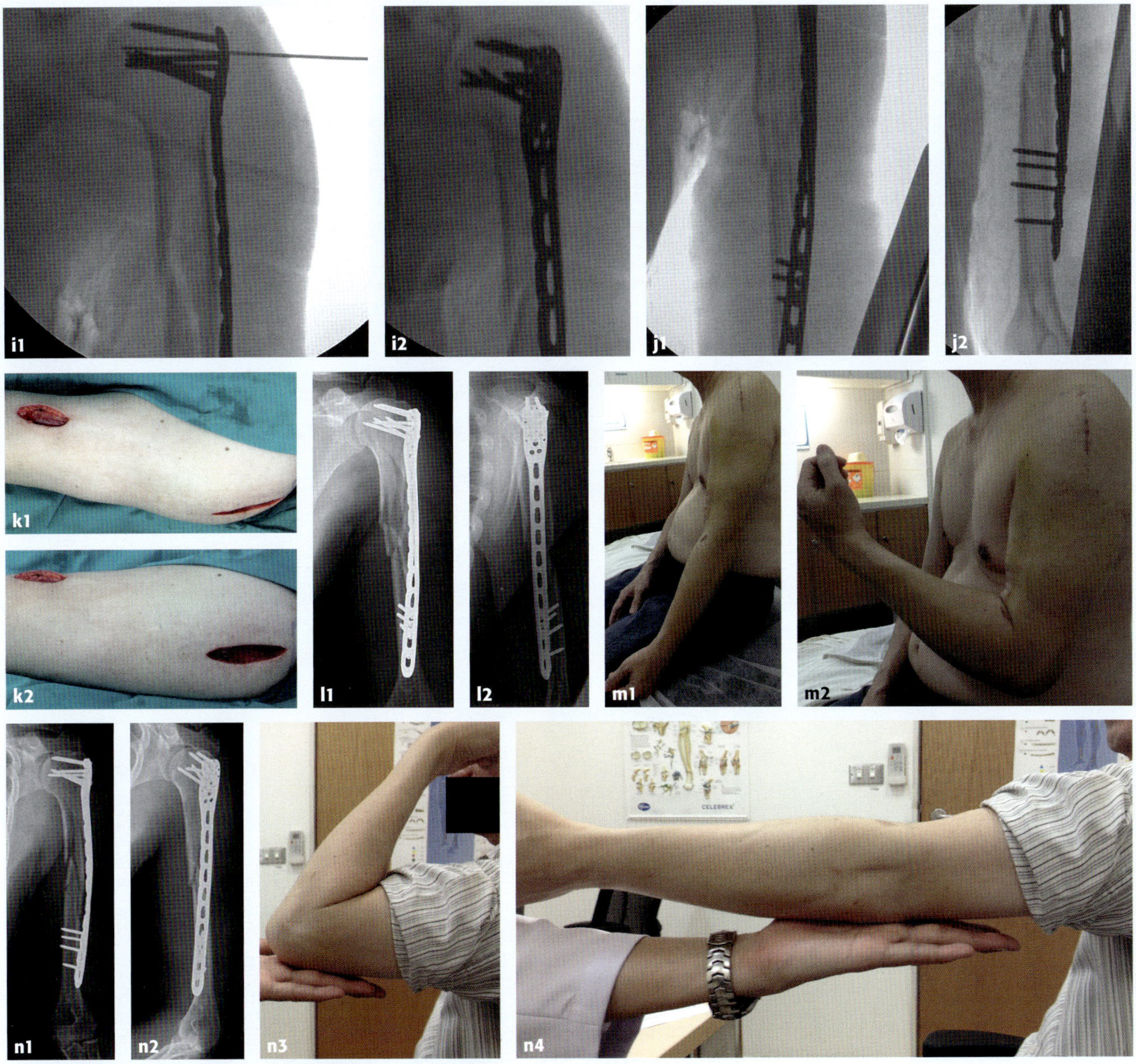


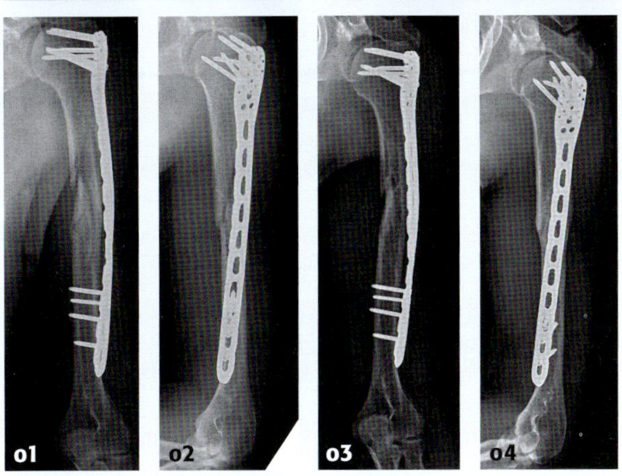


**Fig 3.2-7a–o (cont)** A 57-year-old man with multifragmentary fractures after a low-energy injury.

- **i** Proximal screw fixation was performed. For minimally invasive plate osteosynthesis (MIPO) with PHILOS, the screw fixation was limited above the axillary nerve area, leaving some screw holes empty.
- **j** Distal fixation with positioning screws (cortical screws).
- **k** The skin incisions after fixation from anterior (**k1**) and lateral views (**k2**).
- **l** Immediate postoperative x-rays show proper alignment and good plate positioning as planned preoperatively.
- **m** Wound conditions and active ROM 10 days after MIPO.
- **n** X-rays of the humerus at the 1-month follow-up (**n1–n2**) and clinical photographs showing ROM of the elbow (**n3–n4**). The patient was pain free during continued ROM exercises.
- **o** The follow-up x-rays at 3 months (**o1–o2**) and 9 months (**o3–o4**) show union of the fragments. The patient had no pain at the fracture site and full ROM of the elbow and shoulder.

## 5.6 Antegrade nailing with a long nail—
**Case 8: Fig 3.2-8**

CASE 8

### Patient

An 83-year-old woman had a fall at home and sustained a fracture of the right humerus (**Fig 3.2-8a–c**). One year previously she sustained a pertrochanteric fracture of the left femur, which was treated with a proximal femoral nail.

### Comorbidities

- Alzheimer's disease
- Chronic renal insufficiency
- Depression
- Atrial fibrillation
- Osteoporosis

### Treatment and outcome

Treatment decision—Initial treatment was nonoperative with a plaster cast. Because of the patient's dementia and inability to comply with restrictions, nonoperative treatment was not tolerated.

Closed reduction and internal fixation (using a multilocking nail) was performed (**Fig 3.2-8d–e**). The displacement of the shaft fragment due to the traction of the deltoid muscle was acceptable.

Postoperative x-rays showed that length and rotation were restored; the displacement of the shaft fragment is clearly visible (**Fig 3.2-8f–g**).

At the 5-month follow-up, the patient was satisfied and did not attend further follow-up examinations (**Fig 3.2-8h–i**).

At the 3-year follow-up, the nonreduced shaft fragment healed (**Fig 3.2-8j–l**). The patient had no pain and good function (**Fig 3.2-8m–o**). The x-rays show that the displaced fragment healed completely.

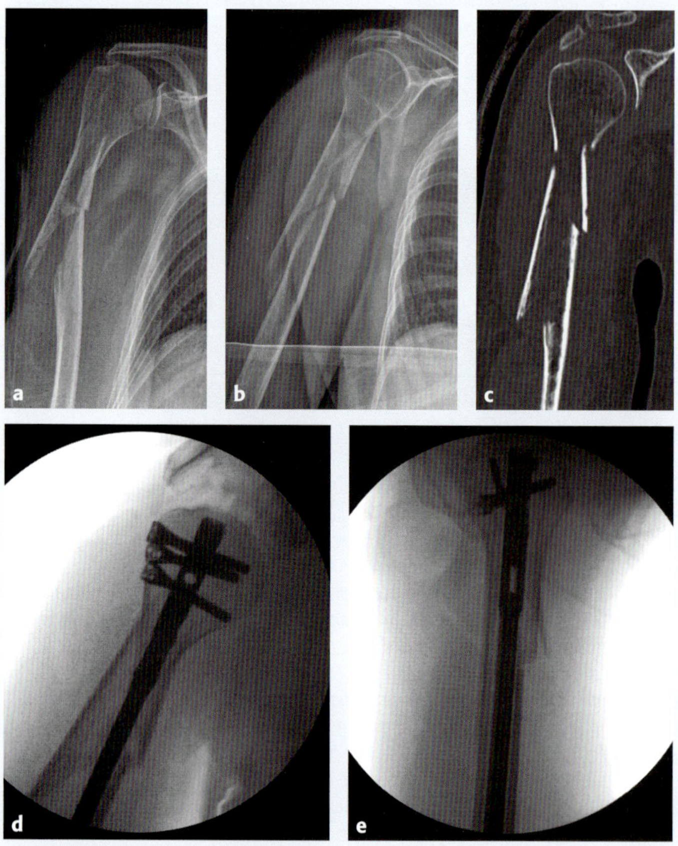


**Fig 3.2-8a–o** An 83-year-old woman with a right humeral fracture.
**a–c** The patient had a multifragmentary fracture type, which involved the proximal humerus (greater tuberosity) with a nondisplaced fracture line demonstrated on the computed tomographic scan (**c**).
**d–e** Closed reduction and internal fixation with a multilocking nail.

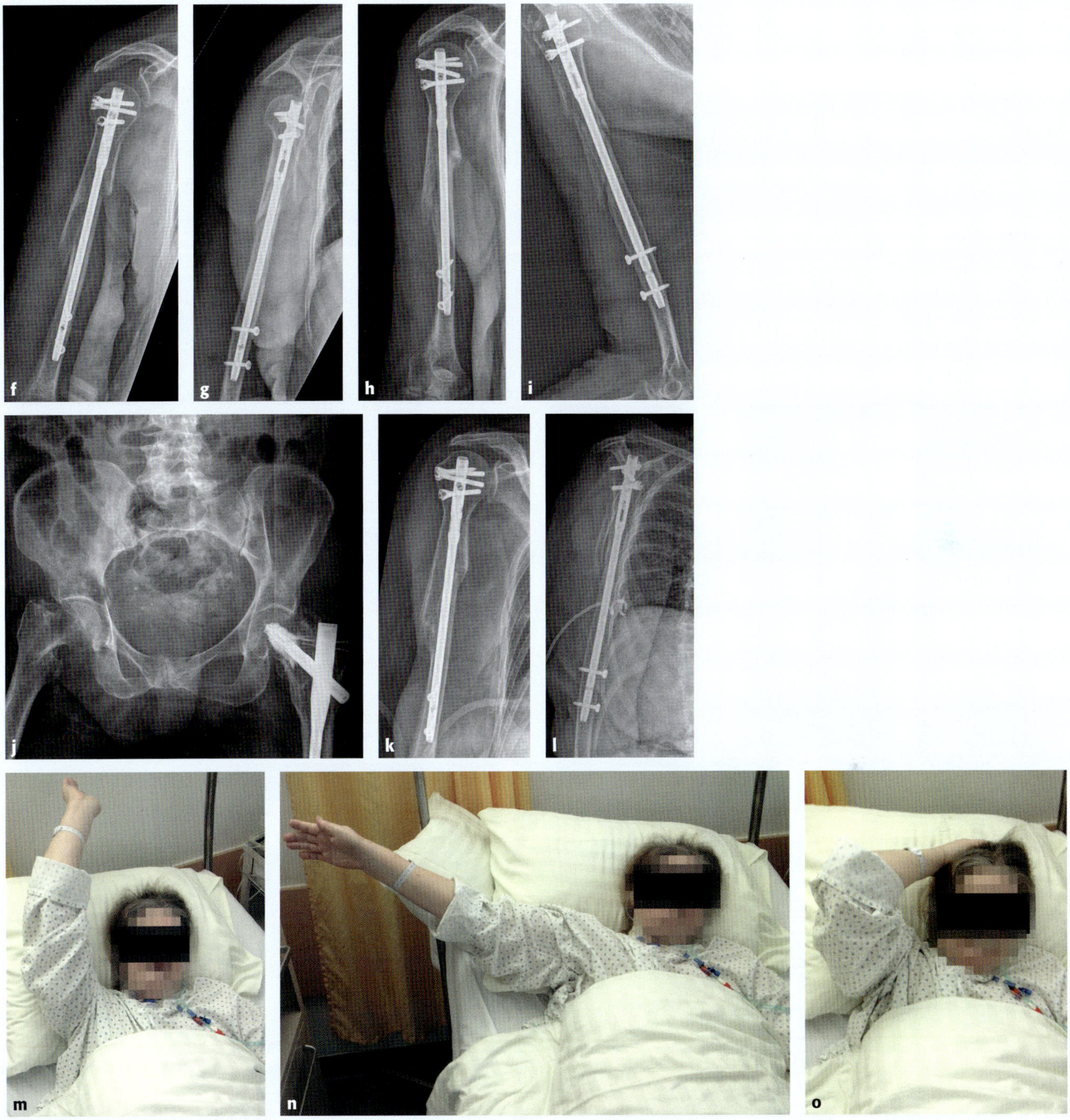

**Fig 3.2-8a–o (cont)** An 83-year-old woman with a right humeral fracture.
**f–g** X-rays taken 2 days after surgery (**f**) and after physical therapy had already started (**g**).
**h–i** These x-rays show that the implant is still in place; there is no loosening and some callus formation.
**j–l** Additional images 3 years postoperatively obtained during evaluation of a pertrochanteric fracture of the right femur.
**m–o** These clinical photographs were taken in bed because of the recent pertrochanteric fracture of the right femur.

## 5.7 Antegrade nailing for segmental fractures—Case 9: Fig 3.2-9

CASE 9

### Patient

An 82-year-old man had a fall on the street. He sustained a fracture of the left humerus at two levels (**Fig 3.2-9a–c**).

### Comorbidities

- Chronic heart failure
- Dementia
- Malnutrition
- Vitamin D deficiency
- Osteoporosis

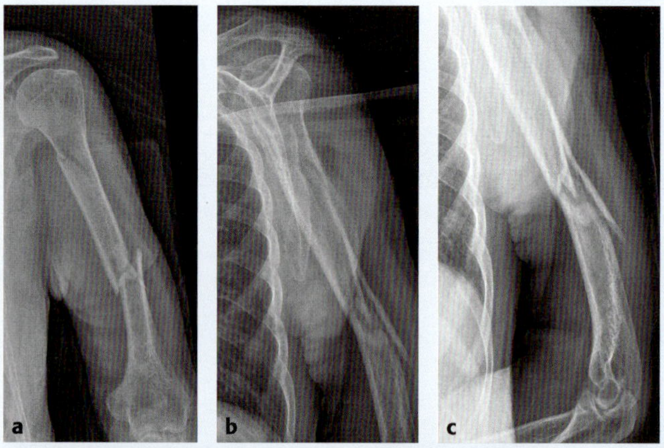


### Treatment and outcome

Preoperative imaging—As the patient was relatively active and would have had difficulty complying with immobilization, operative repair was planned. The surgeon performed antegrade nailing because of its less invasive approach (**Fig 3.2-9a–c**).

Intraoperative imaging—The correct entry point is the key step in intramedullary nailing, and must be checked and documented with intraoperative image intensification in two planes (**Fig 3.2-9d–i**).

Postoperative—The patient had physical therapy during his hospitalization but refused outpatient therapy (**Fig 3.2-9j–k**). His abduction was 110° after 5 weeks and 170° after 3 months.

Six-month follow-up—After 6 months the patient was pain free with full symmetrical function for both upper extremities (**Fig 3.2-9l–m**).

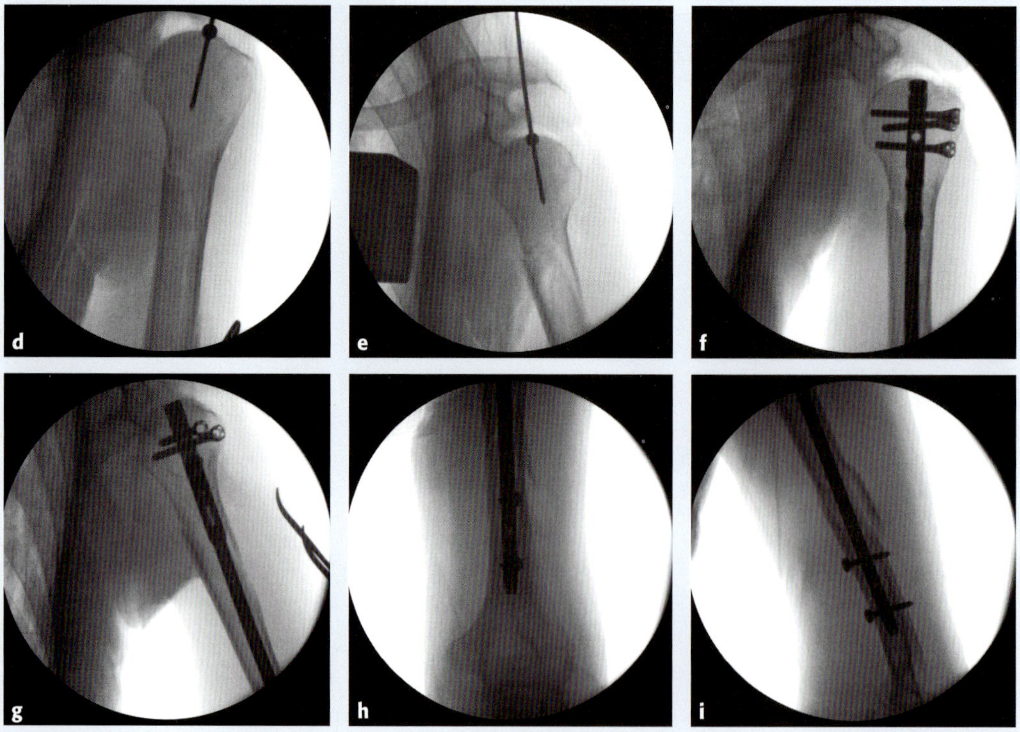


**Fig 3.2-9a–m** An 82-year-old man with a left humeral fracture after a fall.
**a–c** The patient had humeral fractures at two levels, similar to the AO/OTA Fracture and Dislocation Classification 12C2.
**d–i** Intraoperative imaging, AP and lateral views.

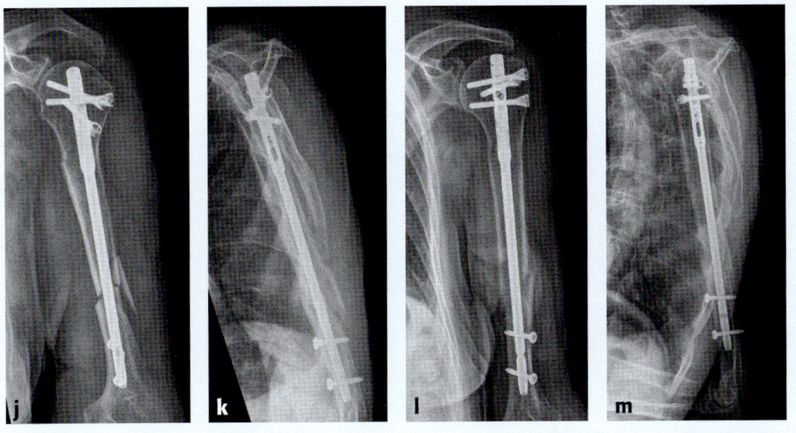


**Fig 3.2-9a–m (cont)** An 82-year-old man with a left humeral fracture after a fall.
**j–k** Postoperative imaging.
**l–m** Postoperative imaging at 6 months.

## 5.8 Antegrade nailing with a very short distal fragment—Case 10: Fig 3.2-10



### Patient

A 75-year-old woman had a fall on the street. She sustained a fracture of the left humerus (**Fig 3.2-10a–b**).

### Comorbidities

- Type 2 diabetes mellitus
- High blood pressure
- Obesity
- Myocardial infarction 16 years ago and on anticoagulation
- Preexisting ipsilateral rupture of the supra- and infraspinatus tendons

### Treatment and outcome

Treatment decision—In this case nonoperative treatment was the initial choice, but neither cast fixation nor bracing were possible due to obesity (**Fig 3.2-10c–d**).

Surgical planning—This very obese patient would have needed a long plate in combination with a large posterior approach to span the whole bone, and eventually two plates. Prone lateral decubitus positioning was not felt to be safe from the anesthesiology consultation, due to the patient's obesity. The surgical team wanted to avoid a large open approach because of the patient's obesity and diabetes.

Alternatively, antegrade nailing (closed reduction and internal fixation) was considered. The sitting beach chair position was advantageous for respiration during anaesthesia.

The challenge for antegrade nailing was locking the nail in the short distal fragment (**Fig 3.2-10e–g**).

Surgery—intraoperative imaging—The intraoperative imaging demonstrates correct length and rotation of the fracture, but the borderline anchoring and locking of the distal nail end; only the most distal screw options were feasible (**Fig 3.2-10h–i**).

Postoperative imaging—The AP projection shows good alignment, the lateral projection again demonstrates the critical implant anchorage (**Fig 3.2-10j–k**).

Aftercare—In this case aftercare was very conservative: The patient was managed in a shoulder sling for 4 weeks because of the short distal fragment, and passive mobilization was performed for 6 weeks. Active exercises were allowed thereafter.

One-year follow-up—The 1-year follow-up x-rays show that the fracture was healed (**Fig 3.2-10l–m**). Clinically, the patient had poor function due to the preexisting rotator cuff tear: abduction 60°, anteversion 60°.

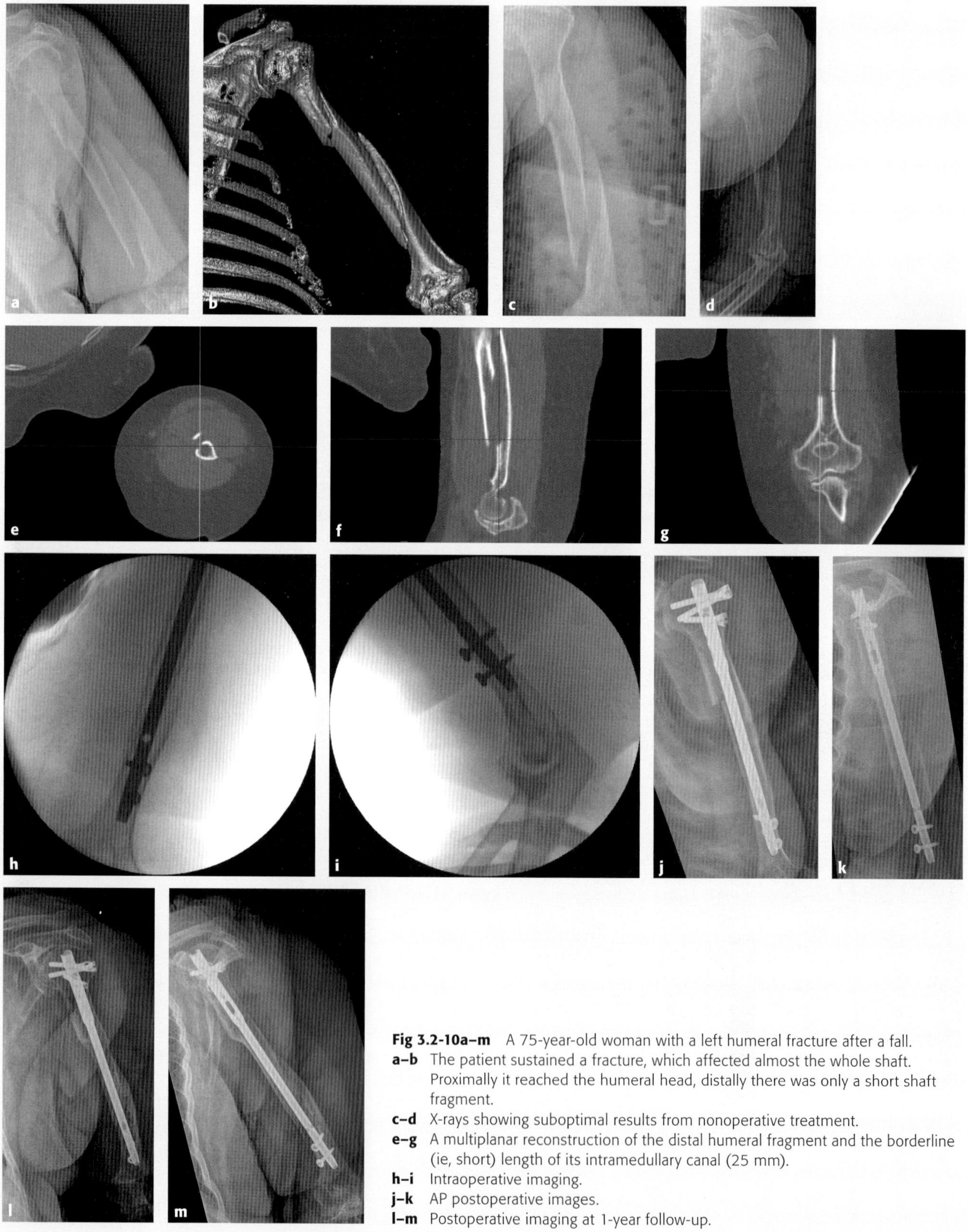

**Fig 3.2-10a–m** A 75-year-old woman with a left humeral fracture after a fall.
**a–b** The patient sustained a fracture, which affected almost the whole shaft. Proximally it reached the humeral head, distally there was only a short shaft fragment.
**c–d** X-rays showing suboptimal results from nonoperative treatment.
**e–g** A multiplanar reconstruction of the distal humeral fragment and the borderline (ie, short) length of its intramedullary canal (25 mm).
**h–i** Intraoperative imaging.
**j–k** AP postoperative images.
**l–m** Postoperative imaging at 1-year follow-up.

## 6 Complications [29, 30]

- Radial nerve injury [26]:
  - The radial nerve is at risk during fracture reduction for both nailing and plating.
  - Screw fixation from anterior to posterior in the humeral midshaft should be avoided to prevent radial nerve injury at the site of its crossing at the posterior cortex.
  - Do not harm the radial nerve by traction, direct or indirect injury during plating, or fixation of locking bolt in the distal shaft.
- Arterial injury can occur with drilling when inserting the locking bolt for IM nailing.
- Shoulder dysfunction in antegrade nailing is of concern, so the approach has to be done properly.
- Loss of fixation is not uncommon in osteoporotic bone (**Fig 3.2-11**):
  - Plate loosening
  - Nail protrusion at entry point
  - Backing out of proximal locking bolts
- Nonunion (**Fig 3.2-12**, **Fig 3.2-13**)
- Refractures after implant removal
- Periimplant fracture:
  - After plating
  - Supracondylar fracture with retrograde nailing
- Infection in open fracture

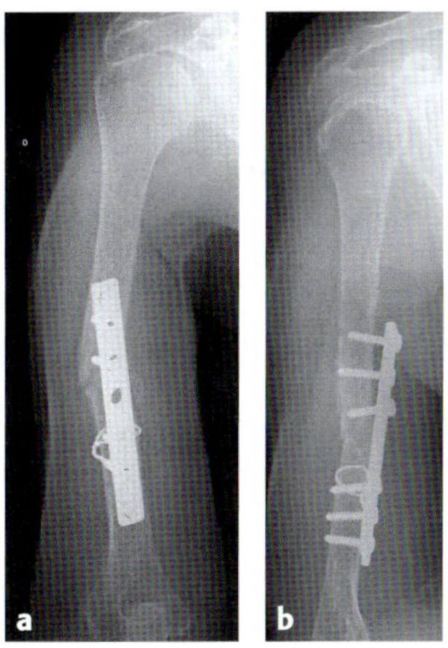

**Fig 3.2-11a–b** A 72-year-old woman after a car accident with a closed fracture of the humeral shaft. The x-rays 1 month after initial fixation with dynamic compression plate show loosening of the screws.

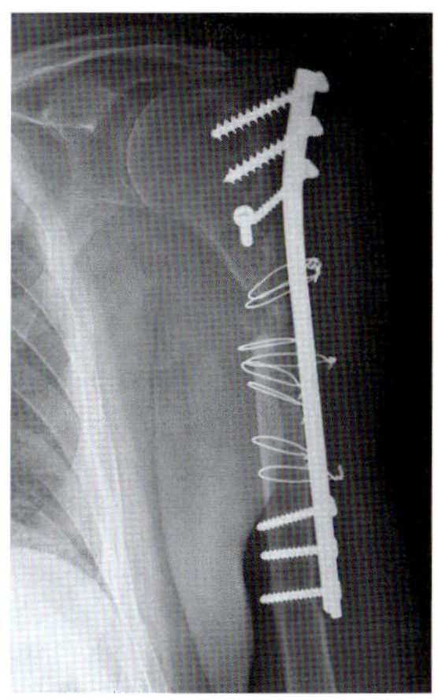

**Fig 3.2-12** These x-rays of a 65-year-old man show failure of fixation after open reduction and internal fixation with multiple wiring and dynamic compression plate. The patient had pain for 10 months following the initial fixation. Note that many wires in the open technique may cause biological disturbance during the healing process.

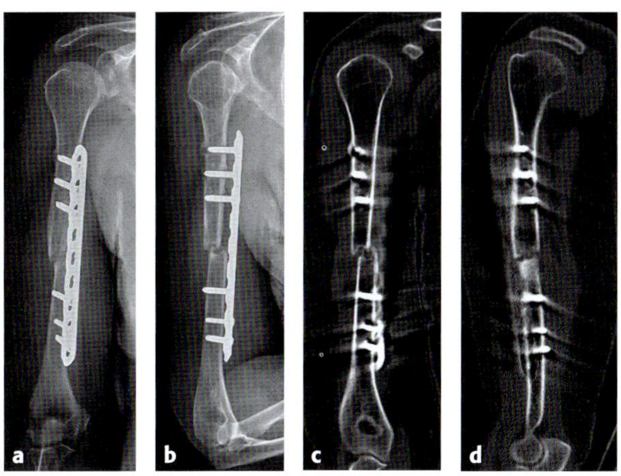

**Fig 3.2-13a–d** A 77-year-old woman with a transverse fracture. The patient was treated with minimally invasive plate osteosynthesis but failure occurred after 5 months. X-rays (**a–b**) and computed tomographic scans (**c–d**) demonstrate a significant gap with nonunion of the fracture site. Reduction by indirect technique left a small gap and created a high strain to reparative tissue which resulted in nonunion.

## 7 References

1. **Ekholm R, Adami J, Tidermark J, et al.** Fractures of the shaft of the humerus. An epidemiological study of 401 fractures. *J Bone Joint Surg Br.* 2006 Nov;88(11):1469–1473.
2. **Bergdahl C, Ekholm C, Wennergren D, et al.** Epidemiology and patho-anatomical pattern of 2,011 humeral fractures: data from the Swedish Fracture Register. *BMC Musculoskelet Disord.* 2016 Apr 12;17:159.
3. **Hu X, Xu S, Lu H, et al.** Minimally invasive plate osteosynthesis vs conventional fixation techniques for surgically treated humeral shaft fractures: a meta-analysis. *J Orthop Surg Res.* 2016 May 11;11(1):59.
4. **Walker M, Palumbo B, Badman B, et al.** Humeral shaft fractures: a review. *J Shoulder Elbow Surg.* 2011 Jul;20(5):833–844.
5. **Jawa A, McCarty P, Doornberg J, et al.** Extra-articular distal-third diaphyseal fractures of the humerus. A comparison of functional bracing and plate fixation. *J Bone Joint Surg Am.* 2006 Nov;88(11):2343–2347.
6. **Cadet ER, Yin B, Schulz B, et al.** Proximal humerus and humeral shaft nonunions. *J Am Acad Orthop Surg.* 2013 Sep;21(9):538–547.
7. **Marti RK, Verheyen CC, Besselaar PP.** Humeral shaft nonunion: evaluation of uniform surgical repair in fifty-one patients. *J Orthop Trauma.* 2002 Feb;16(2):108–115.
8. **Pailhe R, Mesquida V, Rubens-Duval B, et al.** Plate osteosynthesis of humeral diaphyseal fractures associated with radial palsy: twenty cases. *Int Orthop.* 2015 Aug;39(8):1653–1657.
9. **Shao YC, Harwood P, Grotz MR, et al.** Radial nerve palsy associated with fractures of the shaft of the humerus: a systematic review. *J Bone Joint Surg Br.* 2005 Dec;87(12):1647–1652.
10. **Liu GY, Zhang CY, Wu HW.** Comparison of initial nonoperative and operative management of radial nerve palsy associated with acute humeral shaft fractures. *Orthopedics.* 2012 Aug 1;35(8):702–708.
11. **Ekholm R, Ponzer S, Tornkvist H, et al.** Primary radial nerve palsy in patients with acute humeral shaft fractures. *J Orthop Trauma.* 2008 Jul;22(6):408–414.
12. **Pollock FH, Drake D, Bovill EG, et al.** Treatment of radial neuropathy associated with fractures of the humerus. *J Bone Joint Surg Am.* 1981 Feb;63(2):239–243.
13. **Bodner G, Buchberger W, Schocke M, et al.** Radial nerve palsy associated with humeral shaft fracture: evaluation with US—initial experience. *Radiology.* 2001 Jun;219(3):811–816.
14. **Ouyang H, Xiong J, Xiang P, et al.** Plate versus intramedullary nail fixation in the treatment of humeral shaft fractures: an updated meta-analysis. *J Shoulder Elbow Surg.* 2013 Mar;22(3):387–395.
15. **Liu GD, Zhang QG, Ou S, et al.** Meta-analysis of the outcomes of intramedullary nailing and plate fixation of humeral shaft fractures. *Int J Surg.* 2013;11(9):864–868.
16. **Kumar A, Sadiq S.** Non-union of the humeral shaft treated by internal fixation. *International Orthopaedics.* 2002 August 01;26(4):214–216.
17. **Perren SM.** The concept of biological plating using the limited contact-dynamic compression plate (LC-DCP). Scientific background, design and application. *Injury.* 1991;22(Suppl 1):1–41.
18. **Baumgaertel F, Perren SM, Rahn B.** Tierexperimentelle Untersuchungen zur „biologischen" Platten-osteosynthese von Mehrfragment-frakturen des Femurs [Animal experiment studies of "biological" plate osteosynthesis of multi-fragment fractures of the femur]. *Unfallchirurg.* 1994 Jan;97(1):19–27. German.
19. **Apivatthakakul T, Arpornchayanon O, Bavornratanavech S.** Minimally invasive plate osteosynthesis (MIPO) of the humeral shaft fracture. Is it possible? A cadaveric study and preliminary report. *Injury.* 2005 Apr;36(4):530–538.
20. **Carroll EA, Schweppe M, Langfitt M, et al.** Management of humeral shaft fractures. *J Am Acad Orthop Surg.* 2012 Jul;20(7):423–433.
21. **Sarmiento A, Kinman PB, Galvin EG, et al.** Functional bracing of fractures of the shaft of the humerus. *J Bone Joint Surg Am.* 1977 Jul;59(5):596–601.
22. **Ring D.** Current concepts in plate and screw fixation of osteoporotic proximal humerus fractures. *Injury.* 2007 Sep;38(Suppl 3):S59–S68.
23. **Egol KA, Kubiak EN, Fulkerson E, et al.** Biomechanics of locked plates and screws. *J Orthop Trauma.* 2004 Sep;18(8):488–493.
24. **Alonso-Llames M.** Bilaterotricipital approach to the elbow. Its application in the osteosynthesis of supracondylar fractures of the humerus in children. *Acta Orthop Scand.* 1972;43(6):479–490.
25. **Hessmann MH, Ring DC.** Humerus, distal. In: Rüedi TP, Buckley RE, Moran CG, eds. *AO Principles of Fracture Management.* 2nd ed. Switzerland: AO Publishing; 2007:609–625.
26. **Apivatthakakul T.** Humerus, shaft. In: Tong GO, Bavonratanavech S, eds. *Minimally Invasive Plate Osteosynthesis (MIPO).* Switzerland: AO Publishing; 2007:145–179.
27. **Khong KS KR, Ghista DN.** *Mechanobiology.* Switzerland: AO Publishing; 2007.
28. **Fernandez Dell'Oca AA.** The principle of helical implants. Unusual ideas worth considering. *Injury.* 2002 Apr;33 Suppl 1:SA1–27.
29. **Garnavos C.** Humeral shaft fractures. In: Court-Brown CM, Heckman JD, McQueen MM, et al, eds. *Rockwood and Green's Fractures in Adults.* 8th ed. Philadelphia: Wolters Kluwer Health; 2014:1287–1340.
30. **Perez EA.** Fractures of the Shoulder, Arm, and Forearm. In: Azar FM, Beaty JH, Canale ST, ed. *Campbell's Operative Orthopaedics.* 13 ed. Philadelphia: Elsevier Health Sciences; 2017:2927–3016.

# 3.3 Distal humerus

Rohit Arora, Alexander Keiler, Michael Blauth

## 1 Introduction

Distal humeral fractures (DHFs) in adults are complex and technically demanding injuries. In contrast to proximal humeral and distal radial fractures, operative fixation is indicated in most cases due to the impact of limited elbow function on activities of daily living. Many controversial and challenging issues include:

- Difficult exposure (with or without olecranon osteotomy)
- Comminution in the metaphyseal and/or epiphyseal region (with or without bone graft)
- Fixation strategies
- The role of primary total elbow arthroplasty

In order to achieve acceptable function, immobilization of the elbow should generally be avoided or at least limited to 2–3 weeks with intermittent mobilization.

## 2 Epidemiology and etiology

Distal humeral fractures account for 7–8% of all adult fractures in the western world [1]. Of more than 2,000 humeral fractures documented in the Swedish fracture registry between 2011 and 2013, only 8% were of the distal third, 79% of the proximal third, and 13% in the shaft. About 83% of humeral fractures affect patients older than 50 years [2]. Robinson et al [3] estimated an incidence of 5.7 cases per 100,000 people per year with a nearly equal male to female ratio. Of these, approximately 6% are isolated fractures of the capitulum humeri [4].

Looking at patient age reveals a bimodal peak: the first one represents 12–19-year-old men with fractures mostly due to high-energy trauma or athletic activities; the second peak is induced by women typically older than 80 years with osteoporotic bone who sustain the fracture after a ground level fall [5–7]. The latter group of patients demonstrated an increasing prevalence from 11 out of 100,000 in 1970 to 30 out of 100,000 in 1995 [8].

With the nondominant arm being affected in up to 89% of patients [7], the mechanism of injury in this population normally involves falling on the outstretched arm with a direct axial force transmitted to the capitulum humeri via the radial head [9]. The spontaneous reduction of a posterolateral elbow subluxation with shearing or compression force to the capitulum and/or the trochlea humeri represents a variant mechanism of injury [10].

## 3 Classification

In general, we distinguish between extra- and intercondylar DHF as well as capitellar and trochlear fractures. Several classifications of DHFs exist. Fractures are considered "distal" if they are located distal to the fossa olecrani:

- In 2003, Ring et al [11] described five injury patterns based on radiographic and intraoperative findings.
- The most commonly used classification is from the AO Foundation/Orthopaedic Trauma Association (AO/OTA), with letters from A to C for extraarticular, partial articular, and complete articular fractures. To describe the degree of comminution or give a further definition of the fracture location, the classification is further amended with numerals [5].
- Distal coronal fractures (AO/OTA type B3 fractures) are specified and divided in subtypes by Bryan et al and modified by McKee (**Table 3.3-1**) [12].

| Fracture type | Description |
|---|---|
| **I (Hahn-Steinthal)** | Coronal shear fracture resulting in osteochondral fragment extending up to the lateral ridge of the trochlea or minimally over it |
| **II (Kocher-Lorenz)** | Coronal shear fracture resulting in cartilaginous fragment with little or no subchondral bone attached |
| **III** | Fractures resulting in comminution of the capitellar fragment |
| **IV (McKee modification) [13]** | Coronal shear fracture of the capitulum and trochlea as a single fragment |

**Table 3.3-1** Bryan and Morrey classification of capitellar fractures modified by McKee [12, 14].

## 4 Decision making

The combination of complex anatomy, fracture comminution, short distal fracture segment, and osteoporotic bone quality makes these fractures difficult to treat [10, 15]. In older patients, a stable fixation to allow for functional treatment is the most important goal. Smaller gaps or steps in the joint surface are of minor importance. An olecranon osteotomy should be avoided so as not to cause additional problems.

### 4.1 Approach

Numerous approaches to the elbow have been described. Functional outcome does not appear to depend on the approach used [16, 17]. The approaches can be divided into posterior, medial, and lateral approaches. From posterior, we may use an olecranon osteotomy, triceps-splitting, triceps-reflecting [18], and triceps-sparing approaches.

Our preferred approach is the triceps-sparing paratricipital posterior approach according to Alonso-Llames [19]. It allows the surgeon to address medial and lateral aspects of the distal humerus and may be complemented by an olecranon osteotomy if necessary. In older patients, there should always be an attempt to manage fractures without olecranon osteotomy (**Case 1: Fig 3.3-1**). A tourniquet is not applied routinely.

AO/OTA C1 and C2 fractures are addressed via this approach without compromising the quality of reduction. In severely comminuted fractures, olecranon osteotomy may be necessary.

Due to the uncompromised extensor apparatus, immediate postoperative flexion/extension can be encouraged. Furthermore, this approach seems to be associated with fewer wound healing problems, shorter surgery time, and reduced blood loss compared to approaches involving an olecranon osteotomy (**Case 1: Fig 3.3-2**) [20].

In case of coronal fracture types, leaving the anconeus muscle attached to the proximal ulna, an arthrotomy anterior to the collateral ligaments can be performed (**Case 2: Fig 3.3-3**).

## Patient

A 79-year-old woman sustained an AO/OTA type C3 DHF after falling from standing height (**Fig 3.3-1a–b**).

## Comorbidities

- Osteoporosis
- Hypertension
- Insulin-dependent diabetes mellitus

## Treatment and outcome

Surgery was performed in prone position without olecranon osteotomy. Using the bilateral paratricipital approach, the distal fracture fragments were fixed to each other using joysticks. Applying an interfragmentary screw created one joint block, which was then fixed to the radial and ulnar column of the distal humerus using dorsolateral and ulnar plates according to the 90° plating technique. Follow-up at 13 months showed fracture union with active range of motion of 0–15–120° (**Fig 3.3-1c**).

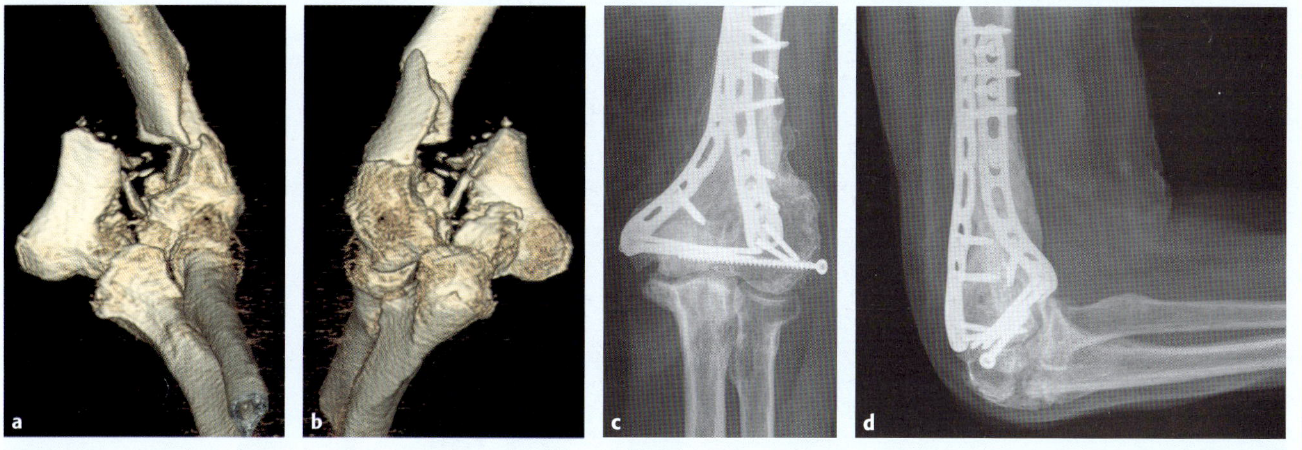


**Fig 3.3-1a–c** Female patient with an AO/OTA type C3 distal humeral fracture.
**a–b** A 3-D computed tomographic scan showing metaphyseal and epiphyseal comminution.
**c–d** The 13-month follow-up x-ray showing fracture union.

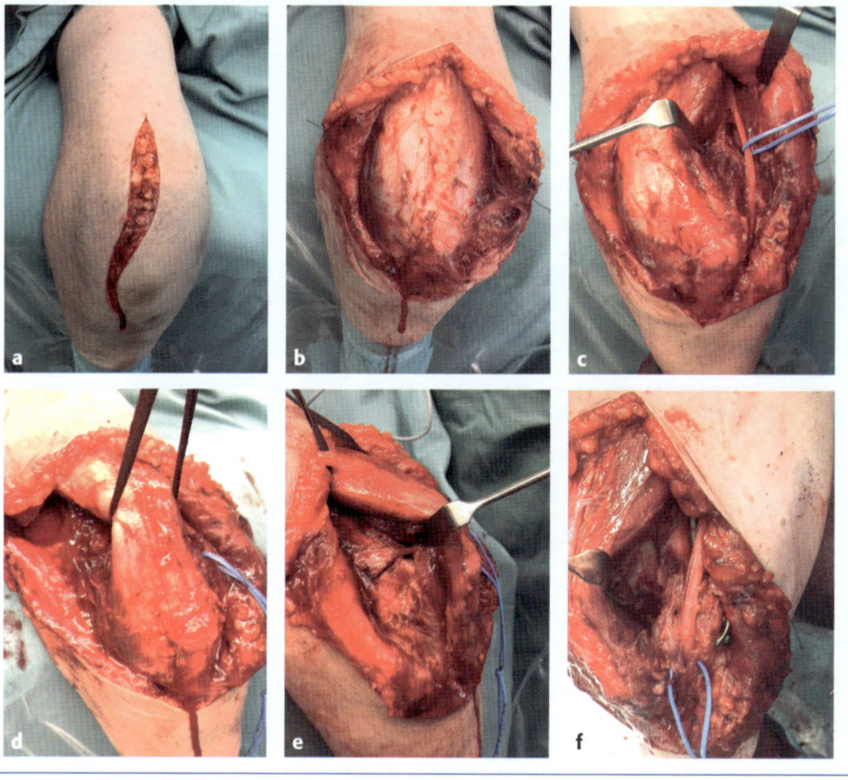


**Fig 3.3-2a–f** Triceps-sparing paratricipital posterior approach. A double curved skin incision is performed (**a**). Ulnar and radial full-thickness skin flaps are created and retracted to expose the triceps tendon (**b**). The ulnar nerve is identified and secured with a vessel loop (**c**). We do not routinely transpose the nerve at the end of surgery. The triceps tendon is mobilized and looped (**d**). Now, the radial and ulnar aspect of the elbow can be addressed alternatively by retracting the triceps tendon (**e–f**).

CASE 2

### Patient

A 75-year-old woman fell on the street from standing height.

### Treatment and outcome

Initial AP and lateral x-rays and 3-D computed tomography identified a dislocated elbow joint fracture with a fracture of the capitellum and trochlea (**Fig 3.3-3a–e**).

An extended lateral approach was performed. Before the lateral collateral ligament complex the already ruptured capsule was dissected and the capitellar fracture fragment addressed (**Fig 3.3-3f**). Because fracture reduction was not possible from the radial approach alone, an additional extended medial approach was performed (**Fig 3.3-3g**).

Before the intermuscular septum, the ruptured joint capsule was detached, and preserving the medial collateral ligament complex, the trochlear fracture fragment was reduced through the medial approach and an ulnar plate was applied to fix the supracondylar fracture (**Fig 3.3-3h**).

The multifragmented capitellar and trochlear fracture was fixed directly using three headless screws. The supracondylar fracture was fixed by posterolateral and medial plates. The fractured radial epicondyle was stabilized with an independent screw. Intraoperative AP and lateral x-rays confirmed correct reduction and fracture fixation. To avoid stress rising at the end of the locking plates the most proximal screw of the ulnar plate was used as a conventional screw (**Fig 3.3-3i–j**).

AP and lateral postoperative x-rays showed acceptable bone union. Range of motion was measured as 0–20–120° with unrestricted pronation and supination (**Fig 3.3-3k–l**).

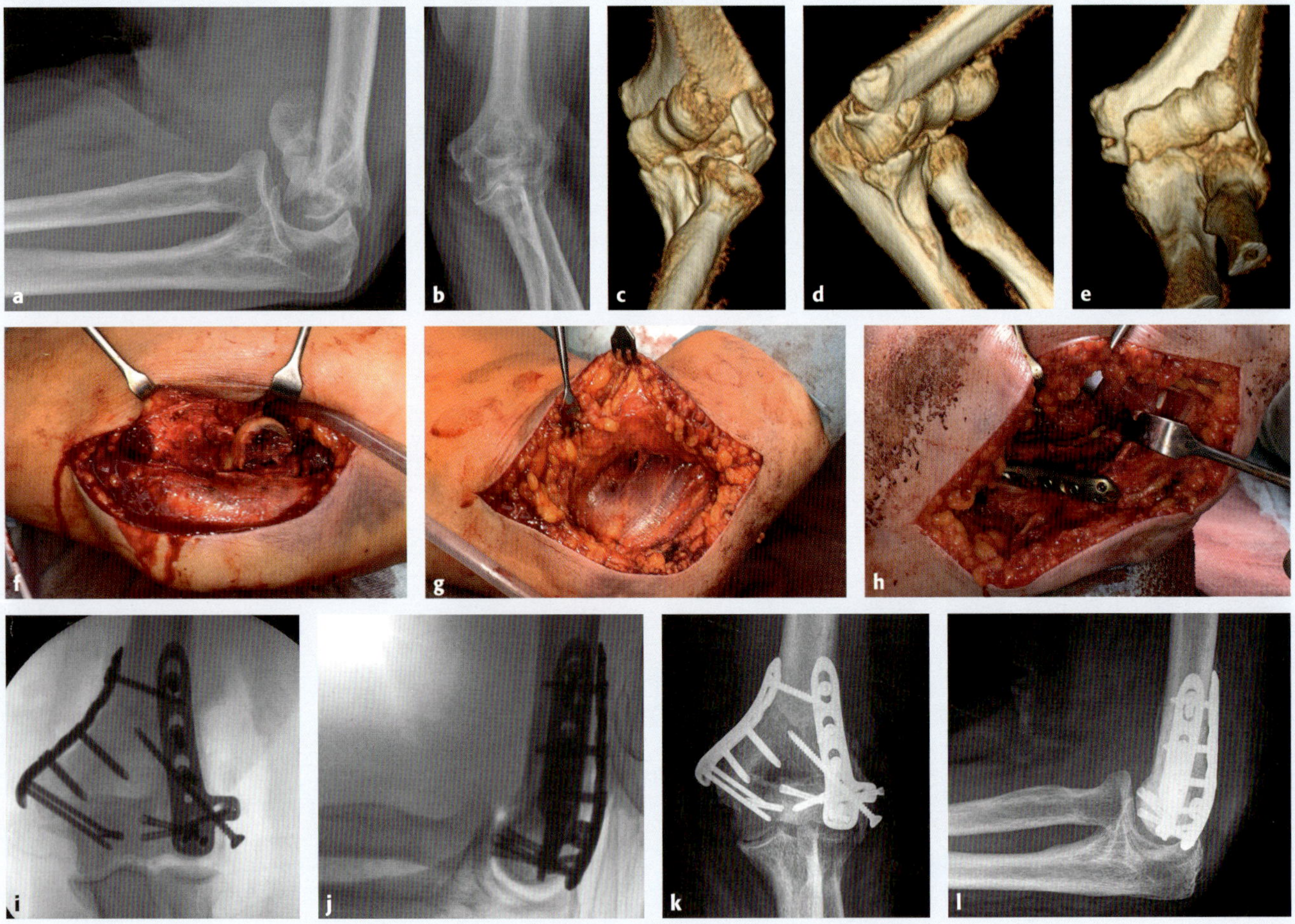


**Fig 3.3-3a–l** A 75-year-old woman with an elbow fracture dislocation and a fracture of the capitellum and trochlea.
**a–e** X-rays images and 3-D computed tomographic scans showing a displaced capitellar and trochlear fracture with epiphyseal/metaphyseal fracture.
**f** Clinical photograph showing the ruptured capsule with the capitellar fracture fragment on the radial side.
**g** Clinical photograph of the ulnar incision.
**h** Fixed ulnar column of the supracondylar fracture by ulnar plate.
**i–j** Intraoperative image intensifier x-rays showing good fracture alignment.
**k–l** Final follow-up x-rays showing fracture union.

### 4.2 Nonoperative treatment

Even initially nondisplaced fractures tend to displace secondarily [15]. These facts render nonoperative treatment of DHF limited primarily to patients with contractures, a short life expectancy, or an abundance of comorbidities that render the surgical intervention life-threatening. It should be noted that plaster immobilization alone usually leads to nonunion (**Case 3: Fig 3.3-4**). In case of nonoperative management, splinting only assists with pain management.

CASE 3

**Patient**

A 92-year-old woman living in a nursing home. Type and time of trauma could not be recalled. Due to mild dementia and multiple falls, she sustained a distal humeral fracture that was initially treated by a general practitioner.

**Comorbidities**

- Mild dementia
- Multiple falls

**Treatment and outcome**

After roughly 3 weeks, the patient presented to our department with a loose plaster splint and few complaints (**Fig 3.3-4a**). Continuation of nonoperative treatment with development of a nonunion (**Fig 3.3-4b**). Two weeks later she sustained a minimal displaced odontoid fracture type II according to Anderson and D'Alonzo (**Fig 3.3-4c**) that was also treated nonoperatively. Three months later a pertrochanteric femoral fracture was fixed (**Fig 3.3-4d**). Mobilization and rehabilitation was not impaired by the humeral nonunion nor did she complain about pain.

**Discussion**

Distal humeral fractures are "absolute" indications for internal fixation. This case impressively demonstrates an exception to the rule. In the geriatric population, there is a fine line between causing additional harm to patients and withholding an invasive treatment step that would help to keep them more autonomous. This patient obviously tolerated the nonunion surprisingly well with a follow-up after half a year.

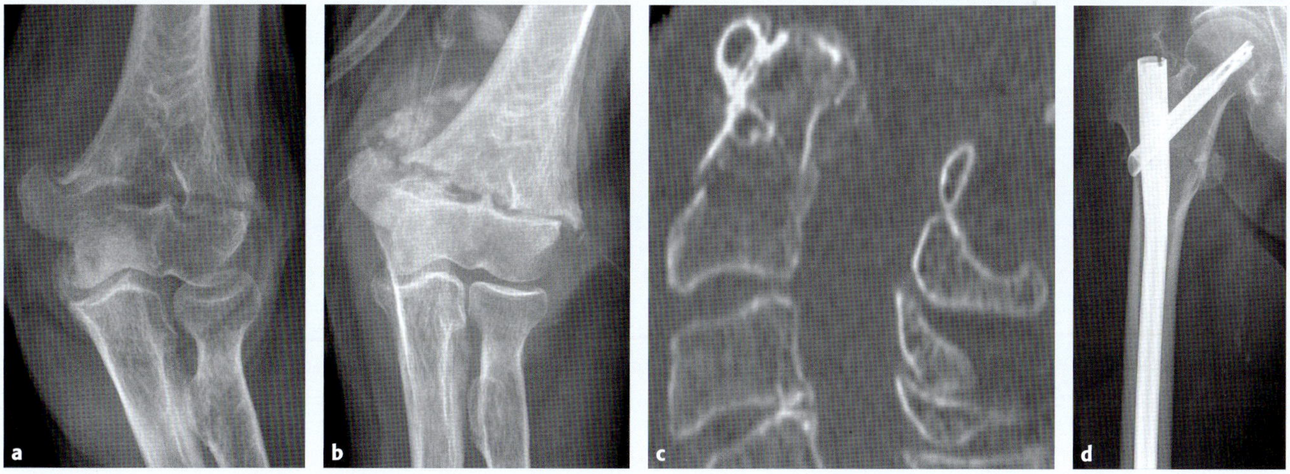


**Fig 3.3-4a–d** A 92-year-old woman with a distal humeral fracture (DHF).
**a** Metaphyseal DHF around 10 days after trauma.
**b** Same patient treated with above-elbow cast at 3 weeks after trauma.
**c** Computed tomographic scan showing displaced odontoid fracture type II according to Anderson.
**d** Intratrochanteric femur fracture treated with long proximal femoral nail antirotation nail with bone union.

### 4.3 Open reduction and internal fixation

Distal humeral fractures almost always require a stable fixation, usually provided by plates and screws (**Case 4: Fig 3.3-5**). We prefer anatomically preshaped locking plates.

Biomechanically, parallel plate configuration is superior to perpendicular positioning in osteoporotic bone [21].

CASE 4

**Patient**

An 80-year-old woman sustained a ground-level-fall with impact on the left hand, with pain at the left elbow, swelling, and no soft-tissue or skin lesions.

**Treatment and outcome**

The patient sustained a displaced, very low fracture of the left distal humerus (**Fig 3.3-5a–d**) and was treated with open reduction and plating of the distal columns (**Fig 3.3-5e–f**). Immediate postoperative mobilization resulted in satisfactory active and passive range of motion and radiological results at the final follow-up at 1 year.

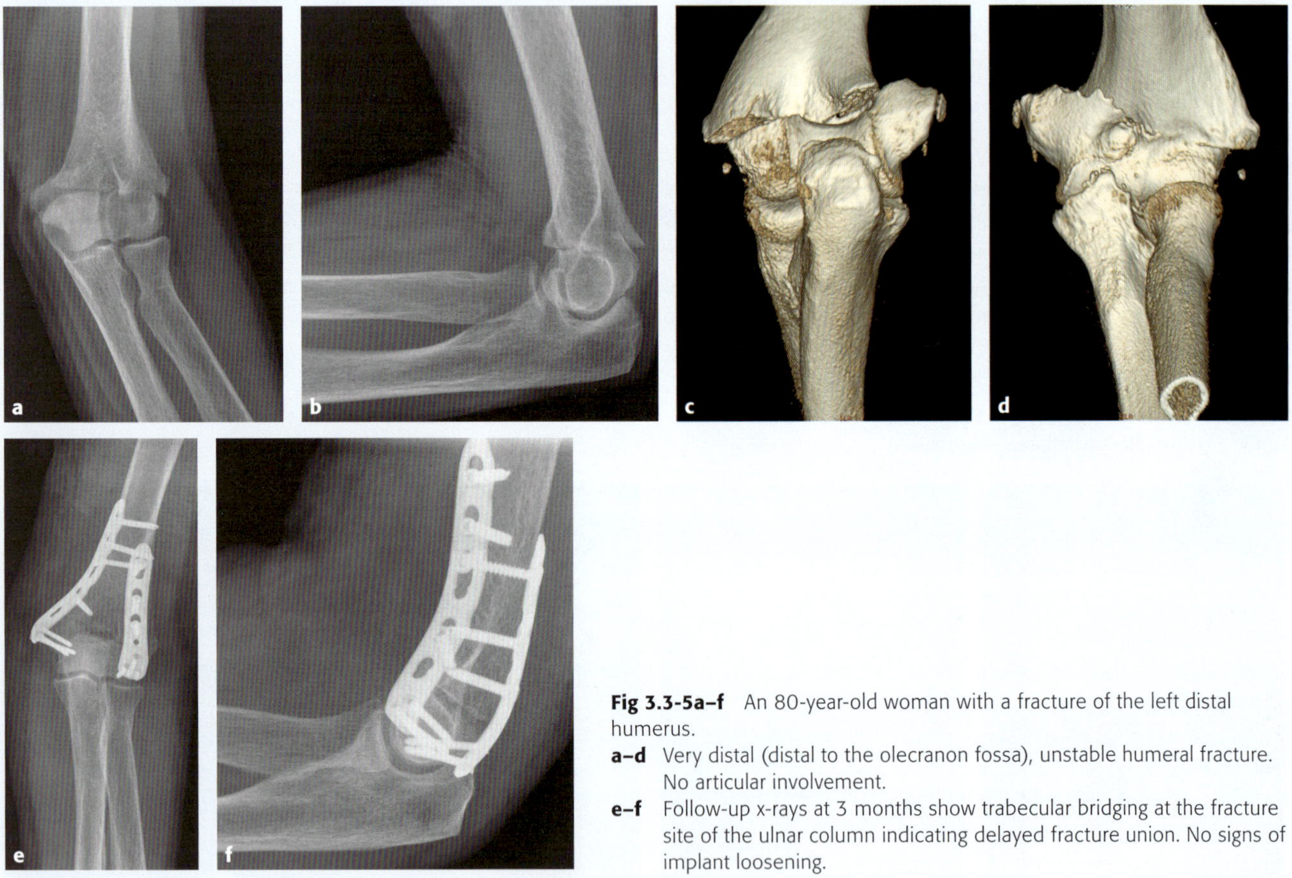


**Fig 3.3-5a–f** An 80-year-old woman with a fracture of the left distal humerus.
**a–d** Very distal (distal to the olecranon fossa), unstable humeral fracture. No articular involvement.
**e–f** Follow-up x-rays at 3 months show trabecular bridging at the fracture site of the ulnar column indicating delayed fracture union. No signs of implant loosening.

Closed reduction and fixation with percutaneous K-wires should no longer be used in older patients because it does not provide enough stability, even with additional plaster immobilization **(Fig 3.3-6)**. Open reduction and osteosynthesis with single screws and/or K-wires regularly leads to a nonunion.

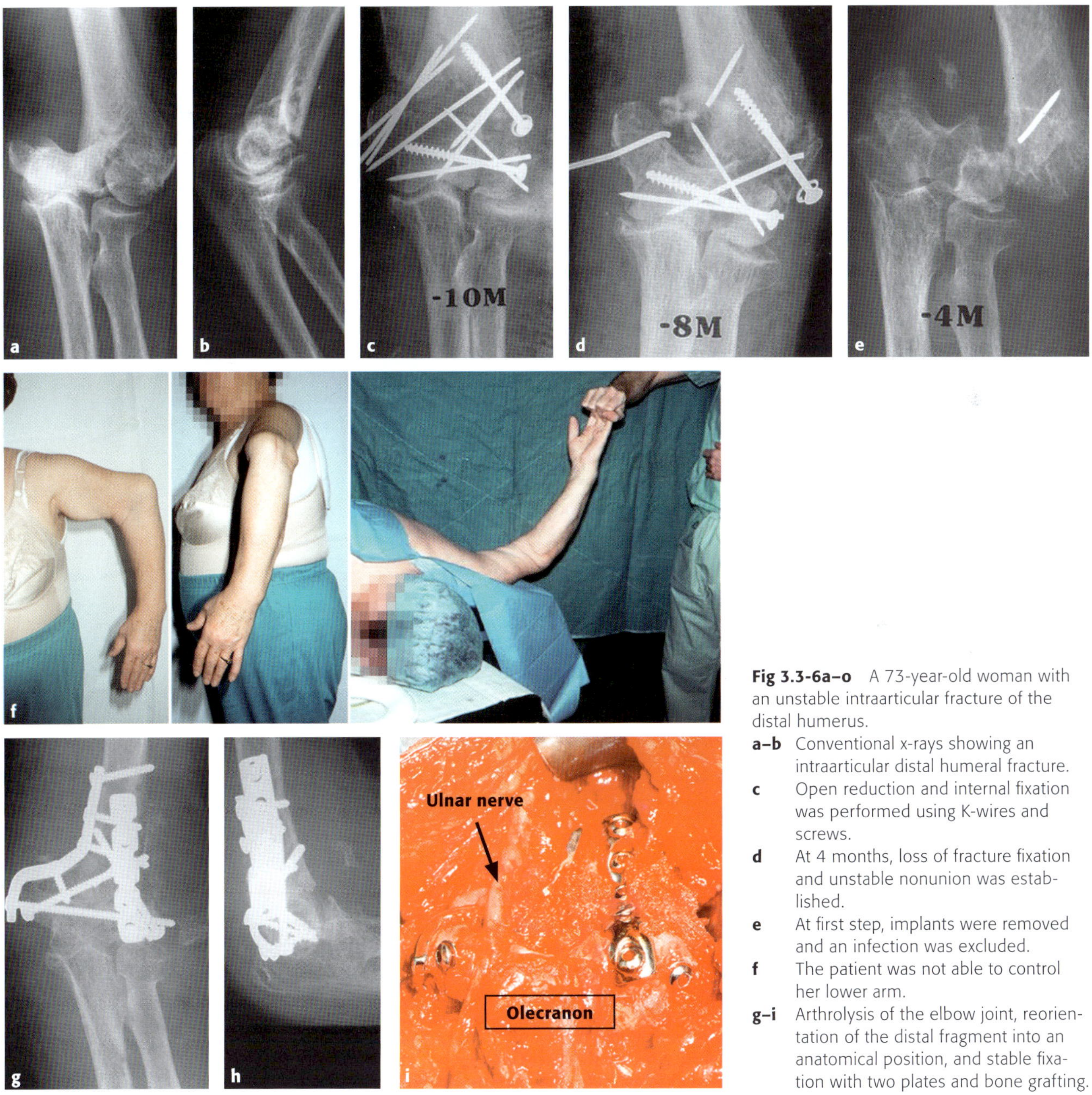


**Fig 3.3-6a–o** A 73-year-old woman with an unstable intraarticular fracture of the distal humerus.

- **a–b** Conventional x-rays showing an intraarticular distal humeral fracture.
- **c** Open reduction and internal fixation was performed using K-wires and screws.
- **d** At 4 months, loss of fracture fixation and unstable nonunion was established.
- **e** At first step, implants were removed and an infection was excluded.
- **f** The patient was not able to control her lower arm.
- **g–i** Arthrolysis of the elbow joint, reorientation of the distal fragment into an anatomical position, and stable fixation with two plates and bone grafting.

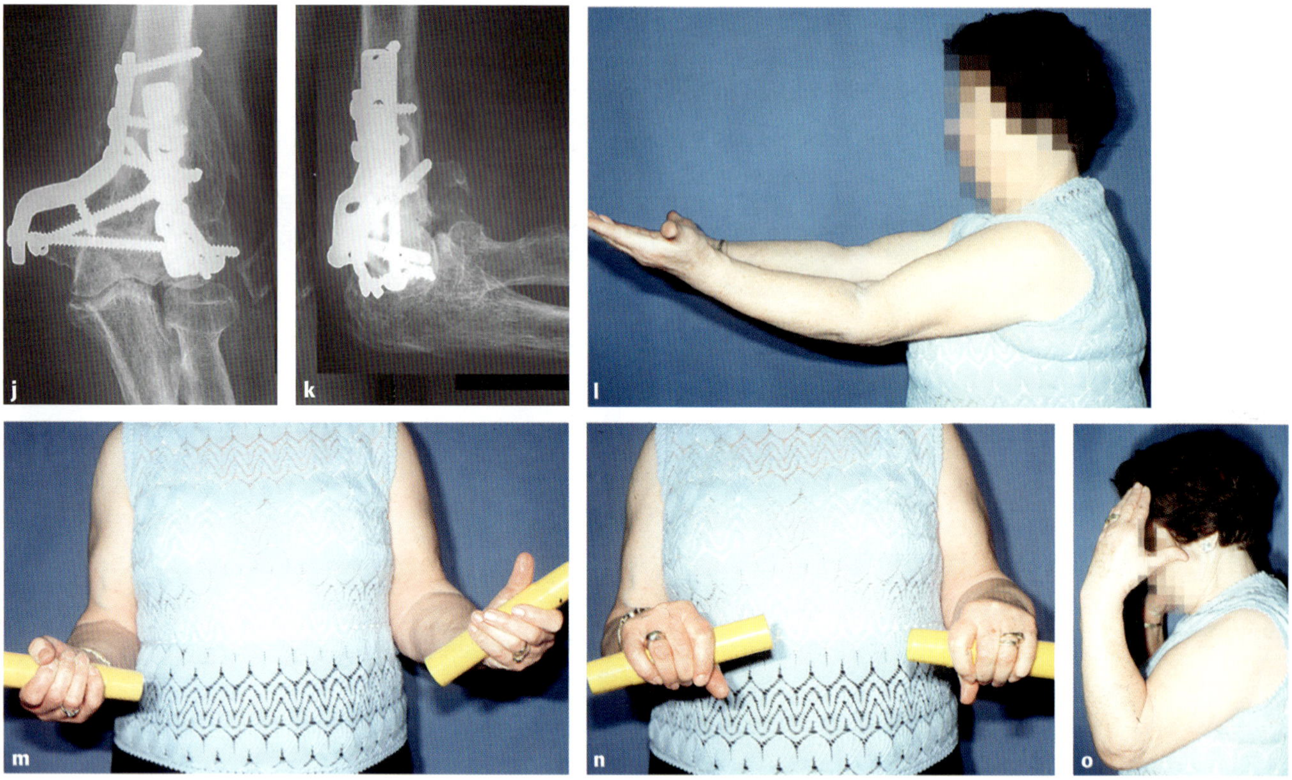


**Fig 3.3-6a–o (cont)** A 73-year-old woman with an unstable intraarticular fracture of the distal humerus.
**j–o** Good functional outcome after treatment. After 3 months uneventful healing with extension–flexion 0–15–130° and pronation–supination 75–0–85° [22].

Occasionally, in patients with significant contraindications to general anesthesia or in extremely frail patients with simple supracondylar fractures, a closed reduction and percutaneous X-type screw fixation can lead to a satisfactory result (**Case 5: Fig 3.3-7**) [23].

**CASE 5**

### Patient

A 93-year-old female patient with supracondylar distal humeral fracture and pronounced osteoporosis (**Fig 3.3-7a–b**).

### Comorbidities

- Osteoporosis

### Treatment and outcome

After closed reduction, two crossing screws were percutaneously inserted (**Fig 3.3-7c–d**). After 6 weeks of immobilization, the fracture was healed (**Fig 3.3-7e–f**).

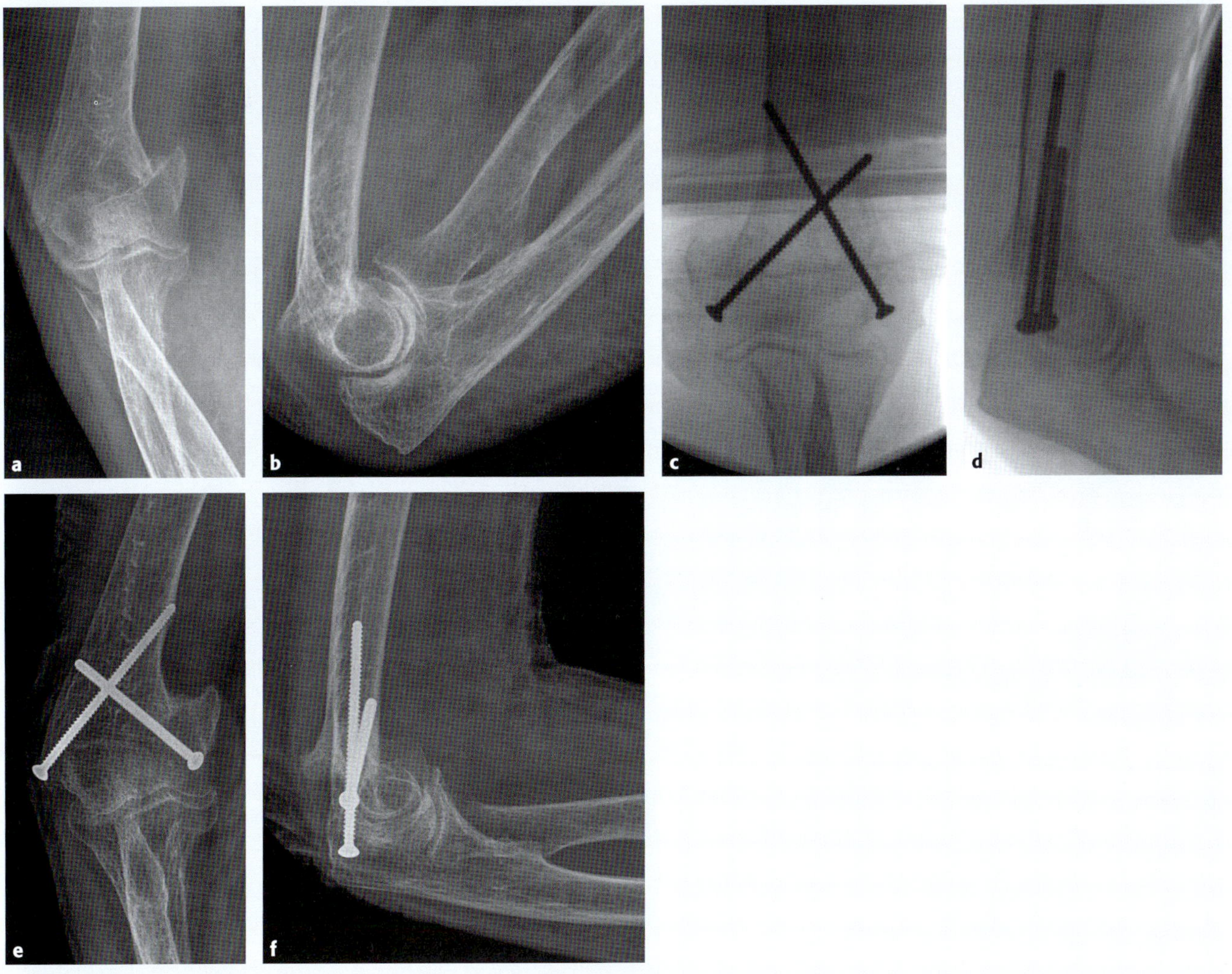


**Fig 3.3-7a–f** A 93-year-old woman with a distal humeral fracture.
**a–b** Conventional x-rays showing a supracondylar extraarticular fracture of the distal humerus.
**c–d** Intraoperative x-rays showing two crossing screws inserted percutaneously after closed reduction. Additionally, an above-elbow splint was applied for 6 weeks.
**e–f** Six-week postoperative x-ray showing healed fracture with minimal varus deformity.

### 4.4 Total elbow arthroplasty

In a multicenter randomized controlled trial of open reduction and internal fixation (ORIF) versus total elbow arthroplasty (TEA) for displaced intraarticular distal humeral fractures, McKee et al [24] concluded that TEA is a preferred alternative for ORIF in older patients with complex distal humeral fractures not amenable to stable fixation (**Case 6: Fig 3.3-8**).

**CASE 6**

#### Patient

A 93-year-old female patient fell while riding her bicycle and sustained a comminuted distal humeral fracture (**Fig 3.3-8a–d**).

#### Comorbidities

- None

#### Treatment and outcome

After intraoperative examination, the decision was taken to replace the elbow joint with a Coonrad-Morrey prosthesis leading to a functional result after 3 months (**Fig 3.3-8e–k**).

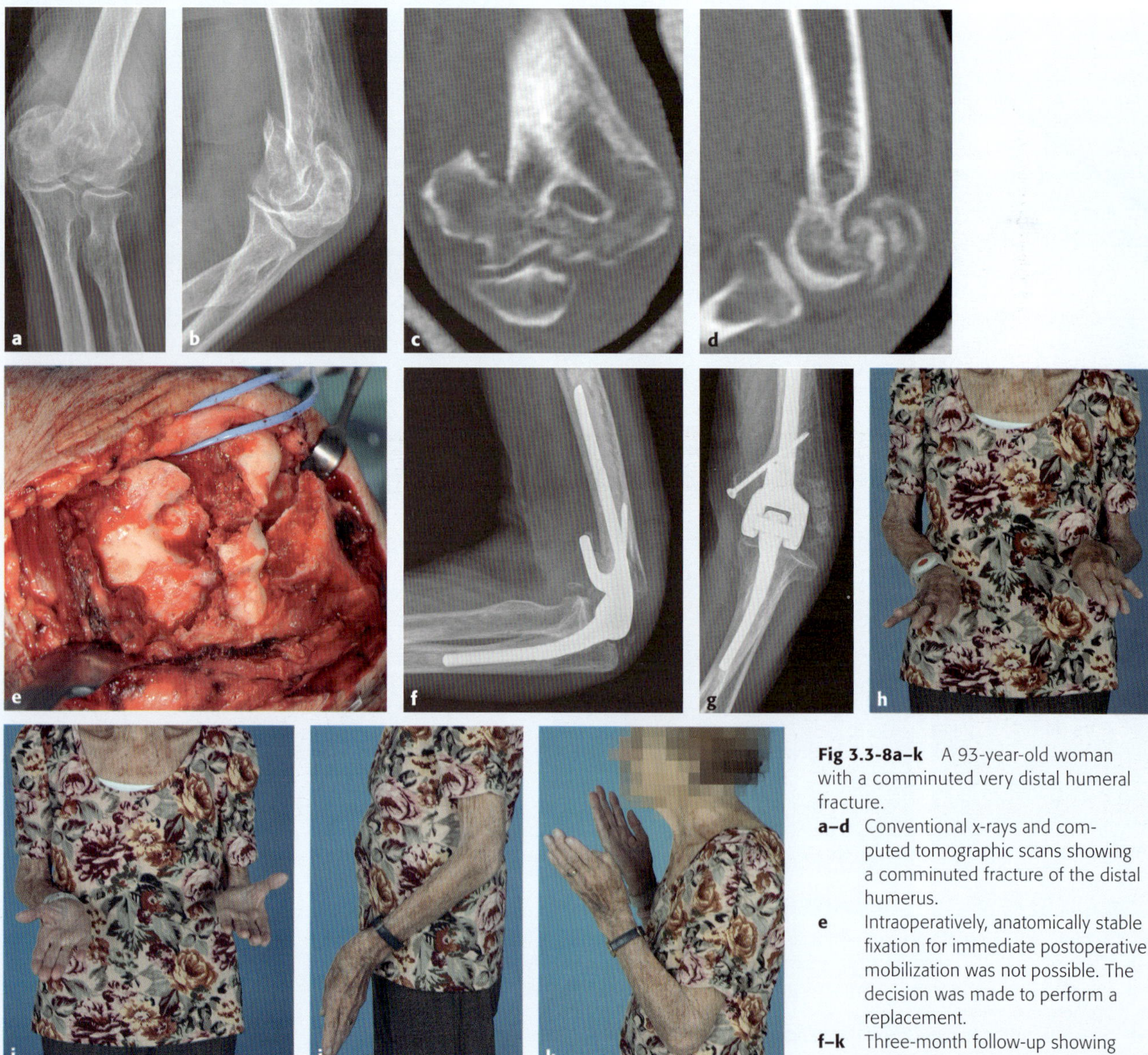

**Fig 3.3-8a–k** A 93-year-old woman with a comminuted very distal humeral fracture.
**a–d** Conventional x-rays and computed tomographic scans showing a comminuted fracture of the distal humerus.
**e** Intraoperatively, anatomically stable fixation for immediate postoperative mobilization was not possible. The decision was made to perform a replacement.
**f–k** Three-month follow-up showing good radiographic and clinical results.

The term "amenable to stable fixation" may be dependent on the experience and skills of the surgeon in charge. According to our own experience, and with the principles mentioned before, most fractures are feasible for ORIF, even with comminution and osteoporosis (**Case 7: Fig 3.3-9**).

CASE 7

**Patient**

A 75-year-old female patient fell while in a bus and sustained an osteoporotic distal humeral fracture with intraarticular component and comminution on the radial side (**Fig 3.3-9a–b**).

**Comorbidities**

- None

**Treatment and outcome**

Open reduction and internal fixation via a posterior approach was performed (**Fig 3.3-9c–g**). No postoperative immobilization with immediate physiotherapy. Excellent functional result after 3 months (**Fig 3.3-9h–k**).

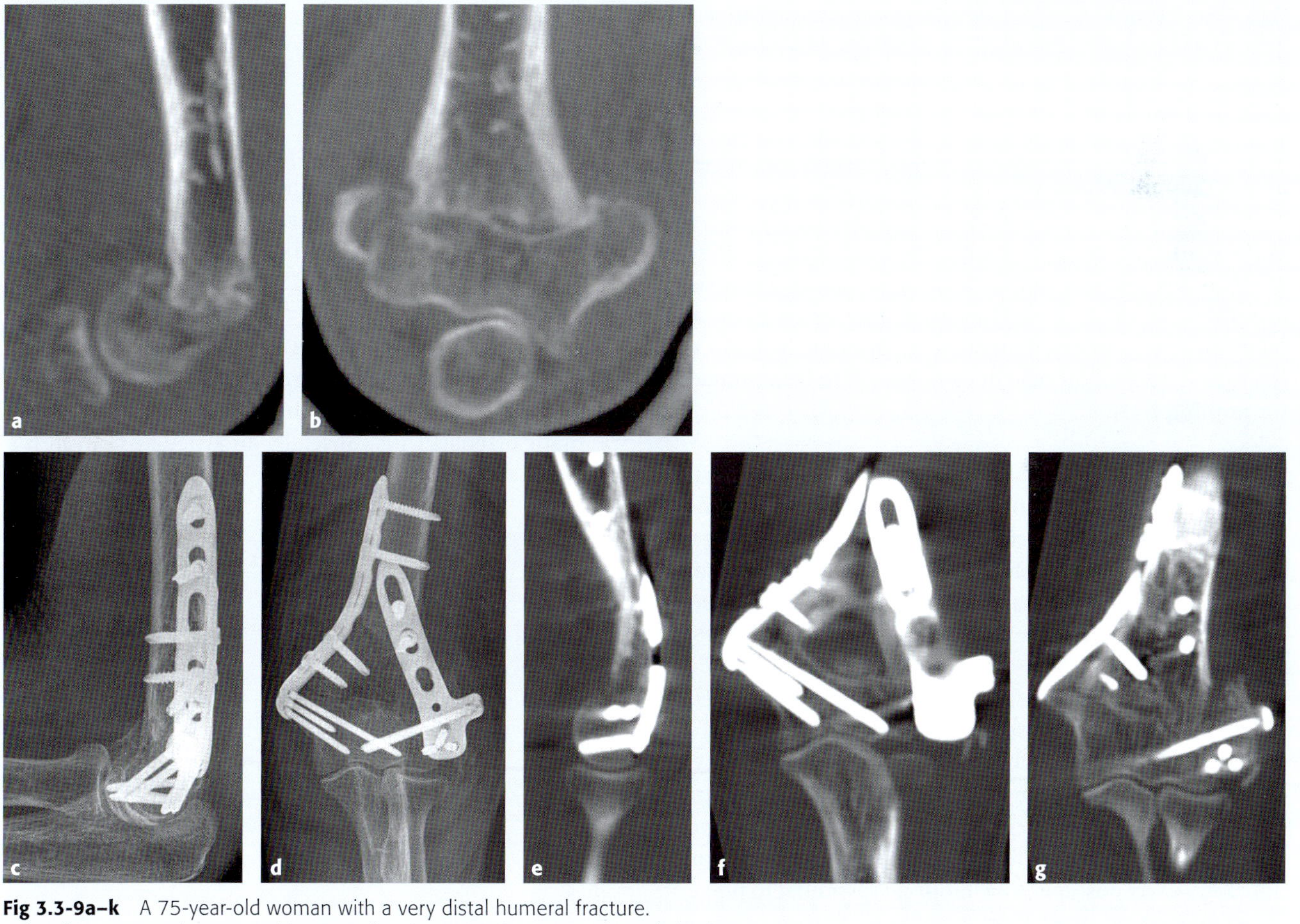


**Fig 3.3-9a–k** A 75-year-old woman with a very distal humeral fracture.
**a–b** The computed tomographic scans showing comminution on the radial column.
**c–g** Six-week postoperative x-rays after fracture fixation with open reduction and internal fixation showing some bone resorption at the radial column.

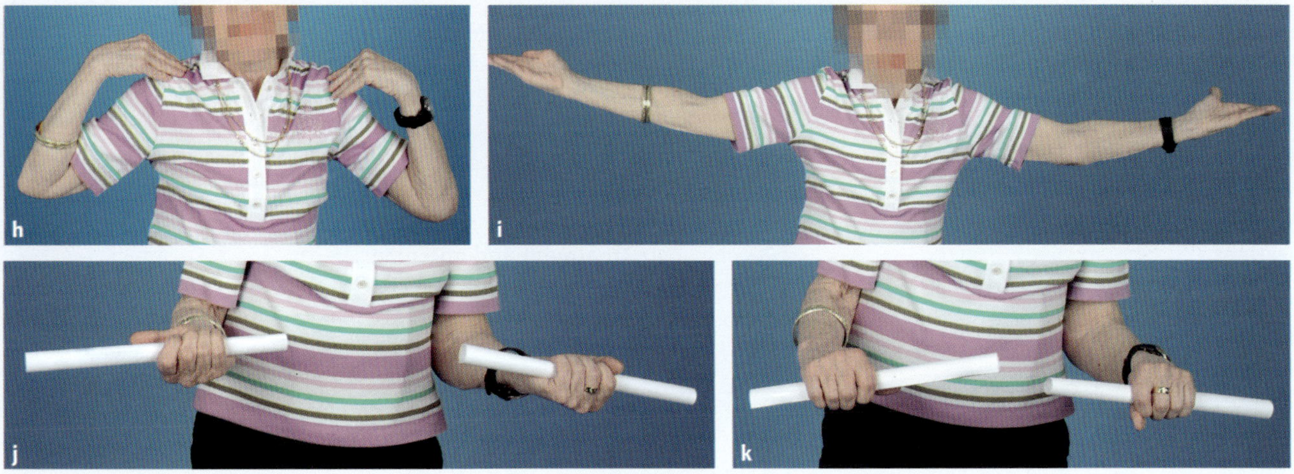

**Fig 3.3-9a–k (cont)** A 75-year-old woman with a very distal humeral fracture.
**h–k** Clinical photographs at 3 months showing good functional results.

## 5 Complications

The risk of complications during the treatment of DHFs in adults is low and uneventful healing is typical. The risk of nonunion seems to be higher after high-energy trauma, open fractures, and nonoperative treatment, whereas the fracture classification type does not seem to be a predictor for nonunion [3].

Fractures of the capitellum and the trochlea may lead to fragments that are devascularized and at high risk of becoming necrotic. The danger of osteonecrosis seems to be especially high in fractures involving both the medial and lateral columns of the distal humerus. Ulnar nerve neuropathy and poor soft-tissue conditions make these fractures challenging [25, 26].

Short-term complications in fracture treatment might consist of joint stiffness or instability. Older patients are in particular danger of developing joint stiffness in the setting of cast fixation longer than 2–3 weeks or with inadequate early functional aftercare, often as a consequence of poor postoperative pain control. To ensure a good functional outcome, early postoperative motion is essential to prevent the elbow joint capsule from developing fibrosis.

For older patients with comminuted displaced intraarticular fractures, primary total arthroplasty may be a superior treatment option, as stable internal fixation is difficult to achieve in osteoporotic bone [5, 27].

Joint instability may originate from associated ligament insufficiency or when the fracture extends beyond the trochlear ridge and leads to ulnohumeral dissociation [7]. Posttraumatic osteoarthritis caused by an articular step-off is a long-term complication [28].

## 6 References


1. **Court-Brown CM, Caesar B.** Epidemiology of adult fractures: a review. *Injury.* 2006 Aug;37(8):691–697.
2. **Bergdahl C, Ekholm C, Wennergren D, et al.** Epidemiology and patho-anatomical pattern of 2,011 humeral fractures: data from the Swedish Fracture Register. *BMC Musculoskelet Disord.* 2016 Apr 12;17:159.
3. **Robinson CM, Hill RM, Jacobs N, et al.** Adult distal humeral metaphyseal fractures: epidemiology and results of treatment. *J Orthop Trauma.* 2003 Jan;17(1):38–47.
4. **Widhalm HK, Seemann R, Wagner FT, et al.** Clinical outcome and osteoarthritic changes after surgical treatment of isolated capitulum humeri fractures with a minimum follow-up of five years. *Int Orthop.* 2016 Dec;40(12):2603–2610.
5. **Nauth A, McKee MD, Ristevski B, et al.** Distal humeral fractures in adults. *J Bone Joint Surg Am.* 2011 Apr 06;93(7):686–700.
6. **Throckmorton TW, Zarkadas PC, Steinmann SP.** Distal humerus fractures. *Hand Clin.* 2007 Nov;23(4):457–469, vi.
7. **Mighell M, Virani NA, Shannon R, et al.** Large coronal shear fractures of the capitellum and trochlea treated with headless compression screws. *J Shoulder Elbow Surg.* 2010 Jan;19(1):38–45.
8. **Palvanen M, Kannus P, Niemi S, et al.** Secular trends in the osteoporotic fractures of the distal humerus in elderly women. *Eur J Epidemiol.* 1998 Feb;14(2):159–164.
9. **Bilsel K, Atalar AC, Erdil M, et al.** Coronal plane fractures of the distal humerus involving the capitellum and trochlea treated with open reduction internal fixation. *Arch Orthop Trauma Surg.* 2013 Jun;133(6):797–804.
10. **Heck S, Zilleken C, Pennig D, et al.** Reconstruction of radial capitellar fractures using fine-threaded implants (FFS). *Injury.* 2012 Feb;43(2):164–168.
11. **Ring D, Jupiter JB, Gulotta L.** Articular fractures of the distal part of the humerus. *J Bone Joint Surg Am.* 2003 Feb;85-A(2):232–238.
12. **Bryan RS, Morrey BF.** Fractures of the distal humerus. In: Morrey BF, ed. *The Elbow and Its Disorders.* Philadelphia: Saunders; 1985:302–339.
13. **McKee MD, Jupiter JB, Bamberger HB.** Coronal shear fractures of the distal end of the humerus. *J Bone Joint Surg Am.* 1996 Jan;78(1):49–54.
14. **Trinh TQ, Harris JD, Kolovich GP, et al.** Operative management of capitellar fractures: a systematic review. *J Shoulder Elbow Surg.* 2012 Nov;21(11):1613–1622.
15. **Srinivasan K, Agarwal M, Matthews SJ, et al.** Fractures of the distal humerus in the elderly: is internal fixation the treatment of choice? *Clin Orthop Relat Res.* 2005 May(434):222–230.
16. **Lee JJ, Lawton JN.** Coronal shear fractures of the distal humerus. *J Hand Surg Am.* 2012 Nov;37(11):2412–2417.
17. **Ljungquist KL, Beran MC, Awan H.** Effects of surgical approach on functional outcomes of open reduction and internal fixation of intra-articular distal humeral fractures: a systematic review. *J Shoulder Elbow Surg.* 2012 Jan;21(1):126–135.
18. **Bryan RS, Morrey BF.** Extensive posterior exposure of the elbow. A triceps-sparing approach. *Clin Orthop Relat Res.* 1982 Jun;(166):188–192.
19. **Alonso-Llames M.** Bilaterotricipital approach to the elbow. Its application in the osteosynthesis of supracondylar fractures of the humerus in children. *Acta Orthop Scand.* 1972;43(6):479–490.
20. **Zhang C, Zhong B, Luo CF.** Comparing approaches to expose type C fractures of the distal humerus for ORIF in elderly patients: six years clinical experience with both the triceps-sparing approach and olecranon osteotomy. *Arch Orthop Trauma Surg.* 2014 Jun;134(6):803–811.
21. **Stoffel K, Cunneen S, Morgan R, et al.** Comparative stability of perpendicular versus parallel double-locking plating systems in osteoporotic comminuted distal humerus fractures. *J Orthop Res.* 2008 Jun;26(6):778–784.
22. **Blauth M, Becker T, Regel G.** Ellbogengelenknahe, transepikondyläre Humeruspseudarthrosen. *Oper Orthop Traumatol.* 1997 Dec;9(4):277–287. German.
23. **Paryavi E, O'Toole RV, Frisch HM, et al.** Use of 2 column screws to treat transcondylar distal humeral fractures in geriatric patients. *Tech Hand Up Extrem Surg.* 2010 Dec;14(4):209–213.
24. **McKee MD, Veillette CJ, Hall JA, et al.** A multicenter, prospective, randomized, controlled trial of open reduction—internal fixation versus total elbow arthroplasty for displaced intra-articular distal humeral fractures in elderly patients. *J Shoulder Elbow Surg.* 2009 Jan-Feb;18(1):3–12.
25. **Wiggers JK, Ring D.** Osteonecrosis after open reduction and internal fixation of a bicolumnar fracture of the distal humerus: a report of four cases. *J Hand Surg Am.* 2011 Jan;36(1):89–93.
26. **Dubberley JH, Faber KJ, Macdermid JC, et al.** Outcome after open reduction and internal fixation of capitellar and trochlear fractures. *J Bone Joint Surg Am.* 2006 Jan;88(1):46–54.
27. **Simone JP, Streubel PN, Sanchez-Sotelo J, et al.** Low transcondylar fractures of the distal humerus: results of open reduction and internal fixation. *J Shoulder Elbow Surg.* 2014 Apr;23(4):573–578.
28. **Giannicola G, Sacchetti FM, Greco A, et al.** Open reduction and internal fixation combined with hinged elbow fixator in capitellum and trochlea fractures. *Acta Orthop.* 2010 Apr;81(2):228–233.

# 3.4 Elbow

Rohit Arora, Kerstin Simon, Marco Keller, Michael Blauth

## 1 Introduction

Older adults with elbow fracture dislocations (EFDs) present with a wide range of functional, physical, and cognitive impairments. Therefore, the surgical solution must be customized and adapted to the functional needs and ability to comply with postoperative care and rehabilitation. The most important goal is a stable joint to allow early postoperative motion [1]. Geriatric patients with a stiff elbow joint may lose independence in activities of daily living.

Geriatric EFD usually occur after low-energy falls from standing height with the elbow joint in extension and abduction, while the forearm is in supination. They are typically associated with poor bone quality [2, 3].

Patients generally present suffering from pain, swelling, and limited range of motion (ROM) of the elbow [4]. In older patients, simple elbow dislocations with ligamentous injuries only are rare because of the reduced bone quality. Elbow dislocations are mostly associated with fractures of the distal humerus or the olecranon [5].

In EFD, the extent of concomitant bony and ligamentous injuries is proportional to the functional outcome and complications [6]. Retrospective studies show primary total elbow replacement in elbow dislocation fractures produces good to excellent results [5, 7]. With the goal of single-shot surgery, the ideal treatment modality is often the one least prone to complications.

## 2 Epidemiology

Elbow dislocations are the most common dislocations after those involving the shoulder, with an incidence of 6–13 cases per 100,000 person-years [8]. A systematic review of elbow dislocations between 2002 and 2006 in 102 hospitals in the US reveal an incidence of 5.21 dislocations per 100,000 person-years, a slight male predominance (53%), with the majority caused by falls and in the home setting (51.5%) [9]. Elbow dislocations account for 11–28% of all elbow injuries and involve the nondominant extremity in approximately 60% of the cases [10–12].

While some authors report concomitant coronoid fractures in about 10% of the elbow dislocations [13], others claim that almost every elbow dislocation is associated with a coronoid fracture as a result of shear forces caused by posterior translation against the humeral trochlea [2] after falls on the outstretched hand [4]. An additional rupture of the anterior bundle causes compression fractures of the radial head [14].

McKee et al [15] demonstrated a lesion of the lateral collateral ligament (LCL) complex in 100% of elbow dislocations and involvement of medial collateral ligament (MCL) complex in 80% of cases.

## 3 Classification

There are three major patterns of traumatic EFD: posterolateral, anterior, and posterior transolecranon fracture dislocations.

### 3.1 Posterolateral instability (terrible triad)

Posterolateral EFD include fractures of the radial head and the coronoid with a rupture of the LCL complex (**Fig 3.4-1**). In most cases, at the time of trauma the elbow pivots around the MCL leaving this ligament complex intact. Posterolateral impaction fractures of the capitellum are frequent [16].

### 3.2 Varus posteromedial instability

This injury is characterized by an anteromedial coronoid fracture with LCL complex rupture. In most cases, the coronoid is fractured at the level of the anteromedial facet, which is also known as the sublime tubercle, where the MCL inserts. The lateral ulnar collateral ligament is mostly avulsed from the dorsal radial epicondyle. The radial head stays intact in most of the cases (**Case 1: Fig 3.4-2**).

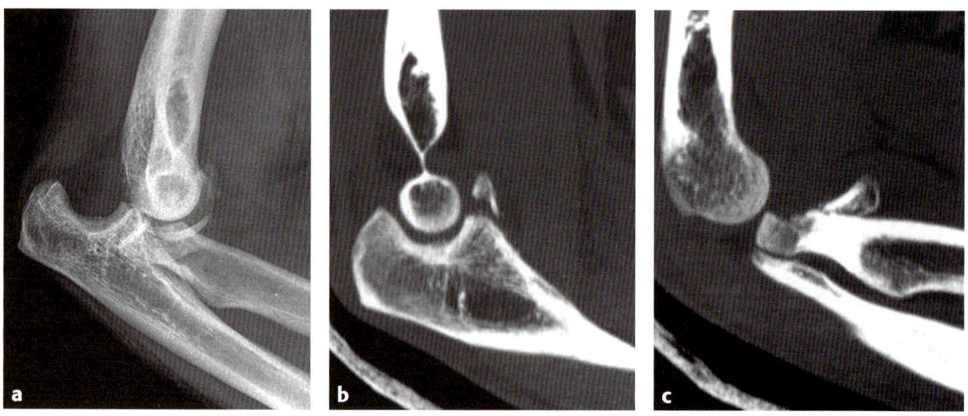


**Fig 3.4-1a–c** Posterior elbow dislocation (**a**) and sagittal computed tomographic scan after closed reduction with coronoid and radial head fractures as patterns of a terrible triad injury (**b–c**).

**CASE 1**

**Patient**

A 75-year-old woman fell at home from standing height and sustained an elbow fracture dislocation with intraarticular fragments (**Fig 3.4-2a–b**).

**Comorbidities**

- Hypertension
- Hypothyroidism

**Treatment and outcome**

The coronoid is fractured with its anteromedial facet (sublime tubercle) as the insertion point of the anterior part of the medial collateral ligament complex. Additionally, the lateral ulnar collateral ligament is avulsed with a bone fragment from the posterolateral aspect of the distal humerus (**Fig 3.4-2c–f**). After closed reduction, the joint was unstable in < 40° of flexion.

Intraoperatively, the lateral ulnar collateral ligament was avulsed with a bony fragment from the posterolateral humeral surface (**Fig 3.4-2g**).

Open reduction and plate fixation of the radial distal humeral column was performed. The ulnar ligament complex was fixed to the plate using fiber wire. This resulted in a stable elbow joint in full extension (**Fig 3.4-2h–j**).

The 12 month follow-up demonstrates concentric reduction of the ulnohumeral joint and a good functional result (**Fig 3.4-2k–p**).

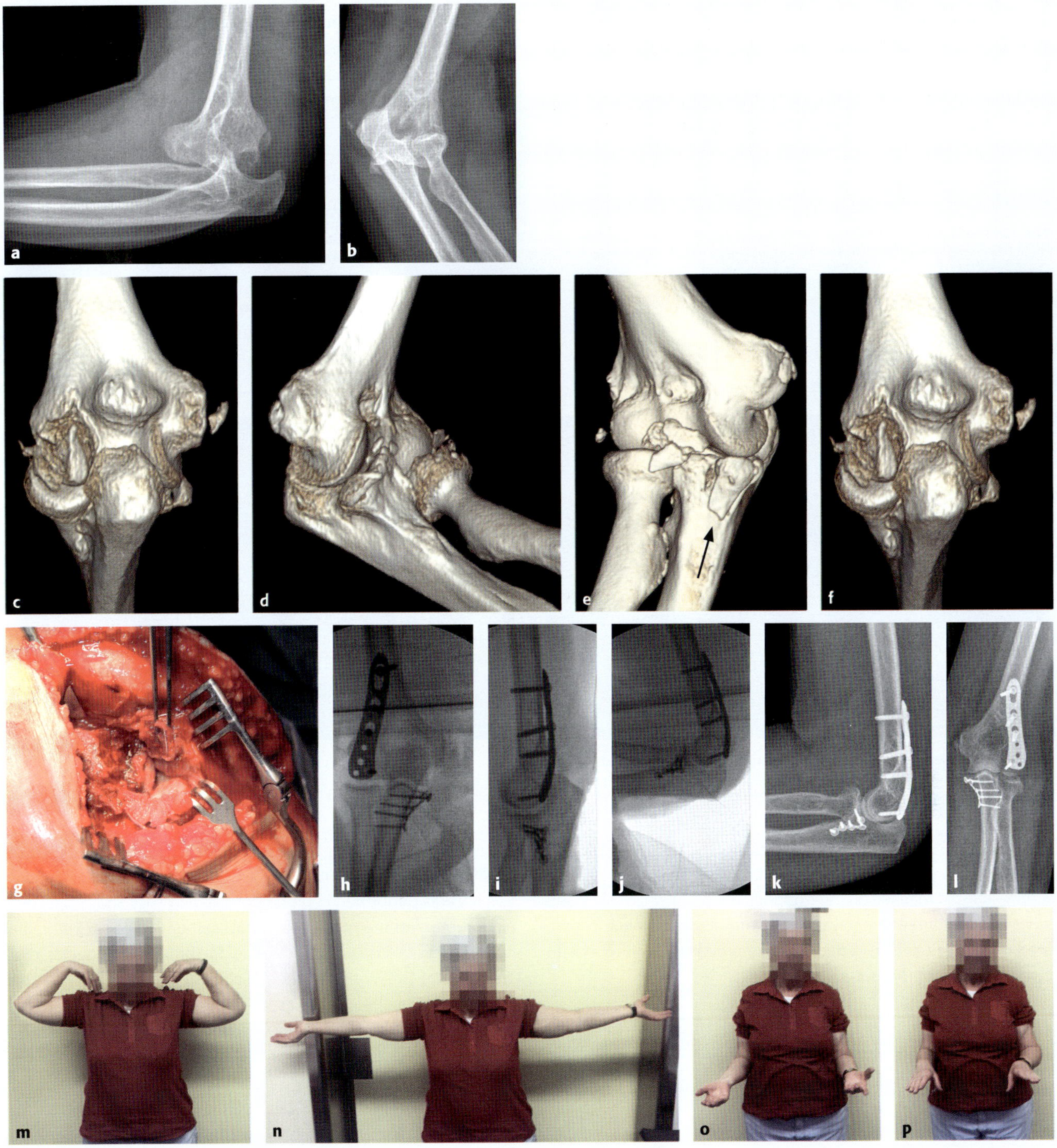

**Fig 3.4-2a–p** Elbow fracture dislocation with intraarticular fragments.
**a–b** Elbow fracture dislocation with intraarticular fragments.
**c–f** The anteromedial facet of the coronoid is fractured (sublime tubercle, black arrow) (**e**) and the lateral ulnar collateral ligament avulsed with a bone fragment (red arrow) (**f**).
**g** Intraoperative clinical photograph showing avulsion of the ulnar collateral ligament with a bony fragment.
**h–j** Plate fixation of the anteromedial fracture fragment and a dorsal plate buttressing the avulsed posterolateral fragment.
**k–l** Twelve-month follow-up x-rays showing concentric reduction of the ulnohumeral joint.
**m–p** Final follow-up with good clinical results.

### 3.3 Anterior transolecranon fracture dislocation

In this pattern, the distal humerus displaces across the facets lunaris of the proximal ulna, fracturing the olecranon with variable involvement of the coronoid or the proximal ulnar shaft, leaving the radial head intact (**Fig 3.4-3**).

### 3.4 Posterior transolecranon fracture dislocation

In this type, the proximal ulnar fractures and the radius dislocate posteriorly leading to shear fractures of the radial head and neck. Coronoid fractures also belong to this type of injury (**Fig 3.4-4**).

In those cases in which the proximal radioulnar joint is disrupted, the subtype is called Monteggia equivalent. The proximal radioulnar dislocation may best be detected on axial computed tomographic (CT) scan views.

Ligaments are avulsed with bone fragments so that bone fixation restores the ligamentous instability (**Case 2: Fig 3.4-5**).

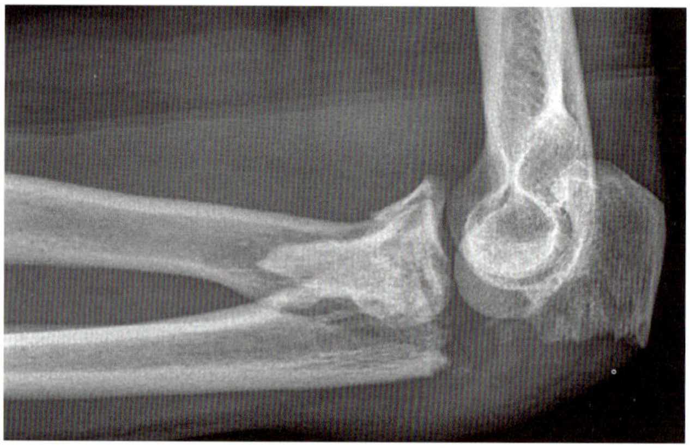

**Fig 3.4-3** Anterior transolecranon fracture dislocation with an anterior displacement of the proximal radius and proximal ulna without a disruption of the proximal radioulnar joint.

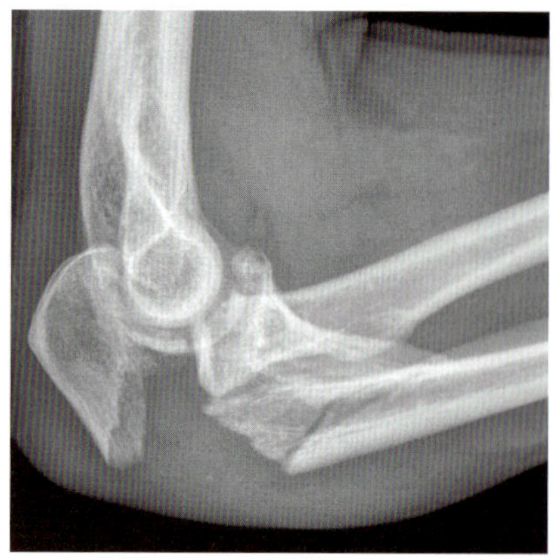

**Fig 3.4-4** Posterior transolecranon fracture dislocation with posterior displacement of the proximal radius and proximal ulna as a unit without disruption of the proximal radioulnar joint. The posterior displacement leads to a radial head and coronoid fracture.

CASE 2

#### Patient

An 83-year-old man fell on the extended right arm while skiing and sustained a Monteggia equivalent fracture dislocation with associated radial head and neck fractures. He presented with moderate swelling and pain (**Fig 3.4-5a–h**).

#### Comorbidities

- No comorbidities were documented

#### Treatment and outcome

Surgery was performed in prone position. Findings showed a complete rupture of the medial collateral ligament complex. The radial head was dislocated posteriorly out of the proximal radioulnar joint. The attempt to reconstruct the radial head and neck failed so the remaining radial head was resected, making the exposure to the fractured coronoid easier. Cannulated screw fixation of the coronoid process and plate fixation of the olecranon was performed. The radial head was replaced by a prosthesis and repair of the lateral collateral ligament complex resulted in a stable condition on the ulnar site. Intraoperative x-rays showed no subluxation or dislocation.

Follow-up x-rays at 16 months showed a concentric radio- and ulnohumeral joint with bone union (**Fig 3.4-5i–j**).

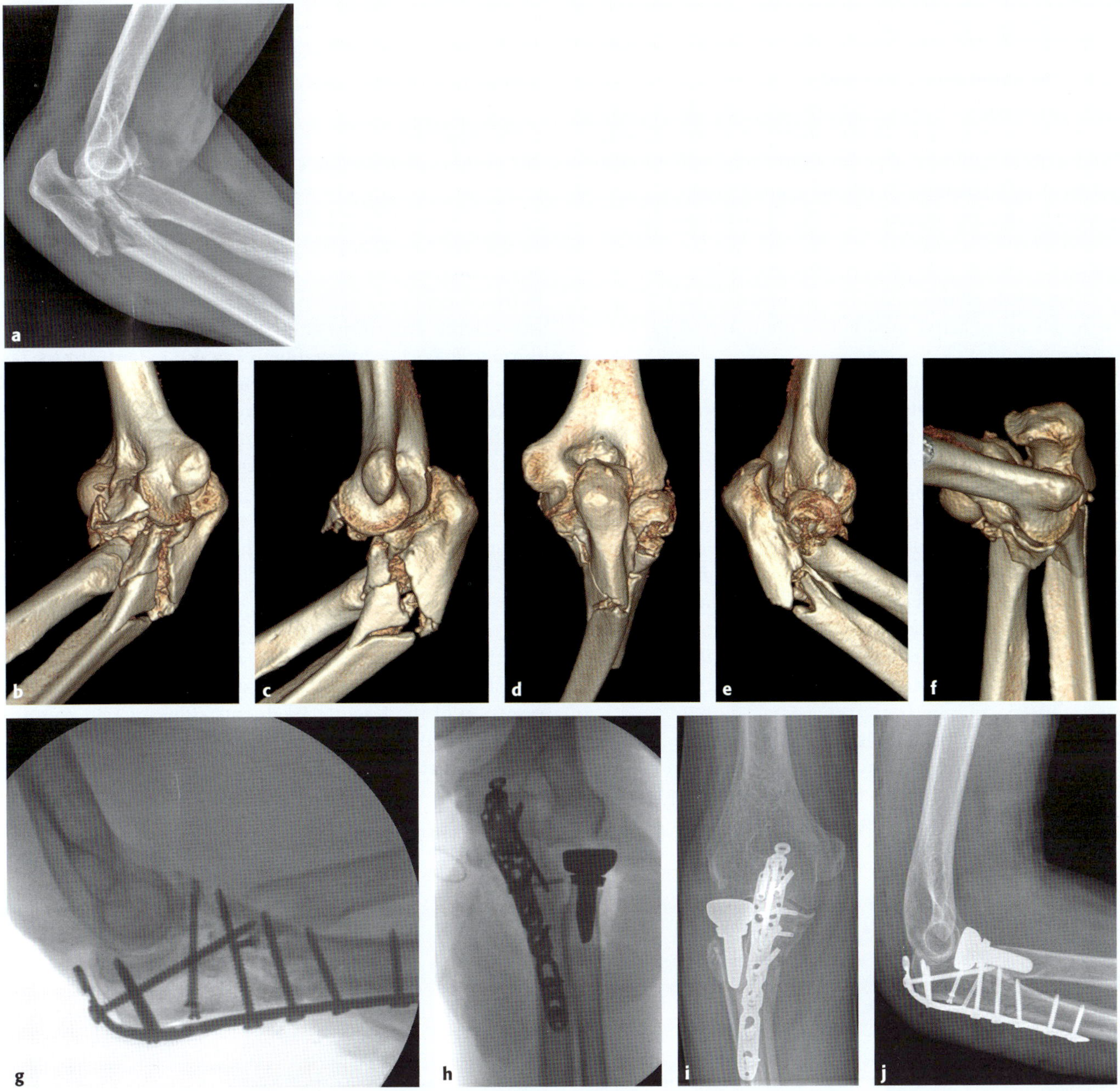

**Fig 3.4-5a–j** An 83-year-old man with a posterior transolecranon fracture dislocation.

**a–f** Posterior transolecranon fracture dislocation with associated radial head and neck fractures.

**g** Intraoperative x-ray showing the radial head resected. Reduction of the coronoid fragment was performed through the radial exposure. The fragment was fixed indirectly with screws from the dorsal aspect of the ulna and the olecranon fixed using a plate.

**h** Intraoperative x-ray showing the final fixation with radial head replacement.

**i–j** Postoperative x-rays taken at 16 months show a concentric radio- and ulnohumeral joint with bone union.

## 4 Therapeutic options

### 4.1 Nonoperative treatment

The majority of EFD are treated operatively to avoid osseous nonunion or recurrent dislocation [17]. Operative intervention restores stability and permits early motion of the elbow. Chan et al [17] demonstrated that a small subset of patients can be treated nonoperatively. Criteria for the nonoperative management include:

- Concentric elbow reduction, documented by CT scan
- Stable arc of active motion to a minimum of 30° extension
- Small and minimally displaced radial head fracture
- Smaller coronoid tip fracture (Regan-Morrey classification types 1 or 2)

In these cases, the elbow fracture dislocation should be reduced and immobilized in an elbow cast with the forearm in neutral rotation for a maximum of 3 weeks. Frequent clinical and x-ray examinations can reveal potential complications like recurrent subluxation or dislocation which must initiate operative fixation. Physiotherapy can be initiated as soon as pain subsides and starts with passive and active exercises around the neutral position.

### 4.2 Operative treatment

For the remaining fracture presentations, nonoperative methods can otherwise lead to recurrent instability and long-term fixation-induced stiffness [18].

The goals of operative treatment are restoration of the osseous anatomy and reconstruction of the ligamentous restraints to provide stability for early motion [2, 19].

#### 4.2.1 Approach

The authors prefer a single dorsal skin incision for all complex elbow fracture dislocations with the patient in prone position. Dissecting radial and ulnar skin flaps exposes the medial und lateral aspects of the elbow joint.

In transolecranon fracture dislocations, the radial skin flap is retracted anteriorly and the radial head is addressed through a Kocher interval between the extensor carpi radialis muscle and the anconeus muscle. The coronoid fragments can usually be exposed through the olecranon fracture site. In anteromedial coronoid fractures the ulnar skin flap is retracted anteriorly and the coronoid fracture is exposed using the flexor carpi ulnaris (FCU) splitting approach. The FCU is split in line with the anterior margin of the medial epicondyle and anterior part of the MCL complex (**Fig 3.4-6**).

In terrible triads, the radial skin flap is retracted anteriorly and the radial head is addressed through the rent of the lateral ligament complex. If the radial head has to be replaced, resection of the fracture fragments allows good exposure and access to the coronoid fracture for fixation. An additional medial approach can be avoided (**Fig 3.4-7**).

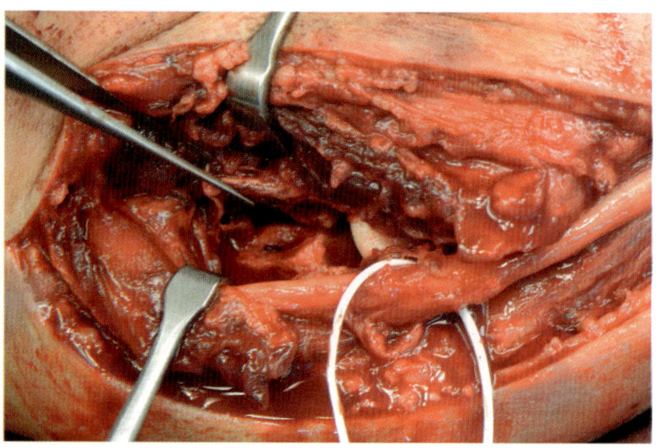

**Fig 3.4-6** Intraoperative image of the flexor carpi ulnaris (FCU) splitting approach (the left of the image is distal and the top is anterior). The ulnar nerve is looped and retracted dorsally. The anterior part of the FCU is retracted anteriorly by the upper Langenbeck retractor. The anteromedial facet of the coronoid (sublime tubercle) is held in the forceps.

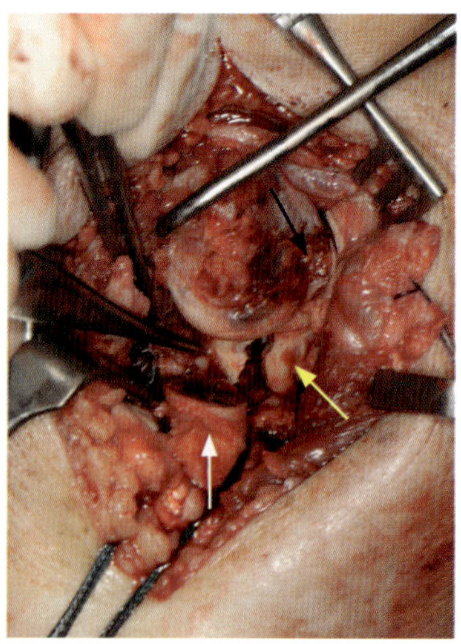

**Fig 3.4-7** Intraoperative image showing the coronoid fracture after the radial head has been resected (white arrow showing the proximal radial shaft stump). The forceps are holding down the tip of the coronoid (yellow arrow showing the base of the coronoid). The origin of the lateral collateral ligament complex (black arrow) has been avulsed from the lateral epicondyle.

### 4.2.2 Radial head

It is important to fix the radial head fracture if technically feasible. In cases of complex elbow instability, partial or entire radial head resection aggravates instability and should not be performed. Replacement is considered for fractures with more than four fragments, and in cases where the radial head fracture has no periosteal contact with the neck [20, 21].

Otherwise, open reduction and internal fixation with plate fixation in the "safe zone" is attempted to avoid impingement. Plating may be associated with impaired forearm rotation; oblique screws may be an alternative. Comminution at the head-neck junction may require corticocancellous bone grafting, for example, from the posterolateral surface of the distal humerus (**Fig 3.4-8**) [22].

### 4.2.3 Coronoid process

The significance of coronoid fractures with regard to elbow stability can be difficult to determine. Some authors tend to ignore fractures affecting less than 30% of the height [23]. In clinical practice, there are more parameters to consider than the size of the coronoid fragment alone. Especially if the fracture contains the anterior and the medial facet of the coronoid process, it should always be fixed. For this reason, each patient with a coronoid fracture must be assessed individually intraoperatively. In valgus posteromedial injuries, the authors fix each coronoid fracture when there is joint incongruity in 90° of flexion or if there is instability under varus stress, regardless of fragment size (**Fig 3.4-9**) [24].

Larger coronoid fragments should be fixed by retrograde cannulated screws (**Fig 3.4-10**). The anteromedial facet fragments are best fixed using buttress plates (**Case 3: Fig 3.4-11**).

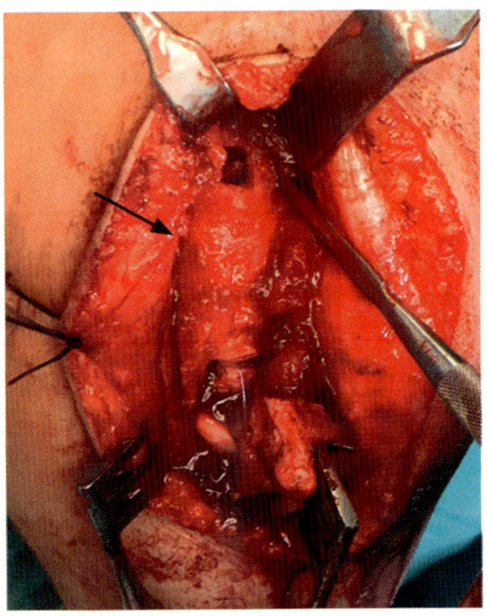

**Fig 3.4-8** Intraoperative situation showing the triceps reflected ulnarly and the radial column of the distal humerus, with the defect (arrow), where the bone graft has been harvested.

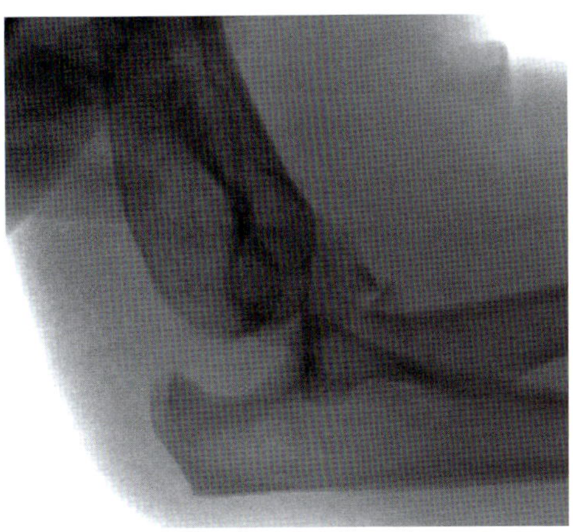

**Fig 3.4-9** Posterior dislocation in 90° flexion, confirming the loss of the buttress function of the fractured coronoid. In these cases, the coronoid should always be fixed regardless of its size.

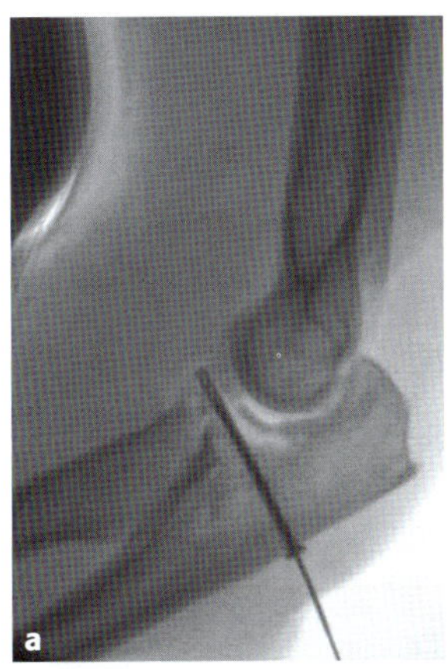

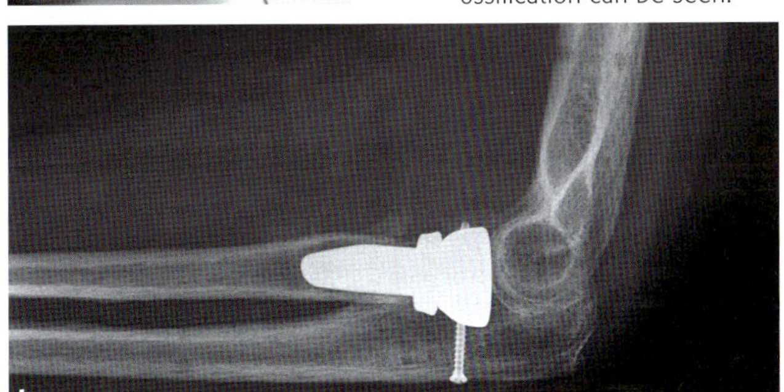

**Fig 3.4-10a–b** Fixation of larger coronoid fragments.

- **a** After resection of the radial head, the coronoid fragment was reduced from the radial side and fixed indirectly using a cannulated screw inserted from the dorsal ulna.
- **b** Follow-up x-ray showing the replaced radial head and anatomically fixed coronoid fragment. Mild anterolateral ossification can be seen.

CASE 3

## Patient

A 71-year-old woman fell down the stairs and presented with moderate swelling but intact perfusion, function, and sensibility after elbow fracture dislocation. Initial x-rays and 3-D computed tomographic scans showed a displaced fracture of the left elbow with coronoid fracture (**Fig 3.4-11a–e**).

## Comorbidities

- Hypertension
- Smoker

## Treatment and outcome

Surgery was performed in prone position: The medial collateral ligament (MCL) complex was partially ruptured, with a multifragmentary coronoid process fracture. The ulnar approach with split of the flexor carpi ulnaris was performed. The anterior part of the MCL was attached to the fracture fragment. The anteromedial fracture fragment was stabilized using two cannulated screws and a plate. For capsule refixation, nonresorbable sutures were used. The lateral ligament complex was fixed through the radial side using bone anchors. Intraoperative extension x-rays demonstrate no tendency for dislocation (**Fig 3.4-11f–h**).

After 14 months, good functional and radiographic results were obtained (**Fig 3.4-11i–n**).

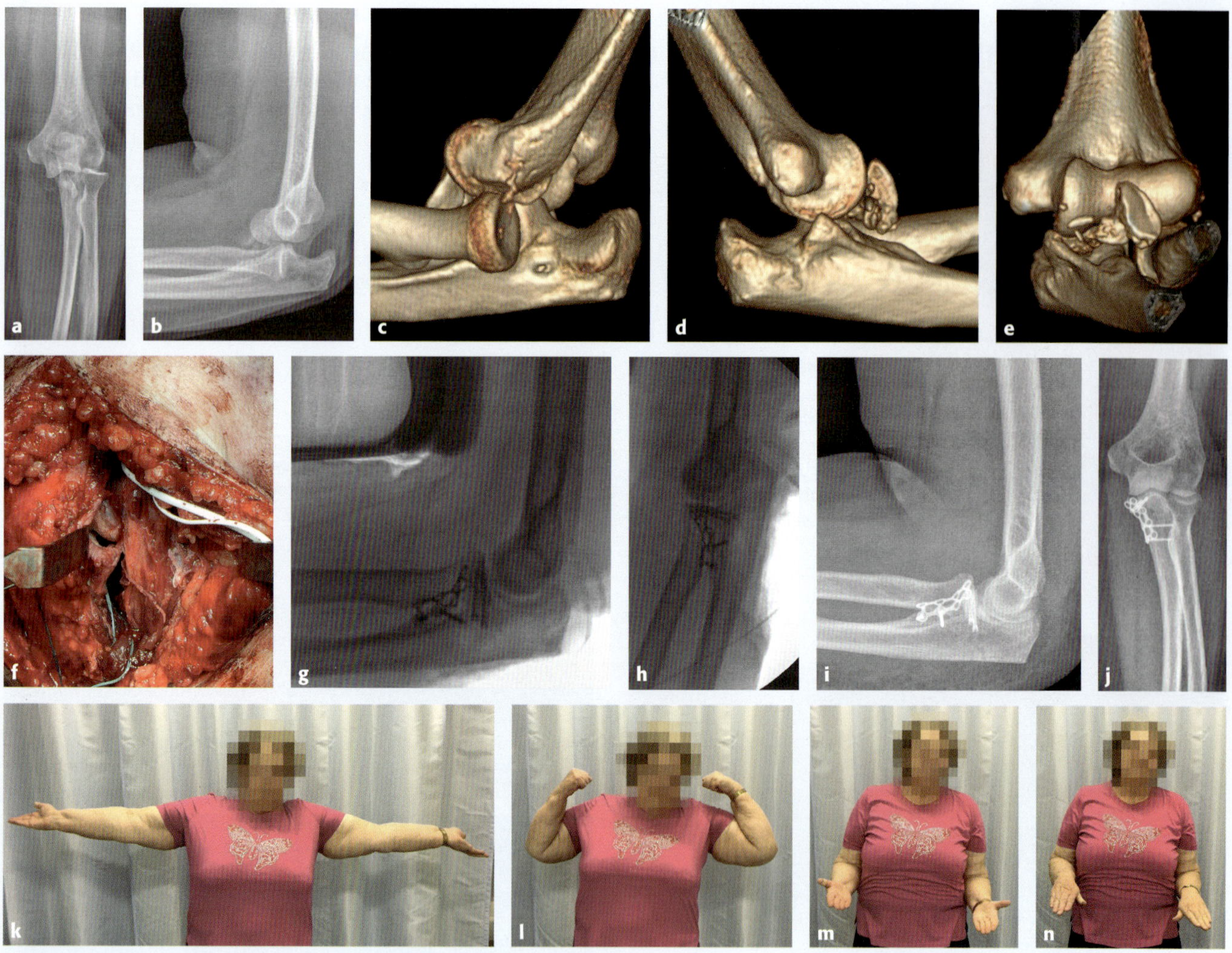


**Fig 3.4-11a–n** A 71-year-old woman with fracture dislocation of the left elbow.
**a–e** X-rays and 3-D computed tomographic scans showing a displaced fracture of the left elbow with a displaced multifragmentary coronoid fracture.
**f** Intraoperative image showing a ruptured medial collateral ligament with a multifragmentary coronoid process fracture.
**g–h** Intraoperative passive extension under image intensifier showed no tendency for instability.
**i–n** X-rays and clinical photographs at 14 months demonstrating good x-rays and functional results.

### 4.2.4 Ligaments

The LCL complex is ruptured in most terrible triad patterns and varus posteromedial injuries. In acute cases, transosseous repair to its origin in the center of the lateral epicondyle using bone anchors with nonabsorbable sutures is sufficient and should always be performed.

The MCL complex is only addressed, if, after reconstruction of the coronoid radial head and LCL complex, the elbow tends to dislocate with passive extension above 60° [24]. In these cases, the MCL complex and the common flexor/pronator muscles are stripped from the origin and are repaired using bone anchors with nonabsorbable sutures.

### 4.2.5 Hinged external fixator

A hinged external fixator should be used in any case of residual instability after reconstruction of all repairable bony and soft-tissue structures. The advantage of a dynamic external fixator applied in the concentric axis of the elbow is the start of early protected motion even in complex instability (**Case 4: Fig 3.4-12**).



**Patient**

An 83-year-old woman fell on her extended arm and was complaining of pain in the elbow and inability to move. Peripheral perfusion and function were found intact. The patient reported a spontaneous reduction of the elbow joint. Fracture of the coracoid process and a displaced radial head fracture were noted (**Fig 3.4-12a–d**).

**Comorbidities**

- Alcohol abuse
- Chronic obstructive pulmonary disease

**Treatment and outcome**

At index surgery, the radial head fragment was fixed with screws (**Fig 3.4-12e–f**). Two days postoperative, increasing pain and redislocation of the elbow joint occurred (**Fig 3.4-12g**).

During the revision surgery no signs of a repair of the lateral ligament complex were found. The lateral collateral ligament complex was avulsed from its origin. The radial head was not amenable for reconstruction. Radial head replacement and reconstruction of the lateral ligament complex using an anchor was performed. As the surgery was done 4 days after the initial procedure, an additional medial approach was avoided for reconstruction of the medial ligament complex. A hinged external fixator for 3 weeks was applied. Mobilization was started immediately after surgery to avoid joint stiffness (**Fig 3.4-12h**).

After 1 year some heterotopic ossification occurred: range of motion extension–flexion was 0–15–120° and pronation–supination was 70–0–60° (**Fig 3.4-12i–j**).

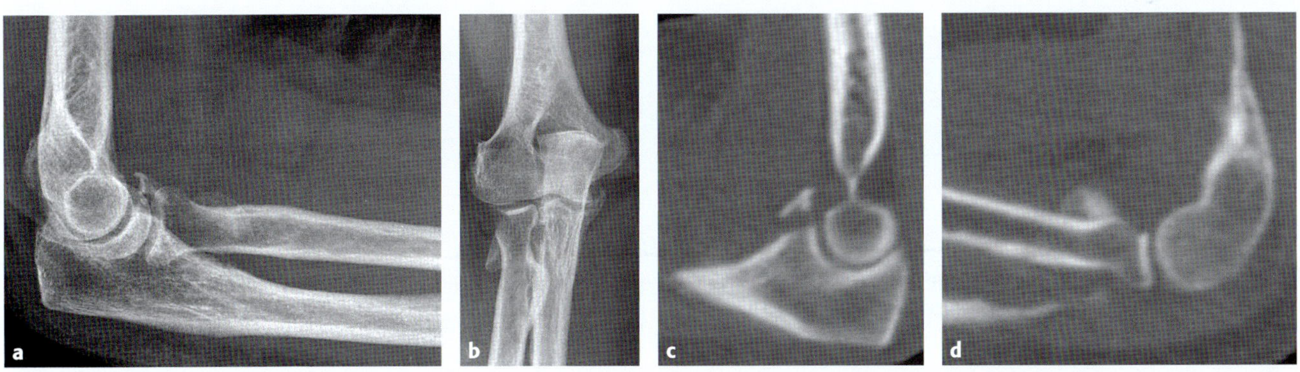


**Fig 4.3-12a–j** An 83-year-old woman with a coracoid process fracture.
**a–d** X-rays showing fracture of the coracoid process and displaced radial head.

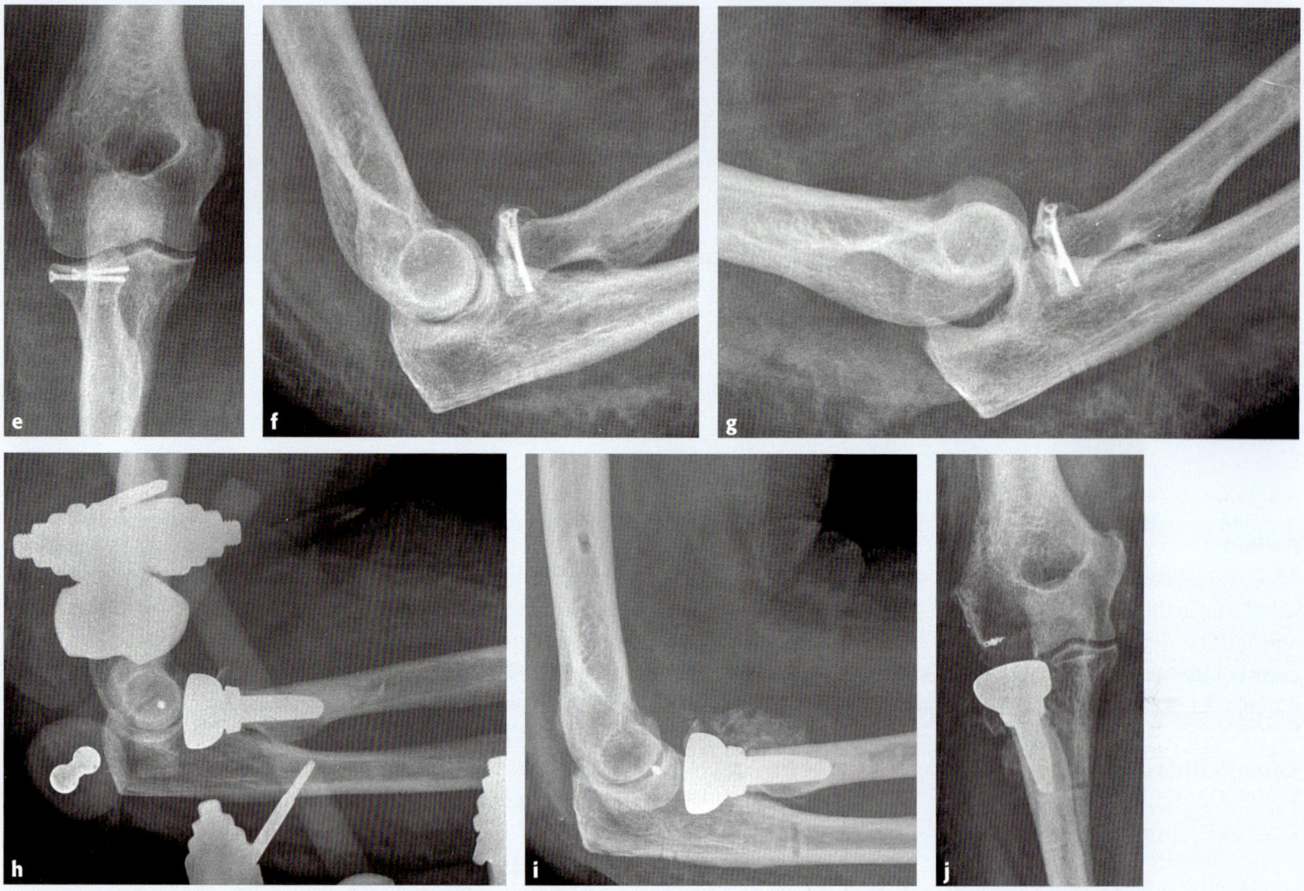


**Fig 4.3-12a–j (cont)** An 83-year-old woman with a coracoid process fracture.
**e–f** Postoperative x-rays showing radial head fragment fixed with screws.
**g** X-ray showing instability of the elbow joint.
**h** X-rays after revision surgery showing the radial head replaced and a hinged external fixator applied. The lateral ligament complex was reattached using a bone anchor.
**i–j** Follow-up x-rays at 1 year demonstrating a concentric elbow joint with some heterotopic ossification.

## 5 Complications

The most common complications after elbow fracture dislocations are chronic instability due to errors in identifying instabililty at the time of initial examination and/or after operative repair (**Case 5: Fig 3.4-13**, **Case 6: Fig 3.4-14**), elbow stiffness due to postoperative pain or immobilization over 2–3 weeks and heterotopic ossification (HO). Risk factors for HO include age, lesions of the central nervous system, burns, and genetic factors. Operative or nonoperative treatment and surgical timing do not seem to influence the occurrence of HO, which can occur in up to 56% of cases. Heterotopic ossification can result in limited ROM due to bony impingement [13, 25–27].

**Patient**

A 78-year-old woman fell on her extended forearm and sustained a terrible triad elbow fracture dislocation. The patient was treated initially at another trauma hospital.

**Comorbidities**

- Mild dementia
- Hypertension
- Parkinson's disease

**Treatment and outcome**

The trauma x-rays showed a posterior elbow dislocation with associated radial head fracture and fracture of the coronoid tip (**Fig 3.4-13a–e**). Initially, the dislocated elbow joint was reduced and fixed in a cast in another hospital.

One month later, at the time of cast removal, the patient did not complain about pain but showed remaining instability with subluxation of the ulnohumeral joint (**Fig 3.4-13f**). To stabilize the elbow joint, closed reduction of the elbow joint was performed and an external fixator applied (**Fig 3.4-13g**). This device was removed after 6 weeks and physiotherapy was initiated.

The patient presented 1.5 years after the trauma at the authors' department. She was unable to move actively and had a painful passive range of motion (ROM) of 0–0–120°. X-rays showed osteoarthritis and a subluxed elbow joint (**Fig 3.4-13h–i**).

Total elbow arthroplasty was performed. The patient presented pain free and satisfied 2 years after trauma and 5 months after elbow joint replacement. Final ROM was 0–15–120° and forearm rotation was 80–0–65° (**Fig 3.4-13j–o**).

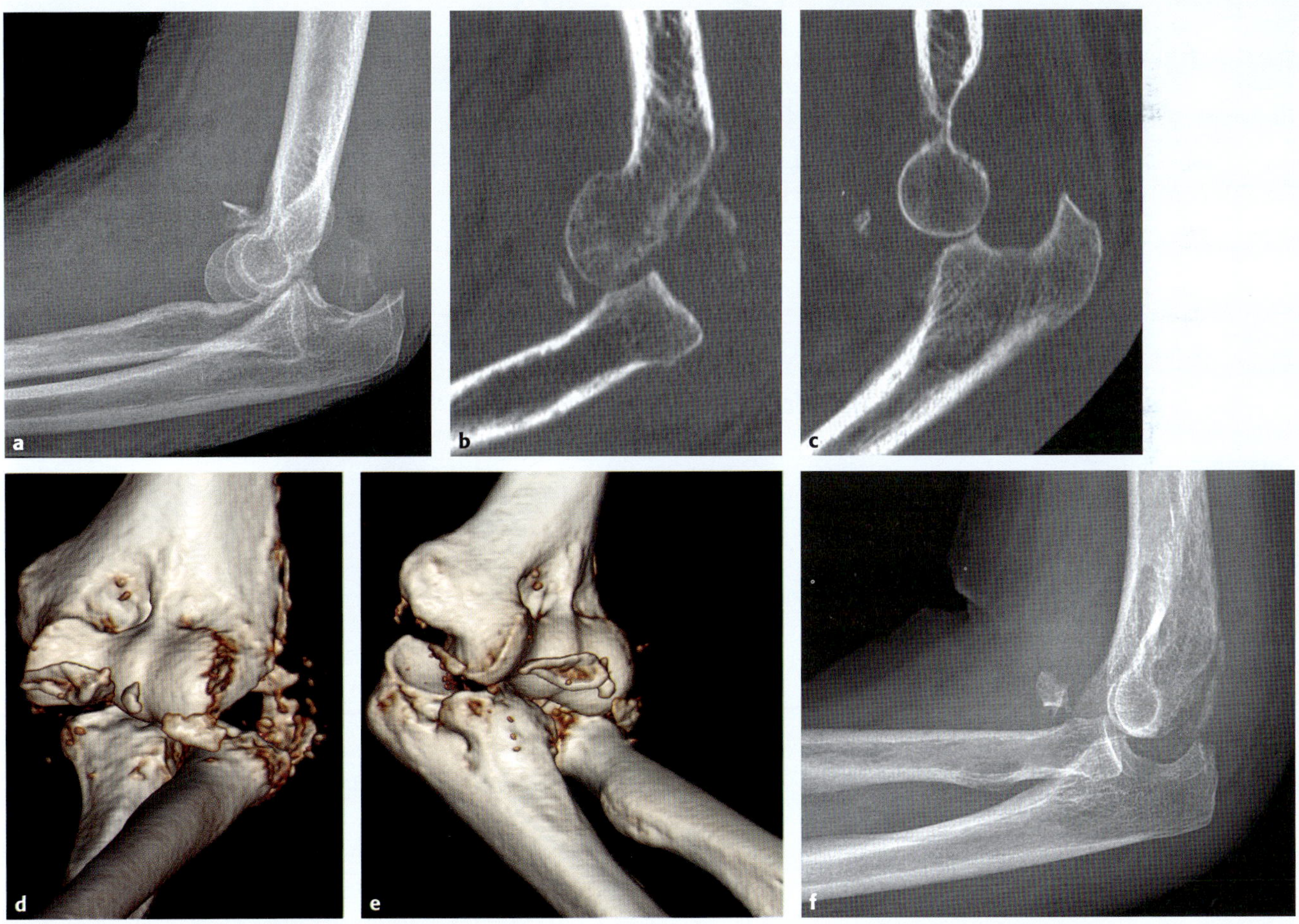


**Fig 3.4-13a–o** A 78-year-old woman with a triad elbow fracture dislocation.
**a–e** X-rays and computed tomographic scans showing a posterior elbow dislocation with associated radial head fracture and fracture of the coronoid tip (terrible triad injury).
**f** X-ray after 4 weeks showing instability with subluxation of the ulnohumeral joint.

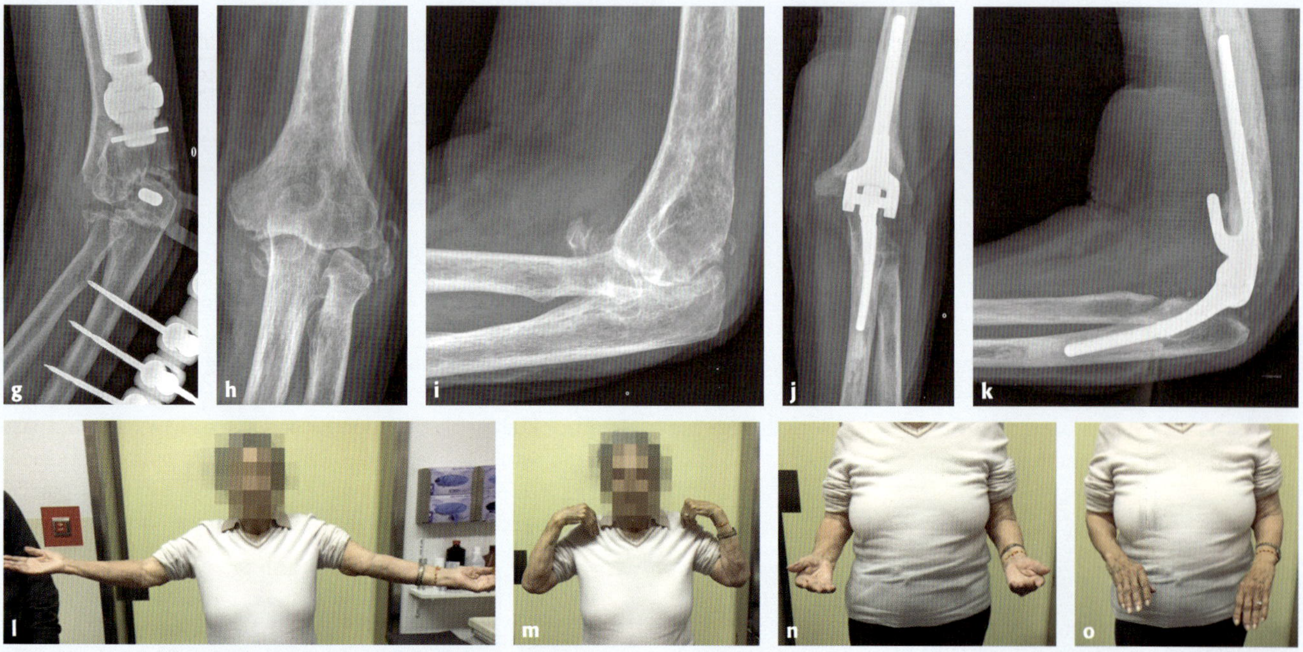

**Fig 3.4-13a–o (cont)** A 78-year-old woman with a triad elbow fracture dislocation.
**g** At 4 weeks, closed reduction was performed and an external fixator applied.
**h–i** After 1.5 years, osteoarthritis and a subluxed elbow joint.
**j–o** X-rays and clinical photographs taken 2 years after trauma and 5 months after elbow joint replacement.

CASE 6

### Patient

A 74-year-old man fell while cycling and sustained a multifragmented fracture of the anteromedial coronoid fragment (**Fig 3.4-14a–b**).

### Comorbidities

- No comorbidities were documented

### Treatment and outcome

Primarily, a nonoperative treatment with cast immobilization was initiated. In the follow-up x-ray after 1 week, ulnohumeral instability with subluxation (drop sign) was recognized (**Fig 3.4-14c**).

The anteromedial coronoid fracture was fixed by buttress plating using the flexor carpi ulnaris splitting approach, and the tip of the coronoid was fixed indirectly using a cannulated screw (**Fig 3.4-14d–f**).

On the first postoperative x-rays after 4 days, a subluxation of the ulnohumeral joint on the lateral x-ray (**Fig 3.4-14g**) was recognized, as well as insufficiency of the lateral ligament complex (widening of the radiohumeral joint on AP x-ray (**Fig 3.4-14h**).

In the revision surgery, an additional posterolateral approach was performed and the posterior part of the lateral collateral ligament complex was fixed to its origin at the lateral epicondyle using bone anchors (**Fig 3.4-14i–j**).

Final follow-up showed a concentrically reduced elbow joint with acceptable range of motion (**Fig 3.4-14k–p**).

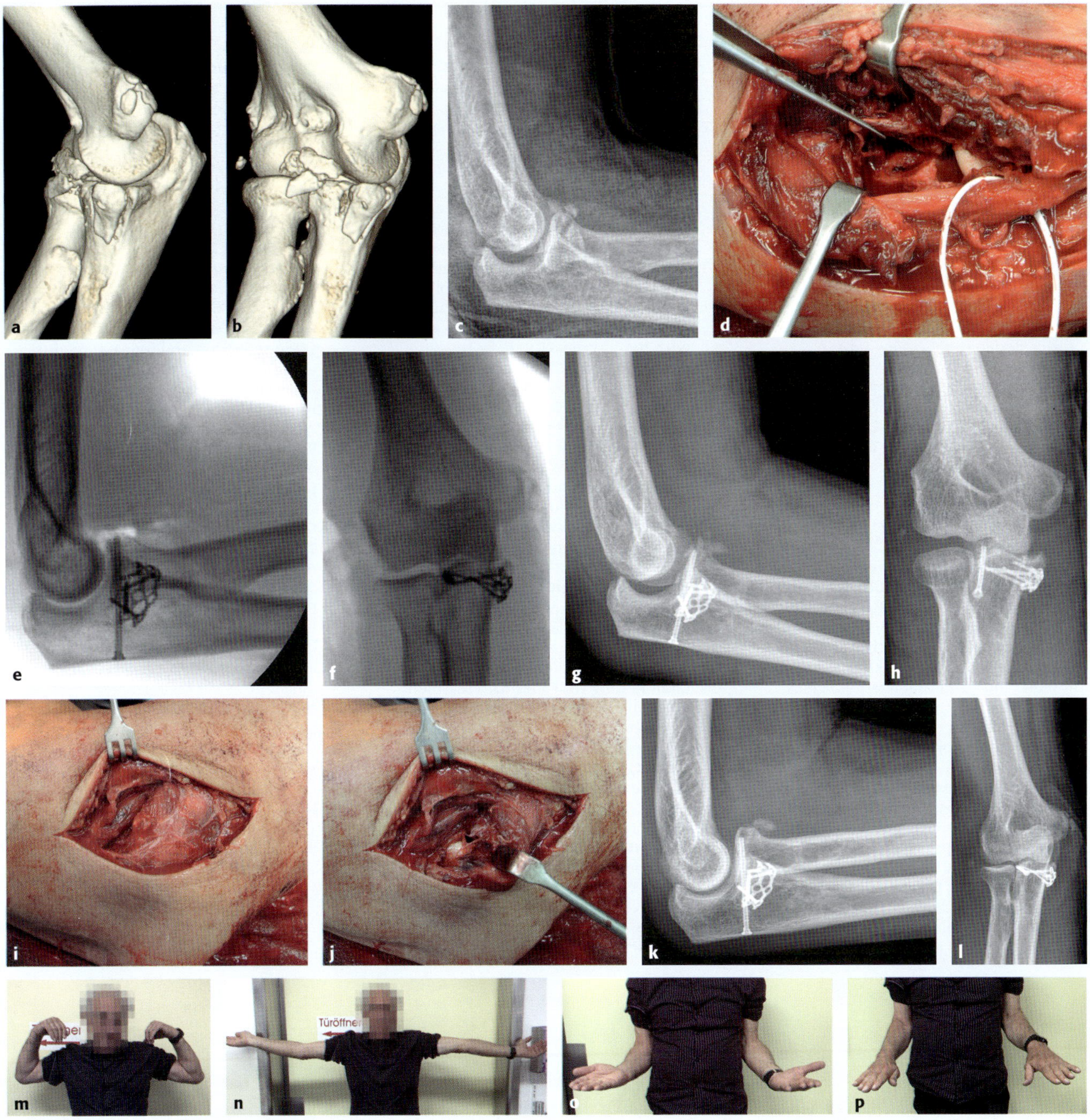

**Fig 3.4-14a–p** A 74-year-old man with a multifragmented fracture of the anteromedial coronoid fragment.

**a–b** Computed tomographic scans showing a multifragmented fracture of the anteromedial coronoid fragment and bony avulsions from the medial and lateral epicondyles.

**c** Follow-up x-ray after 1 week of cast immobilization showing ulnohumeral instability with subluxation.

**d** Intraoperative image showing a medial flexor carpi ulnaris split approach with the anteromedial fracture fragment held by the forceps.

**e–f** Intraoperative image intensification showing buttress plate to fix the anteromedial coronoid fracture and a cannulated screw to fix the tip of the coronoid with concentric reduction of the elbow joint.

**g–h** A subluxation of the ulnohumeral joint on the lateral x-ray (**g**) as well as insufficiency of the lateral ligament complex (widening of the radiohumeral joint on the AP x-ray (**h**) was recognized.

**i–j** Intraoperative images showing the posterior part of the lateral collateral ligament complex avulsed from the lateral epicondyle.

**k–p** Final follow-up x-rays and clinical photographs showing a concentrically reduced elbow joint with acceptable range of motion.

## 6 References

1. **McKee MD, Pugh DM, Wild LM, et al.** Standard surgical protocol to treat elbow dislocations with radial head and coronoid fractures. Surgical technique. *J Bone Joint Surg Am.* 2005 Mar;87(Suppl 1[Pt 1]):22–32.
2. **Bohn K, Ipaktchi K, Livermore M, et al.** Current treatment concepts for "terrible triad" injuries of the elbow. *Orthopedics.* 2014 Dec;37(12):831–837.
3. **Xiao K, Zhang J, Li T, et al.** Anatomy, definition, and treatment of the "terrible triad of the elbow" and contemplation of the rationality of this designation. *Orthop Surg.* 2015 Feb;7(1):13–18.
4. **Chen NC, Ring D.** Terrible Triad Injuries of the Elbow. *J Hand Surg Am.* 2015 Nov;40(11):2297–2303.
5. **Siebenlist S, Stöckle U, Lucke M.** Problematik osteoporotischer Frakturen am Ellenbogen [Osteoporotic fractures of the elbow]. *Obere Extremität.* 2009;4(3):160–167. German.
6. **Siebenlist S, Braun KF.** Ellenbogenluxationsfrakturen [Elbow dislocation fractures]. *Unfallchirurg.* 2017 Jul;120(7):595–610. German.
7. **McKee MD, Veillette CJ, Hall JA, et al.** A multicenter, prospective, randomized, controlled trial of open reduction—internal fixation versus total elbow arthroplasty for displaced intra-articular distal humeral fractures in elderly patients. *J Shoulder Elbow Surg.* 2009 Jan–Feb;18(1):3–12.
8. **Wyrick JD, Dailey SK, Gunzenhaeuser JM, et al.** Management of complex elbow dislocations: a mechanistic approach. *J Am Acad Orthop Surg.* 2015 May;23(5):297–306.
9. **Stoneback JW, Owens BD, Sykes J, et al.** Incidence of elbow dislocations in the United States population. *J Bone Joint Surg Am.* 2012 Feb 01;94(3):240–245.
10. **Hobgood ER, Khan SO, Field LD.** Acute dislocations of the adult elbow. *Hand Clin.* 2008 Feb;24(1):1–7.
11. **Josefsson PO, Johnell O, Wendeberg B.** Ligamentous injuries in dislocations of the elbow joint. *Clin Orthop Relat Res.* 1987 Aug;(221):221–225.
12. **Josefsson PO, Nilsson BE.** Incidence of elbow dislocation. *Acta Orthop Scand.* 1986 Dec;57(6):537–538.
13. **Heck S, Gick S, Dargel J, et al.** Die Behandlung der akuten Luxation und Luxationsfraktur des Ellenbogens – Bewegunsfixateur [External fixation with motion capacity in acute dislocations and fracture dislocations of the elbow. Fixation with motion capacity]. *Unfallchirurg.* 2011 Feb;114(2):114–122. German.
14. **Sheps DM, Kiefer KR, Boorman RS, et al.** The interobserver reliability of classification systems for radial head fractures: the Hotchkiss modification of the Mason classification and the AO classification systems. *Can J Surg.* 2009 Aug;52(4):277–282.
15. **McKee MD, Schemitsch EH, Sala MJ, et al.** The pathoanatomy of lateral ligamentous disruption in complex elbow instability. *J Shoulder Elbow Surg.* 2003 Jul–Aug;12(4):391–396.
16. **Chan K, King GJ, Faber KJ.** Treatment of complex elbow fracture-dislocations. *Curr Rev Musculoskelet Med.* 2016 Jun;9(2):185–189.
17. **Chan K, MacDermid JC, Faber KJ, et al.** Can we treat select terrible triad injuries nonoperatively? *Clin Orthop Relat Res.* 2014 Jul;472(7):2092–2099.
18. **Chen HW, Liu GD, Ou S, et al.** Operative Treatment of Terrible Triad of the Elbow via Posterolateral and Anteromedial Approaches. *PLoS One.* 2015;10(4):e0124821.
19. **Papatheodorou LK, Rubright JH, Heim KA, et al.** Terrible triad injuries of the elbow: does the coronoid always need to be fixed? *Clin Orthop Relat Res.* 2014 Jul;472(7):2084–2091.
20. **Acevedo DC, Paxton ES, Kukelyansky I, et al.** Radial head arthroplasty: state of the art. *J Am Acad Orthop Surg.* 2014 Oct;22(10):633–642.
21. **Iannuzzi NP, Leopold SS.** In brief: the Mason classification of radial head fractures. *Clin Orthop Relat Res.* 2012 Jun;470(6):1799–1802.
22. **Pike JM, Grewal R, Athwal GS, et al.** Open reduction and internal fixation of radial head fractures: do outcomes differ between simple and complex injuries? *Clin Orthop Relat Res.* 2014 Jul;472(7):2120–2127.
23. **Rouleau DM, Sandman E, van Riet R, et al.** Management of fractures of the proximal ulna. *J Am Acad Orthop Surg.* 2013 Mar;21(3):149–160.
24. **Giannicola G, Calella P, Piccioli A, et al.** Terrible triad of the elbow: is it still a troublesome injury? *Injury.* 2015 Dec;46(Suppl 8):S68–S76.
25. **Englert C, Zellner J, Koller M, et al.** Elbow dislocations: a review ranging from soft tissue injuries to complex elbow fracture dislocations. *Adv Orthop.* 2013;2013:951397.
26. **Mittlmeier T, Beck M.** Luxation des Ellenbogengelenks des Erwachsenen [Dislocation of the adult elbow joint]. *Unfallchirurg.* 2009 May;112(5):487–505. German.
27. **Noblin J, Geissler W, Bass D.** The incidence of heterotopic ossification with elbow injuries. *Orthop Trans.* 1995;19:162.

# 3.5 Olecranon

Peter Kaiser, Simon Euler

## 1 Introduction

Olecranon fractures account for 80% of all fractures of the proximal ulna. Similar to distal radius and vertebral fractures, olecranon fractures may serve as a "sentinel fracture" that indicates widespread poor bone quality [1].

There is a steep increase in incidence of proximal ulna fractures in the seventh decade of life with a peak in the ninth decade for both male and female patients. The incidence increases from 12 per 100,000 in the general population to 70–80 per 100,000 in the geriatric population (> 65 years). There seems to be no gender predominance and open fractures are relatively rare [1]. About 25–30% of the patients with a fracture of the proximal ulna sustain a concomitant injury to the ipsilateral limb most frequently a proximal radius fracture followed by a proximal humerus, forearm, metacarpal and classic geriatric hip and pelvic fractures (**Case 3: Fig 3.5-7**, **Case 4: Fig 3.5-8**, **Case 5: Fig 3.5-9**, **Case 15: Fig 3.5-19**) [1, 2].

The most common cause of this type of injury is the direct impact from a fall from standing height [1]. In such cases, the olecranon impacts on the distal humerus, potentially resulting in a comminuted fracture pattern. Indirect trauma as a result of a powerful contraction of the triceps muscle during a fall on the outstretched arm typically results in a simple transverse or oblique fracture pattern [3, 4]. Overall, the simple 2-part fracture represents the most frequent fracture type (Mayo 2A; AO/OTA 2U1B) [1]. Fracture displacement occurs as a result of triceps muscle pull in cases of a ruptured periosteum and triceps aponeurosis, which can lead to a considerable loss of function [3]. However, older patients may demonstrate satisfactory function that meets their personal needs despite gross displacement (**Case 5: Fig 3.5-9**).

Based on a combination of case series review and traditional experience, the standard treatment for displaced olecranon fractures is open reduction and operative fixation including tension band wiring or one of a variety of plate fixation methods [5, 6]. However, due to osteoporotic bone and vulnerable soft-tissue conditions, operative complications are frequently reported at rates up to 70% [7, 8]. Due to the frailty of this group of patients, even displaced olecranon fractures are often treated nonoperatively, leading to reasonable results without the risk of anesthetic or operative complications [1, 9. 10]. This chapter provides an overview and treatment algorithm for olecranon fractures in older adults.

## 2 Diagnostics

Diagnostic and therapeutic recommendations should be based on the unique medical, cognitive, and social conditions as well as the functional needs of each patient. A thorough medical history examination including the patient's general condition and health status, comorbidities as well as functional expectations are mandatory prior to the planning of the individual treatment. Patients should also be carefully reviewed for any cognitive disabilities, as those may limit adequate patient compliance with the treatment course.

### 2.1 Clinical evaluation

The history should ask the following questions:

- How did the injury happen (ie, mechanism of injury)?
- Was it a single injury or are there additional injuries and locations of pain?
- What was the preinjury level of function and activity (eg, independent, walking aids, or bedridden)?
- Was the dominant hand injured?
- What is the level of care available at the patient's current residence (ie, independent, family, or nursing home)?
- What are the patient's medical comorbidities and chronic treatments including anticoagulation?
- What is the patient's mental status and expected ability to comply?

The clinical examination should address the following aspects:

- Fracture crepitus, soft-tissue status, open bursa, or even an open fracture?
- Severe pain or pseudoparalysis?
- Joint stability?
- Active range of motion (ROM)?
- Vascular and neurological status?
- Damage to the ulnar nerve (ie, proximity to the fracture site)?
- Complaints of pain at other locations (ie, concomitant injury)?

## 2.2 Imaging

Plain AP and lateral x-rays are usually sufficient (**Fig 3.5-1**).

A computed tomographic scan should be obtained in cases without adequate conventional x-rays to clearly identify the fracture pattern (**Case 1: Fig 3.5-2**, **Case 2: Fig 3.5-3**). This is especially important for operative planning and for visualization of concomitant fractures of the radial head or the coronoid process.

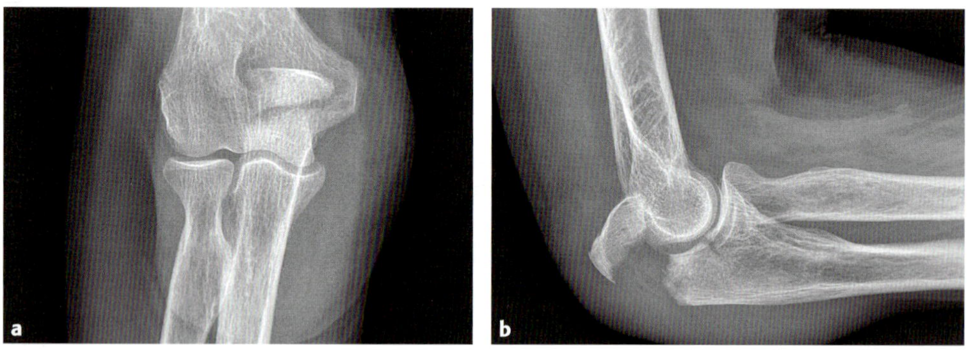


**Fig 3.5-1a–b** Correct AP (**a**) and lateral (**b**) x-rays of a 74-year-old woman with an olecranon fracture after a bike accident.

CASE 1

### Patient

An 87-year-old woman fell down the stairs.

### Comorbidities

- Rheumatoid arthritis
- Degenerative changes of the joint

### Treatment and outcome

Owing to an insufficient view of the fracture on conventional x-rays, a computed tomographic scan was obtained, which revealed a simple Mayo type IA fracture pattern. The patient was treated nonoperatively (**Fig 3.5-2a–b**).

The lateral view 4 months after the initial injury showed a nonunion and destruction of the elbow joint. The patient could reach her mouth but could not perform any overhead activities (range of motion 0–0–90°). However, the patient refused any further treatment and was referred to physical therapy (**Fig 3.5-2c**).

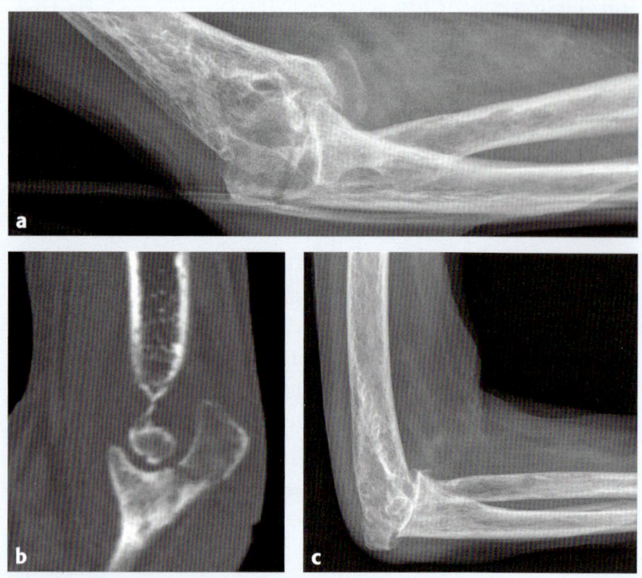


**Fig 3.5-2a–c** An 87-year-old woman after a fall.
**a–b** Computed tomographic scan showing a simple Mayo type IA fracture pattern.
**c** Lateral view 4 months after the initial injury showing a nonunion and destruction of the elbow joint.

**Patient**

A 79-year-old man had a fall while rock climbing.

**Treatment and outcome**

The computed tomographic scan was essential to assess the complete fracture pattern and to accurately plan the surgery (**Fig 3.5-3a–b**).

The patient was treated with open reduction and internal fixation using a locking plate, followed by 3 weeks of cast fixation and physical therapy without cast fixation. Six months after surgery, the patient was satisfied and pain free with almost full range of motion (**Fig 3.5-3c**).

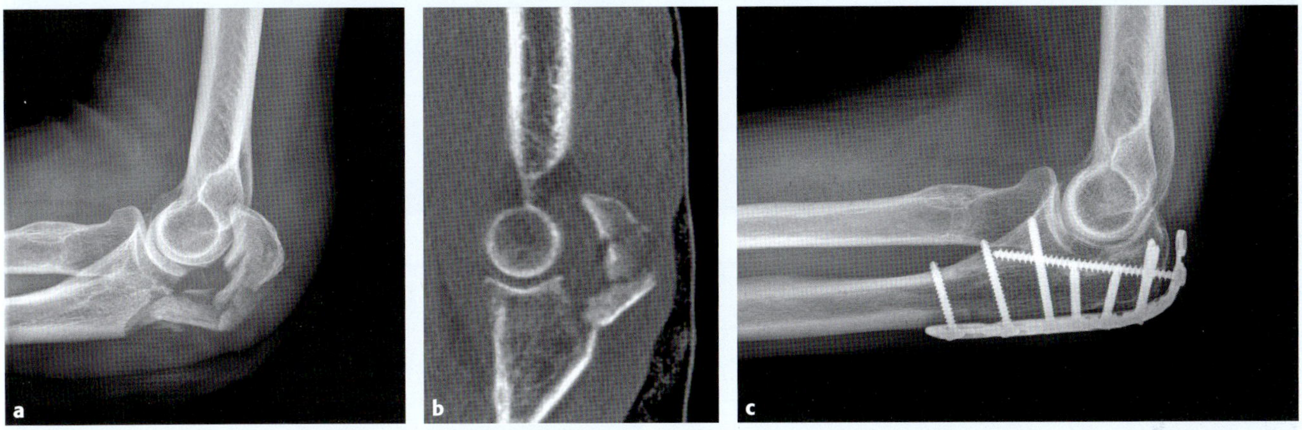


**Fig 3.5-3a–c** A 79-year-old male patient after a rock climbing accident.
**a–b** Computed tomographic scan used to assess the complete fracture pattern and to accurately plan the surgery.
**c** Treatment with open reduction and internal fixation using a locking plate.

## 3 Classification

There are four major classification systems commonly used for olecranon fractures: Colton [11], Mayo [12], Schatzker [13], and the AO/OTA Fracture and Dislocation Classification [14]. They are based on the fracture pattern and do not consider the patient's age or bone quality. Overall, all systems are associated with low reproducibility and none has yet been universally accepted [15, 16].

### 3.1 AO/OTA Fracture and Dislocation Classification

The AO/OTA classification differentiates between the following three types:

- **Type 2U1A**—extraarticular fracture
- **Type 2U1B**—partial articular fracture
- **Type 2U1C**—complete articular fracture, of olecranon and coronoid (C3)

### 3.2 Mayo classification

The system is based on stability, displacement, and comminution (**Fig 3.5-4**) [12, 16]:

- Type I—nondisplaced noncomminuted (IA) and comminuted (IB) olecranon fractures
- Type II—displaced but stable noncomminuted (IIA) and comminuted (IIB) olecranon fractures with more than 3 mm of fragment displacement but intact collateral ligaments and a stable forearm in relation to the humerus
- Type III—displaced and unstable noncomminuted (IIA) and comminuted (IIB) olecranon fractures with an unstable forearm in relation to the humerus (fracture dislocation)

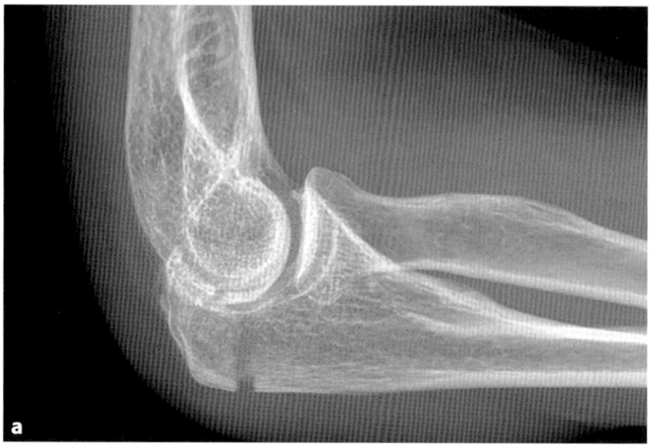

IA—nondisplaced noncomminuted

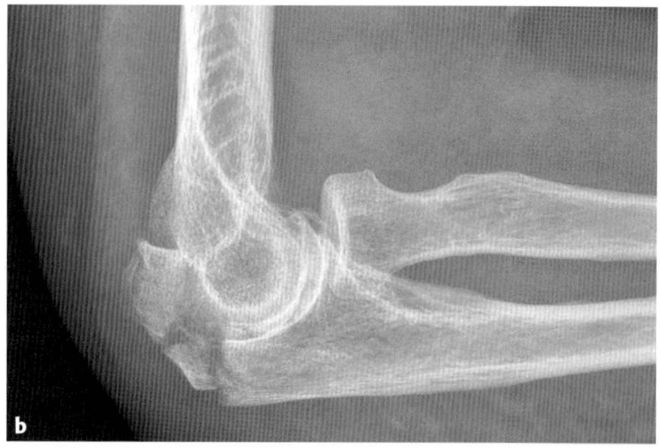

IB—nondisplaced comminuted

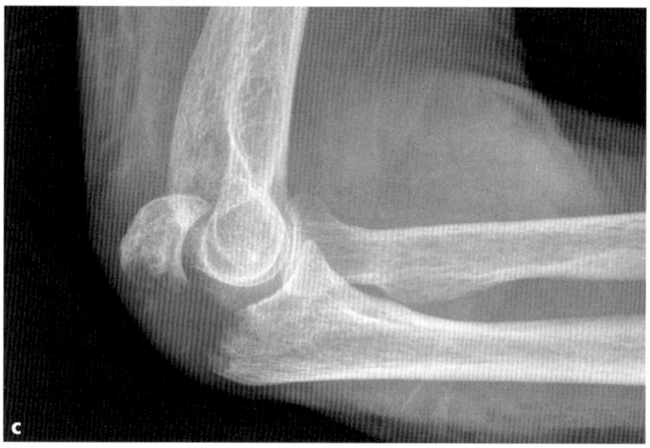

IIA—displaced stable noncomminuted

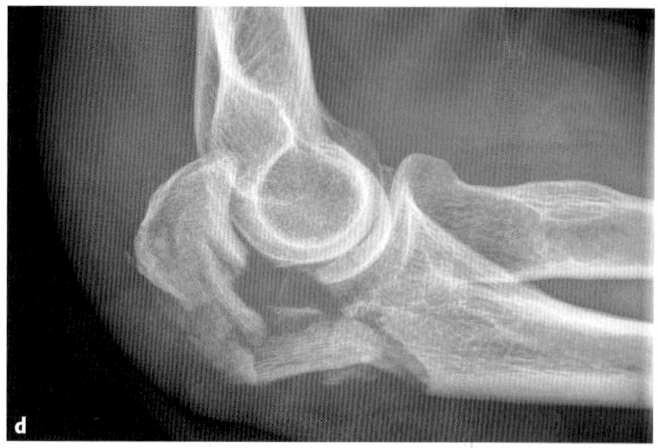

IIB—displaced stable comminuted

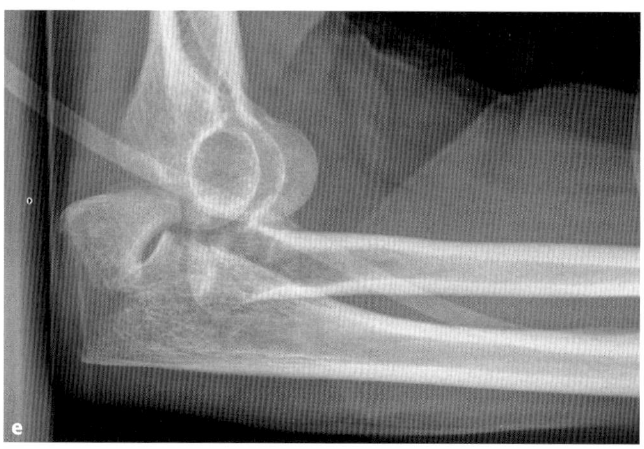

IIIA—displaced unstable noncomminuted

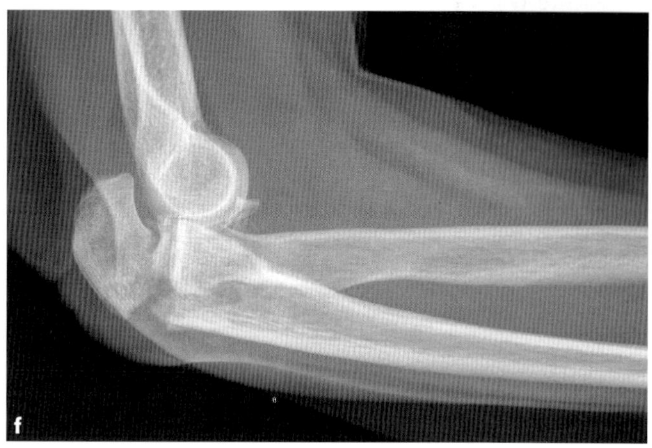

IIIB—displaced unstable comminuted

**Fig 3.5-4a-f** Mayo classification demonstrated with x-ray of mostly geriatric patients.
**a** A 73-year-old woman fell on her right elbow during a cerebral infarction.
**b** A 74-year-old woman slipped and fell directly onto her right elbow.
**c** A 91-year-old woman slipped and fell on the sidewalk.
**d** A 79-year-old man fell while rock climbing.
**e** A 47-year-old woman jumped from the second floor.
**f** A 73-year-old woman collapsed and fell on the floor sustaining a multifragmentary transolecranon fracture dislocation.

## 4 Decision making

Due to the increased risk of anesthetic and operative complications in older adults, nonoperative treatment is a reasonable treatment option in many cases. The American Society of Anesthesiologists (ASA) score is known to correlate with the rate of intraoperative complications as well as the operative outcome [17, 18, 19]. Nondisplaced Mayo type I fractures can be successfully treated nonoperatively and avoid the risk of operative or anesthetic complications. Uneventful fracture healing is frequent, and there remains no significant functional loss even in cases of nonunion.

Displaced Mayo type II fractures remain controversial regarding the treatment of choice. Recent studies demonstrate good clinical outcomes for low-demand geriatric patients with a nonoperative approach [20, 21]. However, displaced fragments may significantly reduce elbow function, leading to a decreased ROM. Furthermore, the overlying skin may be compromised, potentially resulting in severe skin irritation and ulceration. For these cases, the ASA score can predict individual patient's risk for operative treatment. The anticipated functional benefits of surgery should be carefully balanced against the risks in this patient group, with interdisciplinary decision making involving orthopedic surgeons, geriatricians, anesthesiologists, and the patient and family.

The decision for nonoperative or operative treatment can be made depending on the fracture classification and the ASA score (**Fig 3.5-5**). Ideally, the final decision should be made based on an orthogeriatric discussion.

In Mayo type II and III fractures, nonoperative treatment has been shown to provide reasonable clinical results in older, low-demand patients [20, 21].

These fragility fractures have the potential to heal nonoperatively with osseous union (**Case 3: Fig 3.5-7**) or nonunion (**Case 4: Fig 3.5-8**, **Case 6: Fig 3.5-10**). Either way, the clinical outcome is usually satisfactory in older adults, resulting in nearly normal extension and, in the authors' experience, adequate pain control, even in cases with a large displaced fragment (**Case 5: Fig 3.5-9**) or multiple fracture fragments (**Case 4: Fig 3.5-8**).

Displaced fragments can be addressed operatively by tension band wiring, which does have the potential to provide good fracture consolidation and satisfactory clinical outcomes as early as 3 months postinjury (**Case 9: Fig 3.5-13**). However, in cases with poor bone quality, K-wires might loosen and fracture dislocation can occur. In older adults, revision surgery then has to be considered very carefully, as adequate fracture healing, sufficient ROM, and good clinical outcome is still possible without reoperation (**Case 8: Fig 3.5-12**). Even with significant loss of reduction, surgical revision can be avoided in cases of satisfactory elbow function. A more specific indication for operative revision is surgical hardware causing ongoing soft-tissue compromise.

Locking plate fixation with functional aftertreatment is another preferred option in older patients. In our experience, plate fixation often leads to satisfactory results with comparable ROM to the uninjured contralateral extremity (**Case 11: Fig 3.5-15**, **Case 12: Fig 3.5-16**, **Case 14: Fig 3.5-18**). There are various plating systems without evidence of one plate being superior to another [22]. In osteoporotic bone, a locking plate has been shown to be advantageous in various other fracture locations, and should be used in osteoporotic bone to decrease the risk of cut out and secondary fracture dislocation [23–26]. One exception involves Mayo type IIA fractures in which there was no benefit of plate

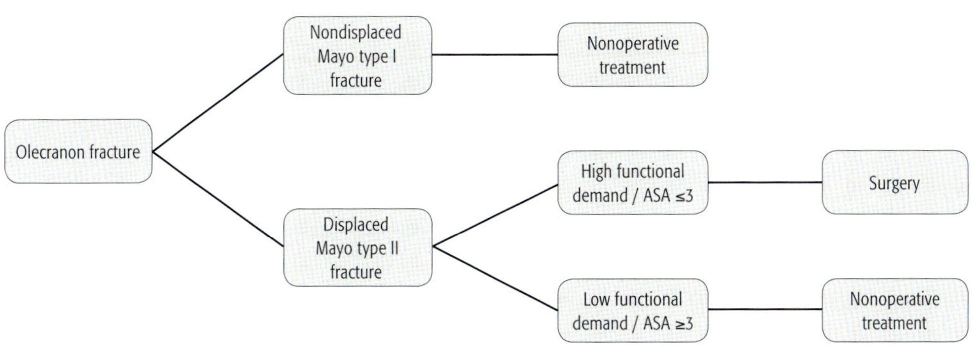


**Fig 3.5-5** Treatment algorithm for olecranon fractures.
Abbreviation: ASA, American Society of Anesthesiologists.

fixation over tension band wiring [27, 28]. In a multifragmentary fracture type Mayo IIB plating offers more options for fragment fixation and provides overall a more stable construct compared to wiring.

Operative treatment of osteoporotic bones is less successful and may lead to complications, potentially resulting in salvage procedures. Because of skin irritation, wound breakdown, or pain, implant removal (**Case 11: Fig 3.5-15**) becomes necessary in up to 80% of all cases following open reduction and internal fixation of olecranon fractures in older adults [29]. Salvage procedures include fragment excision, arthroplasty, or revision surgery with or without bone grafting. In the absence of adequate randomized controlled trials of operative versus nonoperative approaches, the optimal treatment of displaced olecranon fractures remains controversial [6].

## 5 Therapeutic options

There are various nonoperative and operative treatment options, depending on the fracture classification (**Fig 3.5-6**).

### 5.1 Nonoperative treatment

Nonoperative treatment (**Case 3: Fig 3.5-7**, **Case 4: Fig 3.5-8**, **Case 5: Fig 3.5-9**, **Case 6: Fig 3.5-10d-f**) should include initial functional passive physical therapy without limitation and elbow cast fixation for comfort for up to a maximum of 3 weeks depending on the patient's pain level. For nonoperative treatment, suggestions for the maximally acceptable fragment displacement range from 2 mm to 5 mm in the literature [10, 30]. However, even higher degrees of displacement can have the potential for a pain-free result with satisfactory ROM (**Case 5: Fig 3.5-9**).

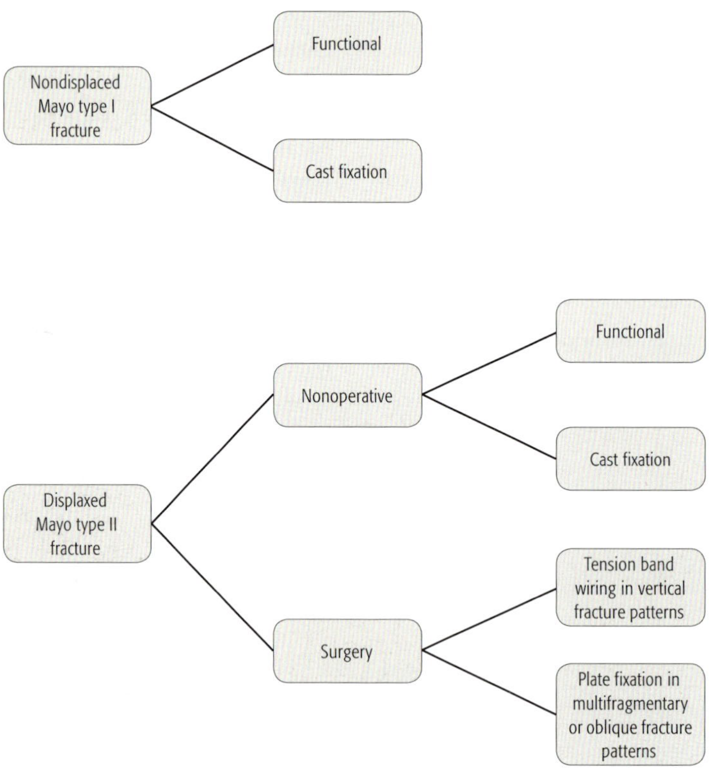


**Fig 3.5-6** Possible therapeutic options for each fracture pattern in olecranon fractures.

**Patient**

A 67-year-old male patient fell at home and sustained a nondisplaced olecranon fracture.

**Treatment and outcome**

X-rays showed a nondisplaced fracture of the olecranon (Mayo type IA) (**Fig 3.5-7a**), accompanied by a distal radial fracture (**Fig 3.5-7b–c**) on the ipsilateral side. For more information on the Mayo classification, see topic 3 in this chapter.

Both fractures were treated nonoperatively (**Fig 3.5-7d–e**). After 3 weeks of elbow cast fixation and initial physical therapy, the patient was pain free. He was dismissed from the outpatient clinic 6 weeks postinjury.

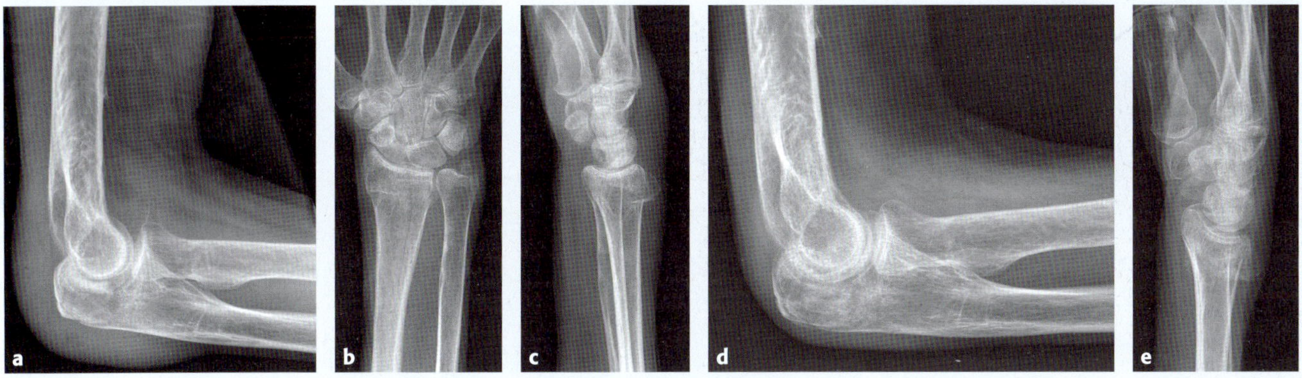


**Fig 3.5-7a–e** A 67-year-old man after a fall.
**a–c** X-rays showing a nondisplaced olecranon fracture (Mayo type IA) (**a**), accompanied by a distal radius fracture (**b–c**) on the ipsilateral side.
**d–e** Nonoperative treatment of both fractures with elbow cast fixation for 3 weeks.



**Patient**

A 95-year-old woman fell in the nursing home. Before the accident, she was fully mobile and independent.

**Treatment and outcome**

The patient sustained a multifragmentary olecranon fracture (**Fig 3.5-8a**), a medial femoral neck fracture, and a superior and inferior pubic ring fracture (**Fig 3.5-8b**). She was treated nonoperatively with cast fixation for the olecranon fracture and operatively with a hemiarthroplasty for the femoral neck fracture.

After 3 weeks, both the fracture gap and the grade of displacement had increased (**Fig 3.5-8c**). However, 7 weeks after the injury, the patient was pain free with an active range of motion of 0–5–150° and was able to manage her activities of daily living independently.

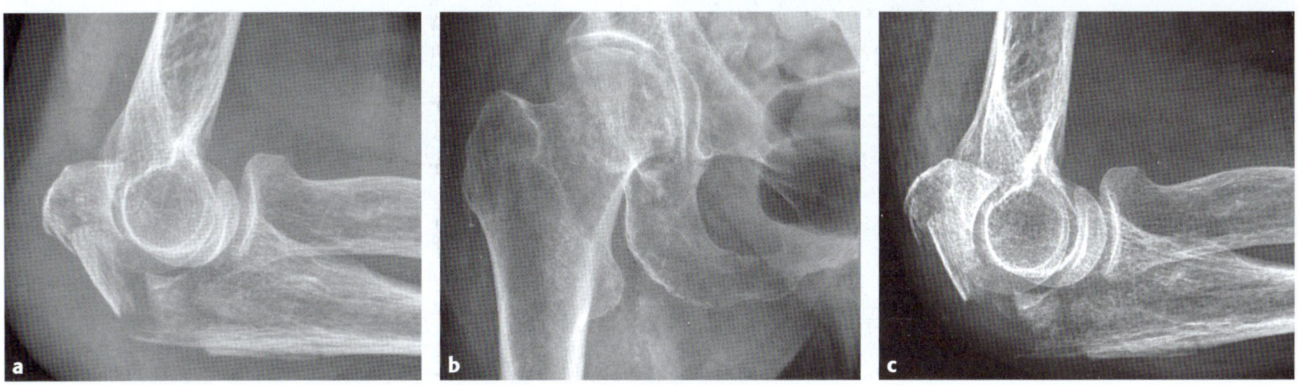


**Fig 3.5-8a–c** A 95-year-old woman after a fall.
**a–b** X-rays showing a multifragmentary olecranon fracture (**a**), a medial femoral neck fracture, and a superior and inferior pubic ring fracture (**b**).
**c** Three-week postoperative x-ray showing increased fracture gap and grade of displacement.

CASE 5

## Patient

A 91-year-old woman sustained a Mayo type IIB fracture after slipping and falling on the sidewalk.

## Treatment and outcome

The patient sustained a Mayo type IIB fracture (**Fig 3.5-9a**) with a concomitant ipsilateral hip fracture (**Fig 3.5-9b**) and proximal humeral fracture (**Fig 3.5-9c**).

Six weeks postinjury, the hip fracture was treated operatively using a trochanteric femoral nail (TFN) and the patient was initially mobilized with a wheeled walker (**Fig 3.5-9d**). Olecranon and proximal humerus were treated nonoperatively (**Fig 3.5-9e**). Active range of motion of the olecranon was 0–5–130°, the patient was pain free and had no complaints. Because of a malrotation of the femur after the initial TFN implantation, the patient underwent revision surgery with a derotation of the femur and new TFN implantation. She was able to walk independently using a walking stick on the injured side 6 weeks after the injury.

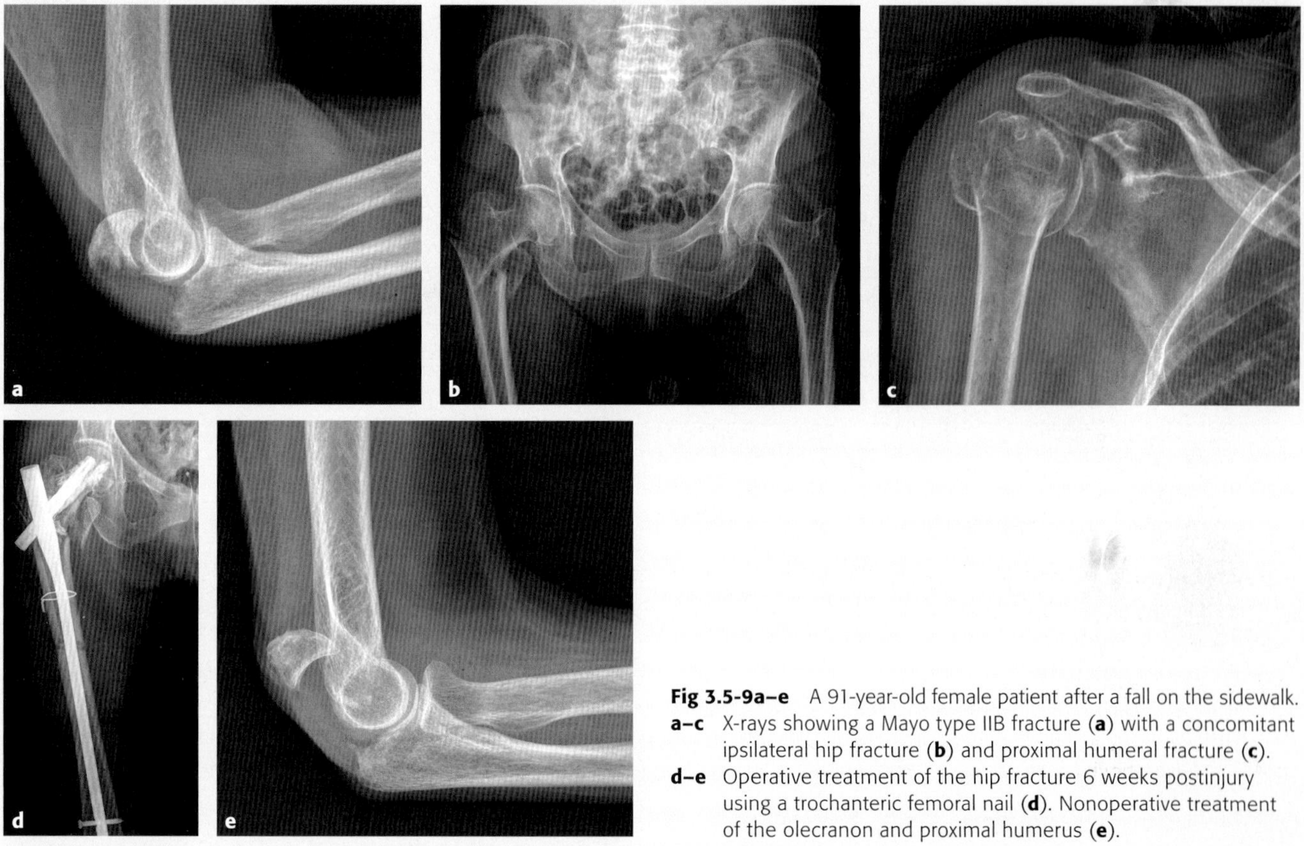


**Fig 3.5-9a–e** A 91-year-old female patient after a fall on the sidewalk.
**a–c** X-rays showing a Mayo type IIB fracture (**a**) with a concomitant ipsilateral hip fracture (**b**) and proximal humeral fracture (**c**).
**d–e** Operative treatment of the hip fracture 6 weeks postinjury using a trochanteric femoral nail (**d**). Nonoperative treatment of the olecranon and proximal humerus (**e**).

**Patient**

A 91-year-old healthy woman fell at home and sustained a Mayo type IIB fracture (**Fig 3.5-10a**).

**Treatment and outcome**

The patient was operated by open reduction and tension band wiring (**Fig 3.5-10b–c**). Two months after surgery the x-ray barely showed the former fracture line. The patient was satisfied and pain free and had a range of motion (ROM) of 0–5–140° and free rotation (**Fig 3.5-10f–g**). The hardware did not bother her at all.

Two years later, this patient fell again in her nursing home and sustained a contralateral Mayo type IA olecranon fracture (**Fig 3.5-10d**). This time, she was treated with an above-the-elbow cast for 2 weeks and functional training thereafter. Three months after the injury, the x-ray showed a tight nonunion. The patient was satisfied, pain free and had a ROM of 0–20–100° on her left side. The extension deficit in comparison to the other side did not bother her (**Fig 3.5-10e–g**).

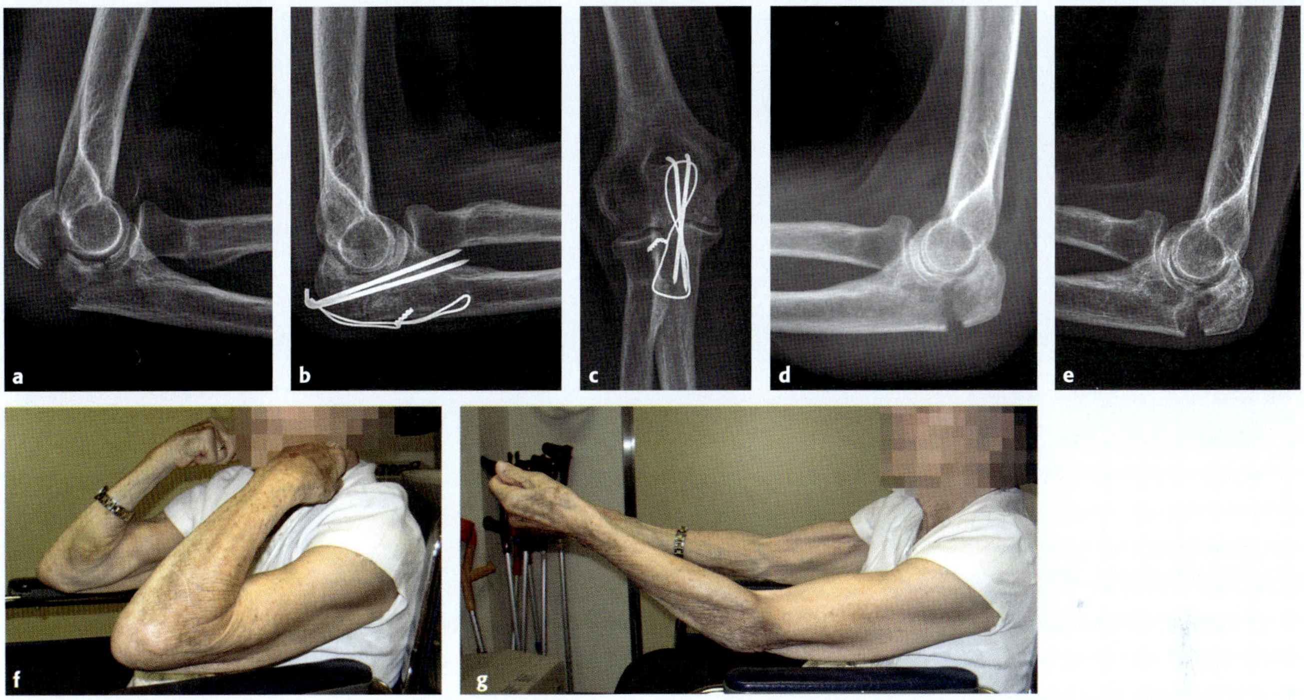

**Fig 3.5-10a–g** A 91-year-old female patient after a fall.

**a–c, f–g** X-rays showing a Mayo type IIB fracture (**a**) that was operated by open reduction and tension band wiring (**b–c**). Two months after surgery, the patient had a range of motion (ROM) of 0–5–140° and free rotation (**f–g**).

**d–f** X-ray showing a contralateral Mayo type IA olecranon fracture sustained 2 years later (**d**). Three-month postinjury x-ray showing a tight nonunion (**e**). Clinical images of the patient with a ROM of 0–20–100° on her left side and an extension deficit in comparison to the other side (**f–g**).

## 5.2 Operative treatment

Operative procedures include tension band wiring, and plate or screw fixation in Mayo type II and III fractures.

### 5.2.1 Tension band wiring

Mayo type IIA and B fractures with a vertical fracture line may be treated successfully using tension band wiring (**Case 6: Fig 3.5-10a-c, Fig 3.5-10f, Case 7: Fig 3.5-11, Case 8: Fig 3.5-12, Case 9: Fig 3.5-13, Case 10: Fig 3.5-14**). Single fragments may additionally be fixed using separate screws (**Case 9: Fig 3.5-13**).

Intraoperatively, implant position needs to be checked carefully. The K-wires should be positioned parallel to the ulnar shaft and just perforating the ventral ulnar cortices. Otherwise, the K-wire might impinge on the radial tuberosity, which can result in pain and a diminished rotation ROM (**Case 10: Fig 3.5-14**).

CASE 7

### Patient

An 89-year-old man slipped and fell on the sidewalk sustaining a Mayo type IIA fracture (**Fig 3.5-11a**).

### Comorbidities

- Hypereosinophilic syndrome
- Coronary heart disease
- Pacemaker
- Status postpulmonary embolism
- Status post total hip arthroplasty

### Treatment and outcome

This Mayo type IIA fracture was treated with tension band wiring (**Fig 3.5-11b**). Following operative treatment, the patient was placed in a cast for 3 weeks and prescribed initial physical therapy. Seven months after the initial injury, the fracture showed substantial bony healing and the patient was pain free with a range of motion of 0–15–110° as well as free rotation.

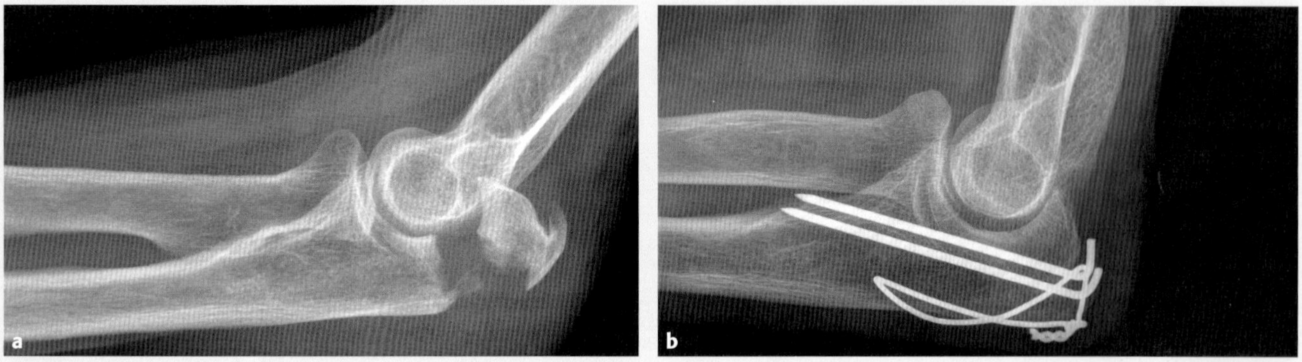


**Fig 3.5-11a–b** An 89-year-old male patient after falling on the sidewalk.
**a** X-ray showing a Mayo type IIA fracture.
**b** Operative fracture treatment with tension band wiring.

CASE 8

### Patient

A 91-year-old woman fell in the nursing home and sustained a Mayo type IIB olecranon fracture (**Fig 3.5-12a**).

### Treatment and outcome

The patient was treated with tension band wiring 1 day after the injury and dismissed after 6 days with a cast fixation (**Fig 3.5-12b**). She presented with a fracture displacement and pin loosening 22 days after surgery (**Fig 3.5-12c**). Because the patient was low-demand, further treatment was chosen to be nonoperative and all material was left in situ. Six months after surgery, the patient was pain free and had a range of motion of 0–10–110°. She had no complaints and the fracture was healed (**Fig 3.5-12d**).

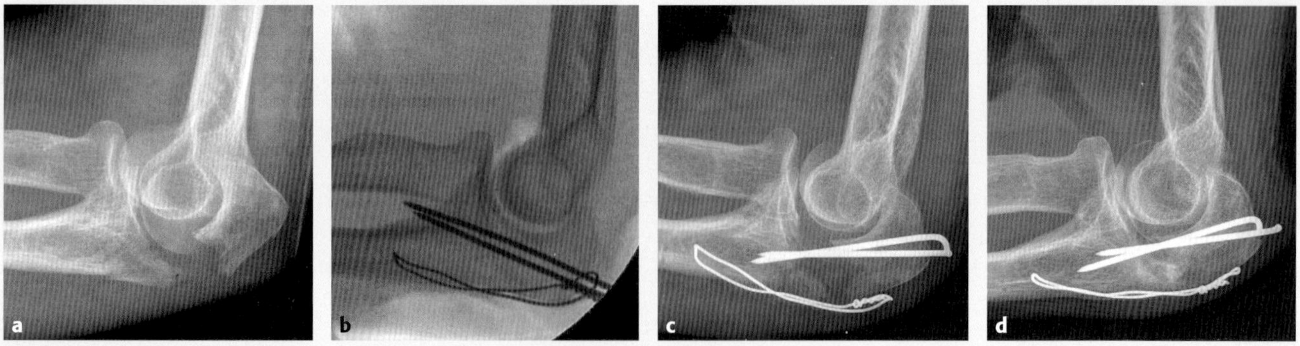


**Fig 3.5-12a–d**
**a** X-ray showing a Mayo type IIB olecranon fracture.
**b** One-day postinjury x-ray of fracture treated with tension band wiring.
**c** X-ray 22 days postoperative showing fracture displacement and pin loosening.
**d** Nonoperative treatment with all material left in situ showing healed fracture 6 months after surgery.

**Patient**

A 91-year old female patient fell from a stair and sustained a Mayo type IIB olecranon fracture (**Fig 3.5-13a**).

**Treatment and outcome**

The patient was treated with tension band wiring and screw fixation (**Fig 3.5-13b**). Three months after surgery, the patient was satisfied and pain free with a range of motion of 0–15–110°. She could handle her activities of daily living in the nursing home without complaints. The fracture had healed by this follow-up.

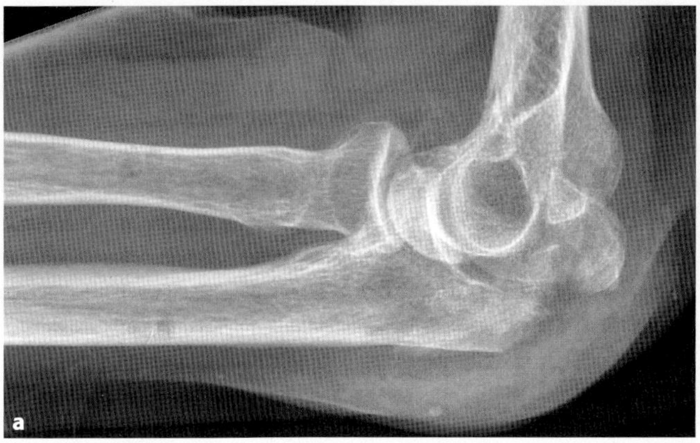


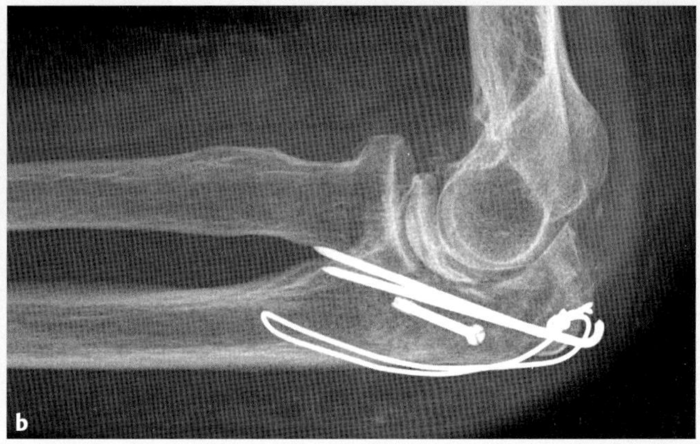


**Fig 3.5-13a–b** A 91-year-old woman after a fall.
**a** X-ray showing a Mayo type IIB olecranon fracture.
**b** Treatment with tension band wiring and screw fixation.



**Patient**

An 86-year-old patient fell while bicycling and sustained a Mayo type IA fracture (**Fig 3.5-14a**).

**Treatment and outcome**

The Mayo type IA fracture (**Fig 3.5-14a**) was treated by tension band wiring (**Fig 3.5-14b–c**). Three weeks after surgery, the patient had persistent complaints and pain with forearm rotation. The x-rays showed the radial K-wire impinging with the radial tuberosity (**Fig 3.5-14c**).

The patient was revised and the radial pin was shortened. Five months after the injury the patient was satisfied, pain free, with free rotation and a range of motion of 0–10–130° (**Fig 3.5-14d–e**). Hardware removal was not necessary.

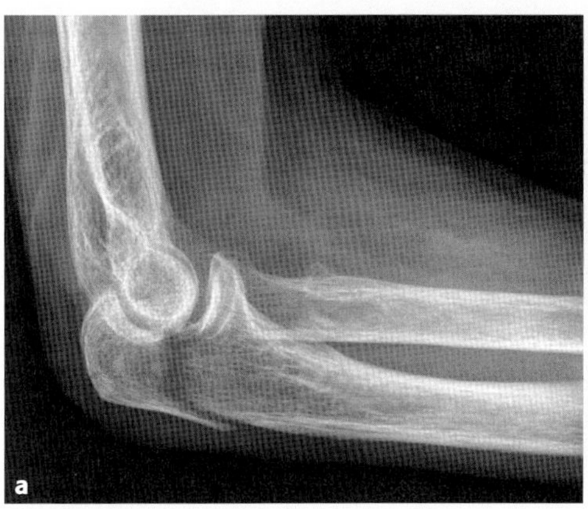


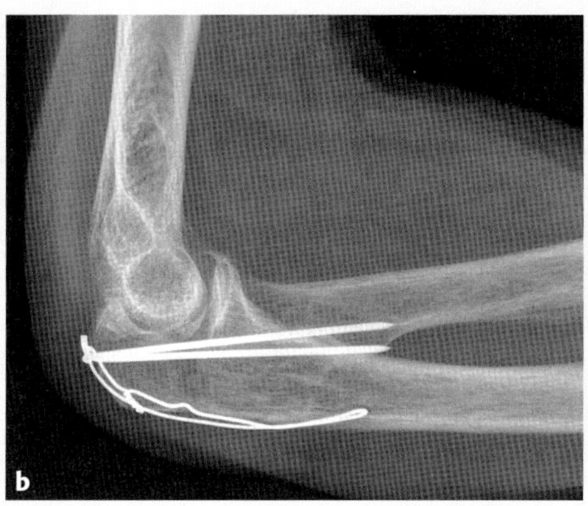


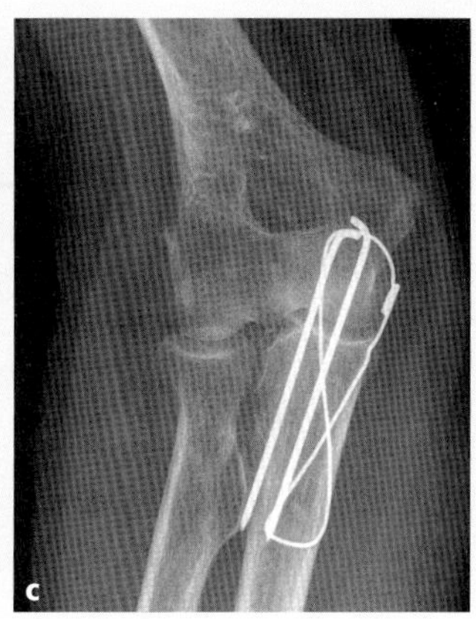


**Fig 3.5-14a–e** A 86-year-old patient after a bicycling accident.
**a–b** X-rays showing a Mayo type IA fracture (**a**), which was treated by tension band wiring (**b–c**).
**c** Three-week postoperative x-ray showing the radial K-wire impinging with the radial tuberosity.

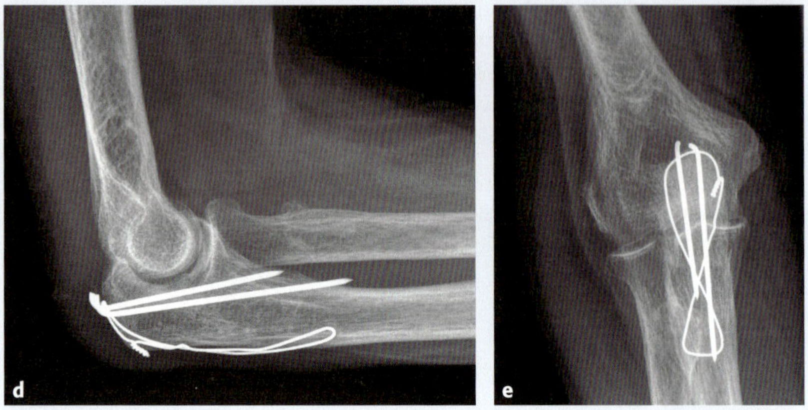


**Fig 3.5-14a–e (cont)**
**d–e** The patient was revised and the radial pin was shortened.

### 5.2.2 Plate fixation

Multifragmentary Mayo type IIB fractures may be treated with open reduction and plate fixation. All fragments can be fixed adequately, resulting in a stable construct. (**Case 11: Fig 3.5-15**, **Case 12: Fig 3.5-16**, **Case 13: Fig 3.5-17**, **Case 14: Fig 3.5-18**, **Case 15: Fig 3.5-19**).

CASE 11

**Patient**

An 87-year-old woman fell down the stairs and sustained a Mayo type IIB fracture (**Fig 3.5-15a**).

**Treatment and outcome**

The patient was treated operatively with open reduction and internal locking plate fixation. Postoperative physical therapy was started immediately without any restrictions. Nine months after surgery, the fracture was healed and the patient was pain free and had a range of motion (ROM) of 0–10–120° (**Fig 3.5-15b**).

However, the skin was irritated by the implant. Therefore, plate removal was conducted with an improvement of range of motion to 0–5–130° and free rotation (**Fig 3.5-15c**).

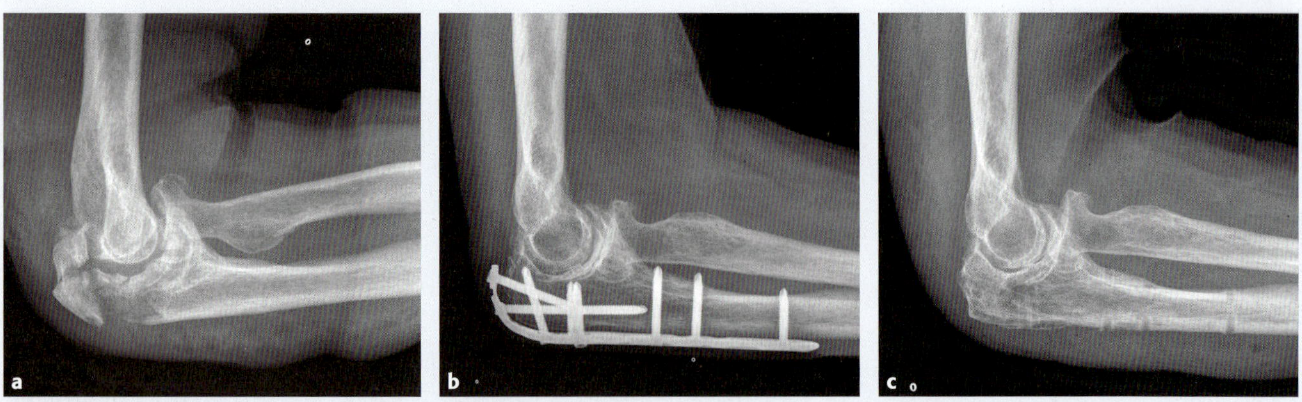


**Fig 3.5-15a–c** A 87-year-old female patient after a fall.
**a–b** X-ray showing a Mayo type IIB fracture (**a**) that was treated operatively with open reduction and internal locking plate fixation. The fracture was healed 9 months postoperatively (**b**).
**c** Plate removal due to skin irritation, which led to better range of motion and free rotation.

CASE 12

**Patient**

A 74-year-old man fell while mountain biking and sustained a Mayo type IIB fracture (**Fig 3.5-16a**).

**Treatment and outcome**

The patient was treated operatively with open reduction and locking plate fixation. Postoperative physical therapy was started immediately without any restrictions. Six weeks after surgery, the patient was satisfied and pain free. He had a range of motion of 0–0–135° and refused any further ambulatory follow-ups (**Fig 3.5-16b**).

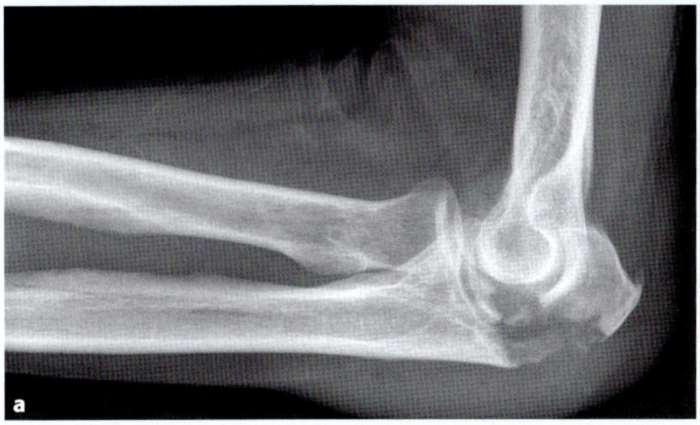


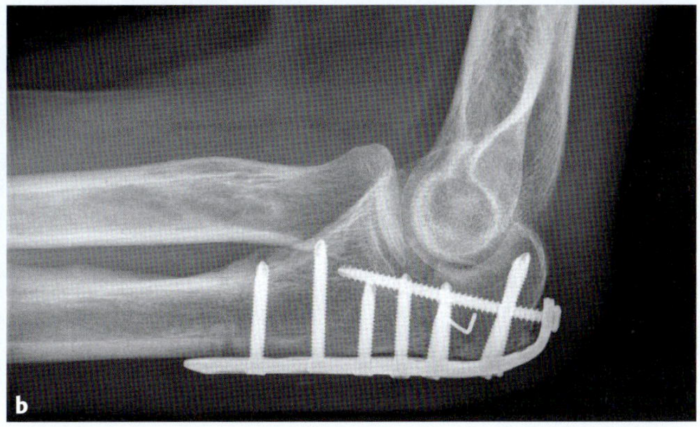


**Fig 3.5-16a–b** X-rays showing a Mayo type IIB fracture (**a**) that was treated operatively with open reduction and locking plate fixation with satisfactory results 6 weeks postoperative (**b**).

Fragments can be approached best from a dorsal position, but this comes with a risk of skin irritation and implant removal. Plate positioning on the lateral side of the ulna is possible in order to avoid skin irritation, but not all fracture fragments may be able to be addressed properly.

CASE 13

**Patient**

A 76-year-old woman fell on the sidewalk and sustained a Mayo type IIB fracture (**Fig 3.5-17a**).

**Treatment and outcome**

The fracture was treated operatively with plate fixation (**Fig 3.5-17b–c**). Two weeks after surgery, she presented with secondary fragment displacement and screw penetration into the joint (**Fig 3.5-17d–e**). Revision surgery using a femoral head allograft was conducted. Three months after the initial injury, the patient was able to manage her activities of daily living sufficiently with some minor functional complaints. Range of motion was 0–20–135° with free rotation (**Fig 3.5-17f**).

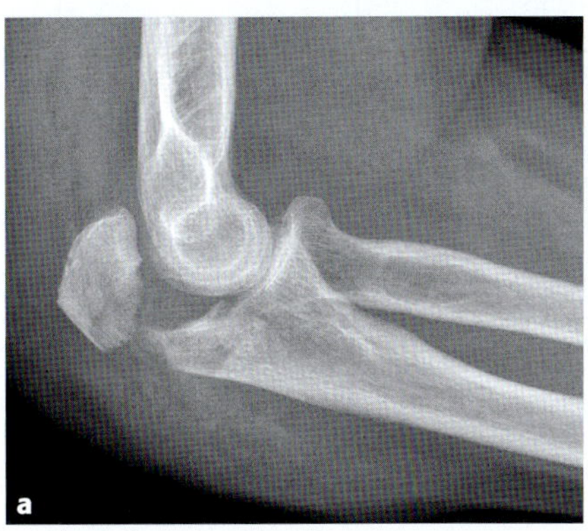


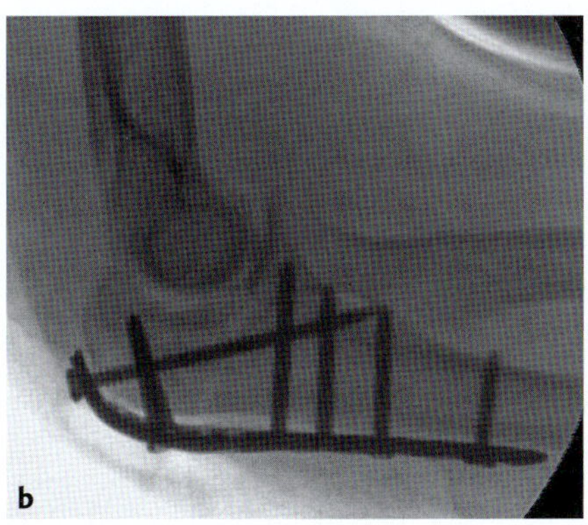


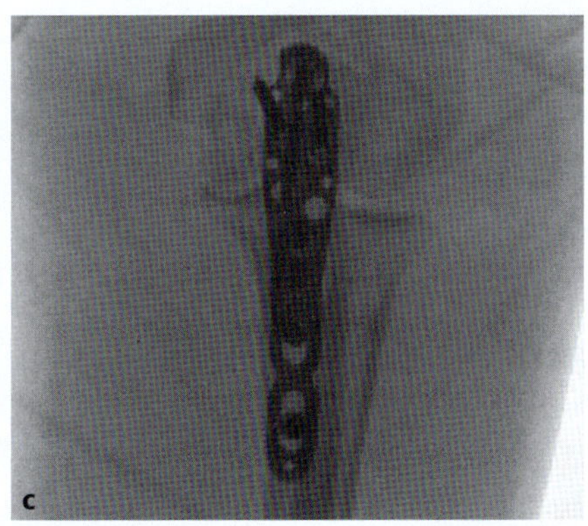


**Fig 3.5-17a–f** X-rays showing a Mayo type IIB fracture (**a**) which was treated operatively with plate fixation (**b–c**).

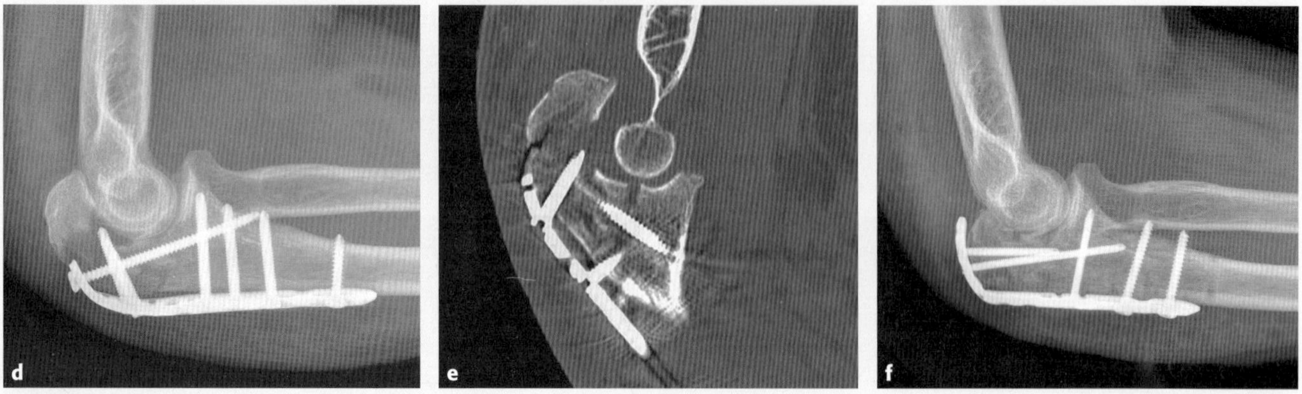

**Fig 3.5-17a–f (cont)** Two-week postoperative x-ray of secondary fragment displacement and screw penetration into the joint (**d–e**). Revision surgery using a femoral head allograft was conducted.

CASE 14

### Patient

An 87-year-old patient fell on the sidewalk and sustained a Mayo type IIA fracture with a concomitant wound dehiscence (tissue separation) (**Fig 3.5-18a**).

### Treatment and outcome

The patient was treated with open reduction and plate fixation. Intraoperative image intensification showed good reduction and fixation (**Fig 3.5-18b**).

However, 4 days after surgery, the x-ray showed cut through, loss of reduction, and fragment redisplacement (**Fig 3.5-18c**).

The injury was revised and the separated fragment was treated by fiberwire tensioning and wire cerclage. Two months after surgery, the patient was pain free and satisfied with a range of motion of 0–5–120°. The x-ray showed fracture healing (**Fig 3.5-18d**).

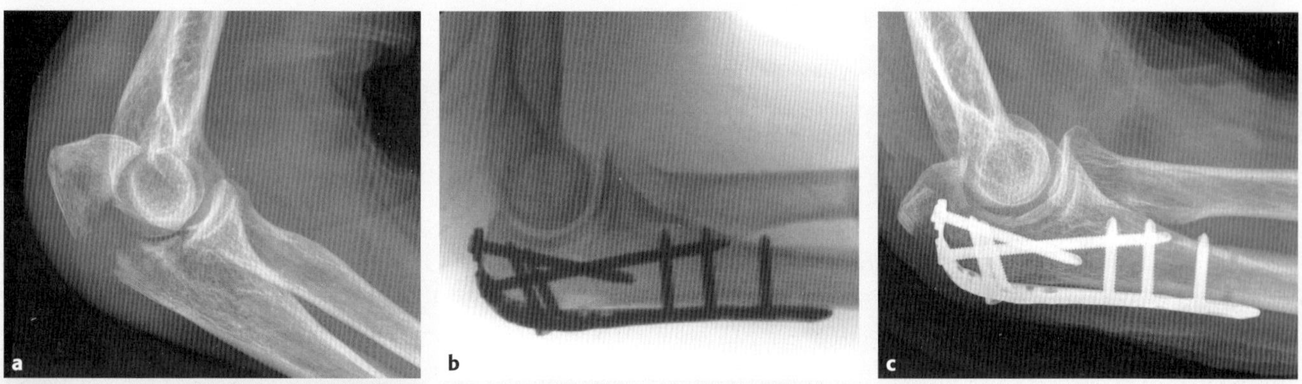

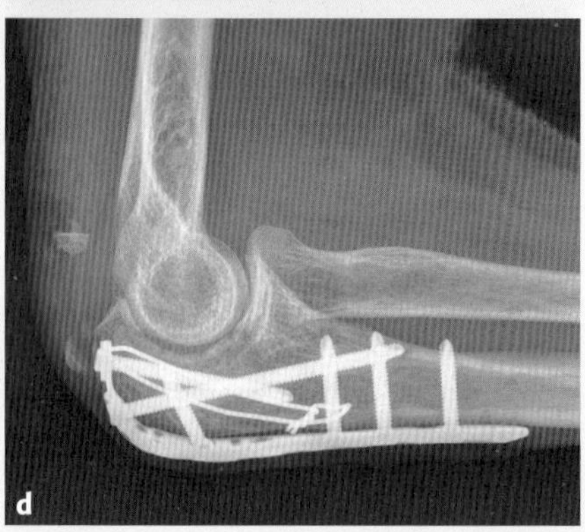

**Fig 3.5-18a–d** An 87-year-old patient after a fall.

- **a** X-ray of a Mayo type IIA fracture with a concomitant wound dehiscence.
- **b** Intraoperative image intensification showing good reduction and fixation after fracture treatment with open reduction and plate fixation.
- **c** Four-day postoperative x-ray showing cut through, loss of reduction, and fragment redisplacement.
- **d** X-ray showing fracture healing after revision of injury and treatment of the separated fragment by fiberwire tensioning and wire cerclage.

The positioning of the plate has to be taken into consideration. The plate must be long enough at the olecranon end to act as a buttress against cut through and secondary displacement. In osteoporotic bone, a plate that is too short at the olecranon might not sufficiently fix the proximal fracture fragment and might more easily result in cut through (**Case 18: Fig 3.5-17**). This can also be the case if the proximal screw does not retain single fragments adequately (**Case 14: Fig 3.5-18**). For these reasons, a long cortical screw should be placed, fixing the proximal fragment with the inserting triceps tendon. In addition, the plate should be long enough in its proximal extension to additionally buttress against proximal fragment dislocation. Additional suture augmentation using nonabsorbable material can be another reasonable option to fix the triceps tendon to the construct and decrease distraction forces by an offloading triceps suture technique [31].

## 5.3 Complications

### 5.3.1 Implant cut out

Beware of screw cut through in osteoporotic bone (**Case 13: Fig 3.5-17**, **Case 14: Fig 3.5-18**, **Case 15: Fig 3.5-19**). Screw fixation can fail in osteoporotic bone. Consider longer cast fixation, especially in patients with impaired ability to comply with activity restrictions, due to a potential stronger triceps pull. Screw loosening and concomitant fracture dislocation can also occur in cases of infection. Revision surgery and delayed treatment of open wounds have an increased risk for infection and wound complications. In cases of failed operative fixation or symptomatic nonunion, a salvage procedure like fragment excision can still result in a satisfactory functional outcome.

**CASE 15**

### Patient

A 68-year-old woman fell and sustained a Mayo type IIA fracture (**Fig 3.5-19a**).

### Comorbidities

- Osteoporosis
- Alcoholic cirrhosis

### Treatment and outcome

The patient sustained a Mayo type IIA fracture (**Fig 3.5-19a**), and periprosthetic femoral (**Fig 3.5-19b**) and pubic fractures (**Fig 3.5-19c**).

Two days postinjury, the fracture was treated operatively with tension band plate fixation (**Fig 3.5-19d–e**). Cut through of the proximal ulnar fragment 5 days after surgery (**Fig 3.5-19f–g**).

Eleven days postinjury, the patient was operatively revised using a "twin" plate fixation (**Fig 3.5-19h–i**). Partial cut through was again detected 4 days after the second surgery, which was not seen during operative image intensification (**Fig 3.5-19j–k**).

In the meantime, the patient developed a wound dehiscence, which resulted in another revision surgery 24 days after the initial injury. Implant removal was conducted, the fracture fragment was excised, tissue samples were acquired, and a negative-pressure wound closure and an external fixator were applied. After antibiotic treatment, the wound healed uneventfully, and the patient was satisfied with a painless active range of motion of 0–20–150°. Compared to the uninjured contralateral side, the elbow extension force was reduced and did not limit the patient (**Fig 3.5-19l–m**).

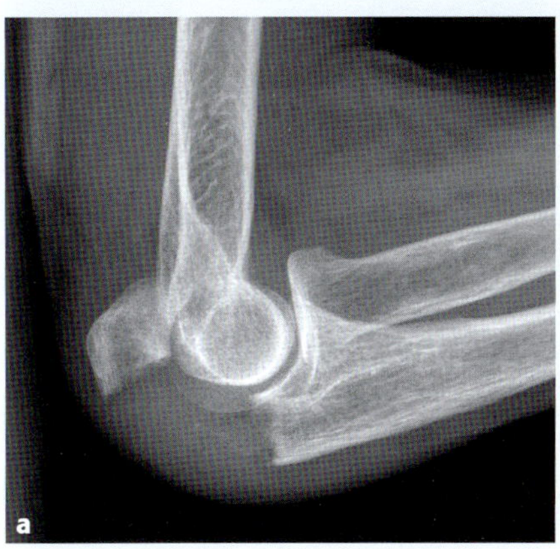


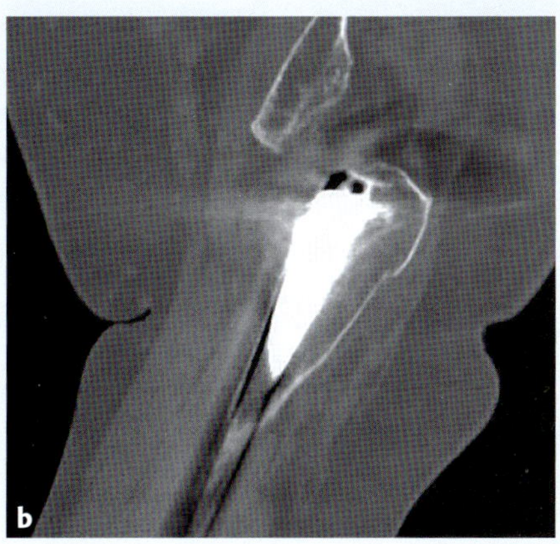


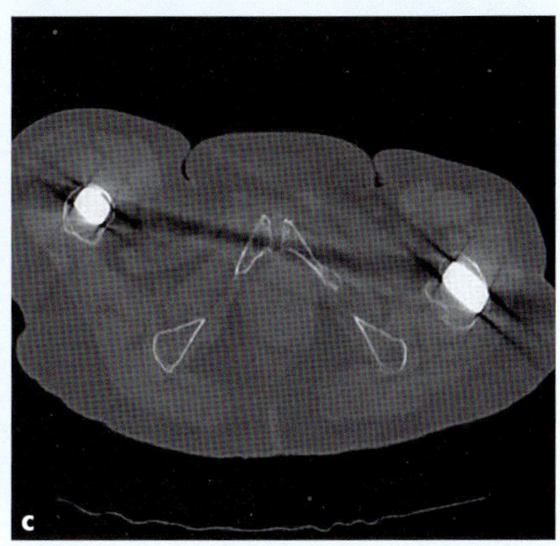


**Fig 3.5-19a–m** A 68-year-old female patient after a fall.
**a–c** X-rays showing a Mayo type IIA fracture (**a**), and periprosthetic femoral (**b**) and pubic fractures (**c**).

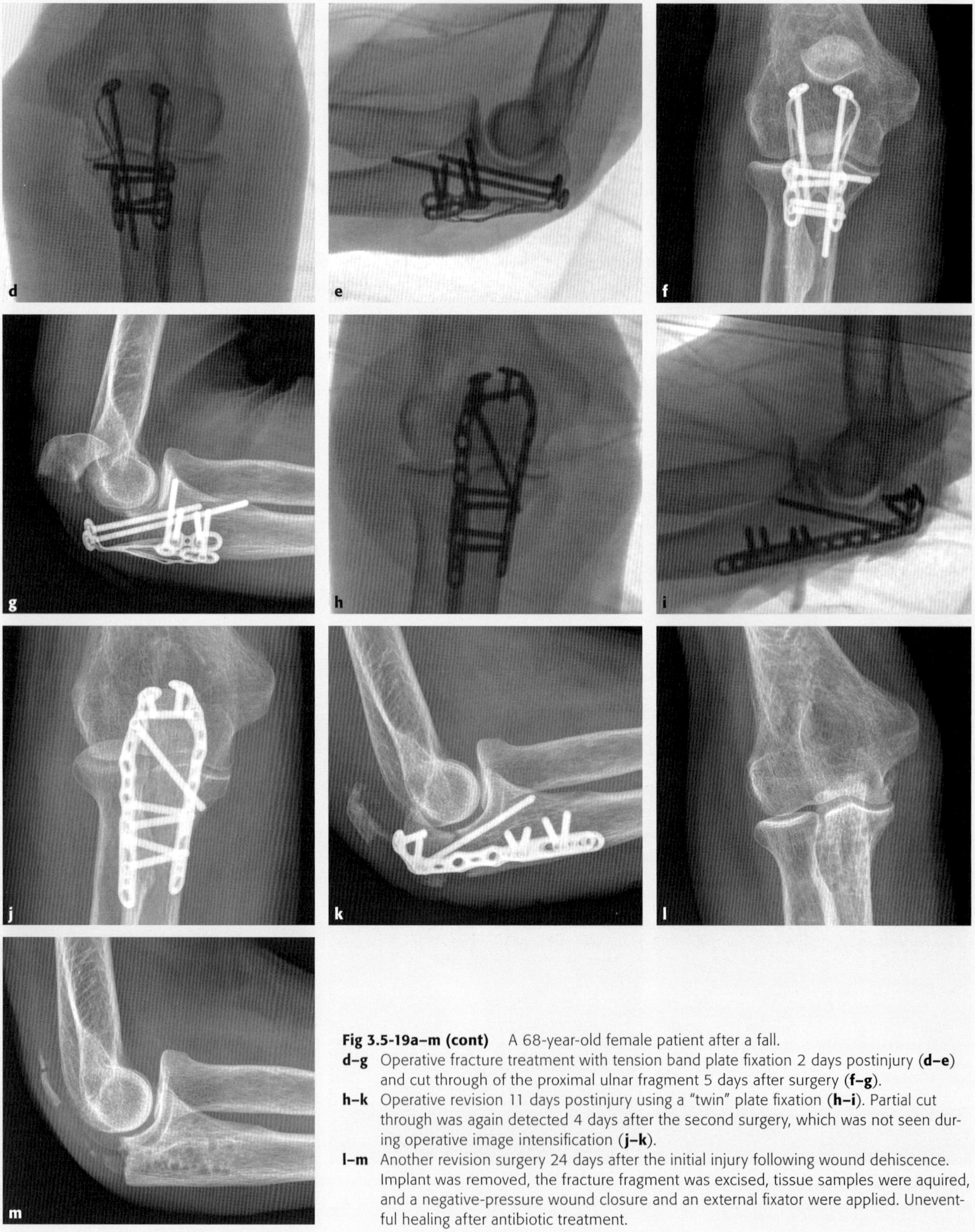


**Fig 3.5-19a–m (cont)** A 68-year-old female patient after a fall.

**d–g** Operative fracture treatment with tension band plate fixation 2 days postinjury (**d–e**) and cut through of the proximal ulnar fragment 5 days after surgery (**f–g**).

**h–k** Operative revision 11 days postinjury using a "twin" plate fixation (**h–i**). Partial cut through was again detected 4 days after the second surgery, which was not seen during operative image intensification (**j–k**).

**l–m** Another revision surgery 24 days after the initial injury following wound dehiscence. Implant was removed, the fracture fragment was excised, tissue samples were aquired, and a negative-pressure wound closure and an external fixator were applied. Uneventful healing after antibiotic treatment.

### 5.3.2 Nonunion

Nonunion of olecranon fractures can occur following both operative and nonoperative treatment [9]. While in the general population 1% of operatively treated olecranon fractures result in a nonunion [32], nonunion rates as high as 78% have been described in the geriatric population [20, 21]. Most nonunions of the olecranon are asymptomatic fibrous nonunions without the need for further treatment (**Case 4: Fig 3.5-8**, **Case 5: Fig 3.5-9**, **Case 6: Fig 3.5-10**, **Case 16: Fig 3.5-20**) [32].

Retrospective analyses of older low-demand patients following nonoperatively treated olecranon fractures have shown that, even in cases of displaced Mayo type II fractures, no patient required operative treatment for a symptomatic nonunion [20, 21]. In the case of symptomatic nonunion in combination with functional loss and extension deficit, pain, or elbow stiffness, operative treatment may be appropriate.

Operative options include fragment excision with triceps tendon reattachment (**Case 15: Fig 3.5-19l–m**), plate fixation, or tension band wiring with or without bone grafting and joint replacement [32].

If the fracture fragment is smaller than 50% of the trochlear articular surface, fragment excision and triceps tendon reattachment may lead to satisfactory results in older adults with minor triceps weakness [33]. However, it is important to rule out any elbow instability prior to excision of the fragment. This technique may also be considered as a salvage procedure in cases of postoperative infection.

If the fragment is larger than 50% with a symptomatic functional deficit, or in cases of an unstable elbow joint, reconstructive measures including bone grafting and total elbow arthroplasty must be considered [29, 32].

**CASE 16**

**Patient**

A 77-year-old patient sustained a Mayo type I fracture (**Fig 3.5-20a**) after slipping and falling down the stairs.

**Comorbidities**

- Alcohol abuse

**Treatment and outcome**

Nonoperative treatment with passive motion exercises was chosen initially. Three months postinjury, there was no bone healing but increased displacement. However, the clinical outcome was satisfactory with a pain-free range of motion of 0–0–130° similar to the contralateral uninjured side (**Fig 3.5-20b**).

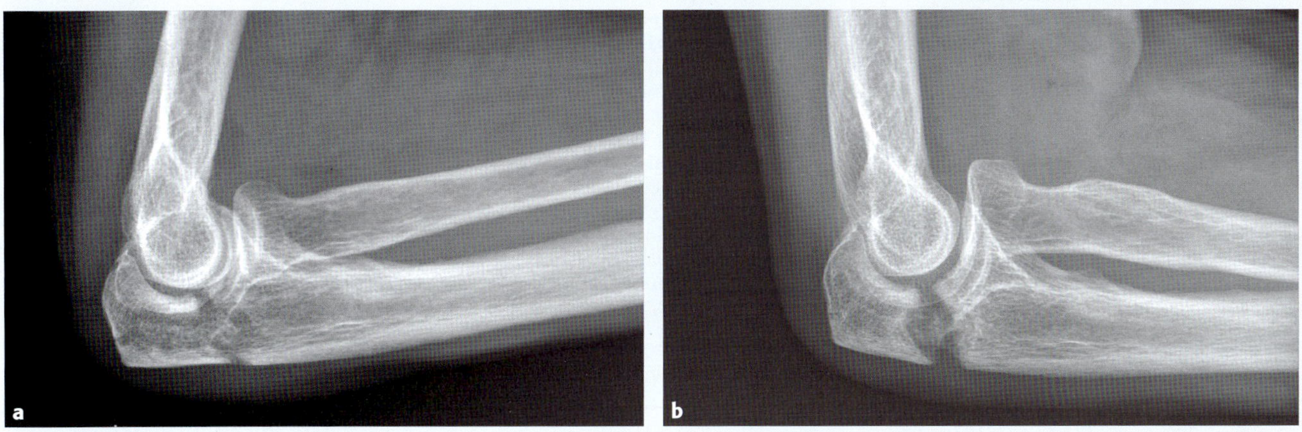


**Fig 3.5-20a–b** A 77-year-old patient after a fall.
**a** X-ray showing a Mayo type I fracture.
**b** X-ray showing no bony healing but increased displacement 3 months after the injury and following nonoperative treatment.

Nonunion following both nonoperative and operative treatments of olecranon fractures in older adults appears to be frequent but mostly asymptomatic. In most cases, no further treatment is necessary as patients typically are pain free with adequate ROM.

## 6 References


1. **Duckworth AD, Clement ND, Aitken SA, et al.** The epidemiology of fractures of the proximal ulna. *Injury.* 2012 Mar;43(3):343–346.
2. **Rommens PM, Kuchle R, Schneider RU, et al.** Olecranon fractures in adults: factors influencing outcome. *Injury.* 2004 Nov;35(11):1149–1157.
3. **Newman SD, Mauffrey C, Krikler S.** Olecranon fractures. *Injury.* 2009 Jun;40(6):575–581.
4. **Sahajpal D, Wright TW.** Proximal ulna fractures. *J Hand Surg Am.* 2009 Feb;34(2):357–362.
5. **Ring D.** Elbow fractures and dislocations. In: Rockwood C, Green D, Buchholz R, eds. *Rockwood and Green's Fractures in Adults.* 7th ed. Philadelphia Lippincott Williams & Wilkins; 2010:905–944.
6. **Symes M, Harris IA, Limbers J, et al.** SOFIE: Surgery for Olecranon Fractures in the Elderly: a randomised controlled trial of operative versus non-operative treatment. *BMC Musculoskelet Disord.* 2015 Oct 27;16:324.
7. **Helm RH, Hornby R, Miller SW.** The complications of surgical treatment of displaced fractures of the olecranon. *Injury.* 1987 Jan;18(1):48–50.
8. **Romero JM, Miran A, Jensen CH.** Complications and re-operation rate after tension-band wiring of olecranon fractures. *J Orthop Sci.* 2000;5(4):318–320.
9. **Danziger MB, Healy WL.** Operative treatment of olecranon nonunion. *J Orthop Trauma.* 1992;6(3):290–293.
10. **Veras Del Monte L, Sirera Vercher M, Busquets Net R, et al.** Conservative treatment of displaced fractures of the olecranon in the elderly. *Injury.* 1999 Mar;30(2):105–110.
11. **Colton CL.** Fractures of the olecranon in adults: classification and management. *Injury.* 1973 Nov;5(2):121–129.
12. **Morrey BF.** Current concepts in the treatment of fractures of the radial head, the olecranon, and the coronoid. *Instr Course Lect.* 1995;44:175–185.
13. **Schatzker J.** *Fractures of the Olecranon (12-B1). The rationale of operative fracture care.* Berlin: Springer; 2005:123–129.
14. **Müller ME, Allgöwer M, Perren S.** *Manual of internal fixation: techniques recommended by the AO-ASIF group.* Berlin: Springer Verlag, 1991.
15. **Tamaoki MJ, Matsunaga FT, Silveira JD, et al.** Reproducibility of classifications for olecranon fractures. *Injury.* 2014 Nov;45 Suppl 5:S18–S20.
16. **Benetton CA, Cesa G, El-Kouba Junior G, et al.** Agreement of olecranon fractures before and after the exposure to four classification systems. *J Shoulder Elbow Surg.* 2015 Mar;24(3):358–363.
17. **Clement ND, Green K, Murray N, et al.** Undisplaced intracapsular hip fractures in the elderly: predicting fixation failure and mortality. A prospective study of 162 patients. *J Orthop Sci.* 2013 Jul;18(4):578–585.
18. **Ginsel BL, Taher A, Ottley MC, et al.** Hospital mortality after arthroplasty using a cemented stem for displaced femoral neck fractures. *J Orthop Surg (Hong Kong).* 2014 Dec;22(3):279–281.
19. **Muller F, Galler M, Zellner M, et al.** The fate of proximal femoral fractures in the 10th decade of life: an analysis of 117 consecutive patients. *Injury.* 2015 Oct;46(10):1983–1987.
20. **Duckworth AD, Bugler KE, Clement ND, et al.** Nonoperative management of displaced olecranon fractures in low-demand elderly patients. *J Bone Joint Surg Am.* 2014 Jan 01;96(1):67–72.
21. **Gallucci GL, Piuzzi NS, Slullitel PA, et al.** Non-surgical functional treatment for displaced olecranon fractures in the elderly. *Bone Joint J.* 2014 Apr;96-B(4):530–534.
22. **Edwards SG, Martin BD, Fu RH, et al.** Comparison of olecranon plate fixation in osteoporotic bone: do current technologies and designs make a difference? *J Orthop Trauma.* 2011 May;25(5):306–311.
23. **Kim T, Ayturk UM, Haskell A, et al.** Fixation of osteoporotic distal fibula fractures: A biomechanical comparison of locking versus conventional plates. *J Foot Ankle Surg.* 2007 Jan–Feb;46(1):2–6.
24. **Ring D, Kloen P, Kadzielski J, et al.** Locking compression plates for osteoporotic nonunions of the diaphyseal humerus. *Clin Orthop Relat Res.* 2004 Aug(425):50–54.
25. **Snow M, Thompson G, Turner PG.** A mechanical comparison of the locking compression plate (LCP) and the low contact-dynamic compression plate (DCP) in an osteoporotic bone model. *J Orthop Trauma.* 2008 Feb;22(2):121–125.
26. **Stoffel K, Booth G, Rohrl SM, et al.** A comparison of conventional versus locking plates in intraarticular calcaneus fractures: a biomechanical study in human cadavers. *Clin Biomech (Bristol, Avon).* 2007 Jan;22(1):100–105.
27. **Amini MH, Azar FM, Wilson BR, et al.** Comparison of Outcomes and Costs of Tension-Band and Locking-Plate Osteosynthesis in Transverse Olecranon Fractures: A Matched-Cohort Study. *Am J Orthop (Belle Mead NJ).* 2015 Jul;44(7):E211–E215.
28. **Schliemann B, Raschke MJ, Groene P, et al.** Comparison of tension band wiring and precontoured locking compression plate fixation in Mayo type IIA olecranon fractures. *Acta Orthop Belg.* 2014 Mar;80(1):106–111.
29. **Baecher N, Edwards S.** Olecranon fractures. *J Hand Surg Am.* 2013 Mar;38(3):593–604.
30. **Veillette CJ, Steinmann SP.** Olecranon fractures. *Orthop Clin North Am.* 2008 Apr;39(2):229–236, vii.
31. **Izzi J, Athwal GS.** An off-loading triceps suture for augmentation of plate fixation in comminuted osteoporotic fractures of the olecranon. *J Orthop Trauma.* 2012 Jan;26(1):59–61.
32. **Papagelopoulos PJ, Morrey BF.** Treatment of nonunion of olecranon fractures. *J Bone Joint Surg Br.* 1994 Jul;76(4):627–635.
33. **Gartsman GM, Sculco TP, Otis JC.** Operative treatment of olecranon fractures. Excision or open reduction with internal fixation. *J Bone Joint Surg Am.* 1981 Jun;63(5):718–721.

# 3.6 Distal forearm

Rohit Arora, Alexander Keiler, Susanne Strasser

## 1 Introduction

Two hundred years ago, Abraham Colles stated that after a distal radial fracture (DRF) "...the limb will again enjoy perfect freedom in all its motions, and be completely free of pain" [1]. From today's point of view, this is not the case. Despite an impressive body of literature and a multitude of technical solutions, we still do not have enough evidence to guide all specific treatment options.

Due to increasing age and activity level of older adults, appropriate management of these fractures is of growing concern. Prevention of wrist arthrosis and restoration of wrist function allowing a rapid return to an active and independent lifestyle are major goals.

In this chapter, we discuss the typical characteristics of this injury, their significance for fragility fracture patients (FFPs), current treatment options, and possible complications. Some of the challenges are:

- The impact on the function of an individual patient is variable and can be difficult to predict. Generally, tolerance for anatomical deviations is higher, mostly due to limited functional needs. The radiographic outcome does not correlate well with the clinical and functional outcome (**Fig 3.6-1**).
- Internal fixation in DRFs with multifragmented intraarticular distal fracture fragments in osteoporotic bone is challenging. Even with the use of locking implants, subsidence of the joint fragments lead to secondary intraarticular screw penetration.
- Due to intraarticular comminution, dorsal metaphyseal instability, and poor bone quality, some DRFs are not restorable. In these cases, arthroplasty of the distal radius may be an alternative treatment option.
- The surgeon needs to closely attend to optimal plate position to minimize the risk of implant removal in the future.
- The differentiation between DRFs and distal forearm fractures (DFFs) is crucial. The treatment options are different in DFFs in which the distal ulnar fracture causes more instability. Additionally, DFFs are often grade 1 or grade 2 open fractures on the ulnar side.
- The treatment of DRF in older adults is controversial. Nondisplaced DRFs are treated nonoperatively, and standard operative fixation is recommended for palmar displaced DRFs (**Fig 3.6-2**), DFFs, open fractures, and fracture dislocations.
- Early functional physical and occupational therapy after operative fixation prevents joint stiffness and improves the clinical outcome significantly.

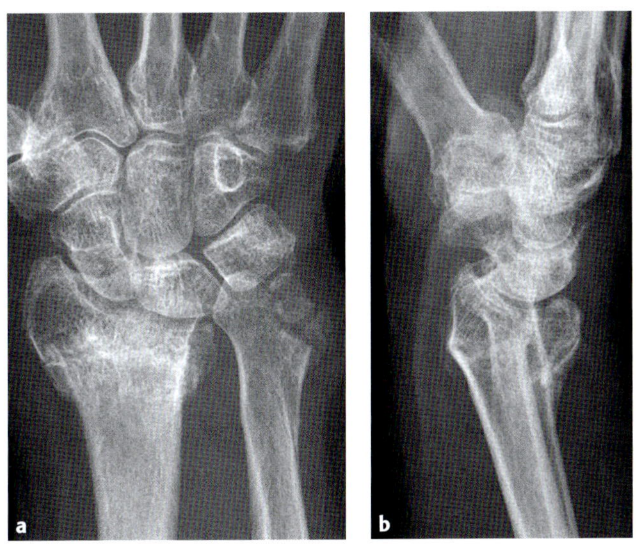


**Fig 3.6-1a–f** An 81-year-old woman with a malunion.
**a–b** AP (**a**) and lateral (**b**) x-ray views of malunion after nonoperatively treated distal radial fracture with loss of dorsal inclination, shortening, and ulnar-plus position.

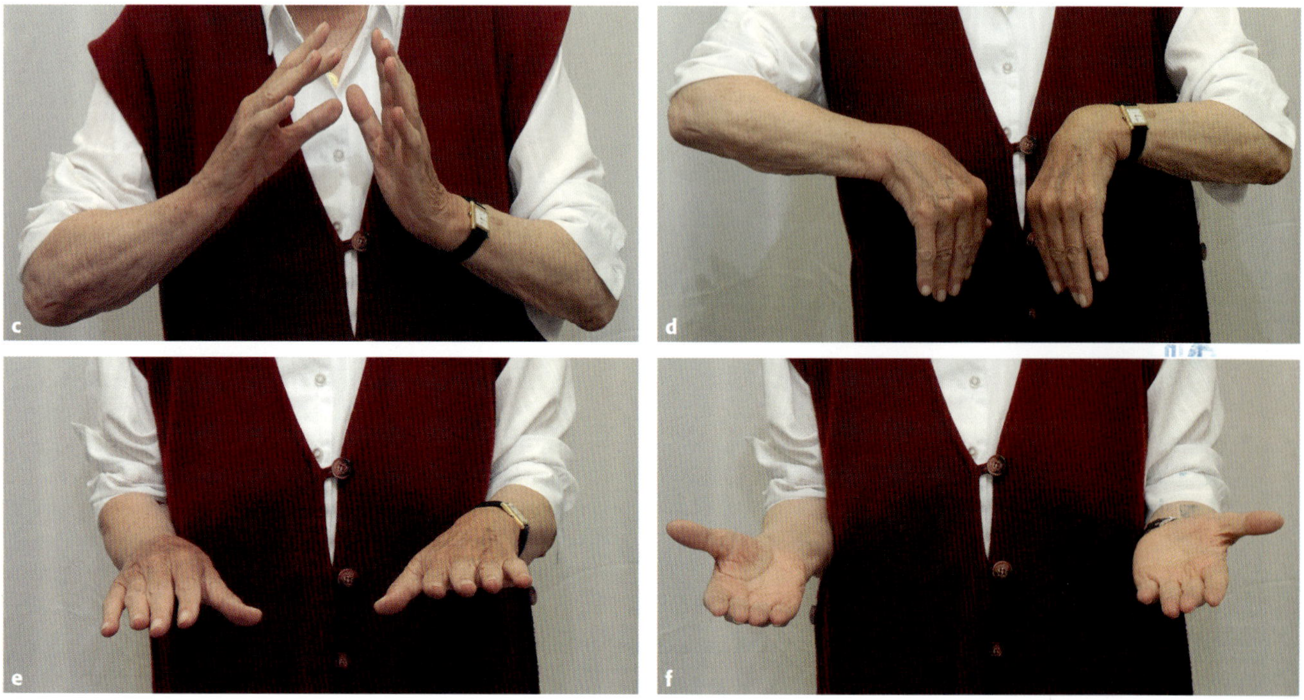


**Fig 3.6-1a–f (cont)** An 81-year-old woman with a malunion.
**c–f** Despite the malunion, there is a good clinical outcome with satisfactory function and without subjective impairment (**c–f**) with an average Disabilities of the Arm, Shoulder and Hand score of 8, Patient-Rated Wrist Evaluation score of 10, Visual Analog Scale for pain of 0 (for no pain), average extension of 50°, flexion of 45°, unrestricted pronation and supination, and a grip strength of 78% of the contralateral side.

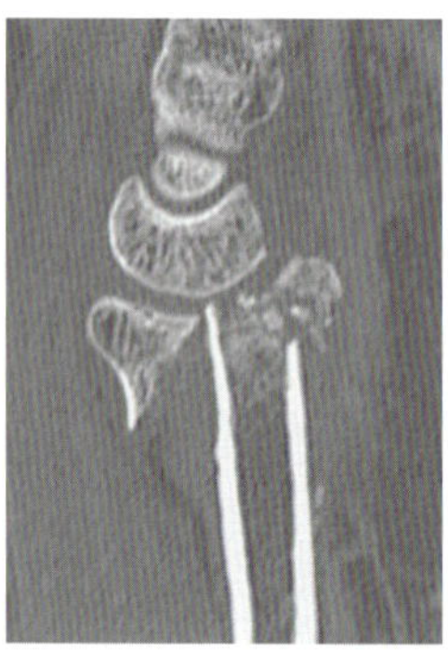

**Fig 3.6-2** Sagittal view of a computed tomographic scan of a 78-year-old female patient suffering from a distal radial fracture with palmar displacement.

## 2 Epidemiology and etiology

Distal radial fractures are the most common upper extremity fractures in individuals aged 65 years and older, ranking second in total fracture frequency after vertebral compression fractures [2]. The overall incidence varies in different countries. In Scandinavia it is about 30 per 10,000 people per year [3]. Across populations there is a bimodal fracture distribution with peaks in young men and older women, with approximately 70% of the fractures of the adults occurring in women between 61 and 69 years [4]. In the younger population, these fractures are most often the result of high-energy trauma or falls from a height. In contrast, in older adults, these fractures mostly result from low-energy trauma from falls from a standing height or lower. Some recent studies identify a correlation between wrist fracture (ie, "indicator fracture") and future osteoporotic fractures at other sites [5, 6]. In women, the risk of a hip fracture increases 1.4–1.8 times after a previous wrist fracture. In older men, the risk of hip fracture increases 2.3–2.7 times [7]. Distal radial fractures have significant associated socioeconomic costs [8].

Epidemiological studies are scarce because only a small proportion of this fracture type requires hospital admission. However, incidence rates of DRF/DFFs have been shown to be comparable to hip fracture incidence rates where data are available [9]. Furthermore, depending on the population investigated, trend analysis on DRF/DFF incidence has shown increases, decreases, or a stable pattern over the period of observation [9–11].

## 3 Diagnostics

Distal radial fractures usually cause immediate pain, tenderness, bruising, and swelling. In most cases, the fracture deformity is visible. For further treatment, it is essential to consider patients' functional lifestyle (eg, practiced sports), the activity of daily living (ADL) needs (eg, living independently or requiring the use of a cane or walking frame), and other functional demands.

### 3.1 Plain x-rays

In simple fracture patterns, plain AP and lateral x-rays are performed before and after reduction.

### 3.2 Computed tomography and magnetic resonance imaging

Computed tomography (CT) is often used in multifragmented intraarticular fractures for preoperative planning to assess associated injuries and sometimes for decision making. Computed tomography scans performed after reduction generally provide more information than those performed while the fracture is displaced. In acute DRFs, magnetic resonance imaging (MRI) examination is not of clinical importance.

### 3.3 Radiographic parameters

Specific radiographic parameters with biomechanical and clinical implications have been developed to assess the radiocarpal joint:

- Palmar tilt—angle subtended by the line perpendicular to the long axis of the radius and a line drawn from the dorsal to palmar cortex of the distal radius (average: 10–12°) (**Fig 3.6-3**).
- Radial inclination—angle between the longitudinal axis of the radius and a line connecting the radial cortex of the apex of the radial styloid and the central point of the sigmoid notch of the distal radius (average: 22–23°) (**Fig 3.6-4**).
- Radial length—distance between the apex of the radial styloid and the level of the ulnar head at the distal radioulnar joint (DRUJ) (average: 11–12 mm) (**Fig 3.6-5**).
- Ulnar variance—difference in axial length between the central point of the ulnar corner of the sigmoid notch of the distal radius and the most distal extension of the ulnar head on the AP view (**Fig 3.6-6**).

### 3.4 Assessment of distal radioulnar joint instability

The distal radioulnar joint is dynamically tested for instability intraoperatively and after anatomical reconstruction of the DRF. In neutral position, the ulna translates in comparison with the uninjured side. The testing of the DRUJ is of high clinical importance, as for example in cases where the DRUJ is stable, the ulnar styloid fracture can be treated nonoperatively.

In stable conditions of the DRUJ, a nonunion of the ulnar styloid is usually asymptomatic. None of the most recent studies demonstrate that acute fixation of ulnar styloid fractures has been beneficial [12]. For very rare cases of chronic ulnar symptoms, results of secondary repair have been encouraging, making late fixation of ulnar styloid in symptomatic patients an acceptable option.

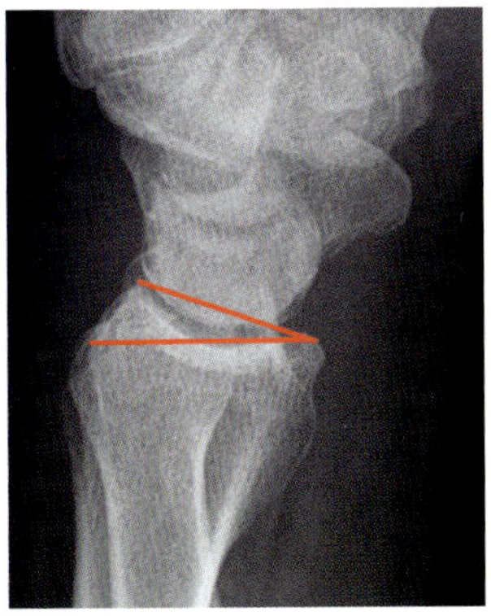

**Fig 3.6-3** Palmar tilt is measured as the angle subtended by the line perpendicular to the long axis of the radius and a second line drawn from the dorsal to palmar cortex of the distal radius.

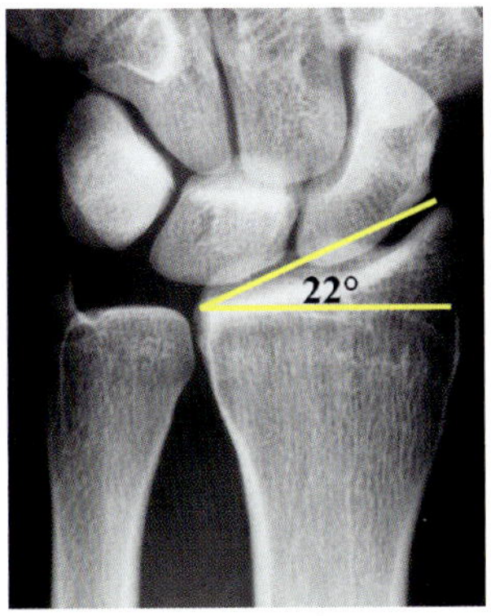


**Fig 3.6-4** Radial inclination is assessed as the angle between the longitudinal axis of the radius and a line connecting the radial cortex of the apex of the radial styloid and the central point of the sigmoid notch of the distal radius.

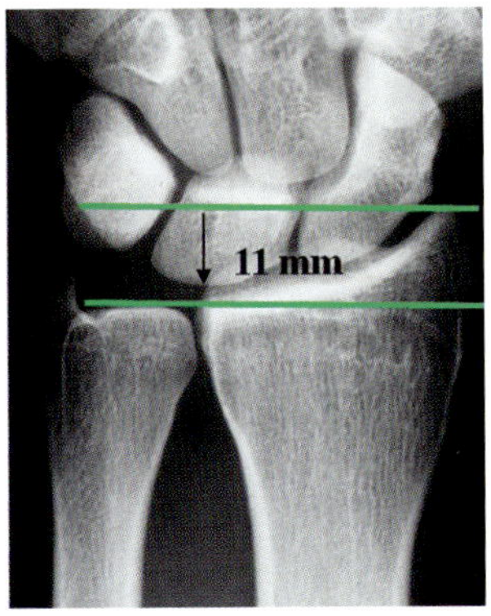


**Fig 3.6-5** Radial length is assessed as the distance between the apex of the radial styloid and the level of the ulnar head at the distal radioulnar joint.

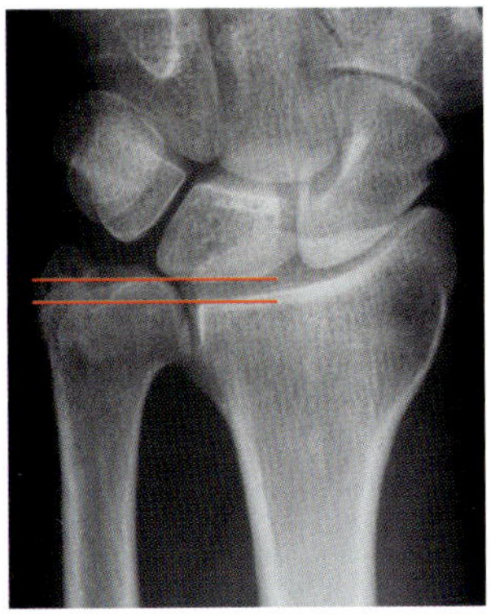

**Fig 3.6-6** Ulnar variance is defined as the difference in axial length between the central point of the ulnar corner of the sigmoid notch of the distal radius and the most distal extension of the ulnar head on the AP view.

## 4 Classification

### 4.1 AO/OTA Fracture and Dislocation Classification and others

There are a number of fracture classifications, such as AO/OTA, Frykman, Melone, Fernandez, Pechlaner, etc, and no single gold standard system. Andersen et al [13] compared the Frykman, Melone, Mayo, and AO/OTA classification systems and reported a low degree of interobserver and intraobserver agreement for plain x-rays. Arealis et al [14] reported that even the use of CT scans does not increase the interobserver or intraobserver reliability for various classification systems.

In scientific papers comparing results of DRFs, the AO/OTA classification is most often used. Eponyms describe the fracture pattern more clearly, as for example a Colles' fracture defined as dorsally and a Smith's fracture as palmarly displaced.

### 4.2 Frequently used eponyms

#### 4.2.1 Colles' fracture

Colles' fracture is a fracture of the distal radius with dorsal and radial displacement of the wrist and hand. Dorsal metaphyseal comminution is typical. The fracture is sometimes referred to as a "dinner fork" or "bayonet" deformity due to the shape of the resultant forearm (**Fig 3.6-7**) [15].

#### 4.2.2 Smith's fracture

This fracture of the distal radius is also sometimes known as a reverse Colles' fracture or Goyrand-Smith's fracture. The distal fracture fragment is displaced palmarly, as opposed to a Colles' fracture where the fragment is displaced dorsally. Depending on the severity of the impact, there may be one or many fragments, and it may or may not involve the articular surface of the wrist joint (**Fig 3.6-8**). Smith's fractures are less common than Colles' fractures [16].

#### 4.2.3 Barton's fracture

This fracture is an intraarticular fracture of the distal radius with dislocation of the radiocarpal joint. There are two types of Barton's fractures, ie, dorsal and palmar, the latter being more common. The Barton's fracture is caused by a fall on an extended and pronated wrist, increasing carpal compression force on the dorsal rim. The intraarticular component distinguishes this fracture from a Smith's or a Colles' fracture (**Fig 3.6-9**) [17].

#### 4.2.4 Chauffeur's fracture

This intraarticular fracture of the radial styloid process with subluxation of the carpus, which is attached to the styloid fracture fragment, is also known as a Hutchinson's fracture or backfire fracture. The radial styloid is within the fracture fragment, although the fragment can vary markedly in size. The fracture extends proximally in a variable oblique direction from essentially transverse to almost sagittal from the distal radial articular surface through the lateral cortex of the distal radius, thus separating the radial styloid from the rest of the radius (**Fig 3.6-10**) [18, 19].

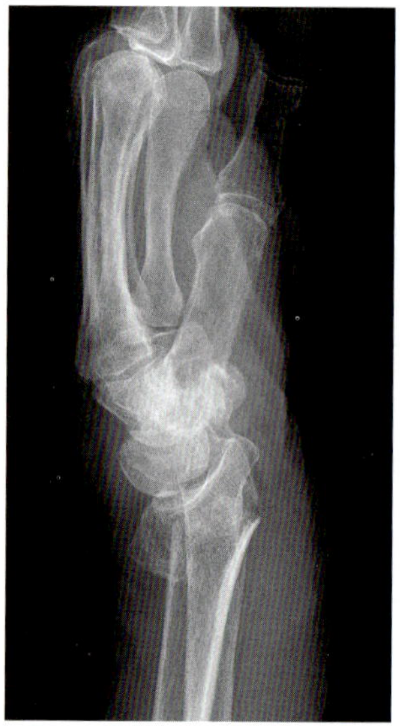

**Fig 3.6-7** Colle's fracture—dorsal displacement of the distal fracture fragment with dorsal metaphyseal comminution.

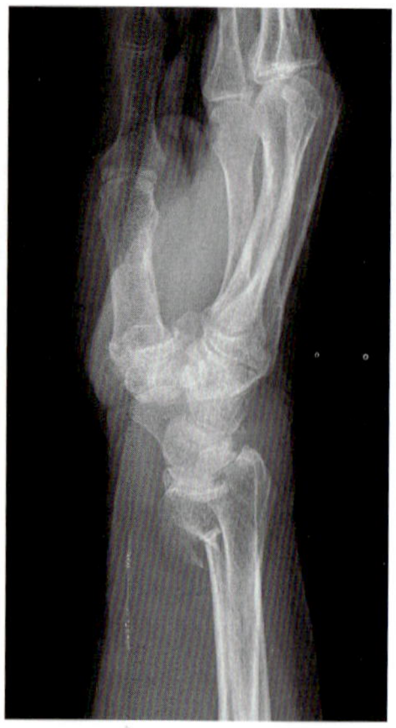

**Fig 3.6-8** Smith's fracture—palmar displacement of the distal fracture fragment.

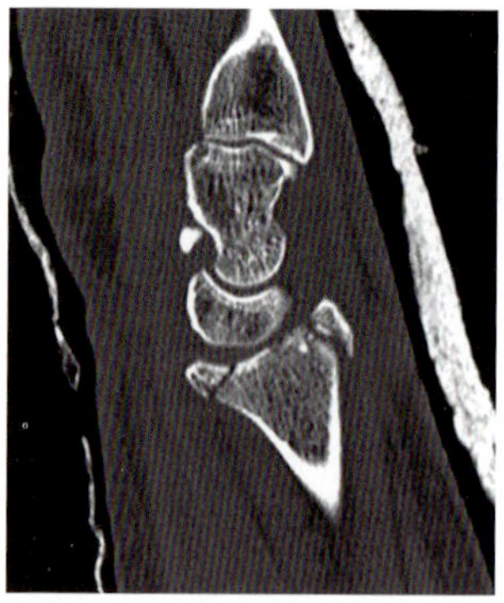

**Fig 3.6-9** Barton's fracture—fracture dislocation with either dorsal or palmar displacement of the carpus together with the fracture fragment.

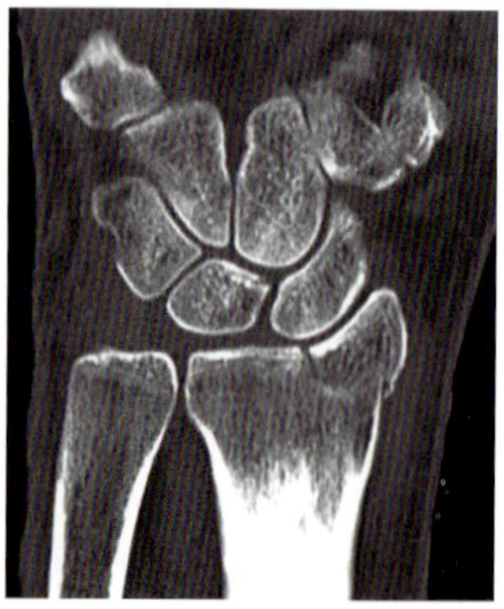

**Fig 3.6-10** Chauffeur's fracture—radial styloid fracture with subluxation of the carpus attached to the styloid fracture fragment.

### 4.3 The three-column concept

This concept by Rikli et al [20] helps understand the fracture pattern in complex and intraarticular DRFs:

- The radial column includes the radial styloid with the scaphoid facet.
- The intermediate column consists of the lunate facet and the sigmoid notch, forming the distal radioulnar joint.
- The ulnar column consists of the distal ulna along with the triangular fibrocartilaginous complex (TFCC).

### 4.4 Distal forearm fractures

Distal ulnar head and/or ulnar neck fractures associated with DRFs are defined as DFFs. Isolated ulnar styloid fractures must be distinguished from distal ulnar fractures (DUF). In 6% of cases, widely displaced DRFs in older adults are associated with DUF [21]. Of those, 13% are grade 1 open fractures according to Gustilo and Anderson, where the distal ulnar shaft penetrates the skin on the ulnar side.

### 4.5 Fracture dislocations

In these fracture patterns, the carpus follows either the palmar or the dorsal fracture fragment (usually the palmar or dorsal rim fragment of the intermediate column, lunate facet fragment) and leads to a carpal subluxation. Fracture dislocations should be treated operatively even in older adults.

### 4.6 Practical approach

Instead of using strict classification systems, we usually describe the following parameters:

- Palmar or dorsal displacement of the distal fracture fragment. As palmarly displaced DRFs, these should be treated operatively.
- Intraarticular or extraarticular fracture characteristics help describe the fracture severity.
- Metaphyseal comminution results in increased instability.
- Palmar or dorsal depression (die-punch fragment) of the intermediate column (lunate facet), the critical corner involving the DRUJ), is a factor (**Fig 3.6-11**).
- Any signs of fracture displacement with small palmar (teardrop) or dorsal rim fracture where the carpus follows the fracture fragment resulting in radiocarpal subluxation (**Fig 3.6-12**).
- Associated fractures of the ulnar column (ie, distal ulnar fracture) (**Fig 3.6-13**). These increase the instability and require treatment of the ulnar column.
- Associated carpal or soft-tissue injuries (**Fig 3.6-14**). These require additional treatment (eg, suture of intrinsic ligaments).

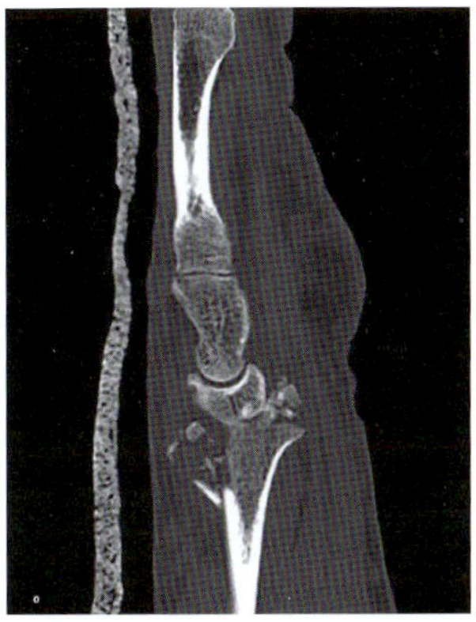

**Fig 3.6-11** Lateral x-ray view of an 89-year-old female patient with palmar and dorsal depression (die-punch fragment) of the intermediate column (lunate facet); the critical corner of the intermediate column is the die-punch fragment which includes the distal radioulnar joint.

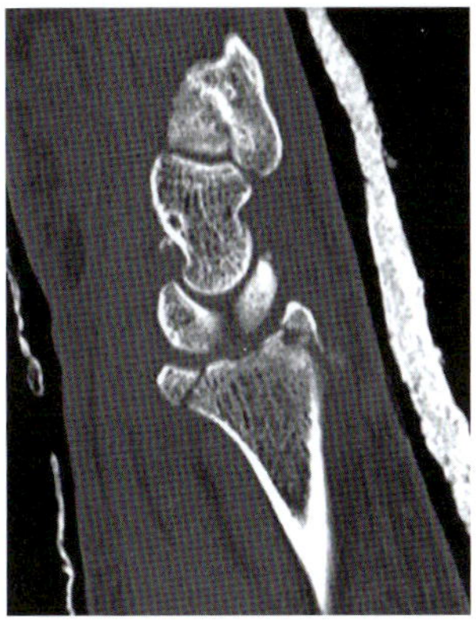

**Fig 3.6-12** Fracture dislocation with small palmar (teardrop) or dorsal rim fracture. The carpus follows the fracture fragment resulting in radiocarpal subluxation.

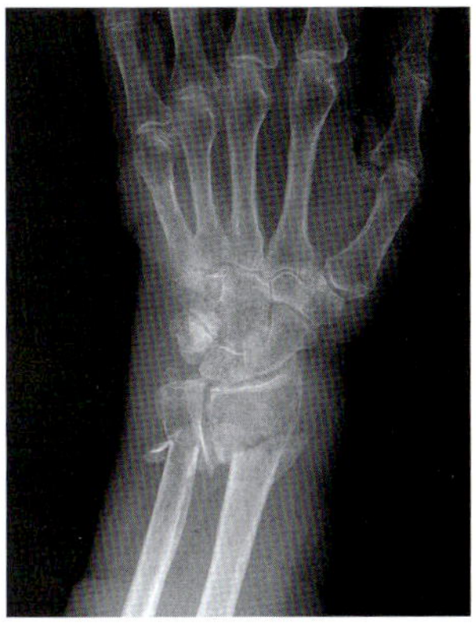

**Fig 3.6-13** AP view of an 84-year-old female patient with distal radial fracture and associated fractures of the ulnar column.

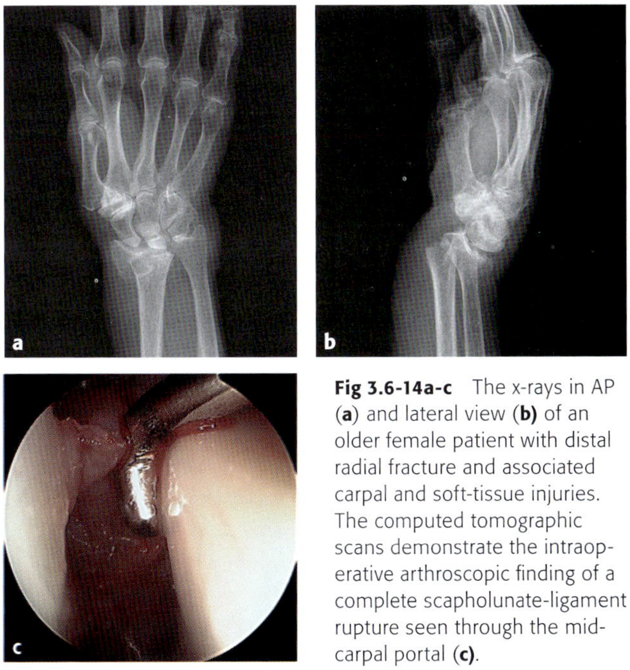


**Fig 3.6-14a-c** The x-rays in AP (**a**) and lateral view (**b**) of an older female patient with distal radial fracture and associated carpal and soft-tissue injuries. The computed tomographic scans demonstrate the intraoperative arthroscopic finding of a complete scapholunate-ligament rupture seen through the midcarpal portal (**c**).

## 5 Decision making

The treatment of DRF in older adults is controversial. Stable fractures can be treated with cast immobilization, usually with satisfactory outcomes. For unstable DRFs in which fracture reduction cannot be maintained with cast immobilization, additional fixation is suggested. Some authors have suggested that unstable DRFs should be managed nonoperatively because fracture reduction and anatomical alignment on x-rays are not correlated with better functional outcomes in older adults. On the other hand, several case series have documented excellent results of internal fixation with very low complication rates of dorsally displaced DRF with the use of locking implants in this population (see Rikli et al [22]).

### 5.1 Fracture manipulation versus splinting

Historically, displaced DRFs were reduced under local or general anesthesia in the emergency department and then immobilized with a below elbow plaster cast. Fracture reduction was assessed using x-rays after closed reduction and cast application. Nowadays it is controversial if acute DRF should be reduced initially in older adults for the following reasons:

- Decreased bone mineral density (BMD) is associated with DRF instability and a 50% risk for secondary displacement after closed reduction and casting [23].
- There is a high incidence in loss of reduction after cast treatment; 30% displace during the first 10 days and another 29% after 10 days [24].
- Closed remanipulation after secondary displacement in patients treated nonoperatively is not successful [25].
- There is no correlation identified between fracture classification, initial displacement, or final radiographic outcome in low demand patients, particularly in those with dementia in nursing homes [26].
- The risk for displacement with an unacceptable radiographic result increases in patients older than 58 years [23].
- Sakai et al [27] reported a significant correlation between increasing displacement of distal fracture fragment and lower BMD.

Patient age has been shown to correlate with fracture instability. Cumulative risk factors for the loss of reduction are:

- Age greater than 60 years
- More than 20° of dorsal angulation or 5 mm of radial shortening
- Dorsal comminution
- Ulnar fracture or intraarticular radiocarpal involvement [28]

Osteoporosis weakens the metaphyseal bone by decreasing trabecular bone volume, commonly resulting in a large metaphyseal void after reduction, which increases fracture instability [29, 30]. Nesbitt et al [23] reported that age is the only significant risk factor in predicting secondary displacement and instability in DRFs treated by closed reduction and immobilization. Considering these outcomes, the question arises whether reduction of displaced DRFs should be attempted. After reduction, the majority of these fractures will lose reduction and go on to radiographic malunion, but without evidence that this reliably leads to poor functional outcome. In our practice closed fracture reduction by fracture manipulation is indicated only in specific situations such as:

- Simple fractures with dorsal angulation less than 20° and radial shortening of less than 5 mm, as fracture manipulation is more likely to lead to better anatomical fracture reduction [31].
- If patients are polytraumatized.
- If surgery is planned, in cases where the soft tissues are at risk or nerves are compressed by fracture fragments.

In most other situations, painful fracture manipulations can be avoided. Finger trap traction and below elbow cast application without any fracture manipulation as initial treatment option for acute DRF is suggested. After decrease of swelling, the cast is changed without any further manipulation. Wrists are immobilized in a short arm cast in a neutral position for 5 weeks. Active finger exercises are started immediately. After cast removal, physiotherapy is recommended.

### 5.2 Operative versus nonoperative

Several studies have demonstrated a high correlation between the anatomical result and the functional outcome in young, active, and high-functioning patients. Malunion of distal radial fractures can result in posttraumatic wrist arthrosis and unsatisfactory functional outcomes with a deformed and painful wrist [32, 33]. Thus, restoring articular congruity and radial length with open reduction and internal fixation (ORIF) is recommended for the treatment of DRFs in younger patients [34, 35].

The therapeutic choice in FFPs is often inappropriately based on the results of fracture treatment in much younger patients [32]. Distal radial fractures are a good example illustrating how decision making in older patients should differ considerably:

- Older patients are a heterogenous group and with diverse demands.
- Comorbidities contribute to increased perioperative risk.
- Consequences of malunited fractures are much less predictable and often clinically insignificant.

Presently, there is no consensus regarding the best treatment for unstable DRFs in the older population [36].

In a single center prospective trial, the authors randomized 73 patients with a displaced and unstable DRF to ORIF with a palmar locking plate or to closed reduction and cast immobilization. There were no significant differences between the groups in terms of the range of motion (ROM) or pain relief during the entire follow-up period ($P > .05$). Patients in the operative group had lower Arm, Shoulder and Hand (DASH) and Patient-Rated Wrist Evaluation (PRWE) scores, indicating better wrist function in the early postoperative time period ($P < .05$), but there were no significant differences between the groups at 6 and 12 months. However, grip strength was significantly better at all times in the operative group ($P < .05$). Furthermore, dorsal radial tilt, radial inclination, and radial shortening were significantly better in the operative than in the nonoperative treatment group at the time of the latest follow-up ($P < .05$). The number of complications was significantly higher in the operative treatment group (thirteen compared with five, $P < .05$). At the 12-month follow-up examination, the ROM, pain rating, and the PRWE and DASH scores were not different between the operative and nonoperative treatment groups (**Case 1: Fig 3.6-15**, **Fig 3.6-16**) [37].

Achieving anatomical reconstruction did not produce any improvement in ROM or ability to perform ADLs [37].

Treatment of DRFs not only depends on patient age but also on geographic variation, local culture, the surgeon's training, or on the surgeon's age [38, 39]. Nelson et al [40] reported that even among highly active older adults, distal radius malunion did not affect functional outcomes.

CASE 1

**Patient**

A 78-year-old woman with a distal radial fracture.

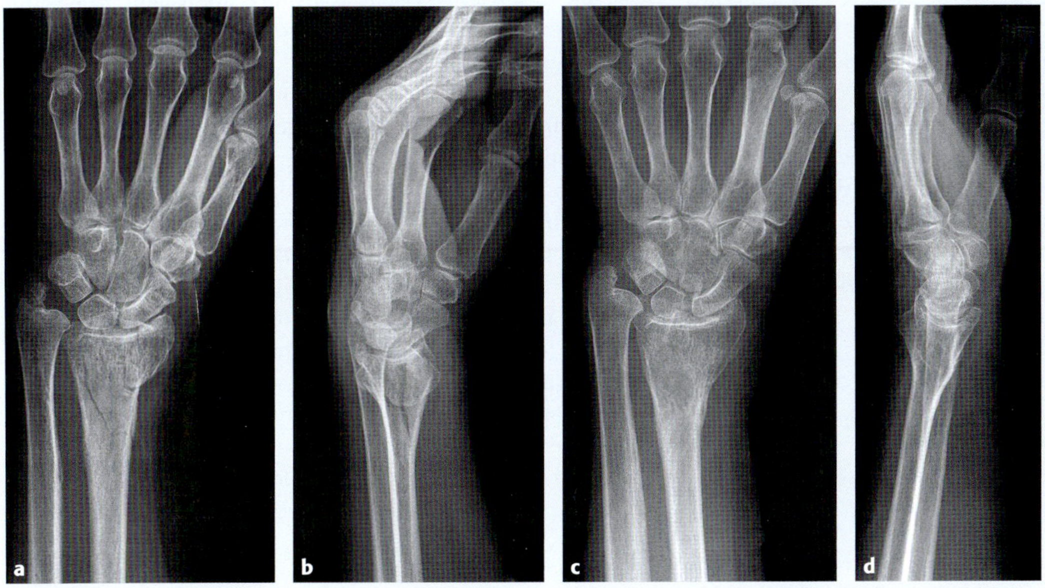


**Fig 3.6-15a–h**

**a–b** Initial x-rays showing AP and lateral views.

**c–d** The radiographic outcome after fracture healing.

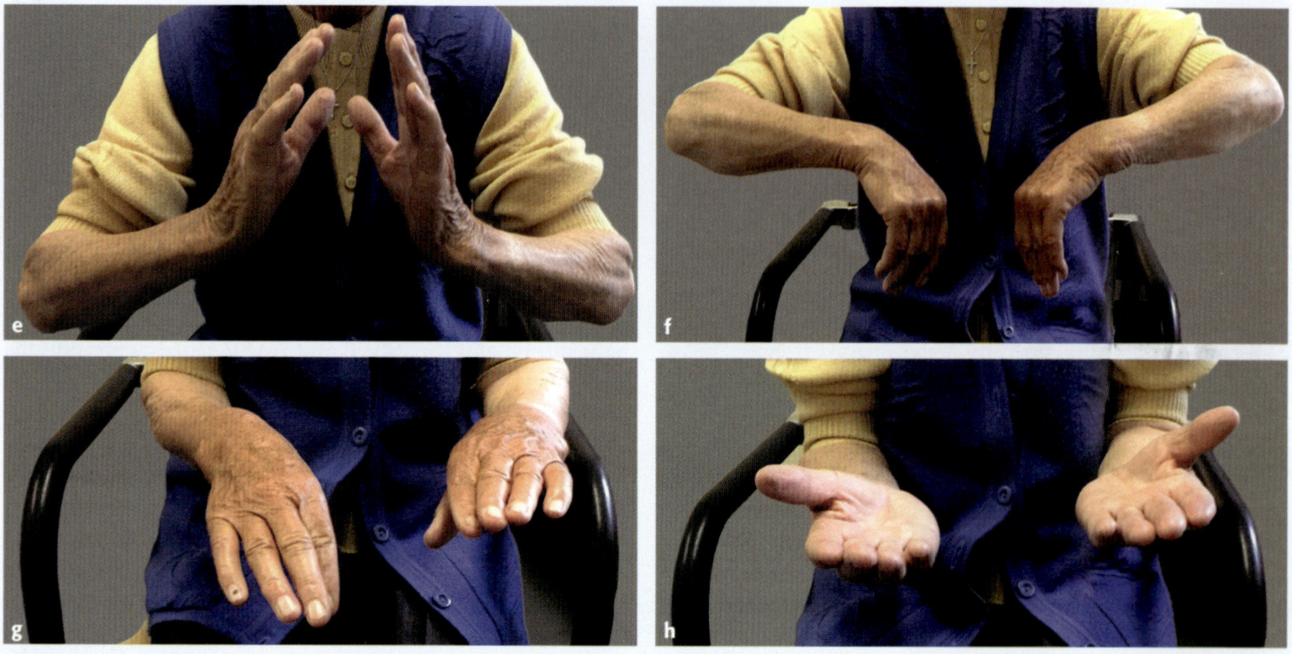

**Fig 3.6-15a–h (cont)** Functional outcome of the same 78-year-old patient in flexion (**e**), extension (**f**), pronation (**g**) and supination (**h**).

Chung et al [41] systematically reviewed the literature for the treatment options of DRFs in patients older than 60 years treated with five common techniques, ie, palmar locking plate system, nonbridging external fixator (EF), bridging EF, percutaneous K-wire fixation and cast immobilization. The authors concluded that despite worse radiographic results in the group with cast immobilization, functional results were not different from those in the operatively treated groups. There were no significant differences for all five treatment groups regarding active ROM, grip strength or the DASH scores though significantly better radiographic results were noticed in the group treated with palmar locking plates. Major complications not requiring reoperation were mostly in the group of bridging EF, whereas major complications requiring secondary surgeries were found in the palmar locking plate group.

The main goal of surgeons treating older adults with DRFs should be a pain-free patient with satisfactory functional hand and wrist motion for performance of ADLs, specifically in hygiene, feeding and mobility.

Decision making for operative or nonoperative treatment must involve the patient. Patients and caregivers should be informed that:

- Nonoperatively treated unstable DRFs will end up in malunion and a visible deformity. Some patients will not accept the visible deformity of malunion and therefore surgery should be considered for them.
- Not all malunions are symptomatic and if there will be a symptomatic malunion, there exist options to treat this condition later [42].

After DRFs, pain, grip strength, and ROM continue to improve for up to 2–4 years. Patients with malunion had more disability at 1 year but showed significant improvement at 2–4 years [43]. The poor correlation between the radiographic and functional outcomes in older adults might be related to decreased functional demand on the wrist associated with aging [44]. In summary, there are no significant differences between long-term functional outcomes after nonoperative or operative treatment of unstable DRFs in older adults, save better grip strength in those treated with palmar locking plates.

### 5.2.1 Fracture-related factors

Nondisplaced DRFs are treated nonoperatively. For the following fracture patterns, we recommend standard operative fixation even in older adults:

- Palmarly displaced DRF where the carpus is malaligned relatively to the forearm shaft (**Fig 3.6-16**) [45].

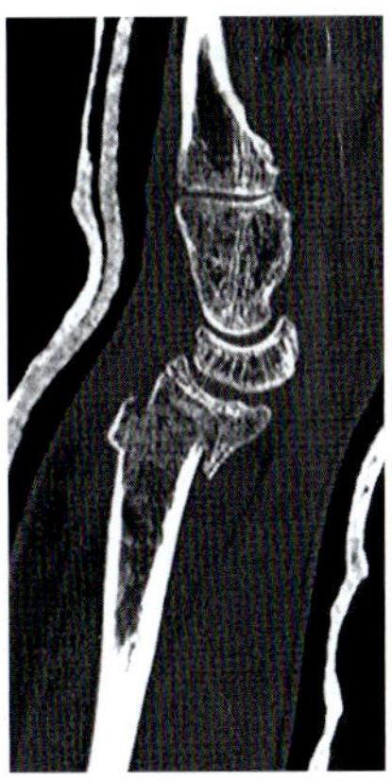

**Fig 3.6-16** The computed tomographic scan in the sagittal plane of a 76-year-old female patient shows a palmarly displaced distal radial fracture.

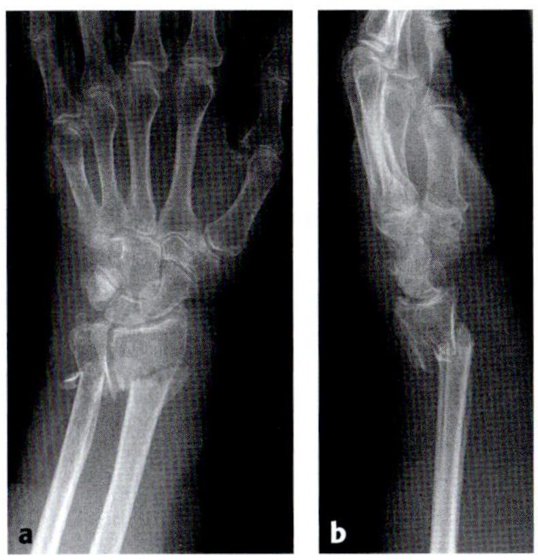

**Fig 3.6-17a–b** AP (**a**) and lateral (**b**) views show a distal radial fracture combined with a distal ulnar fracture. The involvement of all three columns leads to a highly unstable situation.

- Distal radial fracture combined with distal ulnar fracture and involvement of all three columns leads to a highly unstable situation. Nonoperative treatment will end up in severe malunion (**Fig 3.6-17**). Nonoperative treatment of these fractures leads to unpredictable results. Malalignment of the radius and ulna as well as disruption of the DRUJ cause functional impairment of forearm rotation and wrist motion [21]. Failure to achieve stable anatomical reduction and congruity of the DRUJ compromises the ability to reestablish ulnar variance and stability of the DRUJ, which may cause local dysfunction, nonunions of the distal radius and ulna, ulnar-sided wrist pain, and posttraumatic arthritis [46–48]. Malalignment with angular deformity of DUF of more than 10° in any direction, translation of more than half of the ulnar head relative to the radius, and articular displacement are considered to be unstable and ORIF of DUFs is recommended [49].
- For open fractures (**Fig 3.6-18**) and displaced fractures (**Fig 3.6-19**, see topic 4.2.3 in this chapter) operative fixation is recommended.

In unstable DRFs, where fracture reduction cannot be maintained with cast immobilization, additional fixation is suggested [25].

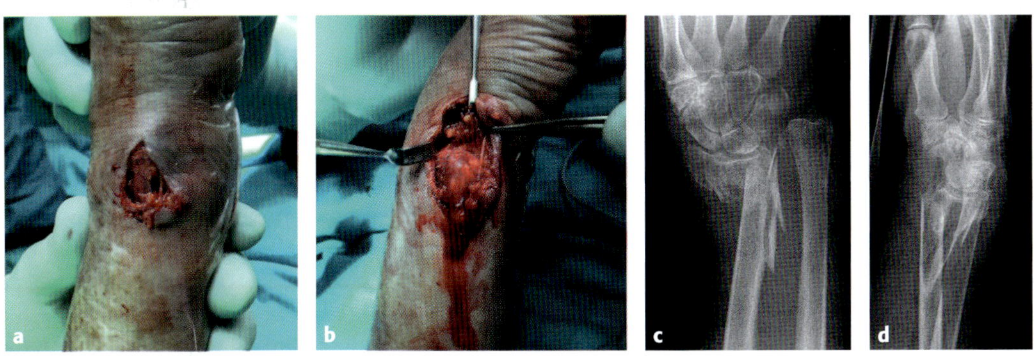

**Fig 3.6-18a–d** Preoperative finding (**a–b**) and an x-ray in AP (**c**) and lateral (**d**) views of an 89-year-old female patient with an open distal radial fracture.

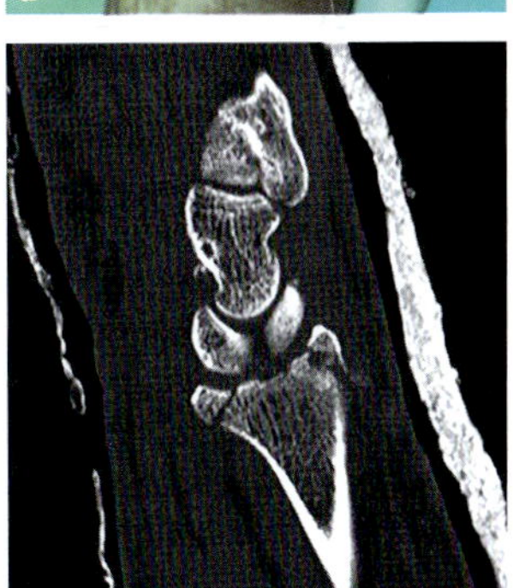

**Fig 3.6-19** The computed tomographic scan of a 76-year-old female patient shows a displaced distal radial fracture after closed reduction (see topic 4.2.3 in this chapter).

### 5.2.2 Patient-related factors

Because of the variabilty in patient demands, functional outcomes, and individual patient perioperative risk, the factors in **Table 3.6-1** should be included in the decision-making process:

| In favor of operative management | In favor of nonoperative management |
|---|---|
| Younger age | Advanced age |
| Short immobilization time | Risk of postoperative delirium |
| High level of acitivity and independence | Low demand with a low level of activity |
| Low Charlson Comorbidity Index | High Charlson Comorbidity Index |
| Early return to daily and sport activities | High degree of osteoporosis |
| Associated fractures | Dementia |
| High cosmetic demand | Frailty |

**Table 3.6-1** Patient-related factors to be included in decision making.

## 5.3 Choice of implants

### 5.3.1 Percutaneous pinning

Pinning alone may not be enough to maintain articular and metaphyseal support, as K-wires are not load-bearing devices. Additionally, a forearm splint is necessary to neutralize the bending forces across the metaphysis. The wires are left up to 4 weeks and the forearm cast is worn for 6 weeks. Percutaneous pinning is a relative simple method of fixation that is recommended for reducible extraarticular and simple intraarticular DRFs without metaphyseal comminution and with good bone quality. In multifragmented intraarticular fractures with impacted joint fragments it is quite difficult to reduce these fragments by percutaneous pinning. In these cases, other procedures like a plate osteosynthesis might be the appropriate therapy option.

Azzopardi et al [50] concluded that percutaneous pinning of unstable, extraarticular DRFs provides only minimal improvement in the radiographic parameters compared with immobilization in a cast alone. This did not correlate with an improved functional outcome in older adults.

### 5.3.2 External fixation

External fixation as a treatment option for DRFs was primarily reserved for highly unstable and severely comminuted fractures where reconstruction of the articular surface seemed impossible, in open fractures with soft-tissue problems, and as a part of orthopedic damage control in polytraumatized patients.

In a prospective randomized study, Roumen et al [51] compared external fixation with closed reduction and immobilization for redisplaced DRFs in patients older than 55 years. Patients treated with EF had significantly better radiographic results with no difference in function.

In general, major complications associated with external fixation and percutaneous pinning are pin-track infection and iatrogenic injury of the superficial radial nerve. Overdistraction of the wrist joint may lead to complex regional pain syndrome (CRPS) [52]. Especially in osteoporotic bone, with weak bony purchase of the pins, additional casting is necessary and loosening of the pins occurs quite early so that they have to be removed before definitive bone healing. Gehrmann et al [53] reported that the risk of pin-track infections is eliminated through the use of ORIF and advises the use of fixed-angle plating of DRF through a palmar approach. Last, adults with cognitive impairment are likely to find it difficult to safely comply with EF and weight bearing or ROM limitations, making complications due to EF more likely. Because of these issues, we no longer use percutaneous K-wire fixation or external fixation as definitive treatment option for treating unstable DRF in the FFP.

### 5.3.3 Plating

Open reduction and internal fixation allows anatomical reduction and stable fixation with early postoperative wrist mobilization. As DRFs are hyperextension injuries and the dorsal cortex of the distal radius is weak, most displace dorsally. Traditionally, all dorsally displaced DRFs were treated through a dorsal approach using a dorsal buttress plate. The problems of dorsal plating are extensor tenosynovitis with tendon rupture due to hardware prominence. To improve this, special low-profile steel plates and dorsal Pi-shaped plates were designed [54]. To adapt to the anatomy of the dorsal distal radius, the Pi-plate was designed to fit close to the dorsal aspect around the Lister's tubercle. However, Campbell [55] reported attrition ruptures of extensor tendons after dorsal Pi-plate application and Kambouroglou and Axelrod [56] described tendon ruptures and failure of the Pi-plate system.

In biomechanical evaluations, the palmar fixed-angle plate is efficient in restoring the normal axial force distribution, superior to conventional palmar and dorsal T-plate fixation [57]. The fixed-angle screws lock into the plate and do not rely on engagement of the screw threads in bone, leading to better fixation especially in osteoporotic bone. The other advantage of locking plates is the good subchondral support of the distal fragments even in very short distal fracture fragments. The latest generation of locking plates offer the option of variable locking screws, which allow a total angulation of 30° for screw placement.

In a prospective multicenter study, Rikli et al [22, 58] did not find that poor bone quality increased the risk of loss of reduction, screw and plate pull-out for patients older than 50 years with DRFs treated with palmar locking plates. In patients with an average low local BMD, the authors showed that treatment with a palmar locking plate was associated with a low risk of complications related to fracture type and implant.

## 6 Therapeutic options—radial fractures

### 6.1 Closed reduction and cast immobilization

Especially in nondisplaced DRF, an obvious hematoma of the third dorsal extensor compartment should be evacuated to avoid secondary rupture of the extensor pollicis longus (EPL) tendon (**Fig 3.6-20**) [59]. We perform finger trap traction and apply a dorsal below elbow splint without any fracture manipulation as initial treatment. After local edema subsides, the fractured wrist is immobilized in a short arm cast in a neutral position for 5 weeks. Active exercises of the fingers are started immediately. After cast removal, physiotherapy is started.

Fracture reduction should always be performed under local anesthesia or under hematoma block in the emergency department, as follows (**Fig 3.6-21**):

- Application of finger traps to the thumb and index finger with the arm put on horizontal traction with 3 kg using countertraction along the upper arm to disimpact the fracture by ligamentotaxis should be used. After 10 minutes of traction, the initial dorsal displacement is exaggerated to mobilize the distal fracture fragment from the shaft. Direct pressure is then applied to the distal fragment to a palmar direction with a counterpressure on the palmar surface of the forearm. During this maneuver, the palmar cortices are reduced and used as a hinge to manipulate the dorsally displaced fragment into neutral wrist position (closed reduction). While still in traction, a well-molded dorsal splint is applied. A circumferential cast is not recommended to avoid cast-induced compartment syndrome.
- After the primary swelling has decreased, the splint is converted to a below elbow cast.
- In total, DRFs are immobilized in a forearm cast in neutral position of the wrist for 5 weeks. No study has been able to show any significant differences between long and short arm cast for the treatment of DRFs. The elbow, fingers, and the thumb should be left free to avoid stiffness.

Secondary loss of primary reduction can occur up to 2 weeks after primary closed reduction. In these cases, repeated manipulation, especially in the osteoporotic bone, is not recommended and has been associated with the development of CRPS type 1 [26].

Active and passive finger motion is encouraged early. If nonoperative treatment is chosen, cast disease, namely atrophy and joint stiffness, must be avoided. Fingers in older adults may be arthritic and are particularly susceptible to detrimental stiffness if the joints are not moved shortly after injury. Finger stiffness is quite avoidable through early identification and prompt physiotherapy referral. A therapy program after cast removal including active-assisted motion of the wrist and grip strengthening is started at 5 weeks after bone healing.

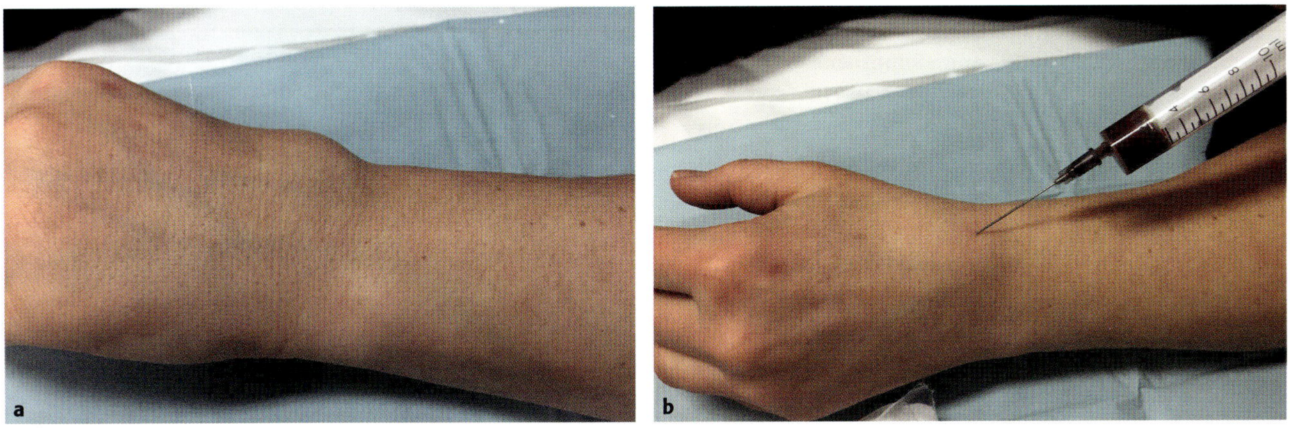

**Fig 3.6-20a–b** Hematoma in the third dorsal extensor compartment before (**a**) and after (**b**) puncture.

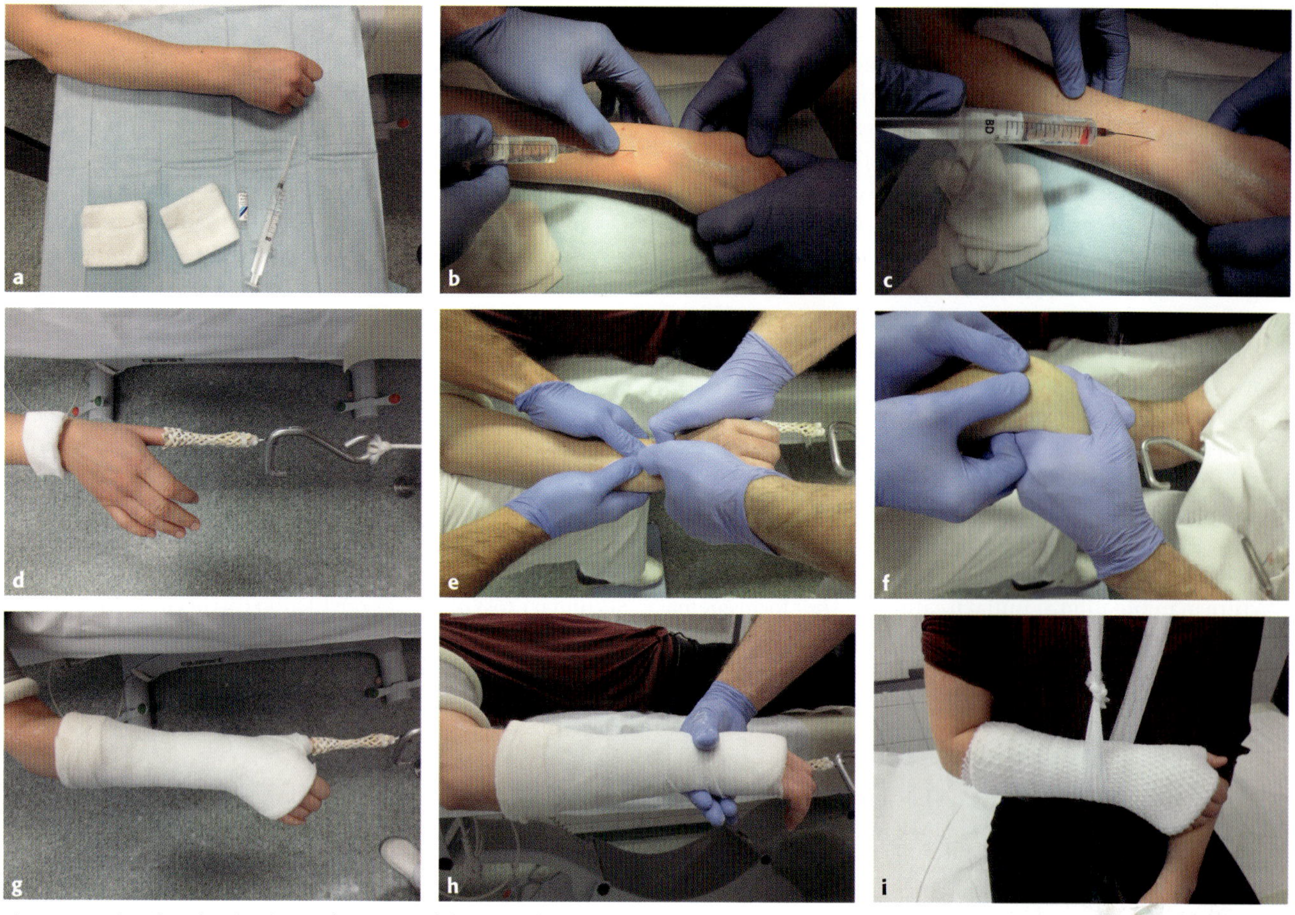

**Fig 3.6-21a–i** Closed reduction and cast immobilization. The fracture hematoma is aspirated to ensure the fracture gap is reached and local anaesthesia is injected (**a–c**). A finger trap is applied and the arm is put on horizontal traction with 3 kg using countertraction along the upper arm to disimpact the fracture by ligamentotaxis (**d**). After traction, the initial dorsal displacement is exaggerated to mobilize the distal fracture fragment from the shaft. Direct pressure is applied to the distal fragment to a palmar direction with a counterpressure on the palmar surface of the forearm. During this maneuver, the palmar cortices are reduced and used as a hinge to manipulate the dorsally displaced fragment into neutral wrist position (**e–f**). While still on traction (**g**), a well-molded dorsal splint is applied (**h–i**).

## 6.2 Palmar locking plate fixation

To overcome the problems that can come with dorsal plating, many authors favor the palmar approach [60]. The most appropriate plates should be selected to correspond with the fracture pattern. There is no single plate that is universally successful or devoid of any potential complications for all types of unstable DRFs, including intraarticular and extraarticular fracture patterns.

Fragment-specific fixation and double plate fixation techniques may be helpful to treat various fracture types, especially intraarticular fractures with a large metaphyseal void (**Fig 3.6-22**):

- Henry palmar approach between the flexor carpi radialis (FCR) tendon and the radial artery.
- The FCR tendon together with the flexor pollicis longus tendon is retracted ulnarly to indirectly protect the median nerve.
- The pronator quadratus muscle is released from its radial insertion and reflected ulnarly to gain access to the fracture site.
- Careful reduction of fracture fragments, as poor bone quality can lead to iatrogenic fractures.

- Insertion of two K-wires from the palmar rim and one percutaneously from the radial styloid under image intensification.
- A fixed-angle plate is first fixed at the gliding hole to allow appropriate plate positioning under image intensifier control proximally to the watershed line, defined as a transverse ridge that closes the concave surface of the palmar radius distally. Distal to this line, the radius slopes in a dorsal-distal direction and becomes prominent palmarly (**Fig 3.6-23**). Plates beyond or distal to the watershed line can exert pressure on the flexor tendons and can cause tendon rupture (**Fig 3.6-24**).
- In intraarticular fractures, wrist arthroscopy detects intraarticular steps and associated soft-tissue injuries.
- In comminuted intraarticular fractures the locking screws are placed in the most distal subcortical position to act as a subcortical buttress against fracture subsidence. The subcortical plate retains greater loading capacity than the osteopenic compressed cancellous metaphyseal bone. Exact drilling with special drill guides that are screwed the distal plate holes is essential to guarantee perfect engagement of the locking screws into the plate. Especially with variable locking plate systems, which allow a range of about 30° of screw insertion, intraarticular screw placement can be performed quite easily. If fracture instability demands distal placement of hardware, close follow-up investigations and hardware removal should be considered at first sign of flexor tendon irritation.
- Intraoperative control with image intensifier is used to check plate and screw position. The lateral tilt x-ray visualizes, with the wrist angulated 20–30°, the articular surface and intraarticular hardware.

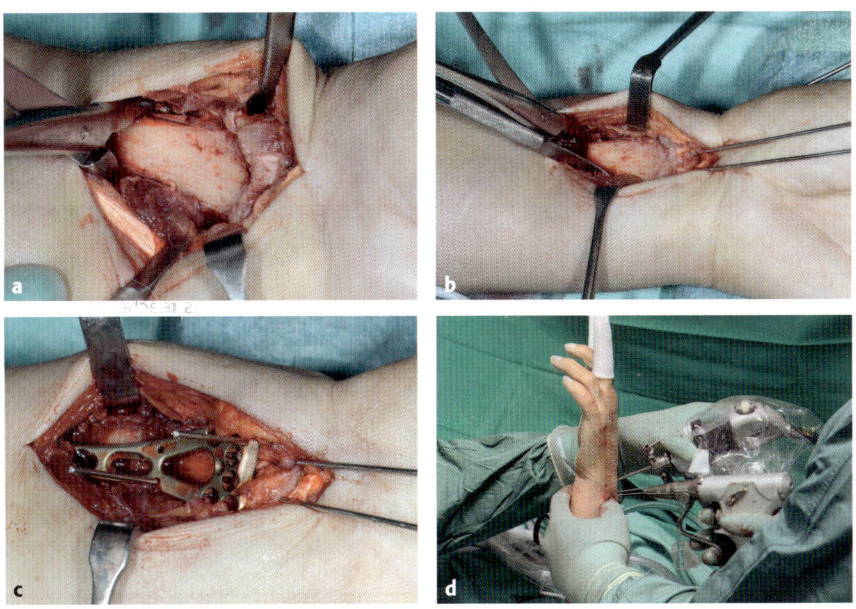

**Fig 3.6-22a–d** After open reduction via a palmar approach (**a**), the fracture is secured with K-wires (**b**) and a palmar distal radial plate is applied (**c**). After an arthroscopic fine-tuning of the articular surface, the plate is adjusted (**d**) and secured by variable angle locking screws.

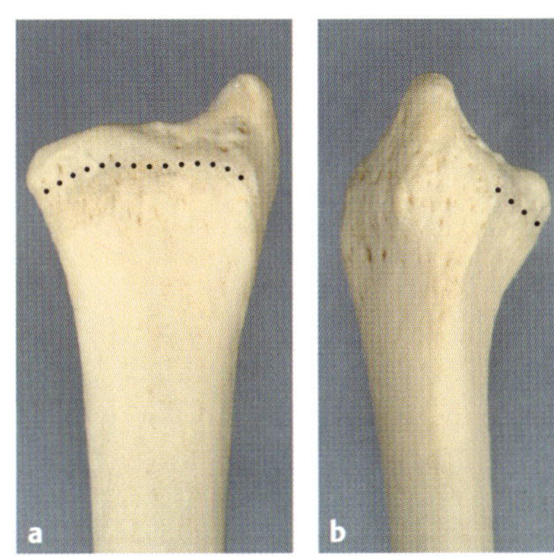

**Fig 3.6-23a–b** The watershed line (black dots) on an anatomical specimen in AP (**a**) and lateral (**b**) views.

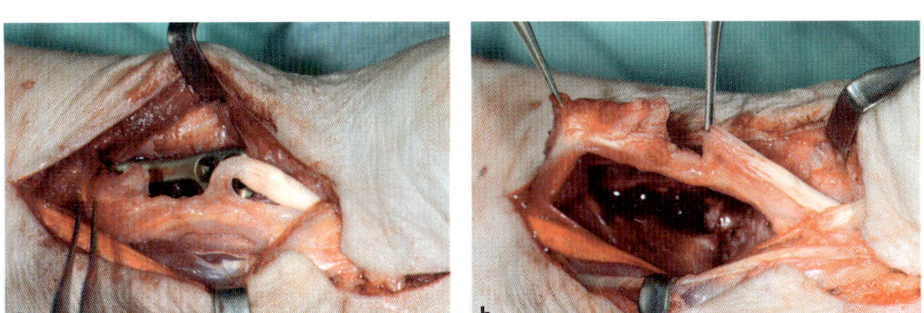

**Fig 3.6-24a–b** Intraoperative situs of a flexor tendon injury of a 70-year-old female patient that occurred 6 months after surgical treatment.

- Extensor tendon ruptures may occur because of excessively long screws overlaying the dorsal cortex (**Fig 3.6-25a**). Because of the triangular shape of the dorsal cortex, the most ulnar and radial screws are typically shorter than the central screws (**Fig 3.6-25b**). The "skyline view" is used to detect excessively long screws penetrating the dorsal cortex (**Fig 3.6-26**) [61].
- Reattachement of the pronator quadratus muscle to protect the flexor tendons (**Case 2: Fig 3.6-27**).

### 6.2.1 Tips and tricks

In comminuted intraarticular and metaphyseal fractures, conventional palmar plates require additional metaphyseal support like bone grafts, bone substitutes, or additional dorsal plates to avoid loss of reduction due to metaphyseal instability. Palmar fixed-angle plates improve mechanical rigidness and make dorsal metaphyseal bone grafting redundant [62]. They act like an internal fixator, unloading the comminuted dorsal metaphyseal bone.

### 6.2.2 Aftercare

Aftercare includes:

- For control of pain and swelling, a below-the-elbow splint can be applied for 1 week. Active digital mobilization is started immediately.
- No immobilization is necessary in extraarticular metaphyseal fractures and in simple intraarticular DRFs where intraoperatively a stable fixation can be achieved.
- Immobilization—in DRFs with metaphyseal void or severe intraarticular involvement, a palmar slab splint is applied for 3 weeks.
- Physiotherapy is helpful. Active and passive wrist mobilization out of the splint can prevent finger and wrist joint stiffness.

## 6.3 Dorsal locking plate fixation

Some fracture patterns require the dorsal approach to address the dorsal ulnar fragment of the lunate fossa as well as a dorsally comminuted fracture. Dorsal plate fixation was associated with higher rates of extensor tendon complications including irritation, synovitis, and rupture due to direct contact with bulky dorsal plates. However, the latest implants are significantly thinner in their profile and the locking mechanism has decreased the number of soft-tissue problems using dorsal plates. Matschke et al [63] compared palmar with dorsal locking plate fixation in DRFs and reported no significant differences in functional results and rate of complications at 2 years.

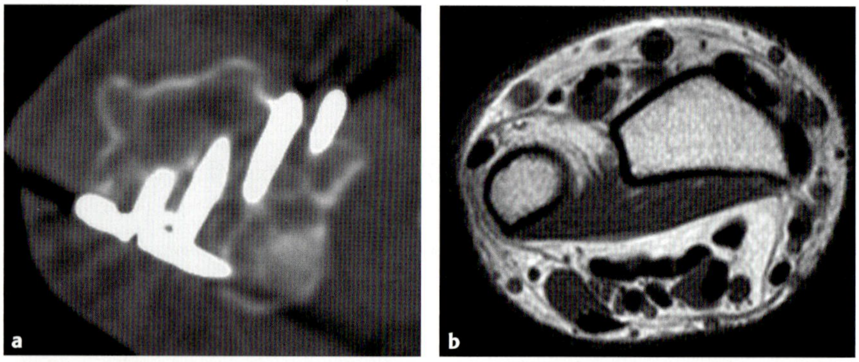


**Fig 3.6-25a–b** Screws are too long, protruding through the dorsal cortex (**a**). Magnetic resonance imaging scan illustrating the triangle shape of the dorsal cortex (**b**).

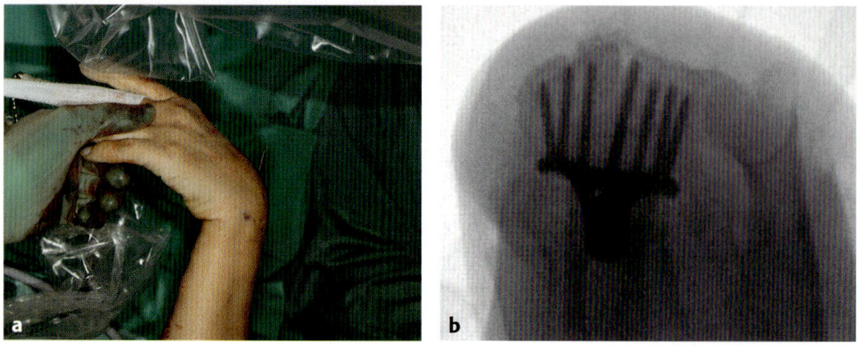


**Fig 3.6-26a–b** Skyline view. The image intensifier is placed on top of the surgical table to perform the skyline views. The elbow is flexed 75° with the forearm in maximum supination and the wrist maximally flexed. Under image intensifier control, the elbow position is changed into flexion or extension until an optimal position is obtained that enables visualization of the dorsal cortex of the radius with its entire width, Lister's tubercle, and the distal radioulnar joint (**a**). In this position screws crossing the dorsal cortex can be visualized and then changed (**b**).

**Patient**

An 86-year-old woman sustained a complex comminuted distal radial fracture with separation of palmar and dorsal articular fragments (**Fig 3.6-27a–d**).

**Treatment and outcome**

To restore the articular surface, a palmar rim plate was used that was covered with a flap of the pronator quadratus muscle (**Fig 3.6-27e–h**). The pronator quadratus muscle was removed on the ulnar side and the plate was attached (**Fig 3.6-27i**). Following anatomical reduction and internal fixation, the pronator quadratus flap was reattached (**Fig 3.6-27j–k**) to protect the flexor tendons (**Fig 3.6-27l**).

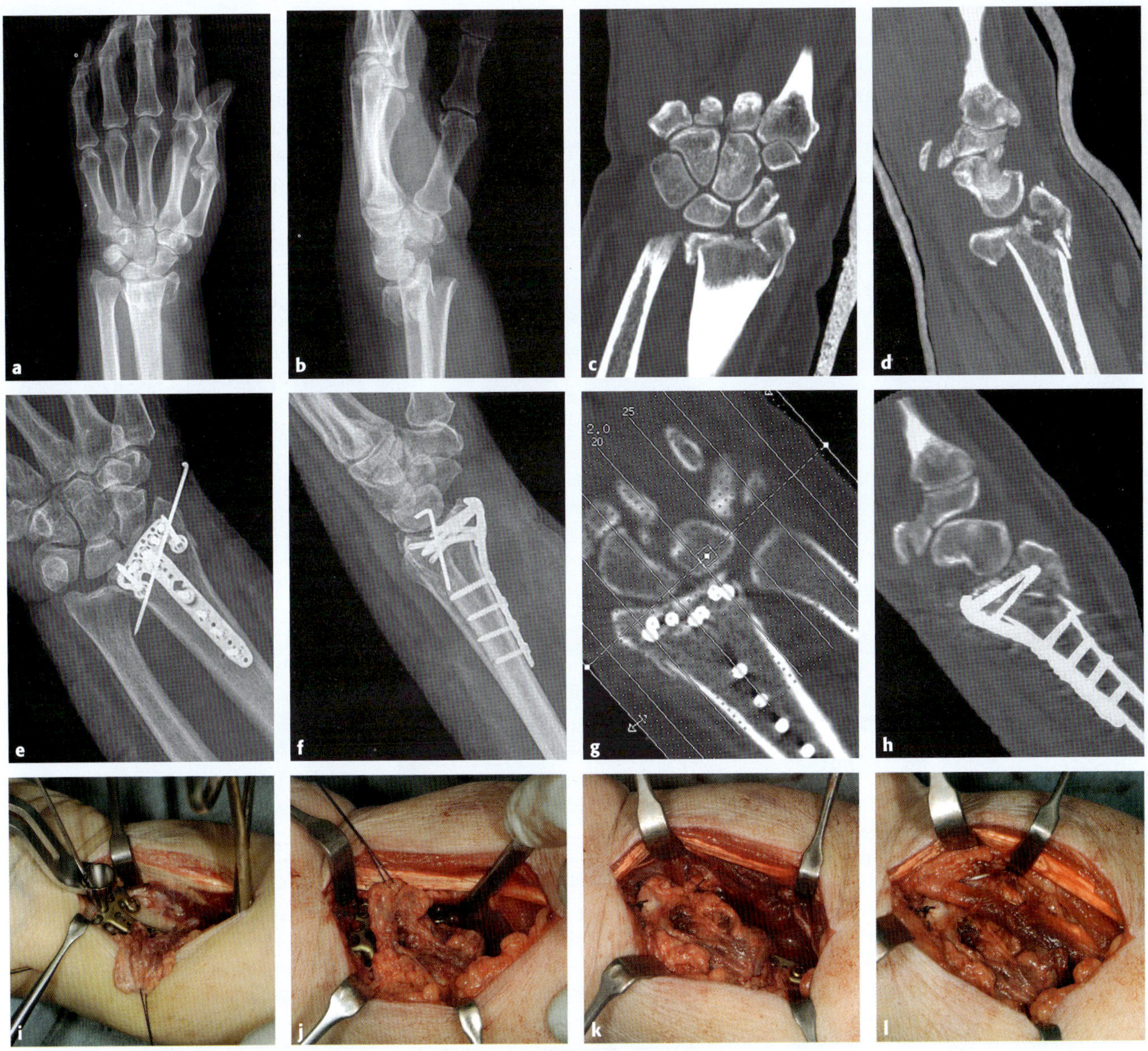


**Fig 3.6-27a–l** An 86-year-old woman with a fracture of the distal radius.
**a–d** X-rays showing a complex comminuted fracture of the distal radius with separated palmar and dorsal articular fragments.
**e–h** Articular surface reconstruction with a palmar rim plate.
**i** Removal of the pronator quadratus muscle on the ulnar side and attachment of the plate.
**j–l** Clinical images showing anatomical reduction and internal fixation followed by reattachment of the pronator quadratus flap (**j–k**) to protect the flexor tendons (**l**).

To prevent extensor tendon problems, a retinaculum flap to cover the implant can be used. In this technique, the extensor retinaculum is divided in two parts, ie, one radially and one ulnarly based. Both flaps are elevated from the fractured Lister's tubercle and the EPL tendon is exposed. After ORIF the ulnarly based retinaculum flap is passed underneath the extensor tendons and is used to cover the distal part of the plate. The radially based flap is fixed ulnarly over the extensor tendons to prevent tendon bowstringing (**Case 3: Fig 3.6-28**, **Case 4: Fig 3.6-29**).

**CASE 3**

### Patient

A 78-year-old man sustained a complex distal radial fracture with comminution and isolated fragments of the radial styloid process together with separation of palmar and dorsal articular fragments (**Fig 3.6-28a–b**).

### Treatment and outcome

As a biological support to avoid loss of reduction due to metaphyseal instability, an allograft was used (**Fig 3.6-28c–d**). One and a half years after surgery, x-ray controls show sufficient healing with incorporation of the graft (**Fig 3.6-28e–f**). Clinically, a very satisfying functional result is seen (**Fig 3.6-28g–j**).

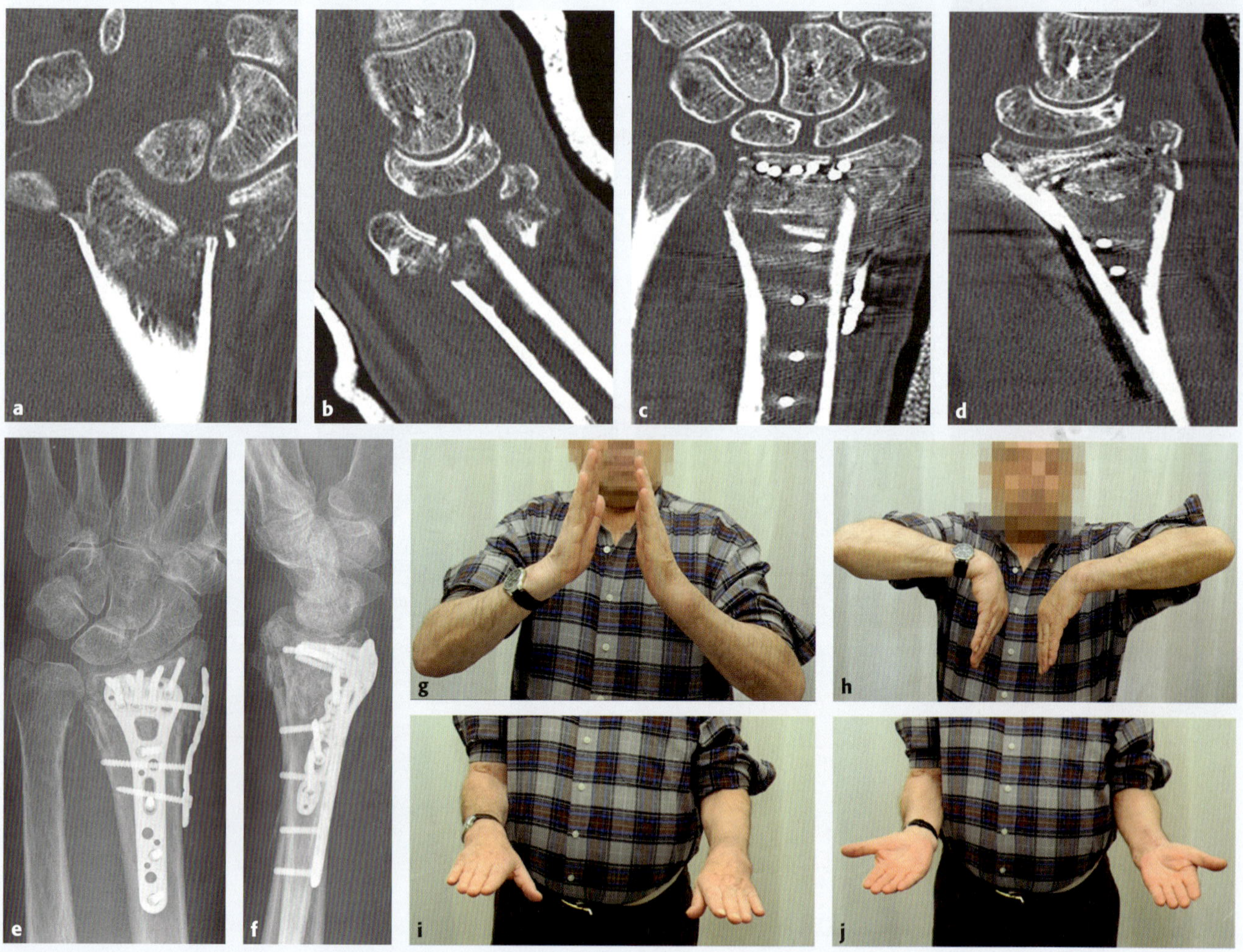


**Fig 3.6-28a–j** A 78-year-old man with a complex distal radial fracture.
**a–b** Complex distal radial fracture with comminution and isolated fragments of the radial styloid process together with separation of palmar and dorsal articular fragments.
**c–d** Use of allograft as a biological support to avoid loss of reduction due to metaphyseal instability.
**e–f** X-rays at 1.5 years postoperative show sufficient healing with incorporation of the graft.
**g–j** Clinical images show a very satisfying functional result.

CASE 4

**Patient**

A 70-year-old man with a multifragmented distal radial fracture with radial impaction and fracture of the styloid process.

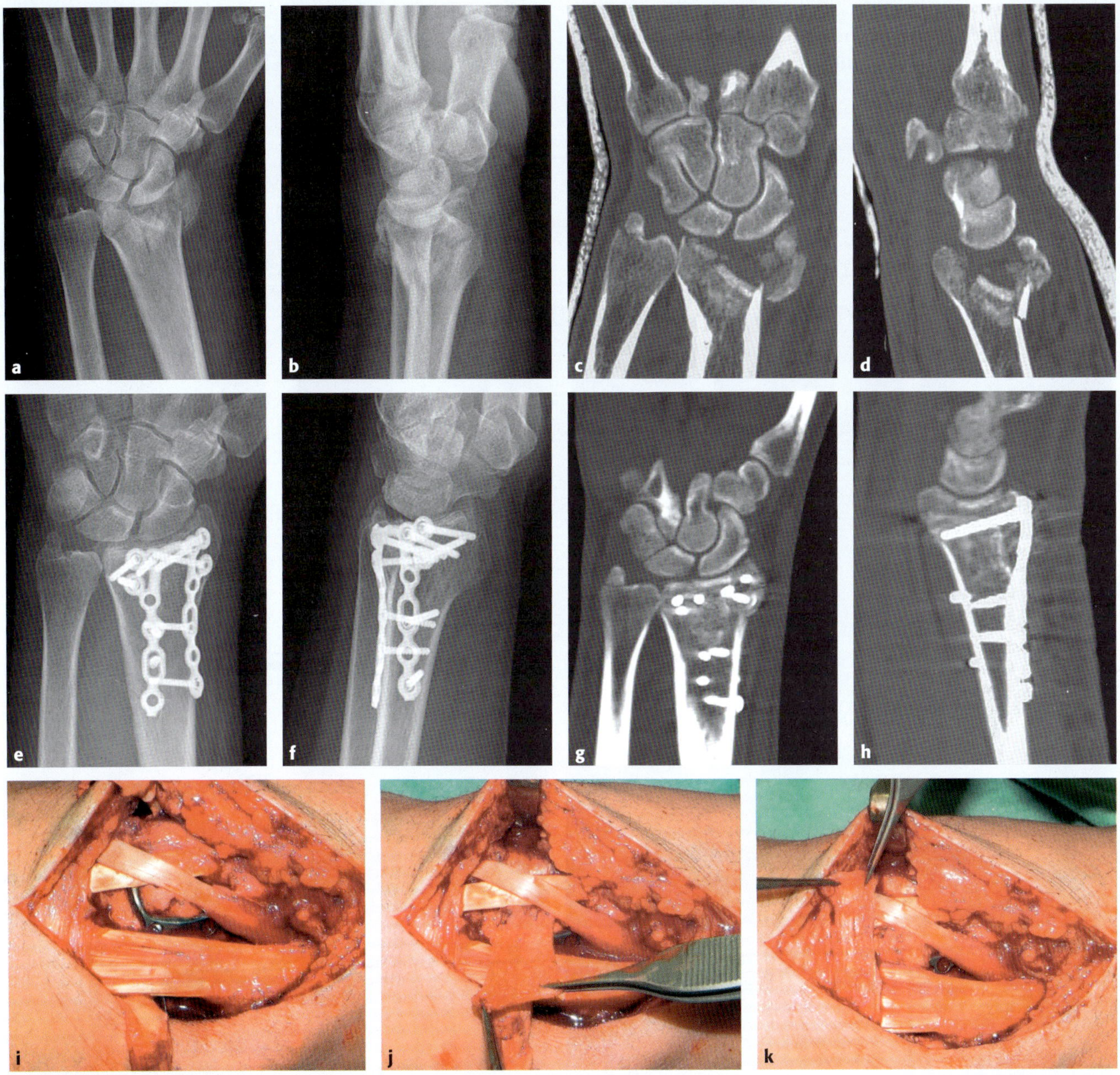


**Fig 3.6-29a–k** Multifragmented distal radial fracture with radial impaction and fracture of the styloid process (**a–d**). For reconstruction, a dorsal plate was applied (**e–h**). To prevent extensor tendon problems, a retinaculum flap to cover the implant was used (**i–j**). The extensor retinaculum was divided in two parts, ie, one radially and one ulnarly based. Both flaps were elevated from the fractured Lister's tubercle and the extensor pollicis longus tendon was exposed (**i**). After open reduction and internal fixation, the ulnarly based retinaculum flap was passed underneath the extensor tendons and was used to cover the distal part of the plate (**j**). The radially based flap was fixed ulnarly over the extensor tendons to prevent tendon bow-stringing (**k**).

## 6.4 Radiocarpal prosthesis

Following the concept of primary joint replacement in proximal and distal humeral fractures in older adults, Herzberg et al [64] described the primary use of wrist hemiarthroplasty in multifragmented, impacted, and irreparable acute DRFs in an older cohort. Participants had an average age of 76 years and some comorbidities but were living at home and were independent in ADLs. Hemiarthroplasty produced earlier return to preinjury independence in daily activities with shorter operative time and fewer complications compared to palmar plating (**Case 5: Fig 3.6-30**) [64].

**CASE 5**

### Patient

A 77-year-old woman with status postmastectomy due to breast cancer sustained a multifragmented, impacted, and irreparable acute distal radial fracture (**Fig 3.6-30a–b**).

### Treatment and outcome

Following the concept of primary replacement, wrist hemiprosthesis was implanted (**Fig 3.6-30c–d**). Ten months after surgery, the patient showed a good clinical outcome and mobility despite a residual lymphatic swelling due to the mastectomy (**Fig 3.6-30e–h**).

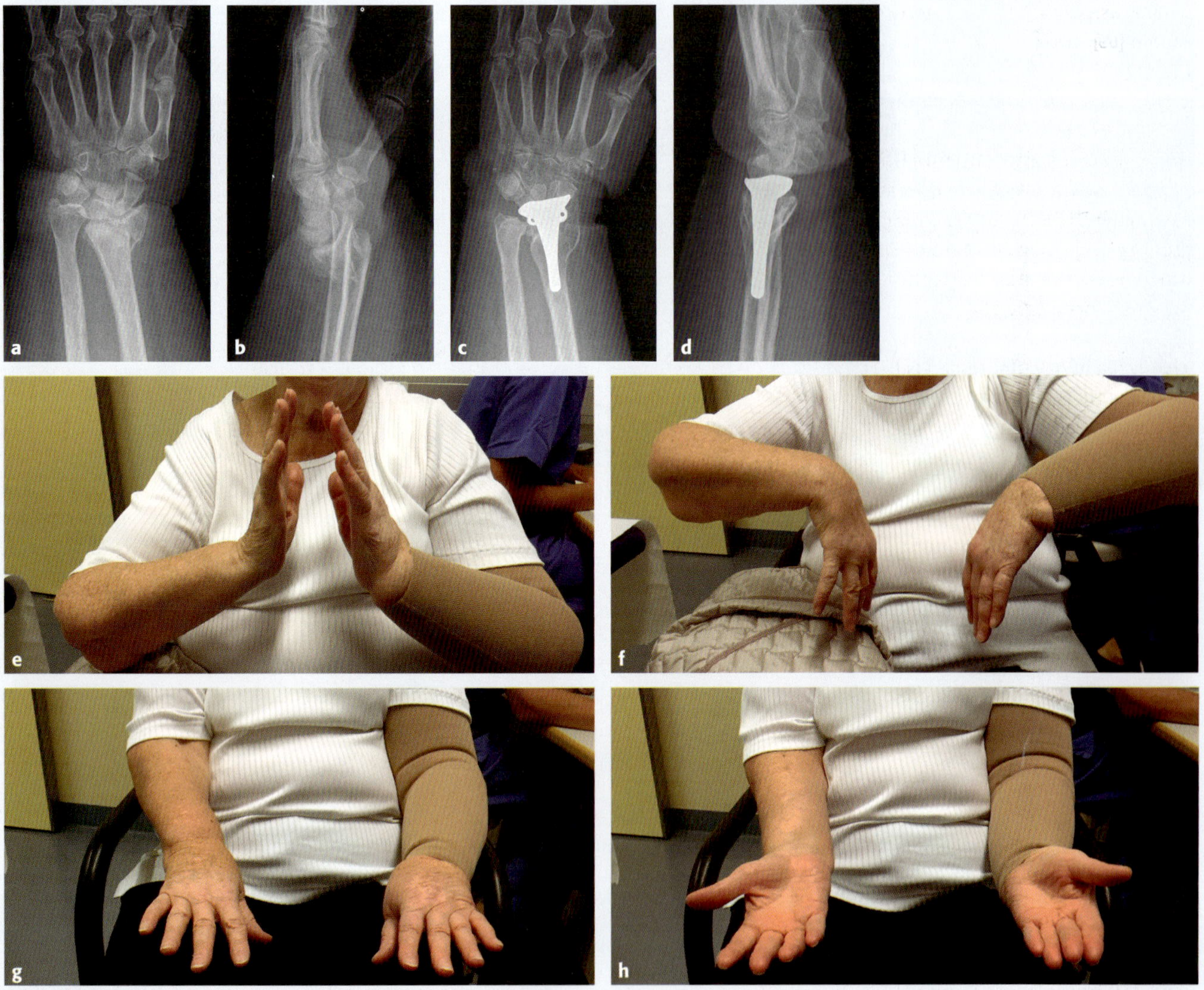


**Fig 3.6-30a–h** A 77-year-old woman with a distal radial fracture.
**a–b** X-rays showing multifragmented, impacted, and irreparable acute fracture of the distal radius.
**c–d** X-rays showing implanted wrist hemiprosthesis.
**e–h** Clinical images at 10 months after surgery showing a good clinical outcome and mobility.

## 7 Therapeutic options—distal forearm fractures

At this time, treatment regimens are controversial and vary from ORIF of the ulna, percutaneous pin fixation and external fixation, or cast immobilization [65–68]. These injury patterns often go hand in hand with large metaphyseal defects in both radius and ulna. A common difficulty in maintaining reduction is the large metaphyseal defect after restoration of the length of radius and ulna. To overcome this, we use corticocancellous iliac bone grafts to restore length and prevent metaphyseal collapse. If bone graft is not available, locking plates can help to maintain radial length. Reduction and fixation of the small fragments of the distal ulna is challenging. After reduction and fixation of DRFs, 75% of the associated ulnar fractures remain displaced or unstable [69].

### 7.1 Nonoperative treatment of the distal ulnar fracture

Biyani et al [21] recommended ORIF of DRF as the standard of care treatment in the operative therapy of DRF associated with DUF. In simple ulnar neck fractures, where after anatomical reconstruction of DRF the ulnar head fractures remains aligned and stable, nonoperative treatment of DUF may be considered [70].

The fovea of the ulnar head is the center of forearm rotation whereas the radius rotates around the ulnar head. In cases of ulnar head fractures, an above elbow cast for 6 weeks is recommended to neutralize the deforming forces during the forearm rotation.

### 7.2 Operative treatment using locking plates

Distal radial fractures are treated using palmar locking plates as described above. In cases with metaphyseal comminution of DRF and DUF, the radius can be primary shortened to overcome the metaphyseal void. The proximal fragment is impacted into the distal fragment to neutralize the metaphyseal defect and avoid secondary axial displacement forces. Fixation of the shortened radius without bone grafting and leaving the ulnar fracture untreated may cause the late development of posttraumatic arthritis, ulnar-sided wrist pain, DRUJ instability, and limited rotation of the forearm.

The advent of low-profile locking plates made early mobilization possible, and good functional results were reported after fixation of these fractures in association with DRFs (see *AO Principles of Fracture Management*) [70, 71].

### 7.3 Bridging plate

Treatment of intraarticular DRFs with extensive comminution extending up to the metaphyseal-diaphyseal junction remains challenging for the following reasons:

- External fixation, which neutralizes compressive forces on the articular segment, may not provide sufficient stability and immobilization to allow healing of the metaphysis to the diaphysis proximally. Using an EF would require a longer working distance for the EF and a prolonged duration of application because the metaphyseal-diaphyseal has a longer healing time than the metaphyseal region.
- Open reduction and internal fixation is challenging too, because the articular fracture is difficult to restore using plates, due to the metaphyseal void with no support of the articular fragments.
- A bridging plate achieves more stability (**Case 6: Fig 3.6-31**), avoiding hybrid options using plate and external fixation or multiple plates [72].

Ligamentotaxis is used to restore radial length and radiocarpal alignment, which can be preserved with the application of a bridging plate. Additional fixation for the articular fragments can be used when necessary to achieve a more anatomical reduction.

The surgery is performed without tourniquet control with the patient lying supine on a radiolucent table. A 4 cm incision is made dorsally over the third metacarpal bone. The extensor tendons at this level are retracted. A second, 4–6 cm incision is made at the dorsal radial aspect of the radius at least 4 cm proximal to the fracture site. According to the fracture pattern, a locking compression plate 3.5 is then passed from distal to proximal along the floor of the fourth dorsal extensor compartment. At the Lister's tubercle, a third 2 cm incision is made to retract the EPL tendon and care is taken to ensure that the plate does not irritate either the EPL or the digital extensor tendon as it is passed proximally under the tendons with use of the plane between the extensor tendons (fourth compartment) and the periosteum and joint capsule. The plate is fixed to the third metacarpal bone, with care taken to drill the holes in the midline of the metacarpal, thereby avoiding subsequent rotatory displacement of the hand relative to the forearm. If the DRUJ is stable postoperatively, no immobilization is used. In cases with comminuted ulnar head fractures, the forearm is maintained in a sugar-tong splint for 4 weeks following stabilization, whereby active digital and elbow movement are initiated immediately. The bridging plate is retained for 3 months and removed after confirmation of bone healing [72].

CASE 6

## Patient

An 83-year-old woman sustained a distal radial fracture.

## Treatment and outcome

Initially, pin fixation was chosen as the operative treatment (**Fig 3.6-31a–b**). Subsequent pin-track infection occurred (**Fig 3.6-31c**). The pins had to be removed, extended operative wound debridement was done (**Fig 3.6-31d**), and an external fixator was applied. Soft-tissue damage was covered by a local flap (**Fig 3.6-31e–f**). Over time, further displacement occurred (**Fig 3.6-31g–h**) and a bridging plate fixation was chosen (**Fig 3.6-31i–j**). The plate was used for 3 months and after bone healing was confirmed the implant was removed (**Fig 3.6-31k–l**). The soft tissue also showed a satisfying healing process (**Fig 3.6-31m–n**).

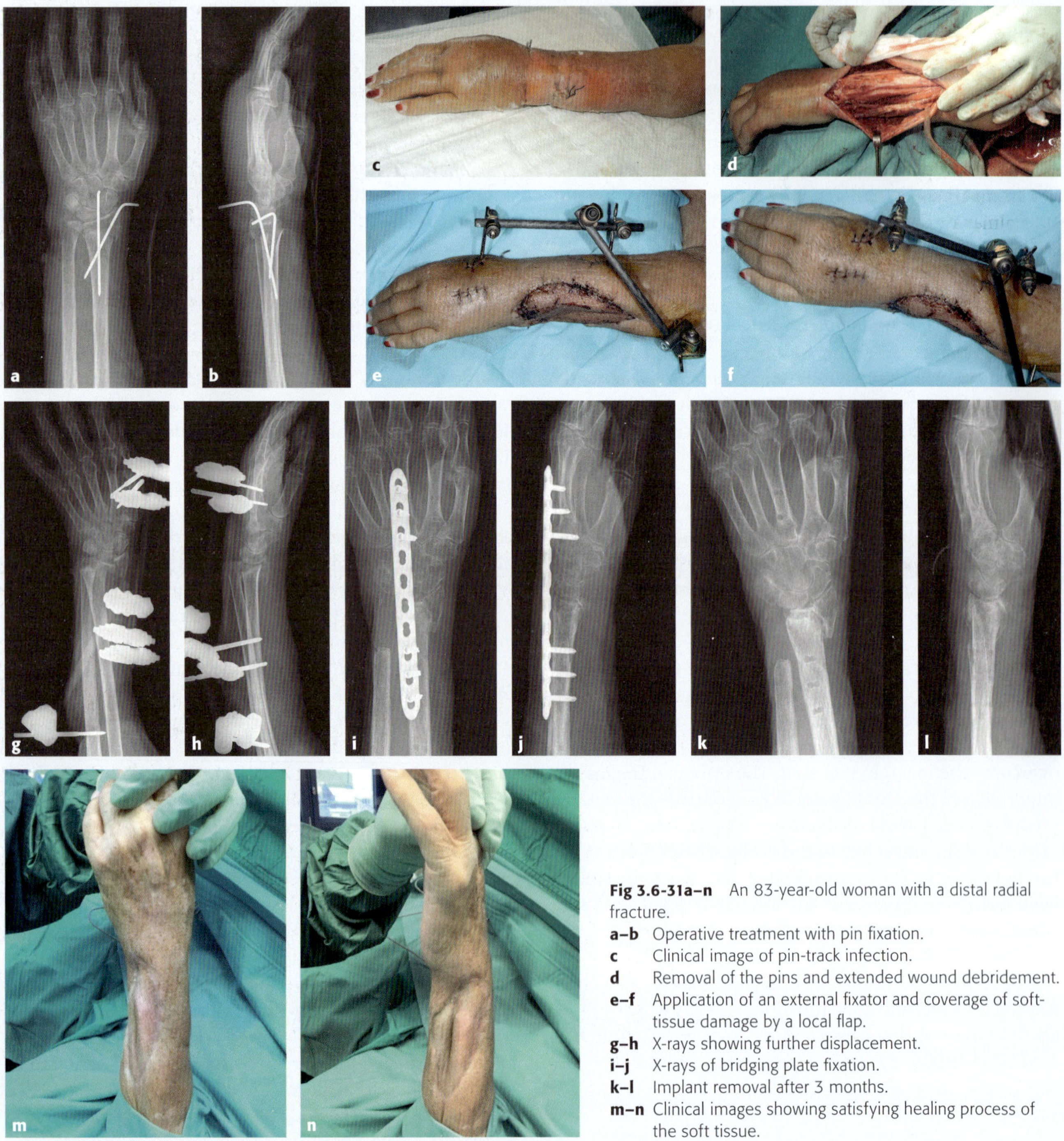


**Fig 3.6-31a–n** An 83-year-old woman with a distal radial fracture.

- **a–b** Operative treatment with pin fixation.
- **c** Clinical image of pin-track infection.
- **d** Removal of the pins and extended wound debridement.
- **e–f** Application of an external fixator and coverage of soft-tissue damage by a local flap.
- **g–h** X-rays showing further displacement.
- **i–j** X-rays of bridging plate fixation.
- **k–l** Implant removal after 3 months.
- **m–n** Clinical images showing satisfying healing process of the soft tissue.

## 8 Therapeutic options—fracture dislocations

Fracture dislocations require operative treatment regardless of the age of the patient. Usually, the palmar ulnar corner of the distal radial joint surface is involved. This fragment is the critical corner and should be stabilized properly. In these cases, it is impossible to fix the fragment using a conventional palmar locking plate placed proximally to the watershed line. The distal screws are too proximal to reach and stabilize the rim fragment.

For these reasons, fragment-specific fixation techniques should be used. Small screws, pin plates, or special hook plates help to fix, buttress and support the palmar rim fragments until bone healing. Appropriate implant position on the palmar rim should be confirmed intraoperatively on true lateral and tilt lateral views. Implant prominence with contact to flexor tendons must be avoided (**Fig 3.6-32**).

In DRFs with small dorsal rim fragments, dorsal plating is performed. In these dorsal shear fractures, mostly the dorsal rim of the lunate facet is displaced. This fragment should be fixed, as it is part of the sigmoid notch forming the DRUJ. Additionally, the dorsal radioulnar ligaments are attached to this fragment.

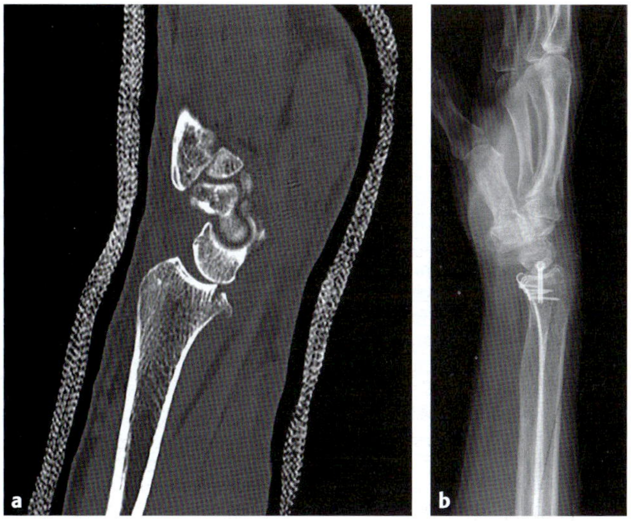


**Fig 3.6-32a–b** The carpus follows the palmar fracture fragment and leads to a carpal subluxation (**a**). Fragment-specific fixation techniques with a small screw and a hook plate were used (**b**).

## 7 References

1. **Abraham A, Handoll HH, Khan T.** Interventions for treating wrist fractures in children. *Cochrane Database Syst Rev.* 2013 Mar 28(3):CD004576.
2. **Chung KC, Spilson SV.** The frequency and epidemiology of hand and forearm fractures in the United States. *J Hand Surg Am.* 2001 Sep;26(5):908–915.
3. **Wilcke MK, Hammarberg H, Adolphson PY.** Epidemiology and changed surgical treatment methods for fractures of the distal radius: a registry analysis of 42,583 patients in Stockholm County, Sweden, 2004–2010. *Acta Orthop.* 2013 Jun;84(3):292–296.
4. **Flinkkila T, Sirnio K, Hippi M, et al.** Epidemiology and seasonal variation of distal radius fractures in Oulu, Finland. *Osteoporos Int.* 2011 Aug;22(8):2307–2312.
5. **Cummings SR, Nevitt MC, Browner WS, et al.** Risk factors for hip fracture in white women. Study of Osteoporotic Fractures Research Group. *N Engl J Med.* 1995 Mar 23;332(12):767–773.
6. **Schousboe JT, Fink HA, Taylor BC, et al.** Association between self-reported prior wrist fractures and risk of subsequent hip and radiographic vertebral fractures in older women: a prospective study. *J Bone Miner Res.* 2005 Jan;20(1):100–106.
7. **Jaglal SB, Weller I, Mamdani M, et al.** Population trends in BMD testing, treatment, and hip and wrist fracture rates: are the hip fracture projections wrong? *J Bone Miner Res.* 2005 Jun;20(6):898–905.
8. **Shauver MJ, Yin H, Banerjee M, et al.** Current and future national costs to medicare for the treatment of distal radius fracture in the elderly. *J Hand Surg Am.* 2011 Aug;36(8):1282–1287.
9. **Dimai HP, Svedbom A, Fahrleitner-Pammer A, et al.** Epidemiology of distal forearm fractures in Austria between 1989 and 2010. *Osteoporos Int.* 2014 Sep;25(9):2297–2306.
10. **Amin S, Achenbach SJ, Atkinson EJ, et al.** Trends in fracture incidence: a population-based study over 20 years. *J Bone Miner Res.* 2014 Mar;29(3):581–589.
11. **Sabesan VJ, Valikodath T, Childs A, et al.** Economic and social impact of upper extremity fragility fractures in elderly patients. *Aging Clin Exp Res.* 2015 Aug;27(4):539–546.
12. **Kramer S, Meyer H, O'Loughlin PF, et al.** The incidence of ulnocarpal complaints after distal radial fracture in relation to the fracture of the ulnar styloid. *J Hand Surg Eur.* 2013 Sep;38(7):710–717.
13. **Andersen DJ, Blair WF, Steyers CM Jr, et al.** Classification of distal radius fractures: an analysis of interobserver reliability and intraobserver reproducibility. *J Hand Surg Am.* 1996 Jul;21(4):574–582.
14. **Arealis G, Galanopoulos I, Nikolaou VS, et al.** Does the CT improve inter- and intra-observer agreement for the AO, Fernandez and Universal classification systems for distal radius fractures? *Injury.* 2014 Oct;45(10):1579–1584.
15. **Solomon LB, Warwick D, Nayagam S.** *Apley's System of Orthopaedics and Fractures.* 9th ed. Boca Raton: Taylor & Francis Group; 2010.
16. **Venes D, Davis FA.** *Taber's Cyclopdic Medical Dictionary.* 22nd ed. Philadelphia: F.A. Davis; 2013.
17. **Wheeless CR.** Distal radius fracture. Available at: www.wheelessonline.com/ortho/12591. Updated August 12, 2013. Accessed April 2017.
18. **Fernandes DL, Jupiter JB.** *Fractures of the Distal Radius. A Practical Approach to Management.* 2nd ed. New York: Springer-Verlag; 2002.
19. **Yochum TR, Rowe LJ.** *Essentials of Skeletal Radiology:* Lippincott Williams & Wilkins; 2005.
20. **Rikli DA, Regazzoni P, Babst R.** Die dorsale Doppelplattenosteosynthese am distalen Radius—ein biomechanisches Konzept und dessen klinische Realisation [Dorsal double plating for fractures of the distal radius—a biomechanical concept and clinical experience]. *Zentralbl Chir.* 2003 Dec;128(12):1003–1007. German.
21. **Biyani A, Simison AJ, Klenerman L.** Fractures of the distal radius and ulna. *J Hand Surg Br.* 1995 Jun;20(3):357–364.
22. **Rikli D, Goldhahn J, Kach K, et al.** The effect of local bone mineral density on the rate of mechanical failure after surgical treatment of distal radius fractures: a prospective multicentre cohort study including 249 patients. *Arch Orthop Trauma Surg.* 2015 Feb;135(2):201–207.
23. **Nesbitt KS, Failla JM, Les C.** Assessment of instability factors in adult distal radius fractures. *J Hand Surg Am.* 2004 Nov;29(6):1128–1138.
24. **Porter M, Stockley I.** Fractures of the distal radius. Intermediate and end results in relation to radiologic parameters. *Clin Orthop Relat Res.* 1987 Jul(220):241–252.
25. **McQueen MM, MacLaren A, Chalmers J.** The value of remanipulating Colles' fractures. *J Bone Joint Surg Br.* 1986 Mar;68(2):232–233.
26. **Beumer A, McQueen MM.** Fractures of the distal radius in low-demand elderly patients: closed reduction of no value in 53 of 60 wrists. *Acta Orthop Scand.* 2003 Feb;74(1):98–100.
27. **Sakai A, Oshige T, Zenke Y, et al.** Association of bone mineral density with deformity of the distal radius in low-energy Colles' fractures in Japanese women above 50 years of age. *J Hand Surg Am.* 2008 Jul–Aug;33(6):820–826.
28. **Lafontaine M, Delince P, Hardy D, et al.** [Instability of fractures of the lower end of the radius: apropos of a series of 167 cases]. *Acta Orthop Belg.* 1989;55(2):203–216. French.
29. **Crilly RG, Delaquerriere Richardson L, Roth JH, et al.** Postural stability and Colles' fracture. *Age Ageing.* 1987 May;16(3):133–138.
30. **Lafontaine M, Hardy D, Delince P.** Stability assessment of distal radius fractures. *Injury.* 1989 Jul;20(4):208–210.
31. **Chang HC, Tay SC, Chan BK, et al.** Conservative treatment of redisplaced Colles' fractures in elderly patients older than 60 years old—anatomical and functional outcome. *Hand Surg.* 2001 Dec;6(2):137–144.
32. **Mackenney PJ, McQueen MM, Elton R.** Prediction of instability in distal radial fractures. *J Bone Joint Surg Am.* 2006 Sep;88(9):1944–1951.
33. **McQueen M, Caspers J.** Colles fracture: does the anatomical result affect the final function? *J Bone Joint Surg Br.* 1988 Aug;70(4):649–651.
34. **Rozental TD, Beredjiklian PK, Bozentka DJ.** Functional outcome and complications following two types of dorsal plating for unstable fractures of the distal part of the radius. *J Bone Joint Surg Am.* 2003 Oct;85-A(10):1956–1960.
35. **Ng CY, McQueen MM.** What are the radiological predictors of functional outcome following fractures of the distal radius? *J Bone Joint Surg Br.* 2011 Feb;93(2):145–150.
36. **Handoll HH, Madhok R.** WITHDRAWN: Surgical interventions for treating distal radial fractures in adults. *Cochrane Database Syst Rev.* 2009 Jul 08(3):CD003209.
37. **Arora R, Lutz M, Deml C, et al.** A prospective randomized trial comparing nonoperative treatment with volar locking plate fixation for displaced and unstable distal radial fractures in patients sixty-five years of age and older. *J Bone Joint Surg Am.* 2011 Dec 07;93(23):2146–2153.

38. **Fanuele J, Koval KJ, Lurie J, et al.** Distal radial fracture treatment: what you get may depend on your age and address. *J Bone Joint Surg Am.* 2009 Jun;91(6):1313–1319.
39. **Waljee JF, Zhong L, Shauver MJ, et al.** The influence of surgeon age on distal radius fracture treatment in the United States: a population-based study. *J Hand Surg Am.* 2014 May;39(5):844–851.
40. **Nelson GN, Stepan JG, Osei DA, et al.** The impact of patient activity level on wrist disability after distal radius malunion in older adults. *J Orthop Trauma.* 2015 Apr;29(4):195–200.
41. **Chung KC, Shauver MJ, Birkmeyer JD.** Trends in the United States in the treatment of distal radial fractures in the elderly. *J Bone Joint Surg Am.* 2009 Aug;91(8):1868–1873.
42. **Pillukat T, van Schoonhoven J, Prommersberger KJ.** Ist die Korrekturosteotomie der fehlverheilten distalen Radiusfraktur auch beim älteren Menschen indiziert? [Is corrective osteotomy for malunited distal radius fractures also indicated for elderly patients?]. *Handchir Mikrochir Plast Chir.* 2007 Feb;39(1):42–48. German.
43. **Brogren E, Hofer M, Petranek M, et al.** Fractures of the distal radius in women aged 50 to 75 years: natural course of patient-reported outcome, wrist motion and grip strength between 1 year and 2–4 years after fracture. *J Hand Surg Eur.* 2011 Sep;36(7):568–576.
44. **Young BT, Rayan GM.** Outcome following nonoperative treatment of displaced distal radius fractures in low-demand patients older than 60 years. *J Hand Surg Am.* 2000 Jan;25(1):19–28.
45. **Marcano A, Taormina DP, Karia R, et al.** Displaced intra-articular fractures involving the volar rim of the distal radius. *J Hand Surg Am.* 2015 Jan;40(1):42–48.
46. **Ring D, Prommersberger KJ, Gonzalez del Pino J, et al.** Corrective osteotomy for intra-articular malunion of the distal part of the radius. *J Bone Joint Surg Am.* 2005 Jul;87(7):1503–1509.
47. **Fernandez DL, Capo JT, Gonzalez E.** Corrective osteotomy for symptomatic increased ulnar tilt of the distal end of the radius. *J Hand Surg Am.* 2001 Jul;26(4):722–732.
48. **Fernandez DL, Ring D, Jupiter JB.** Surgical management of delayed union and nonunion of distal radius fractures. *J Hand Surg Am.* 2001 Mar;26(2):201–209.
49. **Lee SK, Kim KJ, Park JS, et al.** Distal ulna hook plate fixation for unstable distal ulna fracture associated with distal radius fracture. *Orthopedics.* 2012 Sep;35(9):e1358–e1364.
50. **Azzopardi T, Ehrendorfer S, Coulton T, et al.** Unstable extra-articular fractures of the distal radius: a prospective, randomised study of immobilisation in a cast versus supplementary percutaneous pinning. *J Bone Joint Surg Br.* 2005 Jun;87(6):837–840.
51. **Roumen RM, Hesp WL, Bruggink ED.** Unstable Colles' fractures in elderly patients. A randomised trial of external fixation for redisplacement. *J Bone Joint Surg Br.* 1991 Mar;73(2):307–311.
52. **Margaliot Z, Haase SC, Kotsis SV, et al.** A meta-analysis of outcomes of external fixation versus plate osteosynthesis for unstable distal radius fractures. *J Hand Surg Am.* 2005 Nov;30(6):1185–1199.
53. **Gehrmann SV, Windolf J, Kaufmann RA.** Distal radius fracture management in elderly patients: a literature review. *J Hand Surg Am.* 2008 Mar;33(3):421–429.
54. **Carter PR, Frederick HA, Laseter GF.** Open reduction and internal fixation of unstable distal radius fractures with a low-profile plate: a multicenter study of 73 fractures. *J Hand Surg Am.* 1998 Mar;23(2):300–307.
55. **Campbell DA.** Open reduction and internal fixation of intra articular and unstable fractures of the distal radius using the AO distal radius plate. *J Hand Surg Br.* 2000 Dec;25(6):528–534.
56. **Kambouroglou GK, Axelrod TS.** Complications of the AO/ASIF titanium distal radius plate system (pi plate) in internal fixation of the distal radius: a brief report. *J Hand Surg Am.* 1998 Jul;23(4):737–741.
57. **Leung F, Zhu L, Ho H, et al.** Palmar plate fixation of AO type C2 fracture of distal radius using a locking compression plate—a biomechanical study in a cadaveric model. *J Hand Surg Br.* 2003 Jun;28(3):263–266.
58. **Rikli D, Goldhahn J, Kach K, et al.** Erratum to: The effect of local bone mineral density on the rate of mechanical failure after surgical treatment of distal radius fractures: a prospective multicentre cohort study including 249 patients. *Arch Orthop Trauma Surg.* 2015 Jul;135(7):1043.
59. **Hirasawa Y, Katsumi Y, Akiyoshi T, et al.** Clinical and microangiographic studies on rupture of the E.P.L. tendon after distal radial fractures. *J Hand Surg Br.* 1990 Feb;15(1):51–57.
60. **Hove LM, Nilsen PT, Furnes O, et al.** Open reduction and internal fixation of displaced intraarticular fractures of the distal radius. 31 patients followed for 3–7 years. *Acta Orthop Scand.* 1997 Feb;68(1):59–63.
61. **Haug LC, Glodny B, Deml C, et al.** A new radiological method to detect dorsally penetrating screws when using volar locking plates in distal radial fractures. The dorsal horizon view. *Bone Joint J.* 2013 Aug;95-B(8):1101–1105.
62. **Orbay JL, Fernandez DL.** Volar fixed-angle plate fixation for unstable distal radius fractures in the elderly patient. *J Hand Surg Am.* 2004 Jan;29(1):96–102.
63. **Matschke S, Wentzensen A, Ring D, et al.** Comparison of angle stable plate fixation approaches for distal radius fractures. *Injury.* 2011 Apr;42(4):385–392.
64. **Herzberg G, Burnier M, Marc A, et al.** Primary wrist hemiarthroplasty for irreparable distal radius fracture in the independent elderly. *J Wrist Surg.* 2015 Aug;4(3):156–163.
65. **Melamed E, Danna N, Debkowska M, et al.** Complex proximal ulna fractures: outcomes of surgical treatment. *Eur J Orthop Surg Traumatol.* 2015 Jul;25(5):851–858.
66. **Nieto H, Billaud A, Rochet S, et al.** Proximal ulnar fractures in adults: a review of 163 cases. *Injury.* 2015 Jan;46(Suppl 1):S18–S23.
67. **Zumsteg JW, Molina CS, Lee DH, et al.** Factors influencing infection rates after open fractures of the radius and/or ulna. *J Hand Surg Am.* 2014 May;39(5):956–961.
68. **Yi PH, Weening AA, Shin SR, et al.** Injury patterns and outcomes of open fractures of the proximal ulna do not differ from closed fractures. *Clin Orthop Relat Res.* 2014 Jul;472(7):2100–2104.
69. **Walz M, Kolbow B, Mollenhoff G.** Distale Ulnafraktur als Begleitverletzung des körperfernen Speichenbruchs. Minimal-invasive Versorgung mittels elastisch-stabiler intramedullärer Nagelung (ESIN) [Fracture of the distal ulna accompanying fracture of the distal radius. Minimally invasive treatment with elastic stable intramedullary nailing (ESIN)]. *Unfallchirurg.* 2006 Dec;109(12):1058–1063. German.
70. **Dennison DG.** Open reduction and internal locked fixation of unstable distal ulna fractures with concomitant distal radius fracture. *J Hand Surg Am.* 2007 Jul–Aug;32(6):801–805.
71. **Rüedi T, Buckley R, Moran C.** *AO Principles of Fracture Management.* 2nd ed. Stuttgart New York: Thieme Verlag; 2007.
72. **Ruch DS, Ginn TA, Yang CC, et al.** Use of a distraction plate for distal radial fractures with metaphyseal and diaphyseal comminution. *J Bone Joint Surg Am.* 2005 May;87(5):945–954.

# 3.7 Pelvic ring

Pol M Rommens, Michael Blauth, Alexander Hofmann

## 1 Introduction

Pelvic ring disruptions in younger patients are typically high-energy injuries resulting from traffic accidents, falls from great height, or crush traumas. Very often, these patients are multiply injured, need hemodynamic resuscitation and provisional pelvic stabilization with a pelvic binder, clamp or another type of external fixation. Selective angiographic arterial embolization and pelvic packing are often indicated [1].

Fragility fractures of the pelvis present a totally different clinical picture. They occur in frail, older patients and are the result of a low-energy trauma such as a ground-level fall. In some patients, the history of their injuries is not obtainable. Repetitive "harmless" events such as the transfer from the bed to a chair or from a chair to the toilet, sneezing, coughing, which may not be regarded as traumatic, have been described as causing fragility fractures of the pelvis [2].

Pelvic ring injuries in advanced age may also result from a high-energy trauma. A typical accident mechanism is a trauma from being struck by a vehicle while crossing the street. These patients find themselves quickly in a life-threatening situation; resuscitation must follow the rules of advanced trauma life support similar to younger adults [3]. In this chapter, we discuss the characteristics, diagnostic, and therapeutic measures pertaining to fragility fractures of the pelvis. In this chapter, "fragility fractures of the pelvis" is abbreviated as FFP; note that this abbreviation is used for "fragility fracture patient" in other chapters.

## 2 Epidemiology and etiology

In some countries, the incidence of hip fractures is declining while the number of pelvic and acetabular fractures is increasing. In the US, hip fractures peaked in 1996 and declined by 25.7% until 2010. During the same 18-year period, pelvic fractures increased by 24%. Absolute numbers, however, remained different with 167,000 hip fractures and 33,000 pelvic fractures in 2010 [4]. In Finland, the age-adjusted incidence of hip fractures has also steadily declined since 1997. From 1970 to 2013, the number of age-adjusted incidences of pelvic fractures has increased from 73 to 364. The incidence increased in all age groups (ie, ages 80–84 years, 85–89 years, and 90+ years) of women and men during the entire study period. If both the fracture incidence and rate of the aging population continue to rise at the current pace, the number of low-trauma pelvic fractures in Finland will be 2.4 times higher in 2030 than it was in 2013 [5].

Both advancing age and comorbidities are associated with the increase of the risk of suffering a fragility fracture of the pelvic ring (FFP). Many patients have a history of osteoporosis, vitamin D deficiency, long-term immobilization, long-term glucocorticoid use, pelvic irradiation for malignancy, or bone graft harvest at the posterior ilium for lumbar spine surgery (**Fig 3.7-1**) [6].

Fragility fractures of the pelvic ring occur in osteoporotic bone. With increasing age, bone mass is decreasing continuously. Wagner et al [7] demonstrated that this decrease is following a specific and consistent pattern in the sacrum. The sacral body is far less affected than the sacral ala. In advanced cases, areas of very low bone mineral density without any bone, called an alar void, can be seen in the region lateral of the S1 and S2 neuroforamina (**Fig 3.7-2**).

The leading symptom in patients who have suffered an FFP is pain in the pelvic region. Sitting and standing are difficult or impossible, while lying quietly in bed minimizes the pain level. Most patients are unable to walk. A minority are still able to walk short distances with walking aids. Pain typically starts immediately after the fall and has an acute and sharp character. In some patients, history of pain is longer and related to previous events, which have been unrecognized, undiagnosed, or inadequately treated (**Case 1: Fig 3.7-3**).

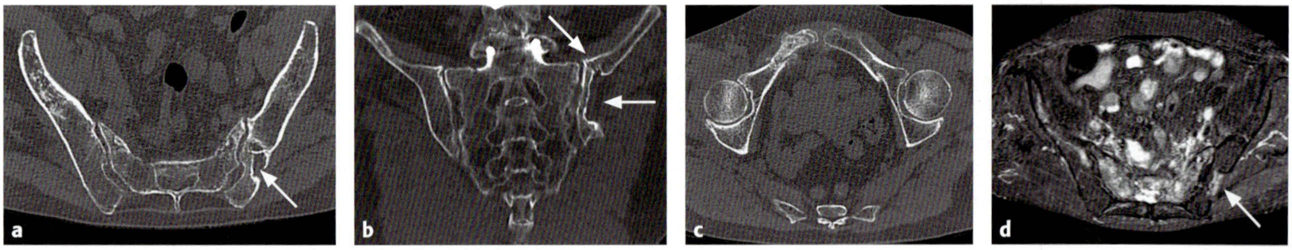


**Fig 3.7-1a–d** A 75-year-old woman with a history of spondylodesis. Cancellous bone grafts were taken from the left posterior ilium.
- **a** Transverse computed tomographic (CT) cut through the posterior pelvic ring showing the bone defect at the left posterior ilium (arrow).
- **b** Coronal CT cut showing the large cortical defect and a fracture line through the ilium (arrows).
- **c** Transverse CT cut through the anterior pelvic ring showing a right superior pubic ramus fracture.
- **d** Transverse magnetic resonance imaging picture showing the bone defect at the left posterior ilium (arrow) and bone bruise in the whole sacrum.

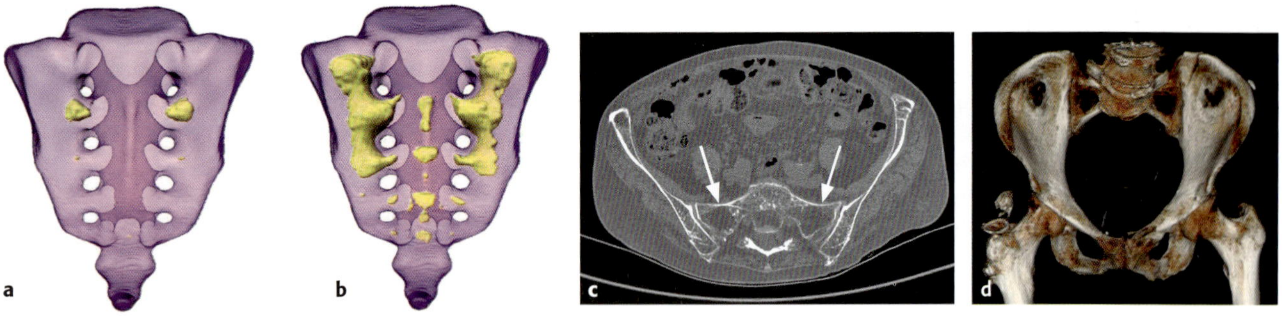


**Fig 3.7-2a–d** Averaged morphology of the nontraumatized sacrum of 92 Europeans, derived from their pelvic computed tomographic data.
- **a** Group of Europeans with bone mineral density above 100 Hounsfield Units (HUs) measured in the center of the L5 vertebral body. There are only small areas with bone mineral density below 0 HUs. They are colored in yellow and situated just lateral and below the neuroforamen S1.
- **b** Group of Europeans with bone mineral density below 100 HUs measured in the center of the L5 vertebral body. There are large areas with bone mineral density below 0 HUs. They are colored in yellow and are situated in the left and right sacral ala and extend from S1–3. There are smaller areas of low bone mineral density in the sacral bodies S2 and S3 (Courtesy of Wagner et al [7]).
- **c** Computed tomographic cut through the posterior pelvis of an 89-year-old woman. Large areas without trabecular bone are visible in the left and right sacral ala (arrows). They are called "alar voids".
- **d** A 3-D reconstruction of the pelvic ring of the same person as in **c**. The alar voids in the sacral ala are clearly visible.

**Patient**

A 75-year-old woman sustained a right anterior pelvic ring fracture after slipping from a chair, 4 weeks before admission.

**Comorbidities**

- No relevant comorbidities

**Treatment and outcome**

The primary x-ray revealed a right superior and inferior pubic rami fracture (**Fig 3.7-3a**). Initially, treatment was nonoperative. But the patient had intractable pain which increased over time. Two months later, bilateral sacral ala fractures and another anterior pelvic ring fracture on the left side were diagnosed on a pelvic computed tomographic scan (**Fig 3.7-3b–d**). She was seen in multiple clinical departments, was bedridden because of pain, and developed pressure ulcers on both heels. She also developed recurrent urinary tract infection and weight loss. Fixation with two iliosacral screws in S1 helped lessen the pain, and mobilization with weight bearing as tolerated was started (**Fig 3.7-3e**). Two months later, the fractures seemed to have healed. The patient was very satisfied, completely pain free, and walked without crutches (**Fig 3.7-3 f**).

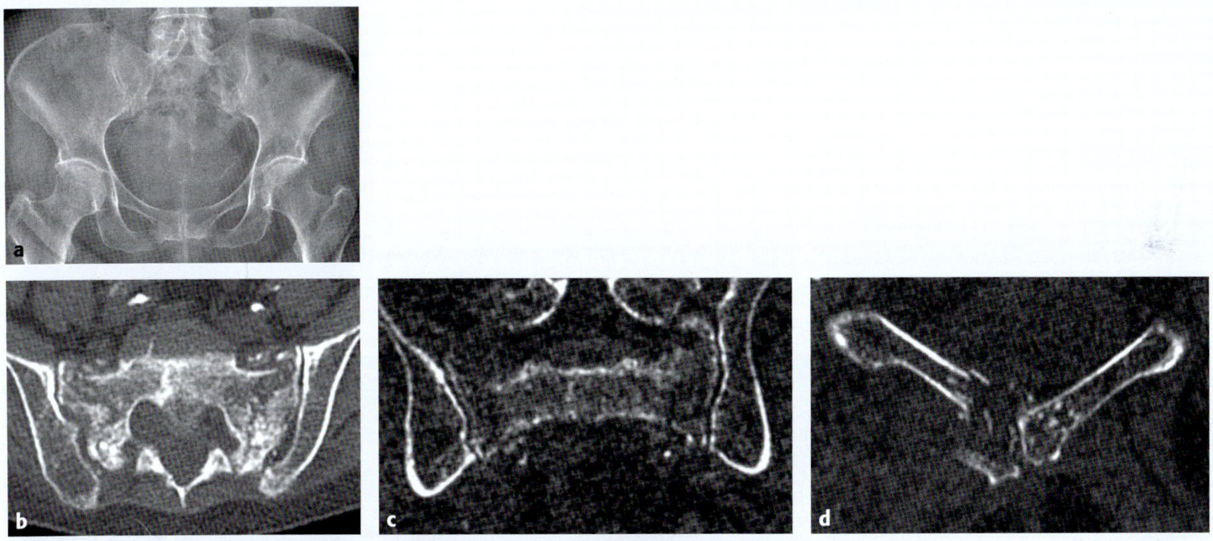

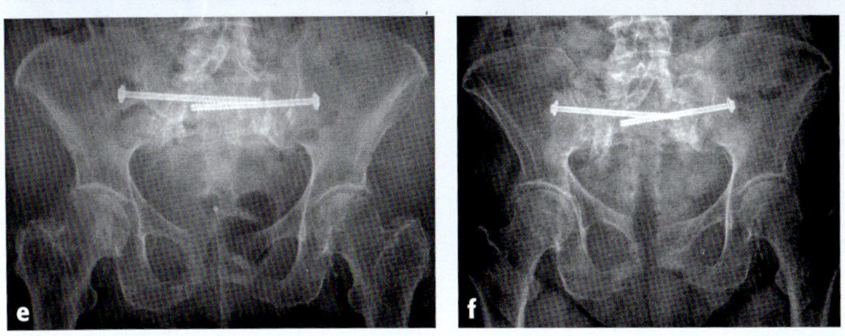

**Fig 3.7-3a–f** A 75-year-old woman with a fracture of the right anterior pelvic ring.
- **a** X-ray showing the right anterior pelvic ring fracture.
- **b–d** Transverse and coronal computed tomographic (CT) cuts through the posterior pelvis and a coronal CT cut through the anterior pelvis.
- **e** AP pelvic x-ray after surgical stabilization.
- **f** AP pelvic x-ray 2 months postoperative showing healed fractures.

## 3 Diagnostics

### 3.1 Physical examination

Pain is localized at the pubic symphysis, the groin, and/or in the posterior pelvis or the low back. In the latter cases, the physician may be confused and focus on diagnostic examinations of the lumbar spine:

- Manual compression on both iliac wings enhances pain intensity dramatically without demonstrating major instability. Direct palpation of the pubic symphysis, the groin, and the sacrum will additionally provoke pain.
- Inspection of the skin and soft tissues around the pelvic ring, including the low back and the perineal region, is necessary to rule out local infections or decubitus ulcers.
- Neurological and vascular status of the lower extremities should be evaluated.

## 3.2 Creeping hemorrhage

Hemodynamic instability due to continuing bleeding after low-energy pelvic trauma is not typical, but has been described [8, 9]. There is an eightfold increase in odds of pelvic hemorrhage in patients older than 55 years (**Case 2: Fig 3.7-4**).

Especially in patients taking anticoagulants, there must be a high index of suspicion for continuing bleeding. Arteriosclerosis impairs the ability of vasospasm with less chance of spontaneous cessation of arterial bleeding.

CASE 2

### Patient

An 81-year-old woman suffered a left superior and inferior pubic rami fracture after a fall at home.

### Comorbidities

- Atrial fibrillation
- Cardiac insufficiency

### Treatment and outcome

Nonoperative treatment with pain medication was started. The hemodynamic situation of the patient deteriorated within the first few hours after admission. A swelling above the pubic symphysis was noticed.

An x-ray of the pelvis showed a slightly displaced superior and inferior pubic ramus fracture (**Fig 3.7-4a**). Transverse computed tomographic cuts through the anterior pelvic ring were performed showing the left-sided superior pubic ramus fracture and a large hematoma inside the small pelvis, which stayed in direct connection with the fracture (**Fig 3.7-4b–c**). The patient was taken to the angiography ward where an active bleeding of the pubic branch of the left inferior epigastric artery was discovered (**Fig 3.7-4d**). A selective embolization and coiling was performed (**Fig 3.7-4e**). The hemodynamic situation of the patient improved. She was taken to the operating room 4 days later for operative removal of the hematoma. The patient recovered well and was discharged 18 days after admission (Courtesy of Dietz et al [9]).

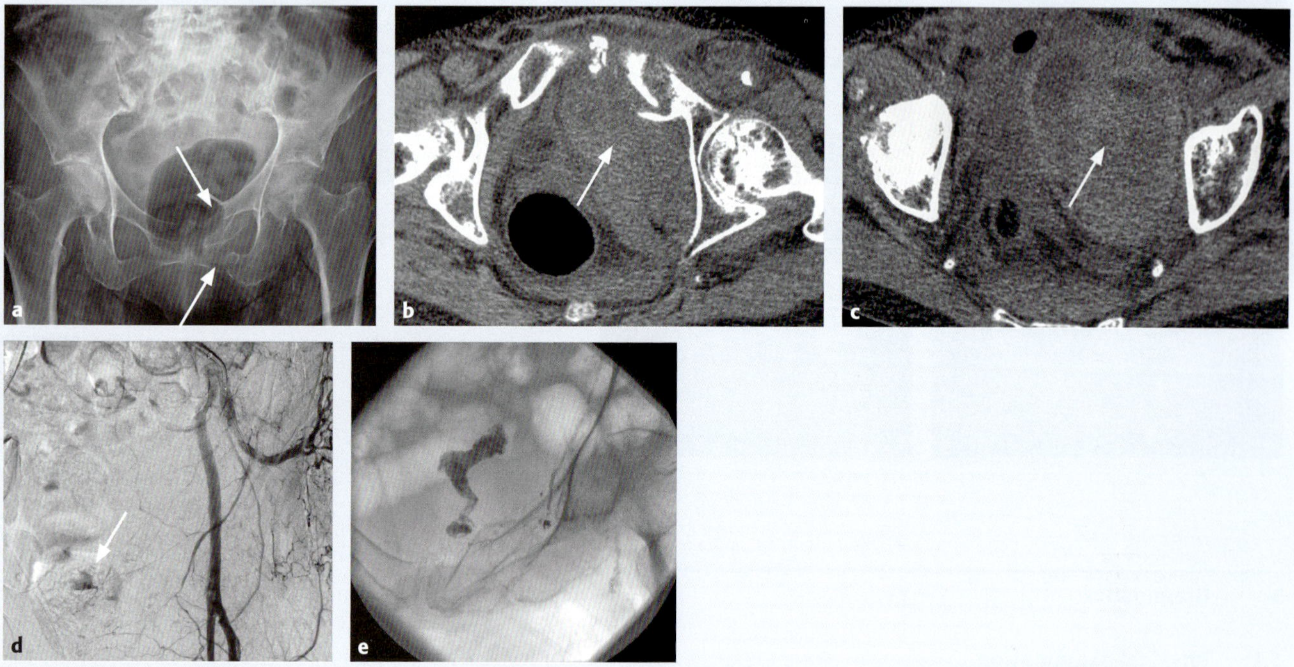


**Fig 3.7-4a–e** An 81-year-old woman with a left superior and inferior pubic rami fracture.
**a** AP x-ray of the pelvis showing a slightly displaced superior and inferior pubic ramus fracture (white arrows).
**b–c** Transverse computed tomographic cuts through the anterior pelvic ring showing the left-sided superior pubic ramus fracture and a large hematoma inside the small pelvis, which stays in direct connection with the fracture (white arrow).
**d** Angiographic image showing where an active bleeding of the pubic branch of the left inferior epigastric artery was discovered (the white arrow shows the contrast flush).
**e** Intraoperative x-ray of the left symphyseal region after coiling.

It is recommended to monitor the hemodynamic condition of these patients for at least 24 hours. A flowchart for early clinical and radiological monitoring of patients with FFP is presented in **Fig 3.7-5** [9]. In case of bleeding, arterial angiography with selective embolization represents a highly effective treatment of choice. Patients are at risk of exsanguinating with delayed diagnosis and undertreatment.

## 3.3 Imaging

### 3.3.1 Plain x-rays

#### AP pelvic x-ray

Fractures of the superior and inferior pubic rami or the pubic bone near the symphysis are easily recognized. In case of a lateral impact, the fracture line at the superior pubic ramus runs horizontally and there is a slight overriding of the fracture fragments, the lateral fracture fragment being displaced medially (**Fig 3.7-6a**).

#### Inlet and outlet views

There is controversy whether inlet and outlet views should be taken in this patient cohort. Some authors recommend taking them as a reference for a later follow-up. Others rely on computed tomographic (CT) scans in case of any fracture visible on the AP pelvic x-ray. Computed tomographic scans may also be added to AP x-rays during follow-up.

The inlet view gives a good idea of the amount and direction of rotation of the innominate bone. Integrity of the inner curve of the innominate bone and the anterior cortex of the sacrum can best be analyzed in the inlet view (**Fig 3.7-6b**). The outlet view gives the best information about the posterior pelvis, the shape and symmetry of the sacrum, the neuroforamina and the sacroiliac joints (**Fig 3.7-6c**). We recommend taking these three views as a reference for later follow-ups.

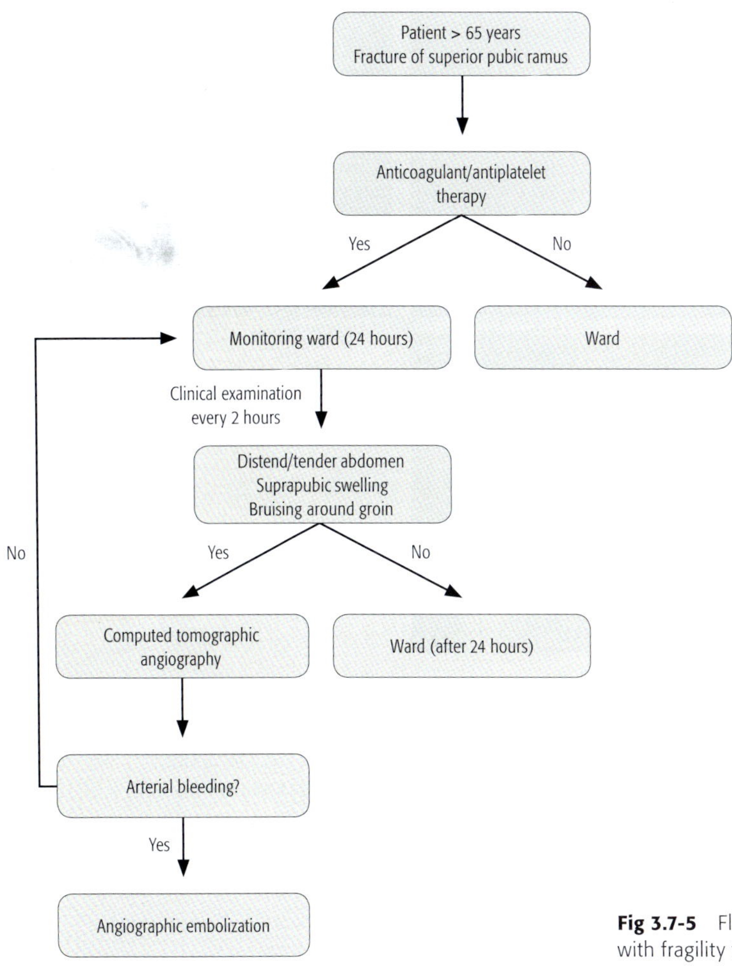


**Fig 3.7-5** Flowchart for clinical and radiological monitoring of patients with fragility fractures of the pelvic ring (Courtesy of Dietz et al [9]).

The large, often obese soft-tissue envelope, bowel content, and bowel gas overlie bony structures and joints. Moreover, due to rarefaction of cortical and cancellous bone, fissures and nondisplaced fractures may not be recognized on plain x-rays. Posterior pelvic ring pathology may be missed with inadequate treatment as consequence [10]. Additional pelvic fractures may occur and enhance complexity and instability (**Fig. 3.7-7**).

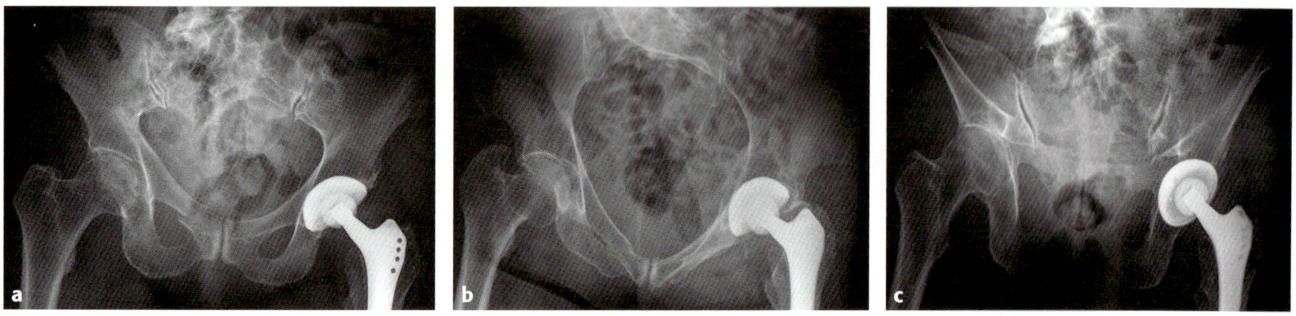


**Fig 3.7-6a–c** A 76-year-old woman sustained a fracture of the right superior pubic ramus after a fall at home.
- **a** AP pelvic x-ray showing the visible horizontal fracture of the right superior pubic ramus.
- **b** Pelvic inlet view showing a slight internal rotation of the right hemipelvis.
- **c** Pelvic outlet view showing a symmetrical posterior pelvis. Fractures, displacement, or dislocations are not visible.

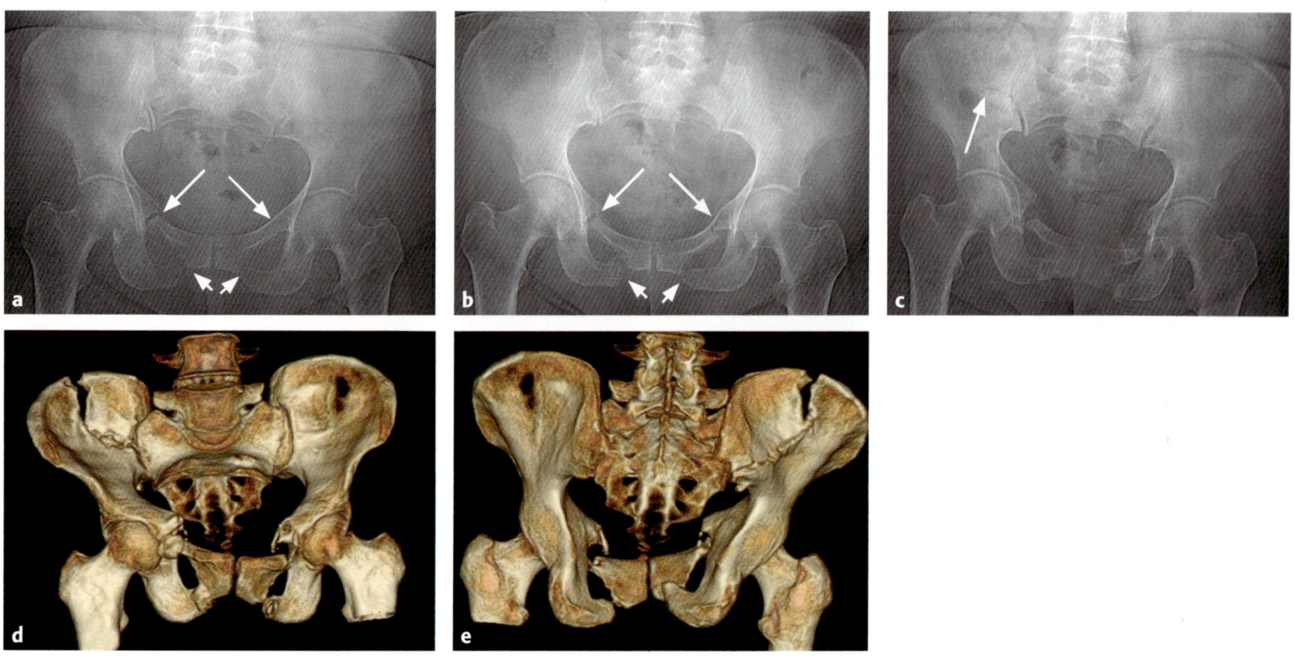


**Fig 3.7-7a–e** A 57-year-old woman with a bilateral pubic rami fracture after a fall at home.
- **a** AP x-ray showing a bilateral, nearly nondisplaced superior and inferior pubic rami fracture (white arrows). The fractures were treated nonoperatively.
- **b** AP pelvic x-ray taken 2 weeks later showing more displacement of the pubic rami fractures on both sides (white arrows).
- **c** AP pelvic x-ray after 3 months showing complete displacement of all fractures. There is also a horizontal fissure in the right ilium starting from the sacroiliac joint (white arrow).
- **d** A computed tomographic scan of the pelvis was only taken 5 months after the fall. The 3-D reconstruction with view from the front showing a complete iliac fracture with displacement and further displacement of the anterior butterfly fragment.
- **e** A 3-D reconstruction with view from the back.

(Images courtesy of Dr Guy Putzeys, AZ Groeninghe, Kortrijk, Belgium.)

### 3.3.2 Computed tomographic scan

A pelvic CT scan is recommended when a lesion of any kind of the pelvic ring has been diagnosed on plain x-rays. In a cohort of 245 patients with FFP, more than 80% had a posterior pelvic ring fracture. When only a plain x-ray is obtained on admission, there is a high risk of missing posterior pelvic ring fractures [11].

In coronal reconstructions, a fracture of the lateral mass of the sacrum is sometimes better seen than in transverse sections. A horizontal sacral fracture with more or less severe angulation can only be recognized in sagittal reconstructions (**Fig 3.7-8**).

In some patients, signs of an older injury may be visible. Bone resorption at a fracture site is a sign of chronic instability, and callus formation is a sign of bone healing. Chronic instabilities at or around a joint may end in bone resorption, joint widening, inclusion of nitrogen bubbles, and free intraarticular or periarticular bone fragments (**Fig 3.7-9**, **Fig 3.7-10**, **Fig 3.7-11**).

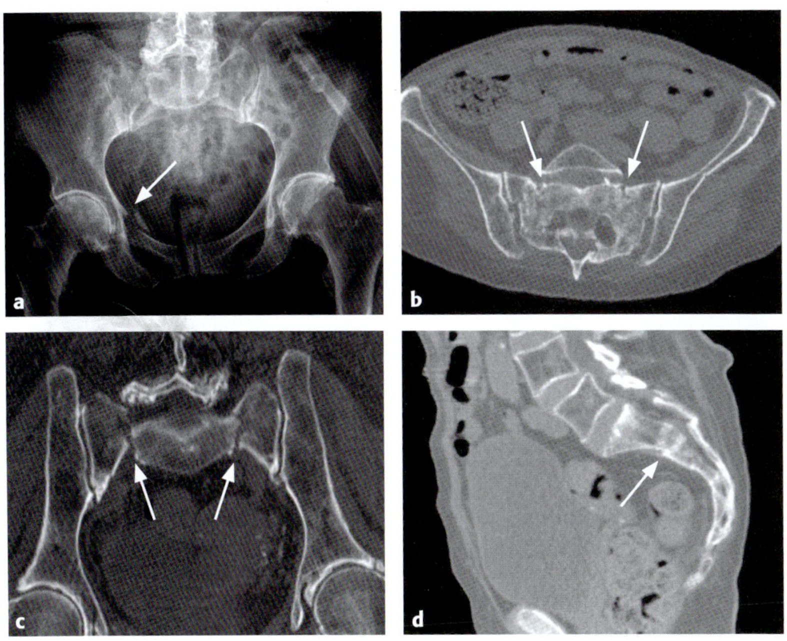


**Fig 3.7-8a–d** An 80-year-old woman with a fracture of the right superior and inferior pubic ramus after a fall.

- **a** AP x-ray of the pelvis showing a superior (white arrow) and inferior pubic ramus fracture on the right.
- **b** Transverse computed tomographic (CT) cut through the posterior pelvis showing a bilateral fracture through the sacral ala (white arrows).
- **c** Coronal CT cut through the sacrum showing bilateral complete and displaced sacral alar fractures (white arrows).
- **d** Sagittal CT cut through the midsacrum showing a horizontal fracture component between S1 and S2 with slight displacement in flexion (white arrow).

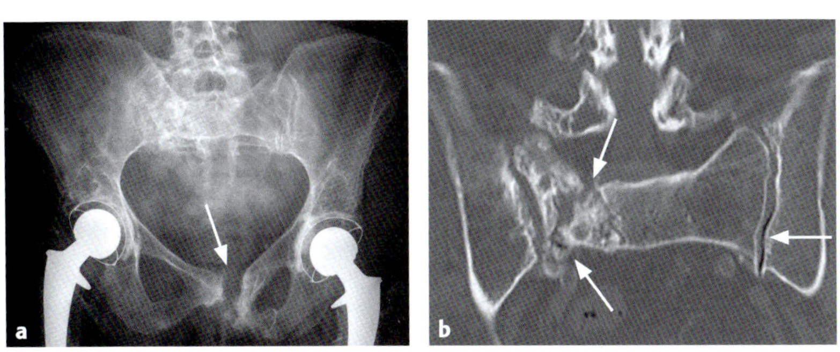


**Fig 3.7-9a–b** A 74-year-old woman with rheumatoid arthritis.

- **a** AP pelvic x-ray showing bone resorption and widening of the pubic symphysis (white arrow) due to chronic instability.
- **b** Coronal computed tomographic cut through the sacrum showing a complete fracture of the right sacral ala, bone resorption, callus formation, and widening of the right sacroiliac joint (white arrows). On the contralateral side, there is nitrogen inside the joint as a sign of instability (white arrow).

### 3.3.3 Magnetic resonance imaging

This is the most sensitive examination and can detect bone bruise within the sacrum, fissures, and fractures before they become visible using other modalities (**Fig 3.7-12**). Magnetic resonance imaging (MRI) may be indicated where conventional diagnostic measures cannot explain the clinical picture or the persistent complaints of pain. If pathology is detected with MRI, it rarely has consequences in terms of an operative treatment. Differentiation between bone marrow edema and malignancy is also possible with MRI [12]. With MRI, studies demonstrate up to 95% involvement of the posterior ring.

## 4 Classification

The Tile [13], AO/OTA Fracture and Dislocation [14], and Young-Burgess [15] classifications have been developed to distinguish different types of high-energy pelvic ring lesions. The Tile [13] and AO/OTA [14] classifications distinguish rotationally unstable from rotationally and vertically unstable injuries after AP, lateral, or vertical impacts. According to the direction of traumatic force, the Young-Burgess classification [15] differentiates AP displacement, lateral compression, vertical shear, and combined pelvic ring injuries. The Denis classification divides the sacrum into three zones. Denis I refers to the sacral ala, Denis II to the zone around the neurforamina and Denis III to the sacral body, medial to the neuroforamina [16].

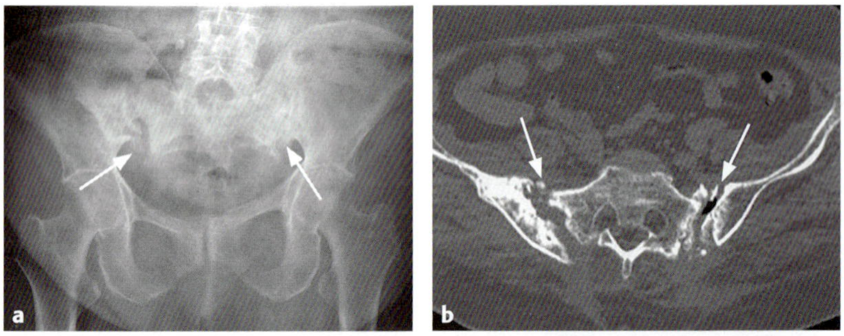

**Fig 3.7-10a–b** A 75-year-old woman with a history of pelvic pain.
- **a** AP x-ray of the patient's pelvis. There is an intrusion of the sacrum into the small pelvis (white arrows).
- **b** Transverse computed tomographic cut through the sacrum showing bilateral bone resorption, joint widening, and intraarticular nitrogen (white arrows).

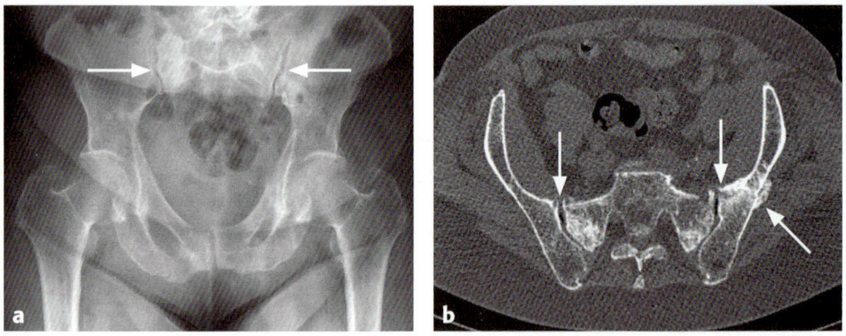

**Fig 3.7-11a–b** A 73-year-old woman with a history of chronic pain after a fall.
- **a** AP x-ray of the pelvis showing bilateral pubic rami fractures with callus formation and bilateral widening of the sacroiliac joints with nitrogen bubbles inside (white arrows).
- **b** Transverse computed tomographic cut through the posterior pelvis revealing a left-sided ilium fracture with bridging callus, bilateral sacral alar fractures, and confirming the nitrogen inside the irregular sacroiliac joints (white arrows).

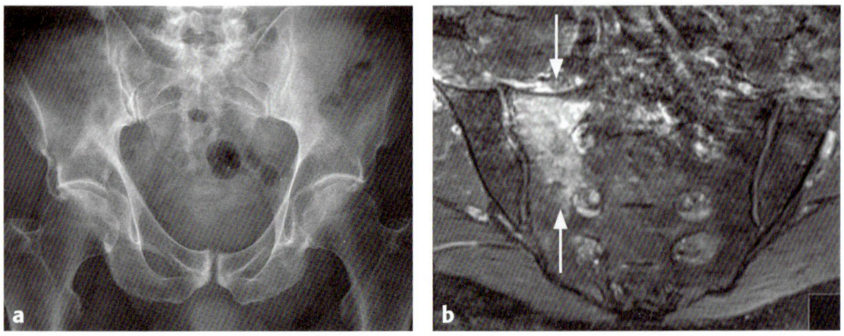

**Fig 3.7-12a–b** A 72-year-old man with bone bruise of the sacral ala.
- **a** AP pelvic x-ray of the patient with chronic pelvic pain after a long walk, showing no fractures, dislocations, or irregularities.
- **b** Magnetic resonance imaging depicting right-sided bone bruise of the sacral ala without fracture.

High-energy pelvic trauma is complicated by additional injuries of neurological and vascular structures, hollow organs, and the skin, with additional impacts on prognosis and outcomes.

In contrast, low-energy FFPs have completely different trauma mechanisms. Concomitant injuries of the soft tissues are rare. It is not the direction of the traumatic impact but the areas of very low bone density that are responsible for the fracture morphology [17]. Instability of FFP may increase over time, when the original lesion has been overlooked or undertreated (**Fig 3.7-7**). This is unique to FFP. The above-mentioned characteristics of FFP led to the development of a new, specific, and comprehensive classification system. The classification of FFP is based on an analysis of both conventional x-rays and CT data of 245 patients, 65 years or older with FFPs [18].

The most important criterion is the degree of instability. Instability is defined as the inability of a structure to withstand physiological loads without displacement. Also in older adults, this criterion is crucial for identifying an indication for surgery. Fracture displacement is the leading hint of instability. Nondisplaced lesions are characterized by a crush zone or a fracture without deformation. Displaced lesions are characterized by a crush or a fracture with deformation of the anatomical landmarks. The second criterion is the localization of the fracture in the posterior pelvis. The localization of the instability determines type and invasiveness of the surgical treatment.

Four different categories with slight, moderate, high, and highest instability were identified, namely types I–IV. The subtypes were characterized by a, b, or c. The main goals of treatment are restoration of prefracture stability and mobility. Due to instability, FFP generates intense pain and immobilization. Immobilization leads to rapid deterioration of the physical condition of the patient with higher morbidity and mortality due to secondary complications. The decision for an operation is needed, and the decision on which type of osteosynthesis should be performed is based on the severity of instability of the pelvic ring. It is therefore of utmost importance to thoroughly analyze the characteristics of the fractures and classify them within the new classification system, as this will ultimately form the basis for decision making.

In the following topics, the different types and subtypes of FFP are presented and a recommendation for treatment is given for all types. The operative techniques to be used are described in topic 7 of this chapter.

### 4.1 Fragility fracture of the pelvis type I

Fragility fractures of the pelvis type I are anterior pelvic ring fractures without involvement of the posterior pelvic ring. These are the lesions with the lowest degree of instability. Type Ia are unilateral (**Fig 3.7-13**) and type Ib are bilateral anterior lesions (**Fig 3.7-14**). The latter is much less frequent. Type I comprised 17.5% of all FFP in the authors' case series. Conversely, more than 80% of patients had a posterior pelvic ring injury. These findings support the use of CT evaluation for all low-energy pelvic ring fractures with anterior pelvic ring fractures, as there is a high risk of a concomitant posterior ring fracture that is often missed on conventional x-rays.

Fragility fracture of the pelvis type I should be treated nonoperatively. The authors hospitalize the patient and perform hemodynamic monitoring for the first 24 hours (see topic 4.2 in this chapter). When mobilization is not possible or delayed due to significant pain, pelvic stability should be reevaluated. If additional fractures are detected or primarily nondisplaced fractures displaced, operative management may be considered. External fixation can be regarded as a minimally invasive stabilization of anterior pelvic ring lesions. But there is little data on morbidity and outcome of pelvic external fixation in older adults. We assume that patients requiring anterior stabilization have posterior pelvic ring instability as well. Secondary fractures of the posterior ring may be induced over time in the stiff, older pelvis after initial anterior disruption (**Fig 3.7-7**).

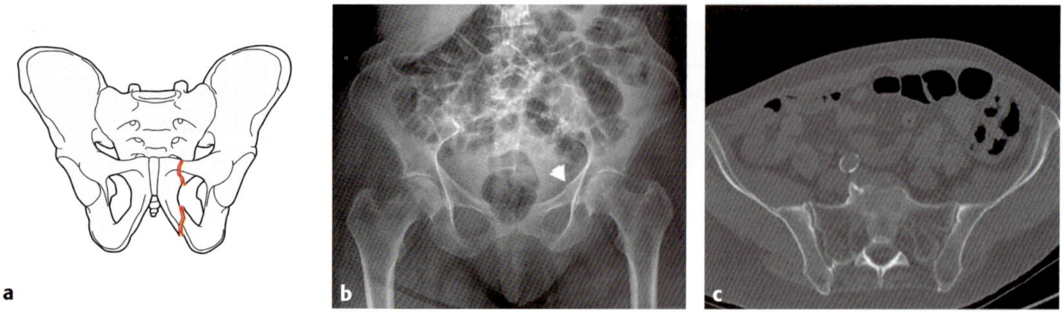

**Fig 3.7-13a–c** Type Ia—unilateral isolated anterior pelvic ring fracture.
**a** Illustration of a type Ia fracture.
**b** Conventional AP pelvic x-ray.
**c** Transverse computed tomographic cut.

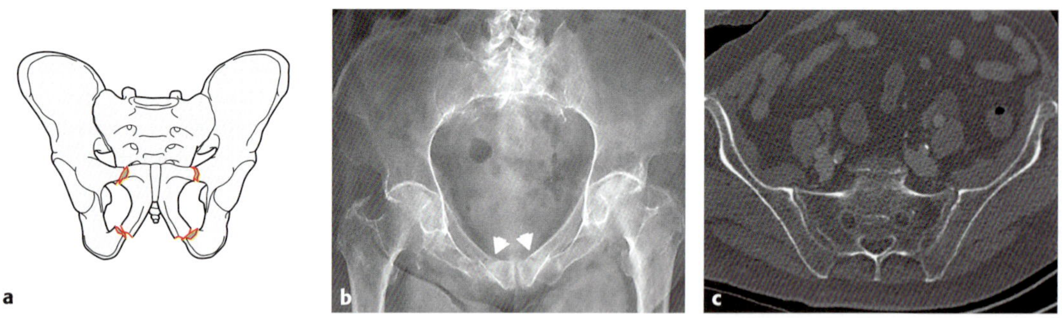

**Fig 3.7-14a–c** Type Ib—bilateral isolated anterior pelvic ring fracture.
**a** Illustration of a type Ib fracture.
**b** Conventional AP pelvic x-ray.
**c** Transverse computed tomographic cut.

### 4.2 Fragility fracture of the pelvis type II

Fragility fractures of the pelvis type II are characterized by nondisplaced posterior pelvic ring fractures. Type II lesions suffer more instability than type I lesions. Type IIa is a nondisplaced isolated posterior pelvic ring fracture (**Fig 3.7-15**), type IIb is a sacral crush with anterior disruption (**Fig 3.7-16**), and type IIc is a nondisplaced sacral, sacroiliac, or iliac fracture with anterior disruption (**Fig 3.7-17**). Type II fractures account for more than half of FFP [18]. Sacral fractures or crush zones of the sacral ala are much more frequent than sacroiliac dislocations or fractures of the posterior ilium. Fractures through the sacrum have unique and consistent fracture patterns [17]. The reason for this is the decrease in bone mass in the sacral ala, lateral to the neuroforamina in older patients. This has been demonstrated in a statistical model of the sacrum by Wagner et al [7, 19] based on CT data of 92 older Caucasians.

Fragility fractures of the pelvis type II must be regarded as posterior pelvic fractures before completion and displacement. They are more unstable than isolated anterior lesions but less unstable than displaced posterior lesions. They are typically associated with anterior instabilities. The traumatizing vector of FFP type IIb and FFP type IIc comes from a lateral direction, reflecting a sideways fall from a standing position with a lateral compression injury.

Nonoperative treatment with weight bearing as tolerated is initiated if patients are able to be mobilized within a few days. As the pelvic ring is broken posteriorly and anteriorly, we expect more pain and a longer rehabilitation time compared to FFP type I. It is important to listen to the complaints of the patient. If, after a maximum of 1 week, the pain is subsiding and the patient is able to mobilize independently, nonoperative therapy is continued. Follow-up x-rays after mobilization, and at 3, 6, and 12 weeks are recommended. Secondary fracture displacement with a higher degree of instability and transformation into a higher FFP type must be ruled out. Displacement of fractures of the posterior pelvic ring leads to a higher degree of instability and to classification in a higher FFP category. Nonoperative therapy must then be switched to operative therapy.

Complaints are another reason for changing therapy. When there is intense pain and patient transfer out of bed is impossible, operative fixation is recommended (**Case 3: Fig 3.7-18**). If the fracture fragments of the posterior pelvic ring are not displaced, percutaneous stabilization techniques such as iliosacral screw fixation seem most useful.

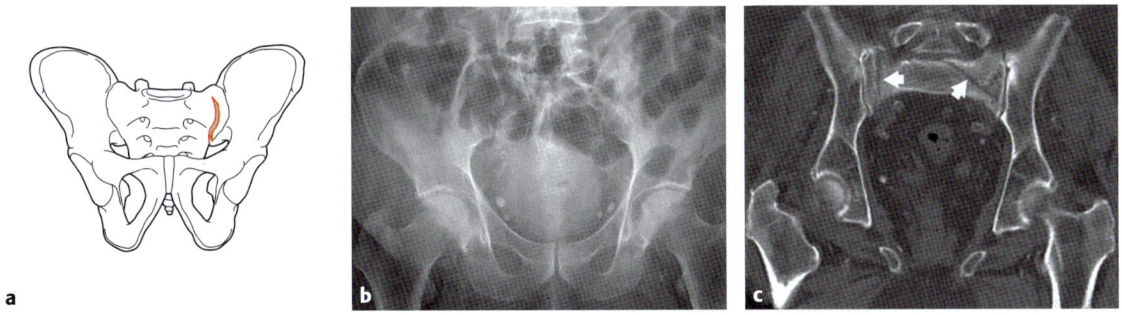


**Fig 3.7-15a–c** Type IIa—nondisplaced isolated posterior pelvic ring injury.
**a** Illustration of a type IIa fracture.
**b** Conventional AP pelvic x-ray.
**c** Coronal computed tomographic cut.

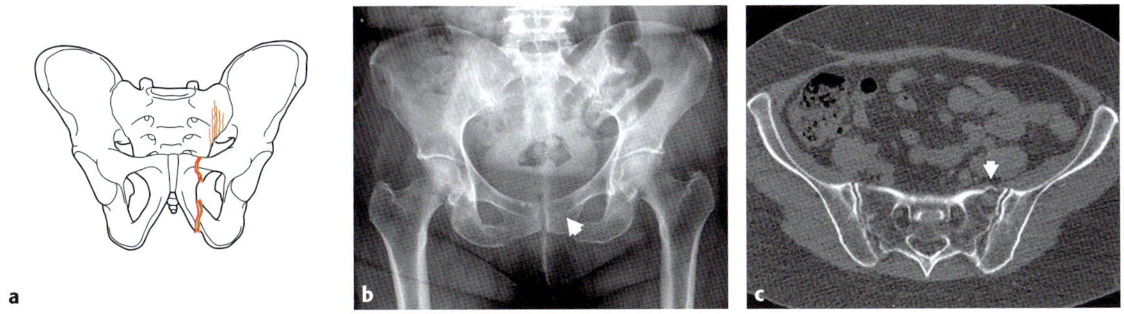


**Fig 3.7-16a–c** Type IIb—sacral crush with anterior pelvic ring fracture.
**a** Illustration of a type IIb fracture.
**b** Conventional AP pelvic x-ray.
**c** Transverse computed tomographic cut.

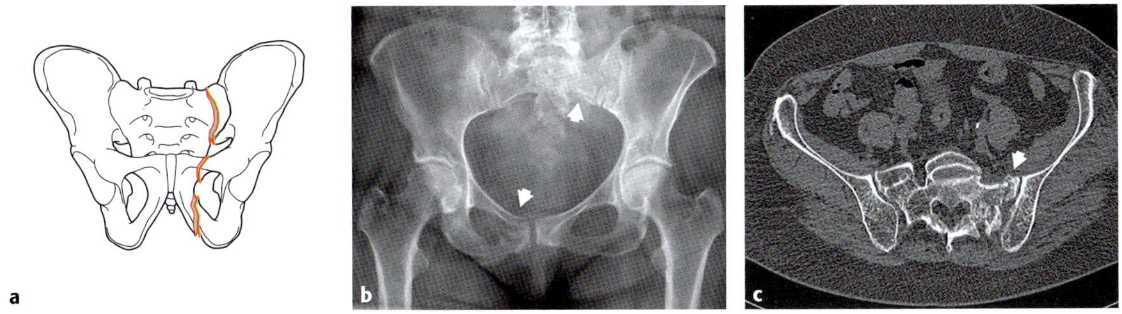


**Fig 3.7-17a–c** Type IIc—nondisplaced sacral fracture, nondisplaced iliosacral or iliac fracture with anterior pelvic ring fracture.
**a** Illustration of a type IIc fracture.
**b** Conventional AP pelvic x-ray.
**c** Transverse computed tomographic cut.

CASE 3

## Patient

An 85-year-old woman had a fall at home and sustained a fragility fracture of the pelvic ring type IIc.

## Comorbidities

- Hypothyreosis
- Arterial hypertension

## Treatment and outcome

The AP x-ray of the pelvis showed a left-sided pubic ramus fracture. Due to intense pain, mobilization was not possible for 3 weeks (**Fig 3.7-18a**). Inlet and outlet views were obtained (**Fig 3.7-18b–c**).

A coronal computed tomographic (CT) cut through the sacrum was performed and showed a complete fracture of the left sacral ala (white arrows in **Fig 3.7-18d**). The transverse CT cut through the anterior pelvic ring showed the left-sided pubic fracture (**Fig 3.7-18e**). After a 3-week nonoperative treatment, operative fixation was performed. The sacral alar fracture was fixed with two iliosacral screws, the pubic ramus fracture with a retrograde transpubic screw. The AP x-ray of the pelvic ring after 2 years showed complete healing of the anterior and posterior pelvic ring (**Fig 3.7-18f**). Another pelvic inlet and outlet view were obtained (**Fig 3.7-18g–h**).

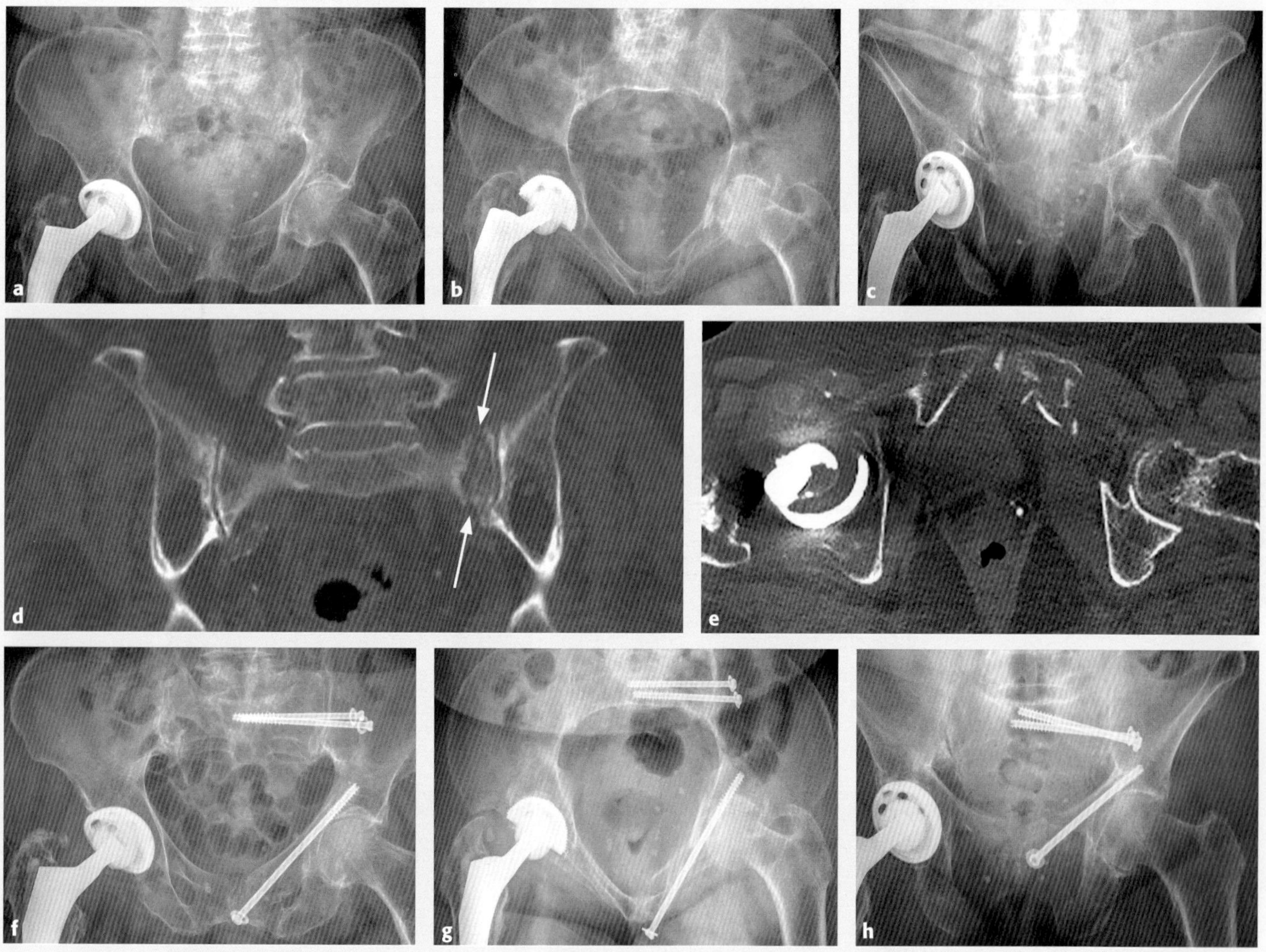


**Fig 3.7-18a–h** Example for change in treatment—an 85-year-old woman with fragility fracture of the pelvis type IIc.

- **a** AP pelvic x-ray of a left-sided pubic ramus fracture.
- **b** Pelvic inlet view.
- **c** Pelvic outlet view.
- **d** Coronal computed tomographic (CT) cut through the sacrum showing a complete fracture of the left sacral ala.
- **e** Transverse CT cut through the anterior pelvic ring showing the left-sided pubic fracture.
- **f** The AP x-ray of the pelvic ring after 2 years showing complete healing of the anterior and posterior pelvic ring. This AP x-ray is showing that the sacral alar fracture is fixed with two iliosacral screws and the pubic ramus fracture with a retrograde transpubic screw.
- **g** Pelvic inlet view.
- **h** Pelvic outlet view.

### 4.3 Fragility fracture of the pelvis type III

Fragility fractures of the pelvis type III are characterized by a displaced unilateral posterior injury combined with an anterior pelvic ring lesion. Displaced unilateral posterior lesions represent the smallest subtype in the group of 245 FFP, occurring in 11% [18]. They have a higher instability than type II lesions. Displacement must be assessed on both CT transections and conventional x-rays. Major displacement in the anterior pelvic ring must always be combined with some displacement in the posterior pelvic ring. Also, larger fracture gaps and changes of anatomical landmarks are signs of displacement.

Fragility fracture of the pelvis type IIIa involves a displaced unilateral ilium fracture (**Fig 3.7-19**).

Fragility fracture of the pelvis type IIIb is a displaced unilateral sacroiliac fracture dislocation (**Fig 3.7-20**).

Fragility fracture of the pelvis type IIIc is a displaced unilateral sacral fracture (**Fig 3.7-21**).

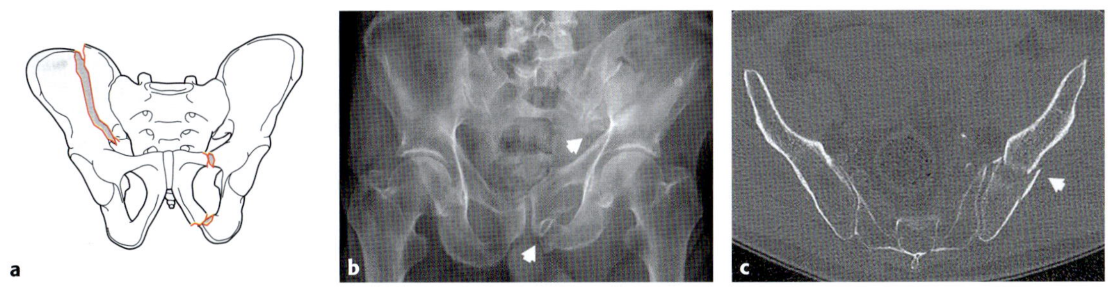


**Fig 3.7-19a–c** Type IIIa—a displaced unilateral iliac fracture with anterior pelvic ring fracture.
**a** Illustration of a type IIIa fracture.
**b** Conventional AP pelvic x-ray.
**c** Transverse computed tomographic cut.

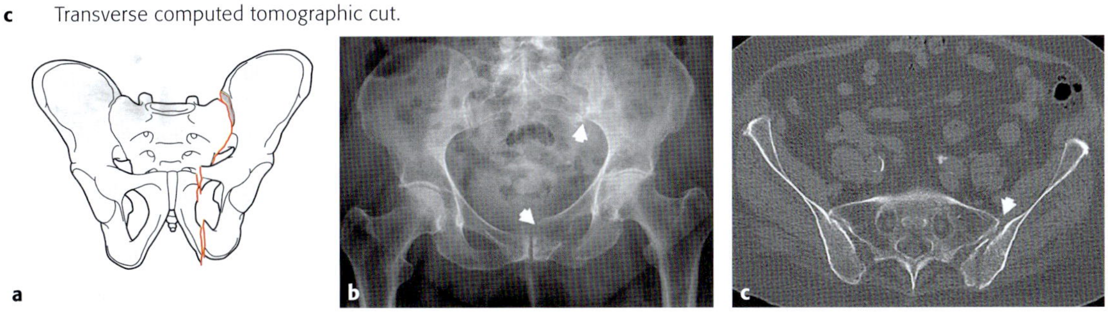


**Fig 3.7-20a–c** Type IIIb—a displaced unilateral sacroiliac fracture-dislocation with anterior pelvic ring fracture.
**a** Illustration of a type IIIb fracture.
**b** Conventional AP pelvic x-ray.
**c** Transverse computed tomographic cut.

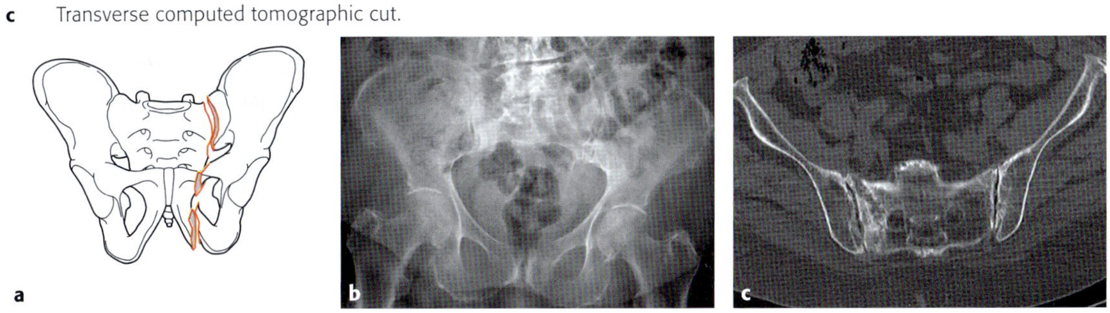


**Fig 3.7-21a–c** Type IIIc—a displaced unilateral sacral fracture with anterior pelvic ring fracture.
**a** Illustration of a type IIIc fracture.
**b** Conventional AP pelvic x-ray.
**c** Transverse computed tomographic cut.

It cannot be expected that these lesions will heal spontaneously. Due to severe pain, the patients are bedridden and mobilization is impossible. Operative treatment is therefore recommended as an urgent procedure. The type of internal fixation depends on the localization of the posterior instability. With limited displacement of the sacrum, sacroiliac joint, or posterior ilium, percutaneous stabilization is possible (**Case 4: Fig 3.7-22**). In case of gross displacement or a fracture through the ilium, an open reduction and internal fixation (ORIF) is required (**Case 5: Fig 3.7-23**).

CASE 4

### Patient

An 85-year-old woman sustained a fragility fracture of the pelvic ring type IIIb lesion after a fall at home.

### Comorbidities

- Hypercholesterolemia
- Arterial hypertension

### Treatment and outcome

The AP x-ray of the pelvis showed a left-sided displaced superior and inferior pubic ramus fracture (**Fig 3.7-22a**). Pelvic inlet and outlet views were obtained (**Fig 3.7-22b–c**). A transverse computed tomographic (CT) cut through the sacrum showed a fracture-dislocation of the left sacroiliac joint (white arrows in **Fig 3.7-22d**) while a transverse CT cut through the anterior pelvic ring revealed the left-sided pubic fracture (**Fig 3.7-22e**). The fracture-dislocation of the sacroiliac joint was fixed with two iliosacral screws and the pubic ramus fracture with a retrograde transpubic screw. The AP x-ray of the pelvic ring after 3 years showed complete healing of the anterior and posterior pelvic ring (**Fig 3.7-22f**). Another inlet and another outlet view of the pelvis were obtained (**Fig 3.7-22g–h**).

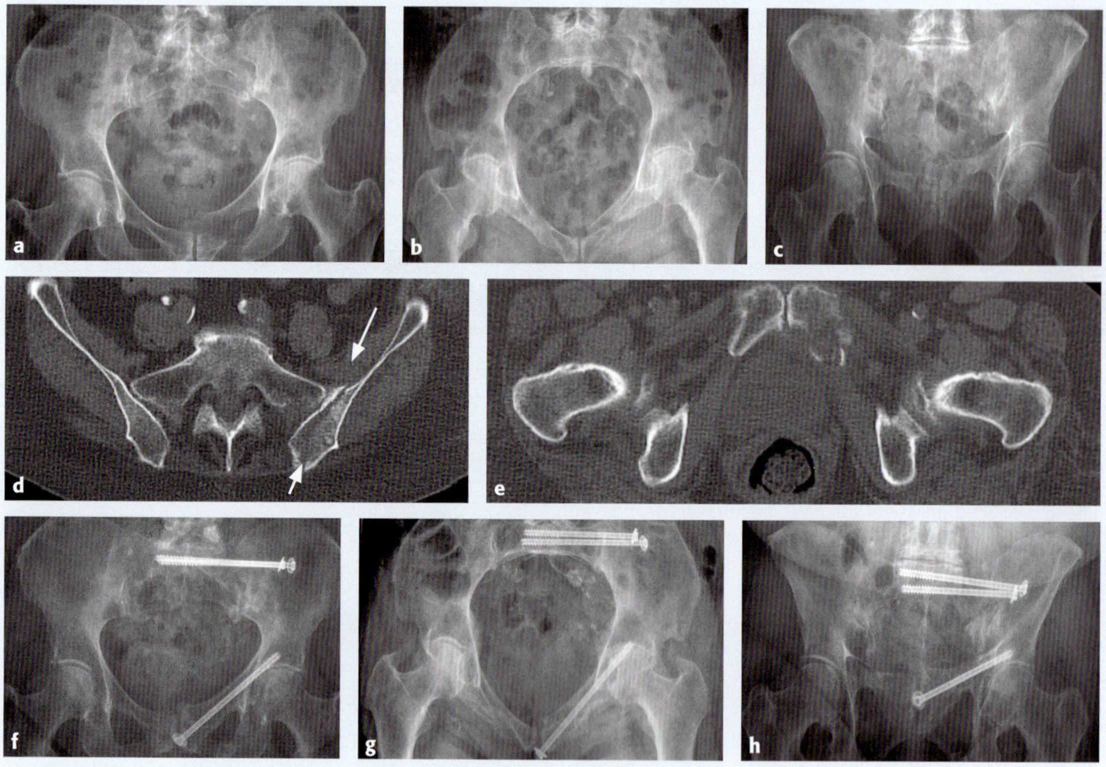


**Fig 3.7-22a–h** Example of a displaced type III fracture in the posterior ilium.
**a** AP pelvic x-ray of a left-sided displaced superior and inferior pubic ramus fracture.
**b** Pelvic inlet view.
**c** Pelvic outlet view.
**d** Transverse computed tomographic (CT) cut through the sacrum showing a fracture dislocation of the left sacroiliac joint (white arrows).
**e** Transverse CT cut through the anterior pelvic ring showing the left-sided pubic fracture.
**f** AP x-ray of the pelvic ring after 3 years showing complete healing of the anterior and posterior pelvic ring.
**g** Pelvic inlet view.
**h** Pelvic outlet view.

**Patient**

An 84-year-old woman fell in a nursing home.

**Comorbidities**

- Type 2 diabetes mellitus
- Renal insufficiency
- Macular degeneration

**Treatment and outcome**

The AP x-ray of the pelvis showed a left-sided fracture through the ilium running from the inner curve to the iliac crest (white arrows) and through the left superior and inferior pubic rami (**Fig 3.7-23a**).

The transverse computed tomographic (CT) cut through the posterior pelvic ring showed the fracture starting near the sacroiliac joint and the transverse CT cut through the ilium revealed the displacement in the fracture site, corresponding to a fragility fracture of the pelvis type IIIa (**Fig 3.7-23b–c**). It was operatively stabilized with an angular stable plate for the iliac fracture and a lag screw along the iliac crest (**Fig 3.7-23d**). Inlet and outlet views of the pelvis were obtained (**Fig 3.7-23e–f**).

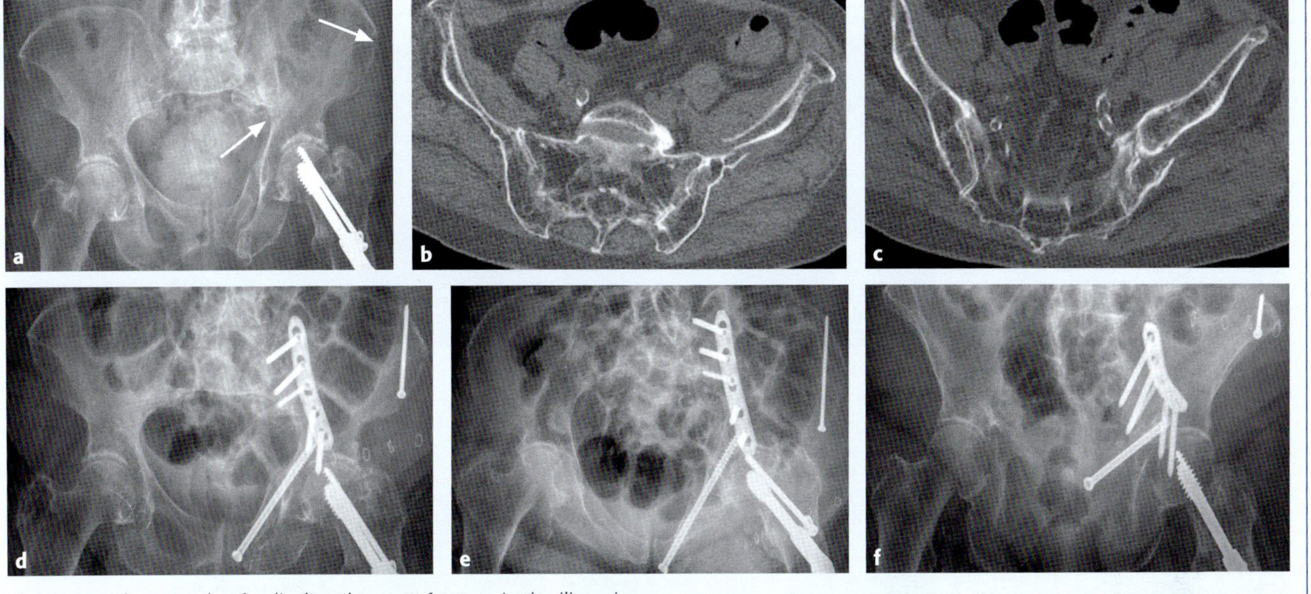


**Fig 3.7-23a–f** Example of a displaced type III fracture in the iliac wing.
- **a** AP x-ray of the pelvis showing a left-sided fracture through the ilium running from the inner curve to the iliac crest (white arrows) and through the left superior and inferior pubic rami.
- **b** Transverse computed tomographic (CT) cut through the posterior pelvic ring showing the fracture starting near to the sacroiliac joint.
- **c** Transverse CT cut through the ilium showing the displacement in the fracture site. It concerns a fragility fracture of the pelvis type IIIa.
- **d** Operative stabilization with angular stable plate for the ilium fracture and lag screw along the iliac crest.
- **e** Pelvic inlet view.
- **f** Pelvic outlet view.

## 4.4 Fragility fracture of the pelvis type IV

Fragility fractures of the pelvis type IV are displaced bilateral posterior injuries. The frequency of H-type sacral fractures (FFP type IVb), which is about 15%, is striking in the case series and was the starting point for the new classification [18]. This fracture morphology can be regarded as the extension of unilateral or bilateral nondisplaced vertical sacral alar fractures, seen in FFP type II lesions [17]. The horizontal component of the fracture is hardly visible on conventional x-rays. Looking at the sagittal reconstructions of CT to detect or exclude this fracture is therefore strongly recommended (**Fig 3.7-8**).

Fragility fracture of the pelvis type IVa has bilateral iliac fractures or bilateral sacroiliac disruptions (**Fig 3.7-24**).

Fragility fracture of the pelvis type IVb is an H-type sacral fracture, containing a bilateral vertical fracture through the sacral ala with a horizontal component connecting them (**Fig 3.7-25**).

Fragility fracture of the pelvis type IVc is a combination of different posterior instabilities (**Fig 3.7-26**).

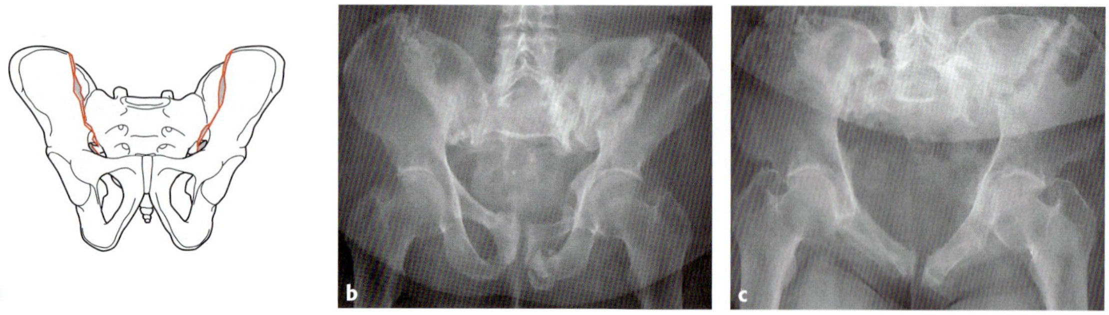

**Fig 3.7-24a–c** Type IVa—bilateral iliac fractures or bilateral sacroiliac disruptions with anterior pelvic ring fracture.
**a** Illustration of a type IVa fracture.
**b** Conventional AP pelvic x-ray.
**c** Pelvic inlet view.

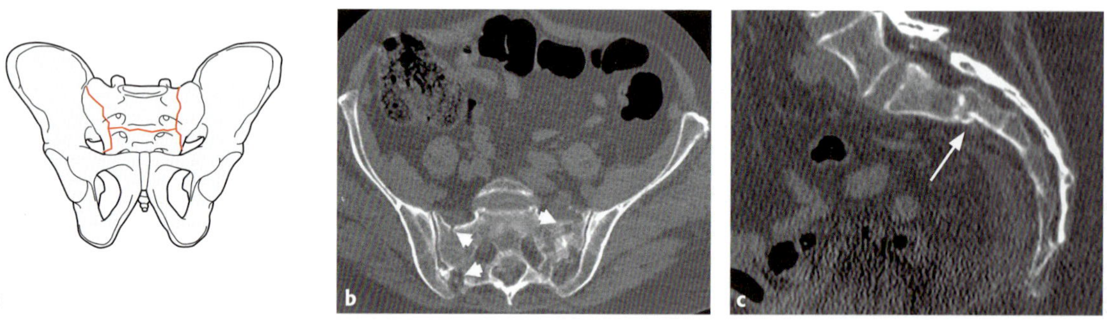

**Fig 3.7.25a–c** Type IVb—H-type sacral fracture with anterior pelvic ring fracture.
**a** Illustration of a type IVb fracture.
**b** Transverse computed tomographic (CT) cut.
**c** Sagittal computed tomographic cut.

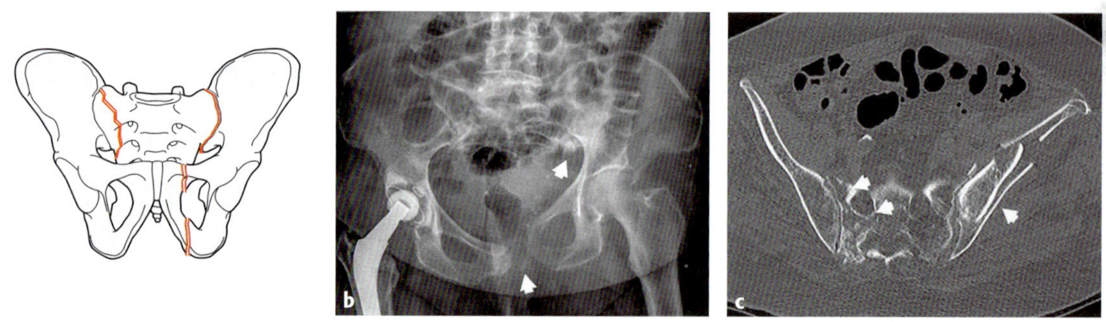

**Fig 3.7-26a–c** Type IVc—combination of different posterior instabilities with anterior pelvic ring fracture.
**a** Illustration of a type IVc fracture.
**b** Conventional AP pelvic x-ray.
**c** Transverse computed tomographic cut.

Fragility fractures of the pelvis possess the highest degree of instability when there is dissociation between the lumbosacral skeleton and the pelvic ring. Operative fixation restores stability and prevents further dislocation of the lumbosacral spine. Operative stabilization connects the lumbar spine to the posterior ilium to prevent intrusion of the lumbosacral spine into the pelvis. Iliolumbar fixation can be performed on both sides separately; alternatively, a transverse rod connects the constructs of both sides. When the lumbopelvic fixation is combined with an iliosacral screw fixation, the construct is described as triangular fixation (**Case 6: Fig 3.7-27**).

**Patient**

A 67-year-old woman with chronic pain in the posterior pelvis. She did not recall any specific trauma.

**Comorbidities**

- Rheumatoid arthritis
- Spinal canal stenosis
- Hypothyreosis
- Cardiac insufficiency
- Vascular dementia
- Glaucoma
- Cataract

**Treatment and outcome**

A coronal computed tomographic (CT) cut through the sacrum displayed bilateral complete fractures of the sacral ala (white arrows in **Fig 3.7-27a**). Transverse CT cut through the sacrum confirmed the fractures in the sacral ala (white arrows in **Fig 3.7-27b**). The transverse CT cut through the anterior pelvic ring showed a right-sided superior pubic ramus fracture (white arrow in **Fig 3.7-27c**).

A sagittal CT cut through the midsacrum revealed a horizontal sacral fracture between S1 and S2 with intrusion of the lumbosacral segment into the small pelvis (white arrow in **Fig 3.7-27d**). There was an H-type fracture of the sacrum and a fracture of the anterior pelvic ring, which corresponded with a fragility fracture of the pelvis type IVb.

The patient was treated with bilateral iliolumbar fixation between L4 and the posterior ilium. Additionally, an iliosacral screw was inserted in S1 on both sides. The fracture of the anterior pelvic ring was stabilized with a retrograde transpubic screw (**Fig 3.7-27e**). Inlet and outlet views of the pelvis were obtained (**Fig 3.7-27f–g**).

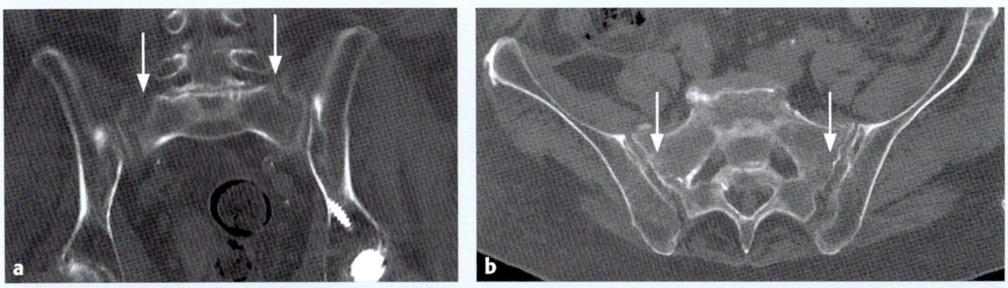


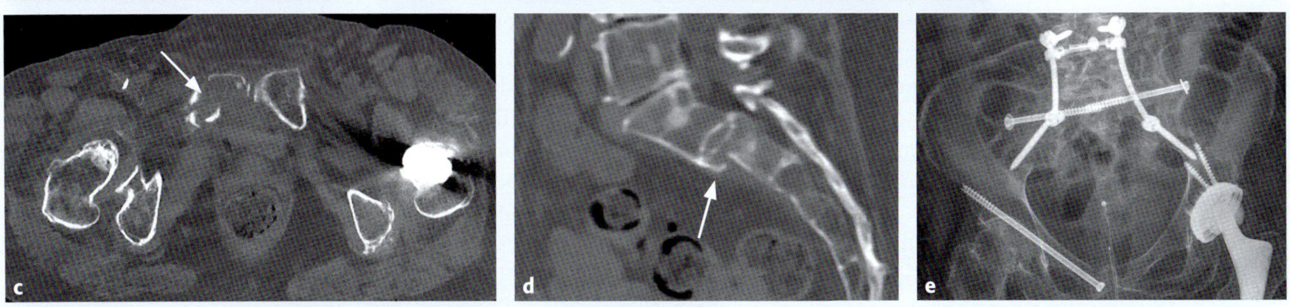


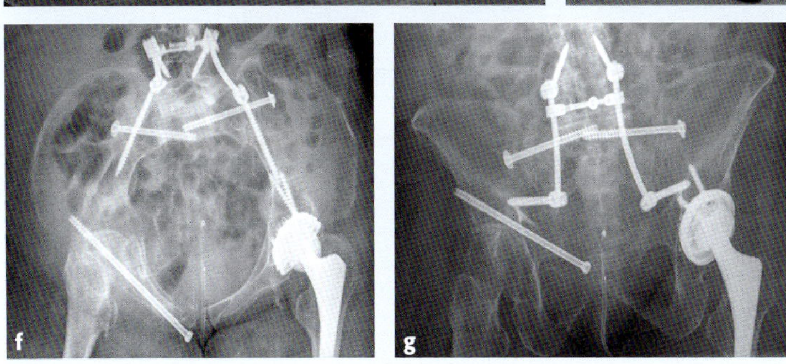


**Fig 3.7-27a–g** Example of a lumbopelvic fixation—a 67-year-old woman with bilateral complete fractures of the sacral ala.

**a** Coronal computed tomographic (CT) cut through the sacrum showing bilateral complete fractures of the sacral ala (white arrows).

**b** Transverse CT cut through the sacrum confirming the fractures in the sacral ala (white arrows).

**c** Transverse CT cut through the anterior pelvic ring showing a right-sided superior pubic ramus fracture (white arrow).

**d** A sagittal CT cut through the midsacrum revealing a horizontal sacral fracture between S1 and S2 with intrusion of the lumbosacral segment into the small pelvis (white arrow).

**e** AP x-ray of the pelvis 3 months after surgery.

**f** Pelvic inlet view.

**g** Pelvic outlet view.

In the vast majority, posterior pelvic ring lesions are associated with anterior pelvic ring lesions and vice versa. When treating the posterior pelvic ring operatively, surgeons should also take fixation of the anterior pelvic ring into consideration. Sole stabilization of the posterior pelvic ring may not restore adequate stability to the whole ring, with a higher risk of implant loosening or secondary fracture displacement due to continuous and repetitive loading during mobilization. Closing the whole ring gives the best support for a quick postoperative pain relief and safe mobilization.

The anterior pelvic ring can be stabilized with an external fixator or with different internal devices [20]. Some techniques of application are percutaneous, others less invasive and still others open. They use a bridging, positioning, or compression principle. The decision on which osteosynthesis is the most appropriate depends on fracture type, extent of displacement, and localization of instability. The different techniques for anterior pelvis fixation, their indications, and limitations will be described in topics 5.2.11–5.2.14 of this chapter.

## 5 Therapeutic options

### 5.1 Nonoperative management

Successful nonoperative management of pelvic ring fractures in older patients requires optimal orthogeriatric comanagement. Meticulous monitoring of pain levels and daily interprofessional and interdisciplinary discussion of the treatment progress with appropriate adaptations can limit the functional decline. Cornerstones of nonoperative treatment are:

- Pain management with oral analgesics, typically routine acetominophen with additional opioid dosing. Often opioids need to be given routinely for patients to be able to be mobilized. Patients are at high risk for severe constipation due to pain, immobility, and opioid therapy, and need to be placed on routine laxatives and monitored for effect. The pain from constipation can be confused with pain related to the fracture (see chapter 1.12 Pain management).
- Physiotherapy starts with the patient still in bed. To prepare the patient for out-of-bed mobilization, breathing therapy and mobilization of the extremities is performed. Once adequate pain control is achieved, the patient will sit up. This is followed by standing and consecutively trying to take first steps with the assistance of a physiotherapist and a walking aid such as a rolling walking frame. The order is always written "weight bearing as tolerated", as this population is not able to successfully observe partial weight bearing.
- Continuous x-ray controls during follow-up evaluate bone healing and rule out further displacement with delayed healing or nonunion. Especially bilateral anterior lesions are prone to secondary displacement due to pulling muscle forces. It is recommended to take conventional pelvic x-rays at 3, 6, and 12 weeks. Alternatively, a pelvic CT control confirms bone healing (**Case 7: Fig 3.7-28**). Some patients develop painful nonunions and need operative fixation.

The patient decides how fast mobilization can take place with regard to pain. It is expected that out-of-bed mobilization is possible within a few days after trauma. When mobilization is successful, discharge with further pain management and physiotherapy can be planned.

In all patients with FFP, being treated nonoperatively or operatively, the underlying bone disease must be diagnosed and treated in accordance with established guidelines [21]. The multidisciplinary team should therefore include geriatricians and specialists in bone metabolism, like endocrinologist and osteologist. Teriparatide can play an important role in accelerating bone healing of osteoporotic pelvic fractures [22, 23] (see chapter 1.10 Osteoporosis).

**Patient**

A 75-year-old woman who was treated nonoperatively for a fragility fracture of the pelvic ring type IIc lesion.

**Comorbidities**

- Degenerative lumbar scoliosis

**Treatment and outcome**

The fracture had healed. A small amount of callus was visible in front of the anterior sacral cortex of the left sacral ala (white arrow in **Fig 3.7-28a**). A coronal computed tomographic (CT) cut showed the healed fracture with a small remaining fissure in the posterior part of the previous fracture line (white arrow in **Fig 3.7-28b**). A transverse CT cut through the anterior pelvic ring showed periosteal callus bridging over the previous fracture site (white arrow in **Fig 3.7-28c**). A transverse CT cut through the inferior pubic ramus showed bridging callus anteriorly and posteriorly (white arrow). The patient was able to walk with full weight bearing and without walking aids (**Fig 3.7-28d**).

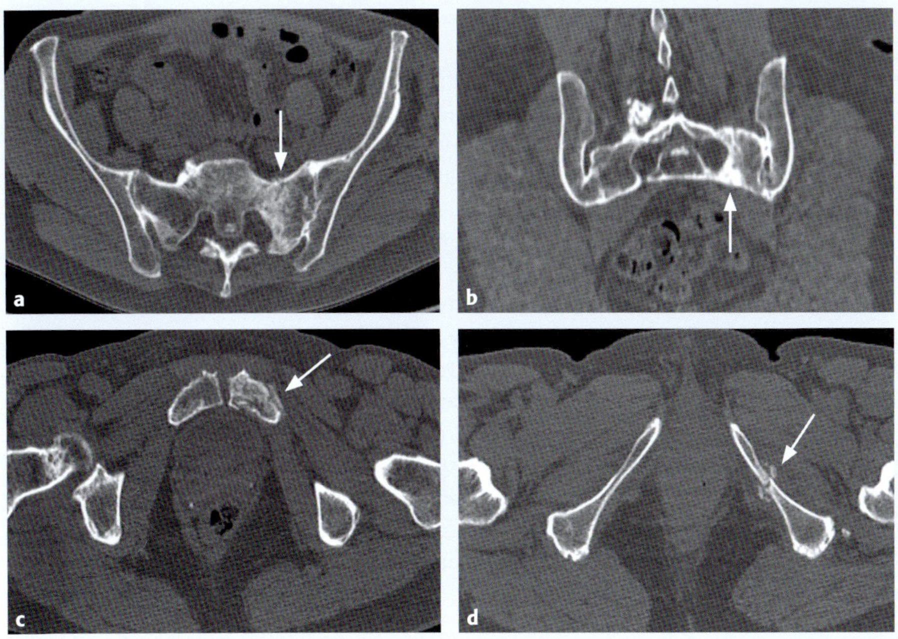


**Fig 3.7-28a–d** Callus formation after nonoperative treatment of a fragility fracture of the pelvis.
**a** Transverse computed tomographic (CT) cut through the sacrum showing a healed fracture with a small amount of callus in front of the anterior sacral cortex of the left sacral ala (white arrow).
**b** Coronal CT cut showing the healed fracture with a small remaining fissure in the posterior part of the previous fracture line (white arrow).
**c** Transverse CT cut through the anterior pelvic ring showing a periosteal callus bridge over the previous fracture site (white arrow).
**d** Transverse CT cut through the inferior pubic ramus showing bridging callus anteriorly and posteriorly (white arrow).

## 5.2 Operative treatment

Multiple techniques for reduction and fixation of posterior and anterior pelvic ring instabilities have been developed for high-energy pelvic trauma. In adolescents and adults, ORIF is more often used than closed reduction and percutaneous fixation. In contrast to FFP in older patients, restoration of the anatomy is of utmost importance for regaining an excellent long-term clinical function.

The principles of operative treatment in fragility fracture patients (see chapter 1.2 Principles of orthogeriatric surgical care) apply also to pelvic ring injuries:

- Precise anatomical reduction is less important than restoring stability for pain control and mobilization.
- Minimally invasive, percutaneous procedures are attractive because they take less time, involve less blood loss, and allow for quick recovery.
- Lengthy and aggressive surgery with higher blood loss and higher risk of infection, heterotopic ossification, and thromboembolism should be avoided [24].

The type of stabilization depends on the individual anatomy of the posterior pelvis, especially the morphology of the sacrum, as well as the characteristics and localization of instability (see topic 4 in this chapter).

Topics 5.2.2–5.2.10 refer to fixation techniques for the posterior pelvic ring, while topics 5.2.11–5.2.14 refer to the anterior pelvic ring.

### 5.2.1 Timing and planning

Patients with FFP are generally hemodynamically stable; there is usually no need for emergency fixation. Timing depends more on the general condition of the patient and patient's preference to reserve operative treatment for failed nonoperative treatment. Preoperative planning must include positioning of the patient, the choice of reduction maneuvers and instruments, the sequence of operative procedures, and the type of implants that will be used. Preoperatively, the bowels should be purged to assure good intraoperative visualization of bony landmarks with image intensification. This is of special interest for all cases in which a percutaneous procedure is planned.

### 5.2.2 Iliosacral screw in supine position

#### Indication

The indications include:

- Sacroiliac dislocations
- Fracture dislocations (crescent fracture)
- Nondisplaced or minimally displaced fractures of the sacral ala or through the neuroforamina (Denis zones I and II) [16]. In the majority of FFPs, the sacral alar fracture is at least one component of the injury.

#### Preoperative computed tomographic evaluation

The pelvic ring is a complex 3-D structure and the morphology varies between individuals. The operative anatomy of the posterior pelvic ring is especially variable. Corridors for exact implant insertion are sometimes narrow or nonexistent. For these reasons it is highly recommended that surgeons analyze the CT data thoroughly before surgery to avoid malposition of implants [18, 25]. Especially in dysmorphic sacra, it is beneficial to use computer navigation for exact screw placement [26].

#### Positioning

When positioning the patient, it is essential that:

- The patient is placed with the injured side on the edge of a radiolucent table enabling free orientation of the drill.
- A large skin area starting from the pubic symphysis and the umbilicus going posteriorly at the gluteal region is draped.
- The lower extremities are not draped, as reduction maneuvers are not necessary.

#### Image intensification

High-quality image intensifier visualization of the injured pelvic side must be assured. Before starting the procedure, a lateral x-ray of the lumbosacral junction is produced. In this x-ray, the ideal insertion point for iliosacral screw insertion in the body of S1 is identified. A small skin incision allows penetration of the drill through the gluteal muscles. Under image intensifier control, the tip of the drill is placed at the ideal insertion point on the outer cortex of the posterior ilium. With a hammer blow or a short drilling, the drill tip perforates this outer cortex. The image intensifier is now turned back for AP x-ray, inlet, and outlet views for further drilling and screw insertion (**Fig 3.7-29**) [27].

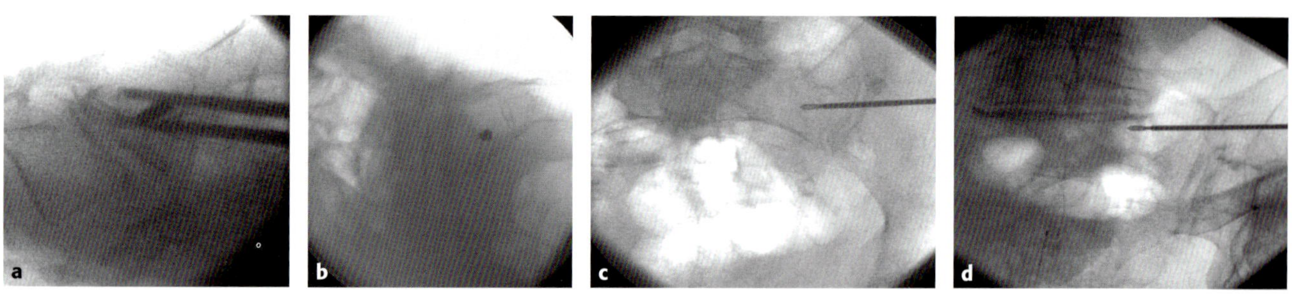


**Fig 3.7-29a–d** Example of optimal placement of screws.
**a** Intraoperative lateral x-ray of the lumbosacral transition. The ideal entry portal is identified under image intensification with the drill bit held in a Kocher clamp.
**b** The drill bit has been drilled through the outer and inner table of the posterior ilium; its position is below the iliac cortical density in the center of the S1 corridor.
**c** Intraoperative pelvic inlet view shows the tip of the drill bit in line with the anterior third of the S1 sacral body.
**d** Intraoperative outlet view. The tip of the drill bit is in line with the superior part of the S1 sacral body.

## Screw fixation

Depending on the diameter of the sacral corridor, insertion of one or two screws will be possible. Biomechanical studies have proven that stability of a sacroiliac fixation is significantly higher with two screws [28, 29]. Screw purchase in FFP is significantly lower in older than in younger patients due to lower trabecular density. A higher risk of implant loosening indicates the need for regular x-ray controls. The following technical tips are important:

- Iliosacral screws are placed perpendicular to the plane of instability, ie, the coronal plane for sacral alar fractures.
- The screws to be used are 7.3 mm or 8 mm cannulated screws with a long or continuous thread.
- The screws cross the midline and reach the opposite ala. This ensures that the thread of the screw is situated in the sacral body, which has the highest trabecular density (Denis zone III) [16]. Screw lengths have to be adapted accordingly [7, 29].
- Washers help to avoid screw perforation through the near cortex.
- Tightening the screws with a long thread will put some compression on the fracture site by direct pressure of the screw head with washer against the lateral cortex of the posterior ilium. The surgeon feels increasing resistance [29].
- In case a screw with continuous thread is used, it is sufficient to insert the screw until its head with washer touches the lateral cortex of the posterior ilium. No compression is obtained; the screw has the function of a positioning screw.
- In case two screws are inserted, their trajectory should be parallel or slightly converging. The tips of both screws are then located in the body of S1 but behind each other. The second screw can also be placed in the body of S2, but the sacral corridor of S2 is smaller than the one in S1.

Although low or no compression is achieved in the fracture gap, iliosacral screw insertion in osteoporotic bone increases local stiffness and diminishes pain (**Case 8: Fig 3.7-30**). But due to low anchorage in trabecular bone, there is a higher risk of secondary screw loosening. Changes in the screw design may help achieve better anchorage.

Perforated cannulated screws allow for cement augmentation. After screw insertion, a few cc of cement with a low viscosity are applied to the cancellous bone around the tip of the screw. The cement interdigitates with the trabecular bone and the pull-out force is much higher than without cement [30]. The cement must not leak into the fracture site, the alar void, the sacral canal, or the canal of the sacral nerve roots of S1. Therefore, cement application has to be done carefully, slowly, and under image intensifier control [31].

An alternative procedure is using nonperforated cannulated iliosacral screws, turning them back for about 1 cm after complete insertion, filling up the canal of the screw with liquid cement and finally reinserting the screws as before [30]. Recently, a combination of sacroplasty with cement-augmented iliosacral screw osteosynthesis has been proposed [32].

Little is known in the literature about results and complications of cement augmentation. Although the first results seem promising, critical analysis is still needed to recommend it as a standard procedure [33].

CASE 8

### Patient

An 82-year-old woman sustained a displaced superior pubic ramus fracture after a fall at home.

### Comorbidities

- No known comorbidities

### Treatment and outcome

The AP x-ray of the pelvis showed a displaced superior pubic ramus fracture on the right side (**Fig 3.7-30a**).

A coronal computed tomographic cut through the sacrum showed a complete fracture of the right sacral ala (white arrows). The lesion corresponded with a fragility fracture of the pelvic ring type IIc. Non-operative treatment was started, but operative therapy was performed 2 weeks later because the patient had intense pain (**Fig 3.7-30b**).

Two iliosacral screws were inserted in S1 to stabilize the sacral alar fracture and a retrograde transpubic screw to stabilize the pubic ramus fracture (**Fig 3.7-30c**). The AP x-ray at the 1-year follow-up showed complete healing of the fracture (**Fig 3.7-30d**).

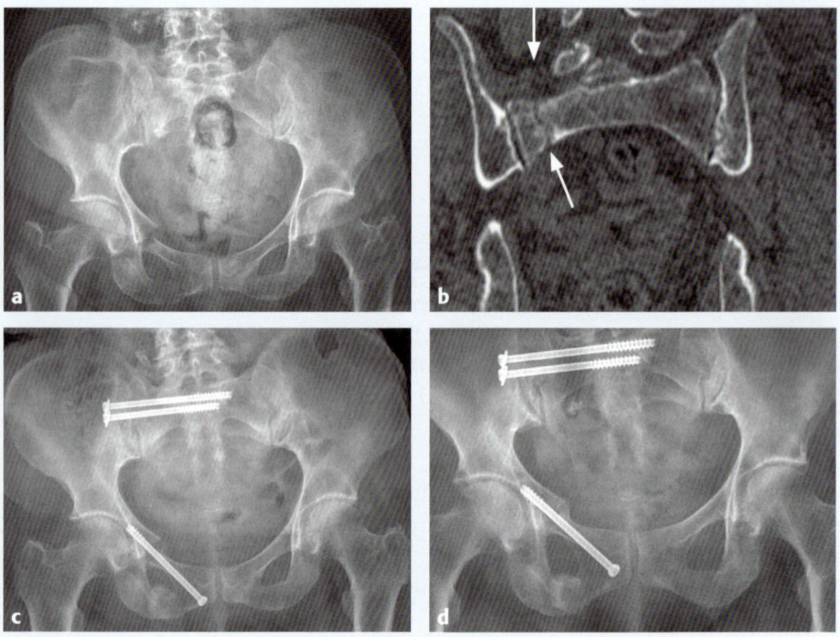


**Fig 3.7-30a–d** Example of a percutaneous sacroiliac fixation.
**a** AP pelvic x-ray of a displaced superior pubic ramus fracture on the right side.
**b** Coronal computed tomographic cut through the sacrum showing a complete fracture of the right sacral ala (white arrows).
**c** Postoperative AP x-ray of the pelvis after insertion of two iliosacral screws in S1 for stabilization of the sacral alar fracture and a retrograde transpubic screw for stabilization of the pubic ramus fracture.
**d** AP pelvic x-ray 1 year later showing complete healing of the fractures.

### 5.2.3 Iliosacral screws in prone position

The prone position has several advantages for iliosacral screw osteosynthesis. The authors recommend using the prone position whenever iliosacral screw fixation in supine position seems to be complicated or other surgeries have to be done in prone position. The main advantages of prone position are:

- Due to gravity, the soft tissues of the buttocks fall down, which makes it easier to access the posterior ilium.
- The distance from skin to bone becomes shorter, which enhances precision of screw placement. In obese people, this is of significant importance.
- The technique corresponds with the one described for the supine position.

### 5.2.4 Anterior plate fixation of the posterior ilium

A minority of patients with FFP have a fracture of the ilium. The fracture typically starts at the inner curve of the innominate bone and runs laterally and proximally through the ilium wing toward the iliac crest (**Case 5: Fig 3.7-23**) [34].

The main steps are:

- The approach should occur via the first window of the ilioinguinal approach and exposes the iliosacral joint medially and the iliopectineal eminence distally.
- Debridement, reduction, and compression of the fracture gap should be performed with the help of one or several reduction forceps. More important than precise reduction is creating sufficient stability.
- Fixation is done with a preshaped and twisted large fragment angular stable plate along the pelvic brim. At least two angular stable screws should be used at each side of the fracture. The screws must take the longest trajectory through the bone possible. The proximal screws are directed parallel to the iliosacral joint and have a length of up to 70 mm, the distal screws are directed toward distal and lateral, taking the longest trajectory in the iliac bone above the acetabular cavity.
- At the iliac crest, the fracture is stabilized with a long small fragment lag screw, which runs parallel to the iliac crest between the inner and outer cortex. Alternatively, a small fragment bridging plate is placed on top of the iliac crest (**Fig 3.7-31**).

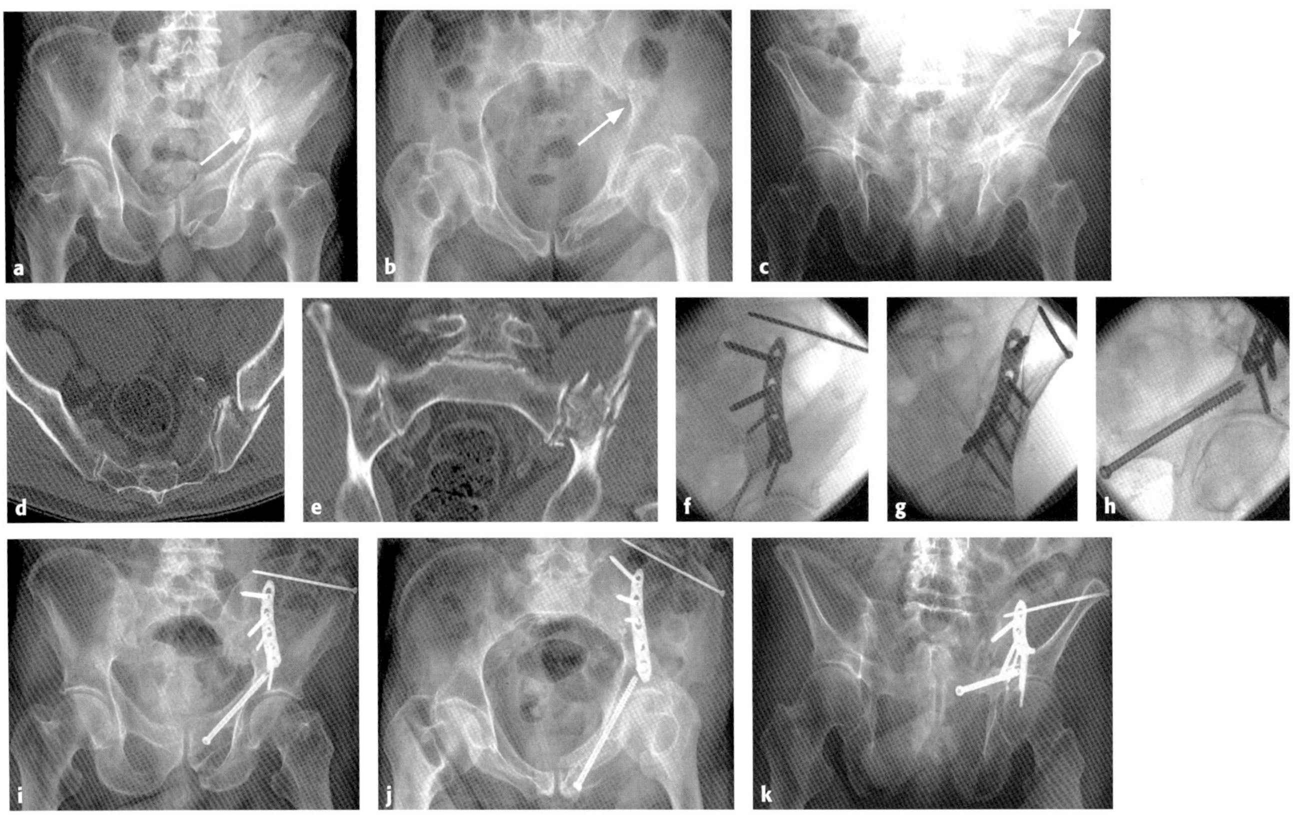

**Fig 3.7-31a–k** Example of plate fixation.

**a** AP x-ray of the pelvis in a 78-year-old man with Alzheimer's disease and recurrent falls. There is a fracture through the ilium starting at the inner curve and running through the iliac wing towards the iliac crest (white arrow). There is also a fracture of the left superior and inferior pubic rami.
**b** Pelvic inlet view shows the fracture at the inner curve (white arrow).
**c** Pelvic outlet view shows the fracture at the iliac crest (white arrow).
**d** Transverse computed tomographic (CT) cut through the ilium shows the left-sided fracture.
**e** Coronal CT cut confirming the iliac fracture near the sacroiliac joint.
**f** Intraoperative alar x-ray of the left ilium showing the position of the angular stable plate.
**g** Intraoperative obturator x-ray of the left ilium.
**h** Intraoperative obturator x-ray of the obturator foramen showing the position of the retrograde transpubic screw.
**i** Postoperative AP x-ray of the pelvis with angular stable plate bridging the left ilium fracture, lag screw along the iliac crest and retrograde transpubic screw.
**j** Postoperative inlet view.
**k** Postoperative outlet view.

### 5.2.5 Sacroplasty

This is a minimally invasive procedure to inject cement into the fractured sacrum [35]. Multiple insertion points for the needle have been described in literature. It can be inserted:

- Directly behind the fracture zone
- In the distal ala through thin soft tissues
- At the typical location used for iliosacral screw insertion [36]

According to the literature, pain intensity reduces significantly and mobilization can be started quickly. Indication may be based on MRI findings only [37] or CT diagnostics [31]. Clearly, the risk of leakage is much higher with cortical fractures in place (**Fig 3.7-32**) [31, 37]. Concerns regarding this technique are:

- The cement behaves as a foreign body between the fracture fragments and may hinder bone healing.
- The fracture plane of the sacral ala is vertical. Vertical loading while standing and walking leads to shearing forces that interfere with bone healing and may not be neutralized by cement augmentation.
- Most fractures of the posterior pelvic ring are combined with fractures of the anterior pelvis. Current literature does not describe what happens with anterior instabilities after sacroplasty.
- Some FFP fractures may evolve from a category of lower to a category of higher instability. It is not clear which operative treatment should be performed in case of contralateral or additional ipsilateral sacral fracture after sacroplasty.
- Little is known about the long-term outcome after sacroplasty. The question which fracture types of FFP benefit the most from sacroplasty remains unsolved. In the authors' opinions, only a minority of FFP are suitable for this technique.

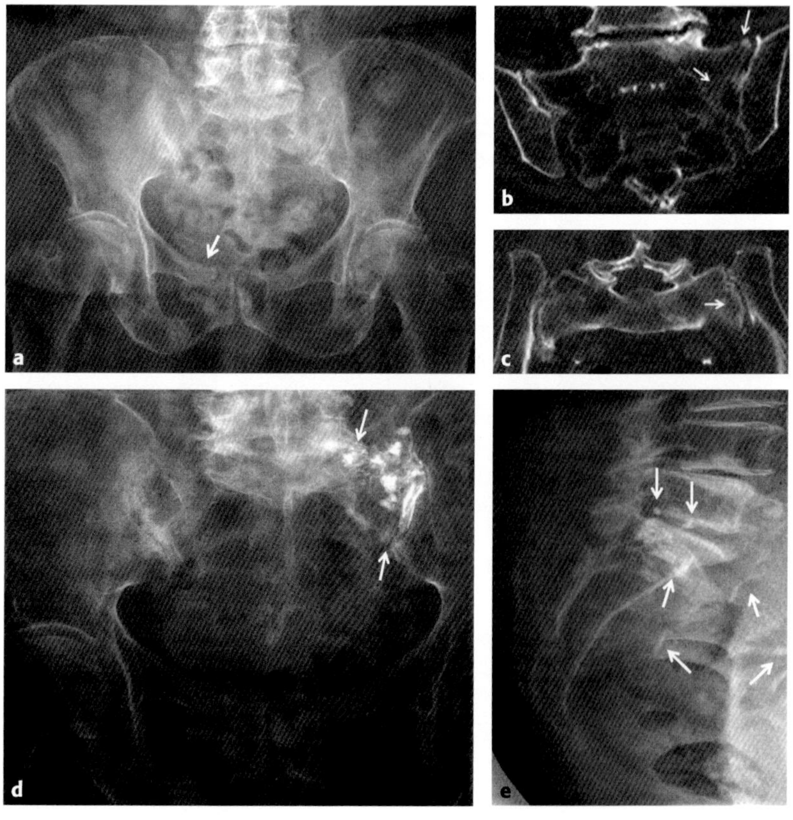


**Fig 3.7-32a–e** An 87-year-old woman with a history of pain in the posterior pelvic region without memorable trauma.

- **a** AP pelvic x-ray showing a right-sided superior and inferior pubic ramus fracture (white arrow). Callus formation indicates that the fractures are older.
- **b** Coronal computed tomographic (CT) cut through the sacrum showing a complete fracture of the sacral ala near the sacroiliac joint (white arrows).
- **c** Transverse CT cut confirming the lateral sacral alar fracture (white arrow).
- **d** Postoperative AP pelvic x-ray after sacroplasty. Besides cement in the sacral ala, there is cement in the sacroiliac joint.
- **e** Lateral x-ray of the sacrum. There is cement extravasation into several presacral veins and through the anterior cortex of the sacral ala (white arrows).

### 5.2.6 Transiliac bars

Transiliac bars bridge the area of instability; in connection with an anterior stabilization, they act as a tension band [38]. Advantages of transiliac bars are:

- It is a less invasive technique.
- They offer high stability with compressive forces perpendicular to the fracture plane(s).
- Bilateral lesions can be treated with one fixation. A bilateral iliosacral screw osteosynthesis with four screws in the sacral corridor S1 or two screws in S1 and two in S2 will probably not provide similar enduring stability in older patients.
- There is no penetration into the sacral bone with reduced risk of damage to neural and vascular structures inside the sacrum or just anterior to it.

Disadvantages include the prominent hardware that can be felt behind the sacrum and may disturb the patient while sitting. In the era of bridging plates and transsacral bars, transiliac bars are used less frequently.

Two incisions are made parallel and just lateral to the posterior iliac crests. The lateral cortex of the posterior ilium is exposed. One fingerbreadth anterior to the crest, a hole of 6 mm is drilled through the posterior ilium. Through the hole, a threaded 6 mm bar is passed in the coronal plane behind the sacrum towards the opposite posterior ilium. A similar hole is drilled and the bar pushed through this second hole. On both sides, nuts are placed over the ends of the threaded bar. Washers are used to prevent perforation of the nuts through the outer cortex. When tightening the nuts, compression is created on the sacral fracture. A second bar may be placed below the first bar using the same technique.

### 5.2.7 Transsacral bars

A threaded bar is inserted through the sacral corridor of S1 [39, 40]. This is only possible if this corridor is available. This fixation stabilizes monolateral or bilateral nondisplaced or minimally displaced fractures of the sacral ala or sacroiliac joint. The technique is demanding and preoperative planning is of utmost importance. A small part of the Caucasian but a larger part of the Asian population has dysmorphic sacra, in which the transsacral corridor is too small or nonexistent [7].

The procedure is performed through small skin incisions, which are placed in line with the central axis of the transsacral corridor of S1. Two incisions of 4–5 cm are sufficient. The horizontal direction of the transsacral bar is perpendicular to the plane of the sacral fractures. Tightening of the nuts and washers creates compression and enhances stability (**Case 9: Fig 3.7-33**). The stability of the construct does not depend on the strength of the cancellous bone in the body of S1, as is the case with iliosacral screw osteosynthesis. The stability depends on the strength of the external cortex of the posterior iliac wing, against which the nuts and washers are tightened. The few outcome data for this technique have been reported as positive [40, 41].

**CASE 9**

**Patient**

A 77-year-old woman with a left superior and inferior pubic ramus fracture after a fall at home.

**Comorbidities**

- Hypercholesterolemia
- Hypothyreosis
- Urinary incontinence

**Treatment and outcome**

The AP x-ray of the pelvis showed a left superior and inferior pubic ramus fracture (**Fig 3.7-33a**). An inlet x-ray of the pelvis was obtained (**Fig 3.7-33b**). A transverse computed tomographic cut through the sacrum showed a bilateral sacral alar fracture that was complete on the right side and incomplete on the left side (white arrows). These fractures corresponded with a fragility fracture of the pelvis type IIc (**Fig 3.7-33c**). The fractures were fixed operatively with a transsacral bar and bilateral iliosacral screws. The pubic ramus fracture was stabilized with a retrograde transpubic screw. The AP pelvic x-ray taken after 2 years showed complete healing of all fractures. There was a slight loosening of the retrograde transpubic screw (**Fig 3.7-33d**). Another inlet and outlet view of the pelvis was taken (**Fig 3.7-33e–f**).

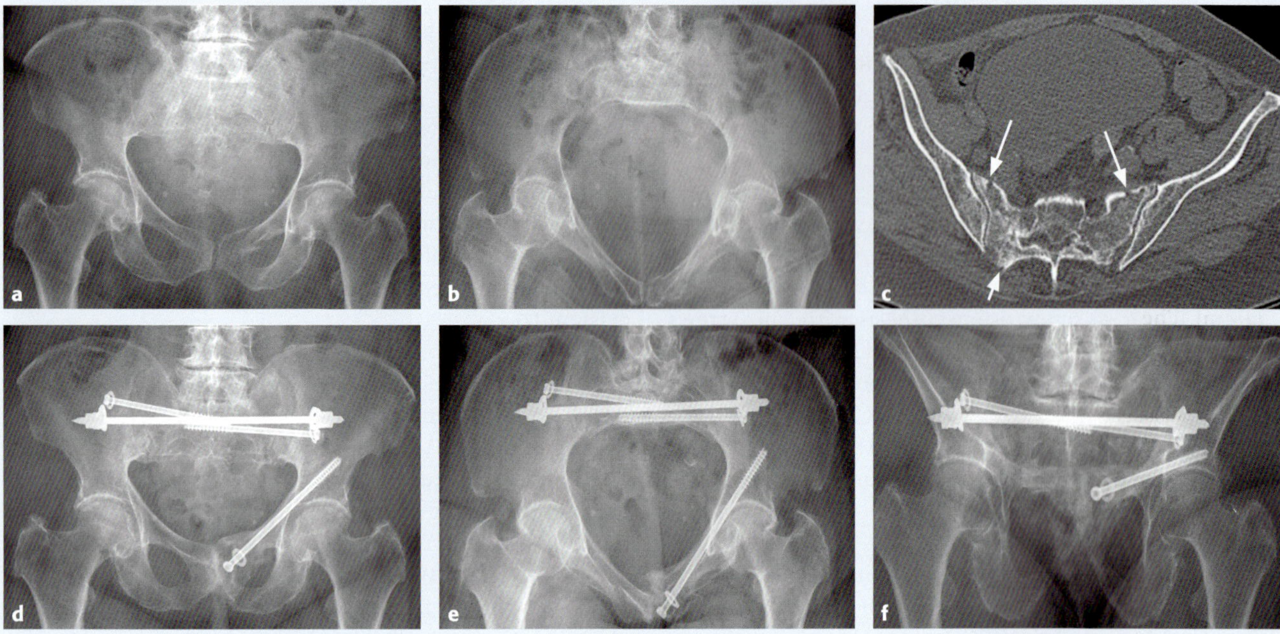


**Fig 3.7-33a–f**. A 77-year-old woman with a fracture of the superior and inferior pubic ramus.

- **a** AP pelvic x-ray of a left superior and inferior pubic ramus fracture.
- **b** Pelvic inlet view.
- **c** Transverse computed tomographic cut through the sacrum showing a bilateral sacral alar fracture, complete on the right side and incomplete on the left side (white arrows).
- **d** AP pelvic x-ray after 2 years showing complete healing of all fractures but a slight loosening of the retrograde transpubic screw.
- **e** Pelvic inlet view.
- **f** Pelvic outlet view.

### 5.2.8 Bridging plate

A plate, which is curved at its ends, is used instead of a transiliac bar. The plate lies posterior to the sacrum and is contoured around the posterior iliac crests near the posterior iliac spines. To prevent placing uncomfortable hardware just below the skin, an osteotomy of the posterior superior iliac spines (PSISs) can be performed and a bone block the width of the plate removed. Once the plate has been inserted, the bone blocks are reinserted and fixed with a small screw [42]. The plate can also be inserted more distally between the notches just below the posterior inferior iliac spines. This distal plate location has the advantage of the implant being very close to the posterior cortex of the sacrum. The plate ends are bowed and fitted against the posterior ilium. Long screws can be inserted through the two marginal plate holes on each side. One screw goes in the anterior direction parallel to the sacroiliac joint, the other screw in the superior direction parallel to the iliac crest.

Bridging plate osteosynthesis can be done as a less invasive procedure. The incisions are similar to those for transiliac bar osteosynthesis. The soft tissues behind the sacrum and between the posterior iliac crests are tunneled for plate positioning [43]. The plate takes the function of a tension band, but it does not create direct compression on the fracture site. With this bridging osteosynthesis, bilateral sacral alar fractures are stabilized in one procedure. In case of unilateral fractures, the bridging plate can prevent development of a contralateral fracture. Combination of iliosacral screws with the posterior plate enhances stability. Specific angular stable plate designs have been developed. They create a higher stability than the nonangular stable fixation [44, 45].

### 5.2.9 Transiliac internal fixator

A minimally invasive alternative to transiliac bars or bridging plate osteosynthesis is the insertion of a transiliac internal fixator. An osteotomy of the PSIS is performed, and a bone block with the width of a pedicle screw head removed. The trajectory for a long pedicle screw is drilled. From the PSIS, this trajectory passes above the greater sciatic notch and goes in the direction of the anterior inferior iliac spine. The screw is located between the inner and outer cortex of the ilium. The pedicle screw has a diameter of up to 7 mm and can have a length of 100 mm. The screw heads are connected with a rod of 5 or 6 mm diameter which is placed in a subcutaneous tunnel (**Case 10: Fig 3.7-34**) [46]. In a biomechanical model with complete iliosacral disruption, stability is as high as anterior plate osteosynthesis of the sacroiliac joint and iliosacral screw osteosynthesis [47]. The experience with transiliac internal fixation of type C lesions in high-energy pelvic trauma is very good, but there are no published data yet on this procedure in FFP.

CASE 10

**Patient**

An 86-year-old woman with a history of several falls and posterior pelvic pain.

**Comorbidities**

- Cardiac insufficiency
- Stenosis of the aortic valve
- Peripheral arterial disease
- Renal insufficiency
- Pneumonia

**Treatment and outcome**

A fracture of the anterior pelvic ring could not be identified (**Fig 3.7-34a**). A transverse computed tomographic (CT) cut through the sacrum revealed a complete fracture of the left sacral ala (white arrows). This lesion corresponded with a fragility fracture of the pelvis type IIa (**Fig 3.7-34b**). A coronal CT cut confirmed the complete fracture of the left sacral ala (**Fig 3.7-34c**). A posterior transiliac internal fixator was inserted (**Fig 3.7-34d**). An inlet and an outlet view of the pelvis were obtained (**Fig 3.7-34e–f**).

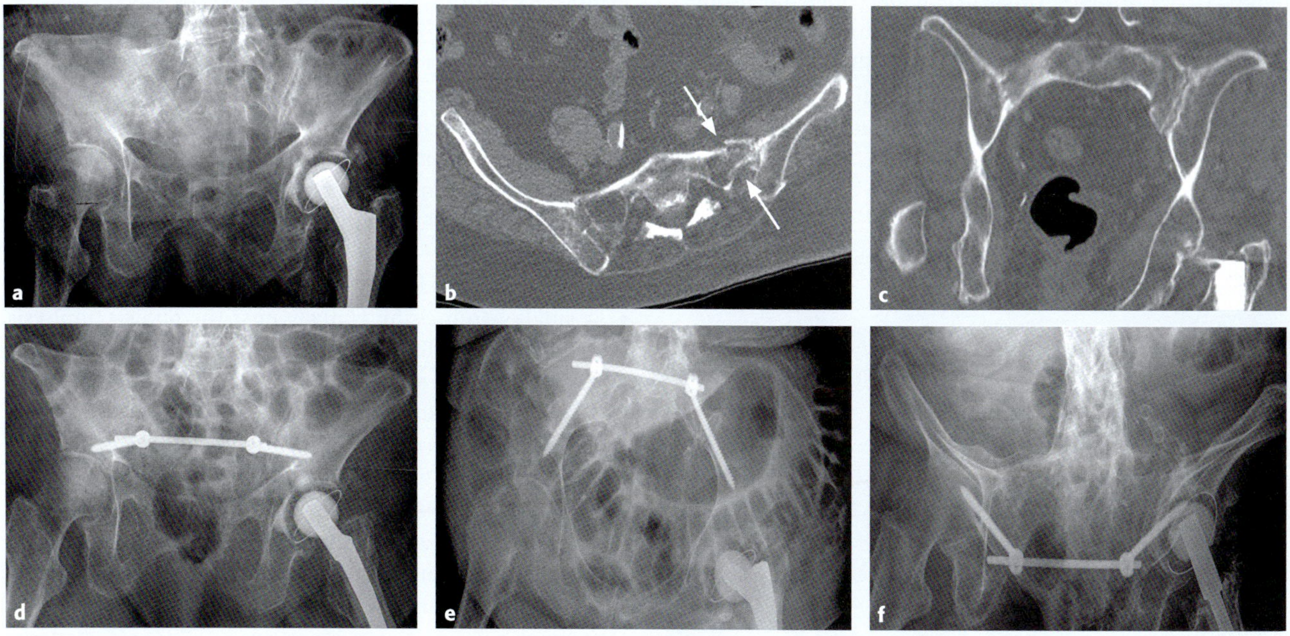


**Fig 3.7-34a–f** An 86-year-old woman with several falls in the past and actual posterior pelvic pain.
**a** AP pelvic x-ray not showing a fracture of the anterior pelvic ring.
**b** Transverse computed tomographic (CT) cut through the sacrum revealing a complete fracture of the left sacral ala (white arrows).
**c** Coronal CT cut confirming the complete fracture of the left sacral ala.
**d** Postoperative AP pelvic x-ray showing the inserted posterior transiliac internal fixator.
**e** Pelvic inlet view.
**f** Pelvic outlet view.

### 5.2.10 Lumbopelvic fixation

With this technique, a tight connection is created between the lumbar spine and the posterior ilium. A vertical incision above the sacrum going up to the level of L4 or L5 is needed. One pedicle screw is placed in the pedicle of L5 at the side of instability. In case of pronounced lordosis, the L4 pedicle is preferred so that a more vertically directed construct is built. The second pedicle screw is inserted in the posterior ilium as described in transiliac internal fixation. A connection rod is inserted between and fixed to the pedicle screws. In case of an H-type sacral fracture, a bilateral lumbopelvic fixation with transverse connection between both rods is performed [48]. The procedure can be performed percutaneously, but more intraoperative image intensification is needed for precise pedicle insertion. Lumbopelvic fixation can be combined with a transverse fixation like iliosacral screws or a transsacral bar. The construct then looks triangular (**Case 6: Fig 3.7-27**) [49].

The advantage of lumbopelvic fixation is its less invasive procedure. The construct controls vertical instability. It is especially recommended in H-type fractures to prevent further intrusion of the lumbosacral segment into the small pelvis. It is a bridging construct, which does not produce fracture compression. Literature of lumbopelvic fixation focuses on the control of vertically unstable pelvic fractures or spondylolisthesis of the lumbosacral junction [48, 50]. Little is known about complications and results in FFP.

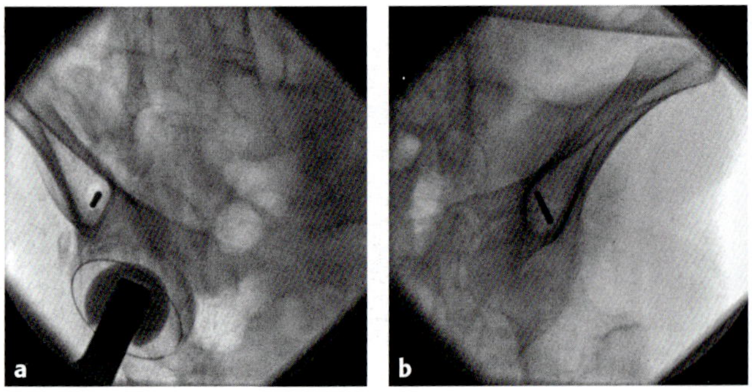


**Fig 3.7-35a–b** Insertion point for supraacetabular external fixator Schanz screw. Under image intensification, the corridor becomes visible in the obturator outlet views as a high triangle above the acetabular cavity.

**a** Image intensification with K-wire inside the triangle.
**b** Image intensification of the contralateral side, also with K-wire inside the triangle. The K-wires will consecutively be replaced by Schanz screws.

### 5.2.11 Supraacetabular external fixation

From each side, one or two Schanz screws are inserted from the anterior inferior iliac spine toward the PSIS (**Fig 3.7-35**). The skin incisions run vertically from the anterior superior iliac spine (ASIS) downward. The trajectory through the soft tissues has to be prepared bluntly. Care has to be taken not to injure the lateral cutaneous femoral nerve, which runs below the inguinal ligament just medial to the ASIS towards distal and lateral. The screws have a length of up to 100 mm. They are connected to each other and to the other side with rods. The frame bridges the anterior pelvis [51–53]. Biomechanical studies have proven that its stability is high enough to control disruptions of the anterior pelvic ring but not of the posterior pelvic ring [54]. If a posterior pelvic ring lesion has been identified, operative stabilization should be considered as well.

### 5.2.12 Retrograde transpubic screw

The optimal indication for retrograde transpubic screw fixation is a superior pubic ramus fracture, which is situated above the obturator foramen or at the anterior rim of the acetabulum. Fractures which are situated more medially, running within the pubic bone and near to the pubic symphysis, cannot be bridged safely with a screw:

- The screw can be inserted with a percutaneous technique if the fracture is minimally displaced.
- Before starting surgery, the level and inclination of the screw are identified under image intensifier control with the help of a long K-wire or drill bit that is placed over the skin of the lower abdomen and moved until it perfectly covers the trajectory of the screw in the superior pubic ramus. This line is marked.
- A small skin incision is made near the pubic symphysis following that line, and the trajectory to the anterior pubic bone is prepared.
- The 2.8 mm drill bit is held in 45° inclination to the frontal and sagittal planes. Under image intensification, the location of the drill tip is adjusted until it lies precisely in line with the optimal trajectory of the screw. The image intensifier is brought into the obturator-outlet and iliac-inlet positions consecutively, while the drill bit enters the canal and is moved cranially and laterally through the superior pubic ramus [55]. Special attention is paid to avoid penetration of the drill bit into the acetabulum. The drilling procedure is continued until the tip of the drill bit reaches and perforates the posterolateral cortex of the iliac body.
- The length of the trajectory in the bone may reach 130 mm [56]. The most anterior part of the trajectory is overdrilled by 4.5 mm. A 7.2 mm cannulated screw of appropriate

length is inserted over the 2.8 mm drill bit. The use of a washer is not absolutely necessary. The screw head lies in the thick tendinous attachment of the adductor muscles at the pubic bone (**Case 3: Fig 3.7-18, Case 9: Fig 3.7-33**).

- The screw primarily splints the superior pubic ramus fracture; it does not achieve strong compression [55]. When the drill bit cannot pass the acetabulum without perforating the joint, a shorter screw must be chosen. It will generate lower stability and have a higher risk of loosening.

When the superior pubic ramus fracture is displaced but appropriate for retrograde transpubic screw fixation, closed or open reduction can be done. The skin incision is the same, but can be smaller than in the case of plate fixation. The displaced superior pubic ramus fracture is reduced by direct means and the trajectory for the screw drilled under control of finger touch and image intensification.

### 5.2.13 Plate fixation

An infraumbilical midline incision or a Pfannenstiel skin incision can be chosen. The linea alba is split above the symphysis and the retropubic space exposed. The anterior curve of the pelvic ring can be exposed further laterally following the modified Stoppa approach. As the instability is not situated in the joint, but close to it, the plate will not be placed strictly above the pubic symphysis but more toward one side. Small fragment curved plates are used, which allow variable screw directions [57, 58]. It is advisable to drill long trajectories in the bone for the screws and use screws as long as possible to obtain good purchase and a high pull-out force. Near the pubic symphysis, screw lengths of 60 mm should be used. The infraacetabular corridor with the screw passing lateral to the obturator foramen and medial to the acetabulum going into the posterior column should be used, if possible. It can have a length of more than 100 mm and has a very good holding power in the strong ischium (**Case 11: Fig 3.7-36**) [59]. When the fracture is situated at the anterior lip of the acetabulum, an infrapectineal plate can be used through a Stoppa approach. The plate is curved and runs from the posterosuperior margin of the pubic bone below the pelvic brim toward the sacroiliac joint. Two or three screws can be placed above the acetabulum, realizing a good anchorage of the plate into the iliac body. Double plate osteosynthesis may be considered in cases of chronic instability, where a high stability over a long healing time is necessary (**Case 12: Fig 3.7-37**).

The approach is very well endured by older adults, as it uses anatomical layers without necessitating muscle or tendon detachment [60]. To date, the literature has not specifically addressed plate fixation or retrograde transpubic screw fixation in the anterior pelvis of a geriatric population.

**CASE 11**

**Patient**

A 75-year-old woman with a history of rheumatoid arthritis.

**Comorbidities**

- Rheumatoid arthritis
- Hodgkin's disease
- Sicca syndrome
- Aortic valve replacement
- Chronic hepatic disease
- Total hip replacements
- Total knee replacement

**Treatment and outcome**

There was bone resorption, bone defect, and instability of the pubic symphysis. Irregular bone architecture was visible at the right sacral ala (**Fig 3.7-36a**). Pelvic inlet and outlet views were obtained (**Fig 3.7-36b–c**). A transverse computed tomographic (CT) cut through the sacrum showed a complete fracture of the right sacral ala with bone defect and connection with the sacroiliac joint (**Fig 3.7-36d**). A coronal CT cut showed the irregular sacral alar fracture with callus formation at the anterior sacral cortex (**Fig 3.7-36e**). A postoperative coronal CT cut through the sacrum revealed that the posterior pelvic ring fracture had been fixed with a transsacral bar and additional iliosacral screw (**Fig 3.7-36f**). The instability of the pubic symphysis was stabilized after debridement of the joint with a long curved plate. The marginal screws used the infraacetabular corridor. All other screws used the longest possible bone trajectory (**Fig 3.7-36g**). Another inlet view of the pelvis and after 3 months another pelvic outlet view were obtained (**Fig 3.7-36h–i**).

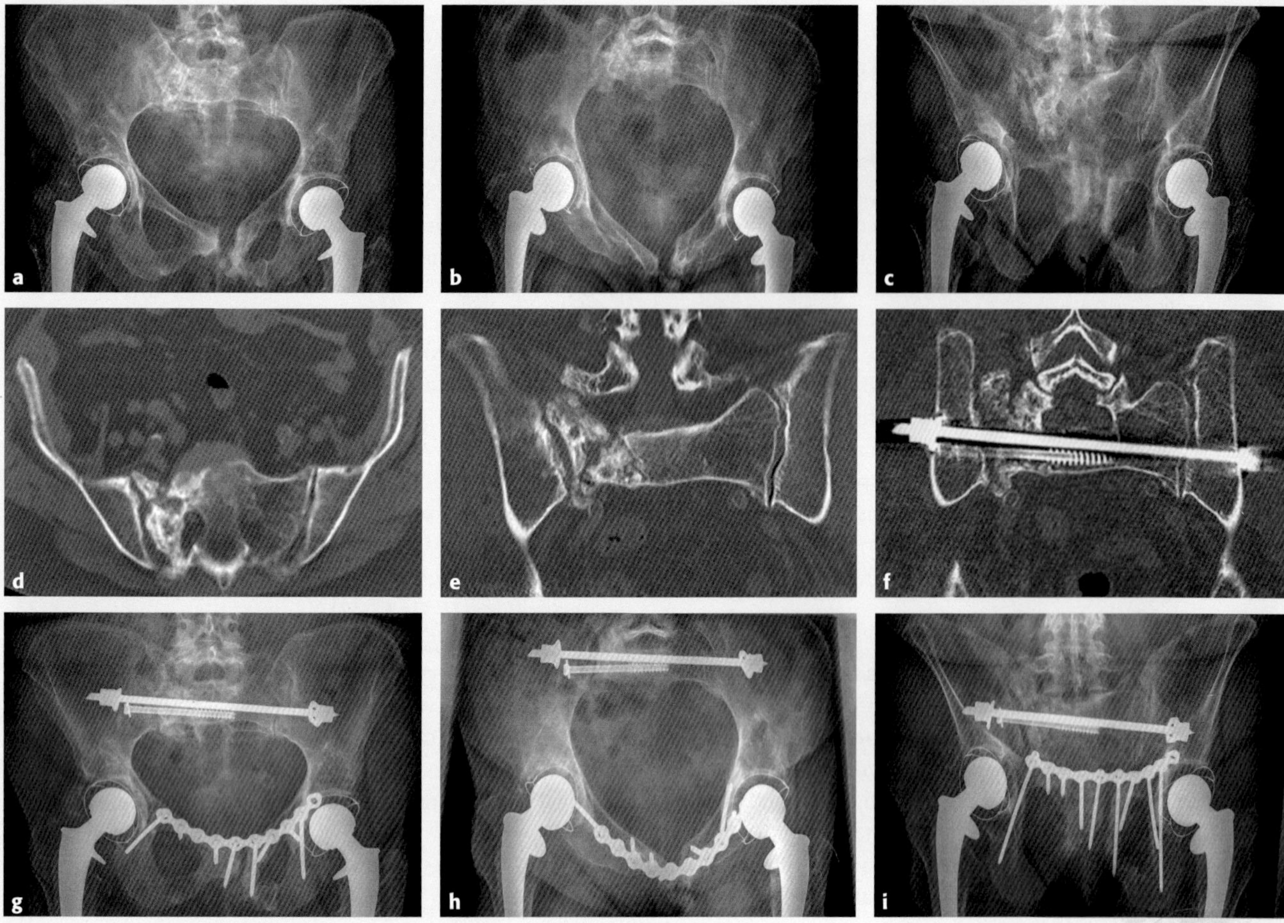


**Fig 3.7-36a–i** A 75-year-old woman with a history of rheumatoid arthritis.

- **a** AP pelvic x-ray showing bone resorption, bone defect, and instability of the pubic symphysis. Irregular bone architecture is visible at the right sacral ala.
- **b** Pelvic inlet view.
- **c** Pelvic outlet view.
- **d** Transverse computed tomographic (CT) cut through the sacrum showing a complete fracture of the right sacral ala with bone defect and connection with the sacroiliac joint.
- **e** Coronal CT cut showing the irregular sacral alar fracture with callus formation at the anterior sacral cortex.
- **f** Postoperative coronal CT cut through the sacrum showing the posterior pelvic ring fracture fixed with a transsacral bar and additional iliosacral screw.
- **g** X-ray showing the pubic symphysis stabilized with a long, curved plate. The marginal screws use the infraacetabular corridor. All other screws use the longest bone trajectory possible.
- **h** Pelvic inlet view.
- **i** Pelvic outlet view 3 months after surgery.

**Patient**

A 77-year-old woman with a history of corticosteroid use.

**Comorbidities**

- Hypothyreosis
- Arterial hypertension

**Treatment and outcome**

The AP x-ray of the pelvis showed instability of the pubic symphysis due to the vertical displacement of the left pubic bone (**Fig 3.7-37a**). A transverse computed tomographic (CT) cut through the sacrum showed a complete and older left sacral alar fracture (**Fig 3.7-37b**). A coronal CT cut through the pubic symphysis showed a small bone defect and irregular margins (**Fig 3.7-37c**). The posterior instability had been treated with a transsacral bar and additional iliosacral screw. The anterior pubic instability had been treated with pubic debridement, tricortical bone grafting, and double plate osteosynthesis, as bony fusion of the pubic symphysis was the therapeutic goal and a longer healing time could be expected (**Fig 3.7-37d**). A pelvic inlet view was obtained (**Fig 3.7-37e**). The pelvic outlet view showed the long marginal screws of the superior plate using the infraacetabular corridors into the ischium. The view was taken 3 months postoperatively (**Fig 3.7-37f**).

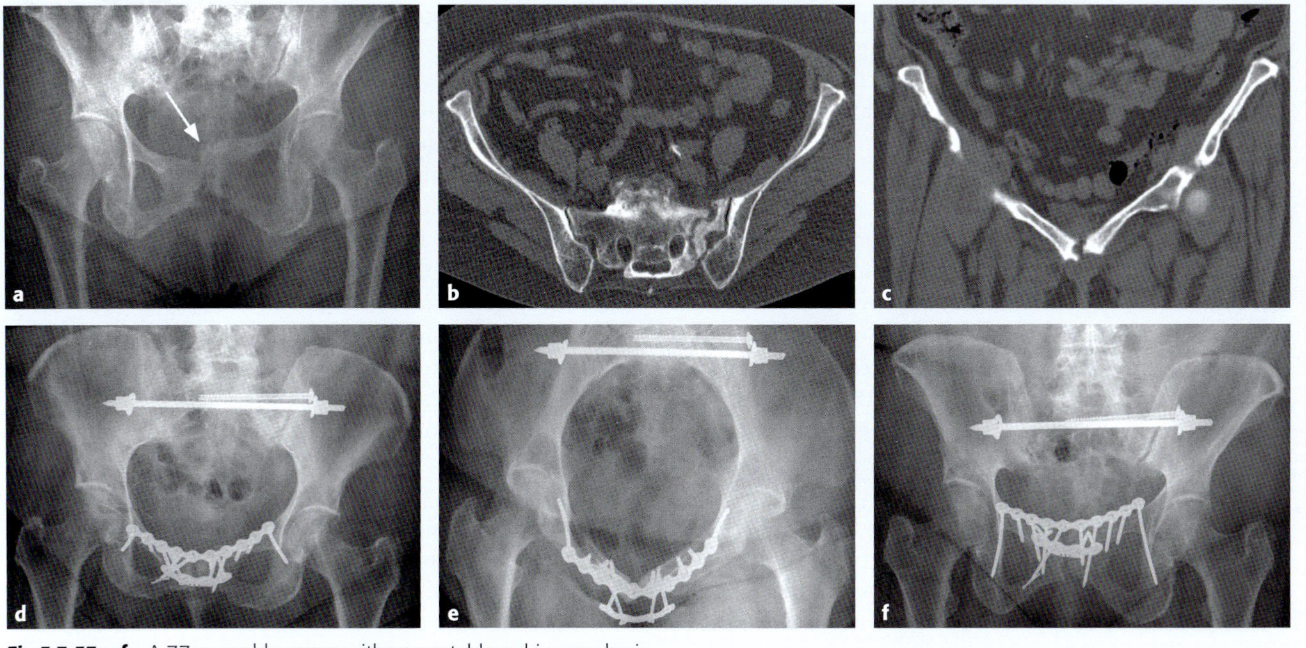


**Fig 3.7-37a–f** A 77-year-old woman with an unstable pubic symphysis.
**a** AP pelvic x-ray showing instability of the pubic symphysis due to the vertical displacement of the left pubic bone.
**b** Transverse computed tomographic (CT) cut through the sacrum showing a complete and older left sacral alar fracture.
**c** Coronal CT cut through the pubic symphysis showing a small bone defect and irregular margins.
**d** Postoperative AP pelvic x-ray.
**e** Pelvic inlet view.
**f** Pelvic outlet view showing the long marginal screws of the superior plate using the infraacetabular corridors into the ischium.

### 5.2.14 Internal fixator

The concept of the internal fixator is similar to that of the transiliac internal fixator on the posterior pelvis. It is a bridging osteosynthesis, which is spanned over the anterior pelvis with the implants being inserted in a less invasive way. Two pedicle screws, ie, one left and one right, are inserted from the anterior inferior iliac spine toward the PSIS. The pathway of the pedicle screws is the same as that of the Schanz screws of the external fixator. The length of the screws is up to 100 mm. A subcutaneous tunnel anterior to the lower abdominal aponeurotic fascia is carefully made between the two screw heads. A bent rod is inserted in this tunnel and locked in both screw heads [61]. The stability of the construct is similar to that of external fixation. As in anteroinferior external fixation, care has to be taken not to injure the lateral cutaneous femoral nerves during preparation of the corridors. When the rod is inserted too deep, it may put direct pressure on the iliopsoas muscle and the femoral nerve. A case series with femoral nerve palsy has been described after anterior internal fixation of the pelvic ring [62, 63].

As the implants are located close to the inguinal region and subcutaneously, implant removal must be considered in patients with complaints of the prominent hardware.

### 5.3 Aftercare

Regardless of the treatment, patients with FFP should receive appropriate analgesia and be mobilized as soon as possible [64] (see chapter 1.12 Pain management). Non-weight bearing is associated with functional decline, complications, and poor outcomes, and patients should be motivated and supported to move and walk as much as possible.

Close clinical supervision is needed to identify patients who are not doing well and express continuing or increasing pain during mobilization [24]. A possible increase of instability must be ruled out with new conventional pelvic x-rays and CT scans.

Patients with FFP type II lesions, who have been treated operatively, and patients with FFP type III and type IV lesions need longer support and rehabilitation. Short transfers, eg, from the bed to a chair or from the bed to the toilet, are allowed immediately. If the patient allows, walking with a rolling walking frame is started. This recommendation has not been proven by clinical studies but is meant to prevent postoperative immobilization with its known complications. Radiological studies after 3, 6, and 12 weeks confirm stability and ongoing fracture healing.

### 5.4 Nonunion

Nonunion of acute fractures or secondary fatigue fractures can occur in the anterior and posterior pelvic ring. With a fracture at one site, the pelvic ring gets more susceptible to fatigue-type fractures at other sites. The FFP then changes from a type of lower instability to one of higher instability. This especially happens in patients who undergo a long period of nonoperative treatment despite continuing complaints. The pelvic ring gradually and progressively fails which finally renders the patient bedridden. Signs of chronic instability can be observed on conventional x-rays and CT scans. Due to continuous motion and wear, bone fragments resorb. Larger fracture gaps and bone defects become visible. In areas with high load, bone resorption is combined with densification of the margins (see **Fig 3.7-9**, **Fig 3.7-10**, **Fig 3.7-11**). At the same time, callus is visible as an attempt of fracture healing. The clinical and radiological picture is that of a nonunion, sometimes stiff, sometimes mobile, but always painful. These situations have to be distinguished from nonunion after operative treatment, which is the consequence of inadequate fixation, implant loosening, and secondary displacement.

#### 5.4.1 Nonunion after nonoperative treatment

Nonunion is the end result of a failed healing process:

- The fracture site represents a high-stress riser along the otherwise stiff pelvic ring. This stress riser impedes healing of a usually benign fracture. The situation is often underdiagnosed.
- Long-standing complaints vary from disabling pain during standing and walking to severe immobilizing pain.
- Operative treatment with restoration of pelvic stability is the only option with a high success rate.
- The type of fixation and the invasiveness of surgery depend on the degree of instability, the localization of the nonunion, and the amount of displacement.

In the posterior pelvic ring, iliosacral screw fixation with or without cement augmentation and transsacral bar osteosynthesis are techniques of choice for nonunions of the sacral ala and the iliosacral joint. They create interfragmentary compression, which is perpendicular to the fracture gap. Open debridement of the nonunion is not needed. In pure iliosacral instabilities, a debridement of the joint is combined with an anterior plate fixation. In case of fractures of the ilium, the technique of osteosynthesis will be the same as in acute lesions. An angular stable plate osteosynthesis provides enough stability for healing.

In anterior pelvic nonunions, high stability is needed for the time of healing. In contrast with the posterior pelvic ring, the bone mass is thin and the corridors for strong implant fixation small. Exposure of the nonunion, debridement, and plate fixation are recommended. As in acute lesions, the plate screws should have the longest trajectory possible in the bone. In case of bone defect, cancellous bone grafting is performed to fill the gap. When a pubic symphysis diastasis with bone defect due to chronic instability is present, a tricortical bone graft is taken from the iliac crest and placed in the defect. The pubic symphysis with tricortical graft is stabilized with a double plate osteosynthesis. The first plate is placed superiorly and the second anteriorly (see **Case 11: Fig 3.7-36**, **Case 12: Fig 3.7-37**).

### 5.4.2 Nonunion after operative treatment

When operative treatment fails, the reasons for failure have to be identified. In addition to metabolic and nutritional contributors to poor bone quality (see chapter 1.10 Osteoporosis), typical mechanical reasons for failure include inadequate stability due to inappropriate fixation, inadequate implants, or low strength of fixation in osteoporotic bone. Depending on the specific problem, implant removal is needed or stability of osteosynthesis enhanced. Internal fixation is always necessary. The most stable osteosynthesis is chosen and the nonunion put under compression. Bone grafting is more often needed as in nonunion after nonoperative treatment. While iliosacral screw osteosynthesis and transsacral bar osteosynthesis are the fixations of choice in the posterior pelvis, it is plate osteosynthesis in the anterior pelvic ring. In all cases of nonunion, an anabolic therapy with teriparatide is strongly recommended to boost fracture healing [22, 23].

## 6 References


1. **Rommens PM, Hofmann A, Hessmann MH.** Management of acute hemorrhage in pelvic trauma: an overview. *Eur J Trauma Emerg Surg.* 2010 Apr;36(2):91–99.
2. **Finiels H, Finiels PJ, Jacquot JM, et al.** Fractures du sacrum par insuffisance osseuse: méta-analyse de 508 cas [Fractures of the sacrum caused by bone insufficiency. Meta-analysis of 508 cases]. *Presse Med.* 1997 Nov 01;26(33):1568–1573. French.
3. **Abdelfattah A, Core MD, Cannada LK, et al.** Geriatric high-energy polytrauma with orthopedic injuries: clinical predictors of mortality. *Geriatr Orthop Surg Rehabil.* 2014 Dec;5(4):173–177.
4. **Sullivan MP, Baldwin KD, Donegan DJ, et al.** Geriatric fractures about the hip: divergent patterns in the proximal femur, acetabulum, and pelvis. *Orthopedics.* 2014 Mar;37(3):151–157.
5. **Kannus P, Parkkari J, Niemi S, et al.** Low-trauma pelvic fractures in elderly Finns in 1970-2013. *Calcif Tissue Int.* 2015 Dec;97(6):577–580.
6. **Rommens PM, Wagner D, Hofmann A.** Surgical management of osteoporotic pelvic fractures: a new challenge. *Eur J Trauma Emerg Surg.* 2012 Oct;38(5):499–509.
7. **Wagner D, Kamer L, Sawaguchi T, et al.** Sacral bone mass distribution assessed by averaged three-dimensional CT models: implications for pathogenesis and treatment of fragility fractures of the sacrum. *J Bone Joint Surg Am.* 2016 Apr 06;98(7):584–590.
8. **Krappinger D, Zegg M, Jeske C, et al.** Hemorrhage after low-energy pelvic trauma. *J Trauma Acute Care Surg.* 2012 Feb;72(2):437–442.
9. **Dietz SO, Hofmann A, Rommens PM.** Haemorrhage in fragility fractures of the pelvis. *Eur J Trauma Emerg Surg.* 2015 Aug;41(4):363–367.
10. **Lau TW, Leung F.** Occult posterior pelvic ring fractures in elderly patients with osteoporotic pubic rami fractures. *J Orthop Surg (Hong Kong).* 2010 Aug;18(2):153–157.
11. **Rommens PM, Ossendorf C, Pairon P, et al.** Clinical pathways for fragility fractures of the pelvic ring: personal experience and review of the literature. *J Orthop Sci.* 2015 Jan;20(1):1–11.
12. **Lyders EM, Whitlow CT, Baker MD, et al.** Imaging and treatment of sacral insufficiency fractures. *AJNR Am J Neuroradiol.* 2010 Feb;31(2):201–210.
13. **Tile M.** Acute pelvic fractures: I. Causation and classification. *J Am Acad Orthop Surg.* 1996 May;4(3):143–151.
14. **Meinberg E, Agel J, Roberts C, et al.** Fracture and Dislocation Classification Compendium—2018. *J Orthopaed Trauma.* 2018 Jan;32(Suppl 1).
15. **Dalal SA, Burgess AR, Siegel JH, et al.** Pelvic fracture in multiple trauma: classification by mechanism is key to pattern of organ injury, resuscitative requirements, and outcome. *J Trauma.* 1989 Jul;29(7):981–1000; discussion 1000–1002.
16. **Denis F, Davis S, Comfort T.** Sacral fractures: an important problem. Retrospective analysis of 236 cases. *Clin Orthop Relat Res.* 1988 Feb;227:67–81.
17. **Linstrom NJ, Heiserman JE, Kortman KE, et al.** Anatomical and biomechanical analyses of the unique and consistent locations of sacral insufficiency fractures. *Spine.* 2009 Feb 15;34(4):309–315.
18. **Rommens PM, Hofmann A.** Comprehensive classification of fragility fractures of the pelvic ring: Recommendations for surgical treatment. *Injury.* 2013 Dec;44(12):1733–1744.
19. **Wagner D, Kamer L, Rommens PM, et al.** 3D statistical modeling techniques to investigate the anatomy of the sacrum, its bone mass distribution, and the trans-sacral corridors. *J Orthop Res.* 2014 Nov;32(11):1543–1548.
20. **Mason WT, Khan SN, James CL, et al.** Complications of temporary and definitive external fixation of pelvic ring injuries. *Injury.* 2005 May;36(5):599–604.
21. **Black DM, Rosen CJ.** Clinical practice. Postmenopausal osteoporosis. *N Engl J Med.* 2016 Jan 21;374(3):254–262.
22. **Peichl P, Holzer LA, Maier R, et al.** Parathyroid hormone 1-84 accelerates fracture-healing in pubic bones of elderly osteoporotic women. *J Bone Joint Surg Am.* 2011 Sep 07;93(17):1583–1587.
23. **Babu S, Sandiford NA, Vrahas M.** Use of Teriparatide to improve fracture healing: What is the evidence? *World J Orthop.* 2015 Jul 18;6(6):457–461.
24. **Rommens PM, Wagner D, Hofmann A.** Fragility fractures of the pelvis. *JBJS Rev.* 2017 Mar 21;5(3).
25. **Goetzen M, Ortner K, Lindtner RA, et al.** A simple approach for the preoperative assessment of sacral morphology for percutaneous SI screw fixation. *Arch Orthop Trauma Surg.* 2016 Sep;136(9):1251–1257.
26. **Zwingmann J, Konrad G, Kotter E, et al.** Computer-navigated iliosacral screw insertion reduces malposition rate and radiation exposure. *Clin Orthop Relat Res.* 2009 Jul;467(7):1833–1838.
27. **Gansslen A, Hufner T, Krettek C.** Percutaneous iliosacral screw fixation of unstable pelvic injuries by conventional fluoroscopy. *Oper Orthop Traumatol.* 2006 Sep;18(3):225–244.
28. **van Zwienen CM, van den Bosch EW, Snijders CJ, et al.** Biomechanical comparison of sacroiliac screw techniques for unstable pelvic ring fractures. *J Orthop Trauma.* 2004 Oct;18(9):589–595.

29. **Bastian JD, Bergmann M, Schwyn R, et al.** Assessment of the breakaway torque at the posterior pelvic ring in human cadavers. *J Invest Surg.* 2015;28(6):328–333.
30. **Oberkircher L, Masaeli A, Bliemel C, et al.** Primary stability of three different iliosacral screw fixation techniques in osteoporotic cadaver specimens—a biomechanical investigation. *Spine J.* 2016 Feb;16(2):226–232.
31. **Bastian JD, Keel MJ, Heini PF, et al.** Complications related to cement leakage in sacroplasty. *Acta Orthop Belg.* 2012 Feb;78(1):100–105.
32. **Collinge CA, Crist BD.** Combined percutaneous iliosacral screw fixation with sacroplasty using resorbable calcium phosphate cement for osteoporotic pelvic fractures requiring surgery. *J Orthop Trauma.* 2016 Jun;30(6):e217–e222.
33. **König MA, Hediger S, Schmitt JW, et al.** In-screw cement augmentation for iliosacral screw fixation in posterior ring pathologies with insufficient bone stock. *Eur J Trauma Emerg Surg.* 2018 Apr;44(2):203–210.
34. **Schildhauer TA, Wilber JH, Patterson BM.** Posterior locked lateral compression injury of the pelvis: report of three cases. *J Orthop Trauma.* 2000 Feb;14(2):107–111.
35. **Garant M.** Sacroplasty: a new treatment for sacral insufficiency fracture. *J Vasc Interv Radiol.* 2002 Dec;13(12):1265–1267.
36. **Ortiz AO, Brook AL.** Sacroplasty. *Tech Vasc Interv Radiol.* 2009 Mar;12(1):51–63.
37. **Kortman K, Ortiz O, Miller T, et al.** Multicenter study to assess the efficacy and safety of sacroplasty in patients with osteoporotic sacral insufficiency fractures or pathologic sacral lesions. *J Neurointerv Surg.* 2013 Sep 01;5(5):461–466.
38. **Gorczyca JT, Varga E, Woodside T, et al.** The strength of iliosacral lag screws and transiliac bars in the fixation of vertically unstable pelvic injuries with sacral fractures. *Injury.* 1996 Oct;27(8):561–564.
39. **Vanderschot P, Kuppers M, Sermon A, et al.** Trans-iliac-sacral-iliac-bar procedure to treat insufficiency fractures of the sacrum. *Indian J Orthop.* 2009 Jul;43(3):245–252.
40. **Mehling I, Hessmann MH, Rommens PM.** Stabilization of fatigue fractures of the dorsal pelvis with a trans-sacral bar. Operative technique and outcome. *Injury.* 2012 Apr;43(4):446–451.
41. **Vanderschot P.** Treatment options of pelvic and acetabular fractures in patients with osteoporotic bone. *Injury.* 2007 Apr;38(4):497–508.
42. **Dolati B, Larndorfer R, Krappinger D, et al.** Stabilization of the posterior pelvic ring with a slide-insertion plate. *Oper Orthop Traumatol.* 2007 Mar;19(1):16–31.
43. **Krappinger D, Larndorfer R, Struve P, et al.** Minimally invasive transiliac plate osteosynthesis for type C injuries of the pelvic ring: a clinical and radiological follow-up. *J Orthop Trauma.* 2007 Oct;21(9):595–602.
44. **Kobbe P, Hockertz I, Sellei RM, et al.** Minimally invasive stabilisation of posterior pelvic-ring instabilities with a transiliac locked compression plate. *Int Orthop.* 2012 Jan;36(1):159–164.
45. **Humphrey CA, Liu Q, Templeman DC, et al.** Locked plates reduce displacement of vertically unstable pelvic fractures in a mechanical testing model. *J Trauma.* 2010 Nov;69(5):1230–1234.
46. **Dienstknecht T, Berner A, Lenich A, et al.** A minimally invasive stabilizing system for dorsal pelvic ring injuries. *Clin Orthop Relat Res.* 2011 Nov;469(11):3209–3217.
47. **Dienstknecht T, Berner A, Lenich A, et al.** Biomechanical analysis of a transiliac internal fixator. *Int Orthop.* 2011 Dec;35(12):1863–1868.
48. **Schildhauer TA, Bellabarba C, Nork SE, et al.** Decompression and lumbopelvic fixation for sacral fracture-dislocations with spino-pelvic dissociation. *J Orthop Trauma.* 2006 Jul;20(7):447–457.
49. **Schildhauer TA, Josten C, Muhr G.** Triangular osteosynthesis of vertically unstable sacrum fractures: a new concept allowing early weight-bearing. *J Orthop Trauma.* 1998 Jun–Jul;12(5):307–314.
50. **Roetman B, Schildhauer TA.** Lumbopelvine Stabilisierung bei bilateraler lumbosakraler Instabilität. Indikationen und Technik [Lumbopelvic stabilization for bilateral lumbosacral instabilities: indications and techniques]. *Unfallchirurg.* 2013 Nov;116(11):991–999. German.
51. **Gansslen A, Pohlemann T, Krettek C.** Der einfache supraazetabuläre Fixateur externe für die Behandlung von Beckenfrakturen [A simple supraacetabular external fixation for pelvic ring fractures]. *Oper Orthop Traumatol.* 2005 Sep;17(3):296–312. German.
52. **Lidder S, Heidari N, Gansslen A, et al.** Radiological landmarks for the safe extra-capsular placement of supra-acetabular half pins for external fixation. *Surg Radiol Anat.* 2013 Mar;35(2):131–135.
53. **Gansslen A, Hildebrand F, Kretek C.** Supraacetabular external fixation for pain control in geriatric type B pelvic injuries. *Acta Chir Orthop Traumatol Cech.* 2013;80(2):101–105.
54. **Bircher MD.** Indications and techniques of external fixation of the injured pelvis. *Injury.* 1996;27(Suppl 2):B3–B19.
55. **Gansslen A, Krettek C.** Retrograde transpubic screw fixation of transpubic instabilities. *Oper Orthop Traumatol.* 2006 Oct;18(4):330–340.
56. **Rommens PM.** Is there a role for percutaneous pelvic and acetabular reconstruction? *Injury.* 2007 Apr;38(4):463–477.
57. **Acklin YP, Zderic I, Buschbaum J, et al.** Biomechanical comparison of plate and screw fixation in anterior pelvic ring fractures with low bone mineral density. *Injury.* 2016 Jul;47(7):1456–1460.
58. **Grimshaw CS, Bledsoe JG, Moed BR.** Locked versus standard unlocked plating of the pubic symphysis: a cadaver biomechanical study. *J Orthop Trauma.* 2012 Jul;26(7):402–406.
59. **Culemann U, Marintschev I, Gras F, et al.** Infra-acetabular corridor—technical tip for an additional screw placement to increase the fixation strength of acetabular fractures. *J Trauma.* 2011 Jan;70(1):244–246.
60. **Bastian JD, Ansorge A, Tomagra S, et al.** Anterior fixation of unstable pelvic ring fractures using the modified Stoppa approach: mid-term results are independent on patients' age. *Eur J Trauma Emerg Surg.* 2016 Oct;42(5):645–650.
61. **Hiesterman TG, Hill BW, Cole PA.** Surgical technique: a percutaneous method of subcutaneous fixation for the anterior pelvic ring: the pelvic bridge. *Clin Orthop Relat Res.* 2012 Aug;470(8):2116–2123.
62. **Hesse D, Kandmir U, Solberg B, et al.** Femoral nerve palsy after pelvic fracture treated with INFIX: a case series. *J Orthop Trauma.* 2015 Mar;29(3):138–143.
63. **Apivatthakakul T, Rujiwattanapong N.** "Anterior subcutaneous pelvic internal fixator (INFIX), Is it safe?" A cadaveric study. *Injury.* 2016 Oct;47(10):2077–2080.
64. **Bukata SV, Digiovanni BF, Friedman SM, et al.** A guide to improving the care of patients with fragility fractures. *Geriatr Orthop Surg Rehabil.* 2011 Jan;2(1):5–37.

# 3.8 Acetabulum

Dietmar Krappinger, Richard A Lindtner, Herbert Resch

## 1 Introduction

The treatment of geriatric acetabular fractures (GAFs) presents a challenge for orthopedic surgeons for the following reasons:

- Despite an increasing incidence over the last few decades, GAF are infrequent injuries and overall personal experience of the treating surgeon is usually low.
- There are important treatment differences with regard to fracture type, degree of instability, and accompanying injuries such as femoral head impaction, preexisting osteoarthritis, comorbidities and functional demands of the patients.
- Treatment options range from nonoperative treatment to internal fixation and hip arthroplasty and even internal fixation and arthroplasty.
- Internal fixation and hip arthroplasty are performed using different approaches, techniques, and implants depending on the surgeon's preferences and abilities.
- There is a lack of controlled studies comparing different treatment options. Most studies typically describe case series limited by small sample sizes and lack of appropriate comparison groups.

## 2 Epidemiology and etiology

The incidence of GAF have shown a marked increase during the last two decades [1]. An overall increase in life expectancy as well as a higher activity level of octogenarians may account for these findings. In 2005, Cornell [2] predicted that geriatric patients may soon be the most typical age group to present with acetabular fractures. Ochs reported an increase in the mean age of patients with acetabular fractures from 43.0 (± 19.1) years in the period from 1991–1993 to 52.7 (± 19.8) years between 2005–2006 [3]. While the group of patients aged between 20–30 years were the most frequent age group in the first study period (1991–1993), the group between 60–70 years represented the peak age group in the second period (2005–2006) [3]. Ferguson et al [4] observed a 2.4-fold increase of the acetabular fracture incidence in patients > 60 between 1980 and 2007 and Sullivan [5] reported an 67% increase of GAF between 1998 and 2010. It is reasonable to assume that this trend will continue during the next few decades. While the overall majority of patients with acetabular fractures are male, women are more frequently represented in the geriatric group [3].

Acetabular fractures in younger patients usually result from high-energy trauma and frequently occur in polytraumatized patients. In older adults, acetabular fractures typically result from ground level-level falls and are either isolated injuries or combined with other osteoporotic fractures such as proximal humeral or distal radial fractures. The fracture type is mainly determined by the position of the hip joint during trauma. In younger patients, the so-called "dashboard mechanism" is a characteristic injury mechanism with the knee and hip joint in flexion and load transmission via the femoral shaft. This results in a posterior fracture dislocation with the involvement of the posterior wall and/or column ("posterior dislocation"). In geriatric patients, the hip joint is usually in extension during the fall on the involved side with load transmission via the greater trochanter and the femoral neck (**Fig 3.8-1**). Given the anteversion of the femoral neck, the anterior column and/or wall as well as the quadrilateral plate are generally involved in GAF with medial protrusion of the femoral head ("central dislocation") [2, 3, 6].

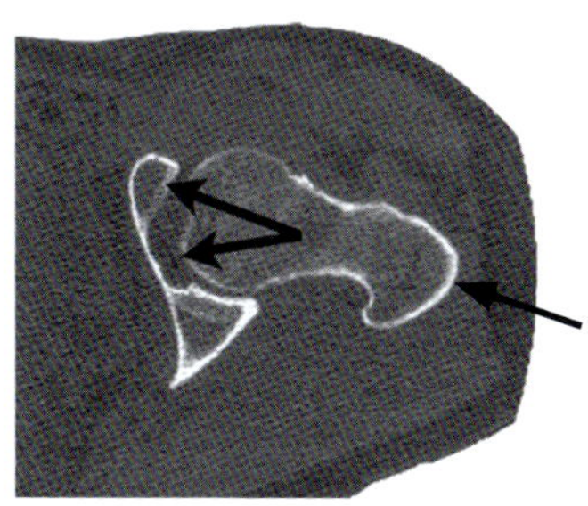

**Fig 3.8-1** Typical mechanism of injury of acetabular fractures in geriatric patients is load transmission via the greater trochanter, involvement of the anterior column and the quadrilateral plate due to the anteversion of the femoral neck (central dislocation).

## 3 Diagnostics

### 3.1 Clinical evaluation

In GAF, individual goals of treatment and the approach largely depend on patient-related factors, so the clinical evaluation must extend beyond the routine history and physical examination. The following patient-related factors should be thoroughly assessed before treatment options are considered:

- Preinjury ambulatory status
- Functional demands
- Independence in activities of daily living
- Medical comorbidities
- Cognitive status
- Bone quality
- Preexisting osteoarthritis of the affected hip
- Concomitant injuries, especially those with an impact on postoperative mobilization plans

The optimal treatment strategy for an individual patient must be chosen considering factors related to both fracture and patient to provide the best possible clinical outcome. The primary goals in the treatment of GAF are prompt and adequate single-staged treatment ("single-shot surgery") allowing for early mobilization and avoiding morbidity and mortality associated with prolonged bed rest and subsequent revision surgery.

### 3.2 Imaging

#### 3.2.1 Plain x-rays

The three standard acetabular views include the AP view of the pelvis, the obturator oblique view (with the pelvis rotated 45° towards the uninjured side) and the iliac oblique view (with the pelvis rotated 45° towards the injured side). According to the authors' experience, however, AP views of the pelvis with an initial CT scan are sufficient to rule out medialization of the femoral head in GAF. Impaction of the subchondral bone of the superomedial acetabular dome may be visible as a double arc on plain radiographs ("gull sign") (**Case 3: Fig 3.8-4, Case 5: Fig 3.8-6**) and is associated with a poor prognosis after nonoperative treatment or internal fixation [7].

#### 3.2.2 Computed tomographic scan

Computed tomography (CT) is the gold standard for the evaluation of acetabular fractures, and multiplanar CT reconstructions are mandatory for understanding the exact acetabular fracture pattern [8, 9]. CT imaging of the pelvis allows for proper assessment of the following parameters:

- Detailed fracture line characteristics and type of acetabular fracture (**Case 1: Fig 3.8-2**)
- Extent of anterior and posterior wall comminution and/or marginal impaction
- Impaction of the weight-bearing acetabular dome and of the femoral head (**Case 3: Fig 3.8-4, Case 5: Fig 3.8-6**)
- Articular surface congruity
- Subtle subluxation/medialization of the femoral head (**Case 3: Fig 3.8-4**)
- Intraarticular bony fragments

Furthermore, modern CT permits manual multiplanar 2-D reconstruction in any arbitrary plane. Additional manual reconstructions complement the information gained from standard axial, coronal, and sagittal planes.

#### 3.2.3 Three-dimensional reconstruction

Three-dimensional surface-rendered CT images from different regions are of great help for enhancing the surgeon's understanding of the acetabular fracture and spatial relationship of fracture fragments as well as for planning the operative approach. Three-dimensional CT allows for subtraction of the femoral head and enables the surgeon to view the complex 3-D anatomy of the fractured acetabulum from any perspective, including the intraoperative view. Furthermore, 3-D CT helps to improve the accuracy and interobserver reliability of acetabular fracture classification especially in surgeons with limited experience [10, 11]. Three-dimensional CT images complement the 2-D images, as the latter more accurately depict fracture details such as marginal and acetabular dome impaction, column comminution, small intraarticular fragments and subtle fracture lines.

#### 3.2.4 Magnetic resonance imaging

In general, magnetic resonance imaging (MRI) is of limited value in the routine assessment of GAF. High-resolution MRI allows for imaging of the acetabular labrum and cartilage. In geriatric patients MRI may be helpful to rule out occult acetabular, femoral head or femoral neck fractures, which may not be visible on x-rays or CT scans.

## 4 Classification

### 4.1 Classification of Letournel and Judet

The classification system of Letournel and Judet is the most widely used and represents an anatomical and radiographic description of acetabular fracture patterns [12]. This system divides acetabular fractures into two groups, ie, basic and associated fractures, with five fracture subtypes in each group. Basic fracture patterns include posterior wall fractures, posterior column fractures, anterior wall fractures, anterior column fractures, and transverse fractures. Associated fracture patterns include T-shaped fractures, posterior column with posterior wall fractures, transverse with posterior wall fractures, anterior column with posterior hemitransverse fractures and two-column fractures. While the AO/OTA or Tile classification of pelvic ring injuries is limited in its use for the assessment of geriatric pelvic ring injuries (see chapter 3.7 Pelvic ring), the commonly used classification systems for acetabular fractures (Letournel and AO/OTA classifications) are valuable for the assessment of GAF as well. The distribution of acetabular fracture patterns in older adults differs significantly from younger patients, with fracture types involving the anterior column being much more common (**Fig 3.8-1**).

### 4.2 AO/OTA Fracture and Dislocation Classification

The alphanumeric AO/OTA classification of acetabular fractures is based on the classification of Letournel and Judet, but includes additional modifiers, making it more complex and less commonly used in daily practice. The AO/OTA classification distinguishes between type A (partial articular fractures with one column involved: A1, posterior wall; A2, posterior column; A3, anterior wall or anterior column), type B (a portion of the acetabular articular surface is in osseous continuity with the iliac bone: B1, transverse; B2, T-shaped; B3, anterior column and posterior hemitransverse) and type C (fracture patterns with no osseous continuity between the acetabular articular surface and the iliac bone: different subtypes of two-column fractures).

### 4.3 Typical fracture types in geriatric patients

Geriatric acetabular fractures show less variation than acetabular fractures in younger patients due to more uniform injury mechanisms. The incidence of anterior column and wall fractures as well as anterior column with posterior hemitransverse fractures is significantly higher in these patients than in younger populations [4]. Additionally, radiographic findings associated with poor outcome, such as superomedial dome impaction (gull sign) (**Case 3: Fig 3.8-4, Case 5: Fig 3.8-6**), comminution, and marginal impaction in posterior wall fractures and femoral head impactions are more commonly seen in geriatric patients [4].

A characteristic fracture type in geriatric patients is the anterior column with posterior hemitransverse fracture (**Case 1: Fig 3.8-2, Case 3: Fig 3.8-4, Case 5: Fig 3.8-6, Case 6: Fig 3.8-7, Case 8: Fig 3.8-9**). In these fractures the anterior column is often multifragmentary or comminuted (**Case 5: Fig 3.8-6**), while the posterior hemitransverse fracture is simple and frequently undisplaced (**Case 1: Fig 3.8-2**). The quadrilateral plate is generally in osseous continuity with the posterior column (**Case 5: Fig 3.8-6**). Due to the medial protrusion of the femoral head with medialization of the quadrilateral plate, the posterior column is typically internally rotated. This mechanism is comparable to the opening of a swinging door by the femoral head and is called "open door injury" by the authors in analogy to the "open book injury" of the pelvic ring.

## 5 Decision making

### 5.1 General remarks

In younger patients, we strive for fracture healing in an anatomical position. Thus, displaced fractures generally require open reduction and internal fixation. The overall goals in the treatment of GAF are as follows:

- Rapid restoration of the hip function by an adequate single-staged treatment (single-shot surgery) to allow for early mobilization with weight bearing as tolerated
- Avoidance of the morbidity and mortality associated with bed rest and/or revision surgery [13, 14]

Treatment options for GAF include:

- Nonoperative treatment (**Case 1: Fig 3.8-2, Case 2: Fig 3.8-3**)
- Internal fixation (**Case 4: Fig 3.8-5**)
- Hip arthroplasty (**Case 3: Fig 3.8-4, Case 5: Fig 3.8-6**)
- Combinations of internal fixation and arthroplasty (**Case 6: Fig 3.8-7, Case 7: Fig 3.8-8**)

The exact roles of the different treatment strategies have not yet been clearly defined as there is a paucity of adequately powered randomized or other prospective studies. Parameters which need to be addressed during decision making include fracture type, age, comorbidities, activity level, osteoporosis, and preexisting osteoarthritis. Orthogeriatric comanagement is necessary for optimal practice. Generally, the delay between trauma and operative intervention should be minimized. The operative treatment of GAF, however, requires special skills and an appropriate level of experience. A delay until operative treatment may be justified if no experienced surgeon is immediately available [13, 14].

### 5.2 Nonoperative versus operative treatment

The appraisal of joint instability, rather than joint congruency in younger patients, represents an important factor in the decision-making process. Instability is often positively correlated with pain and the inability to ambulate. In unclear situations, an attempt to mobilize the patient with adequate pain management and close monitoring is often made. Failure makes a strong case for operative stabilization (**Case 3: Fig 3.8-4**).

For the assessment of fracture stability, it is more important to assess the acetabular columns rather than the acetabular walls. While displaced acetabular walls need operative intervention in young patients, this may not be true for geriatric patients. A displacement of a few millimeters may be tolerated if the femoral head remains centered during weight bearing (**Case 1: Fig 3.8-2**). Regular follow-up x-rays are therefore necessary in these cases in order to detect additional displacement (**Case 3: Fig 3.8-4**). A displacement of only a few millimeters of the acetabular columns is relevant and indicates a higher degree of instability. These fractures typically require operative treatment (**Case 7: Fig 3.8-8**). Nondisplaced fractures of the columns as well as nondisplaced transverse or hemitransverse fractures may be treated nonoperatively with weight bearing as tolerated (**Case 1: Fig 3.8-2, Case 2: Fig 3.8-3**). Operative treatment is usually indicated in fractures with subluxation or dislocation of the hip joint, even in patients in a poor general condition, in order to facilitate nursing care and mobilization (**Case 3: Fig 3.8-4, Case 5: Fig 3.8-6**). Nonoperative treatment of unstable fractures with prolonged bed rest or skeletal traction leads to poor functional results and complications due to immobilization and should be avoided in the treatment of GAF [15].

### 5.3 Internal fixation versus arthroplasty

Due to a lack of adequate trial data, the decision to employ internal fixation or arthroplasty mainly depends on the surgeon's preference, experience, and personal skills [16-18]. New prosthetic fixation concepts for the acetabular components, such as angular stable reinforcement rings (**Case 3: Fig 3.8-4, Case 5: Fig 3.8-6, Case 8: Fig 3.8-9**), and their further development will increase the relevance of primary arthroplasty for GAF.

A 2-stage procedure with initial internal fixation and secondary hip arthroplasty after osseous consolidation of the fracture in the situation of symptomatic posttraumatic osteoarthritis is a standard procedure in the treatment of acetabular fractures in nongeriatric patients. In geriatric patients, however, the concept of single-shot surgery, ie, a single operative intervention in the first days after trauma as a definitive solution, should be applied in order to reduce the number of operative interventions and the overall rehabilitation time. Accordingly, primary hip arthroplasty is an enticing concept for the treatment of geriatric acetabular fractures. The major challenge of primary total hip arthroplasty (THA) is the fixation of the cup in the fractured acetabulum. Revision cups and acetabular reinforcement rings and combinations with internal fixation are frequently required.

Primary arthroplasty may be considered in the following situations:

- Fragile patients with limited mobility (**Case 3: Fig 3.8-4**)
- Comminuted fractures (**Case 5: Fig 3.8-6**)
- Impaction zones of the acetabular dome (gull sign) (**Case 3: Fig 3.8-4, Case 5: Fig 3.8-6**)
- Severe osteoporosis (**Case 8: Fig 3.8-9**)
- Preexisting osteoarthritis (**Case 7: Fig 3.8-8**)
- Fractures that would require extensive surgery or combined approaches (**Case 5: Fig 3.8-6**)
- Acetabular fractures after femoral hemiarthroplasty (**Case 8: Fig 3.8-9**)
- Periprosthetic acetabular fractures (**Case 9: Fig 3.8-10**)

## 6 Therapeutic options

### 6.1 Nonoperative treatment

Nonoperative treatment includes weight bearing as tolerated, using walking aids, and pain medication (**Case 1: Fig 3.8-2, Case 2: Fig 3.8-3**). Nonsteroidal antiinflammatory drugs are often avoided in geriatric patients because of their renal, gastric, and cardiac toxicity. Regular x-ray follow-ups are mandatory in order to rule out secondary displacement. In cases of worsening medial protrusion of the femoral head and/or increasing pain during mobilization, operative intervention may be considered (**Case 3: Fig 3.8-4**).

## Nonoperative treatment

### Patient

A 76-year-old cooperative male patient living with his wife and able to ambulate independently. He sustained a ground-level fall while walking onto his right hip. The initial x-ray showed a minimally displaced fracture without medial protrusion of the femoral head and preexisting radiological signs of hip osteoarthritis. The patient had no relevant hip pain before trauma (**Fig 3.8-2a**). The computed tomographic scan showed an anterior column with incomplete posterior hemitransverse fracture without articular displacement or subluxation (**Fig 3.8-2b–f**).

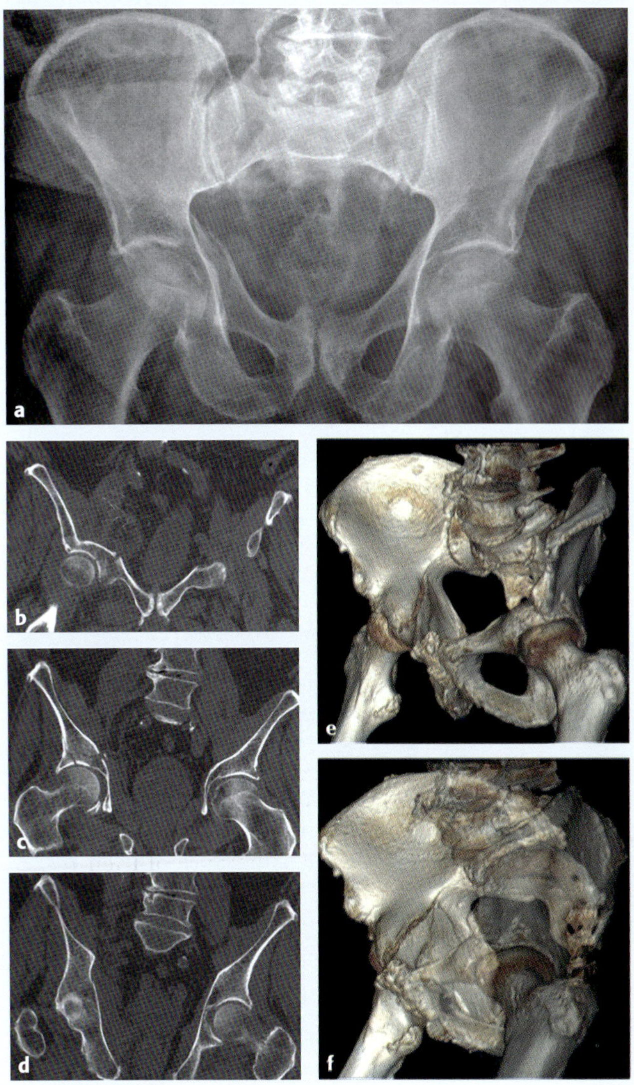

### Comorbidities

- Carotid artery stenosis
- No history of cardiac disease
- Osteoporosis (first diagnosed during the treatment of the acetabular fracture)
- Vitamin D deficiency 25-hydroxyvitamin D3: 9.2 ng/mL (23 nmol/L)

### Fracture type

Anterior column with incomplete posterior hemitransverse fracture (AO/OTA 62B3), no articular displacement, and no medial protrusion of the femoral head (**Fig 3.8-2a-f**).

### Treatment and outcome

Pain management and mobilization were started on the first day after admission. Weight bearing was performed as tolerated by the patient using crutches. Full weight bearing (FWB) was achieved on the fifth day with subsequent discharge after an x-ray follow-up. Vitamin D was given orally. At the final follow-up after 12 months, the patient had no relevant hip pain with complete functional recovery. X-ray follow-up showed mild radiologic progression of the osteoarthritis of the hip but no medial protrusion of the femoral head (**Fig 3.8-2g**).

### Discussion

In stable fractures without displacement of the columns and without medial protrusion of the femoral head, nonoperative treatment is a viable option even in the presence of displacement of the acetabular walls of a few millimeters. Geriatric patients are typically not able to perform partial weight bearing due to frailty, weakness, and preexisting gait disorders. Accordingly, weight bearing should be performed as tolerated by the patient using walking aids. Full weight bearing should not be prohibited. Regular follow-up x-rays are important in the first few weeks. In this case, FWB was achieved on day 5.

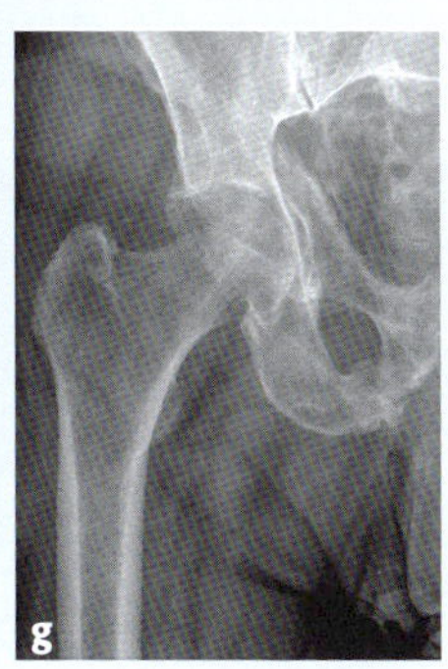

**Fig 3.8-2a–g** A 76-year-old man after a fall.

**a** X-ray showing a minimally displaced acetabular fracture, no medial protrusion of the femoral head, and preexisting signs of hip osteoarthritis.

**b–f** Computed tomographic scan with coronal and 3-D reconstructions showing anterior column with incomplete posterior hemitransverse fracture, no articular displacement, no medial protrusion of the femoral head.

**g** X-ray after 12 months showing mild radiological progression of the osteoarthritis, no medial protrusion of the femoral head, functional recovery.

CASE 2

## Secondary arthroplasty after nonoperative treatment

### Patient

A 79-year-old cooperative female patient was living with her husband and able to ambulate independently. She fell onto her right hip while hiking. The initial x-ray showed a consolidated fracture of the anterior pelvic ring and hip osteoarthritis. The patient had no relevant hip pain before the trauma. While the fracture was not visible on x-ray, the computed tomographic scan showed a nondisplaced transverse fracture of the right acetabulum (**Fig 3.8-3a–b**).

### Comorbidities

- Insulin-dependent diabetes mellitus
- Osteoporosis that was first diagnosed after an anterior pelvic ring fracture and treated with vitamin D3 and calcium
- No history of cardiac disease

### Fracture type

Nondisplaced transverse fracture (AO/OTA 62B1), no articular step-off, and no medial protrusion of the femoral head (**Fig 3.8-3a–b**).

### Treatment and outcome

Nonoperative treatment as described in case 1 was performed with discharge after 7 days. Alendronate (70 mg once a week) was added to her basic osteoporosis treatment. There was an uneventful further course with full functional recovery by 6 months and minimal need for ongoing pain medication. The patient resumed hiking and performed all activities of daily living by herself. Subsequently, however, the patient developed increasing pain in the right hip. An x-ray after 10 months showed progression of the hip osteoarthritis (**Fig 3.8-3c**). Total hip arthroplasty was performed after 12 months with an uncemented press-fit cup. The further course was uneventful (**Fig 3.8-3d**).

### Discussion

This case is similar to the case in **Case 1: Fig 3.8-2**. Rapid mobilization and early discharge from hospital after nonoperative treatment was feasible with an uneventful course during the first 6 months. There was no prolonged period of immobilization and pain, which is a major goal in geriatric fracture treatment. Total hip arthroplasty (THA) after osseous consolidation of the fracture without acetabular deformity supersedes the need for a revision cup or an acetabular reinforcement ring and enables the use of a cementless press-fit cup. The long-term survival rate of patients with secondary THA after consolidated minimally or nondisplaced acetabular fractures is expected to be comparable with the survival rate of patients with primary THA due to osteoarthritis of the hip or THA after femoral neck fractures [19, 20]. Indications for early operative treatment are impaired mobilization due to severe pain and increasing displacement of the fracture. An additional indication for an early THA is persistent pain in the first 6 months after trauma, while patients with an interim pain-free period may be treated with secondary THA as shown in the case above.

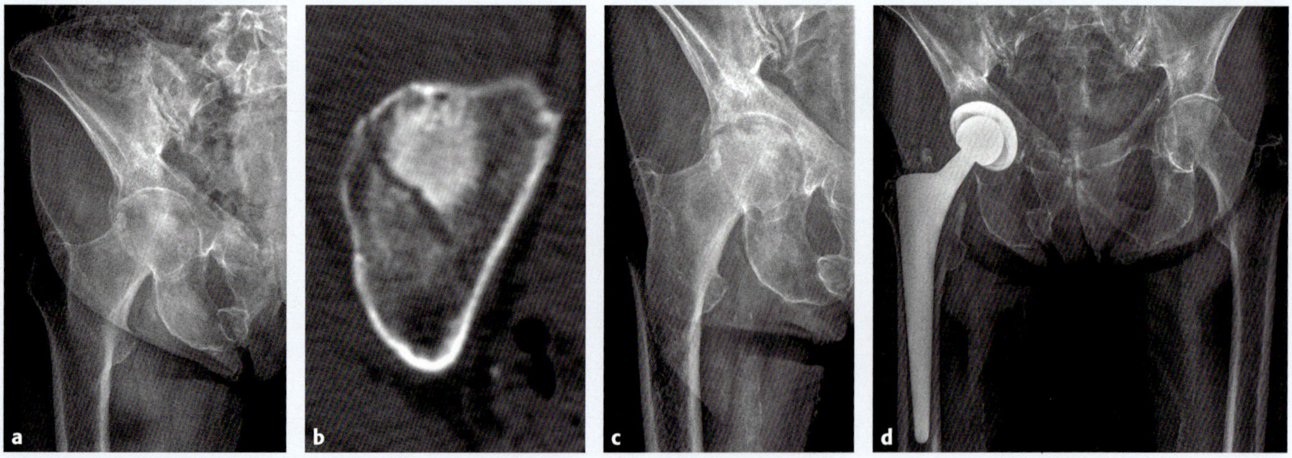


**Fig 3.8-3a–d** A 79-year-old woman after a fall on her hip.
**a** X-ray showing hip osteoarthritis but no visible fracture.
**b** Computed tomographic scan with transverse reconstruction showing a nondisplaced transverse fracture of the right acetabulum.
**c** X-ray after 10 months showing the healed fracture and radiological progression of hip osteoarthritis.
**d** Total hip arthroplasty with uncemented press-fit cup.

## Primary arthroplasty after nonoperative treatment

### Patient

An 81-year-old female patient with severe dementia, living in a nursing home, with very limited mobility and using a walking frame. She was found lying on the floor of the nursing home. The patient was not able to describe the injury. The initial x-ray showed an anterior column fracture with superomedial dome impaction (gull sign) (**Fig 3.8-4a**). The computed tomographic scan revealed an additional undisplaced posterior hemitransverse fracture (**Fig 3.8-4b–d**).

### Comorbidities

- Severe dementia
- Cervical carcinoma
- Severe osteoporosis (receiving drug therapy)
- Congestive heart failure

### Fracture type

Anterior column with undisplaced posterior hemitransverse fracture (AO/OTA 62B3) and superomedial dome impaction (gull sign) (**Fig 3.8-4a–d**).

### Treatment and outcome

Due to her poor general condition and increased operative risks, nonoperative treatment with pain management and mobilization was initially conducted. However, the patient complained of increasing pain in the first days of attempts to mobilize her. An x-ray obtained on day 7 revealed increasing displacement and medial protrusion of the femoral head (**Fig 3.8-4e**). Primary hip arthoplasty with no additional internal fixation was performed on day 11 via a lateral approach in a lateral decubitus position using an angular stable reinforcement ring with a cemented polyethylene cup. This type of cup was used due to her low demand, her sarcopenia, and her dementia in order to reduce the risk of hip dislocation. The reinforcement ring was fixed to the supraacetabular bone using multiple small-fragment locking screws. Bone graft from the femoral head was used to fill the fracture gaps and to avoid cement penetrating into the lesser pelvis. No attempt was made to reduce the medial wall. The postoperative mobilization included full weight bearing with a walking frame. Wound drainage during the fourth postoperative week was successfully managed with a single soft-tissue revision and antibiotic treatment for 6 weeks. The x-rays at 3 months showed a healed acetabular fracture without signs of component loosening (**Fig 3.8-4f**). The patient continued to reside in the nursing home, reached her former level of mobility, and did not have residual hip pain.

### Discussion

At this point, operative repair remains controversial in patients with significantly poor functional status. Typically, such cases are discussed and decided by an interdisciplinary team. Due to her decreased life expectancy, limited general mobility, and the presence of a radiographic feature indicating poor outcome after internal fixation (gull sign), total hip arthroplasty was performed. Osseous continuity between the supraacetabular bone and the sacroiliac joint is mandatory to use this type of reinforcement ring without additional internal fixation of the acetabular columns. The fractured acetabulum is simply bridged. In fractures with extensions to the iliac crest and to the supracetabular bone, additional internal fixation may be considered (**Case 6: Fig 3.8-7, Case 7: Fig 3.8-8**). The major advantage of this type of reinforcement ring is the use of multiple locking screws in different directions for better screw purchase in osteoporotic bone. While techniques for fixation of revision cups and reinforcement rings are in general similar for the treatment of acetabular fractures and acetabular bone defects, there is one major difference, ie, bone defects need to be bridged permanently, while acetabular fractures heal within a few weeks resulting in an overall increased stability and decreased load to the implant.

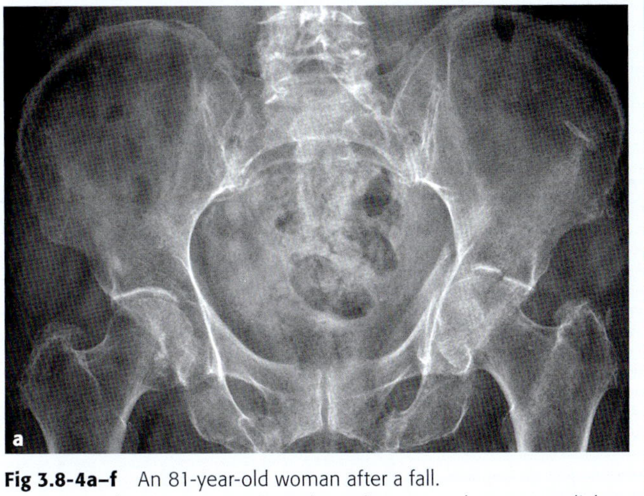


**Fig 3.8-4a–f** An 81-year-old woman after a fall.
**a** X-ray showing an anterior column fracture and superomedial dome impaction (gull sign).

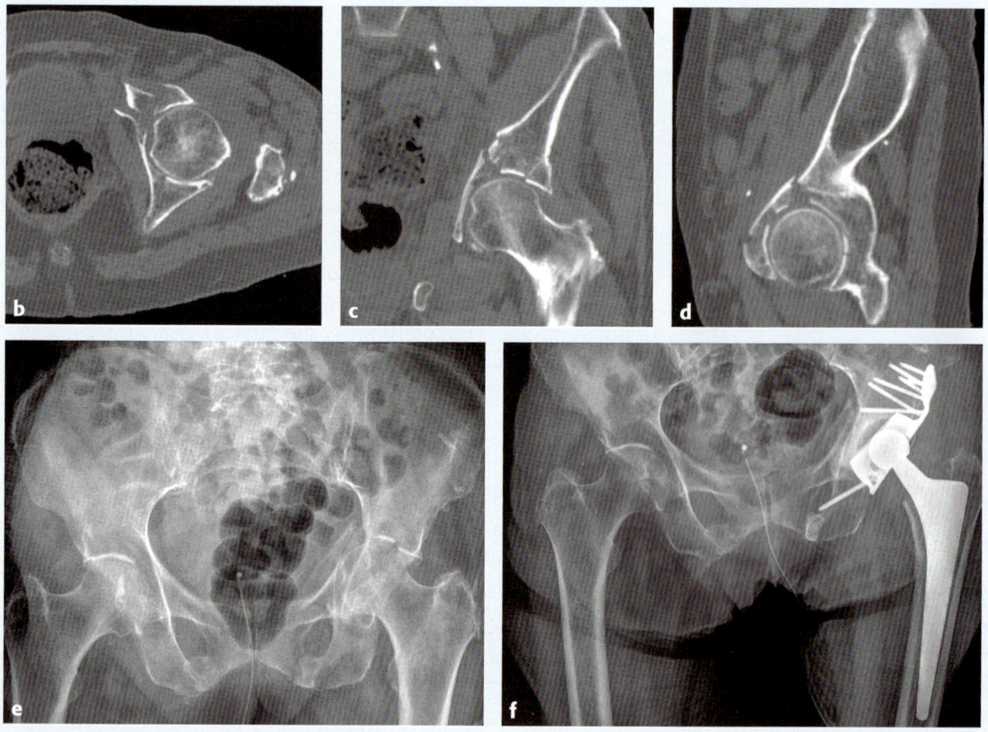


**Fig 3.8-4a–f (cont)** An 81-year-old woman after a fall.
**b–d** Computed tomographic scan with transverse, coronal, and sagittal reconstructions showing no relevant medial protrusion of the femoral head, mild gull sign, and incomplete posterior hemitransverse fracture.
**e** X-ray after 7 days showing increasing displacement and medial protrusion of the femoral head.
**f** X-ray after 3 months showing healed acetabular fracture without signs of component loosening.

## 6.2 Internal fixation

Internal fixation of GAF follows similar principles used for internal fixation of younger patients in terms of reduction and fixation techniques. There are, however, some differences. The workhorse anterior approaches are the ilioinguinal and the Stoppa approaches, while the Kocher-Langenbeck approach is the standard posterior approach. Combined and extensive approaches should be avoided (**Case 4: Fig 3.8-5**). Given the higher incidence of anterior column fractures and medial protrusion of the femoral head, anterior approaches are more frequently used in geriatric patients. The Stoppa approach as an "intrapelvic approach" allows for direct reduction and fixation of the quadrilateral plate, which is crucial to restore the buttress function of the medial wall [21, 22]. The Stoppa approach may be combined with the lateral window of the ilioinguinal approach (Olerud window) to stabilize high anterior column fractures and fractures of the iliac crest (**Case 4: Fig 3.8-5**). Alternatively, the quadrilateral plate may be addressed through the two lateral windows of the ilioinguinal approach and fixed with long cortical screws [23]. Conventional pelvic reconstruction plates may be used for fixation, while future developments will allow the use of angular stable and anatomically pre-shaped plates.

## Internal fixation

### Patient

A 76-year-old cooperative male patient. He was very active and in good general health. An x-ray of the hip obtained two years previously after a simple fall showed joint space narrowing (**Fig 3.8-5a**). The patient, however, did not complain about hip pain at that time. Subsequently, he had a fall from an approximately 3-meter high tree and sustained a two-column fracture of the left acetabulum (**Fig 3.8-5b-c**).

### Comorbidities

- Benign prostatic hypertrophy

### Fracture type

High two-column fracture of the left acetabulum (AO/OTA 62C1) (**Fig 3.8-5b-c**).

### Treatment and outcome

Internal fixation via a midline Stoppa approach with an additional iliac window was performed. The posterior column was indirectly reduced and fixed with a lag screw crossing both columns from anterior to posterior [24]. A posterior approach was not used. Partial weight bearing using crutches was advised for 6 weeks. An x-ray follow-up after 3 years showed osseous consolidation of the fracture and only mild progression of the hip osteoarthritis (**Fig 3.8-5d**). The patient was satisfied with the functional result. There was no need for secondary total hip arthroplasty (THA) at this point.

### Discussion

This is not a typical geriatric fracture despite the patient's age for the following reasons. First, there was a higher-energy trauma. Second, the patient was very active with no relevant comorbidities or osteoporosis. Third, this fracture type typically results from high-energy trauma in nongeriatric patients, while anterior column with posterior hemitransverse fractures are more common in geriatric patients. Accordingly, internal fixation was performed via an anterior approach and primary hip arthroplasty was not considered. Primary arthroplasty in two-column fractures without additional internal fixation is not advisable in general, as these fracture types are defined by an osseous separation of the two columns from the iliac bone, which impedes fixation of the acetabular component. In younger patients, however, the posterior wall fragment may have been addressed directly via a posterior approach in order to prevent or at least delay symptomatic posttraumatic osteoarthritis. In this case, secondary arthroplasty was considered to be necessary given the radiological finding of osteoarthritis already present prior to the injury (**Fig 3.8-5a**). Fortunately, at 3 years the clinical result was satisfactory and secondary THA was not needed.

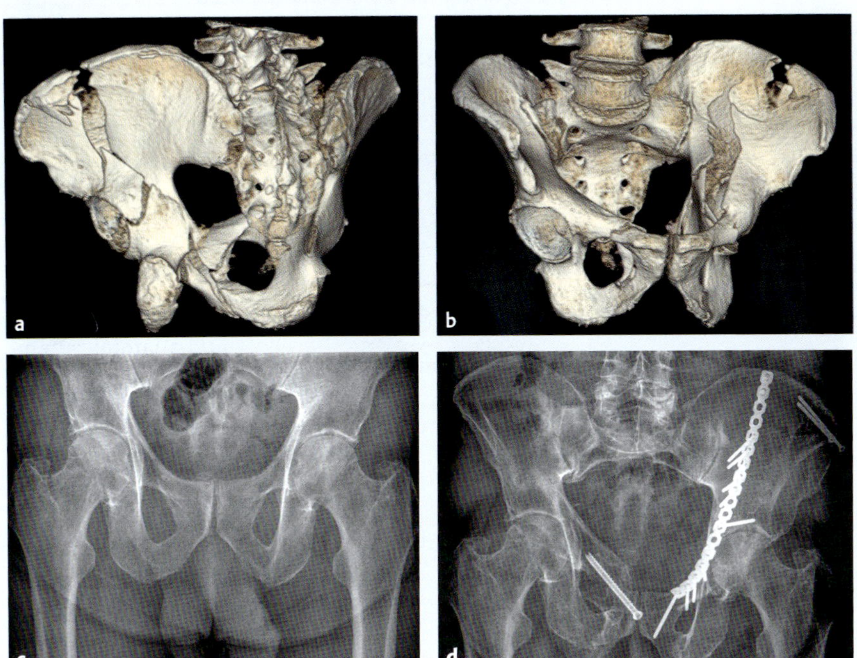

**Fig 3.8-5a–d** A 76-year-old man with a two-column fracture of the left acetabulum.
- **a** X-ray 2 years before trauma showing mild signs of hip osteoarthritis.
- **b** Computed tomographic scan with 3-D reconstruction (view from anterior) showing a two-column fracture of the left acetabulum.
- **c** Computed tomographic scan with 3-D reconstruction (view from posterior) showing a two-column fracture of the left acetabulum.
- **d** X-ray after 3 years showing mild progression of the hip osteoarthritis.

### 6.3 Arthroplasty

The major challenge of primary hip arthroplasty is the fixation of the cup in the fractured acetabulum. Revision cups (**Case 7: Fig 3.8-8, Case 9: Fig 3.8-10**) and acetabular reinforcement rings (**Case 3: Fig 3.8-4, Case 5: Fig 3.8-6, Case 8: Fig 3.8-9**) often need to be employed. These implants were mainly developed for the treatment of acetabular bone defects and cup loosening in revision hip arthroplasty and were later adopted for the treatment of GAF. There are several reports describing primary hip arthroplasty using different approaches and implant types and in a small number of patients [16, 20, 25–28]. However, there is a lack of randomized or prospective studies, and the level of evidence is low. Recent developments include reinforcement rings with angular stable fixation of the ring in the supraacetabular bone using multiple locking screws (**Case 3: Fig 3.8-4, Case 5: Fig 3.8-6, Case 6: Fig 3.8-7, Case 8: Fig 3.8-9**). These rings were primarily developed for the treatment of GAF in osteoporotic bone without additional internal fixation of the fractures. The first results in a series of 30 patients showed promising results with no implant-related failures (publication in progress).

**CASE 5**

## Primary arthroplasty

### Patient

An 81-year-old cooperative female patient. After a stroke in 2006, she recovered sufficiently and was able to walk short distances without walking aids. She had a fall while walking on the street and sustained an acetabular fracture on the left side. The trauma x-ray showed medial protrusion of the femoral head (central dislocation) (**Fig 3.8-1**) and a superomedial dome impaction (gull sign) (**Fig 3.8-6a**). Three-dimensional reconstructions showed a multifragmentary fracture of the anterior column (**Fig 3.8-6b**) and a simple fracture of the posterior column with the quadrilateral plate in osseous continuity with the posterior column (**Fig 3.8-6c**).

### Comorbidities

- Ischemic heart disease
- Prior stroke in 2006 with incomplete functional recovery
- Depression

### Fracture type

Anterior column with posterior hemitransverse fracture (AO/OTA 62B3) and superomedial dome impaction (gull sign) (**Fig 3.8-6a-c**).

### Treatment and outcome

With relevant displacement of the posterior column and the quadrilateral plate and medial protrusion of the femoral head, operative treatment was indicated after initial closed reduction and traction. The surgery was performed on the third day after trauma, using an angular stable reinforcement ring (**Fig 3.8-4f**) with a cemented polyethylene cup via a lateral approach. There was no attempt to reduce the quadrilateral plate (**Fig 3.8-6d**). One year postoperatively, the fracture had healed and there was no component loosening (**Fig 3.8-6e**). The patient had reached her previous activity level.

### Discussion

This case shows a typical geriatric acetabular fracture pattern, ie, an anterior column with posterior hemitransverse fracture. The fracture of the anterior column is multifragmentary while the posterior hemitransverse fracture is simple. The quadrilateral plate is in osseous continuity with the posterior column, which is internally rotated (open door injury). There is a superomedial dome impaction (gull sign), which is a poor prognostic parameter after internal fixation. Accordingly, primary total hip arthroplasty was performed via a single approach with an uneventful postoperative course and functional recovery.

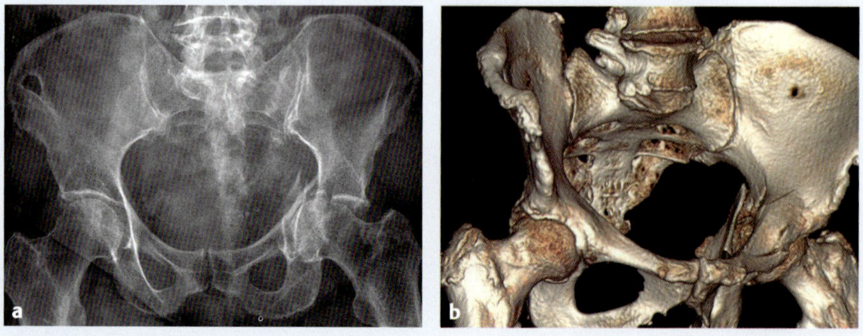


**Fig 3.8-6a–e** An 81-year-old woman with an acetabular fracture on her left side.
- **a** X-ray showing medial protrusion of the femoral head and superomedial dome impression.
- **b** Computed tomographic scan with 3-D reconstruction (view from oblique anterior) showing multifragmentary fracture of the anterior column.

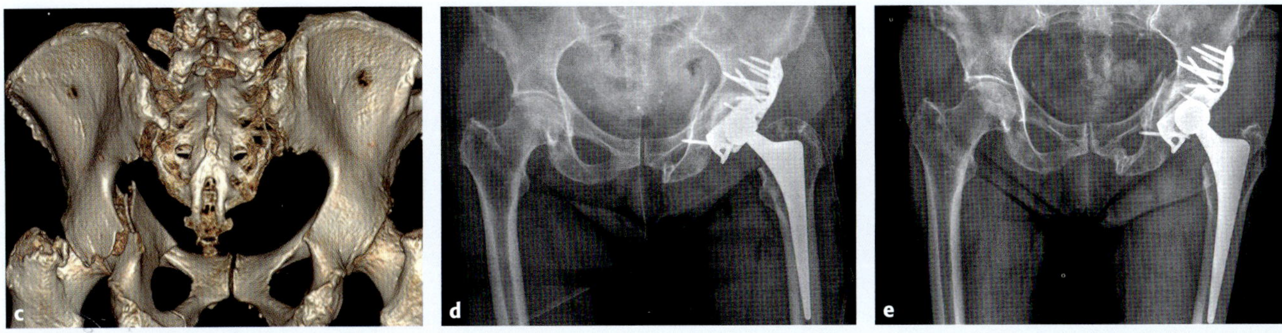

**Fig 3.8-6a–e (cont)** An 81-year-old woman with an acetabular fracture on her left side.
**c** Computed tomographic scan with 3-D reconstruction (view from posterior) showing a simple hemitransverse fracture of the posterior column, quadrilateral plate in osseous continuity with the posterior column.
**d** Postoperative x-ray showing total hip arthroplasty using an angular stable reinforcement ring with a cemented polyethylene cup via a lateral approach.
**e** X-ray after 1 year showing healed acetabular fracture without signs of component loosening.

## 6.4 Internal fixation and arthroplasty

If primary hip arthroplasty is deemed to be the best treatment option for GAF, additional internal fixation may be considered. Internal fixation allows for an easier fixation of revision cups and reinforcement rings by reducing major displacement and adding stability to the acetabular columns. A perfectly anatomical reduction is not essential. The acetabular walls do not need to be addressed in combined procedures. Additionally, it is not necessary to perform internal fixation of both columns in combined procedures. Internal fixation in these cases may be performed via either an anterior (**Case 6: Fig 3.8-7**) or posterior (**Case 7: Fig 3.8-8**) approach. The latter approach allows for fixation and arthroplasty via the same approach with an overall reduced operation time and blood loss. Some case reports in the literature describe combined procedures of internal fixation and arthroplasty, but the overall quality of evidence for this combination is low [2, 28–30].

CASE 6

## Internal fixation via an anterior approach and primary arthroplasty

### Patient

An 83-year-old cooperative female patient, who was living alone and did not use any walking aids, sustained a fall in a bus due to an unexpected emergency braking. The trauma x-ray (**Fig 3.8-7a**) and computed tomographic scan (**Fig 3.8-7b**) showed a multifragmentary anterior column fracture with an additional simple posterior hemitransverse fracture. Additionally, there was a fracture extension to the iliac crest (arrow in **Fig 3.8-7b**).

### Comorbidities

- Hypertension
- No history of cardiopulmonary events

### Fracture type

Anterior column with posterior hemitransverse fracture (AO/OTA 62B3) and fracture extension to the iliac crest (**Fig 3.8-7a-b**).

### Treatment and outcome

Primary arthroplasty was considered as the better treatment option compared to internal fixation due to the age of the patient and the multifragmentary fracture pattern. In order to address the fracture extension to the iliac crest, plate fixation of the anterior column was performed via a midline Stoppa approach in supine position followed by total hip arthroplasty via a lateral approach in lateral decubitus position using an angular stable reinforcement ring. The subsequent course was uneventful. The fracture healed, there was no component loosening (**Fig 3.8-7c**). The patient was able to walk independently again.

### Discussion

In the first step of the decision-making process, operative treatment was deemed to be the best treatment option for this patient due to the multifragmentary fracture pattern and the medial protrusion of the femoral head. In a second step, arthroplasty was favored as described above. The decision for an additional internal fixation was made due to the fracture extension to the iliac crest. The plate bridges the anterior column but does not address the quadrilateral plate. The sole use of a revision cup or a reinforcement ring would not have bridged the fracture extension. The major disadvantage is the need for two approaches with additional operative time and blood loss, which ideally should be minimized in geriatric patients.

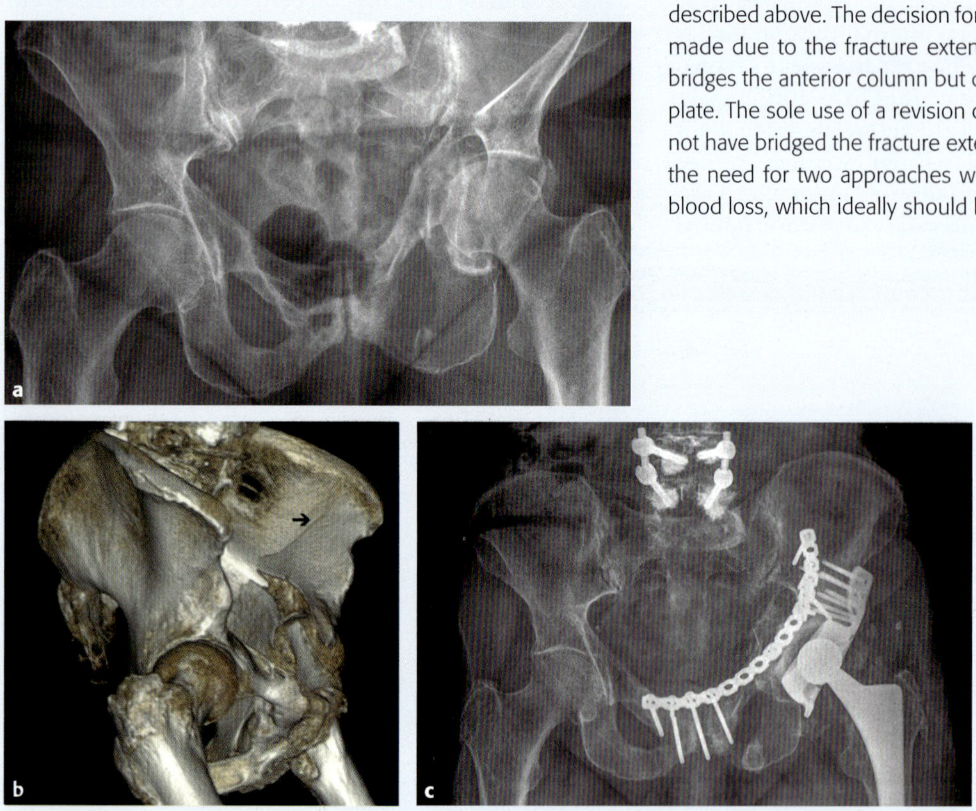


**Fig 3.8-7a–c** An 83-year-old woman with a multifragmentary anterior column fracture.
**a** X-ray showing a multifragmentary anterior column fracture with medial protrusion of the femoral head.
**b** Computed tomographic scan with 3-D reconstruction (view from lateral oblique) showing a multifragmentary anterior column fracture with a simple posterior hemitransverse fracture and fracture extension to the iliac crest (arrow).
**c** X-ray after osseous healing: plate fixation of the anterior column via a midline Stoppa approach in supine position followed by total hip arthroplasty via a lateral approach in lateral decubitus position using an angular stable reinforcement ring.

## Internal fixation via a posterior approach and primary arthroplasty

### Patient

A 78-year-old male patient who was able to walk independently sustained a simple fall while walking. The initial x-ray (**Fig 3.8-8a**) and computed tomographic scan (**Fig 3.8-8b–c**) showed an incomplete low two-column fracture with displacement of the posterior column and a fracture extension to the supraacetabular region (arrows in **Fig 3.8-8b–c**). Additionally, there were signs of preexisting osteoarthritis (ie, narrowing of the joint space and subchondral bone cysts).

### Comorbidities

- Hypertension
- Vitamin D deficiency (25-hydroxyvitamin D3: 8.4 ng/mL [21 nmol/L])
- Anticoagulation for atrial fibrillation

### Fracture type

Incomplete low two-column fracture (AO/OTA 62C2), major displacement of the posterior column (**Fig 3.8-8a**), and fracture extension to the supraacetabular region (arrows in **Fig 3.8-8b–c**).

### Treatment and outcome

Primary arthroplasty was considered as the better treatment option than internal fixation mainly because of the preexisting and symptomatic osteoarthritis. In order to address the fracture extension to the supraacetabular bone, open reduction and plate fixation of the posterior column was performed via a Kocher-Langenbeck approach in a lateral decubitus position followed by total hip arthroplasty using the same approach. A cementless revision cup was used. The further course was uneventful (**Fig 3.8-8d**).

### Discussion

This case is similar to the one in **Case 6: Fig 3.8-7**. The major displacement of the posterior column and the fracture extension, however, can be addressed via a posterior approach. Arthroplasty was performed using the same approach, which eliminated the need for a second approach and reduced the overall operative time. The fracture pattern is not multifragmentary as in **Case 6: Fig 3.8-7** due to the better bone quality in this case. Accordingly, a revision cup with conventional screws was used.

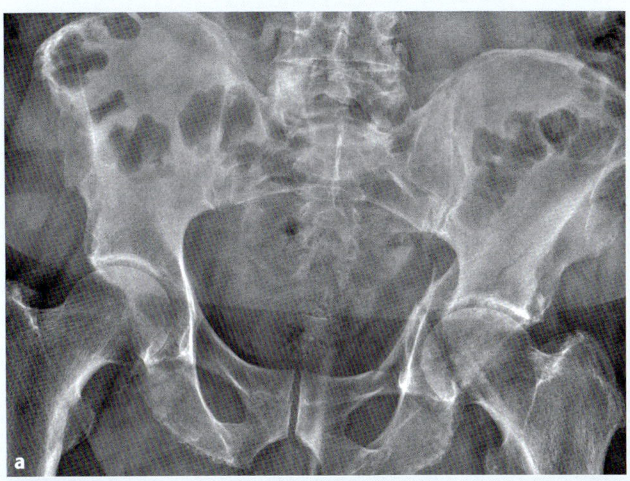

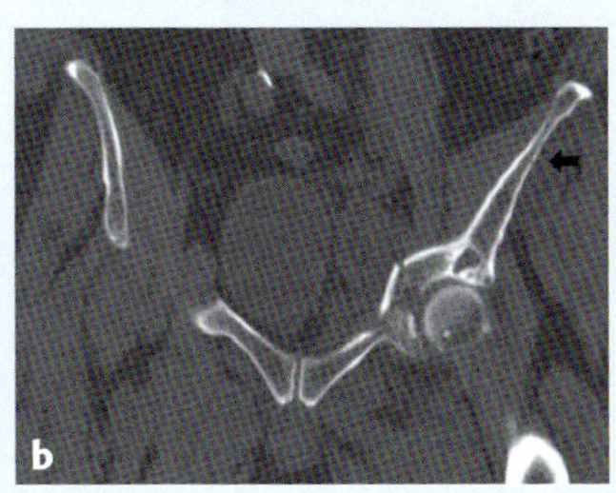

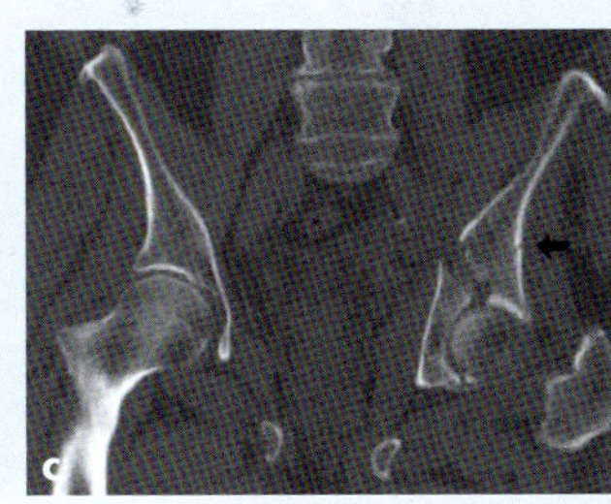

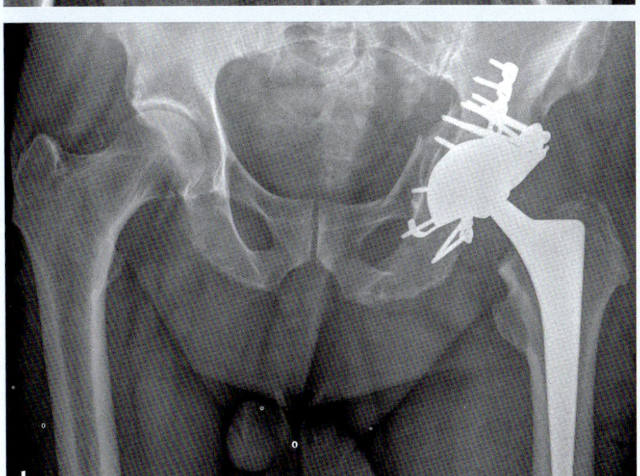

**Fig 3.8-8a–d** A 78-year-old man with a low two-column fracture after a fall.

**a** X-ray showing an incomplete two-column fracture and major displacement of the posterior column.

**b–c** Computed tomographic scan with coronal reconstructions showing fracture extension in the supraacetabular region (arrows).

**d** X-ray after 6 weeks showing open reduction and plate fixation of the posterior column via a Kocher-Langenbeck approach with total hip arthroplasty using a cementless revision cup via the same approach.

CASE 8

## Acetabular fracture after femoral hemiarthroplasty

### Patient

An 88-year-old female nursing home resident who required a walking frame for ambulation sustained a femoral neck fracture 8 years previously, which was treated with femoral hemiarthroplasty. She had a ground-level fall in the nursing home and sustained an anterior column with posterior hemitransverse fracture of the right acetabulum (**Fig 3.8-9a–b**). There was no femoral component loosening of the prosthesis or additional femoral periprosthetic fracture.

### Comorbidities

- Diabetes mellitus
- Renal insufficiency
- Peripheral neuropathy
- Congestive heart failure
- Osteoporosis
- Atrial fibrillation

### Fracture type

Anterior column with posterior hemitransverse fracture (AO/OTA 62B3) and no femoral component loosening or periprosthetic femoral fracture (**Fig 3.8-9a–b**).

### Treatment and outcome

The initial treatment included closed reduction and the application of traction (**Fig 3.8-9c**). Surgery was performed via a lateral approach using an angular stable reinforcement ring with a cemented polyethylene cup. There was no reduction or internal fixation of the acetabular fracture. Bone grafting to fill the fracture gap was not performed, as there was no femoral head available. The further course was uneventful. The patient returned to the nursing home and reached her former mobility level again. An x-ray follow-up after 2 years showed no component loosening and osseous consolidation of the fracture despite the lack of bone grafting (**Fig 3.8-9d**).

### Discussion

Internal fixation of acetabular fractures after femoral hemiarthroplasty is not advisable in general. In this case, an angular stable reinforcement ring with a cemented cup was used due to the frailty of the patient and the poor bone quality. The fracture was not further addressed but healed. The operative procedure took approximately 1 hour and allowed for immediate postoperative full weight bearing, both of which are major goals in geriatric fracture management.

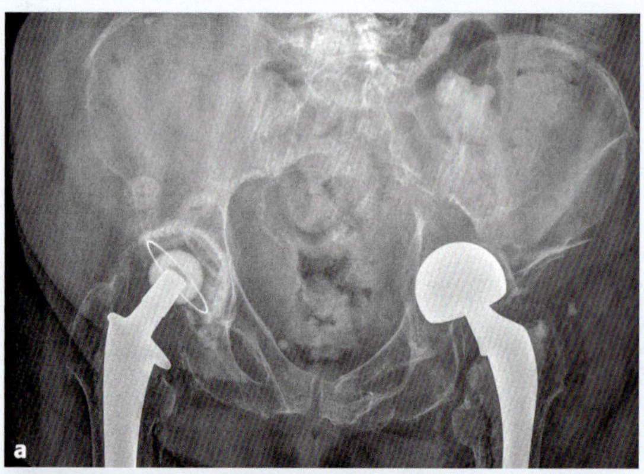


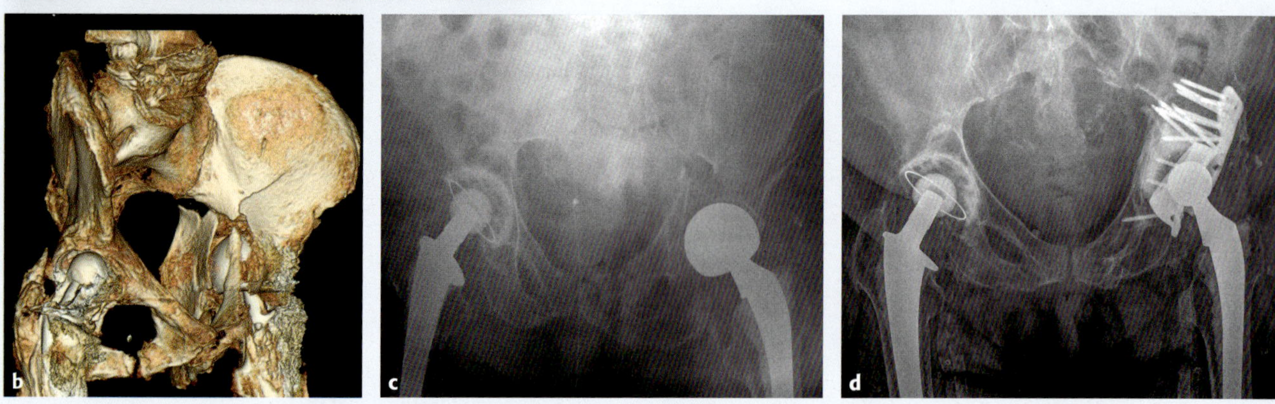


**Fig 3.8-9a–d** An 88-year-old woman with an anterior column fracture after a fall.

**a** X-ray showing an acetabular fracture after femoral hemiarthoplasty.

**b** Computed tomographic scan with 3-D reconstruction (view from anterior oblique) showing the anterior column with posterior hemitransverse fracture, no femoral component loosening or periprosthetic femoral fracture.

**c** X-ray after closed reduction and the application of traction.

**d** X-ray after 2 years showing no component loosening and osseous consolidation of the fracture.

## Periprosthetic acetabular fracture

### Patient

A 71-year-old cooperative female patient able to ambulate independently. Total hip arthroplasty was performed 2 years before due to hip osteoarthritis via a minimally invasive anterior approach. She had a simple fall on her left hip and sustained a periprosthetic transverse fracture of the acetabulum with cup loosening (**Fig 3.8-10a**). There was no loosening of the shaft or periprosthetic femoral fracture.

### Comorbidities

- Hypertension
- Vitamin D deficiency (25-hydroxyvitamin D3: 6.8 ng/mL [17 nmol/L])

### Fracture type

Periprosthetic transverse fracture with cup loosening (AO/OTA 62B1) (**Fig 3.8-10a**).

### Treatment and outcome

Surgery was performed via a posterior Kocher-Langenbeck approach. In a first step, the cup was removed via a posterior arthrotomy. Then the posterior column was reduced and fixed with a pelvic reconstruction plate. The quadrilateral plate was not addressed. A cementless revision cup was used. The further course was uneventful as the x-ray after 6 weeks shows (**Fig 3.8-10b**).

### Discussion

There is no alternative option to revision arthroplasty in this case. In order to facilitate cup fixation in the presence of a transverse fracture, a posterior approach was applied, the posterior column was stabilized, and a revision cup was inserted through the same approach. Due to her younger age, good health status, and better bone quality (**Case 8: Fig 3.8-9**), a revision cup with conventional screws was used.

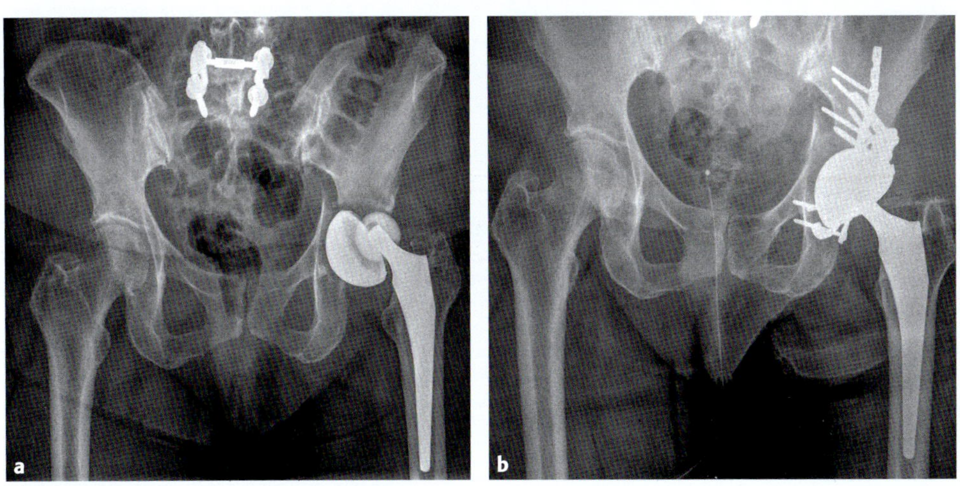


**Fig 3.8-10a–b** A 71-year-old woman after a fall on her left hip.
**a** X-ray showing periprosthetic transverse fracture with cup loosening.
**b** X-ray after 6 weeks showing posterior approach and plate fixation of the posterior column as well as cementless revision cup.

## 7 References


1. **Mears DC.** Surgical treatment of acetabular fractures in elderly patients with osteoporotic bone. *J Am Acad Orthop Surg.* 1999 Mar–Apr;7(2):128–141.
2. **Cornell CN.** Management of acetabular fractures in the elderly patient. *HSS J.* 2005 Sep;1(1):25–30.
3. **Ochs BG, Marintschev I, Hoyer H, et al.** Changes in the treatment of acetabular fractures over 15 years: Analysis of 1266 cases treated by the German Pelvic Multicentre Study Group (DAO/DGU). *Injury.* 2010 Aug;41(8):839–851.
4. **Ferguson TA, Patel R, Bhandari M, et al.** Fractures of the acetabulum in patients aged 60 years and older: an epidemiological and radiological study. *J Bone Joint Surg Br.* 2010 Feb;92(2):250–257.
5. **Sullivan MP, Baldwin KD, Donegan DJ, et al.** Geriatric fractures about the hip: divergent patterns in the proximal femur, acetabulum, and pelvis. *Orthopedics.* 2014 Mar;37(3):151–157.
6. **Hessmann MH, Nijs S, Rommens PM.** Acetabulumfrakturen im Alter. Ergebnisse eines differenzierten Behandlungskonzeptes [Acetabular fractures in the elderly. Results of a sophisticated treatment concept]. *Unfallchirurg.* 2002 Oct;105(10):893–900. German.
7. **Anglen JO, Burd TA, Hendricks KJ, et al.** The "Gull Sign": a harbinger of failure for internal fixation of geriatric acetabular fractures. *J Orthop Trauma.* 2003 Oct;17(9):625–634.
8. **Ohashi K, El-Khoury GY, Abu-Zahra KW, et al.** Interobserver agreement for Letournel acetabular fracture classification with multidetector CT: are standard Judet radiographs necessary? *Radiology.* 2006 Nov;241(2):386–391.
9. **O'Toole RV, Cox G, Shanmuganathan K, et al.** Evaluation of computed tomography for determining the diagnosis of acetabular fractures. *J Orthop Trauma.* 2010 May;24(5):284–290.
10. **Hufner T, Pohlemann T, Gänsslen A, et al.** Die Wertigkeit der CT zur Klassifikation und Entscheidungsfindung nach Acetabulumfrakturen. Eine systematische Analyse [The value of CT in classification and decision making in acetabulum fractures. A systematic analysis]. *Unfallchirurg.* 1999 Feb;102(2):124–131. German.
11. **Garrett J, Halvorson J, Carroll E, et al.** Value of 3-D CT in classifying acetabular fractures during orthopedic residency training. *Orthopedics.* 2012 May;35(5):e615–e620.
12. **Letournel E.** Acetabulum fractures: classification and management. *Clin Orthop Relat Res.* 1980 Sep(151):81–106.
13. **Moed BR, WillsonCarr SE, Watson JT.** Results of operative treatment of fractures of the posterior wall of the acetabulum. *J Bone Joint Surg Am.* 2002 May;84-A(5):752–758.
14. **Mears DC, Velyvis JH, Chang CP.** Displaced acetabular fractures managed operatively: indicators of outcome. *Clin Orthop Relat Res.* 2003 Feb(407):173–186.
15. **Spencer RF.** Acetabular fractures in older patients. *J Bone Joint Surg Br.* 1989 Nov;71(5):774–776.
16. **Ward AJ, Chesser TJ.** The role of acute total hip arthroplasty in the treatment of acetabular fractures. *Injury.* 2010 Aug;41(8):777–779.
17. **Gary JL, VanHal M, Gibbons SD, et al.** Functional outcomes in elderly patients with acetabular fractures treated with minimally invasive reduction and percutaneous fixation. *J Orthop Trauma.* 2012 May;26(5):278–283.
18. **Li YL, Tang YY.** Displaced acetabular fractures in the elderly: results after open reduction and internal fixation. *Injury.* 2014 Dec;45(12):1908–1913.
19. **Toro JB, Hierholzer C, Helfet DL.** Acetabular fractures in the elderly. *Bull Hosp Jt Dis.* 2004;62(1-2):53–57.
20. **Makridis KG, Obakponovwe O, Bobak P, et al.** Total hip arthroplasty after acetabular fracture: incidence of complications, reoperation rates and functional outcomes: evidence today. *J Arthroplasty.* 2014 Oct;29(10):1983–1990.
21. **Hirvensalo E, Lindahl J, Bostman O.** A new approach to the internal fixation of unstable pelvic fractures. *Clin Orthop Relat Res.* 1993 Dec(297):28–32.
22. **Laflamme GY, Hebert-Davies J, Rouleau D, et al.** Internal fixation of osteopenic acetabular fractures involving the quadrilateral plate. *Injury.* 2011 Oct;42(10):1130–1134.
23. **Culemann U, Holstein JH, Kohler D, et al.** Different stabilisation techniques for typical acetabular fractures in the elderly– a biomechanical assessment. *Injury.* 2010 Apr;41(4):405–410.
24. **Gansslen A, Krettek C.** Osteosynthese von Zwei-Pfeiler-Frakturen des Azetabulums über den ilioinguinalen Zugang [Internal fixation of acetabular both-column fractures via the ilioinguinal approach]. *Oper Orthop Traumatol.* 2009 Sep;21(3):270–282. German.
25. **Romness DW, Lewallen DG.** Total hip arthroplasty after fracture of the acetabulum. Long-term results. *J Bone Joint Surg Br.* 1990 Sep;72(5):761–764.
26. **Hoellen IP, Mentzel M, Bischoff M, et al.** Acetabulumfraktur beim alten Menschen. Primäre endoprothetische Versorgung [Acetabular fractures in elderly persons. Primary endoprosthetic treatment]. *Orthopade.* 1997 Apr;26(4):348–353. German.
27. **Borens O, Wettstein M, Garofalo R, et al.** Die Behandlung von Acetabulumfrakturen bei geriatrischen Patienten mittels modifizierter Kabelcerclage und primärer Hüfttotalprothese. Erste Ergebnisse [Treatment of acetabular fractures in the elderly with primary total hip arthroplasty and modified cerclage. Early results]. *Unfallchirurg.* 2004 Nov;107(11):1050–1056. German.
28. **Rickman M, Young J, Trompeter A, et al.** Managing acetabular fractures in the elderly with fixation and primary arthroplasty: aiming for early weightbearing. *Clin Orthop Relat Res.* 2014 Nov;472(11):3375–3382.
29. **Guerado E, Cano JR, Cruz E.** Surgical technique: intraacetabular osteosynthesis with arthroplasty for acetabular fracture in the octogenarian. *Injury.* 2012 Apr;43(4):509–512.
30. **Saxer F, Studer P, Jakob M.** Offene Stabilisierung und Endoprothetik bei geriatrischen Patienten mit acetabulären Frakturen [Open stabilization and primary hip arthroplasty in geriatric patients with acetabular fractures: combination of minimally invasive techniques]. *Unfallchirurg.* 2011 Dec;114(12):1122–1127. German.

# 3.9 Femoral neck

Simon C Mears, Stephen L Kates

## 1 Introduction

Femoral neck fracture is a common injury in older adults, which typically requires both hospitalization and surgery. Successful management of the femoral neck fracture patient requires an understanding of the basic geriatric principles, ie, early operative intervention, managing the osteoporotic bone, and avoiding adverse events including reoperation, and how to apply them:

- Nearly all femoral neck fractures require surgery to return patients as close as possible to their former level of function.
- Better outcomes occur when surgery is performed rapidly after the injury. Earlier surgery has been shown to reduce the risk of mortality and morbidity even when factors such as patient comorbidities are controlled. Surgery within 12 hours of the injury may give the best results.
- Most femoral neck fractures are unstable fractures; arthroplasty allows for immediate weight bearing.
- A truly nondisplaced or stable impacted fracture may be treated with internal fixation techniques.
- Displaced and angulated fractures are best treated with arthroplasty. Internal fixation of displaced fractures leads to an unacceptable rate of reoperation (ie, about 40%) [1–3].
- Arthroplasty technique is dependent on patient factors and surgeon factors. Infirm patients do well with hemiarthroplasty, while active, cognitively intact patients do better with total hip arthroplasty (THA).
- The ideal stem and cup design characteristics are unknown. However, a higher rate of periprosthetic fractures occurs after uncemented stem fixation.
- The goal of surgery is immediate full weight bearing and mobilization. Early rehabilitation allows for maximal return of function.
- Early surgery requires a coordinated approach to care with medical and orthopedic services working together for optimal outcomes.
- The team also includes the emergency department team, medical doctors, anesthesiologists, nurses, therapists, and hospital administrators. All must be fully committed to early surgery and mobilization to achieve the best results.

The goal of this chapter is to present the basics of femoral neck fracture management using case presentations.

## 2 Epidemiology and etiology

Hip fractures are a common injury and femoral neck fractures represent about half of these fractures [4, 5]. The prevalence of femoral neck fracture is increasing worldwide as a result of the aging population. If osteoporosis is effectively treated, the incidence of fractures can be reduced [5].

Femoral neck fractures are usually the result of falls on mechanically weakened bone. Osteoporosis results in bones with thinner cortices and reduced quantity and quality of cancellous bone. Osteoporotic bones are wider in diameter and more susceptible to fracture. Osteoporotic patients also tend to fall more frequently due to poor balance, sarcopenia, visual problems, and comorbid conditions [6]. The rise in frequency of falls increases the likelihood of a catastrophic fall with fracture. Femoral neck fractures often occur in patients with multiple comorbidities. They are more common in women than men, although men experience higher complication rates after a fracture than women.

## 3 Diagnostics

Preoperative evaluation should be streamlined and standardized. Emergency department physicians should quickly evaluate for fracture using plain x-rays and rapidly assess the patient and consult the orthopedic surgeon and medical specialist. Standardization of orders and protocols should allow for quick admission and limited medical testing with a goal of early surgery [7].

### 3.1 Clinical evaluation

Patients with femoral neck fractures typically present with acute hip pain after injury and are unable to bear weight on the injured extremity. Physical examination findings typically demonstrate pain with hip motion. With a displaced fracture, the leg will be shortened and externally rotated. Nondisplaced fractures may present without shortening and the practitioner needs to have a low threshold for imaging to rule out fracture. Patients are often not reliable regarding their history of injury. They may be able to lift their leg and even walk around. If they have a nondisplaced femoral neck fracture, the fracture can displace in the next week or two. For information regarding medical assessments and optimization for surgery, see chapter 1.4 Preoperative risk assessment and preparation.

### 3.2 Imaging

An AP pelvis and AP and lateral views of the affected hip should be performed. A true AP view is needed to visualize the entire femoral neck. Rotated or oblique views may fail to visualize the fracture. A pelvis view is helpful to look for associated injuries or prior surgical implants. It is also used for preoperative planning. Care should be taken to place the uninjured leg in a neutral position while imaging. If the x-rays are normal and examination of the hip produces pain, a fracture is still likely. Further imaging is then required to rule out fracture.

Magnetic resonance imaging is the best test to look for bone edema, nondisplaced or stress fractures [8]. A computed tomographic (CT) scan with thin cuts through the femoral neck is the second best test. This will diagnose most, but not all femoral neck fractures. It is also the most appropriate to evaluate nonunions after fixation attempts.

## 4 Classification

Femoral neck fracture classifications include many different systems of varying complexity [9]. The most commonly used is the Garden system that uses AP hip x-rays and classifies femoral neck fractures into four types. Types 1 and 2 are nondisplaced or minimally displaced and types 3 and 4 are displaced. Discrimination between type 1 and 2 fractures or type 3 and 4 fractures limited by high interobserver variability [10]. Because of this, fractures are termed stable or unstable. In nondisplaced fractures it is important to evaluate the lateral view as well as the AP view. Displacement on the lateral view alone may lead to a higher rate of failure with internal fixation [11]. Stable fractures are either nondisplaced or detectable only by advanced imaging or are valgus-impacted fractures with no displacement on the lateral view. Displaced fractures are any fracture with displacement on lateral x-rays and/or varus displacement.

## 5 Decision making

### 5.1 Operative versus nonoperative

Most patients with femoral neck fractures are treated operatively. A minority may be considered for nonoperative treatment [12]. Generally, this applies to a patient who cannot tolerate any type of surgery or is truly at the end of life. Some patients with dementia may have severe contractures that would make operative repair almost impossible. In these cases, patients may be mobilized as tolerated, and pain control and pressure sore prevention efforts are of utmost importance. A palliative care consult is often useful and consideration should be given to hospice care.

### 5.2 Fixation versus arthroplasty

#### 5.2.1 Stable fractures

Nondisplaced fractures are often considered for internal fixation (**Case 1: Fig 3.9-1**) [13]. It is critical that the fracture is "truly stable". Any displacement on the lateral view generally means instability. Fixation may be performed with cannulated screws or with a sliding hip screw using standard image intensification on a fracture table.

For positioning of cannulated screws, three screws are commonly used and an inverted triangle formation had been shown to lead to fewer nonunions [14]. This has also been shown to be more stable. It is essential to keep the lateral screw entry point above the level of the lesser trochanter [15]. Multiple entry holes should also be avoided to prevent creation of a stress riser and subsequent subtrochanteric femoral fracture [16].

The use of arthroplasty for the treatment of stable fractures is controversial. Arthroplasty has some advantages. It presents no significant risk for poor healing, the development of avascular necrosis, or nonunion or malunion of the fracture. Patients treated with arthroplasty have fewer reoperations, less pain, and higher quality of life than patients treated with fixation [17]. The surgery, however, has risk associated with arthroplasty and leads to slightly higher blood loss [18]. Further studies are required to determine the best treatment for stable femoral neck fractures.

## Stable fracture treated with screw fixation

### Patient

A 93-year-old woman sustained a low-energy fall. She lived with her granddaughter at home and could ambulate independently.

### Comorbidities

- Hypertension
- Mild cognitive dysfunction

### Treatment and outcome

The patient's x-rays in the emergency department revealed a right-sided valgus-impacted femoral neck fracture (**Fig 3.9-1a**). This appeared well aligned on the lateral view (**Fig 3.9-1b**). She underwent screw fixation in situ, which was found to be stable under image intensification (**Fig 3.9-1c–d**). She was mobilized and allowed to bear weight, and the fracture showed evidence of radiographic and clinical healing at 3 months (**Fig 3.9-1e**).

Nine months later she had a similar fall and sustained a similar injury on the contralateral side (**Fig 3.9-1f**), despite the use of intravenous bisphosphonate therapy to manage osteoporosis after the first fracture. This was also treated with screw fixation (**Fig 3.9-1g**). Her second fracture also went on to uneventful healing (**Fig 3.9-1h**).

### Discussion

This patient sustained sequential bilateral stable femoral neck fractures. Both were treated successfully with internal fixation. The patient was allowed to bear weight as tolerated after both surgeries, which was crucial for early rehabilitation and return to function.

Operative fixation options here included the use of internal fixation or arthroplasty. Unstable fracture patterns have more reoperations when internal fixation is used than stable fracture patterns. Determination of the stability of the fracture can be assessed using x-rays with AP and lateral views. There may be a role for the use of computed tomographic scanning to help in this determination [19]. Another possible option is to use image intensification in the operating room to assess stability with range of motion of the hip. This does require extra operating time as this must be done prior to positioning the patient for either internal fixation or hemiarthroplasty. Two image intensifiers can also help in positioning the screws during surgery.

If internal fixation is chosen, various options exist. It is unclear if screw fixation or sliding hip screw with side plate is the best option [20]. Currently, the results of the trial by fixation using alternative implants for the treatment of hip fractures investigators, which seeks to answer this question, are nearing publication [21]. Arthroplasty, while a longer surgery, may provide better results long term with less reoperations and higher patient satisfaction [18]. Another controversial topic within this case is the prevention of second osteoporotic fractures. The rate of a second fracture is particularly high in female patients with advanced age and multiple comorbidities [22]. The exact pharmacological treatment of osteoporosis in geriatric patients or near the end of life is controversial. Treatments that take time to work may not be worthwhile. Bisphosphonate therapy is thought to be cost-effective in patients up to age of 90 years [23]. Fall prevention strategies and supplementation with calcium and vitamin D are worthwhile. Patients with femoral neck fractures should be assessed and treated for osteoporosis after fracture. Despite treatment with intravenous bisphosphonate, this patient sustained a second fragility fracture.

### Key points

- Stable femoral neck fractures with no displacement or with stable valgus impaction can be treated with internal fixation.
- Screws should be carefully positioned in an inverted triangle to give the best chance of fracture healing with internal fixation.
- If the fracture is noted to be unstable on evaluation with image intensifier, strong consideration should be given for arthroplasty rather than internal fixation.

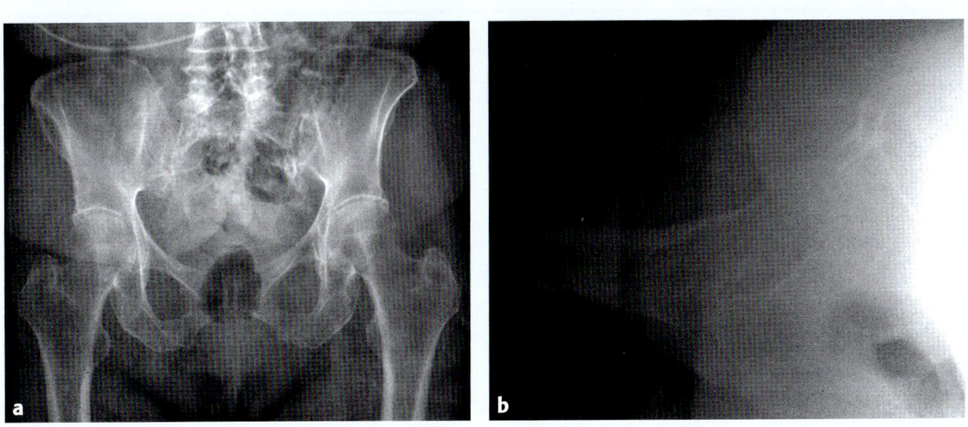


**Fig 3.9-1a–h** A 93-year-old independent woman after several falls.

- **a** AP injury x-ray of the pelvis showing a valgus-impacted right femoral neck fracture.
- **b** The lateral view showing good alignment of the neck and head.

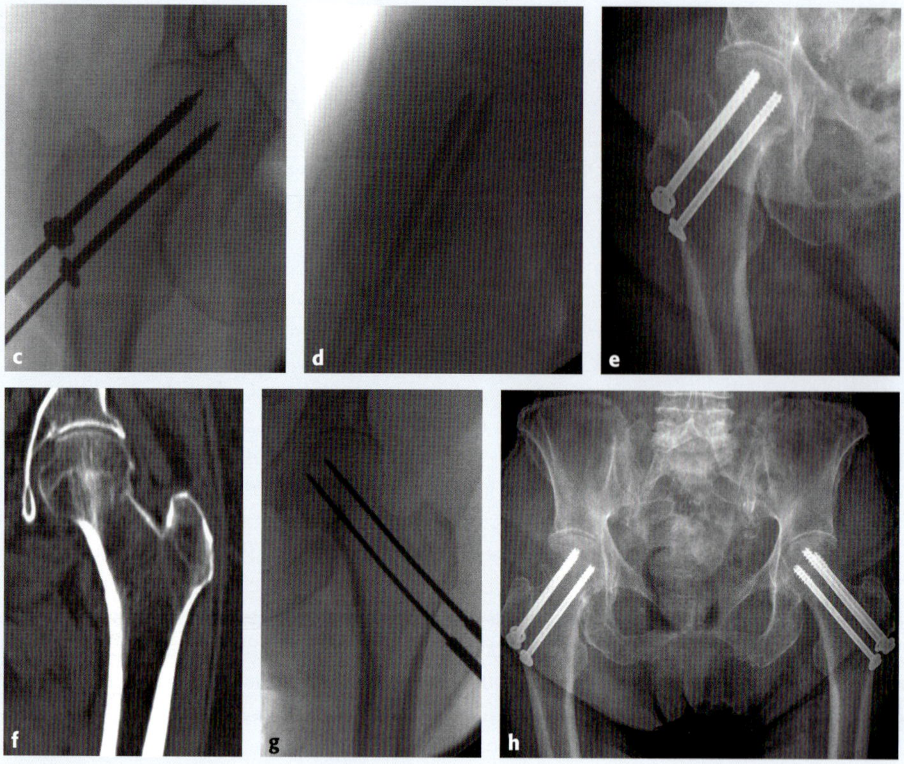

**Fig 3.9-1a–h (cont)** A 93-year-old independent woman after several falls.
- **c** AP view of the hip with image intensification showing the position of the guide wires in the femoral head across the fracture.
- **d** The intraoperative lateral view under image intensification showing the alignment of the guide wires in the lateral plane.
- **e** AP x-ray of the hip showing the fracture fixation at 3 months after the injury. The fracture position is unchanged and there is no change in the position of the screws.
- **f** Coronal computed tomographic scan of the hip showing the contralateral fracture with a very similar pattern to the initial fracture.
- **g** AP intraoperative view with image intensification showing excellent positioning of the guide wires for the screw fixation.
- **h** Both fractures seemed to be radiographically healed and in excellent alignment 3 months after the second fracture.

### 5.2.2 Unstable fractures

Most femoral neck fractures are displaced and are best treated with arthroplasty. In several studies, internal fixation had a significantly higher reoperation rate for nonunion, malunion, shortening, or avascular necrosis [1–3]. (**Case 2: Fig 3.9-2**). A treatment algorithm or femoral neck fracture treatment is seen in **Fig 3.9-3**.

CASE 2

## Unstable fracture treated with fixation

### Patient

A 72-year-old woman with a history of stroke and left-sided weakness. Twenty years earlier, she had sustained a distal femoral fracture treated with a retrograde nail. She was minimally ambulatory getting from bed to chair and always used a walker. The patient fell from a seated position and sustained a displaced femoral neck fracture with x-rays demonstrating a low femoral neck fracture (**Fig 3.9-2a**). The intramedullary rod extended to below the lesser trochanter. After discussion with the patient and family the decision was made to attempt fracture fixation, as arthroplasty would have required removal of the nail.

### Treatment and outcome

Fracture fixation was performed using a 4-hole sliding hip screw with side plate to overlap the nail (**Fig 3.9-2b–c**). The fracture was unstable at the time of fixation and a derotation pin was placed during insertion of the hip screw. The pin was removed after screw placement. The bone quality was extremely poor. After surgery, the patient had increasing pain and at 2 weeks the fracture fixation was seen to have slipped with migration of the screw (**Fig 3.9-2d**). Two weeks later the screw had cut out through the head and pain was worse (**Fig 3.9-2e**).

The patient wanted to try to walk again and elected to have the hardware removed with conversion to a hip arthroplasty. During surgery the hip screw was removed and the hip was found to be stiff. The nail was then removed. The bone of the distal femur had grown in to the nail, and some of the intramedullary bone of the distal femur came out with the nail, weakening the distal bone.

During further hip exposure the distal femur fractured (**Fig 3.9–2f**). The intraoperative decision was made to treat the distal femoral fracture with a long locking plate and the femoral head was removed (**Fig 3.9-2g**). The distal femoral fracture healed and the patient went on to use a motorized wheelchair for ambulation. At 3 months after surgery, the hip was much less painful and she was satisfied with the result (**Fig 3.9-2h–i**).

**Discussion**

Decision making is important in the minimally ambulatory patient. In this situation arthroplasty was fraught with difficulty with the in situ hardware and the extremely poor bone stock. Removal of the retrograde femoral nail was difficult, and the unstable nature of the fracture made fixation challenging. While the sliding hip screw was placed with a low tip-apex distance, the bone quality was so poor that fixation was not sufficient. Perhaps initial hip resection or non-operative care would have led to the same results but with much less morbidity than the two operations that were performed.

Another option for difficult cases with poor bone is the use of cement augmentation. This is not approved for use by the Food and Drug Administration in the United States but is commonly used in Europe [24]. Cement is carefully placed within the femoral head prior to placement of the hip screw. Great care must be taken to prevent cement from entering the joint and if penetration of the femoral head has occurred with the guide wire, cement should not be used.

**Key points**

Unstable fractures have a high rate of failure with internal fixation. Some patients with complex problems and minimal ambulation may be better treated with hip resection or nonoperative treatment. Older adults with hip fractures have little reserve, and very little margin exists for both operative and medical errors. The best results should be achieved in the first surgery to prevent complications, morbidity, and mortality.

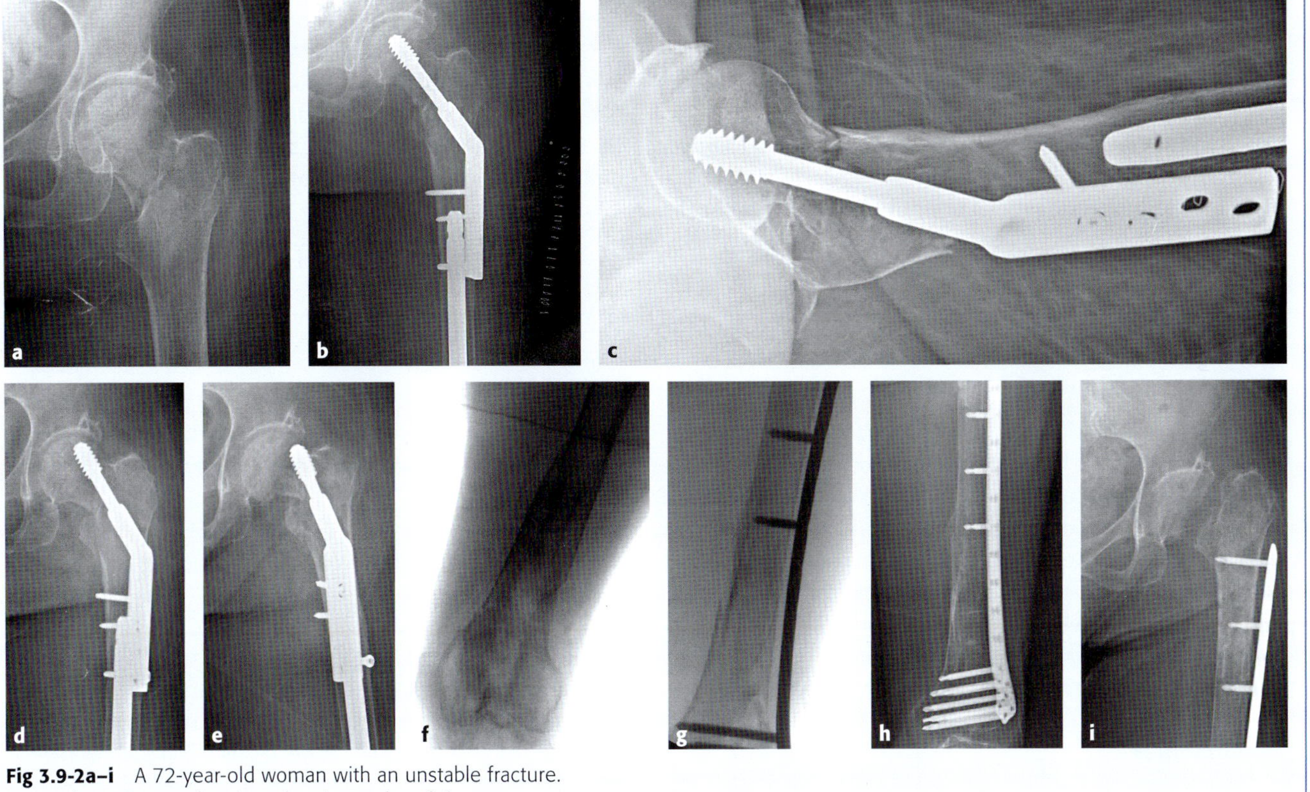


**Fig 3.9-2a–i** A 72-year-old woman with an unstable fracture.

- **a** Injury AP x-ray showing a low femoral neck fracture.
- **b** AP x-ray showing a 2-hole sliding hip screw with side plate placed above the existing retrograde nail.
- **c** Lateral x-ray showing that the reduction was not completely anatomical.
- **d** At 2 weeks after surgery the hip screw had migrated superiorly into the femoral head.
- **e** At 4 weeks the fixation has completely failed and the head screw had penetrated the femoral head.
- **f** Intraoperative image intensification showing an AP view of the distal femur. The fracture line is visible at the supracondylar level.
- **g** Intraoperative x-ray showing plate fixation of the femur.
- **h** Three months after surgery, an AP x-ray shows healing at the fracture site.
- **i** AP view of the hip showing the femoral head resection and the plate extending up to the proximal femur.

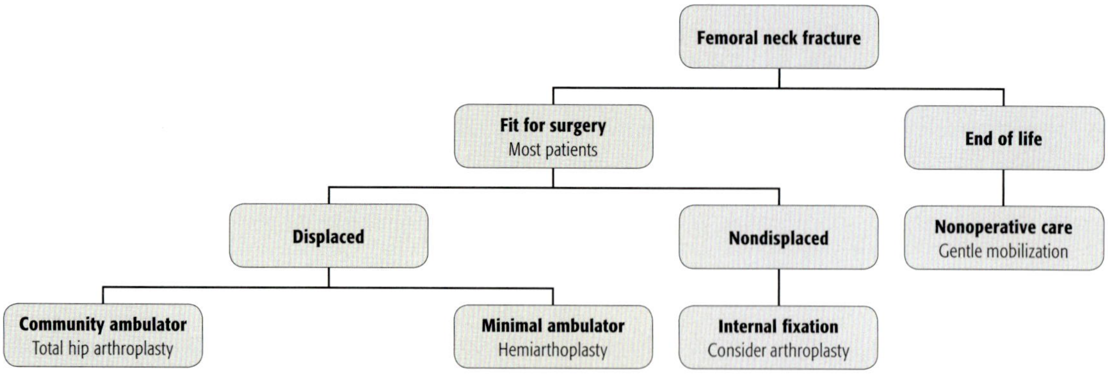


**Fig 3.9-3** An algorithm for treatment of femoral neck fractures [25].

### 5.2.3 Timing

Timing of treatment is critical for the best outcomes. There is debate about the best time to fix hip fractures but clearly, early surgery is better. Longer delays give the patients more days in pain, are expensive, and lead to higher morbidity and mortality rates. The American Academy for Orthopaedic Surgery's (AAOS) *Hip Fracture Clinical Practice Guidelines* give a moderate recommendation for surgery within 48 hours [26]. By implementation of a hip fracture audit including a requirement for hip fracture repair within 36 hours of fracture, mortality rates have been reduced nationwide in the UK from 10.9% to 8.5% (for more information on hip fracture audit, see chapter 2.9 Use of registry data to improve care) [27]. There is some data that extremely rapid repair, ie, less than 12 hours, may have the best results [28, 29].

### 5.2.4 Hemiarthroplasty or total arthroplasty

With arthroplasty, there are several decisions to make. One is whether to perform partial or THA. As a rule, age greater than 80 years, low functional status, and multiple comorbidities all support hemiarthroplasty (**Case 3: Fig 3.9-4**).

CASE 3

## Cemented hemiarthroplasty

### Patient

An 83-year-old man with a history of Parkinson's disease and multiple comorbidities. He had sustained a previous hip fracture on the contralateral side 2 years before. He had a fall 8 weeks back and was in the emergency department with knee pain. The x-rays of the knee at that time did not reveal any acute injury (**Fig 3.9-4a**). He was having difficulty walking and was transferred to a nursing home. His pain continued until he became unable to transfer himself independently. He was found to have knee pain with hip motion, and x-rays revealed a nonunion of a femoral neck fracture (**Fig 3.9-4b–c**).

### Comorbidities

- Multiple comorbidities including deafness and blindness

### Treatment and outcome

He was admitted from the emergency department and evaluated by the medical service. He was believed to be medically optimized for surgery, and cemented hemiarthroplasty was performed using a posterior approach the following day. After surgery he struggled to regain function due to overall weakness and poor mobility. Six weeks after surgery, his pain was greatly improved. The x-rays showed his hemiarthroplasty to be in good position (**Fig 3.9-4d–e**).

At this point the family found it difficult to come in for follow-up and requested that he should only return to the clinic if he had a problem with the hip.

### Discussion

On initial presentation to the emergency department, the diagnosis of femoral neck fracture was missed. The patient complained of knee pain, and the knee x-rays were negative. Hip pain often refers to the knee and any older patient with a fall should be thoroughly evaluated. Any pain on hip examination requires an x-ray to rule out hip fracture. In this case, treatment was delayed by several weeks and this resulted in further deconditioning and worsened functional status for the patient.

The patient had multiple comorbidities but was ambulatory prior to the injury. Cemented hemiarthroplasty allowed for immediate weight bearing and reduced risks of periprosthetic fracture. Despite the length of time until fracture fixation, no arthritic changes were seen on the acetabular side of the hip allowing for hemiarthroplasty. If degenerative changes were seen, total hip arthroplasty (THA) should be considered. With the history of Parkinson's disease, an anterolateral operative approach could be considered to reduce the risk of hip instability.

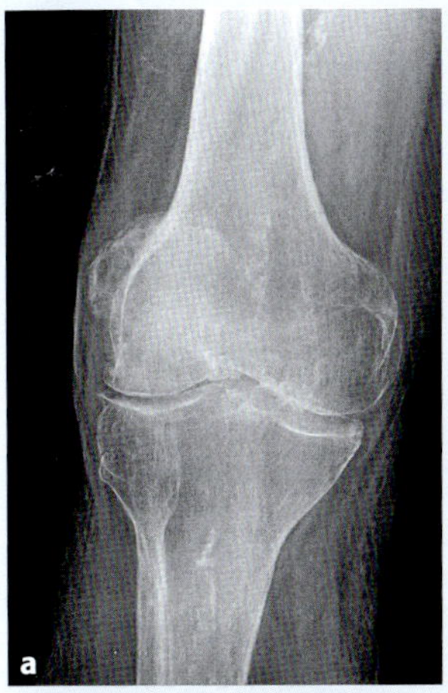


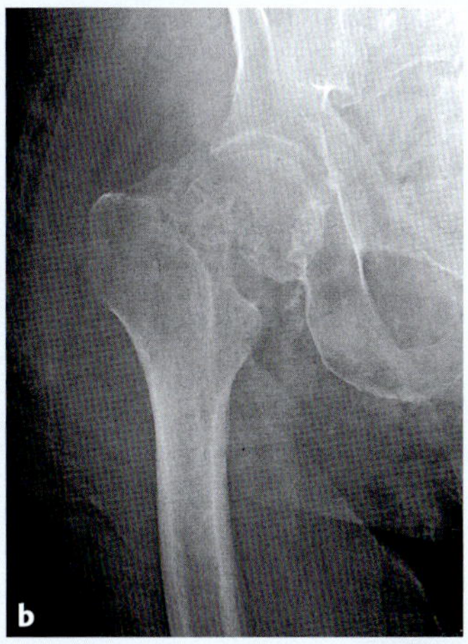


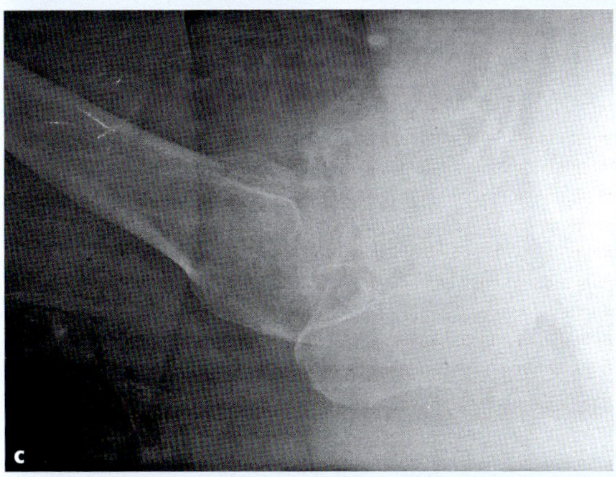


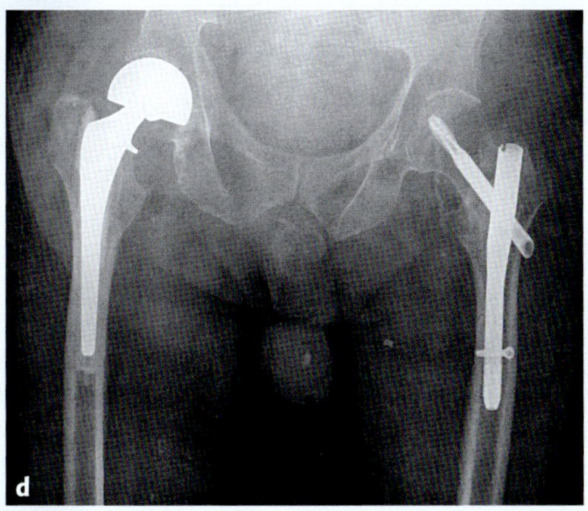


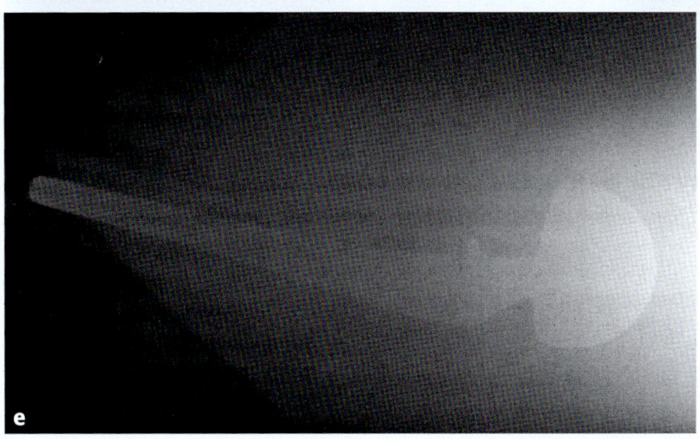


**Key points**

Clinical and radiographic examinations after a fall in an older patient needs to include examination of the hip. Hip pain may radiate to the knee and confuse the evaluation, resulting in a missed diagnosis. Cemented hemiarthroplasty is an excellent treatment option for the medically complex and minimally active patient.

Patients who are active and cognitively intact have more pain from hemiarthroplasty than with THA (**Case 4: Fig 3.9-5**) [30, 31]. However, THA has a higher rate of dislocation than hemiarthroplasty. With partial hip replacement, no functional differences have been found between a unipolar and a bipolar prosthesis [32]. To try to reduce dislocation after THA, some authors have utilized a constrained liner or a dual mobility head. The dual mobility head has a small metal head inside of a large polyethylene head. This articulates with a metal acetabular shell. Good results have been shown with both approaches although long-term results are unknown [33–35].

**Fig 3.9-4a–e** An 83-year-old male patient with Parkinson's disease.

- **a** AP x-ray of the knee taken at the initial injury revealing no fracture. Unfortunately, the hip injury was missed as the pain radiated from the hip to the knee.
- **b** AP x-ray of the hip revealing an unstable chronic femoral neck fracture.
- **c** Lateral x-ray showing the displaced fracture.
- **d** AP pelvis x-ray at 6 weeks after surgery showing a cemented hemiarthroplasty on the right side. The left side had a previous intertrochanteric fracture that has healed with cephalomedullary fixation.
- **e** The lateral x-ray showing good alignment of the femoral stem.

CASE 4

## Total hip arthroplasty

### Patient

A 66-year-old healthy woman fell from a standing position and sustained a displaced femoral neck fracture (**Fig 3.9-5a–b**). She was living with her husband, ambulated independently, and enjoyed gardening and walking.

### Treatment and outcome

She was admitted to the hospital, medically assessed, and optimized for surgery. She underwent total hip arthroplasty (THA) with an anterior approach. The patient was mobilized that evening and allowed to bear weight as tolerated. The following day, physical therapy was initiated and she was able to ambulate about 30 meters. She met criteria for hospital discharge and went home with her family. She did well after surgery and followed a self-directed exercise program. At the 1-month follow-up, she was not using an ambulatory aid and had little pain. The x-rays showed her uncemented hip replacement in excellent position and alignment (**Fig 3.9-5c–d**).

### Discussion

The active patient with a displaced femoral neck fracture should be considered for THA. Total hip arthroplasty has been shown to have less pain and fewer reoperations in active patients. Total replacement does have a higher dislocation rate than hemiarthroplasty and the surgeon should be skilled in arthroplasty to prevent complications. This may present a dilemma over a weekend if a surgeon who routinely performs THA is not available. The risks of operative delay must then be weighed against the potential upside of total versus hemiarthroplasty.

This patient underwent ultra-early fracture repair. Two studies [36, 37] have shown that ultra-early surgery (< 12 hours from admission) may give better results. This patient was treated with a quick mobilization protocol that is often used for total joint replacement patients with hip arthritis. The patient was in good physical shape and had excellent family support. This allowed for early and safe hospital discharge.

### Key points

- Total hip arthroplasty should be utilized in patients with displaced femoral neck fracture and high prefracture activity levels.
- Ultra-early surgery (ie, < 12 hours) may lessen operative morbidity and mortality.
- Rapid recovery protocols can be implemented in active patients with hip fracture.
- At the follow-up, this patient should be assessed and treated for her osteoporosis. This will help to reduce the risk of subsequent fractures as she ages.

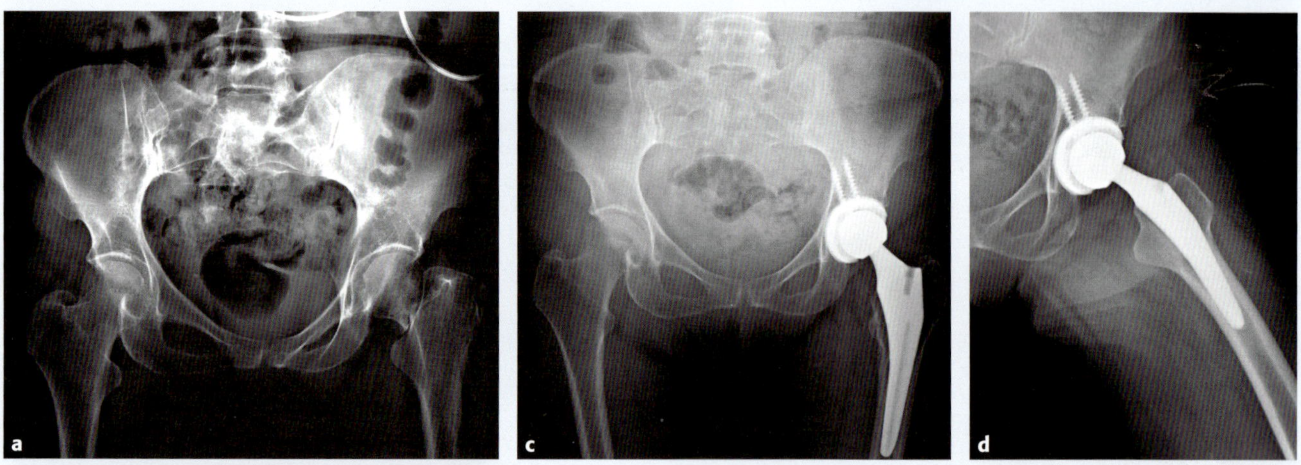

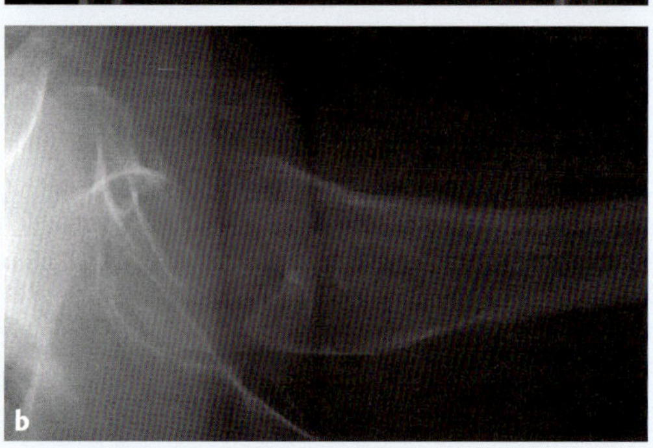

**Fig 3.9-5a–d** Active 66-year-old woman falling from standing height.
**a** Injury AP pelvis x-ray showing a displaced left femoral neck fracture. Bone quality appears to be good.
**b** The lateral x-ray showing the displaced and unstable fracture.
**c** AP pelvis x-ray at 1 month after surgery showing the uncemented implants in good position that appear to be incorporating.
**d** The lateral view showing appropriate anteversion of the cup.

### 5.2.5 Operative approach

Each approach (ie, anterior, anterolateral, or posterior) has risks and benefits. An elevated risk of hip dislocation is associated with THA for fracture [38]. It has been suggested that an anterolateral approach is better, as the risk of dislocation is lower for both hemiarthroplasty [39–41] and THA [42]. This should be strongly considered in patients with neuromuscular disorders or Parkinson's disease, who may be more susceptible to postoperative dislocation. Minimally invasive approaches for hip replacement have not been associated with differences in 1-year outcomes [43]. Minimally invasive techniques should only be used by surgeons with extensive arthroplasty experience.

### 5.2.6 Type of prosthesis

Use of uncemented femoral prostheses is associated with a higher rate of periprosthetic fractures than use of cemented devices [44–47]. These studies have led to AAOS guideline recommendations for the use of cemented femoral stems [26]. Good results have also been shown even in very osteoporotic femora with several types of uncemented stem designs including tapered flat, tapered, rectangular, and fully coated designs. Cemented designs are associated with a low but real rate of acute intraoperative hypotension and mortality [48]. Cementation should be performed carefully without overpressurization.

## 6 Therapeutic options

### 6.1 Initial treatment

A standardized pathway for admission will help get the patient to an appropriate floor bed and off of the hard stretcher in the chaotic environment of the emergency department. The iliac fascia or femoral nerve blocks are helpful to alleviate pain and to minimize the risk of delirium [49]. No benefit has been found with the use of skin or boot traction and this can lead to skin problems or pressure ulceration [50].

### 6.2 Rehabilitation

Maintaining mobility and preparing for rehabilitation of the patient starts on presentation to the emergency department. Adequate pain control will allow less narcotic pain medicine. Nerve blocks given in the emergency department decrease pain and may allow for the patient to be comfortable or to even sit up in the preoperative period.

Early surgery is essential to early rehabilitation. Rehabilitation should be started as soon as possible with an order for weight bearing as tolerated. With fast recovery protocols, patients may be mobilized on the day of surgery. Getting up to the side of the bed or to a chair will begin this process. Continued mobilization and physical therapy will allow the patient to continue the process of rehabilitation. Many patients are functionally impaired before surgery and may be debilitated. This reduces the likelihood of a return to independent living after fracture. For more details, see chapters 1.8 Postoperative surgical management and 1.9 Postacute care.

## 7 Operative complications

Short-term or long-term operative complications impact the outcomes of older fragility fracture patients (FFPs) dramatically and often result in a much worse outcome than in those with a successful index surgery. This is mainly due to the frailty and limited compensatory capacity, ie, reserves, of FFPs. Avoiding complications by any means has a high priority. In case of a complication, a targeted and timely intervention is mandatory to avoid further unnecessary deviations. These situations require excellent co-management and communication within the team.

### 7.1 Failure of screw fixation

Early or late failure of internal fixation is a common complication after treatment of femoral neck fractures. Early failure is from loss of fixation or nonunion. Late failure may be from aseptic necrosis, osteoarthritis, or malunion. Treatment of failure is typically managed with conversion to a hip replacement. This may be a hemiarthroplasty or a THA. Decision making is based on the status of the acetabular cartilage and the patient activity level (**Case 5: Fig 3.9-6**).

The screw holes may weaken the greater trochanter and care should be taken not to break the trochanter. The femoral head should be dislocated first prior to removal of the screw fixation to help prevent intraoperative fracture. The stem should be checked with an intraoperative x-ray to assure that it is not incorrectly placed through the screw holes and not down the shaft of the femur. If a cemented stem is used, the cement may flow out of the screw holes and these should be manually plugged during cementation.

CASE 5

## Conversion to total hip arthroplasty after screw failure—late periprosthetic fracture

### Patient

A 77-year-old woman with Parkinson's disease presented with a previous hip fracture treated with screw fixation 2 years prior. She had developed progressive hip pain and difficulty walking. Her examination revealed a hip with painful range of motion and an antalgic gait. Her Parkinson's disease was managed with medications and she was living at home using a walker for ambulation.

### Treatment and outcome

The x-rays revealed failure of screw fixation with a collapse of the femoral head and secondary arthritic change of the hip joint. From the AP and lateral views the three screws had not been inserted in an inverted triangle configuration (**Fig 3.9-6a–b**). Her bone quality was thought to be poor with a stovepipe-shaped femur and thinning of cortices on both the AP and lateral views. She chose to undergo hip replacement and an uncemented fully coated prosthesis was used due to her poor bone quality. She recovered well from surgery but had a fall 2 months later and sustained a periprosthetic femoral fracture at the tip of the prosthesis (**Fig 3.9-6c**). The prosthesis appeared to be well fixed. This was treated with plate fixation using unicortical screws and cables proximally. Three months after surgery she was bearing weight and there appeared to be callus at the fracture site (**Fig 3.9-6d–e**).

### Discussion

Fracture fixation: It is unknown if the femoral neck fracture was displaced or nondisplaced at the time of the original surgery. Initial hemiarthroplasty, while a larger procedure, would have prevented the osteonecrosis of the femoral head that occurred. Even if fracture fixation was used, a better pattern of screw placement may have given better fixation but may not have prevented aseptic necrosis of the femoral head.

Hip replacement: A fully coated stem was used due to the patient's osteoporotic femoral bone quality. Another option could have been a cemented stem. It is possible that a cemented device would have produced less of a stress riser at the tip of the stem. However, a fall may result in a periprosthetic fracture with any stem design.

Fracture fixation: While an open approach was used for fracture fixation, with current plate design and locking attachment plates for condylar plates, it is possible to use a smaller approach and still achieve excellent fracture fixation. The placement of screws should also be considered. If locking screws are placed just distal to the fracture, a cortical screw will give a less rigid construct. Proximally, locking attachment plates now available may offer improved screw fixation around the stem. For more details on periprosthetic fixation, see chapter 3.13 Periprosthetic fractures around the hip.

### Key points

- Internal fixation has a higher failure rate and need for reoperation than arthroplasty. Arthroplasty should be favored over internal fixation in older patients with displaced femoral neck fractures.
- Uncemented implants have a higher rate of periprosthetic fractures than cemented implants.
- Careful thought to implant construct and screw position should be given in the case of osteoporotic patients with periprosthetic fractures.

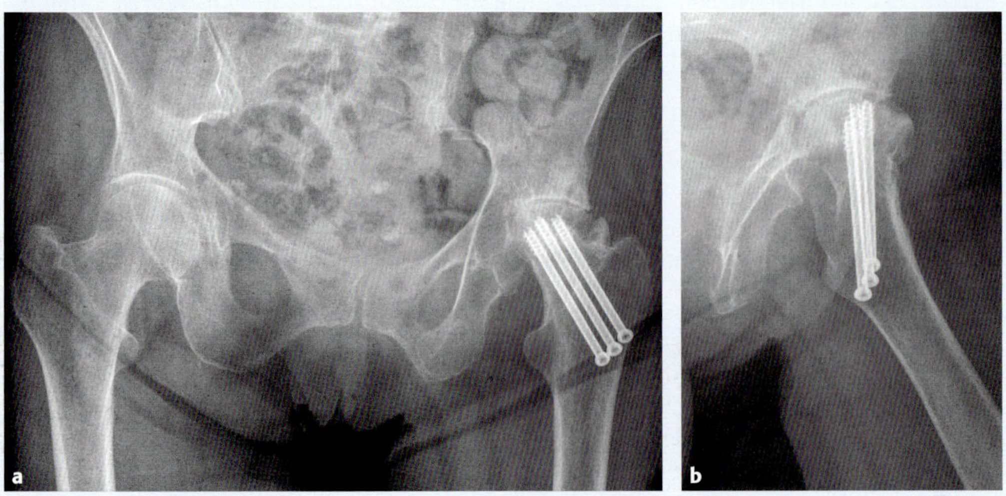


**Fig 3.9-6a–e** A 77-year-old woman with poor bone quality.
**a** AP x-ray showing collapse of the femoral head after screw fixation of a femoral neck fracture.
**b** Lateral x-ray showing the three screws used in a vertical alignment, not in an inverted triangle.

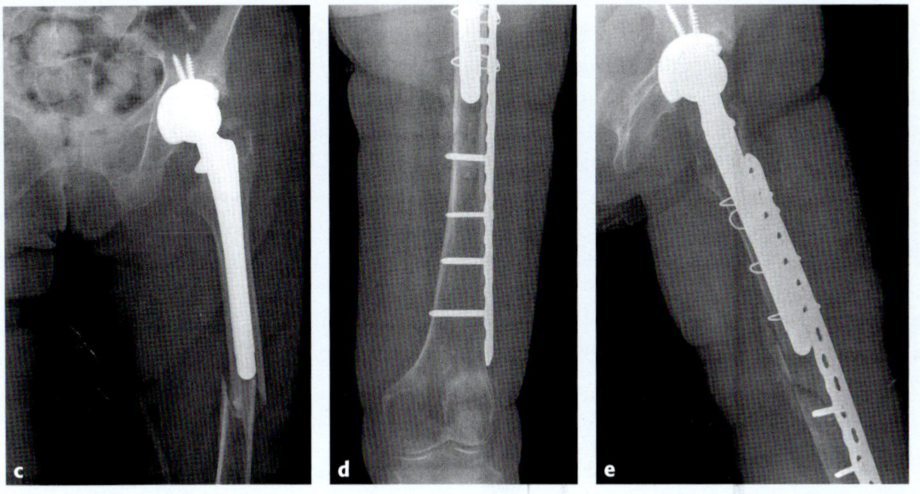


**Fig 3.9-6a–e (cont)** A 77-year-old woman with poor bone quality.
- **c** Injury x-ray showing the total hip arthroplasty with well-fixed stem and a fracture at the tip of the stem.
- **d** AP x-ray at 3 months showing the plate construct with callus formation at the fracture site.
- **e** Lateral x-ray at 3 months after fracture.

## 7.2 Failure of hemiarthroplasty

Hemiarthroplasty has been shown to have excellent implant longevity in hip fracture patients [51]. Implants may fail from erosion of the acetabular cartilage. Risk factors include preexisting osteoarthritis, damage to the labrum during placement of the replacement, or high activity level of the patient. Selection of the wrong size femoral head may cause premature cartilage wear. Typically these patients present with activity-related groin pain. The x-rays will show narrowing of the acetabular cartilage. Treatment of acetabular erosion is best accomplished with conversion to a THA. Another cause of failure is polyethylene wear within a bipolar hemiarthroplasty. This may lead to osteolysis similar to that seen in THA [52].

## 7.3 Failure of total arthroplasty—intraoperative acetabular failure

Placement of the acetabular component can be challenging in very osteoporotic bone. There is a tendency for rapid advancement of the reamer after it goes through the cartilage. This can lead to over medialization of the cup. Even worse is if this over reaming is eccentric and the posterior wall is weakened or removed. This eliminates that ability to get a press fit. The surgeon has several options if this occurs. One is placement of a cemented acetabular component. Another is the use of an augment either autograft from the existing femoral head or the use of a metal augment [53]. This can reconstruct the posterior/superior wall and enable the surgeon to establish a press fit of the cup. The final option is the use of a cage construct [54]. These are complex techniques that require an experienced hip surgeon. If an unexperienced surgeon sees that a stable cup cannot be placed, the best option may be to close the patient without implant placement and immediate referral to a revision hip expert.

## 7.4 Periprosthetic fracture

A common complication of hip replacement surgery is periprosthetic fracture. This may occur during surgery or later from subsequent trauma. Intraoperative fractures typically occur with uncemented components during final component impaction. Treatment is with cerclage wires or cables of the proximal femur. Often the same implant can be used. If the fracture results in an unstable femoral implant situation, conversion to a more distally fixed femoral component is very successful [55]. Later periprosthetic fractures are managed using the Vancouver algorithm [56]. If the component is loose, then it must be revised to a revision implant. If the component is stable, internal fixation is the preferred treatment. For more detailed information, see chapter 3.13 Periprosthetic fractures around the hip.

### 7.5 Dislocation

Dislocation is more common with a THA than with hemiarthroplasty when used for femoral neck fracture. The rate of dislocation in one study was 8.1% [38]. It is unclear why the rate of dislocation is higher when a THA is used for a fracture as opposed to osteoarthritis but it is thought to be due to lack of capsular contracture in the fracture patient. It also may result from patients with cognitive impairment in the perioperative period, a common problem in FFPs. The type of approach is also thought to play a role, with anterolateral approaches more stable than posterior approaches [25]. Dislocation is often the result of incorrect component placement. Careful attention needs to be made to both acetabular and femoral component orientation.

With a hemiarthroplasty, this is most commonly incorrect anteversion of the femoral component. This may depend on the approach [57]. With a posterior approach, retroversion will lead to posterior dislocation. With an anterior or anterolateral approach, excessive anteversion may lead to anterior hip dislocation. The appropriate amount of anteversion is felt to be about 20° [58]. This can be treated with revision of the femoral implant and correction of the malrotation. If the implant is retained and converted to a THA, dislocation will still occur.

Another cause for dislocation of hemiarthroplasty is the lack of a true "suction fit" of the head in the acetabulum. This can result from:

- Retained bony or cement fragments in the acetabulum and/or damage to the labrum of the hip during exposure. The solution is to be certain the acetabulum is free of debris and soft tissue prior to reduction.
- A lack of a hemispherical acetabulum due to deformity, arthritis, or an inverted flap of capsule retained in the acetabulum when the head is reduced. In case of a non-hemispherical acetabulum, the surgeon needs to convert to THA.
- An inappropriately sized head, ie, too large or too small. Obviously, it is essential to achieve a correct head size based on measurement of the extracted head and trial reduction of the trial implant in the acetabulum.

Treatment for component malalignment is correction of the incorrect implant positioning. The femoral component should be in anteversion and the acetabular component with correct anteversion and abduction angle using the safe zone. Most commonly, the dislocation is posterior with deep flexion but anterior dislocation may occur if components are too anteverted. If implant position is correct and dislocation still occurs then the use of a constrained liner should be considered.

Technical tips to avoid dislocation:

- Use a more stable approach for patients prone to dislocation; anterior lateral is the preferred approach.
- Take care not to damage the labrum on approach to leave its suction fit effect on the prosthetic head.
- Make sure that the femoral implant is placed in anteversion and is not retroverted.

### 7.6 Prosthetic joint infection

Infection is the second most common major complication after arthroplasty for hip fracture [59] and problematic for the debilitated FFP. The rate of infection is thought to be higher after arthroplasty for a diagnosis of fracture compared to osteoarthritis [60].

Deep periprosthetic infection should be promptly recognized and treated. Clinical findings may be a painful arthroplasty, wound redness, or drainage. Diagnosis is with arthrocentesis and culture. Options for treatment include surgical debridement and antibiotics or removal of implants and either a 1- or 2-stage approach to treatment [61]. Suppressive treatment with antibiotics alone works poorly. Treatment is difficult and should be tailored to the patient, especially in the very old and fragile patient [61, 62]. The most moribund patients may be treated with implant removal alone and permanent resection arthroplasty (**Case 6: Fig 3.9-7**).

## Infected and dislocated bipolar hemiarthroplasty

### Patient
An 84-year-old woman with dementia sustained a displaced femoral neck fracture.

### Treatment and outcome
She was treated at another hospital with hemiarthroplasty. Two weeks after surgery, she dislocated her hip while sitting up. The hip was managed with closed reduction, but she subsequently dislocated it two more times. She underwent revision surgery to a total hip arthroplasty (THA) using a constrained liner. The original femoral stem was retained.

Subsequently, she dislocated the THA when getting up. The x-rays revealed that the cup had fractured through the acetabulum and the constrained liner was intact (**Fig 3.9-7a–b**). She was transferred into a tertiary referral center for further care. At that time, she was found to be draining serosanguinous fluid from her hip incision. She was acutely delirious on admission, experienced severe hip pain, and was unable to ambulate. Before these events, she had been living at home.

After discussion with her caregivers, the best option was thought to be treatment of her hip infection with removal of all hip implants and debridement. During surgery it was found that the screws in her cup had pulled through the entire posterior acetabulum giving a larger posterior wall/column fracture (**Fig 3.9-7c–d**). The stem was removed and found to have been placed in retroversion. A nonarticulating spacer was placed and she was treated with intravenous antibiotics. Cultures did not grow an organism. After surgery her delirium worsened and she became highly agitated. Geriatric consultation was requested for pharmacological treatment of her delirium/dementia. She required one further surgical debridement to get the wound to heal.

After a long hospital course, her delirium persisted and she was placed in long-term care at a nursing home. At the 6-week follow-up she was found to be comfortable and had no desire to ambulate. She was not considered a good candidate for reimplantation surgery.

### Discussion
The patient was initially treated with hemiarthroplasty, however, her implants were poorly placed. Retroversion of the femoral stem led to posterior hip dislocation. This was then treated with conversion to a constrained THA without correction of the femoral component malposition. The same forces producing the dislocation of her hemiarthroplasty occurred and the implant fractured through her pelvis. Revision surgery for a dislocating hemiarthroplasty is difficult and a thorough evaluation of the stem should be performed. A well cemented stem can be revised by recementing a smaller stem into the existing cement mantle with correct anteversion. With multiple surgeries and infection, this patient's delirium worsened. Ultimately, this led to long-term nursing home placement. Complications and reoperations must be avoided to give good results in the older adult population.

Treatment of an infected total hip prosthesis in the debilitated hip fracture patient is challenging. In this case, due to her poor functional status, a permanent resection arthroplasty was chosen. In a more active patient, a 2-stage approach with reimplantation could have been considered.

### Key points
- The femoral stem must be placed with correct anteversion to prevent hip dislocation.
- Constrained implants play a role in instability treatment only when the implant position is correct. Their use can almost always be avoided.
- All efforts must be made to avoid reoperation in the femoral neck fracture patient; "single-shot surgery" is best.
- Treatment of infection after femoral neck repair is challenging and often requires implant removal.

In a healthier patient, the implants may be directly revised or an antibiotic-impregnated cement spacer may be placed. A course of 6 weeks of pathogen-specific intravenous antibiotics is used after implant removal. If the infection appears to be eradicated the spacer may be removed and a second hip replacement placed. Surgical treatment is required in all deep prosthetic joint infections. Prosthetic joint infections should never be treated with antibiotics alone. It is mandatory to comanage these patients with an infectious disease physician. The orthopedic surgeon should not attempt to manage these patients alone.

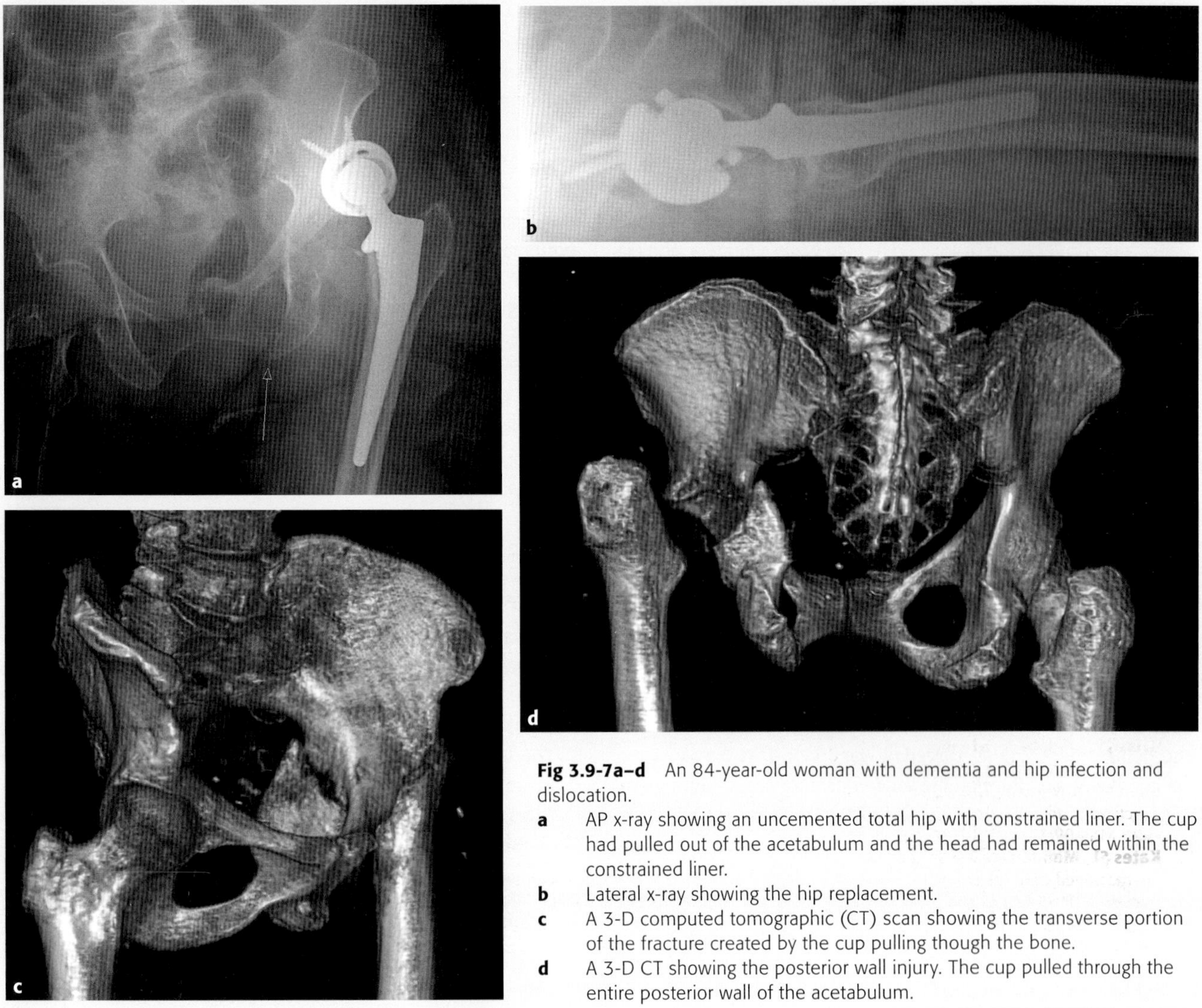


**Fig 3.9-7a–d** An 84-year-old woman with dementia and hip infection and dislocation.

- **a** AP x-ray showing an uncemented total hip with constrained liner. The cup had pulled out of the acetabulum and the head had remained within the constrained liner.
- **b** Lateral x-ray showing the hip replacement.
- **c** A 3-D computed tomographic (CT) scan showing the transverse portion of the fracture created by the cup pulling though the bone.
- **d** A 3-D CT showing the posterior wall injury. The cup pulled through the entire posterior wall of the acetabulum.

## 8 References


1. **Gjertsen JE, Vinje T, Engesaeter LB, et al.** Internal screw fixation compared with bipolar hemiarthroplasty for treatment of displaced femoral neck fractures in elderly patients. *J Bone Joint Surg Am.* 2010 Mar;92(3):619–628.
2. **Hedbeck CJ, Inngul C, Blomfeldt R, et al.** Internal fixation versus cemented hemiarthroplasty for displaced femoral neck fractures in patients with severe cognitive dysfunction: a randomized controlled trial. *J Orthop Trauma.* 2013 Dec;27(12):690–695.
3. **Waaler Bjornelv GM, Frihagen F, Madsen JE, et al.** Hemiarthroplasty compared to internal fixation with percutaneous cannulated screws as treatment of displaced femoral neck fractures in the elderly: cost-utility analysis performed alongside a randomized, controlled trial. *Osteoporos Int.* 2012 Jun;23(6):1711–1719.
4. **Johnell O, Kanis J.** Epidemiology of osteoporotic fractures. *Osteoporos Int.* 2005 Mar;16 Suppl 2:S3–S7.
5. **Amin S, Achenbach SJ, Atkinson EJ, et al.** Trends in fracture incidence: a population–based study over 20 years. *J Bone Miner Res.* 2014 Mar;29(3):581–589.
6. **Grisso JA, Kelsey JL, Strom BL, et al.** Risk factors for falls as a cause of hip fracture in women. The Northeast Hip Fracture Study Group. *N Engl J Med.* 1991 May 09;324(19):1326–1331.
7. **Kates SL, Mendelson DA, Friedman SM.** Co-managed care for fragility hip fractures (Rochester model). *Osteoporos Int.* 2010 Dec;21(Suppl 4):S621–S625.
8. **Haubro M, Stougaard C, Torfing T, et al.** Sensitivity and specificity of CT- and MRI-scanning in evaluation of occult fracture of the proximal femur. *Injury.* 2015 Aug;46(8):1557–1561.
9. **Mears SC.** Classification and surgical approaches to hip fractures for nonsurgeons. *Clin Geriatr Med.* 2014 May;30(2):229–241.
10. **van Embden D, Rhemrev SJ, Genelin F, et al.** The reliability of a simplified Garden classification for intracapsular hip fractures. *Orthop Traumatol Surg Res.* 2012 Jun;98(4):405–408.
11. **Palm H, Gosvig K, Krasheninnikoff M, et al.** A new measurement for posterior tilt predicts reoperation in undisplaced femoral neck fractures: 113 consecutive patients treated by internal fixation and followed for 1 year. *Acta Orthop.* 2009 Jun;80(3):303–307.
12. **Hossain M, Neelapala V, Andrew JG.** Results of non-operative treatment following hip fracture compared to surgical intervention. *Injury.* 2009 Apr;40(4):418–421.
13. **Cserhati P, Kazar G, Manninger J, et al.** Non-operative or operative treatment for undisplaced femoral neck fractures: a comparative study of 122 non-operative and 125 operatively treated cases. *Injury.* 1996 Oct;27(8):583–588.
14. **Yang JJ, Lin LC, Chao KH, et al.** Risk factors for nonunion in patients with intracapsular femoral neck fractures treated with three cannulated screws placed in either a triangle or an inverted triangle configuration. *J Bone Joint Surg Am.* 2013 Jan 02;95(1):61–69.
15. **Kloen P, Rubel IF, Lyden JP, et al.** Subtrochanteric fracture after cannulated screw fixation of femoral neck fractures: a report of four cases. *J Orthop Trauma.* 2003 Mar;17(3):225–229.
16. **Oakey JW, Stover MD, Summers HD, et al.** Does screw configuration affect subtrochanteric fracture after femoral neck fixation? *Clin Orthop Relat Res.* 2006 Feb;443:302–306.
17. **Gjertsen JE, Fevang JM, Matre K, et al.** Clinical outcome after undisplaced femoral neck fractures. *Acta Orthop.* 2011 Jun;82(3):268–274.
18. **Lin JC, Liang WM.** Outcomes after fixation for undisplaced femoral neck fracture compared to hemiarthroplasty for displaced femoral neck fracture among the elderly. *BMC Musculoskelet Disord.* 2015 Aug 19;16:199.
19. **Du CL, Ma XL, Zhang T, et al.** Reunderstanding of garden type I femoral neck fractures by 3-dimensional reconstruction. *Orthopedics.* 2013 Jun;36(6):820–825.
20. **Watson A, Zhang Y, Beattie S, et al.** Prospective randomized controlled trial comparing dynamic hip screw and screw fixation for undisplaced subcapital hip fractures. *ANZ J Surg.* 2013 Sep;83(9):679–683.
21. **FAITH.** Fixation using alternative implants for the treatment of hip fractures (FAITH): design and rationale for a multi-centre randomized trial comparing sliding hip screws and cancellous screws on revision surgery rates and quality of life in the treatment of femoral neck fractures. *BMC Musculoskelet Disord.* 2014 Jun 26;15:219.
22. **Moll MA, Bachmann LM, Joeris A, et al.** Parameters pointing at an increased risk for contralateral hip fractures: systematic review. *Geriatr Orthop Surg Rehabil.* 2016 Mar;7(1):45–61.
23. **Pham AN, Datta SK, Weber TJ, et al.** Cost-effectiveness of oral bisphosphonates for osteoporosis at different ages and levels of life expectancy. *J Am Geriatr Soc.* 2011 Sep;59(9):1642–1649.
24. **Neuburger J, Currie C, Wakeman R, et al.** The impact of a national clinician-led audit initiative on care and mortality after hip fracture in England: an external evaluation using time trends in non-audit data. *Med Care.* 2015 Aug;53(8):686–691.
25. **Rogmark C, Leonardsson O.** Hip arthroplasty for the treatment of displaced fractures of the femoral neck in elderly patients. *Bone Joint J.* 2016 Mar;98-B(3):291–297.
26. **Roberts KC, Brox WT.** AAOS Clinical Practice Guideline: management of hip fractures in the elderly. *J Am Acad Orthop Surg.* 2015 Feb;23(2):138–140.
27. **Neuburger J, Currie C, Wakeman R, et al.** The impact of a national clinician-led audit initiative on care and mortality after hip fracture in England: an external evaluation using time trends in non-audit data. *Med Care.* 2015 Aug;53(8):686–691.
28. **Uzoigwe CE, Burnand HG, Cheesman CL, et al.** Early and ultra-early surgery in hip fracture patients improves survival. *Injury.* 2013 Jun;44(6):726–729.
29. **Bretherton CP, Parker MJ.** Early surgery for patients with a fracture of the hip decreases 30-day mortality. *Bone Joint J.* 2015 Jan;97-B(1):104–108.
30. **Blomfeldt R, Tornkvist H, Eriksson K, et al.** A randomised controlled trial comparing bipolar hemiarthroplasty with total hip replacement for displaced intracapsular fractures of the femoral neck in elderly patients. *J Bone Joint Surg Br.* 2007 Feb;89(2):160–165.
31. **Baker RP, Squires B, Gargan MF, et al.** Total hip arthroplasty and hemiarthroplasty in mobile, independent patients with a displaced intracapsular fracture of the femoral neck. A randomized, controlled trial. *J Bone Joint Surg Am.* 2006 Dec;88(12):2583–2589.
32. **Raia FJ, Chapman CB, Herrera MF, et al.** Unipolar or bipolar hemiarthroplasty for femoral neck fractures in the elderly? *Clin Orthop Relat Res.* 2003 Sep;(414):259–265.

33. **Hernigou P, Filippini P, Flouzat-Lachaniette CH, et al.** Constrained liner in neurologic or cognitively impaired patients undergoing primary THA. *Clin Orthop Relat Res.* 2010 Dec;468(12):3255–3262.
34. **Nich C, Vandenbussche E, Augereau B, et al.** Do dual-mobility cups reduce the risk of dislocation in total hip arthroplasty for fractured neck of femur in patients aged older than 75 years? *J Arthroplasty.* 2016 Jun;31(6):1256–1260.
35. **Adam P, Philippe R, Ehlinger M, et al.** Dual mobility cups hip arthroplasty as a treatment for displaced fracture of the femoral neck in the elderly. A prospective, systematic, multicenter study with specific focus on postoperative dislocation. *Orthop Traumatol Surg Res.* 2012 May;98(3):296–300.
36. **Uzoigwe CE, Burnand HG, Cheesman CL, et al.** Early and ultra-early surgery in hip fracture patients improves survival. *Injury.* 2013 Jun;44(6):726–729.
37. **Bretherton CP, Parker MJ.** Early surgery for patients with a fracture of the hip decreases 30-day mortality. *Bone Joint J.* 2015 Jan;97-B(1):104–108.
38. **Poignard A, Bouhou M, Pidet O, et al.** High dislocation cumulative risk in THA versus hemiarthroplasty for fractures. *Clin Orthop Relat Res.* 2011 Nov;469(11):3148–3153.
39. **Rogmark C, Fenstad AM, Leonardsson O, et al.** Posterior approach and uncemented stems increases the risk of reoperation after hemiarthroplasties in elderly hip fracture patients. *Acta Orthop.* 2014 Feb;85(1):18–25.
40. **Biber R, Brem M, Singler K, et al.** Dorsal versus transgluteal approach for hip hemiarthroplasty: an analysis of early complications in seven hundred and four consecutive cases. *Int Orthop.* 2012 Nov;36(11):2219–2223.
41. **Skoldenberg O, Ekman A, Salemyr M, et al.** Reduced dislocation rate after hip arthroplasty for femoral neck fractures when changing from posterolateral to anterolateral approach. *Acta Orthop.* 2010 Oct;81(5):583–587.
42. **Hailer NP, Weiss RJ, Stark A, et al.** The risk of revision due to dislocation after total hip arthroplasty depends on surgical approach, femoral head size, sex, and primary diagnosis. An analysis of 78,098 operations in the Swedish Hip Arthroplasty Register. *Acta Orthop.* 2012 Oct;83(5):442–448.
43. **Imamura M, Munro NA, Zhu S, et al.** Single mini-incision total hip replacement for the management of arthritic disease of the hip: a systematic review and meta-analysis of randomized controlled trials. *J Bone Joint Surg Am.* 2012 Oct 17;94(20):1897–1905.
44. **Langslet E, Frihagen F, Opland V, et al.** Cemented versus uncemented hemiarthroplasty for displaced femoral neck fractures: 5-year followup of a randomized trial. *Clin Orthop Relat Res.* 2014 Apr;472(4):1291–1299.
45. **Parker MJ, Gurusamy KS, Azegami S.** Arthroplasties (with and without bone cement) for proximal femoral fractures in adults. *Cochrane Database Syst Rev.* 2010 Jun 16(6):CD001706.
46. **Viberg B, Overgaard S, Lauritsen J, et al.** Lower reoperation rate for cemented hemiarthroplasty than for uncemented hemiarthroplasty and internal fixation following femoral neck fracture: 12- to 19-year follow-up of patients aged 75 years or more. *Acta Orthop.* 2013 Jun;84(3):254–259.
47. **Taylor F, Wright M, Zhu M.** Hemiarthroplasty of the hip with and without cement: a randomized clinical trial. *J Bone Joint Surg Am.* 2012 Apr 04;94(7):577–583.
48. **Gjertsen JE, Lie SA, Vinje T, et al.** More re-operations after uncemented than cemented hemiarthroplasty used in the treatment of displaced fractures of the femoral neck: an observational study of 11,116 hemiarthroplasties from a national register. *J Bone Joint Surg Br.* 2012 Aug;94(8):1113–1119.
49. **Mouzopoulos G, Vasiliadis G, Lasanianos N, et al.** Fascia iliaca block prophylaxis for hip fracture patients at risk for delirium: a randomized placebo-controlled study. *J Orthop Traumatol.* 2009 Sep;10(3):127–133.
50. **Handoll HH, Queally JM, Parker MJ.** Pre-operative traction for hip fractures in adults. *Cochrane Database Syst Rev.* 2011 Dec 07(12):CD000168.
51. **von Roth P, Abdel MP, Harmsen WS, et al.** Cemented bipolar hemiarthroplasty provides definitive treatment for femoral neck fractures at 20 years and beyond. *Clin Orthop Relat Res.* 2015 Nov;473(11):3595–3599.
52. **Coleman SH, Bansal M, Cornell CN, et al.** Failure of bipolar hemiarthroplasty: a retrospective review of 31 consecutive bipolar prostheses converted to total hip arthroplasty. *Am J Orthop (Belle Mead NJ).* 2001 Apr;30(4):313–319.
53. **Nehme A, Lewallen DG, Hanssen AD.** Modular porous metal augments for treatment of severe acetabular bone loss during revision hip arthroplasty. *Clin Orthop Relat Res.* 2004 Dec;(429):201–208.
54. **Makinen TJ, Kuzyk P, Safir OA, et al.** Role of cages in revision arthroplasty of the acetabulum. *J Bone Joint Surg Am.* 2016 Feb 03;98(3):233–242.
55. **Springer BD, Berry DJ, Lewallen DG.** Treatment of periprosthetic femoral fractures following total hip arthroplasty with femoral component revision. *J Bone Joint Surg Am.* 2003 Nov;85-A(11):2156–2162.
56. **Duncan CP, Masri BA.** Fractures of the femur after hip replacement. *Instr Course Lect.* 1995;44:293–304.
57. **Enocson A, Lapidus G, Tornkvist H, et al.** Direction of hip arthroplasty dislocation in patients with femoral neck fractures. *Int Orthop.* 2010 Jun;34(5):641–647.
58. **van Embden D, van Gijn W, van de Steenhoven T, et al.** The surgeon's eye: a prospective analysis of the anteversion in the placement of hemiarthroplasties after a femoral neck fracture. *Hip Int.* 2015 Mar–Apr;25(2):127–130.
59. **Leonardsson O, Karrholm J, Akesson K, et al.** Higher risk of reoperation for bipolar and uncemented hemiarthroplasty. *Acta Orthop.* 2012 Oct;83(5):459–466.
60. **Sassoon A, D'Apuzzo M, Sems S, et al.** Total hip arthroplasty for femoral neck fracture: comparing in-hospital mortality, complications, and disposition to an elective patient population. *J Arthroplasty.* 2013 Oct;28(9):1659–1662.
61. **Kapadia BH, Berg RA, Daley JA, et al.** Periprosthetic joint infection. *Lancet.* 2016 Jan 23;387(10016):386–394.
62. **De Angelis G, Mutters NT, Minkley L, et al.** Prosthetic joint infections in the elderly. *Infection.* 2015 Dec;43(6):629–637.

# 3.10 Trochanteric and subtrochanteric femur

Carl Neuerburg, Christian Kammerlander, Stephen L Kates

## 1 Introduction

Trochanteric femoral fractures are the most frequent and typical major injuries in fragility fracture patients (FFPs). These fractures are mainly caused by a simple fall onto the hip [1]. In a number of cases the fracture is just the tip of the iceberg due to the patient's comorbid conditions such as cardiovascular diseases or sarcopenia. In order to allow a remobilization, most of these patients have to undergo surgical repair with the following major treatment goals:

- Operative fixation as early as possible, with active reversal of anticoagulation if necessary
- Expedited, stepwise mobilization with weight bearing as tolerated (WBAT), starting the day of, or first day after, surgery

To reduce complications in these fragile patients, we propose the use of standardized procedures for fracture treatment.

## 2 Epidemiology and etiology

The expected increase in these fractures is predominantly due to demographic changes of our aging population with a high prevalence of osteopenia and osteoporosis:

- The worldwide incidence of hip fractures was estimated to be 1.7 million per year in 1990 and is expected to increase to 6.3 million per year in 2050 [2].
- There are wide variations in hip fracture rates worldwide, with a positive correlation between rates of urbanization and hip fractures [3].
- The 1-year mortality after hip fracture is substantially higher in men (9.4–37.1%) than women (8.2–12.4%) [4].
- In stable urban populations, hip fracture rates remain constant or have decreased, perhaps due to the influence of factors such as birth cohort effects, improvements in bone mineral density, body mass index, osteoporosis medication use, and/or lifestyle interventions such as smoking cessation, improvement in nutritional status, and fall prevention [3].
- In western nations, 10–20% of previously independent hip fracture patients need to move to a nursing home for long-term care following hip fracture [5].

## 3 Diagnostics

### 3.1 Clinical evaluation

Precise preoperative patient assessment with a detailed review of the medical history is essential. Clinical examination should assess blood loss, evaluate the vascular, muscular, and neurological status of the extremity, and identify soft-tissue injuries or any infections (eg, chest infection). The preoperative evaluation should be done in a comanaged system together with a physician with experience in geriatrics and perioperative medical care, and is described in detail in chapter 2.4 Elements of an orthogeriatric comanaged program.

### 3.2 Imaging

#### 3.2.1 Plain x-rays

Two plain views and a pelvic view are the minimum set of radiographic images to understand the fracture, plan the surgery, and select the implant.

#### 3.2.2 Computed tomographic scan

Computed tomographic (CT) scans are helpful to assess more bony and soft-tissue details [6].

## 4 Classification

The AO/OTA Fracture and Dislocation Classification is recommended for trochanteric and subtrochanteric fractures and will be used in this chapter [7]. Pertrochanteric fractures are the most common variant and run from proximal-lateral to distal-medial (AO/OTA Fracture and Dislocation Classification A1, A2). Intertrochanteric or reverse obliquity fractures run from medial-proximal to lateral-distal (AO/OTA A3) [1]. Subtrochanteric fractures are located approximately 5 cm distal from the lesser trochanter [1].

## 5 Decision making

The major goals for the treatment of trochanteric fractures are:

- Single-shot surgery—this means that revision or additional surgeries should be avoided as they are known to worsen the overall outcome.
- Minimal surgical exposure—FFPs are prone to surgical site infections and extended approaches prolong the remobilization phase.
- Immediate mobilization and WBAT—mobilization is one essential issue in older adults to prevent complications; in addition, many are not able to comply with weight-bearing restrictions.

### 5.1 Operative versus nonoperative management

Given the high tensile forces acting on the trochanteric area of the proximal femur [8] and the overall complication rates with bed rest and immobility, treatment should almost always be operative. Nonoperative management is associated with higher mortality and serious functional loss [9]. For these reasons operative fracture fixation is generally recommended in almost all geriatric patients, including bedridden patients, to facilitate nursing care, positioning, and pain relief.

### 5.2 Intramedullary versus extramedullary device

Extramedullary and intramedullary (IM) fixation devices are available for hip fracture fixation. Correct identification of the fracture pattern should influence the choice of implant as recommended by the American Academy of Orthopaedic Surgeons and should be based on a cost-effective implant selection.

There is limited evidence for superiority of either implant based upon randomized trials, and the discussions remain controversial. Recent studies reported that the dynamic hip screw (DHS) was tolerated better by young patients with stable fractures while IM devices such as the proximal femoral nail antirotation (PFNA) had better outcomes with osteoporotic patients, weak bone mass, and reverse oblique fractures [10]. Furthermore, IM fixation can be minimally invasive, which appears to benefit older trauma patients.

A study investigating markers of muscle damage (serum creatine phosphokinase) associated with the surgical approach revealed that intertrochanteric fractures stabilized by a DHS experienced greater soft-tissue injury when compared to patients whose fracture was stabilized by a nail [11].

More studies have compared outcome parameters of intra- versus extramedullary fixation:

- Reduced blood loss and costs were observed in a comparative analysis from France in patients being treated with a DHS [12].
- Operative time appears to be longer in the DHS group, the surgical incision needs to be bigger and convalescence to early full weight bearing (FWB) was achieved at a later stage in patients being treated with a DHS [13].
- A relevant disadvantage of extramedullary fixation with a DHS appears to be the higher risk of femoral neck shortening. However, radiographic findings which favor IM fixation did not correlate with improved functional outcomes as shown in a comparative study [14].
- The additional use of a trochanteric stabilizing plate and a tension band wire with the DHS may be required when the greater trochanter is affected. However, additional implant stabilization of the greater trochanter can be bulky.
- It has been proposed to use a sliding hip screw in stable fractures with intact lesser trochanter and lateral wall of the greater trochanter and to prefer intramedullary systems in all other cases.

Intramedullary nailing seems to be less invasive than DHS placement. In a randomized study of 186 fractures treated by gamma nail or dynamic hip screw, gamma nails were implanted with significantly shorter operation times, smaller incisions, and less intraoperative blood loss. The gamma nail group had a shorter convalescence and earlier FWB, but there was no significant difference in mortality at 6 months, postoperative mobility, or hip function at review [13].

### 5.3 Blade versus screw

Biomechanically, a helical blade improves rotational stability of the construct [15] by compacting the bone around the implant and provides additional purchase in less dense bone [16] (see topic 7.2 in this chapter).

### 5.4 Fixation versus joint replacement

The mainstay of treatment of pertrochanteric fractures is internal fixation [17]. Yet, optimal treatment of unstable trochanteric fractures is controversial due to the variation of available implants and no clear evidence-based guidelines. Potential complications associated with osteosynthesis of proximal femoral fractures include cut-out of the screw or blade (see topic 7.1 in this chapter), loss of reduction, and nonunion.

An investigation of 91 patients treated with a cemented hemiarthroplasty for an unstable pertrochanteric fracture described an operative revision rate of 3.3% and a 30-day mortality of 5.5%. The authors concluded that hemiarthroplasty was a safe treatment strategy for unstable trochanteric fractures in older adults and allows early FWB [18]. A recent age-, gender-, and fracture type-matched case-controlled study conducted by Fichman et al [19] revealed a major complication rate of 3.4% in fracture patients treated with arthroplasty, significantly lower than the complication rate of 20.7% reported with cephalomedullary nailing. In this study, no significant difference was noted between the groups with regard to blood loss, operative time, hospitalization time, discharge destination to rehabilitation, or clinical outcome [19].

Acute prosthetic replacement may be considered but has not yielded broader acceptance and is generally more reserved for revision surgeries [20].

In severe ipsilateral arthritis of the hip, avascular necrosis of the femoral head (**Case 1: Fig 3.10-1**), and in selected unstable pertrochanteric fractures, arthroplasty may be a reasonable option for primary treatment.

CASE 1

**Patient**

An 80-year-old woman had severe hip pain after a fall on her right hip. Until her fall, the patient was mobile, walking with crutches, and managed her daily living independently.

**Comorbidities**

- Chronic obstructive pulmonary disease with a history of glucocorticoid therapy
- Persistent nicotine use (30 pack years)
- Hypertension

**Treatment and outcome**

Primary hemiarthroplasty was performed because of the advanced degree of destruction of the hip joint; the refixation of the greater trochanter was challenging (**Fig 3.10-1a–d**). Yet, reconstruction of the greater trochanter was crucial to maintain function of the affected hip [21]. Reconstruction with cerclage wires or a trochanter stabilizing plate would have been desirable, and total arthroplasty surgery may have been favorable due to the massive arthritic destruction of the acetabular component.

**Key points**

- Total or hemiarthroplasty is an option in case of preexisting arthritis in hip fracture patients.
- Reconstruction of the greater trochanter may be crucial to maintain function of the affected hip [21].

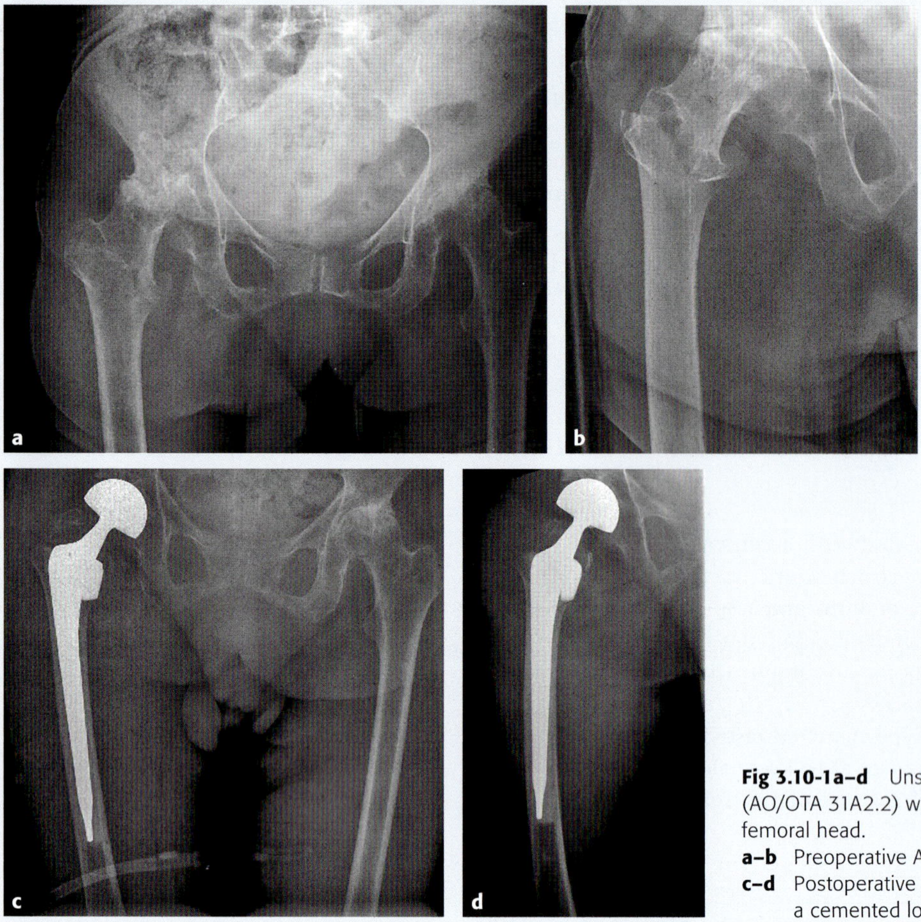


**Fig 3.10-1a–d** Unstable pertrochanteric fracture (AO/OTA 31A2.2) with ipsilateral avascular necrosis of the femoral head.
**a–b** Preoperative AP (**a**) and lateral (**b**) x-rays.
**c–d** Postoperative x-rays following primary treatment with a cemented long-stem hemiprosthesis.

## 5.5 Augmented fixation versus nonaugmented fixation

Polymethylmethacrylate (PMMA) has been used successfully to augment different implants in fixation of osteoporotic fractures [22, 23]. Treatment of trochanteric fractures with a dynamic hip screw and additional PMMA augmentation or an absorbable bone cement based on calcium phosphate has produced faster pain relief and improved fracture healing compared to controls [23]. Augmentation of the head-neck element (blade) following IM PFNA fixation increases the implant-bone interface and therefore strengthens fixation [22, 24]. Cyclic loading of osteoporotic trochanteric fractures treated with a cement-augmented PFNA is notable for significantly more cycles to failure compared to specimens treated with a noncemented PFNA [25], but comparative clinical studies are rare.

Biomechanical findings related to the standardized augmentation of the PFNA:

1. Better anchorage of the blade in osteoporotic bone is the main advantage [26].
2. The use of small amounts of PMMA, ie, 1–2 mL, significantly improves load cycles to cut-out of the PFNA blade [27].
3. Cement positioning at the tip and the cranial side of the blade was found to be most favorable [28].
4. Temperatures higher than 45° C were not measured in the bone cement interface region outside of the cement [29] if up to 6 mL of PMMA cement was used and therefore this procedure is not associated with thermal bone necrosis.

Major advantages of implant augmentation with PMMA are:

- Increased bone-implant interface—implants fail in metaphyseal fractures at the interface with surrounding bony structures, ie, trabeculae. Trabeculae are rarefied and thinned in osteoporotic bone with broken interconnections. Augmentation increases the implant-bone contact by increasing the contact surface area.
- Procedural safety—in a prospective study of 64 patients with trochanteric fractures treated with a PMMA-augmented DHS, no complications such as an avascular necrosis of the femoral head were reported [30]. Another study on augmentation use with the PFNA showed no complications related to the cement especially the exothermic reaction while hardening is not exceeding temperatures above 42° C [31].
- Procedural flexibility—cement is applied through small perforations of the fixation device once it has been inserted. The decision on whether or not to augment can be made only at the end of the operative procedure.

Clinically, there is no contraindication to perform augmentation with reduction and fixation of the fracture, so the decision to use additional augmentation can be taken at the end of the operative procedure.

The use of augmentation is an individual decision. The following factors may suggest a benefit from augmentation:

- Risk of cut-out or device instability due to poor bone quality
- Additional injuries of the upper extremities
- Less than optimal implant placement, mostly combined with malreduction (tip-apex distance [TAD])
- Exchange of blade
- Pathological fractures
- Haptics of helical blade insertion suggesting little resistance and osteoporotic bone conditions

## 6 Therapeutic options in acute fractures

### 6.1 Preoperative treatment

- A preoperative femoral nerve block is helpful to reduce pain before, during, and after the procedure; the risk of complications such as nerve palsy, bleeding, or infection is rare but should be considered [32].
- Additionally, routine acetaminophen and intermittent opioids are recommended for perioperative analgesia throughout the typical hospital course [33] (see also chapter 1.12 Pain management).

Skin traction of the affected femur may also be considered preoperatively, ie, if surgical delay is unavoidable and traction is necessary, although this may not be well tolerated by frail older adults or those with cognitive impairment.

### 6.2 Intraoperative imaging

It is of utmost importance to use standardized x-ray planes intraoperatively and to achieve an optimal anatomical reduction before inserting the nail. In particular, a true lateral view, where the femoral shaft is in one line with the head-neck-fragment, is the only projection to accurately assess the implant position. With excessive anterior bowing of the femur, insertion of a long screw or nail device may be impossible without perforating the anterior cortex of the femoral shaft or causing a fracture [34]. In such a case, a shorter nail or a long bent nail may be used.

### 6.3 Reduction

Reduction is an important step prior to nail insertion and should be oriented towards the opposite side. Closed reduction is performed on a traction table with 10° of adduction and rotation of the foot, if needed. Malrotation of the affected leg must be excluded. The patella should point directly upwards.

If acceptable reduction cannot be achieved with closed reduction, minimally invasive procedures are performed prior to nail insertion. The most commonly used reduction aids for fracture reduction are retractors, bone hooks, collinear clamps, blocking screws, Schanz screws, or the femoral distractor [35].

### 6.4 Intramedullary fixation

Despite the existence of various IM implants, their impact on outcomes is unclear [36]. The basic concepts of IM fixation are discussed in the following pages.

### 6.4.1 Position of the head-neck element

To obtain the best stability, orientation of the lag screw or blade within the dead center of the femoral head in both views is important. In a retrospective analysis, Turgut et al [37] investigated the frequency of cut-out and found that correct reduction of the fracture and proper positioning of the helical blade or screw in the center of the femoral head-neck fragment are associated with the lowest risk of cut-out [37].

A correct TAD has been shown to be associated with a reduced risk of implant failure in hip fractures treated with a DHS [38]. The TAD (**Fig 3.10-2**), which was first described by Baumgaertner et al [38], denotes the sum of the distance (in millimeters) from the tip of the lag screw to the apex of the femoral head, as measured on an AP x-ray and that distance as measured on a lateral x-ray [39]. According to clinical data, the TAD should be < 25 mm to significantly reduce the risk of failure following fracture fixation [40].

### 6.4.2 Nail length

There is ongoing debate about the nail length for IM nailing of trochanteric fractures. Several reports found no difference in union and complication rates for long versus short nails [41, 42]. There was a significantly shorter operative time, estimated blood loss, and transfusion requirements in patients treated with short intramedullary nails [41]. However, in patients older than 65 years with intertrochanteric fractures (AO/OTA 31A3), long nails were associated with reduced implant failure rate 1 year after surgery as well as less hip pain compared to patients treated with short IM nails [43].

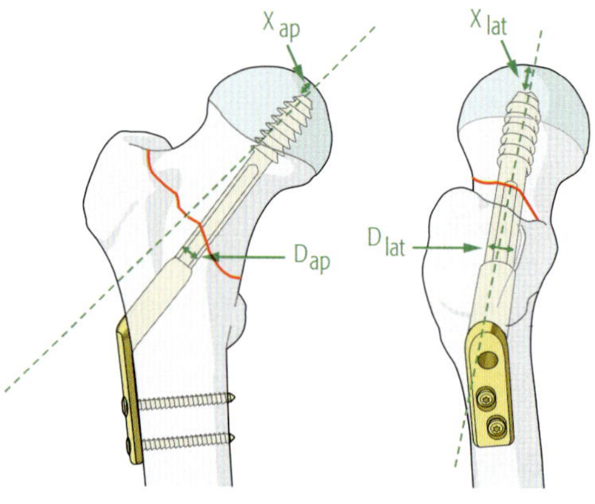


$$TAD = \left(X_{ap} \times \frac{D_{true}}{D_{ap}}\right) + \left(X_{lat} \times \frac{D_{true}}{D_{lat}}\right)$$

**Fig 3.10-2** Technique for calculating the tip-apex distance (TAD) in AP and lateral x-rays was introduced by Baumgaertner et al [39].

### 6.4.3 Reversed type of fractures

The biomechanics of reverse oblique trochanteric fractures differ from those of typical pertrochanteric fractures. They are characterized with a transverse fracture line in the intertrochanteric region and known to have a high level of instability [8]. Accordingly, the use of IM nails is recommended for fixation of reverse oblique trochanteric fractures. The risk of lateral cortical notching should be taken into consideration, in which the lag screw or blade of the intramedullary implant hinders the axial compression while mobilization as it bears on the lateral cortex. Thus, removal of the lateral cortex just distally to the lag screw or blade should be considered in order to allow sliding [44].

### 6.4.4 Subtrochanteric fractures

Besides the use of long IM nails for fixation of subtrochanteric fractures, anatomical reduction is also recommended for optimal outcomes. Some subtrochanteric fractures can be successfully treated with indirect reduction alone. If the fracture cannot be reduced well, an open reduction should be performed, and cerclage wires can be used to achieve better fracture reduction [45].

## 6.5 Standardized implant augmentation

Due to the reduced bone quality and fracture healing in older adults, there is increased use of augmentation techniques in geriatric patients [22, 23]. Polymethylmethacrylate can be used in fracture fixation in different ways:

- Void filler—composite fixation of pathological fractures and fractures in the setting of severe osteoporosis in a nonstandardized fashion has been used for many years with different implants [22, 23].
- Reinforcement of cancellous bone—typically, this technique is used for kyphoplasty in osteoporotic vertebral fractures.
- Implant augmentation—in recent years, methods have been developed to enhance implant purchase in osteoporotic bone. Ideally, this method should be applied in a standardized fashion as shown in **Case 2: Fig 3.10-3**.

### Patient

A 75-year-old woman with minor comorbidities was hit by a strong gust of wind and fell from standing height on her left side, sustaining a reverse oblique trochanteric fracture (AO/OTA 31A3.1).

### Comorbidities

- Hypertension
- Type 2 diabetes mellitus

### Treatment and outcome

Closed reduction on a traction table failed and consequently minimally invasive open reduction was performed using a collinear reposition clamp (**Fig 3.10-3a–f**). The blade was inserted with very little resistance and no predrilling. Therefore, it was decided intraoperatively to use cement augmentation. The side-opening cannula and plunger for controlled cement injection was inserted into the blade via the protection sleeve to rule out leakage into the joint using a water-soluble contrast dye. Thereafter, 3.5 mL of bone cement was applied.

### Key points

- In proximal femoral nail antirotation nailing, predrilling before inserting the blade in an osteoporotic bone should be avoided.
- Augmentation at the end of the operation should be performed.
- Decision for augmentation can be made during the operative procedure after ruling out that there is no perforation of the femoral head into the hip joint using a contrast dye.

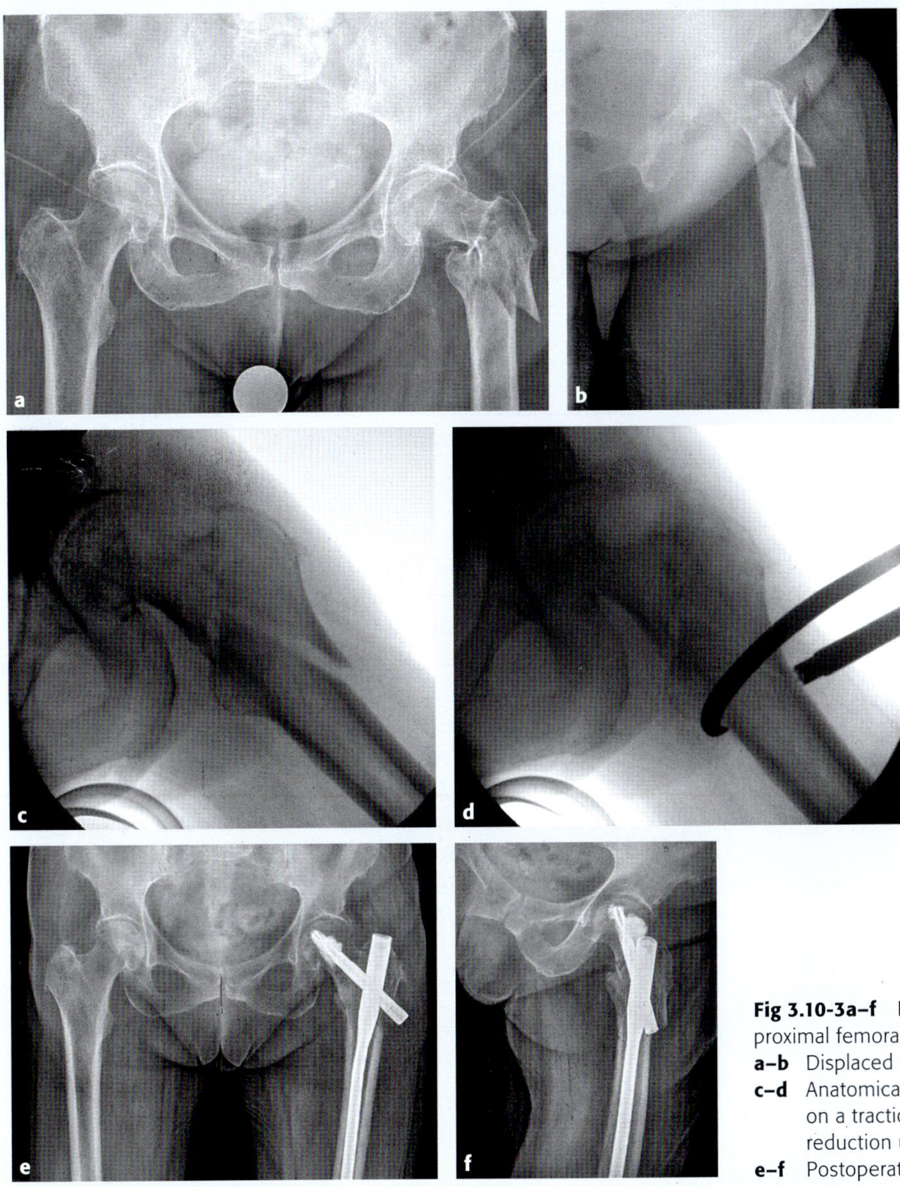

**Fig 3.10-3a–f** Fracture reduction with an augmented proximal femoral nail antirotation (PFNA).
**a–b** Displaced reverse oblique intertrochanteric fracture.
**c–d** Anatomical fracture reduction could not be achieved on a traction table and minimally invasive open reduction using a collinear clamp was necessary.
**e–f** Postoperative x-rays with a long augmented PFNA.

### 6.5.1 Technical aspects

The use of a special bone cement with long-lasting high viscosity applied through the PFNA blade is a prerequisite for a standardized and safe augmentation of IM fixation, following testing for intraarticular leakage with a contrast agent (**Fig 3.10-4**). It is important to note that intraoperative distribution of cement appears to be determined by the osseous microarchitecture of the osteoporotic bone, and controlled guidance of cement distribution is hardly possible.

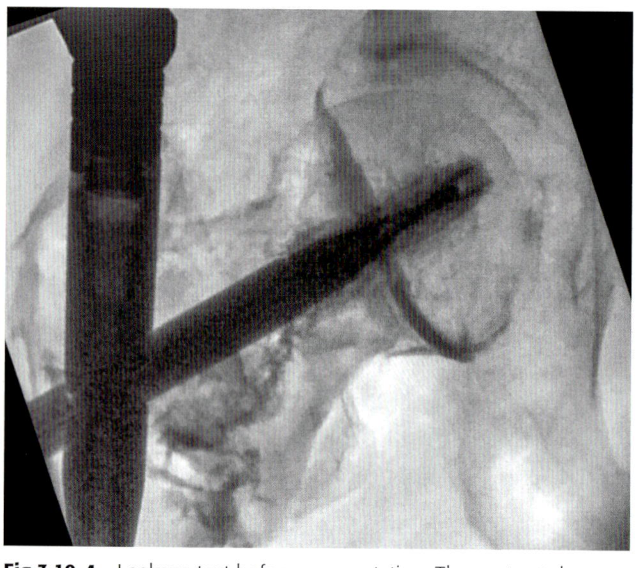

**Fig 3.10-4** Leakage test before augmentation. The contrast dye always follows the path of least resistance; in case of joint perforation, the contrast agent spreads into the articular cavity (producing a crescent sign) and cement augmentation must not be performed. Normally, the contrast dye should distribute within the femoral head, the fracture zone, and the soft tissues.

### 6.6 Postoperative treatment

Key elements of postoperative management:

- Weight bearing as tolerated begins as early as possible. Despite patient limitations in performing FWB, restricted weight bearing can delay the functional recovery and return to independence of geriatric patients [46] (see also chapter 1.8 Postoperative surgical management).
- Regarding the length of venous thromboembolism (VTE) prophylaxis, there have been investigations reporting on a persistent risk that can remain elevated for up to 3 months after fracture repair [47]. It is recommended that duration of anticoagulation be tailored to each patient considering their risks/benefits of anticoagulation. See chapter 1.6 Anticoagulation in the perioperative setting regarding VTE prophylaxis.
- Orthogeriatric comanagement to prevent and treat postoperative complications (see chapter 1.7 Postoperative medical management). Follow-ups at 4 and 12 months postoperatively [33].
- Secondary fracture prevention is generally recommended including strengthening of muscles and metabolic bone workup and osteoporosis treatment according to guidelines (see chapters 1.10 Osteoporosis and 2.7 Protocol and order set development for details).

## 7 Complications

### 7.1 Cut-out

Cut-out is defined as perforation of the helical blade or lag screw through the superior cortex of the femoral head or neck, followed by rotation or varus collapse of the head-neck fragment [48]. Poor reduction of the trochanteric fracture, especially a varus malalignment, appears to be the major risk factor for cut-out [37, 48]. Brunner et al [48] retrospectively analyzed patients following nailing of trochanteric fractures using PFNA or trochanteric fixation nail and found 29 patients who suffered a cut-out and 28 patients who suffered a cut-through (see topic 7.3 in this chapter). Of these, nine fractures were classified as type A1, 34 as type A2, and 14 as type A3, whereas initial operative fixation was performed with PFNA in 47 cases and with trochanteric fixation nail in 10 cases [48]. Second, correct positioning of the screw or blade within the femoral head-neck fragment is important, thus the TAD has proved to be a strong predictor of cut-out in hip fracture treatment [49]. In a retrospective investigation by Lobo-Escolar et al [49] that investigated patients having suffered cut-out after trochanteric fixation, a mean time from surgery to hardware failure of 84 days was observed, indicating that cut-out complications predominantly occur in the early postoperative course, ie, within the first 3 months after surgery.

In these cases with failed fracture fixation, different strategies for revision surgery can be considered and arthroplasty is typically the most reasonable salvage operation. The majority of cut-out complications observed by Brunner et al [48] were treated with an arthroplasty (n = 21) as also shown in **Case 3: Fig 3.10-5**, whereas blade exchange (n = 4), renailing (n = 3), or a Girdlestone treatment were performed in the other cases [48].

**CASE 3**

### Patient

A 75-year-old man presented with an immobilizing pain in his hip 9 months after a reverse oblique trochanteric fracture. At that stage the patient required the use of a walking frame (Charlson Comorbidity Index 2).

### Treatment and outcome

Radiographic course—The initial x-rays showed severe displacement of a reverse oblique trochanteric fracture (AO/OTA 31A3). Six weeks after surgery no implant migration was seen. Three months after surgery, a relevant dislocation could already be seen with a progressive collapse of the medial fragment, but the findings at that stage were unfortunately misinterpreted. Finally, 9 months after surgery a cut-out was seen with perforation of the acetabulum and the decision for endoprosthetic replacement was made (**Fig 3.10-5a–h**).

Postoperative reconsiderations—Compared to a caput-collum-diaphyseal (CCD) angle of 135° of the contralateral hip, the postoperative CCD angle following fracture reduction showed a persisting varus malreduction of the affected hip of 10°. As varus malreduction has shown to be the major cause of implant failure in trochanteric fractures [37, 40, 45]; more distraction of the ipsilateral hip on a fracture table may have been an approach to obtain improved fracture reduction. The tip-apex distance (TAD) was 26 mm, whereas Kraus et al [50] stated that a TAD < 30 mm was favorable according to a retrospective analysis. Last, the use of cerclage wires should have been considered as it may have restricted circulation of the proximal femoral fragment.

Revision surgery—Due to the destruction of the hip, prosthetic replacement was performed with autogenous spongiosa grafts and a modular hip arthroplasty. Postoperative x-rays revealed good implant anchorage and replacement of the joint (**Fig 3.10-5i–k**).

### Key points

- Implant migration following fracture fixation should be carefully diagnosed to avoid complications associated with a collapse and cut-out.
- Endoprosthetic surgery remains the most promising salvage technique following failed fixation of trochanteric fractures.

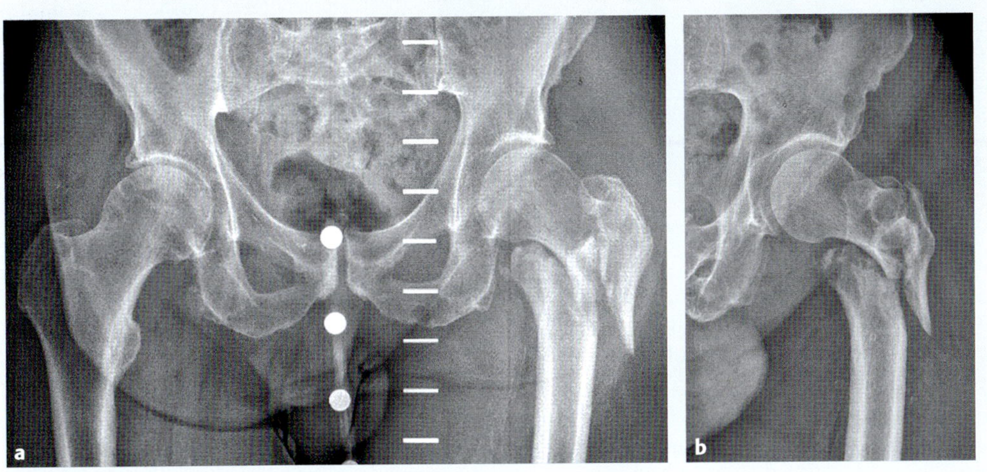

**Fig 3.10-5a–k** Endoprosthesis for salvage following secondary dislocation.
**a–b** Preoperative x-rays showing severe displacement of a reverse oblique trochanteric fracture.

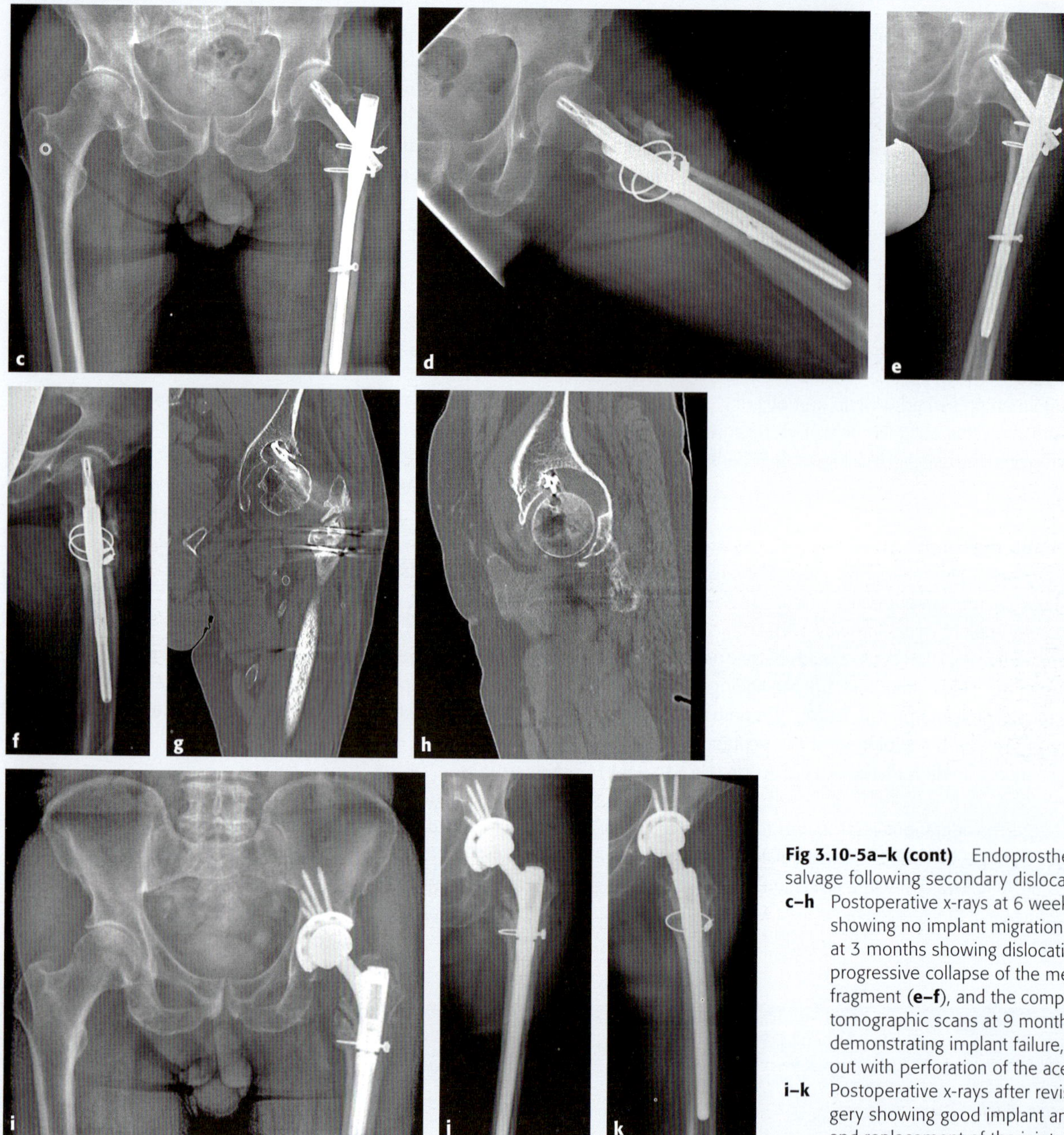


**Fig 3.10-5a–k (cont)** Endoprosthesis for salvage following secondary dislocation.
**c–h** Postoperative x-rays at 6 weeks showing no implant migration (**c–d**), at 3 months showing dislocation with progressive collapse of the medial fragment (**e–f**), and the computed tomographic scans at 9 months (**g–h**) demonstrating implant failure, ie, cut-out with perforation of the acetabulum.
**i–k** Postoperative x-rays after revision surgery showing good implant anchorage and replacement of the joint.

## 7.2 Cut-through

Cut-through is defined as medial perforation of the blade through the cortex of the femoral head, without loss of reduction of the head-neck fragment [48]. Unlike in cut-out, where varus malreduction appears to be the major cause for failure, in the retrospective analysis by Brunner et al [48] the 28 cases of cut-through were associated with significantly lower mean TAD values than cases of cut-out (see also **Fig 3.10-6**). In addition, the number of American Society of Anesthesiologists type four patients was significantly higher in cases experiencing cut-through compared to cut-out [48].

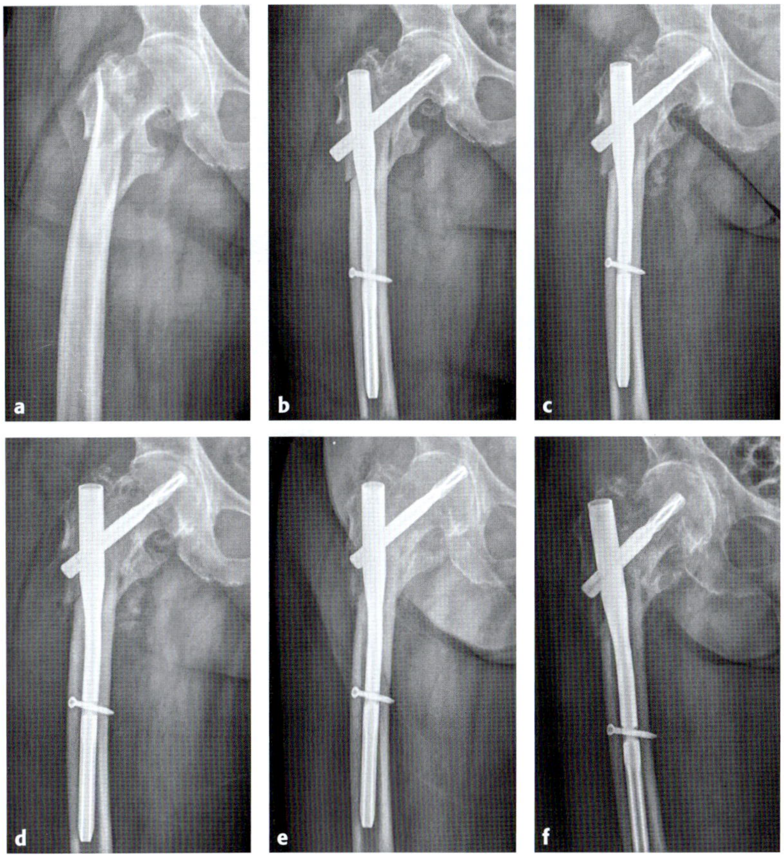

**Fig 3.10-6a–f** An 84-year-old woman with a type A2 fracture (**a**) that was treated with a proximal femoral nail antirotation (**b**) according to Brunner et al [48]. The blade is very close to the joint. Four weeks postoperative, a cut-through of the helical blade was noted (**c**). The blade was replaced (**d**). Four months after revision surgery the patient presented with groin pain. The x-ray (**e**) revealed a repeat perforation of the blade. The blade was exchanged again. The fracture finally healed 4 weeks after the second revision (**f**).

## 7.3 Periimplant fracture

Successfully treated FFPs are at high risk of subsequent fracture, due to persistent gait instability, reduced bone quality, and frailty. The 1-year risk of a secondary fracture is 2.7% and 8.4% for a major or any (nonhip) fracture, respectively, and increases to 14.7% and 32.5% after 5 years [51]. Secondary fracture prevention is important (see **Case 4: Fig 3.10-7**).

**CASE 4**

### Patient

A 94-year-old relatively healthy woman (Charlson Comorbidity Index 1).

### Treatment and outcome

The woman was treated with an augmented proximal femoral nail antirotation (PFNA) due to a pertrochanteric femoral fracture (AO/OTA 31A2.2). After a satisfactory postoperative course (**Fig 3.10-7a–d**), she was discharged to a rehabilitation unit where she sustained another fall 3 weeks after index surgery and presented with a periimplant fracture of the ipsilateral femur (**Fig 3.10-7e–f**).

The perioperative images showed that the blade was positioned inadequately in the ventral aspect of the femoral head-neck fragment. Despite various attempts to reposition the guide wire to achieve best positioning of the blade, the preexisting bone cement prevented a new position of the guide wire. In the end, fracture fixation was achieved with a long PFNA, reaugmentation of the blade and an additional cerclage in the subtrochanteric fracture side (**Fig 3.10-7g–l**).

### Key point

- The use of a long nail is a salvage option for the treatment of periimplant fractures. While reaugmentation worked in this case, repositioning of the guide wire following previous augmentation can be difficult.

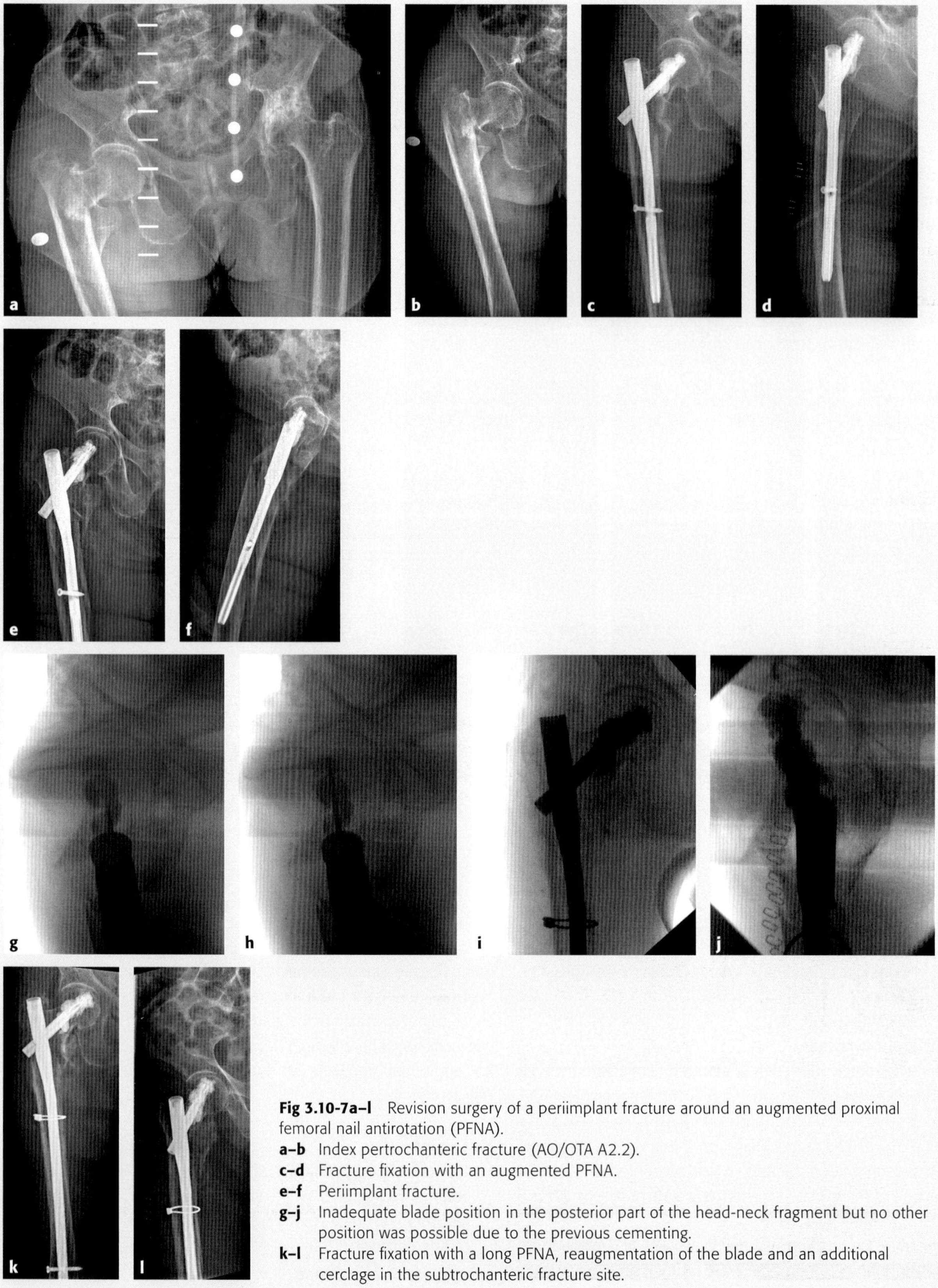

**Fig 3.10-7a–l** Revision surgery of a periimplant fracture around an augmented proximal femoral nail antirotation (PFNA).

**a–b** Index pertrochanteric fracture (AO/OTA A2.2).
**c–d** Fracture fixation with an augmented PFNA.
**e–f** Periimplant fracture.
**g–j** Inadequate blade position in the posterior part of the head-neck fragment but no other position was possible due to the previous cementing.
**k–l** Fracture fixation with a long PFNA, reaugmentation of the blade and an additional cerclage in the subtrochanteric fracture site.

## 7.4 Infection

Infection occurs in 1.1–3.2% of patients with pertrochanteric fractures treated with IM nailing [52]. Deep infection following IM nailing as shown in **Case 5: Fig 3.10-8** should be considered on a case-by-case basis. The antimicrobial immune response is profoundly reduced after surgery in orthogeriatric patients, with altered serum cytokine measurements for up to 7 days postoperatively [53]. Identifying patients at high risk for infection, including urinary, respiratory tract, and wound infection is important, as such infectious complications contribute to poor outcomes in frail older patients.

There is little published literature on early postoperative infection after any internal fixation of a fracture; operative debridement, antibiotic treatment, and retention of stable hardware are recommended until fracture union occurs [54]. In these situations, an interdisciplinary approach with surgeons, microbiologists, geriatricians, and an infection specialist is important to determine the optimal treatment for each patient.

CASE 5

### Patient

An 87-year-old woman suffered a fall in her nursing home and was admitted to hospital 1 day later.

### Comorbidities

- Stroke 10 years before
- Cerebral vasculitis treated with low-dose glucocorticoids
- Chronic pain syndrome following a 360° fusion of the lumbar spine
- Mobile with a walker (Charlson Comorbidity Index 2)

### Treatment and outcome

Right trochanteric fracture (AO/OTA 31A2.3) with a subtrochanteric extension (**Fig 3.10-8a–b**).

Closed reduction and fixation with a short proximal femoral nail antirotation (PFNA). Varus malalignment was accepted with the tip of the blade located in the upper one-third of the femoral head. Thereafter, full weight bearing (FWB) was allowed although the patient complained of persistent hip pain. Two weeks after surgery implant migration became obvious and of the fracture so revision surgery was planned (**Fig 3.10-8c–f**).

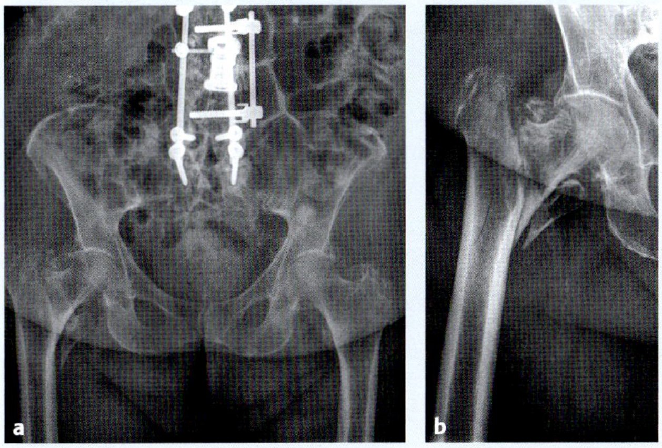


After removal of the implants, open reduction and reimplantation of the PFNA was performed. A subfascial drainage was performed 48 hours after surgery (**Fig 3.10-8g–j**).

Postoperative mobilization with FWB was allowed. The patient developed persistent drainage with elevated C-reactive protein level and leukocyte count. The patient reported increasing pain. Furthermore, radiographic images indicated a progressive fracture displacement with dislocation of the greater trochanter and subsequent implant migration due to the unstable situation.

Resection arthroplasty was performed with identification of *Enterococcus faecalis.* After nine revision surgeries including implantation of a polymethylmethacrylate spacer, the patient was discharged with a greatly reduced functional status and with a local fistula (**Fig 3.10-8k–m**).

### Key points

- The present case demonstrates the importance of single-shot surgery due to the limited reserves of orthogeriatric patients. Thus, precise fracture reduction should be achieved by traction and probably open reduction to prevent fracture displacement and subsequent revision surgery. In the present case cerclage wires may have been desirable in addition to correct the varus malredution.
- Endoprosthetic replacement following failure of internal fixation remains the treatment of choice in these situations [48].
- Immediate and aggressive surgical debridement is appropriate to address the deep infection. Additionally, a prolonged antimicrobial therapy and frequent reevaluations are mandatory.

**Fig 3.10-8a–m** Deep infection following failed revision surgery of a trochanteric fracture.
**a–b** The x-rays showing the fracture of the right hip with a subtrochanteric fracture line.

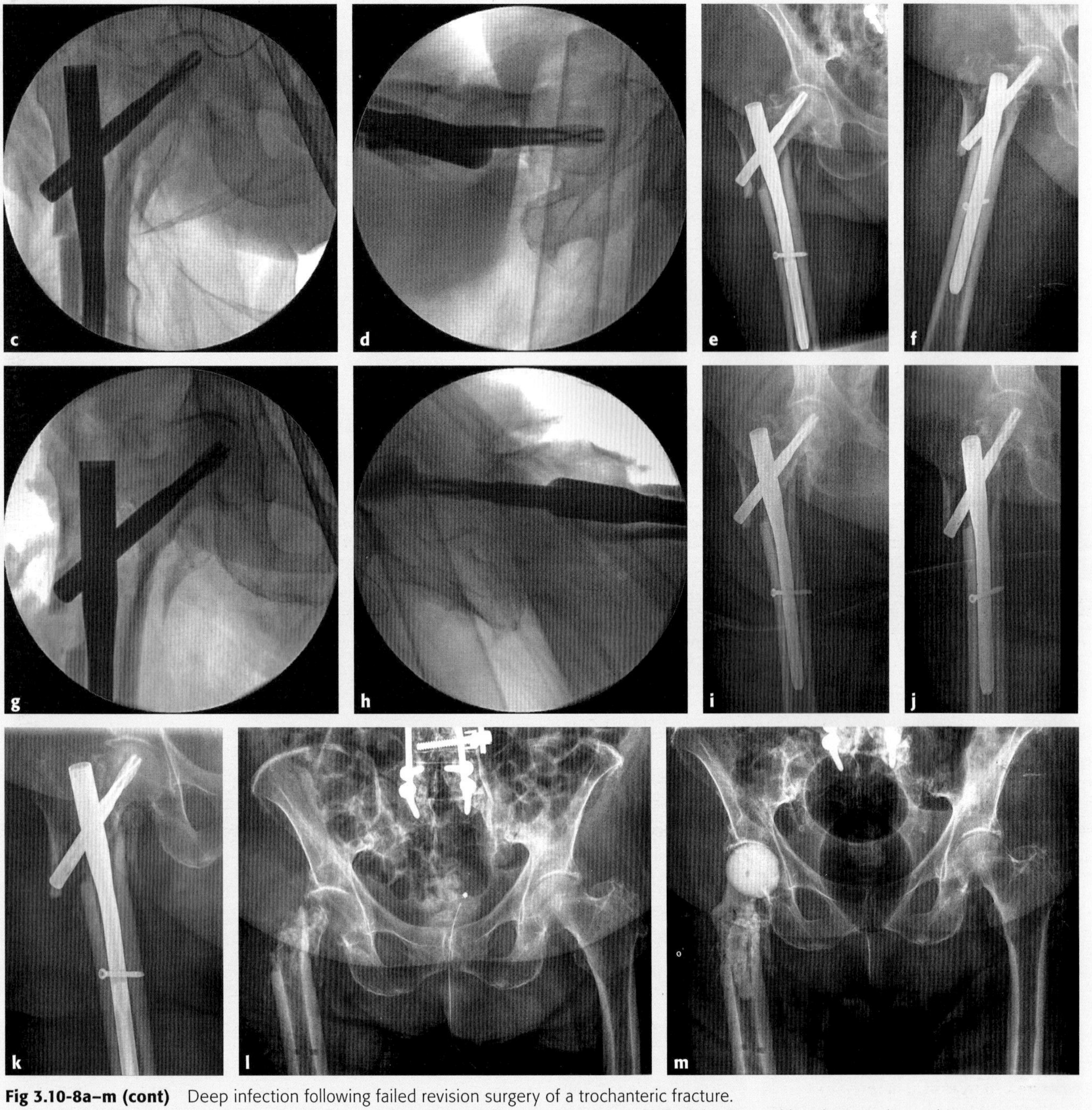


**Fig 3.10-8a–m (cont)** Deep infection following failed revision surgery of a trochanteric fracture.

**c–f** The intraoperative x-ray showing the tip of the blade located in the upper one-third of the femoral head (**c**). Radiographic images at 2 weeks after surgery indicating implant migration and malrotation of the femoral head-neck fragment (**e–f**).

**g–j** The intraoperative (**g–h**) and postoperative (**i–j**) x-rays showing the result after open reduction and reimplantation of the proximal femoral nail antirotation.

**k–m** The radiographic images indicating a progressive fracture displacement with dislocation of the greater trochanter and subsequent implant migration (**k**). At this stage the femoral nail had to be removed due to a deep infection (**l**) and was ultimately replaced with a cement spacer (**m**).

## 8 References


1. **Wagner S, Ruter A.** Per- und subtrochantäre Femurfrakturen [Per- and subtrochanteric femur fractures]. *Unfallchirurg.* 1999 Mar;102(3):206–222. German.
2. **Friedman SM, Mendelson DA.** Epidemiology of fragility fractures. *Clin Geriatr Med.* 2014 May;30(2):175–181.
3. **Ballane G, Cauley JA, Luckey MM, et al.** Secular trends in hip fractures worldwide: opposing trends East versus West. *J Bone Miner Res.* 2014 Aug;29(8):1745–1755.
4. **Sterling RS.** Gender and race/ethnicity differences in hip fracture incidence, morbidity, mortality, and function. *Clin Orthop Relat Res.* 2011 Jul;469(7):1913–1918.
5. **Dyer SM, Crotty M, Fairhall N, et al.** A critical review of the long-term disability outcomes following hip fracture. *BMC Geriatr.* 2016 Sep 2;16:158.
6. **Isida R, Bariatinsky V, Kern G, et al.** Prospective study of the reproducibility of X-rays and CT scans for assessing trochanteric fracture comminution in the elderly: a series of 110 cases. *Eur J Orthop Surg Traumatol.* 2015 Oct;25(7):1165–1170.
7. **Mattos CA, Jesus AA, Floter Mdos S, et al.** Reproducibility of the Tronzo and AO classifications for transtrochanteric fractures. *Rev Bras Ortop.* 2015 Aug 15;50(5):495–500.
8. **Bonnaire F, Lein T, Bula P.** Pertrochantäre Femurfrakturen. Anatomie, Biomechanik und Wahl der Implantate [Trochanteric femoral fractures: anatomy, biomechanics and choice of implants]. *Unfallchirurg.* 2011 Jun;114(6):491–500. German.
9. **Yoon BH, Baek JH, Kim MK, et al.** Poor prognosis in elderly patients who refused surgery because of economic burden and medical problem after hip fracture. *J Korean Med Sci.* 2013 Sep;28(9):1378–1381.
10. **Kumar R, Singh RN, Singh BN.** Comparative prospective study of proximal femoral nail and dynamic hip screw in treatment of intertrochanteric fracture femur. *J Clin Orthop Trauma.* 2012 Jun;3(1):28–36.
11. **Wagman Y, Segal O, Dudkiewicz I, et al.** Markers of muscle damage for comparing soft tissue injury following proximal femur nail and dynamic hip screw operations for intertrochanteric hip fractures. *Injury.* 2016 Dec;47(12):2764–2768.
12. **Giraud B, Dehoux E, Jovenin N, et al.** Comparaison vis-plaque dynamique et ostéosynthèse intra-médullaire antérograde dans les fractures pertrochantériennes: Une étude prospective randomisée [Pertrochanteric fractures: a randomized prospective study comparing dynamic screw plate and intramedullary fixation]. *Rev Chir Orthop Reparatrice Appar Mot.* 2005 Dec;91(8):732–736. French.
13. **Leung KS, So WS, Shen WY, et al.** Gamma nails and dynamic hip screws for peritrochanteric fractures. A randomised prospective study in elderly patients. *J Bone Joint Surg Br.* 1992 May;74(3):345–351.
14. **Reindl R, Harvey EJ, Berry GK, et al.** Intramedullary versus extramedullary fixation for unstable intertrochanteric fractures: a prospective randomized controlled trial. *J Bone Joint Surg Am.* 2015 Dec 2;97(23):1905–1912.
15. **Al-Munajjed AA, Hammer J, Mayr E, et al.** Biomechanical characterisation of osteosyntheses for proximal femur fractures: helical blade versus screw. *Stud Health Technol Inform.* 2008;133:1–10.
16. **Goffin JM, Pankaj P, Simpson AH, et al.** Does bone compaction around the helical blade of a proximal femoral nail anti-rotation (PFNA) decrease the risk of cut-out?: A subject-specific computational study. *Bone Joint Res.* 2013;2(5):79–83.
17. **Makinen TJ, Gunton M, Fichman SG, et al.** Arthroplasty for pertrochanteric hip fractures. *Orthop Clin North Am.* 2015 Oct;46(4):433–444.
18. **Grote S, Stegmeyer F, Bogner V, et al.** Behandlungsergebnisse nach zementierter Hemiprothese zur Versorgung instabiler pertrochantärer Femurfrakturen alter Patienten [Treatment results after cemented hemiprosthesis for care of unstable pertrochanteric femoral fractures in the elderly]. *Unfallchirurg.* 2012 Mar;115(3):234–242. German.
19. **Fichman SG, Makinen TJ, Safir O, et al.** Arthroplasty for unstable pertrochanteric hip fractures may offer a lower re-operation rate as compared to cephalomedullary nailing. *Int Orthop.* 2016 Jan;40(1):15–20.
24. **Haentjens P, Casteleyn PP, De Boeck H, et al.** Treatment of unstable intertrochanteric and subtrochanteric fractures in elderly patients. Primary bipolar arthroplasty compared with internal fixation. *J Bone Joint Surg Am.* 1989 Sep;71(8):1214–1225.
20. **Laffosse JM, Molinier F, Tricoire JL, et al.** Cementless modular hip arthroplasty as a salvage operation for failed internal fixation of trochanteric fractures in elderly patients. *Acta Orthop Belg.* 2007 Dec;73(6):729–736.
21. **Babst R, Renner N, Biedermann M, et al.** Clinical results using the trochanter stabilizing plate (TSP): the modular extension of the dynamic hip screw (DHS) for internal fixation of selected unstable intertrochanteric fractures. *J Orthop Trauma.* 1998 Aug;12(6):392–399.
22. **Kammerlander C, Erhart S, Doshi H, et al.** Principles of osteoporotic fracture treatment. *Best Pract Res Clin Rheumatol.* 2013 Dec;27(6):757–769.
23. **Mattsson P, Alberts A, Dahlberg G, et al.** Resorbable cement for the augmentation of internally-fixed unstable trochanteric fractures. A prospective, randomised multicentre study. *J Bone Joint Surg Br.* 2005 Sep;87(9):1203–1209.
25. **Fensky F, Nuchtern JV, Kolb JP, et al.** Cement augmentation of the proximal femoral nail antirotation for the treatment of osteoporotic pertrochanteric fractures—a biomechanical cadaver study. *Injury.* 2013 Jun;44(6):802–807.
26. **Neuerburg C, Mehaffey S, Gosch M, et al.** Trochanteric fragility fractures: Treatment using the cement-augmented proximal femoral nail antirotation. *Oper Orthop Traumatol.* 2016 Jun;28(3):164–176.
27. **Sermon A, Boner V, Schwieger K, et al.** Biomechanical evaluation of bone-cement augmented proximal femoral nail antirotation blades in a polyurethane foam model with low density. *Clin Biomech (Bristol, Avon).* 2012 Jan;27(1):71–76.
28. **Sermon A, Hofmann-Fliri L, Richards RG, et al.** Cement augmentation of hip implants in osteoporotic bone: how much cement is needed and where should it go? *J Orthop Res.* 2014 Mar;32(3):362–368.
29. **Fliri L, Lenz M, Boger A, et al.** Ex vivo evaluation of the polymerization temperatures during cement augmentation of proximal femoral nail antirotation blades. *J Trauma Acute Care Surg.* 2012 Apr;72(4):1098–1101.
30. **Gupta RK, Gupta V, Gupta N.** Outcomes of osteoporotic trochanteric fractures treated with cement-augmented dynamic hip screw. *Indian J Orthop.* 2012 Nov;46(6):640–645.

31. **Kammerlander C, Doshi H, Gebhard F, et al.** Long-term results of the augmented PFNA: a prospective multicenter trial. *Arch Orthop Trauma Surg.* 2014 Mar;134(3):343–349.
32. **Ritcey B, Pageau P, Woo MY, et al.** Regional nerve blocks for hip and femoral neck fractures in the emergency department: a systematic review. *CJEM.* 2016 Jan;18(1):37–47.
33. **Prestmo A, Hagen G, Sletvold O, et al.** Comprehensive geriatric care for patients with hip fractures: a prospective, randomised, controlled trial. *Lancet.* 2015 Apr 25;385(9978):1623–1633.
34. **Rüedi TP, Murphy WM.** *AO Principles of Fracture Management.* 1st ed. Stuttgart New York: Thieme; 2000.
35. **Riehl JT, Widmaier JC.** Techniques of obtaining and maintaining reduction during nailing of femur fractures. *Orthopedics.* 2009 Aug;32(8):581.
36. **Queally JM, Harris E, Handoll HH, et al.** Intramedullary nails for extracapsular hip fractures in adults. *Cochrane Database Syst Rev.* 2014 Sep 12(9):CD004961.
37. **Turgut A, Kalenderer O, Karapinar L, et al.** Which factor is most important for occurrence of cutout complications in patients treated with proximal femoral nail antirotation? Retrospective analysis of 298 patients. *Arch Orthop Trauma Surg.* 2016 May;136(5):623–630.
38. **Baumgaertner MR, Curtin SL, Lindskog DM, et al.** The value of the tip-apex distance in predicting failure of fixation of peritrochanteric fractures of the hip. *J Bone Joint Surg Am.* 1995 Jul;77(7):1058–1064.
39. **Parmar V, Kumar S, Aster A, et al.** Review of methods to quantify lag screw placement in hip fracture fixation. *Acta Orthop Belg.* 2005 Jun;71(3):260–263.
40. **Kane P, Vopat B, Heard W, et al.** Is tip apex distance as important as we think? A biomechanical study examining optimal lag screw placement. *Clin Orthop Relat Res.* 2014 Aug;472(8):2492–2498.
41. **Boone C, Carlberg KN, Koueiter DM, et al.** Short versus long intramedullary nails for treatment of intertrochanteric femur fractures (OTA 31-A1 and A2). *J Orthop Trauma.* 2014 May;28(5):e96–e100.
42. **Hou Z, Bowen TR, Irgit KS, et al.** Treatment of pertrochanteric fractures (OTA 31-A1 and A2): long versus short cephalomedullary nailing. *J Orthop Trauma.* 2013 Jun;27(6):318–324.
43. **Li Z, Liu Y, Liang Y, et al.** Short versus long intramedullary nails for the treatment of intertrochanteric hip fractures in patients older than 65 years. *Int J Clin Exp Med.* 2015;8(4):6299–6302.
44. **Biber R, Bail HJ, Stedtfeld HW.** Lateral cortical notching in specific cases of delayed unions or nonunions after intertrochanteric and reversed fractures. *Arch Orthop Trauma Surg.* 2013 Apr;133(4):495–501.
45. **Hoskins W, Bingham R, Joseph S, et al.** Subtrochanteric fracture: the effect of cerclage wire on fracture reduction and outcome. *Injury.* 2015 Oct;46(10):1992–1995.
46. **Koval KJ, Sala DA, Kummer FJ, et al.** Postoperative weight-bearing after a fracture of the femoral neck or an intertrochanteric fracture. *J Bone Joint Surg Am.* 1998 Mar;80(3):352–356.
47. **Bjornara BT, Gudmundsen TE, Dahl OE.** Frequency and timing of clinical venous thromboembolism after major joint surgery. *J Bone Joint Surg Br.* 2006 Mar;88(3):386–391.
48. **Brunner A, Buttler M, Lehmann U, et al.** What is the optimal salvage procedure for cut-out after surgical fixation of trochanteric fractures with the PFNA or TFN?: A multicentre study. *Injury.* 2016 Feb;47(2):432–438.
49. **Lobo-Escolar A, Joven E, Iglesias D, et al.** Predictive factors for cutting-out in femoral intramedullary nailing. *Injury.* 2010 Dec;41(12):1312–1316.
50. **Kraus M, Krischak G, Wiedmann K, et al.** Klinische Evaluation des PFNA® und Zusammenhang zwischen Tip-Apex-Distanz und mechanischem Versagen [Clinical evaluation of PFNA(R) and relationship between the tip-apex distance and mechanical failure]. *Unfallchirurg.* 2011 Jun;114(6):470–478. German.
51. **Gibson-Smith D, Klop C, Elders PJ, et al.** The risk of major and any (non-hip) fragility fracture after hip fracture in the United Kingdom: 2000–2010. *Osteoporos Int.* 2014 Nov;25(11):2555–2563.
52. **Mavrogenis AF, Panagopoulos GN, Megaloikonomos PD, et al.** Complications after hip nailing for fractures. *Orthopedics.* 2016 Jan–Feb;39(1):e108–116.
53. **Sutherland AG, Cook A, Miller C, et al.** Older patients are immunocompromised by cytokine depletion and loss of innate immune function after HIP fracture surgery. *Geriatr Orthop Surg Rehabil.* 2015 Dec;6(4):295–302.
54. **Berkes M, Obremskey WT, Scannell B, et al.** Maintenance of hardware after early postoperative infection following fracture internal fixation. *J Bone Joint Surg Am.* 2010 Apr;92(4):823–828.

# 3.11 Femoral shaft

Elizabeth B Gausden, Dean G Lorich

## 1 Introduction

A significant proportion of femoral shaft fractures (FSFs) occur in older adults presenting unique issues for medical and surgical management. These features are similar to those typically considered for other fragility fractures of the hip, spine, and wrist. Approximately one-third of all FSFs are the result of low-energy trauma [1] typically a ground level fall, with poor bone quality presenting a specific challenge [1–3]. In addition, pathological lesions cause approximately 15% of nonhip femoral fractures [4].

The incidence of FSF decreases from 20 years to middle age, then following a small rise, markedly increases after the age of 75 years [5]. The average age of FSF following low-energy injury is 65 years [3]. Over 90% of FSFs in patients between the ages of 17 and 29 years are related to traffic accidents, but in patients older than 70 years, 65% of FSFs are related to ground level falls [6]. The majority of patients with low-energy FSFs have at least one comorbidity or risk factor, such as age, diabetes mellitus, or chronic obstructive pulmonary disease, predisposing them to osteopenia [3].

There is no one optimal treatment option for older patients with an FSF. Specific treatment recommendations depend on both patient factors and fracture characteristics, in addition to the surgeon's experience and preference. For patients with the types of physique and fracture patterns that are amenable to intramedullary (IM) nailing, nonunion and overall complication rates have declined in the past few decades likely secondary to improved instrumentation and techniques. Malrotation and malalignment continue to be problems. The advent of locked plating has improved outcomes following plate osteosynthesis in osteoporotic patients with FSFs. This chapter provides a summary of the various techniques currently in practice for treating FSFs in older patients.

## 2 Diagnostics

An FSF is defined as a fracture between the region 5 cm below the lesser trochanter to 8 cm proximal to the adductor tubercle [7].

### 2.1 Clinical evaluation

A complete history is an essential part of the clinical evaluation of the patient and should be obtained from the patient if possible and family members when necessary. Specific items include:

- Level of function prior to injury
- Occupation
- History of malignancy
- History of osteoporosis
- History of bisphosphonate use (may be inferred based on the fracture pattern)
- History of fracture
- History of cognitive impairment

There is evidence that geriatric patients with fractures distal to the hip display functional, cognitive, and comorbidity profiles similar to those of geriatric hip fracture patients [8]. In addition to fracture pattern analysis, the patient's functional needs, rehabilitation potential (based on functional and cognitive status), and overall medical status are essential to define during initial evaluation. So-called atypical femoral fractures related to bisphosphonate use are discussed in more detail in chapter 3.18 Atypical fractures.

### 2.2 Imaging

Although patients with FSFs may present with obvious deformities, the fractures must be assessed with a true AP view and a cross-table lateral view of the full femur. Additionally, an AP pelvis x-ray as well as orthogonal hip and knee x-rays should be obtained to assess for concomitant injuries, degenerative changes, or adjacent arthroplasties.

Pain should be appropriately treated prior to any imaging, with a femoral nerve block being a good option. In patients with a history of bisphosphonate use and suspected atypical fracture, the contralateral limb should be imaged to screen for lesions that could indicate impending fractures [9]. Additionally, traction views are valuable for comminuted fractures or fractures with gross angulation [10].

Computed tomography (CT) may be useful in preoperative planning for complex comminuted fractures at the metadiaphyseal junction. An additional benefit of obtaining a CT scan is its ability to infer bone quality based on Hounsfield Units [11–13].

Any patient with a low-energy femoral fracture should be referred for workup of osteoporosis with a dual-energy x-ray absorptiometry study and metabolic bone studies following acute treatment of the fracture.

## 3 Classification

The AO/OTA Fracture and Dislocation Classification is the mainstay for classifying FSFs and can help detail injury severity and identify concomitant injuries. The Winquist and Hanson classification has four grades and is based on the degree of fracture comminution; this can be useful in assessing fracture stability [14]. While transverse FSF in the midshaft is the most common fracture across the entire population, older women more frequently sustain long oblique fractures [15].

## 4 Decision making

The overwhelming majority of FSFs will require operative treatment, even when the patient has significant comorbidities. When deciding on the initial treatment, the surgeon needs to take into consideration options such as pain control, traction, or external fixation.

### 4.1 Pain management

Pain management is essential, as this can reduce the adrenergic stress on the limited cardiopulmonary and cognitive reserves of most geriatric patients. Recently, studies have investigated the potential benefits of preoperative regional anesthesia for controlling pain while the patient awaits surgery [16, 17].

### 4.2 Traction

In patients with shortened or angulated FSFs, traction may be applied to the lower extremity to temporarily improve alignment, lengthen the muscles, and reduce spasm while a patient awaits definitive fixation. In a randomized prospective study, there was no difference in pain medication requirements or Visual Analog Scale scores comparing patients who underwent skeletal traction to those who underwent cutaneous traction [18]. Our preference is cutaneous traction for most patients. Adequate padding of the cutaneous traction apparatus is crucial in older patients who are at high risk for pressure ulcers and skin breakdown.

### 4.3 External fixation

The need for external fixation of FSFs has become less common as the techniques of IM nailing and submuscular plating have improved and their complication rates declined [10]. External fixation is still used as temporary fixation in unstable patients as part of a damage-control approach [19], in patients with an ipsilateral arterial injury that requires repair, and in patients with soft-tissue contamination who will require multiple debridements [20].

### 4.4 Consideration for nonoperative management

Nonoperative management may be considered in moribund patients with a life expectancy of days to weeks, as long as pain can be controlled. In this case, the injured leg is only positioned in a foam splint or in cutaneous traction for comfort. All other patients should be fixed operatively.

## 5 Therapeutic options

### 5.1 Intramedullary nailing

Generally, nailing is preferred in FSFs whenever technically feasible. It is a minimally invasive technique that allows for immediate full weight bearing as tolerated. Additionally, the femoral neck may be preventively addressed.

#### 5.1.1 Reduction techniques

Femoral shaft fractures at the isthmus may be treated via closed reduction with the passage of an IM nail. However, more comminuted or complex fracture patterns may require open reduction prior to passing the nail. Surgeons may employ the use of the finger, the "F-tool" (ie, a bar with two attached rods in the shape of an "F" that can be adjusted to accommodate the patient's leg and assist in reduction of femoral fractures), Schanz pins, blocking screws, or a ball spike pusher to aid in gross reduction of the fracture in order to pass a guide wire (**Case 1: Fig 3.11-1**, **Case 2: Fig 3.11-2**).

## Patient

A 63-year-old woman sustained a ground-level fall when a co-worker bumped into her.

## Comorbidities

- Diabetes mellitus
- Hypertension
- Osteoporosis
- Hyperlipidemia with previous bisphosphonate use

## Treatment and outcome

The patient sustained a transverse midshaft bisphosphonate-related femoral shaft fracture (**Fig 3.11-1a–d**). Beaking of the cortical bone at the level of the fracture could be best seen on the AP view (**Fig 3.11-1d**), and it was consistent with this patient's history of bisphosphonate use.

Given the transverse nature and the poor bone quality of the patient, the optimal treatment option was an antegrade femoral nail (AFN) that reduced and controlled the fracture and also provided femoral neck protection. Antegrade intramedullary nailing of the left femur was performed in sloppy lateral position and with the standard starting point for a trochanteric entry nail via an open incision. The fracture was reduced with the use of two Schanz pins, one placed in the distal and proximal fragment in order to manipulate the fragments. Once the femur was aligned, a guide wire was passed to the level of the superior patella and measured. Reaming was then performed sequentially from a 9 mm to a 13.5 mm diameter. A 12 mm nail was implanted (**Fig 3.11-1e–i**).

Uneventful healing in anatomical alignment occurred. The authors usually refer patients to a metabolic bone specialist, who may consider use of teriparatide in such patients depending on the results of their metabolic analysis (**Fig 3.11-1j–l)**.

## Key points

- Consider lateral positioning of patients for passing AFNs.
- The use of Schanz pins can obviate the need for open reduction of femoral shaft fractures in certain cases.
- In bisphosphonate-related fractures, bilateral femoral x-rays are necessary to look for pathological changes or evidence of impending fracture, even in the absence of symptoms.
- Referral to a metabolic bone specialist is recommended in all patients with bisphosphate-related fractures.

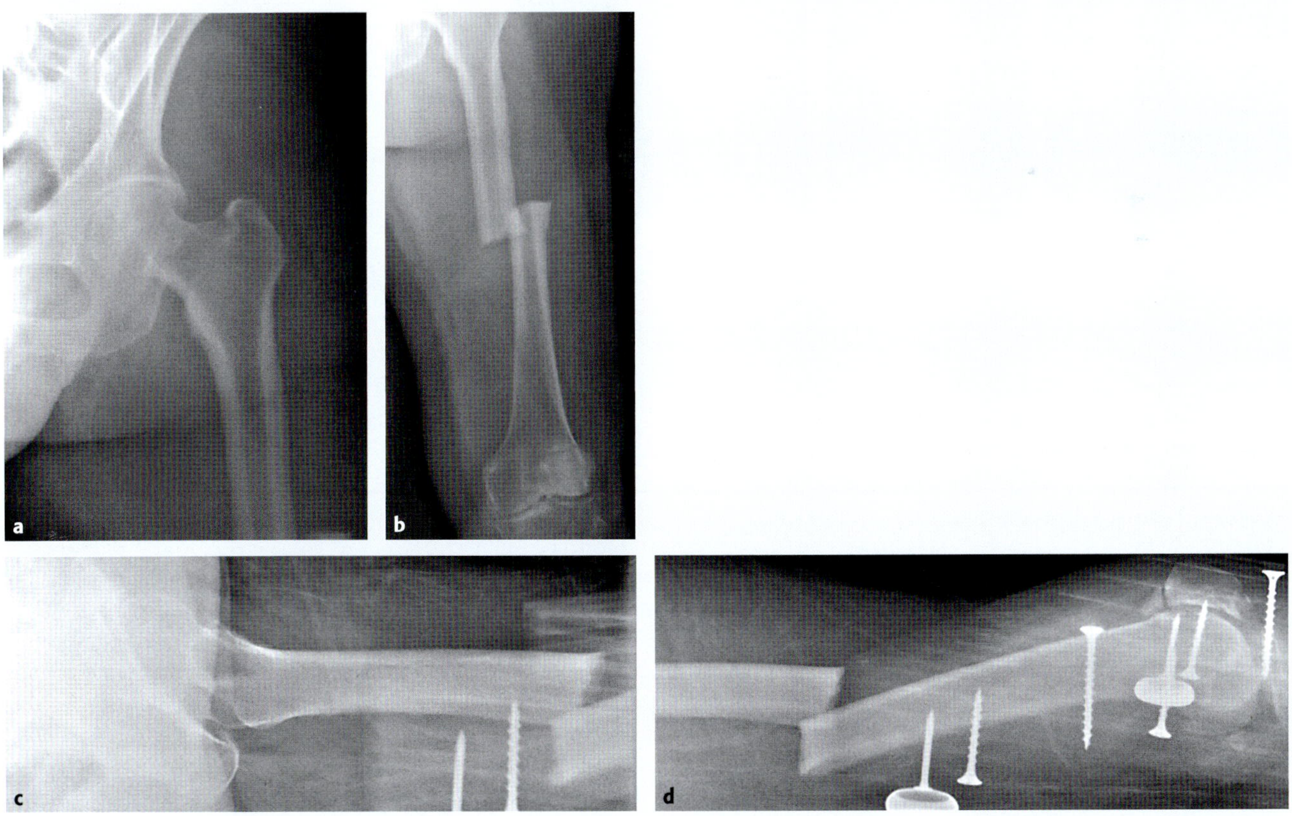

**Fig 3.11-1a–l** A 63-year-old female patient with a femoral shaft fracture after a ground-level fall.
**a–d** Transverse midshaft femoral shaft fracture. The AP view (**b**) showing beaking of the cortical bone at the fracture level.

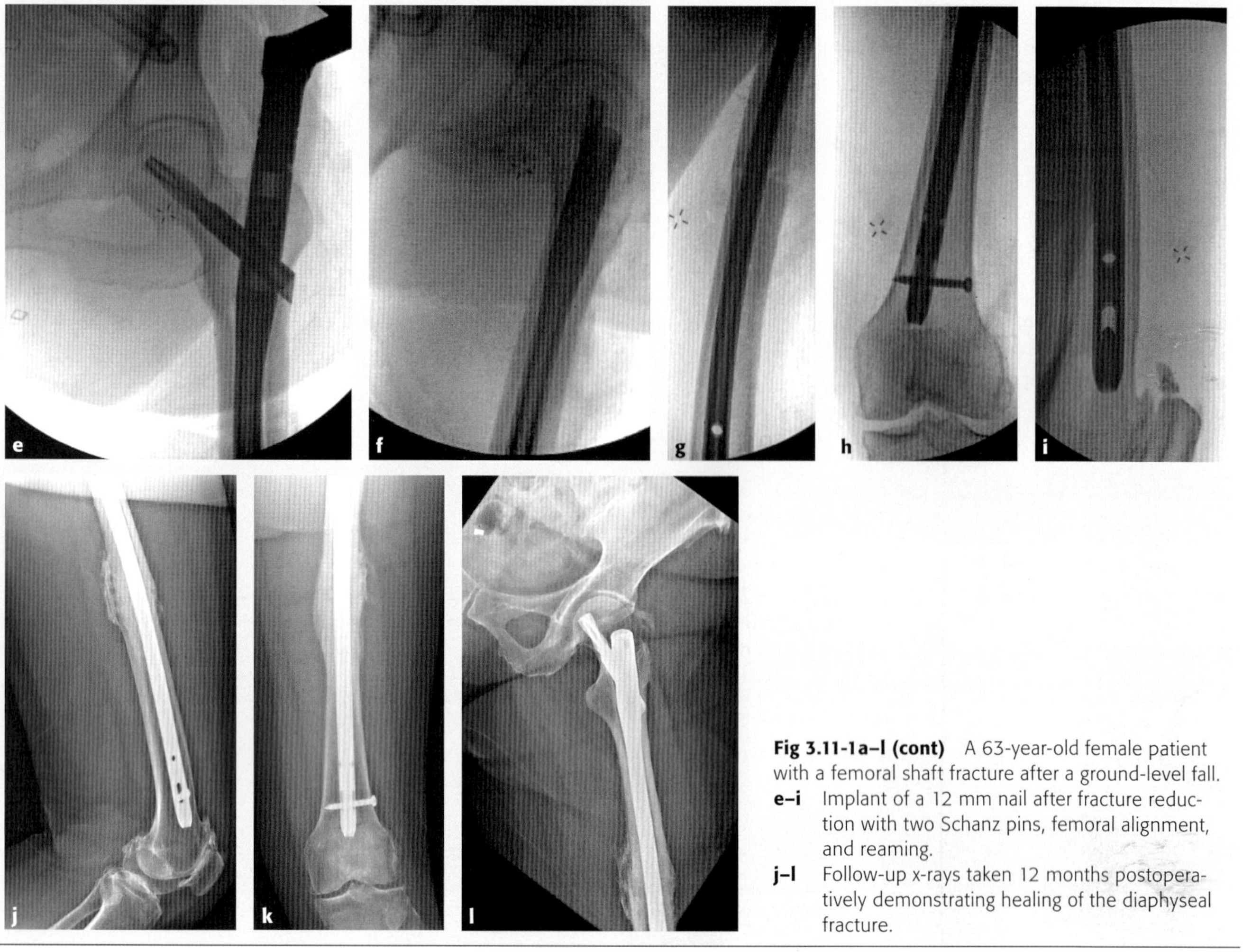


**Fig 3.11-1a–l (cont)** A 63-year-old female patient with a femoral shaft fracture after a ground-level fall.
**e–i** Implant of a 12 mm nail after fracture reduction with two Schanz pins, femoral alignment, and reaming.
**j–l** Follow-up x-rays taken 12 months postoperatively demonstrating healing of the diaphyseal fracture.

CASE 2

### Patient

A 67-year-old woman with no history of cognitive impairment. She drank 2 units of alcohol daily, which equals about a glass of wine, beer, or one shot of alcohol, and was living alone. She tripped on a curb sustaining a ground-level fall onto her left lower extremity.

### Comorbidities

- Atrial fibrillation (not on anticoagulation)
- Asthma and chronic obstructive pulmonary disease
- Previous right lung lower lobectomy
- Depression

### Treatment and outcome

The AP and cross-table lateral views of the left femur demonstrated a spiral fracture involving the distal third of the diaphysis (**Fig 3.11-2a–d**). The spiral oblique fracture of the distal femoral diaphysis from a low-energy injury resulted in shortening and posterior displacement of the distal femur. Nailing and plating were the two options for fracture fixation:

- Nailing—given the distal location of this fracture, retrograde nailing was the preferred technique for controlling the fracture.
- Plating—another option was the lateral approach to the femur and either direct or submuscular plating.

Retrograde nailing was performed via a paramedical patellar incision. As the fracture was widely displaced, in this case a separate incision was made and Weber clamps were used to perform fracture reduction. The canal was reamed and a 14 mm diameter, 400 mm long retrograde nail was inserted. To augment the fixation, two 1.6 mm braided cables were placed as cerclage wires (**Fig 3.11-2e–h**). Six months after intramedullary nailing, the fracture had healed (**Fig 3.11-2i–l**).

**Key point**

- While many diaphyseal femoral fractures can be reduced grossly with the finger, some require minimally invasive or open reduction techniques.

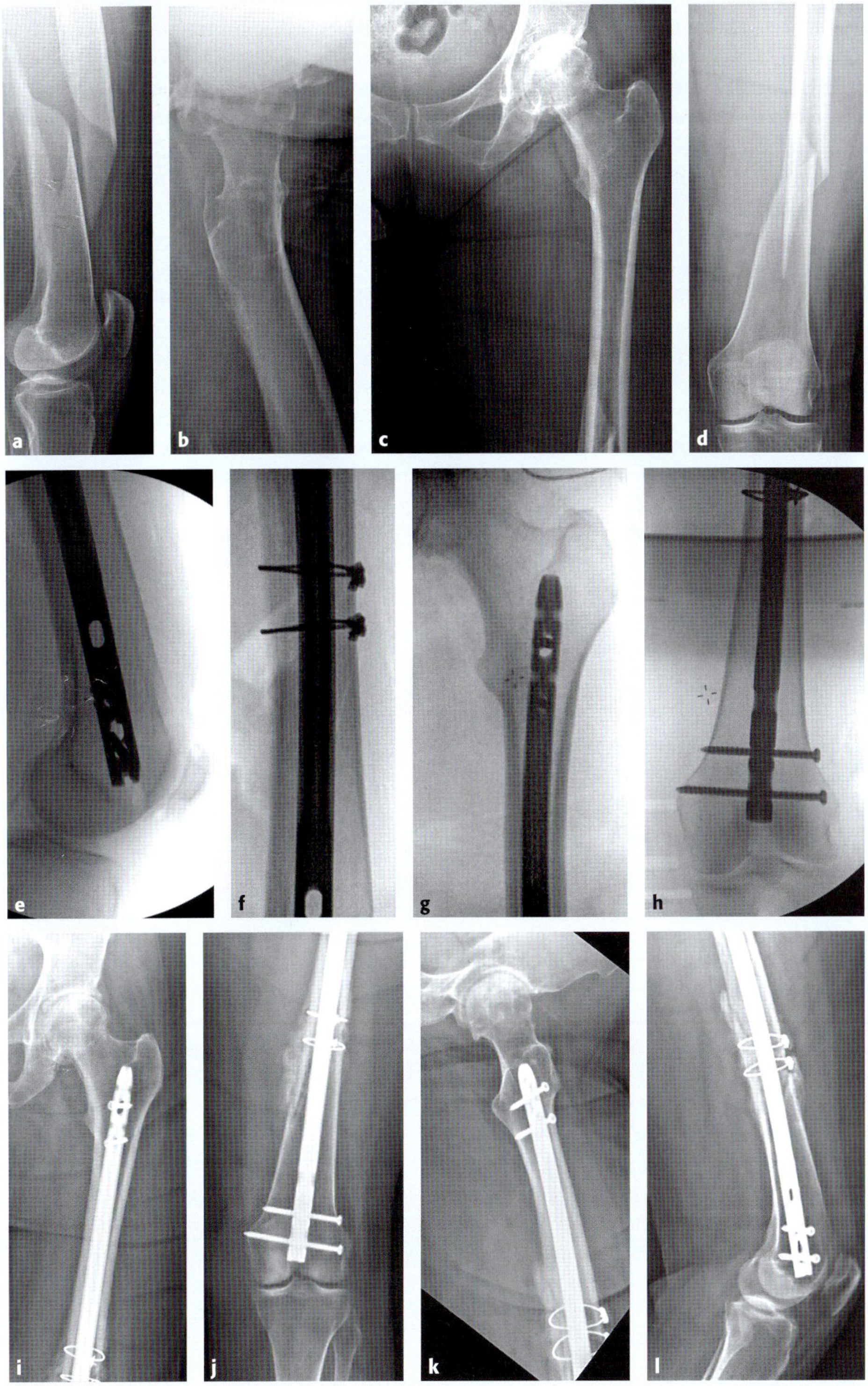


**Fig 3.11-2a–l** A 67-year-old woman sustained a spiral fracture of the left femur.

**a–d** AP and lateral views showing a spiral fracture of the femur including the distal third of the diaphysis.

**e–h** The fracture was cabled, the canal reamed, and a retrograde nail inserted.

**i–l** X-rays showing interval healing 6 months postoperative.

### 5.1.2 Reaming

Reaming can be used in geriatric FSFs on a limited basis to size the canal in order to insert a nail of optimal diameter. We have found that reaming aggressively is generally not required in geriatric stovepipe-type fractures given the generally large diameter IM canal in patients of advanced age. While reamed nails compared to unreamed nails have a shorter time to radiographic union, the risks of reaming are higher in many older, highly comorbid patients. These risks include elevation in IM pressure leading to embolization of fat and bone marrow, stimulation of inflammatory response, and impairment of the immune response [21].

The anterior bow of the femur should be assessed preoperatively with a cross-table lateral x-ray of the entire femur. There is an increased risk of anterior perforation, as the anterior cortex thins in the distal femur in this older population [22].

### 5.1.3 Antegrade intramedullary nailing

Antegrade femoral nails (AFNs) are indicated for patients with a proximal third FSF, as this construct optimizes the short-segment fixation length relative to a retrograde nail.

The two options for points of entry for AFNs are the piriformis fossa and the greater trochanter. Nails that offer the option to protect the femoral neck either with a blade or screw are preferred in older patients with poor bone quality. Nails designed for a greater trochanter entry often offer a larger diameter proximal component that can accommodate a large diameter screw or blade to protect the femoral neck. The sloppy lateral position is preferred for positioning piriformis entry nailing in order to facilitate radiographic confirmation of the starting point as well as ease of fracture reduction.

Rotational malalignment, specifically in internal rotation, is a typical complication of IM nailing and can result in a considerable impact on postoperative mobilization and gait. Head-neck implants, such as recon screws for the lateral femoral nail or the blade in case of proximal femoral nail antirotation, feature a 10° angle to the distal locking screw in the transversal plane. Thus, if the posterior condylar tangential line runs parallel to the axes of the hole of the distal locking screw, the rotation or anteversion of the femur is equal to the angle between the head-neck implant and the distal locking screw, which is 10° [23].

### 5.1.4 Retrograde intramedullary nailing

Recent reports have found comparable results in terms of union and malunion rates between retrograde and antegrade nails in younger patients, likely a result of improvements in technique and reaming [24]. Retrograde femoral nails are indicated in distal third femoral shaft fractures, as they optimize the shorter fracture segment length relative to the antegrade nail, thus providing a better biomechanical construct for fixation (**Case 3: Fig 3.11-3**). It is important to note that IM nailing may not provide adequate fixation in distal third metadiaphyseal fractures in older patients with wide canals and thin cortices (**Case 4: Fig 3.11-4**). In such cases where stability is not achieved with a nail, the fixation can be augmented with cables or plating. Relative indications for retrograde femoral nailing of the femur also include cases in which the proximal entry point is contraindicated or undesirable, such as the case in patients with ipsilateral acetabular or pelvic injury in which an antegrade entry point may violate the surgical approach [25]. Access to the proximal femur can also be difficult in morbidly obese patients, and retrograde femoral nailing may be considered for such patients. Retrograde nailing also allows for immediate weight bearing as tolerated. A propagation of the fracture at the knee must be ruled out with a CT scan. Rotation control is accomplished with a comparison to the contralateral leg, which should be prepared operatively as well as in supine position.

## Patient

A 67-year-old woman sustained an oblique midshaft femoral fracture with posterior comminution after a fall from standing height (**Fig 3.11-3a–c**). She had a left lower extremity operation for a tibial fracture over 30 years prior to this fall.

## Comorbidities

- No comorbidities and no medication use were reported

## Treatment and outcome

For this oblique midshaft femoral fracture with posterior comminution, the treatment options included retrograde nailing, antegrade nailing, and plate osteosynthesis. Since the fracture was slightly distal in the diaphysis, retrograde nailing was preferred in this case. Intraoperative image intensification demonstrated placement of a retrograde femoral nail with cerclage wire at the fracture site maintaining reduction. A spiral blade and a screw were used distally to lock the nail (**Fig 3.11-3d–i**). The follow-up x-rays showed healing of the fracture and anatomical alignment (**Fig 3.11-3j–m**).

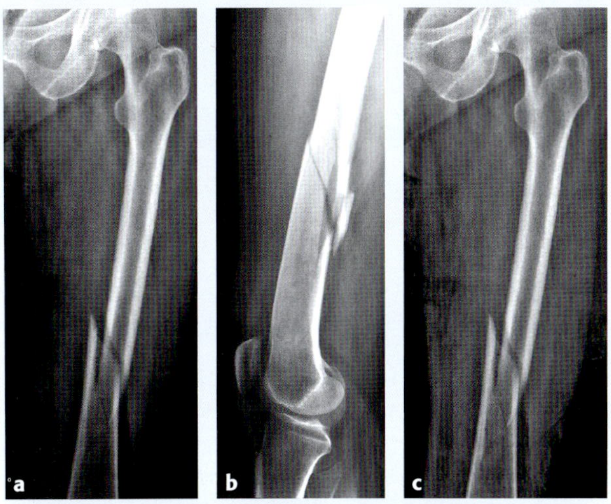


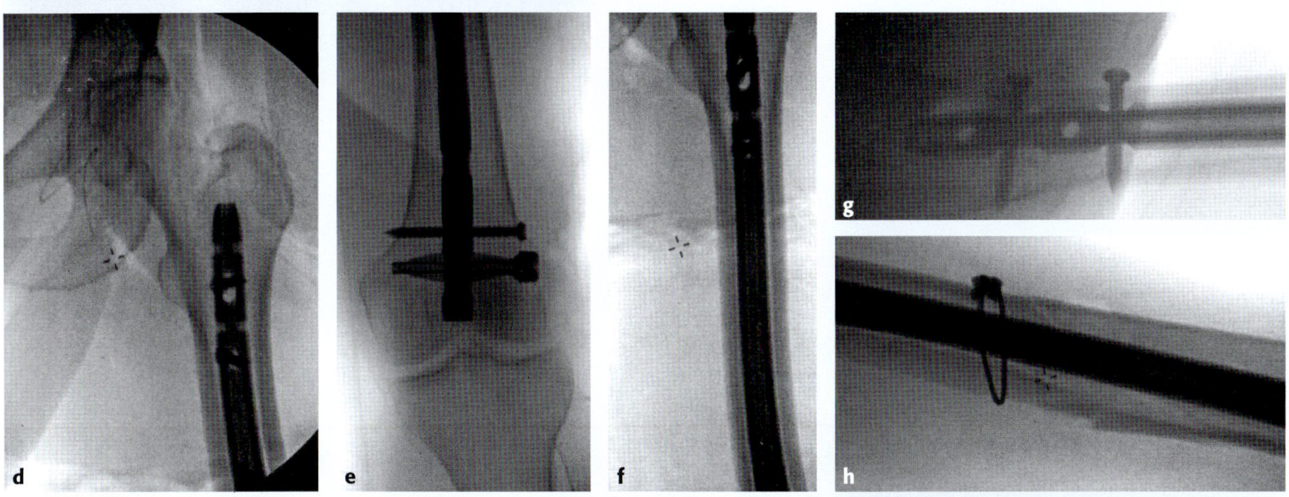


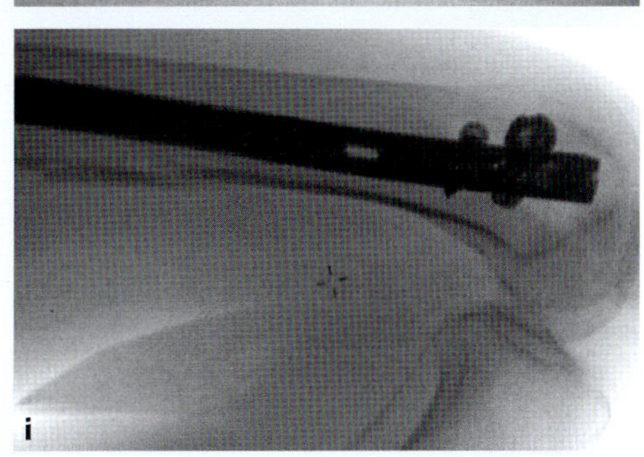


**Fig 3.11-3a–m** A 67-year-old woman with an oblique midshaft femoral fracture.
**a–c** The x-rays showing the midshaft femoral fracture with posterior comminution.
**d–i** Intraoperative image intensification showing retrograde femoral nail placement with cerclage wire. The nail was locked distally with a spiral blade and a screw.

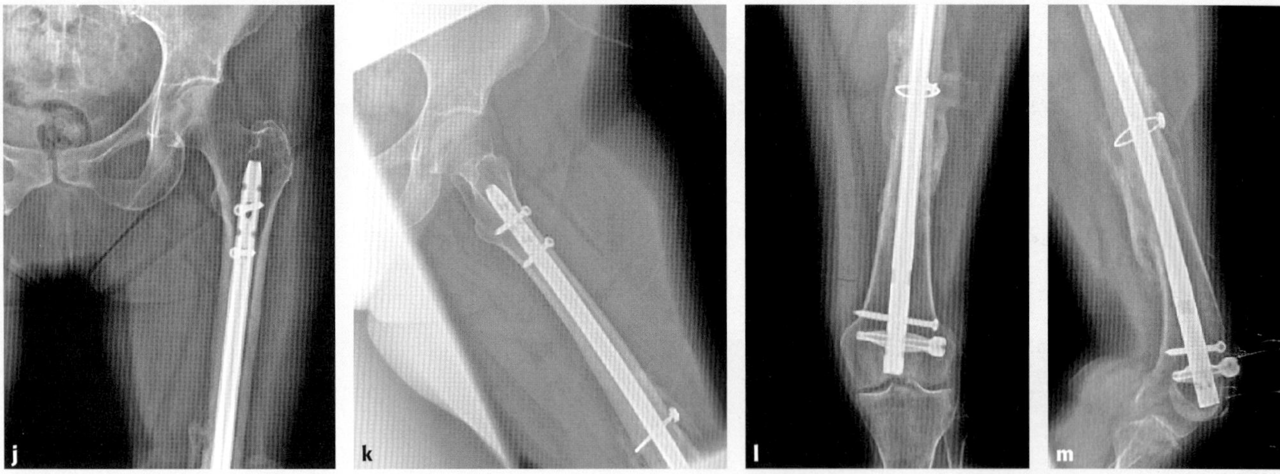

**Fig 3.11-3a–m (cont)** A 67-year-old woman with an oblique midshaft fracture of the femur.
**j–m** Fracture healing and anatomical alignment at the 3 months follow-up.

CASE 4

## Patient

An 88-year-old woman was living in a residential home. She was always walking with a cane.

## Comorbidities

- Dementia
- Hypertension

## Treatment and outcome

The nondisplaced lateral femoral neck fracture and the fracture of the tip of the greater trochanter were fixed with 2-hole dynamic hip and antirotation screws (**Fig 3.11-4a–b**). Six months later the patient sustained a spiral fracture of the same femur with a third fragment (**Fig 3.11-4c–d**). Hardware was removed and antergrade intramedullary nailing with two recon screws performed (**Fig 3.11-4e–f**). The x-rays after 1 week demonstrated major instability and malalignment in the coronal plane (**Fig 3.11-4g**), which could not be improved by additional plaster fixation (**Fig 3.11-4h–i**). Pressure ulcers formed on the heel and over the achilles tendon, which required rotational flaps (**Fig 3.11-4j–l**). The fracture healed in severe valgus malalignment, turning the patient into a bedridden and chair-ridden nursing home patient (**Fig 3.11-4m–o**).

## Key point

- Antegrade femoral nailing does not offer enough stability in fractures distal to the femoral isthmus. Stability must be tested intraoperatively, and extramedullary fixation preferably with a locking plate construct must be added right away.

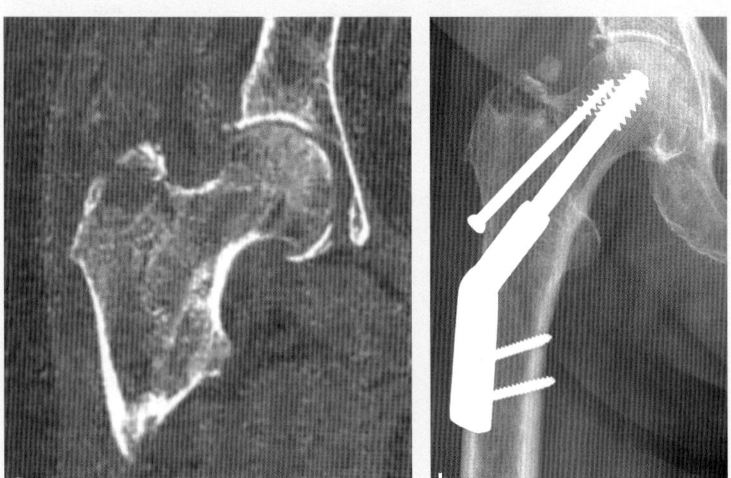

**Fig 3.11-4a–o** An 88-year-old woman with fractures of the lateral femur and the tip of the greater trochanter.
**a–b** The computed tomographic scan (**a**) and x-ray (**b**) showing a nondisplaced lateral femoral neck fracture and a fracture of the tip of the greater trochanter fixed with 2-hole dynamic hip and antirotation screws.

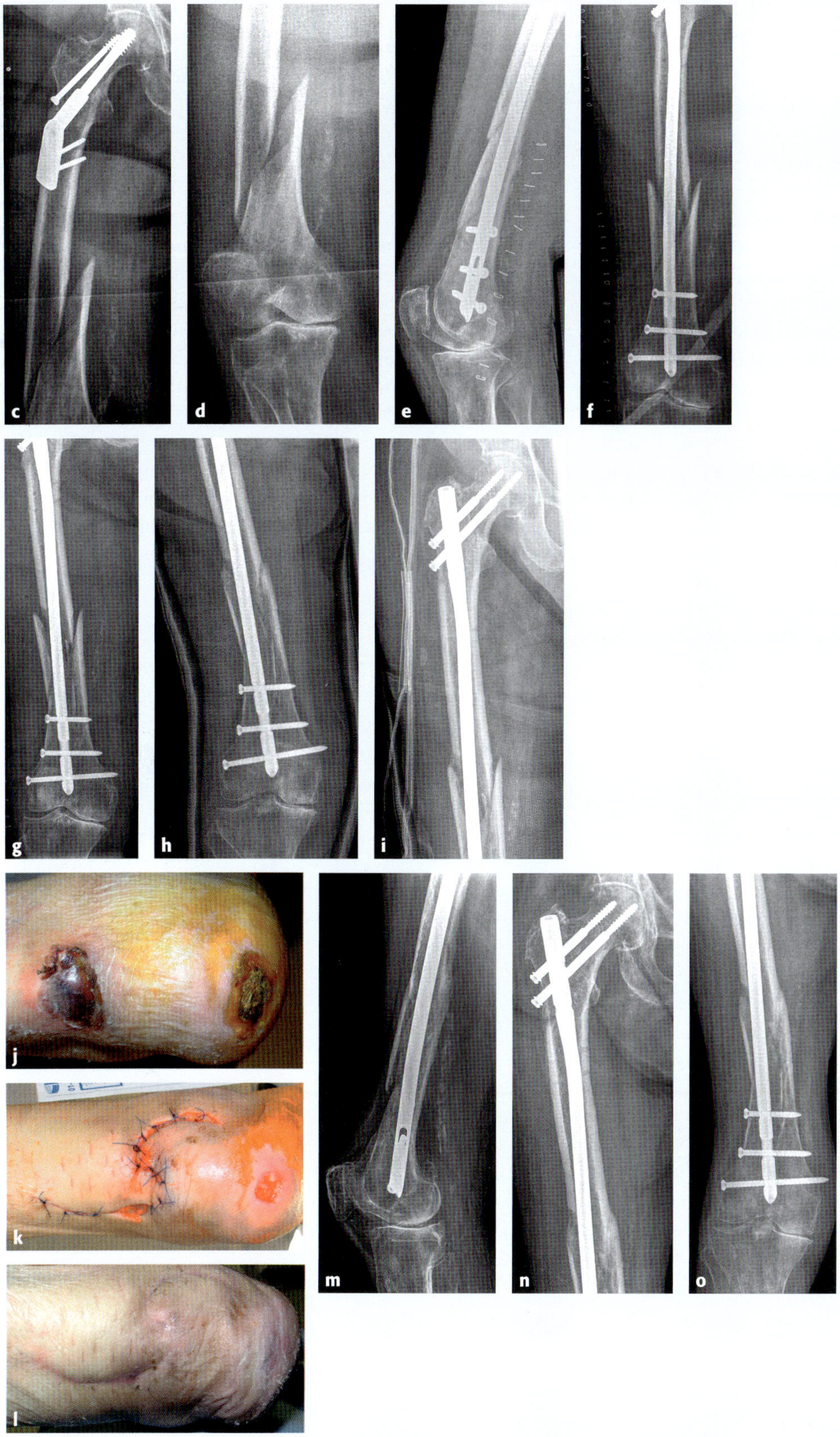

**Fig 3.11-4a–o (cont)** An 88-year-old woman with fractures of the lateral femur and the tip of the greater trochanter.

**c–d** A spiral fracture of the same femur with a third fragment.

**e–f** Antegrade intramedullary nailing with two recon screws after hardware removal.

**g–i** Instability and malalignment in the coronal plane (**g**) was unsuccessfully improved by plaster fixation (**h–i**).

**j–l** Pressure ulcers required rotational flaps.

**m–o** Fracture healing with severe valgus malalignment.

(Case courtesy of the University Department of Trauma Surgery, Innsbruck, Austria.)

### 5.1.5 Protecting the femoral neck

The decision to use an implant for IM nailing of the femur to protect the femoral neck from a periimplant fracture remains controversial, and the literature investigating the issue is limited. Classic teaching suggests that in older patients, particularly those with severe osteopenia or osteoporosis, the entire femur should be protected including the femoral neck. The rate of subsequent femoral neck fracture following FSF in women older than 60 years may be as high as 26%, [26] indicating that protecting the neck with either a cephalomedullary implant or a retrograde reconstruction nail with supplementary fixation for the neck should be strongly considered for such patients. However, a recent retrospective review of patients treated with IM nailing for pathological fractures of the femoral diaphysis or for impending fractures of the diaphysis found no subsequent femoral neck fractures in cases where the neck was not protected [27]. The additional cost of using a reconstruction nail with the option of femoral neck fixation is between USD 260.00 and USD 1,282.00, and a recent decision analysis concluded that empiric neck fixation of all diaphyseal femoral fractures was not a cost-effective strategy unless the rate of subsequent femoral neck fracture is greater than 7% [28]. Therefore, protecting the neck should only be considered in patients at risk for subsequent.

### 5.1.6 Locking

Locking the nail with interlocking screws restores the length and rotational stability of diaphyseal femoral fractures. However, the decision to lock nails and how many screws to use varies based on surgeon preference. Our preference is to use two distal interlocking screws in antegrade nails and two free-hand screws in retrograde nails.

There is biomechanical evidence that two screws provide greater stability, particularly in distal third or proximal third diaphyseal fractures of the femur [29]. When possible, multiplanar locking options are preferred to ensure greater stability. In older patients with thinner cortices and larger diameter IM canals, ensuring adequate fixation with appropriate length interlocking screws is essential. Biomechanically, angular stable locking screws have shown to allow for more cycles to failure in cadaveric osteoporotic tibiae. The clinical impact of using these screws is not clear.

## 5.2 Plate fixation

The relative indications for plate fixation of FSFs include an extremely narrow femoral canal precluding IM nailing, previous nonunion or malunion, and fractures that extend into the pertrochanteric or distal femoral metaphyseal region [10].

Submuscular plating is also a consideration for certain femoral shaft fractures in older patients. Unlike in younger patients, retrograde nailing may not provide appropriate fixation and deformity correction for distal third fractures (**Case 5: Fig 3.11-5**). Submuscular plating or combining plating with IM nailing improves the stability and strength of fixation. Supplementing fixation by adding bone graft to plate constructs may be essential in the geriatric patient with poor bone quality. The lateral fixed angle constructs that are typically utilized for stabilizing distal femoral diaphyseal and metaphyseal fractures often fail to stabilize the medial column.

For femoral shaft fractures with extension into the distal femur, an endosteal fibular allograft positioned in the IM canal in combination with a lateral locking plate can augment stability by providing mechanical support of the medial column and increasing bone stock [30]. Endosteal implants in combination with a laterally based plate create a trestle to support the distal femur (**Case 6: Fig 3.11-6**).

## Patient

An 86-year-old woman sustained an unwitnessed fall at home and was found on the floor by her daughter approximately 2 hours later. At baseline the patient was able to ambulate with a walker.

## Comorbidities

- Dementia
- Mild aortic stenosis with normal left ventricular function
- Diastolic dysfunction
- Osteoarthritis
- Osteoporosis
- Status post pacemaker placement

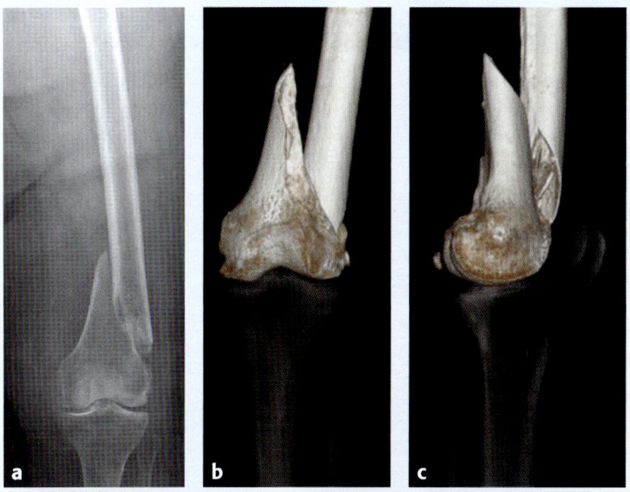

## Treatment and outcome

The radiographic and reconstructed computed tomographic images showed a distal diametaphyseal oblique femoral fracture (**Fig 3.11-5a–c**). The main treatment options for this diametaphyseal oblique femoral shaft fracture included retrograde nailing and osteosynthesis with plate fixation.

The patient was positioned supine and the original plan was to combine a retrograde intramedullary (IM) nail with a medial plate. A standard medial parapatellar approach to the knee was taken and a 15 mm drill bit was used to create a pilot hole for the nail. Then a medial approach to the femur was used and the fracture was reduced with a combination of Weber clamps and traction. At this point a guide wire was placed and the canal was reamed. A 10-hole reconstruction plate 3.5 was used to hold the reduction and secure across the obliquity of the fracture. The nail was then inserted, but the fracture remained grossly unstable due to the patient's osteoporosis. The nail was then removed and a lateral approach was used to apply a lateral locking plate. Demineralized bone matrix was used at the fracture site (**Fig 3.11-5d–h)**. The fracture was healing in anatomical alignment 3 months postoperative (**Fig 3.11-5i–m**).

## Key point

- In patients with severe osteoporosis, IM nails do not provide stability for nonisthmic femoral shaft fractures.

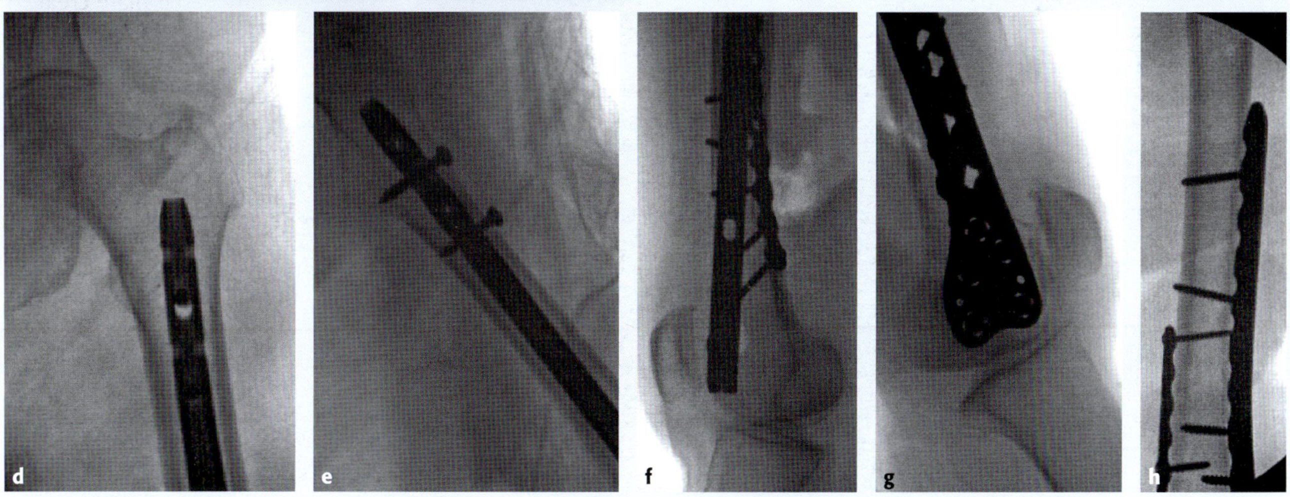

**Fig 3.11-5a–m** An 86-year-old woman sustained a diametaphyseal oblique femoral shaft fracture.
**a–c** Injury x-ray and 3-D computed tomographic scans demonstrating the distal diametaphyseal oblique femoral fracture.
**d–h** Intraoperative image intensification demonstrating the use of a lateral locking plate in addition to a posteromedial reconstruction plate to stabilize the medial column.

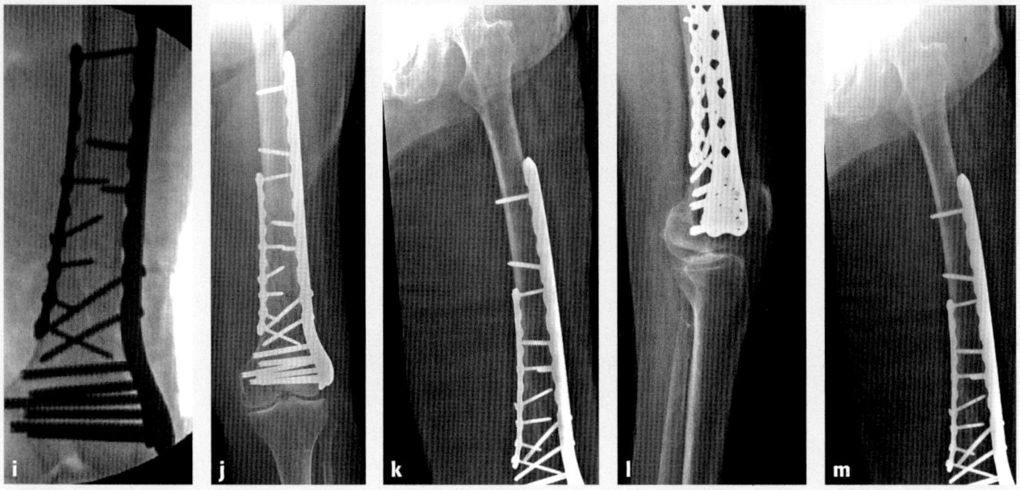


**Fig 3.11-5a–m (cont)** An 86-year-old woman sustained a diametaphyseal oblique femoral shaft fracture.
**i–m** Postoperative x-rays at 3 months showing healing of the fracture in anatomical alignment.

CASE 6

## Patient

A 73-year-old woman with cold agglutinin disease, who had recently undergone right total hip arthroplasty, sustained a mechanical fall from standing. She had a history of intermittent steroid use.

## Comorbidities

- Cold agglutinin disease
- Previous right total hip arthroplasty and recent revision surgery
- Bilateral knee arthroscopy
- Baker cyst removal

## Treatment and outcome

This patient sustained a distal femoral diaphyseal spiral fracture. Normally, a retrograde nail would have been considered, but this was contraindicated in this patient given her total hip prosthesis. In this case, plate fixation was the only viable option. Augmentation of her fixation with bone graft should have been considered.

The x-rays demonstrated a distal femoral diaphyseal spiral fracture with a well-fixed cemented stem of the total hip arthroplasty (**Fig 3.11-6a–d**).

Images were taken intraoperatively with the image intensifier. A swashbuckler incision (ie, a modified anterior approach) was used [31]. An intramedullary allograft was inserted to augment the bone quality and provide additional stability. This was secured with a lateral locking plate that was slid underneath the vastus proximally and positioned on the condyles of the distal femur. The proximal screw was placed into the cement mantle distal to the prosthesis. Multiple screws captured the allograft (**Fig 3.11-6e–j**). The x-rays taken 12 months following osteosynthesis demonstrated interval healing (**Fig 3.11-6k–n**).

## Key point

- In cases of periprosthetic femoral fractures, a locking plate can be secured around a prosthesis with either cables or screws anterior or posterior to the implant.

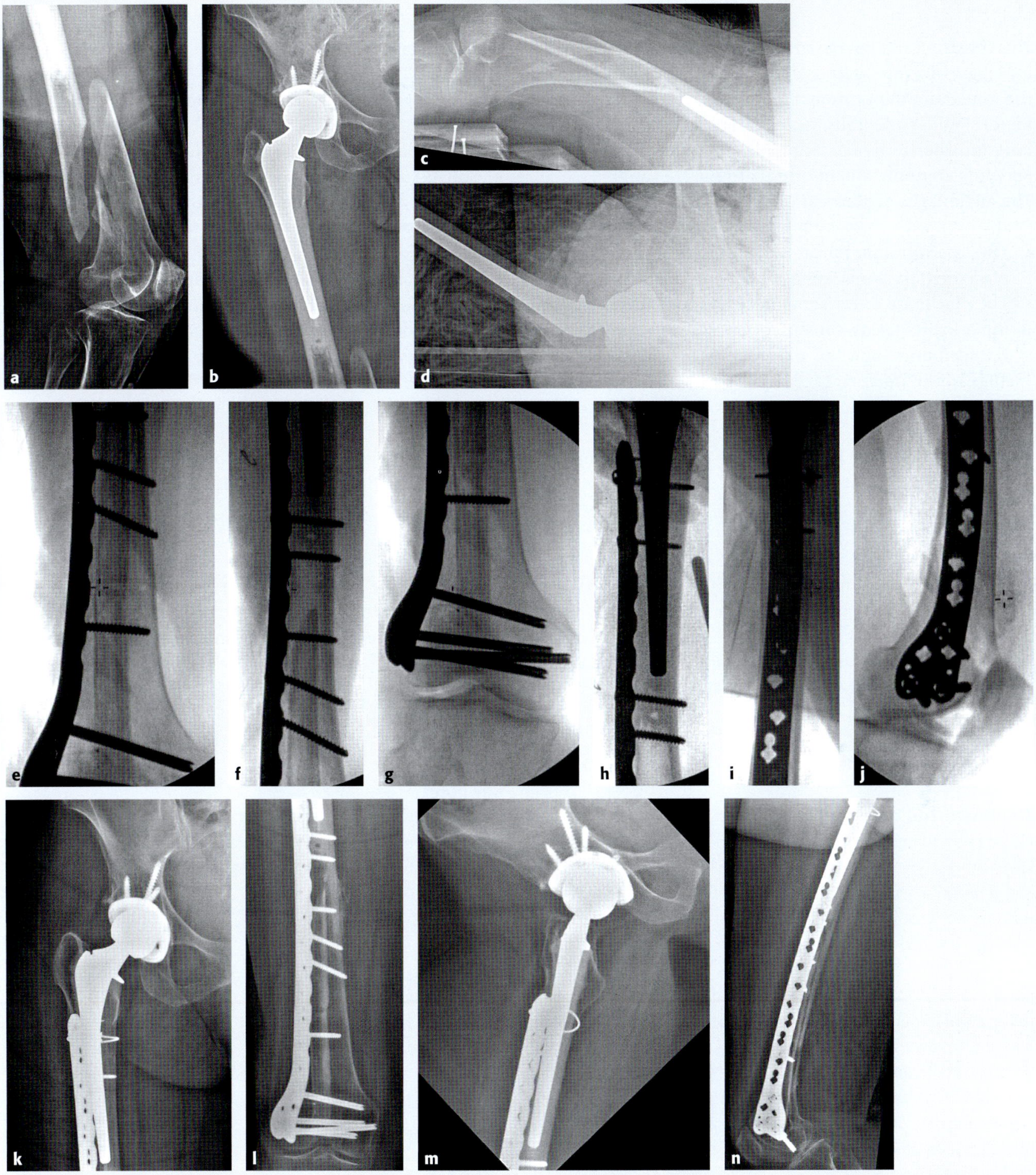


**Fig 3.11-6a–n** A 73-year-old woman sustained a distal femoral diaphyseal spiral fracture.

**a–d** The x-rays showing a distal femoral diaphyseal spiral fracture. The cemented stem of the total hip arthroplasty was well fixed.

**e–j** Intraoperative images taken with the image intensifier showing intramedullary allograft used for stability and secured with a lateral locking plate under the vastus proximally and placed on the condyles of the distal femur. The proximal screw was placed into the cement mantle distal to the prosthesis and multiple screws captured the allograft.

**k–n** The x-rays taken 12 months following osteosynthesis demonstrated interval healing.

This construct also has the advantage of decreasing the working length of screws, as the screws pass from the plate through the fibula and then through the medial cortex of the distal femur. Fibular allografts, which can be as large as 18–21 cm long in order to bypass a fracture, may be shaped to the patient's anatomy and inserted into the IM canal.
The advantages of plates are:

- They permit anatomical reduction with strategic plate placement in simple spiral or oblique fracture patterns.
- They facilitate interfragmentary fixation, thereby creating a load-sharing construct between the anatomically reduced bone and the strategically placed plate at the apex of the fracture.
- There is no additional trauma to the femoral neck or distal femur.
- They are preferred in cases where prostheses limit ability to access the IM canal.

The disadvantages of plates are:

- It requires a more extensile approach with increased blood loss.
- There is a higher risk of infection.
- Soft-tissue can be harmed (quadriceps scarring).
- There is a decreased vascularity of the femur and stress shielding of the bone.

Open reduction and internal fixation of femoral shaft fractures is associated with rates of nonunion as high as 23% and infection rates as high as 28%. Submuscular plating is associated with less soft-tissue stripping and in theory promotes superior healing and lower risk of infection **[32]**. In a recent series that incorporated fibular allograft into a plate construct, the rate of osseous union was 92% by 17 weeks **[30]**. An attempt should be made to address the whole femur also with plate fixation (**Case 7: Fig 3.11-7**).

CASE 7

### Patient

A 46-year-old healthy man with 3 weeks of right knee pain felt his leg give way while jogging. He sustained a spiral fracture of the distal femoral diaphysis with extension into the metaphysis (**Fig 3.11-7a–b**). The computed tomographic scan also demonstrated the distal extent of the fracture (**Fig 3.11-7c–f**).

### Comorbidities

- No active comorbidities

### Treatment and outcome

He had had surgery for a deviated septum and had undergone left knee arthroscopy in the past. Denied previous use of steroids. He had a history of multiple fractures in the past, including a clavicle fracture, rib fractures, and a wrist fracture. Of note, his vitamin D level was low during his hospitalization (66 nmol/L [26.4 ng/mL]).

For this distal diaphyseal spiral fracture of the femur with extension to the distal femur, the main treatment options included plate fixation and retrograde nailing. Sloppy lateral position and lateral approach to the femoral shaft was used. No obvious pathological lesion was noted. The fracture was reduced with a combination of Weber clamps and a reduction was then held with a 16-hole reconstruction plate 3.5 placed posteriorly on the femur (**Fig 3.11-7g–i**).

Given the unusual nature of a 46-year-old person with a low-energy femoral fracture, prophylactic treatment of the entire femur was performed using a distal femoral locking compression plate extending from the knee to the hip. This was placed proximally beneath the vastus lateralis muscle. Demineralized bone matrix was used in the fracture site, which the authors tend to use in cases where there is severe comminution or bone loss (**Fig 3.11-7j–m**).

### Key point

- Low-energy fractures that raise suspicion in younger patients should be treated like osteoporotic fractures in older adults. A full metabolic workup may reveal laboratory abnormalities that should be corrected.

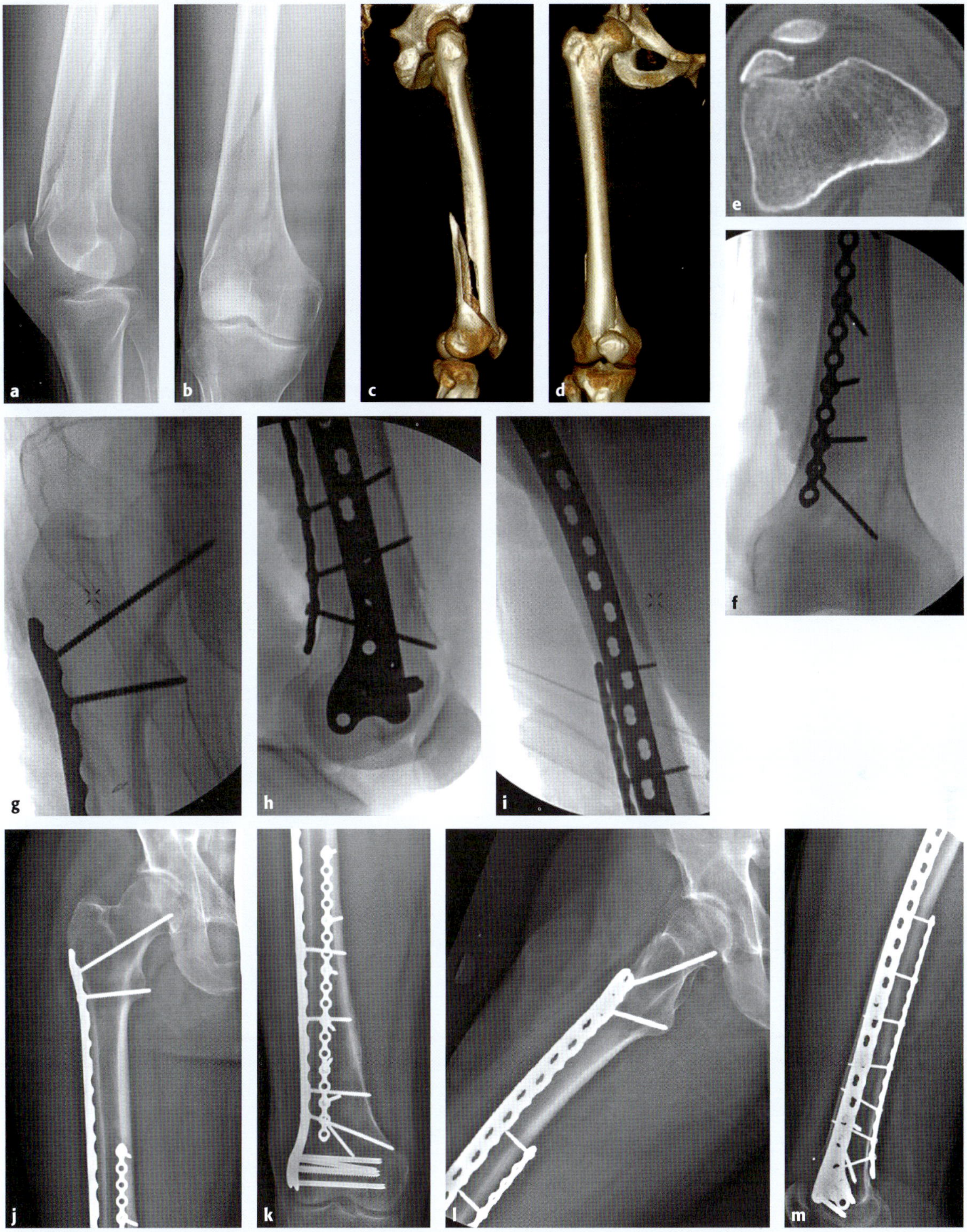


**Fig 3.11-7a–m** A 46-year-old man with a fracture of the distal femoral diaphysis extending into the metaphysis.
**a–b** The x-rays show a spiral fracture of the distal femoral diaphysis that extends into the metaphysis.
**c–f** The computed tomographic scans show the distal extent.
**g–i** Intraoperative image intensification showing the use of a medial plate in addition to a lateral locking plate to reduce and transfix the fracture.
**j–m** The follow-up images demonstrate the position of the lateral locking plate and the reconstruction plate.

## 6 Outcomes

The incidence of malunion, nonunion, deep vein thrombosis (DVT), and infection in patients following IM nailing of femoral shaft fractures is not significantly different between older and younger patients. However, older patients have higher mortality rates, knee pain, loss of motion, and increased postoperative functional dependence following IM nailing compared with younger patients [33]. The mortality rate in older patients following FSFs is reported between 16% and 26% [33, 34]. Within the first 60 days following injury, the mortality rate is 10% [35]. Complications following FSF in older adults include shortening, malalignment, DVT, and infection. Malrotation is a concerning complication that may occur in any patient following IM nailing of the femur. Malrotation represents the most common complication following FSF and the most difficult to prevent. The prevalence of malrotation following IM nailing of FSFs is reported between 2.3% and 27.6% [36].

## 7 References


1. **Arneson TJ, Melton LJ 3rd, Lewallen DG, et al.** Epidemiology of diaphyseal and distal femoral fractures in Rochester, Minnesota, 1965–1984. *Clin Orthop Relat Res.* 1988 Sep;(234):188–194.
2. **Enninghorst N, McDougall D, Evans JA, et al.** Population-based epidemiology of femur shaft fractures. *J Trauma Acute Care Surg.* 2013 Jun;74(6):1516–1520.
3. **Salminen S, Pihlajamaki H, Avikainen V, et al.** Specific features associated with femoral shaft fractures caused by low-energy trauma. *J Trauma.* 1997 Jul;43(1):117–122.
4. **Ng AC, Drake MT, Clarke BL, et al.** Trends in subtrochanteric, diaphyseal, and distal femur fractures, 1984–2007. *Osteoporos Int.* 2012 Jun;23(6):1721–1726.
5. **Hedlund R, Lindgren U.** Epidemiology of diaphyseal femoral fracture. *Acta Orthop Scand.* 1986 Oct;57(5):423–427.
6. **Kootstra G.** *Femoral shaft fractures in adults: a study of 329 consecutive cases with a statistical analysis of different methods of treatment.* Thesis. Assen: van Gorcum; 1973.
7. **Bostman O, Varjonen L, Vainionpaa S, et al.** Incidence of local complications after intramedullary nailing and after plate fixation of femoral shaft fractures. *J Trauma.* 1989 May;29(5):639–645.
8. **Della Rocca GJ, Uppal HS, Copeland ME, et al.** Geriatric patients with fractures below the hip are medically similar to geriatric patients with hip fracture. *Geriatr Orthop Surg Rehabil.* 2015 Mar;6(1):28–32.
9. **Edwards MH, McCrae FC, Young-Min SA.** Alendronate-related femoral diaphysis fracture—what should be done to predict and prevent subsequent fracture of the contralateral side? *Osteoporos Int.* 2010 Apr;21(4):701–703.
10. **Nork S.** Femoral shaft fractures. In: Court-Brown CM, Heckman JD, McQueen MM, et al, eds. *Rockwood and Green's Fractures in Adults.* 8th ed. Philadelphia: Wolters Kluwer Health; 2014:2149–2228.
11. **Emohare O, Wiggin M, Hemmati P, et al.** Assessing bone mineral density following acute hip fractures: the role of computed tomography attenuation. *Geriatr Orthop Surg Rehabil.* 2015 Mar;6(1):16–21.
12. **Marinova M, Edon B, Wolter K, et al.** Use of routine thoracic and abdominal computed tomography scans for assessing bone mineral density and detecting osteoporosis. *Curr Med Res Opin.* 2015;31(10):1871–1881.
13. **Kim YS, Lee S, Sung YK, et al.** Assessment of osteoporosis using pelvic diagnostic computed tomography. *J Bone Miner Metab.* 2016 Jul;34(4):457–463.
14. **Winquist RA, Hansen ST Jr.** Comminuted fractures of the femoral shaft treated by intramedullary nailing. *Orthop Clin North Am.* 1980 Jul;11(3):633–648.
15. **Dencker H.** Femoral shaft fracture and fracture of the neck of the same femur. *Acta Chir Scand.* 1965 Jun;129:597–605.
16. **Hanna L, Gulati A, Graham A.** The role of fascia iliaca blocks in hip fractures: a prospective case-control study and feasibility assessment of a junior-doctor-delivered service. *ISRN Orthop.* 2014;2014:191306.
17. **Black KJ, Bevan CA, Murphy NG, et al.** Nerve blocks for initial pain management of femoral fractures in children. *Cochrane Database Syst Rev.* 2013 Dec 17(12):CD009587.
18. **Even JL, Richards JE, Crosby CG, et al.** Preoperative skeletal versus cutaneous traction for femoral shaft fractures treated within 24 hours. *J Orthop Trauma.* 2012 Oct;26(10):e177–e182.
19. **Pape HC, Hildebrand F, Pertschy S, et al.** Changes in the management of femoral shaft fractures in polytrauma patients: from early total care to damage control orthopedic surgery. *J Trauma.* 2002 Sep;53(3):452–461; discussion 461–452.
20. **Iannacone WM, Taffet R, DeLong WG Jr, et al.** Early exchange intramedullary nailing of distal femoral fractures with vascular injury initially stabilized with external fixation. *J Trauma.* 1994 Sep;37(3):446–451.
21. **Bagheri F, Sharifi SR, Mirzadeh NR, et al.** Clinical outcome of ream versus unream intramedullary nailing for femoral shaft fractures. *Iran Red Crescent Med J.* 2013 May;15(5):432–435.
22. **Ostrum RF, Levy MS.** Penetration of the distal femoral anterior cortex during intramedullary nailing for subtrochanteric fractures: a report of three cases. *J Orthop Trauma.* 2005 Oct;19(9):656–660.
23. **Hoigne D, Hauck R, Babst R.** Technique for intraoperative determination of femoral rotation with a lateral femur nail (LFN, Synthes, Oberdorf, Switzerland). *Arch Orthop Trauma Surg.* 2011 Dec;131(12):1649–1654.
24. **Tornetta P 3rd, Tiburzi D.** Antegrade or retrograde reamed femoral nailing. A prospective, randomised trial. *J Bone Joint Surg Br.* 2000 Jul;82(5):652–654.
25. **Sanders R, Koval KJ, DiPasquale T, et al.** Retrograde reamed femoral nailing. *J Orthop Trauma.* 1993;7(4):293–302.
26. **Patton JT, Cook RE, Adams CI, et al.** Late fracture of the hip after reamed intramedullary nailing of the femur. *J Bone Joint Surg Br.* 2000 Sep;82(7):967–971.
27. **Moon B, Lin P, Satcher R, et al.** Intramedullary nailing of femoral diaphyseal metastases: is it necessary to protect the femoral neck? *Clin Orthop Relat Res.* 2015 Apr;473(4):1499–1502.
28. **Faucett SC, Collinge CA, Koval KJ.** Is reconstruction nailing of all femoral shaft fractures cost effective? A decision analysis. *J Orthop Trauma.* 2012 Nov;26(11):624–632.
29. **Karuppiah SV, Johnstone AJ.** Distal locking in femoral intramedullary nailing system: Is one cross screw sufficient? *J Biomed Sci Eng.* 2012 Oct;5(10):593–596.
30. **Lazaro LE, Warner SJ, Helfet DL, et al.** Favorable outcomes using endosteal medial strut support to augment lateral locking plate fixation for periprosthetic fractures of the distal femur. *J Orthop Trauma.* In press.
31. **Starr AJ, Jones AL, Reinert CM.** The "swashbuckler": a modified anterior approach for fractures of the distal femur. *J Orthop Trauma.* 1999 Feb;13(2):138–140.
32. **Zlowodzki M, Vogt D, Cole PA, et al.** Plating of femoral shaft fractures: open reduction and internal fixation versus submuscular fixation. *J Trauma.* 2007 Nov;63(5):1061–1065.
33. **Elmi A, Rohani AR, Tabrizi A, et al.** Comparison of outcome of femoral shaft fracture fixation with intramedullary nail in elderly patient and patients younger than 60 years old. *Arch Bone Jt Surg.* 2014 Jun;2(2):103–105.
34. **DeCoster TA, Miller RA.** Closed locked intramedullary nailing of femoral shaft fractures in the elderly. *Iowa Orthop J.* 2003;23:43–45.
35. **Boyd AD Jr, Wilber JH.** Patterns and complications of femur fractures below the hip in patients over 65 years of age. *J Orthop Trauma.* 1992;6(2):167–174.
36. **Lindsey JD, Krieg JC.** Femoral malrotation following intramedullary nail fixation. *J Am Acad Orthop Surg.* 2011 Jan;19(1):17–26.

# 3.12 Distal femur

Jong-Keon Oh, Christoph Sommer

## 1 Introduction

Poor bone quality due to osteoporosis creates significant surgical challenges both in fracture reduction and stabilization of distal femoral fractures (DFFs) (**Case 1: Fig 3.12-1**):

- Fracture margins are often too fragile to manipulate directly without further breakage. Reduction clamps can penetrate the bone, making reduction and maintenance quite difficult.
- Provisional fixation often fails.
- Achieving stability, especially around the distal condylar area, is difficult.
- Pronounced varus and anterior angulation malalignment in older patients cause implant-bone mismatch, reduce fixation strength in plating, and makes nailing cumbersome.

Surgeons need to be aware of these difficulties in reduction and fixation when they plan preoperatively. Pitfalls and technical tips to overcome these challenges will be discussed, together with illustrative cases.

CASE 1

**Patient**

A 73-year-old woman sustained a simple spiral distal femoral fracture (DFF) (AO/OTA 33A2.1) after getting up from the floor (**Fig 3.12-1a–b**). She lived alone in an apartment and walked with a cane.

**Comorbidities**

- Osteoarthritis of both knees
- Untreated osteoporosis

**Treatment and outcome**

The fracture was reduced with a collinear clamp, but the fracture gap was still visible. There was no further attempt to anatomically reduce the fracture due to concerns about further bone fractures (**Fig 3.12-1c–d**). The collinear clamp hindered plate positioning (**Fig 3.12-1e**). The fracture was preliminarily fixed with two positioning screws across the fracture site. Washers were used due to poor bone quality. The reduction was not anatomical (**Fig 3.12-1f–h**). Further reduction with the hammer was needed and further adjustment in the coronal plane was performed with the pulling device (whirly-bird) and the less invasive stabilization system (**Fig 3.12-1i–k**). The follow-up x-rays at 18 months after plating showed solid healing with abundant callus bridging, which means the screws did not have real purchase. All seven screw holes at the plate head were filled with locking head screws due to significant osteoporosis (**Fig 3.12-1l–m**).

**Discussion**

Standard minimally invasive plate osteosynthesis technique can be applied in the management of the osteoporotic DFF. It is necessary to create a balanced, flexible fixation construct with proper working length over the fracture span. Placing screws across the fracture level is not routinely recommended as it may hinder fracture-site motion and in turn fracture healing. The immediate intraoperative loss of reduction after insertion of two positioning screws illustrates technical problems at the osteoporotic metaphyseal bone.

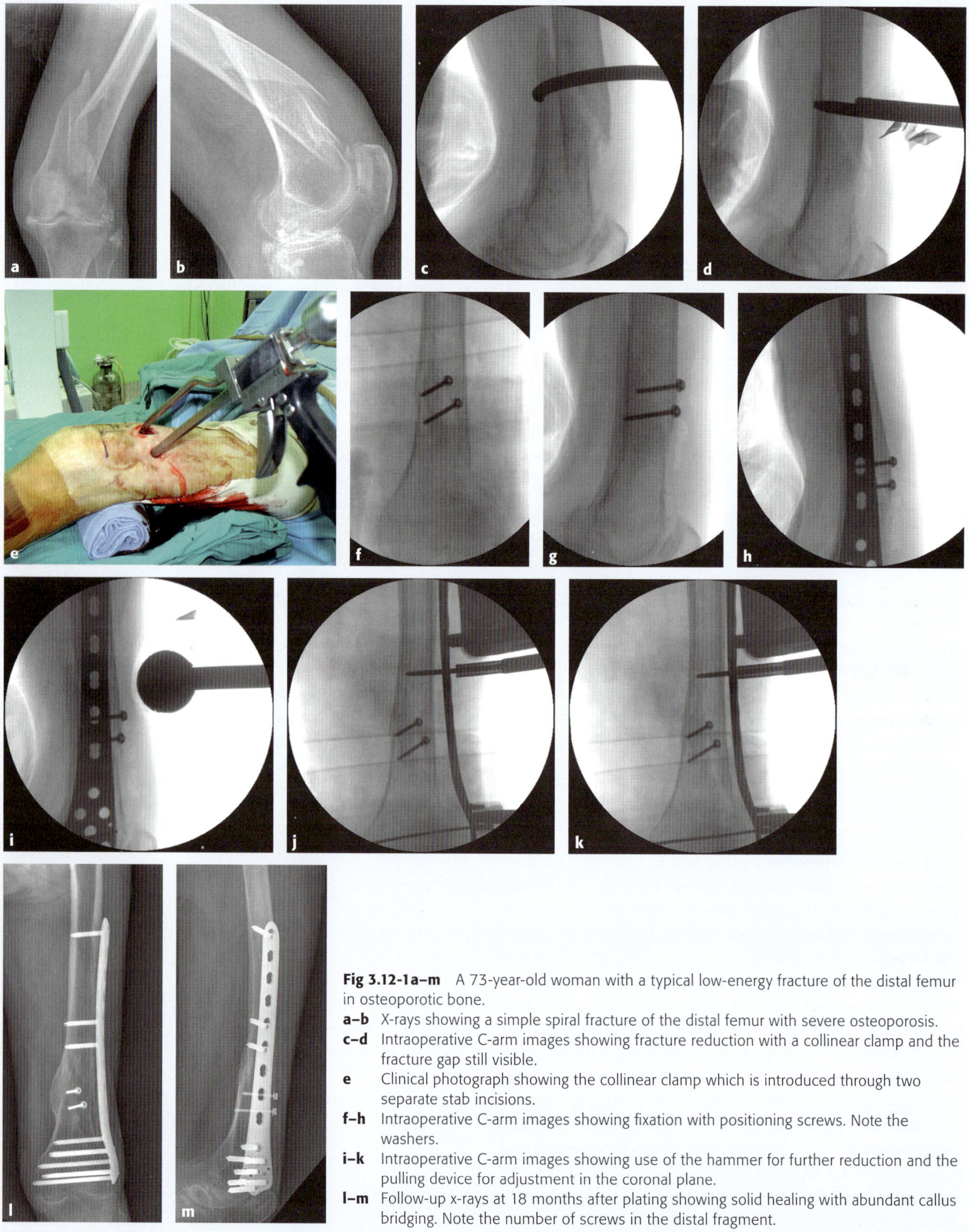


**Fig 3.12-1a–m** A 73-year-old woman with a typical low-energy fracture of the distal femur in osteoporotic bone.
**a–b** X-rays showing a simple spiral fracture of the distal femur with severe osteoporosis.
**c–d** Intraoperative C-arm images showing fracture reduction with a collinear clamp and the fracture gap still visible.
**e** Clinical photograph showing the collinear clamp which is introduced through two separate stab incisions.
**f–h** Intraoperative C-arm images showing fixation with positioning screws. Note the washers.
**i–k** Intraoperative C-arm images showing use of the hammer for further reduction and the pulling device for adjustment in the coronal plane.
**l–m** Follow-up x-rays at 18 months after plating showing solid healing with abundant callus bridging. Note the number of screws in the distal fragment.

## 2 Epidemiology and etiology

Distal femoral fractures represent about 3% of all femoral fractures. They occur in older adults mostly in osteoporotic bone after low-energy trauma and are more common in women (female:male ratio is 2:1). Mean age at fracture is 61 years, with patients older than 65 years in more than half of the cases [1].

## 3 Diagnostics and classification

AP and lateral x-rays of both femurs, including the adjacent joints, must be obtained in addition to well-dedicated views of the knee joint. Computed tomographic (CT) scans are indicated in the following scenarios:

- Intraarticular fracture to assess articular involvement
- Extraarticular fractures when they are mainly centered around the supracondylar area

The Unified Classification System (UCS) has gained popularity among surgeons in recent years. For more information on the UCS, see chapter 3.14 Periprosthetic fractures around the knee and Schütz and Perka [2].

## 4 Decision making

While there is little uncertainty about the necessity of the surgical fixation of DFF even in older patients, there are controversies about the procedure choice between plating and nailing.

Lateral locked plating has been the dominant fixation option for the past 20 years. Retrograde nailing has become more common recently because of improved design and better fixation options around the distal fragment. To improve distal fixation on osteoporotic bone, it is recommended to use the blade and angular stable locking system (ASLS) which enables surgeons to achieve an angular stable construct in osteoporotic bone. Some DFFs at the metadiaphyseal junction can be treated with antegrade nailing [2].

A nail can be inserted through incisions even smaller than those associated with minimally invasive plate osteosynthesis (MIPO) plating. This is especially true in morbidly obese patients. Nails are centrally located and therefore potentially load sharing with a better fatigue life under bending forces than lateral locked plating.

The decision making should be tailored to each fracture and each patient. It also depends on the surgeon's experience and preference. In general, there are certain factors favoring locked plating:

1. In very distal fractures, a locking plate offers the insertion of more screws, ie, at least four to five are necessary, compared to the two to three locking bolts of a nail.
2. In osteoporotic bone, a plate with many locking screws (up to seven) in the distal bloc provides stronger anchorage than a nail with two or three locking bolts or one blade with one or two locking bolts. The risk of cut-through into the joint is less in a locking plate compared to a nail, where the protruding nail can damage intraarticular structures like the patellar intercondylar notch and/or the cruciate ligaments (see **Case 4: Fig 3.12-4j–l**).
3. A torsional fracture pattern in osteopenic bone with a large medullary canal is better stabilized by a locked plate. A nail can toggle easily due to a loose fit in this large cavity, although the stability might be improved by using blocking screws at the correct position in the metaphysis.
4. A periprosthetic or periimplant fracture sometimes does not allow for the use of a nail and therefore requires a locking plate. In particular, an in situ proximal femoral nail or stem should be overlapped more than 7 cm with a distal femoral locked plate. A retrograde nail, nearly touching the proximal nail, should be avoided (see **Case 6: Fig 3.12-6**).

On the other hand, a more proximal fracture at the metadiaphyseal junction, a more oblique or transverse fracture pattern, and good bone quality are factors favoring a nail as primary implant of choice.

## 5 Preoperative planning

Patient positioning, specific reduction technique, and step-by-step description of the whole procedure should all be planned when either nailing or plating (**Case 2: Fig 3.12-2**). Considerations include:

- Selecting the proper length of the implants.
- In periprosthetic fractures with possible loosening, revision prosthesis should be available.
- The type of femoral component in total knee arthroplasty (TKA) should be carefully examined. Closed box-type femoral components preclude retrograde nailing and also limit the locking screw placement to the distal fragment in lateral locked plating. Variable angle locking function is typically beneficial in this situation.

- In retrograde nailing, the size of the distal fragment should be carefully examined to estimate the number of interlocking screws/blades that can be placed.
- In both plating and nailing, separate lag screws for the Hoffa and sagittal plane articular fractures should be placed carefully so as not to interfere with either locking screws for the plating or interlocking screws/blade in nailing.
- The nail insertion depth is based upon the distal fragment size. Underinserting a nail can result in catastrophic articular destruction of the patellofemoral joint, and overinserting a nail may cause the interlocking screw to get too close to the facture site, leaving distal fixation suboptimal.

CASE 2

### Patient

A 70-year-old physically fit and independent woman had a fall on an inclined road. She had undergone total knee replacement 3.5 years prior to injury and has taken oral bisphosphonates for the last 4 years.

### Comorbidities

- None

### Treatment and outcome

The initial x-rays showed a Unified Classification System B1 stable prosthesis (**Fig 3.12-2a–b**). The anterior cortical wedge (**Fig 3.12-2b**) resulted in a secondary notching effect on the femoral component.

The patient was set up and both legs draped, which facilitated lateral imaging and assessment of rotational alignment (**Fig 3.12-2c**). A bump was placed under the distal femur to lessen the flexion deformity of the distal fragment and length was restored with gentle manual traction. Then, sagittal plane reduction was done with leverage technique using the Cobb elevator. The anterior cortical wedge was lifted simultaneously with the Cobb elevator (**Fig 3.12-2d–e**).

Once the sagittal plane alignment was reduced, proper plate length was determined to allow the plate to splint the entire femur and prevent a future fracture around the plate tip and the proximal femur. The plate was inserted through the lateral incision with assistance from the image intensifier. This provisional elastic plate positioning at both ends of the plate would later allow for minor adjustment in alignment and even plate positioning. The final adjustment in the coronal plane was done with a collinear clamp introduced through the separate incision in the middle. Then the locking screws were placed accordingly with working length and screw densities kept in mind.

To accommodate the trochanteric ridge, the plate was bent at the tip (**Fig 3.12-2f–i**). The plate position was checked and provisionally attached to the main fragments with K-wires through the drill sleeve, attached to the plate.

X-rays taken 2 years after plating showed soild healing with good alignment (**Fig 3.12-2j–k**) and with a balanced bridge plating construct with proper working length and screw density at the proximal fragment (4/9 = 0.44).

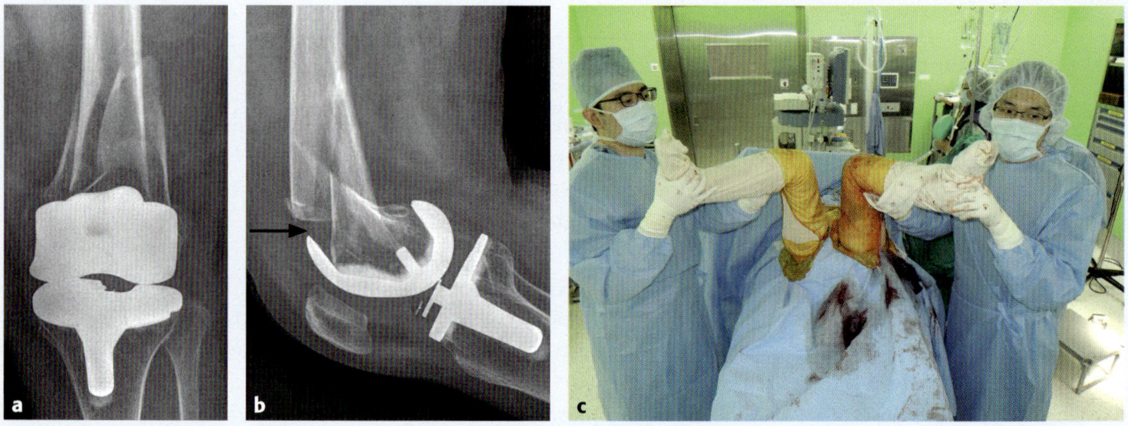


**Fig 3.12-2a–k** A 70-year-old woman with a distal femoral periprosthetic fracture with multiple wedges.
**a–b** Initial x-rays showing a Unified Classification System B1 stable prosthesis. The anterior cortical wedge (arrow in **b**) results in a secondary notching effect on the femoral component.
**c** Setting up the patient for surgery. Note the symmetrical internal rotation of both hips that indicates proper rotational alignment.

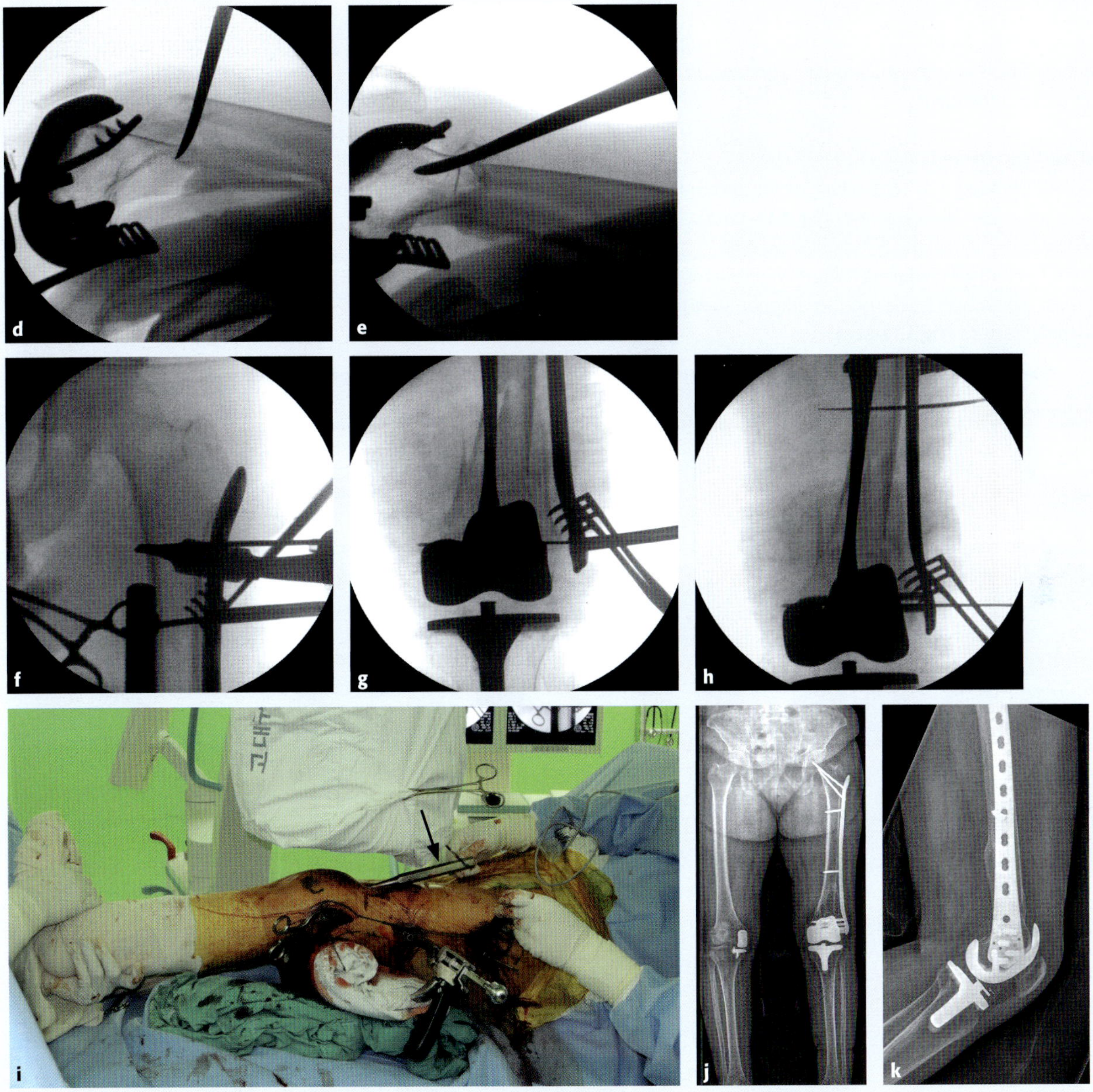

**Fig 3.12-2a–k (cont)** A 70-year-old woman with a distal femoral periprosthetic fracture with multiple wedges.
**d–e** Intraoperative C-arm images showing sagittal plane reduction with leverage technique using the Cobb elevator.
**f–i** Intraoperative C-arm images showing the plate bent at the tip to accommodate the trochanteric ridge (**f–h**), proximal shaft fragment drawn to the plate with collinear clamp to adjust the coronal alignment (**h–i**), and plate provisionally attached to the main fragments with K-wires through the drill sleeve (white arrows in **i**). The Cobb elevator used for leverage is indicated with a black arrow (**i**).
**j–k** X-rays 2 years after plating showing solid healing with good alignment. Note the anterior cortical wedge healed in reduced position in comparison to the initial x-ray.

CASE 3

## Patient

A 63-year-old woman slipped on a wet floor sustaining a distal femoral fracture. She has been treated for hypertension but was otherwise fit and independent.

## Treatment and outcome

The initial x-rays showed a spiral fracture of the distal diaphysis extending into the metadiaphyseal level (**Fig 3.12-3a–b**).

The main spiral fracture was reduced, using a Weber clamp through a small incision which was made on the anterior surface at the level of the spiral fracture (**Fig 3.12-3c–e**).

The x-rays taken 9 months after nailing showed complete healing with callus bridging in good alignment. The angular stable locking systems (ASLSs) were used for distal interlocking. Placing of an ASLS to the dynamic hole may not be recommended routinely as there is no evidence to support this modification. The entire femur was successfully splinted in this patient to prevent future fractures around the hip joint (**Fig 3.12-3f–g**).

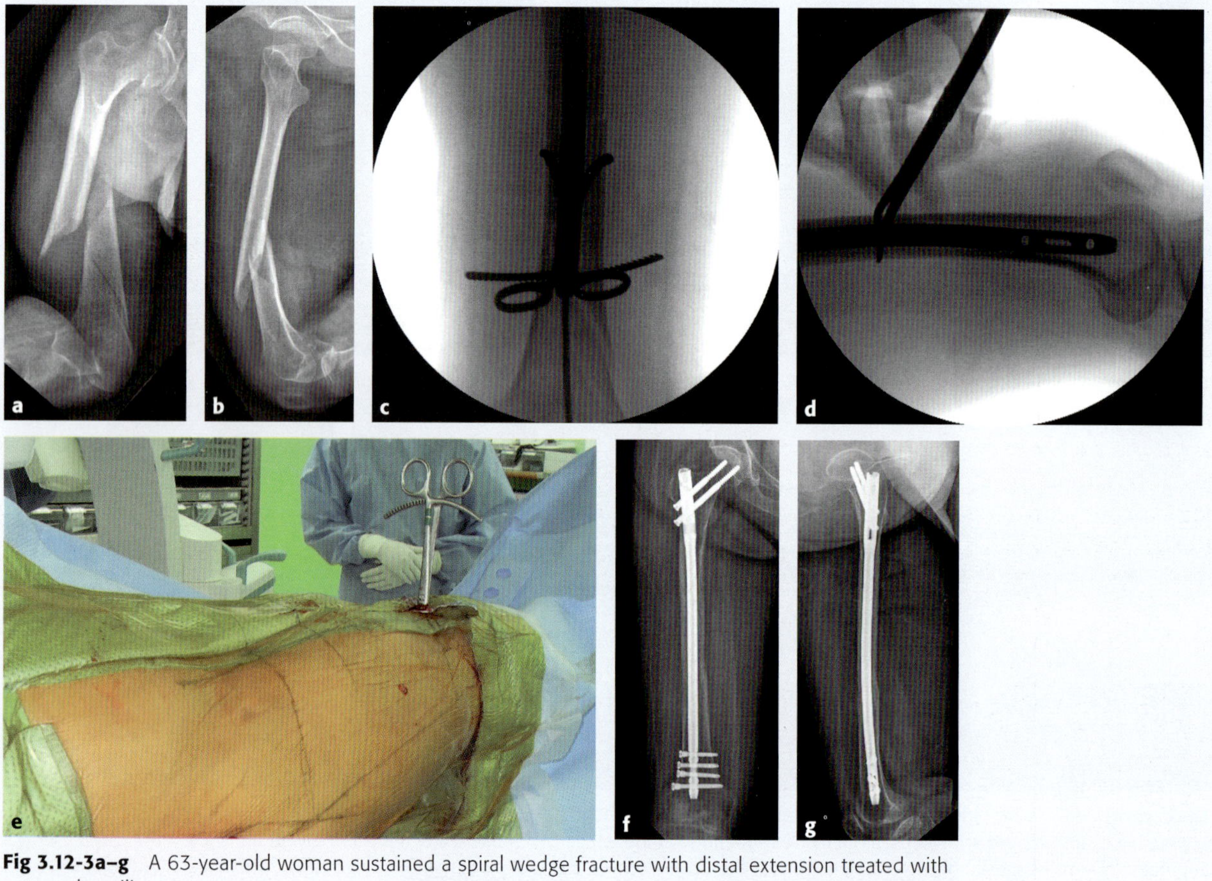


**Fig 3.12-3a–g** A 63-year-old woman sustained a spiral wedge fracture with distal extension treated with antegrade nailing.
**a–b** X-rays showing a spiral fracture of the distal diaphysis extending into the metadiaphyseal level.
**c–e** Reduction of the main spiral fracture with a Weber clamp inserted through a small incision.
**f–g** Nine-month follow-up x-rays showing complete healing with callus bridging in good alignment.

## Patient

A 90-year-old woman was living independently in an apartment with stairs, able to ambulate independently without walking aids. When she fell after slipping on the wet ground, she sustained a distal femoral and two stable lumbar spinal fractures.

## Comorbidities

- Arterial hypertension
- Vascular disease including bilateral moderate stenosis of carotid arteries
- Previous osteoporotic fractures of both distal radii. Osteoporosis treated with vitamin D3 and calcium for more than 10 years and with bisphosphonates for 5 years.

## Treatment and outcome

The patient sustained a distal torsional diaphyseal femoral fracture with a nondisplaced and possibly incomplete fissure line towards the intercondylar notch. A computed tomographic scan was not performed but would have been necessary to document the full extension of this fissure line (**Fig 3.12-4a–c**).

Intraoperative image intensification demonstrated a complete but nondisplaced fissure line into the joint. Prior to insertion of the central guide wire, a large reduction forceps was applied percutaneously to prevent a displacement of this fissure. The wire had to be placed correctly in the center of the intercondylar notch in both planes, which was in line with the femoral shaft (**Fig 3.12-4d–e**).

Retrograde nailing with a distal femoral nail was performed (**Fig 3.12-4f–g**). The nail was a bit short but seemed sufficient in this case due to quite thick cortical bone in the diaphysis. The more osteoporotic the bone, the longer the nail should be to prevent a future femoral fracture at the proximal end of the nail. Distal locking was performed with a locking bolt and a spiral blade, as recommended for osteoporotic bone. Importantly, the distal end of the nail was well below the cartilage surface of the intercondylar notch. This was visualized in the lateral view (**Fig 3.12-4i**), where the distance between the so-called Blumensaat's line (red dotted line in **Fig 3.12-4h–i**) and the nail should be at least 5–10 mm. It is important to get a true lateral view, which is best obtained intraoperatively under image intensification. Only then can the distance between the end of the nail and the bone surface be assessed properly. The postoperative x-rays are often not true lateral (as in this case) and therefore do not allow a perfect visualization of this important detail. In cases of severe osteoporosis, there is a risk of a slow ongoing cut-through process of the locking blade/bolt through the femoral metaphysis with secondary penetration of the nail into the knee joint .

The x-rays of a different 75-year-old woman (**Fig 3.12-4j–l**) show that the nail had moved distally by cut-through of the two locking bolts through the osteoporotic bone. The nail protruded into the intercondylar notch anteriorly (Blumensaat's line, red dotted line in **Fig 3.12-4k**) and damaged the cartilage of the patella (red dotted arrow in **Fig 3.12-4l**). This complication could have been avoided by inserting the nail initially well below the Blumensaat's line and by using a spiral blade distally with less risk of cut-through (**Fig 3.12-4i**).

The 4-month x-rays showed a healed situation and unchanged position of the nail and locking implants (**Fig 3.12-4m–n**). The patient was walking around pain free and nearly as well as before the injury. Further follow-up was not planned and implant removal was not advised.

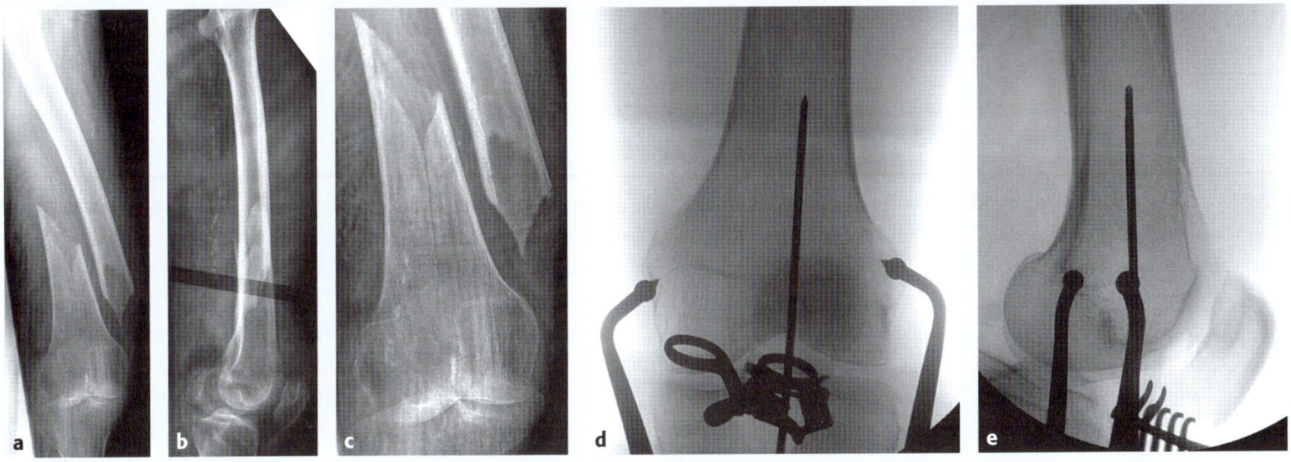


**Fig 3.12-4a–n** A 90-year-old woman with a distal diaphyseal torsional fracture in osteoporotic bone.
**a–c** X-rays showing a distal torsional fracture of the femur with a nondisplaced and possibly incomplete fissure line toward the intercondylar notch.
**d–e** Intraoperative image intensification demonstrating a complete but nondisplaced fissure line into the joint.

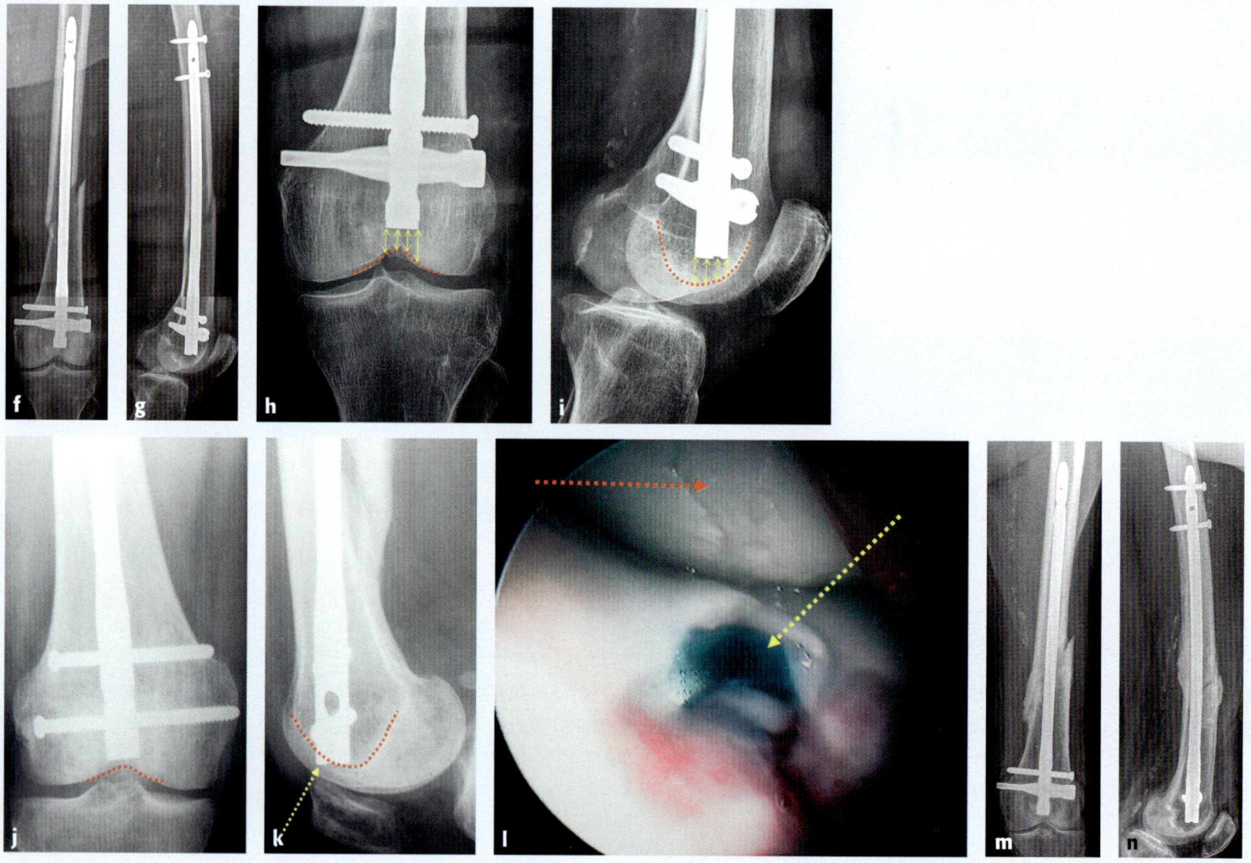


**Fig 3.12-4a–n (cont)** A 90-year-old woman with a distal diaphyseal torsional fracture in osteoporotic bone.
**f–i** Postoperative x-rays after retrograde nailing with a distal femoral nail.
**j–l** X-rays (of a different patient) showing the nail having moved distally by cut-through of the two locking bolts through the osteoporotic bone, having protruded into the intercondylar notch anteriorly (Blumensaat's line, red dotted line in **k**) and then damaged the cartilage of the patella (red dotted arrow in **l**).
**m–n** The 4-month follow-up x-rays showing healed fracture and unchanged position of the nail and locking implants.

## 6 Surgical techniques for reduction and fixation

In general, early definitive fixation as soon as medically optimized is preferable, as immobilization with skeletal traction in older patients frequently induces other complications such as deep vein thromboembolism, muscle wasting, pressure ulcers, and loss of functional status.

### 6.1 Reduction

In general, the authors aim for correct functional alignment (length, rotation, and axis in both planes). This can mostly be achieved in a minimally invasive fashion using different indirect and direct reduction tools and tricks.

In a simple fracture pattern, as is often the case in low-energy fractures in osteoporotic bone, the goal of functional alignment corresponds to a (near) anatomical reduction. Furthermore, we know from experience that simple fractures treated with an implant providing relative stability must be accurately reduced without larger interfragmentary gaps or distraction. This is true for bridge plating as well as for nailing. With a nail fitting well in the small intramedullary canal, this reduction occurs automatically by virtue of the nail itself. But since in most osteoporotic bones the medullary canal is much wider than the chosen nail (especially in fractures at the metadiaphyseal junction), the fracture must be reduced prior to nail or plate insertion. In long spiral or oblique fracture patterns, percutaneously applied cerclage wires and/or reduction forceps allow for minimally invasive (near) anatomical reduction, independent of the chosen implant (nail or plate) (**Case 1: Fig 3.12-1, Case 3: Fig 3.12-3**). These maneuvers must be done gently and are usually combined with indirect reduction techniques such as manual traction on the leg and/or the use of distraction devices as femoral distractor or temporary external fixator.

In more complex fracture patterns, these tools do not help and the reduction is usually achieved over the implant itself. Details are mentioned in the following subchapters.

### 6.1.1 Flexion/extension

For correct alignment, the radiographic shape of the opposite leg is very helpful. Usually, if the leg is positioned horizontally, hyperextension occurs by pulling the gastrocnemius muscles on the distal femur. A roll under the knee (resulting in slight knee flexion) helps to prevent this malalignment. As in all minimally invasive plating procedures, the plate is first aligned in the periarticular (distal) part centrally on the bone and fixed with an initial screw. The next step is the alignment of the other plate end centrally onto the bone and, after correct length and rotation are confirmed, fixation of the plate to the bone either with a drill bit or K-wire (left in situ) or a definitive screw. With a second (preliminary) fixation distally (K-wire or drill bit), a relatively stable situation is achieved, which allows the surgeon to clinically check the flexion/extension accuracy by gently lifting the leg at the foot and extending the knee using the gravity. A straight knee then confirms the correct alignment in this lateral aspect. This has to be compared to the healthy opposite leg (to check for preexisting hyperextension). If a sagittal malalignment is detected, it can be corrected by rotating the distal articular bloc around the already inserted distal central interlocking screw. This can be achieved manually by bending or extending the fracture over a rolled towel until correct alignment is reached. Only then are further screws applied distally as well as proximally.

Aneja et al [4] described the following operative technique to address the problems in controlling the flexion deformity of the distal articular block with a Schanz screw placed in the sagittal plane. Once the articular reduction is done, the compression screws are placed bicortically and 0.5 mm apart in the sagittal plane. Following reconstruction of the articular block, a 4 mm Schanz pin is unicortically placed between the two bicortical screws in an anterior-to-posterior direction on the condylar segment. The Schanz pin is then levered up to correct the sagittal plane deformity. This creates a stronger lever arm construct that can be used to reduce the osteoporotic distal bone fragment with less risk of the Schanz pin wallowing out or even cut-out.

### 6.1.2 Varus/valgus

Malalignment in the frontal plane is common. It can be prevented in light of the fact that in most preshaped distal femoral locking plates the central screw has a fixed angle of 95° in relation to the plate. Aligning this screw parallel to the distal femoral joint line, which connects the lateral and the medial condyles, ensures a correct axial alignment. Before drilling for this first central distal screw, correct parallelism has to be checked. This axis can also be assessed using the so-called cable method, ie, using the electrocautery cable and image intensification to assess a straight line from the center of the femoral head over the center of the knee to the center of the ankle. Malalignment of the distal femur to the plate in this aspect has to be corrected prior to drilling for the first central screw. This can be done either manually by valgus or varus pressure of the lower leg or by an inserted Schanz screw in the distal articular bloc, which can ideally be placed from medially, to avoid interfering with the laterally placed plate.

### 6.1.3 Length alignment

The primary goal is to achieve correct femoral length. In simple fracture patterns, especially short oblique or transverse fractures, the assessment of correct length is easily done by image intensifier control at the fracture site. In long spiral or comminuted fractures, image intensification does not help much and an unacceptable length discrepancy can occur when relying on x-ray alone. In this situation, the length has to be checked with the opposite leg/femur using first the clinical aspect (full leg length) and better, under image intensification with the use of a semiradiolucent ruler. This instrument is usually used in nailing procedures but can also be stored in the hospital separately in a sterile package. In certain rare circumstances, a slight shortening of the fracture zone may be an option (see topic 6.2.1 in this chapter).

### 6.1.4 Rotational alignment

Rotational malreduction is one of the most common technical errors in MIPO of the distal femur [5] and radiographic and clinical assessment is necessary to avoid it. Both assessments are done after preliminary distal and proximal fixation of the implant, still allowing easy correction if necessary. Radiographically, the aspect of the proximal femur of the contralateral side is compared to the injured side in the same

AP projection of the distal femur (patella must be placed centrally). The aspect/size of the lesser trochanter is specifically used for comparison ("trochanter sign"). Clinically, the amount of rotational movement of the femur in a 90–90° position (hip and knee flexed in a right angle) is compared again to the contralateral healthy side (**Case 2: Fig 3.12-2c**).

At the end of the surgery, this rotation is clinically checked again. If there is any doubt about the rotational alignment, the authors advise a postoperative CT scan for measurement. A rotational malalignment of > 10–15° is an indication for operative correction if it is clinically noticeable. Correction is best done soon after primary surgery (days later).

## 6.2 Minimally invasive lateral plating

Lateral locked plating for osteoporotic distal femoral periprosthetic fractures is a viable option if the principles of biological plating are carefully applied with the technical details kept in mind [6, 7].

The minimally invasive plating concept and surgical techniques can also be applied in periprosthetic fractures with osteoporosis. The locking attachment plate improves stability by tangential bicortical locked fixation [8].

### 6.2.1 Primary shortening using lateral plating

Although the usual goal of functional alignment is to achieve correct length, rotation, and axis in both planes, it may be helpful to slightly shorten the fracture zone intentionally. In the case of a small bone defect, especially in an open fracture or a comminution zone, the fracture heals faster and more substantially when it is shortened (**Case 5: Fig 3.12-5**).

CASE 5

#### Patient

An 81-year-old woman living independently in an apartment had a simple fall resulting in a low-energy trauma. She sustained a distal intraarticular femoral fracture (second degree open anterolateral) and lost about 1 L of blood at home. She was hemodynamically stable at the emergency department.

#### Comorbidities

- Arterial hypertension
- Osteoporosis known for 6 years and treated with bisphosphonates (alendronate) over a 5-year period (currently stopped)

#### Treatment and outcome

The x-rays showed a distal femoral fracture with simple articular extension (split in the middle) and metaphyseal comminution (AO/OTA 33C2). Some detached small fragments lay in the subcutaneous area close to the anterolateral wound (second degree open fracture) (**Fig 3.12-5a–b**).

In anticipation of more blood loss, the patient received preoperative blood transfusion and had close monitoring for postoperative anemia. Goal hemoglobin levels in the postoperative geriatric patient are 8 gm/dL or higher, as long as the patient is not symptomatic or unstable. A lateral subvastus approach was performed with debridement of damaged muscle and removal of all devascularized (ie, fully detached) bony fragments, followed by jet lavage using 6 L of saline (**Fig 3.12-5c–e**). The size of the anterior bone defect was decreased by a slight shortening of the femur (about 1 cm). No bone graft was used. The two most proximal screws were placed percutaneously (**Fig 3.12-5c**).

After 2 months (**Fig 3.12-5f–g**), nice bridging callus formation medially and posteriorly was visible, which allowed the patient to fully bear weight (**Fig 3.12-5f–g**). The femur was well aligned and slightly shortened (1 cm) with a remaining semicircular anterior bone defect. The fracture had been bridged (relative stability) with as many screws distally as possible (the plate could have been placed slightly more proximally and anteriorly, which would have allowed for the insertion of even more screws). The plate length was at its minimum: The plate-span ratio (ie, length of plate to length of fracture) should be at least 3. Here it might have been 2.5. The bridging length was correct, with the inner screws as close to the fracture as possible. The number of the proximal screws was also kept to the minimum. Three bicortical locking head screws are usually sufficient in moderate to good bone quality in the diaphysis, as was true in this case. After 3.5 months (**Fig 3.12-5h–i**) increasing bridging callus was visible. The patient was pain free under full weight bearing when using a walking aid. Therefore, no further follow-up was planned.

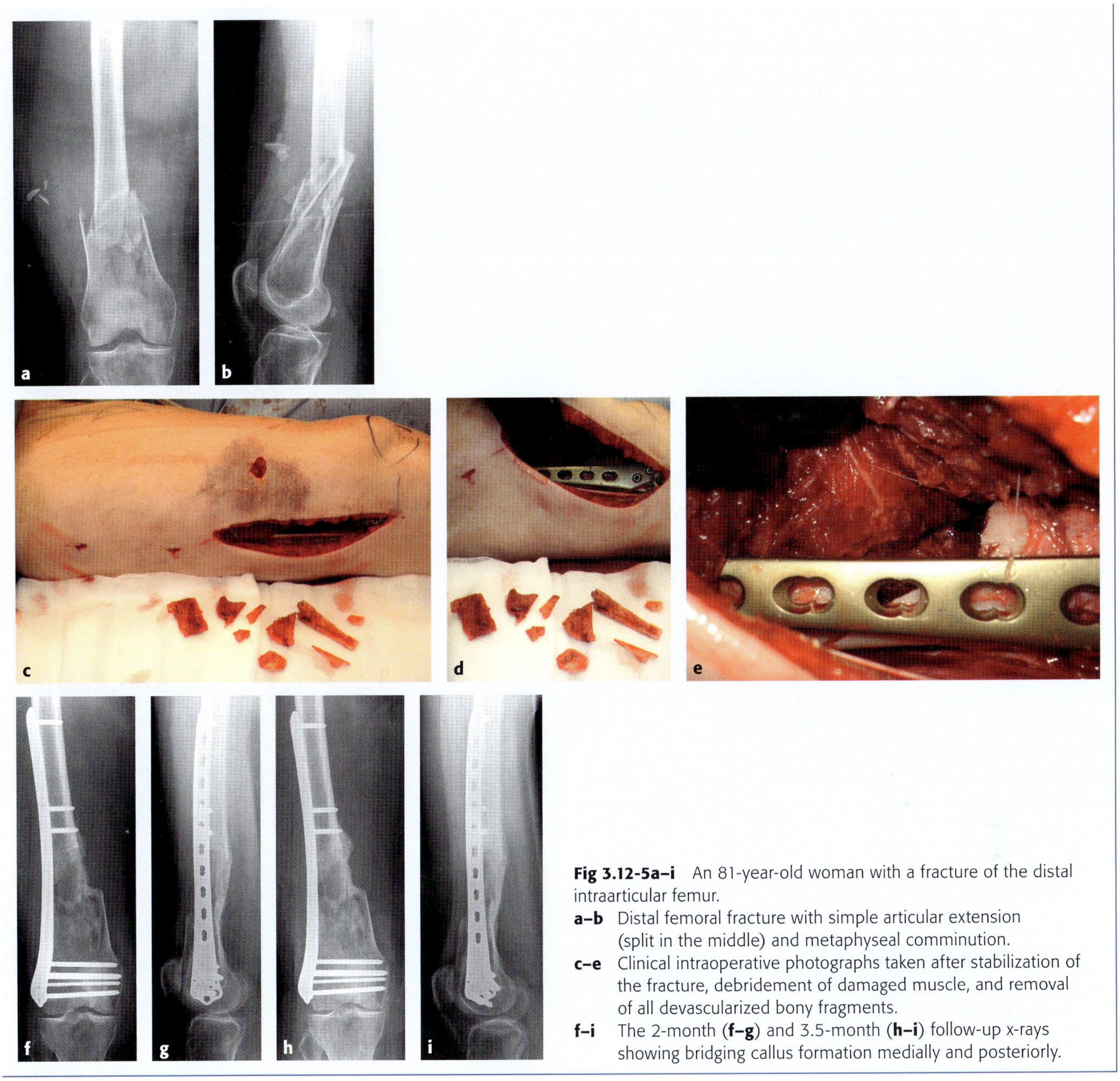

**Fig 3.12-5a–i** An 81-year-old woman with a fracture of the distal intraarticular femur.
**a–b** Distal femoral fracture with simple articular extension (split in the middle) and metaphyseal comminution.
**c–e** Clinical intraoperative photographs taken after stabilization of the fracture, debridement of damaged muscle, and removal of all devascularized bony fragments.
**f–i** The 2-month (**f–g**) and 3.5-month (**h–i**) follow-up x-rays showing bridging callus formation medially and posteriorly.

### 6.2.2 Use of counter-nuts

In the case of a very distal fracture or extreme osteoporosis, the mechanical fixation of the lateral locked plate can be increased using counter-nuts with washers or small plates (as washers) onto the distal screws medially. A similar technique was described by Garnavos et al [9] using independent compression bolts combined with retrograde nailing (**Case 6: Fig 3.12-6**).

CASE 6

## Patient

An 83-year-old woman was living at home with daily nursing help. Walking was severely impaired but still possible on flat ground inside the house with a walking aid. She fell after slipping on a carpet and sustained a distal femoral fracture (DFF). Three years after total hip arthroplasty (THA) and 10 years after a femoral shaft fracture, the DFF healed in 15° of varus. Osteoarthritis was radiographically severe but mildly symptomatic with tolerable pain. Primary replacement instead of osteosynthesis could have been a choice if the symptom (pain) would have been severe before this injury.

## Comorbidities

- Severe osteoporosis for more than 30 years, treated with vitamin D3, calcium (orally), and bisphosphonates for more than 5 years
- History of multiple osteoporotic fractures over these 30 years (ie, right proximal tibia, left distal radius, right distal femur, left distal radius)
- Ten years previously, the patient had survived a central pulmonary embolism with cardiopulmonary resuscitation; since then, she was on long-term warfarin

## Treatment and outcome

Conventional x-rays showed a distal intraarticular, bicondylar femoral fracture, probably simple intraarticular and extraarticular with extreme osteoporosis and THA in situ. There was a history of diaphyseal fractures with malunion in varus position and severe degenerative knee osteoarthritis (**Fig 3.12-6a–c**).

Computed tomographic scans with 2-D reconstruction demonstrated this 3-part fracture that was very distally located with separation of both condyles through the intercondylar notch. No additional fracture in the frontal plane (Hoffa fracture) was visible (**Fig 3.12-6d–g**).

Counter-nuts ± washer are available for different screw types, such as "old" nuts for traditional 4.5 mm cortex screws (**Fig 3.12-6h**) and "new" nuts for 5.0 mm locking head screws (**Fig 3.12-6h–i**).

The 6-month postoperative x-rays showed a healed situation with intact and stable implants (**Fig 3.12-6j–k**). The DFF was well aligned and fixed with a long reversed distal femoral locking compression plate (LCP-DF) 4.5/5.0, which was bent intraoperatively to better fit the varus-deformed diaphysis. It was overlapping the tip of the proximal stem sufficiently (more than 7 cm is recommended). Distally, the intercondylar fracture plane was first compressed over the plate using three cortex screws in the most distal plate holes with old counter-nuts on the medial side. To the most distal screw a washer was applied; to the next more proximal screws a one-third tubular plate (three holes) was added. Both washer and the small plate sank below the bone surface when tightening the screws due to the extreme osteoporosis (for details see also **Fig 3.12-6l**). The patient regained her preinjury level of impaired walking and implant removal was not advised.

The compressive effect by adding the counter-nuts is better visible in **Fig 3.12-6l–m**. As a rule, the compression has to be achieved first, and only then are locking screws applied to keep this compression and to provide angular stability along the plate. Counter-nuts can be applied on both sides, medially and laterally, depending on the location of the screw insertion (**Fig 3.12-6m**, different patient).

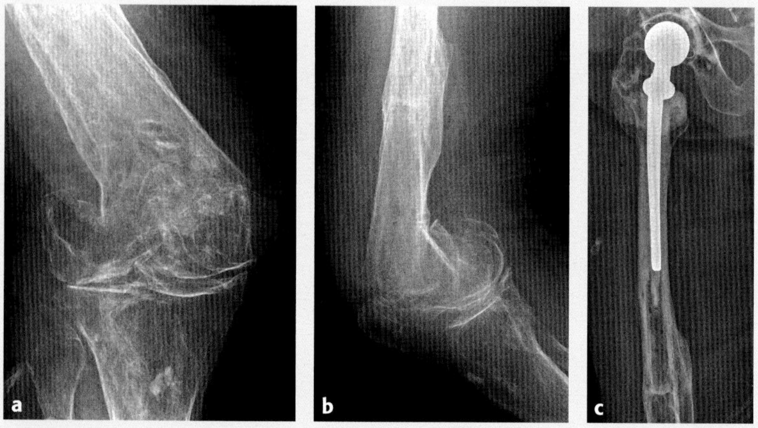


**Fig 3.12-6a–m** An 83-year-old woman with a distal fracture in severely osteoporotic bone.
**a–c** X-rays showing a distal intraarticular, bicondylar fracture of the femur.

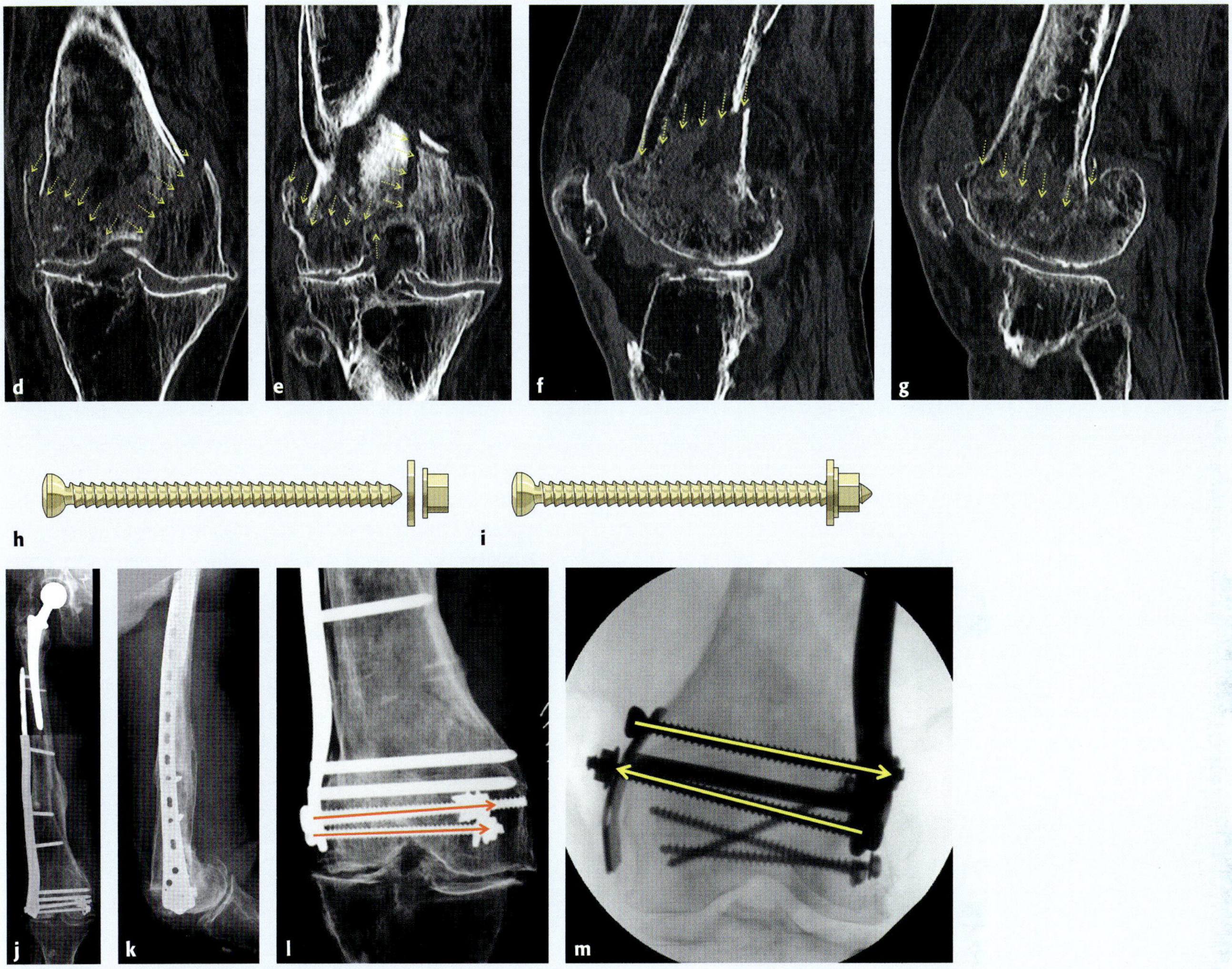


**Fig 3.12-6a–m (cont)** An 83-year-old woman with a distal fracture in severely osteoporotic bone.
**d–g** Very distally located 3-part fracture with the intercondylar notch separating both condyles.
**h–i** Different counter-nuts and washer for different screw types.
**j–k** The 6-month follow-up x-rays showing a healed and well-aligned fracture with intact and stable implants.
**l–m** Conventional x-rays showing the compressive effect by adding the counter-nuts medially and/or laterally.

## 6.3 Medial plating

Most of the DFFs are successfully managed with lateral locked plating alone when plating is chosen (**Case 7: Fig 3.12-7**). Some selective cases need double plating which will be discussed in topic 6.4 of this chapter. There is one specific fracture pattern that may benefit from medial plating. This may be called a "reverse obliquity fracture" of the distal femur. We believe this specific fracture pattern needs special attention by the surgeon as lateral locked plating frequently leads to failures.

CASE 7

### Patient

A 76-year-old woman sustained a distal femoral periprosthetic fracture after a simple fall at home. She had undergone bilateral total knee arthroplasty 15 years ago and was able to ambulate independently with a cane.

### Comorbidities

- None

### Treatment and outcome

The level of fracture was very low, involving the bed of the prosthesis (Unified Classification System type B). The fracture line ran obliquely from the medial metadiaphyseal junction almost down to the lateral epicondylar level, and the distal fragment was displaced superomedially due to the pull of adductor muscles. This fracture orientation leaves limited space for screw placement to the articular fragment without crossing the fracture line.

The cluster of locking screws from the head of the lateral locked plate needs to resist the significant pull-out deforming force if lateral locked plating is chosen (**Fig 3.12-7a–b**). The bone stock and quality in the condylar area were very poor.

This specific fracture pattern poses a risk of failure by pulling out of all locking screws together with the plate distally when it is fixed with a lateral locked plating alone (similar to **Case 9: Fig 3.12-9a–q**).

Considering all these risk factors, the authors recommend the stronger biomechanical option of positioning the plate on the medial side, because there is little pull-out stress on the plate head and more pull-out resistance at the shaft level where the bicortical purchases are possible.

A medial subvastus approach was performed to expose the fracture site directly. The prosthesis was tested and looked stable (**Fig 3.12-7c**), and direct anatomical reduction was achieved with a collinear reduction clamp (**Fig 3.12-7d**). Neutralization plating was done with a reverse proximal tibial variable locking plate and a separate lag screw was placed posterior to the plate. A longer plate length than originally planned was chosen to address this diaphyseal extension (**Fig 3.12-7e–f**). Stability was good enough to allow immediate joint motion. Range of motion exercises with continuous passive motion was commenced 3 days after plating (**Fig 3.12-7g–h**). Follow-up x-rays taken 4 months after plating showed solid union. Primary healing took place at the diaphyseal linear fracture line (**Fig 3.12-7I–j**).

### Discussion

It is critical to recognize this specific fracture pattern as a reverse oblique distal femoral fracture because it carries high risk of failure if treated with lateral locked plating alone.

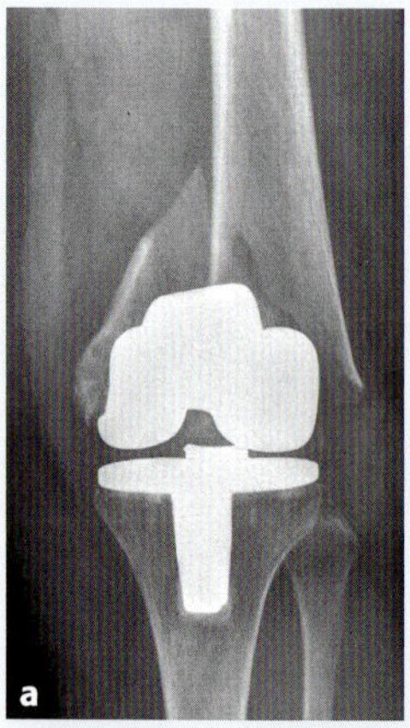
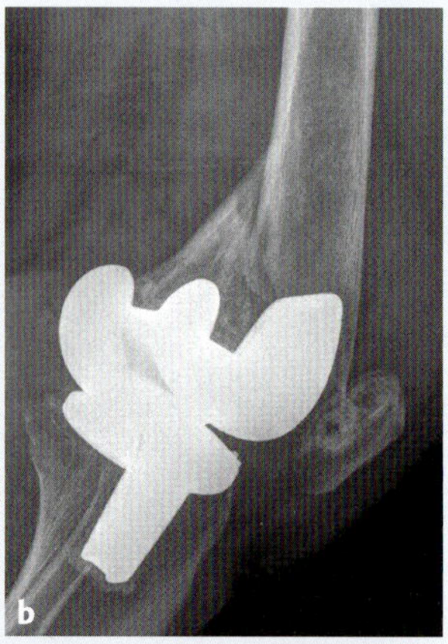
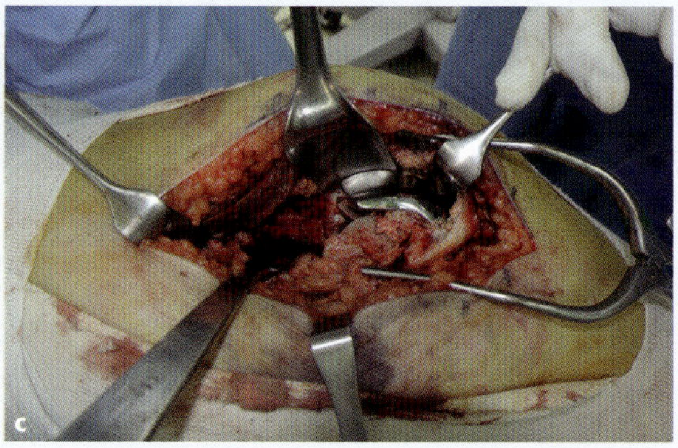
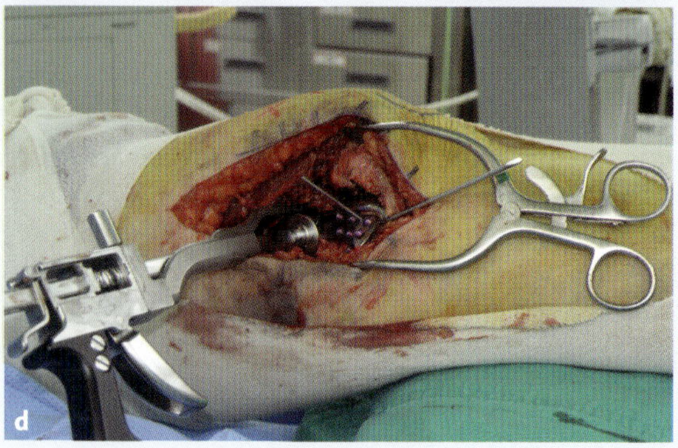

**Fig 3.12-7a–j** A 76-year-old woman with a distal femoral periprosthetic fracture (Unified Classification System type B).
**a–b** X-rays showing a simple oblique periprosthetic distal femoral fracture. The direction of displacement is superomedial.
**c** Intraoperative photograph showing the medial side of the fracture and the prosthesis through the medial subvastus approach.
**d** Intraoperative photograph showing the reduction and plate positioning using a collinear clamp. A reverse proximal tibial variable locking plate was used.

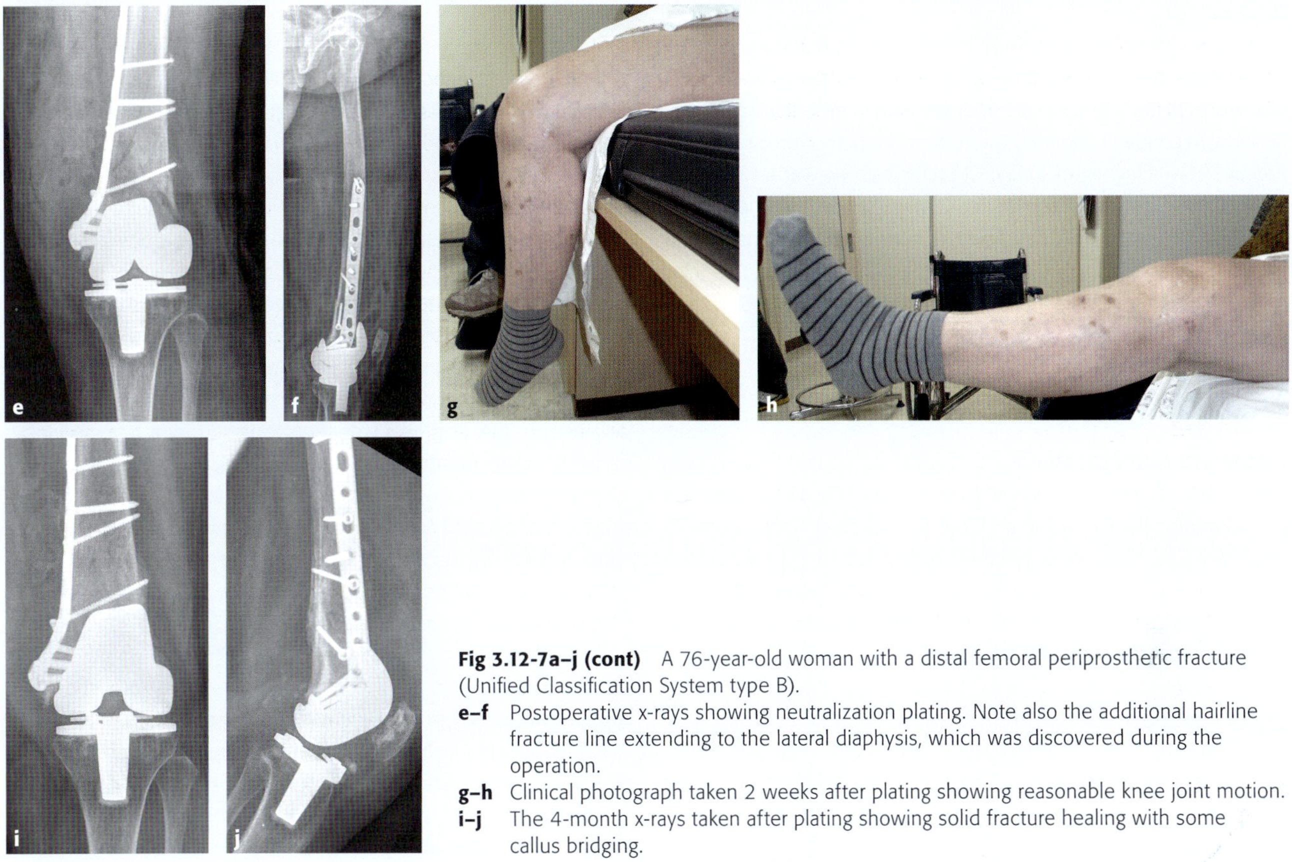

**Fig 3.12-7a–j (cont)** A 76-year-old woman with a distal femoral periprosthetic fracture (Unified Classification System type B).

**e–f** Postoperative x-rays showing neutralization plating. Note also the additional hairline fracture line extending to the lateral diaphysis, which was discovered during the operation.

**g–h** Clinical photograph taken 2 weeks after plating showing reasonable knee joint motion.

**i–j** The 4-month x-rays taken after plating showing solid fracture healing with some callus bridging.

## 6.4 Double plating

A second small medial plate helps with reduction and fixation of very distal intraarticular (and extraarticular) fractures especially in poor quality bone. Preexisting knee flexion impairment after a previous injury can cause difficulty in treating very distal flexion type fractures (**Case 8: Fig 3.12-8**).

CASE 8

## Patient

A 56-year-old active and athletic man fell down the stairs, landing on his flexed knee, sustaining a very distal intraarticular femoral fracture (AO/OTA 31C3). One year previously the patient had sustained a bicondylar multifragmented intraarticular proximal tibial fracture from a high-speed ski injury. This fracture was successfully treated in the authors' hospital in a 2-stage procedure and double plating. A recent follow-up before the current fall demonstrated a well-healed fracture but an obviously limited flexion up to 110° and marked osteopenic bone.

## Comorbidities

- Healthy man but a heavy smoker (35 pack years)

## Treatment and outcome

Conventional x-rays demonstrated the injury (**Fig 3.12-8a–b**), the postoperative (**Fig 3.12-8c–d**) and 9-month follow-up (**Fig 3.12-8e–f**) situations of the ipsilateral proximal tibial fracture the patient had sustained 1 year before the new ipsilateral distal femoral fracture. Due to a long period of limited weight bearing, the bone showed severe osteopenia at the last follow-up.

Conventional x-rays showed a very distal Y-shaped intraarticular distal femoral fracture in valgus deformity due to a lateral metaphyseal comminution (**Fig 3.12-8g–h**). Both condyles were separately fractured and flexed. On the lateral side, a possible nondisplaced Hoffa component was suspected. Consolidated proximal tibial fracture with intact bone and implants is also visible. The bone structure was rarified with very thin cortical bone at the femur and tibia as well as tiny subchondral bone lamella.

After performing a lateral and medial subvastus approach, the medial condyle was first reduced by indirect and direct maneuvers and preliminarily fixed with two K-wires. Reduction was assessed visually and controlled by image intensification. First, a slightly contoured locking compression plate (LCP) T-plate 3.5 was placed at the apex of the fracture of the medial condyle and fixed with a cortical screw in a buttress (or antiglide) function (**Fig 3.12-8i–j**). After image intensifier control of the ideal position, it was definitively fixed with two monocortical locking head screws in the distal diaphysis. The condyle itself was also addressed with two screws. Due to the very poor bone quality, only locking screws could be used to prevent a very early loss of fixation (**Fig 3.12-8k–l**). Only then was the lateral condyle assessed: There was no Hoffa component detected intraoperatively. The disrupted line described above in the injury picture (**Fig 3.12-8h**) corresponded to a localized stable edgy impaction of the cartilage and underlying bone. Therefore, an additional AP fixation (or posterolateral plate) was not necessary. The definitive stabilization to the diaphysis was then achieved by a reversed distal femoral locking compression plate (LCP-DF) 4.5/5.0 in a submuscular minimally invasive technique. The plate was aligned correctly which was checked by a K-wire inserted through an inserted drill threaded drill sleeve into the most distal central hole. This wire has to be parallel to the horizontal joint line in the AP view (**Fig 3.12-8m**). The small intracondylar articular step was accepted.

Intraoperative x-rays at the end of the surgery are shown in **Fig 3.12-8n–o**. Except for the small intracondylar step, the fracture was anatomically reduced and correctly aligned. The main lateral plate (LCP-DF) was slightly too anterior, but the three screws in the diaphysis had been confirmed to be bicortical. Distally, as many screws as possible were placed to optimize the fixation to the articular block in this poor quality bone. Additional augmentation by bone cement did not seem to be necessary and was not intended in this middle-aged male patient.

The 5-month follow-up x-rays show the healed fracture in the same position as the postoperative and stable implants (**Fig 3.12-8p–u**). The bone density was improving. The patient could fully bear weight but could only walk for 15 minutes due to severe muscular atrophy in the thigh. Range of motion was 3–0–100°.

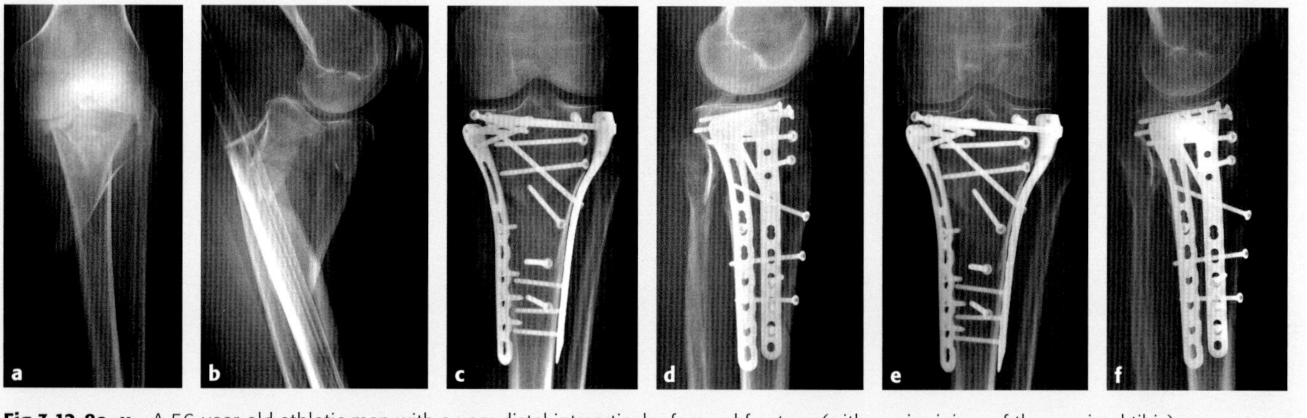


**Fig 3.12-8a–u** A 56-year-old athletic man with a very distal intraarticular femoral fracture (with a prior injury of the proximal tibia).
**a–f** Injury (**a–b**), postoperative (**c–d**), and 9-month follow-up (**e–f**) x-rays of the ipsilateral proximal tibial fracture.

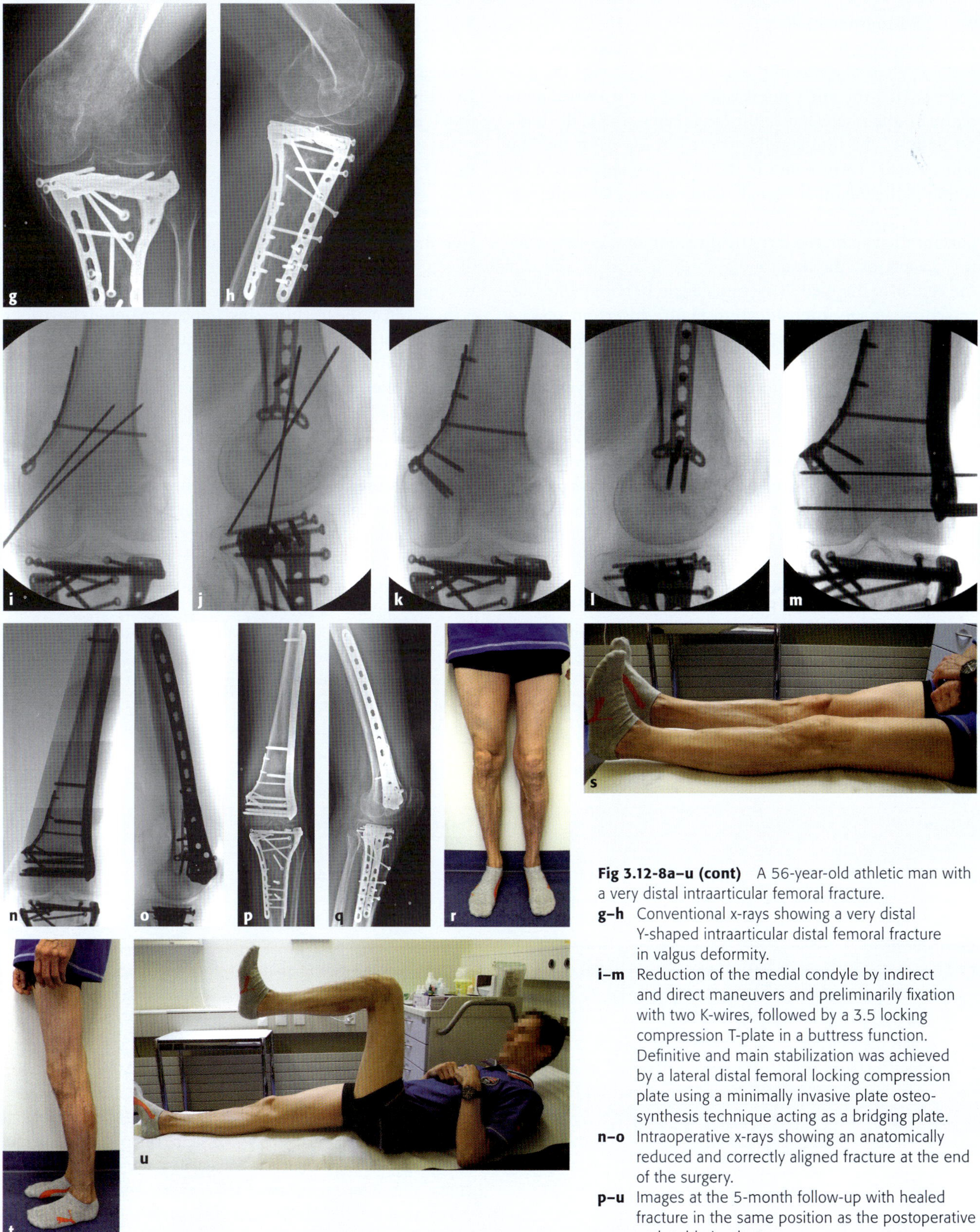


**Fig 3.12-8a–u (cont)** A 56-year-old athletic man with a very distal intraarticular femoral fracture.

**g–h** Conventional x-rays showing a very distal Y-shaped intraarticular distal femoral fracture in valgus deformity.

**i–m** Reduction of the medial condyle by indirect and direct maneuvers and preliminarily fixation with two K-wires, followed by a 3.5 locking compression T-plate in a buttress function. Definitive and main stabilization was achieved by a lateral distal femoral locking compression plate using a minimally invasive plate osteosynthesis technique acting as a bridging plate.

**n–o** Intraoperative x-rays showing an anatomically reduced and correctly aligned fracture at the end of the surgery.

**p–u** Images at the 5-month follow-up with healed fracture in the same position as the postoperative and stable implants.

### 6.5 Retrograde nailing

As with nailing of other anatomical areas, making the correct entry portal is one of the most critical parts of the procedure. First the entry point is located at the lowest point of the Blumensaat's line in the lateral view and at the highest point of the intercondylar notch in the AP view. This point usually corresponds to the distal prolongation of the center of the medullary canal in both planes. Once the correct entry point is found with the guide wire, similar importance has to be given to the direction of the wire when it is drilled into the distal metaphysis: It must be aimed at the center of the medullary canal again in both planes, assessed by image intensification before insertion (**Case 4: Fig 3.12-4**). Only then can the portal be created by drilling with the corresponding cannulated drill bit over the guide wire. The fracture reduction is then usually achieved either by the inserted nail itself (in unreamed nailing technique) or by the inserted long guide wire for reaming in case of reamed nailing. With a correct entry portal, the axial alignment is automatically given over the nail. Correct rotation and length still have to be assessed and corrected when the nail is inserted, using the different tricks mentioned above.

### 6.6 Antegrade nailing

As mentioned in **Case 3: Fig 3.12-3**, some DFFs at the metadiaphyseal junction can be treated with antegrade nailing especially with the help of ASLS [3].

## 7 Failures and nonunions

Locked plating of the distal femur with excessively rigid constructs has been recognized as a cause of impaired healing [10]. It is important to make the balanced bridge plating construct with proper working length and screw density (**Case 9: Fig 3.12-9**, **Case 10: Fig 3.12-10**).

Various mechanical factors that may cause nonunion after DFF fixation have been reported. Mechanical factors that dictate the rigidity of the construct may indirectly influence the mechanical impact on the healing environment, which is the strain at the fracture gaps. Implant materials have long been a point of controversy as to whether they affect fracture healing. Gaines et al [11] reported that the lateral locked plating with titanium plate yielded lower nonunion rates compared to the lateral locked plating with the stainless plate. In a recent multicenter study retrospectively analyzing the results of lateral locked plating of DFFs, Rodriguez at al [12] proposed a rigidity score concept. In this scoring system, the use of a stainless steel plate has two advantages. In their study, the primary significant independent predictor of nonunion was plate design/material. Fixation crossing the fracture was correlated with a higher rate of nonunion, but it did not reach statistical significance. The authors reported no significant differences with respect to number of proximal screws, plate length, total screw density, or proximal screw density, between healed fractures and those with nonunion. Oh et al [13] also reported that a screw across the fracture site can be a cause for nonunion by hindering fracture-site motion.

**CASE 9**

#### Patient

A 64-year-old woman fell down stairs and sustained bilateral interprosthetic distal metaphyseal femoral fractures. She was receiving long-standing calcium and vitamin D supplements for osteoporosis.

#### Comorbidities

- A 35-year history of rheumatoid arthritis treated with corticosteroids for more than 20 years; now she is taking additional immunosuppressive medication
- Diabetes mellitus and obesity (body mass index 31)
- Previous surgeries included bilateral total hip arthroplasty (THA) 15 years ago, and bilateral total knee arthroplasties (TKA) 11 years ago

#### Treatment and outcome

The x-rays showed a distal femoral fracture above a stable TKA (confirmed with a computed tomographic [CT] scan) with severe metaphyseal comminution (AO/OTA 33A3) (**Fig 3.12-9a–b**). The marked thinning of the cortical bone at the distal metaphysis and shaft suggested poor local bone quality in that region, although the authors did not have objective bone density measurements at that time.

Stabilization was achieved using a reversed distal femoral locking compression plate 4.5/5.0 inserted with a minimally invasive plate osteosynthesis technique (**Fig 3.12-9c–d**). Distally, as many screws as possible were inserted in the weak bone and proximally, a minimal number of screws were used, with an additional locking attachment plate around the tip of the stem. There was a slight medial offset probably due to the forced shortening of the fracture. Stress concentration was avoided by overlapping the plates over the stem of the THA by 3–4 cm, although this was less than the desirable overlap length of > 6 cm.

After 6 months, x-rays showed a secondary loss of reduction without evidence of bony healing, necessitating a reoperation despite the absence of pain and instability (**Fig 3.12-9e–f**). The distal bone-screw interface failed due to the poor bone quality.

The CT scan demonstrated the medial shift of the distal femur in relation to the distal end of the plate (**Fig 3.12-9g–h**). The knee prosthesis still seemed to be stably anchored. There were minimal signs of bone healing, possibly due to the immunosuppressive medication. There will be a need for bone grafting at revision surgery.

Reoperation was performed in two stages. First, atrophic scar tissue from the delayed union site was excised for microbiological cultures leaving a large bone defect. All the distal locking head screws were removed without changing anything proximally (**Fig 3.12-9i**). This allowed for reduction of the distal joint block to the plate. A second plate (reversed anterolateral proximal tibial locking compression plate 3.5) was inserted percutaneously on the medial side from distal to proximal. After preliminary supracondylar fixation with a 3.5 mm locking head screw, a large reduction clamp was placed onto both plates (acting as large washers) to accomplish the final reduction (**Fig 3.12-9j**).

X-rays taken after the 2-stage revision surgery (**Fig 3.12-9k–n**) showed that all the distal screws had been augmented with polymethylmethacrylate (red cylinders in **Fig 3.12-9m–n**). Six days after the first surgery, after receiving negative tissue culture results, the large bone defect was filled with a mixture of autogenous bone graft (from posterior iliac crest) and allograft (green area in **Fig 3.12-9m–n**).

Only 16 months after injury (and 10 months after revision) the patient was pain free and ambulated using only two elbow crutches, similar to her prefracture function (**Fig 3.12-9o–q**). The fracture was healed in good alignment, and the prostheses and implants appeared radiographically stable. Implant removal was not advised.

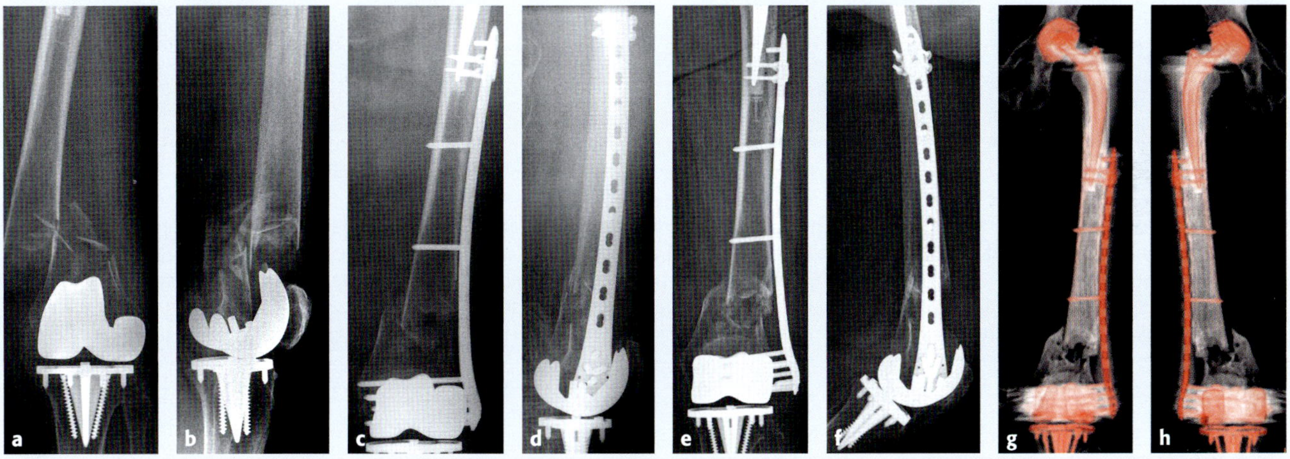


**Fig 3.12-9a–q** A 64-year-old woman with bilateral interprosthetic distal metaphyseal femoral fractures.
**a–b** The x-rays showing a fracture of the distal femur with severe metaphyseal comminution above a stable total knee arthroplasty.
**c–d** Postoperative x-rays after stabilization with a reversed distal femoral locking compression plate 4.5/5.0.
**e–f** Six-month x-rays showing secondary loss of reduction without evidence of bony healing.
**g–h** Computed tomographic scans showing the medial shift of the distal femur in relation to the distal end of the plate but with knee prosthesis still stably anchored.

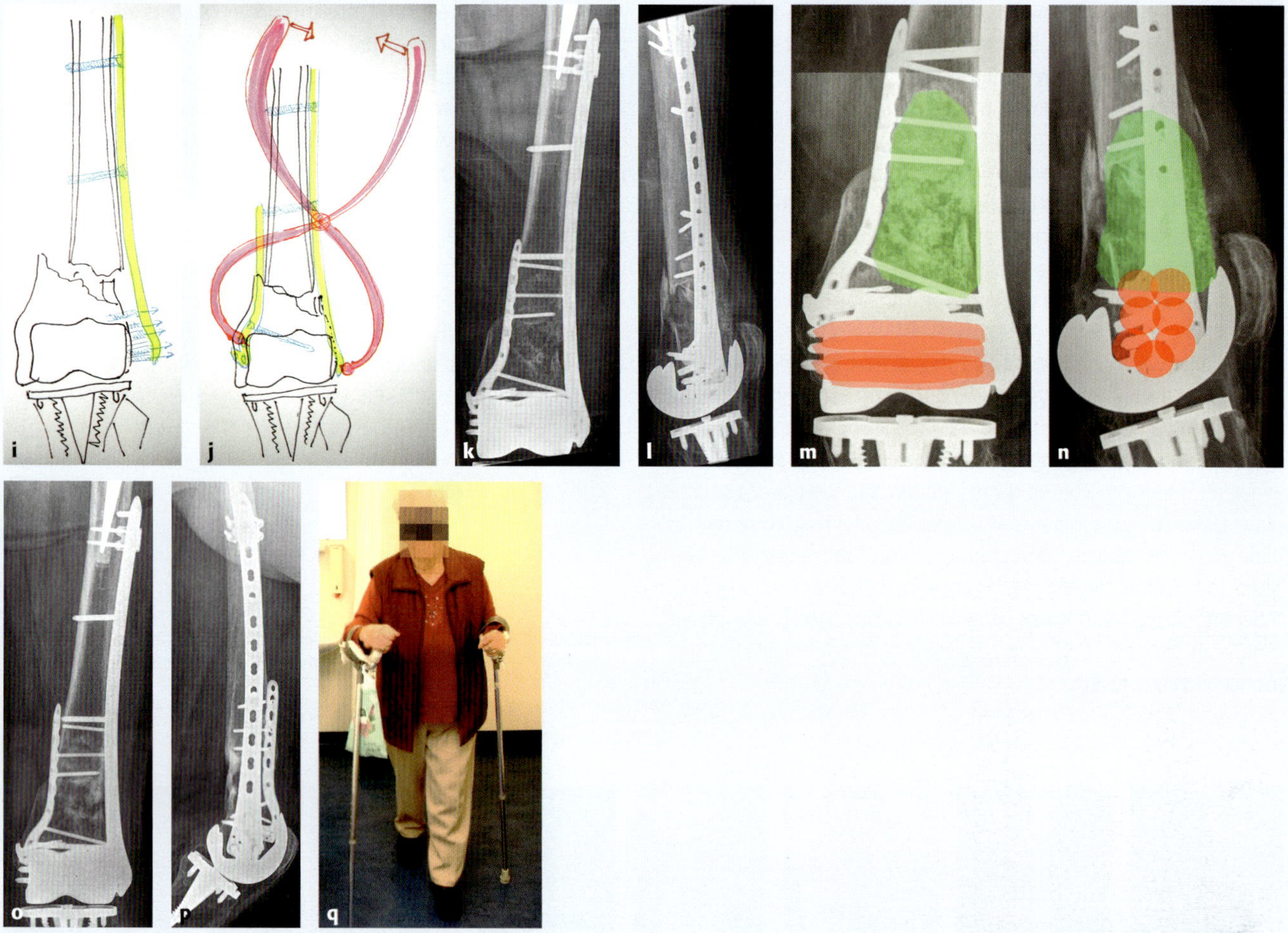

**Fig 3.12-9a–q (cont)** A 64-year-old woman with bilateral interprosthetic distal metaphyseal femoral fractures.
**i–j** Removal of all distal screws and achievement of fracture reduction using a large King-Kong forceps, medially placed onto a newly inserted small fragment locking compression plate (proximal lateral tibial plate) that is acting as a large "washer" to prevent the arm of the forceps sinking into the soft bone.
**k–n** Postoperative x-rays after the 2-stage revision surgery showing polymethylmethacrylate-augmented distal screws (red cylinders in **m–n**) and the large bone defect filled with a mixture of autogenous bone graft (from posterior iliac crest) and allograft (green area in **m–n**).
**o–q** Images taken 16 months after injury (and 10 months after revision) showing the healed and well-aligned fracture with radiographically stable prostheses and implants.

CASE 10

### Patient

A 70-year-old woman was injured in a car accident (low-speed frontal impact), sustaining an isolated closed left distal femoral fracture (DFF) with minor soft-tissue trauma and superficial abrasions over the patellar region. She was referred for evaluation the day after injury.

### Comorbidities

- None recorded

### Treatment and outcome

The x-rays showed a DFF with simple articular extension (split in the middle) and metaphyseal comminution (AO/OTA 33C2) (**Fig 3.12-10a–b**).

After stabilizing the fracture, a lateral minimally invasive plate osteosynthesis approach was performed without visualization of the fracture zone. Alignment was checked by intraoperative image intensification. On images **Fig 3.12-10c–d**, the valgus malalignment was not visualized intraoperatively, although it could have been detected primarily as demonstrated retrospectively (valgus 11°) (**Fig 3.12-10e**).

Five weeks after surgery, valgus malalignment was clinically obvious and documented on x-ray (**Fig 3.12-10f**). Preoperative planning for open-wedge correction was performed (**Fig 3.12-10g**): The mechanical axis crossed the lateral plateau 25 mm off the midline (red line). Anatomical axis (green line) using the opposite side (yellow line) indicated the desired position of the ankle. The level of the osteotomy was planned through the original, partially healed metaphyseal fracture. The center of rotation was drawn (blue circle) and the correction angle was 11°.

At the end of the revision surgery (**Fig 3.12-10h–k**), the existing less invasive stabilization system (LISS) plate was removed, intraoperatively bent 11° at the level of the planned open-wedge plane (red circle) and replaced using the same distal screw holes and screws (**Fig 3.12-10i** shows green line: original form of the LISS; red line: new form of the LISS after bending; blue circle: center of rotation using the soft bridging callus as a medial hinge). The correct axis at the end of the operation was assessed using the "cable-method" (**Fig 3.12-10h–j**). Under image intensifier control the electrocautery cable confirmed the inline position of the center of the femoral head, the knee, and the ankle. No bone graft was used.

After axial correction, postoperative x-rays were taken (**Fig 3.12-10l–m**). Radiographic and clinical outcomes 6 months after correction (**Fig 3.12-10n–p**) showed the healed fracture with only a small remaining lateral defect, which may fill up in coming months. Left leg length and axis were identical to the healthy right side. The patient complained of irritation of the iliotibial tract at the distal end of the plate. Implant removal was recommended no sooner than 1 year after this surgery.

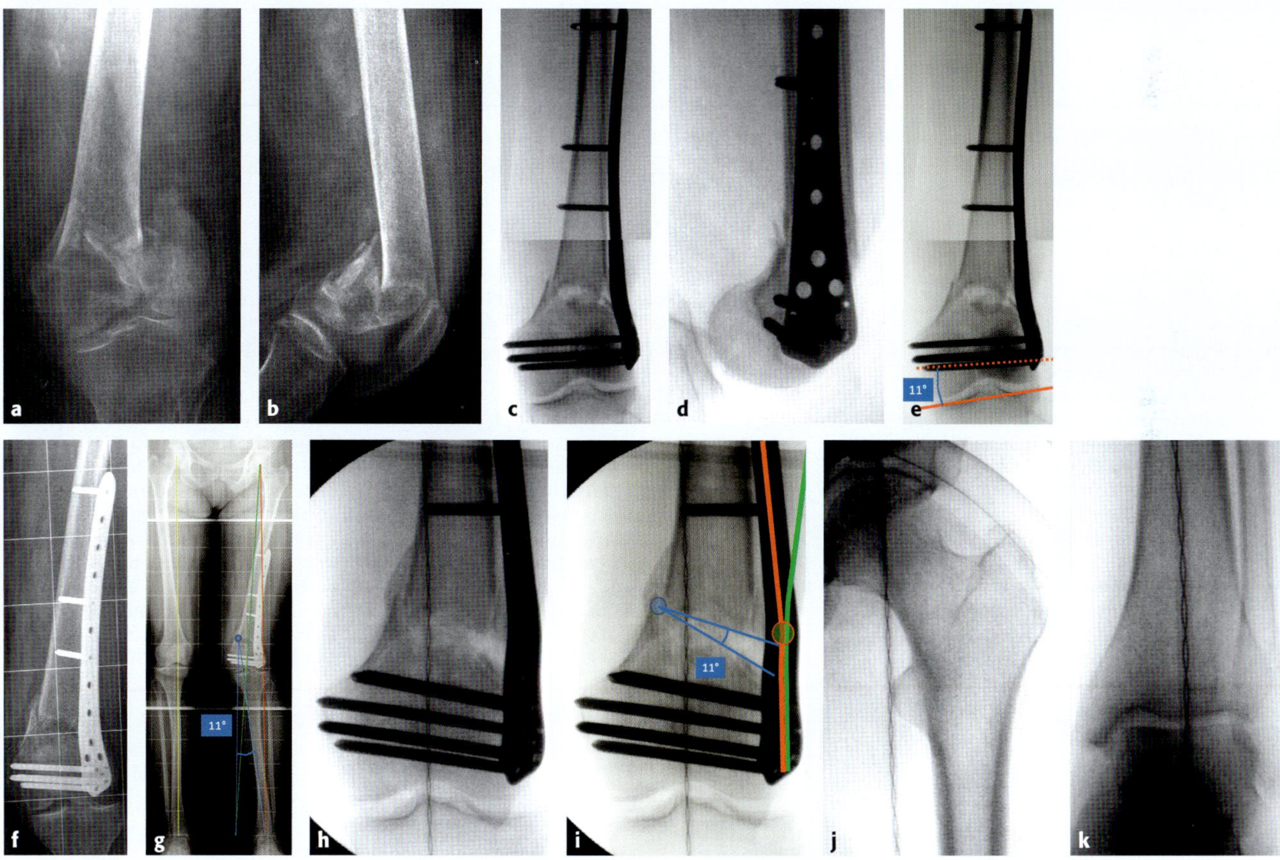


**Fig 3.12-10a–p** A 70-year-old woman with an isolated closed fracture of the left distal femur.
**a–b** X-rays of a distal femoral fracture with simple articular extension and metaphyseal comminution.
**c–e** Intraoperative x-ray after fracture stabilization showing valgus malalignment (valgus 11°) that was not detected during surgery.
**f–g** X-rays taken 5 weeks after surgery showing valgus malalignment.
**h–k** X-rays after revision surgery.

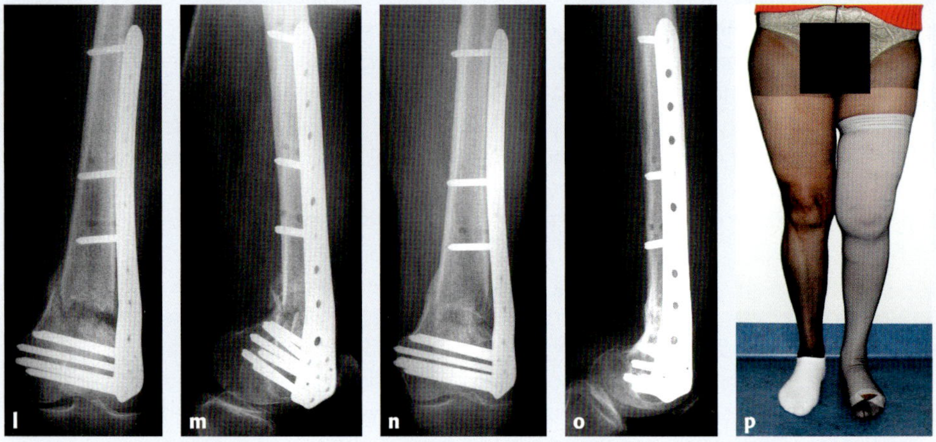


**Fig 3.12-10a–p (cont)** A 70-year-old woman with an isolated closed fracture of the left distal femur.
**l–m** Postoperative x-rays after axial correction.
**n–p** Radiographic and clinical outcome 6 months after correction.

## 8 References

1. **Court-Brown CM, Caesar B.** Epidemiology of adult fractures: a review. *Injury.* 2006 Aug;37(8):691–697.
2. **Schütz M, Perka C.** *Periprosthetic Fracture Management.* Stuttgart: Thieme Publishing; 2013.
3. **Zlowodzki M, Bhandari M, Marek DJ, et al.** Operative treatment of acute distal femur fractures: systematic review of 2 comparative studies and 45 case series (1989 to 2005). *J Orthop Trauma.* 2006 May;20(5):366–371.
4. **Aneja A, Brown JT, Graves M.** A stronger construct for manipulating osteoporotic bone fragments in a distal femur fracture model. *Tech Orthop.* 2015;30(2):125–130.
5. **Buckley R, Mohanty K, Malish D.** Lower limb malrotation following MIPO technique of distal femoral and proximal tibial fractures. *Injury.* 2011 Feb;42(2):194–199.
6. **Raab GE, Davis CM 3rd.** Early healing with locked condylar plating of periprosthetic fractures around the knee. *J Arthroplasty.* 2005 Dec;20(8):984–989.
7. **Ruchholtz S, Tomas J, Gebhard F, et al.** Periprosthetic fractures around the knee-the best way of treatment. *Eur Orthop Traumatol.* 2013 Jun;4(2):93–102.
8. **Lewis GS, Caroom CT, Wee H, et al.** Tangential bicortical locked fixation improves stability in Vancouver B1 periprosthetic femur fractures: a biomechanical study. *J Orthop Trauma.* 2015 Oct;29(10):e364–370.
9. **Garnavos C, Lygdas P, Lasanianos NG.** Retrograde nailing and compression bolts in the treatment of type C distal femoral fractures. *Injury.* 2012 Jul;43(7):1170–1175.
10. **Henderson CE, Lujan TJ, Kuhl LL, et al.** 2010 mid-America Orthopaedic Association Physician in Training Award: healing complications are common after locked plating for distal femur fractures. *Clin Orthop Relat Res.* 2011 Jun;469(6):1757–1765.
11. **Gaines R, Sanders R, Sagi H, et al.** Titanium versus stainless steel locked plates for distal femur fractures: is there any difference? *OTA Abstract.* 2008;55:8.
12. **Rodriguez EK, Zurakowski D, Herder L, et al.** Mechanical construct characteristics predisposing to non-union after locked lateral plating of distal femur fractures. *J Orthop Trauma.* 2016 Aug;30(8):403–408.
13. **Oh JK, Hwang JH, Lee SJ, et al.** Dynamization of locked plating on distal femur fracture. *Arch Orthop Trauma Surg.* 2011 Apr;131(4):535–539.

# 3.13 Periprosthetic fractures around the hip

Steven Velkes, Karl Stoffel

## 1 Introduction

Almost 60 years after Sir John Charnley established total hip arthroplasty (THA) as a procedure that can be performed safely and reproducibly, THA continues to keep its place among the leading operative procedures that afford a significant improvement in quality of life. The procedure has been labeled the "operation of the century" as a result of the relatively low complication rate versus the enormous gains in pain relief and function. Despite this, the procedure is not risk-free, and devastating complications can occur. One potential complication is fracture around the hip implant. In older adults, this complication is similar in morbidity, mortality, and functional impairment to fractures of the proximal femur. The ultimate outcome is typically inferior to revision hip arthroplasty for aseptic loosening or instability. The absolute numbers of THA continue to increase, with both younger active and older patients being offered the procedure. This has created a large pool of patients living with THA, with a related rise in number of patients who will suffer a periprosthetic hip fracture (PPHF) [1–5]. Factors associated with PPHFs include:

- Low-energy falls in older adults
- Osteoporosis
- High-energy trauma in younger active patients
- Revision arthroplasty techniques transferring energy to the tip of the implant stem, such as impaction allograft and cementless press-fit stems
- Cementless procedures in the older osteoporotic patients [6]
- Osteolysis associated with implant loosening
- Independent risk factors such as low body mass index, female gender, advanced age, and rheumatoid arthritis [3, 7, 8]
- Extruded cement and varus stem position [9–11]

Periprosthetic hip fractures can occur at the time of surgery or as a separate event many years later. Fractures during surgery occur in 1% of primary arthroplasties and up to 4% in revision arthroplasty; pathological bone (osteoporosis and osteolysis) have a confounding effect on the incidence. The management of these fractures in the older adult is extremely challenging given the medical fragility of the patient and the complexity of the decision-making and operative procedures involved. These patients demand a team approach, with internists, geriatricians, and arthroplasty and orthopedic trauma surgeons among the medical team members.

## 2 Diagnostics

### 2.1 Clinical evaluation

A detailed assessment of the patient prior to treatment is essential to maximize the chances of a good outcome. The basic diagnosis of PPHF relies on:

- Clinical history of the mechanism of injury (high-energy versus low-energy trauma)
- Pain
- Preinjury functional decline or joint pain. This may indicate loosening or infection. It is important to ask the patient about the function of the joint before the injury, was it a "happy joint" (ie, a joint that functions well with no pain) or not?

The initial examination should include:

- General skin condition and location of previous scars
- Examination of the knee
- Assessment of leg lengths
- Neurovascular status

## 2.2 Imaging

### 2.2.1 Plain x-rays

Images should be reviewed thoroughly to ascertain the type of fracture and the stability of the implant. It is one of the major challenges and tasks to find out if the implant is stable or not. Conventional x-rays should include the following high-quality views:

- AP pelvis, centered over the symphysis
- The affected hip joint in a second plane
- The whole femur in two planes. It is important that the full length of the femur is imaged and the x-rays scrutinized (both the stem and cup) to fully appreciate the entire extent of the fracture, as well as the presence, status, and type of any associated knee implants.

The following details need to be assessed:

- Total hip arthroplasty components for loosening. Careful assessment of the stability of implants in the femur and acetabulum
- Fracture location in relation to the type of implant. Depending on the type of stem, fracture location may indicate loosing even without clear signs of loosening [12].
- Acetabular wear signs
- Available bone stock

High-quality x-rays are essential to look for radiolucent lines around the prosthesis or cement, indicating periacetabular osteolysis. The magnification of the image can be measured by placing a radiopaque calibration object of known dimension at the same plane as the hip joint. If the size of the previously implanted femoral head or cup is known and the border clearly detectable, it can be used also as a scaling marker.

Additional important assessment features include:

- The fracture geometry and any change in implant positioning
- Proximal femoral varus remodeling (**Fig 3.13-1**)
- Femoral shaft deformity
- Presence of an implant below the hip implant, eg, a total knee implant of the revision type

Important factors which may influence the decision making for fracture fixation versus revision arthroplasty include polyethylene wear, acetabular shell position, large osteolytic lesions [13, 14], significant osteoporosis [3, 7], as well as debonding of the cement from the implant and/or extensive cement fracture [15].

### 2.2.2 Computed tomographic scan

More accurate assessment of fracture configuration, osteolysis, and visualization of radiolucent lines around the prosthesis or cement mantle can be made with computed tomography (CT). However the interpretation of some radiolucency around the stem must be made with caution as similar findings can be produced by artifact.

## 2.3 Chronic infection

Trauma and fracture can elevate inflammatory markers (ie, C-reactive protein, erythrocyte sedimentation rate, white blood cell count) making the positive predictive value of these tests for periprosthetic joint infection poor [16]. If the history or the x-ray is suspicious for a periprosthetic joint infection, further diagnostic tests such as bone scintigraphy or a joint aspiration should be performed. The joint aspiration needs to be done preoperatively under sterile conditions prior to skin incision, and may result in surgical delay. Joint aspiration results obtained after the patient has already received antibiotics need to be interpreted with caution as this may obscure identification of pathogens.

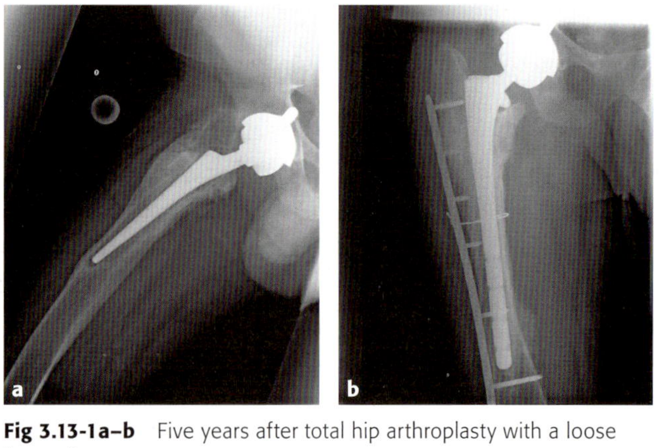


**Fig 3.13-1a–b** Five years after total hip arthroplasty with a loose femoral component.

- **a** Preoperative lateral view of the hip showing encroachment of stem to femoral cortex, a high-risk situation for false route, and femoral fracture at revision.
- **b** Postrevision view. As predicted, a false route occurred and the femoral fracture was fixed with a long elastic plate.

## 3 Classification

Many classification systems of PPHFs have been developed [17–21] but most are only descriptive or do not provide information regarding treatment strategy. The most often used classification systems today are the Johansson [19] and Vancouver classifications [17]. While the Johansson classification focuses only on the location of the fracture in relation to the prosthesis, the Vancouver Classification takes also the surrounding femoral bone stock and the stability of the prosthesis into consideration and can be more useful for devising a treatment strategy.

### 3.1 Vancouver Classification

The Vancouver Classification is the most widely accepted classification system of total PPHFs used today, based on the three most important factors for management: fracture location, stem stability, and quality of the remaining bone stock. This classification divides the femur into three anatomical zones: trochanteric region (A), diaphysis (B), including or just distal to the tip of the prosthesis, and diaphysis well distal to the tip of the prosthesis (C). The Vancouver Classification is both reliable and valid, shows good correlation between radiographic evaluation and intraoperative findings [22, 23], fits all common and uncommon fracture patterns, and has been recently extended to apply to all periprosthetic fractures, regardless of which joint or bone is involved [21].

### 3.2 Unified Classification System

The Unified Classification System (UCS) (**Fig 3.13-2**) combines the original Vancouver Classification with the AO/OTA Fracture and Dislocation Classification with proven excellent agreement among independent observers [24]. The USC uses as standard coding scheme:

- Roman numerals to represent joints, with the hip joint identified as number IV.
- Numbers to represent the bone involved (pelvis 6, femur 3).
- Letters to represent the type of fracture.

Fracture types are defined as follows:

- Type A (apophyseal) are fractures of the greater trochanter (GT) or lesser trochanter (LT). Most often these fractures are associated with some localized osteopenia or osteolysis.
- Distal of the GT to the prosthesis tip or just below is a type B fracture (around the implant). These fractures can further be divided into subtypes: B1 referring to a stable prosthesis suitable for an osteosynthesis, B2 is adjacent to a loose stem with sufficient bone stock for a straightforward revision surgery, and B3 referring to loose stem and inadequate bone stock and marked osteopenia/osteolysis requiring complex revision with possible bone graft. The precise identification of postoperative femoral Vancouver type B1 fractures is an important step in fracture management [17, 25].
- Those fractures that are located well below the prosthetic socket belong to the type C fractures (clear of or distant to the implant). Their treatment is independent of the THA with exception of some special techniques to fix the plate around the proximal stem. This type of fracture accounts for approximately 10% of the fractures around a hip prosthesis [4].
- Type D fractures represent interprosthetic fractures, dividing two implants.
- Type E fractures describe a floating joint with each of the two bones supporting one joint replacement.
- Type F represents fractures articulating or facing a hemiarthroplasty.

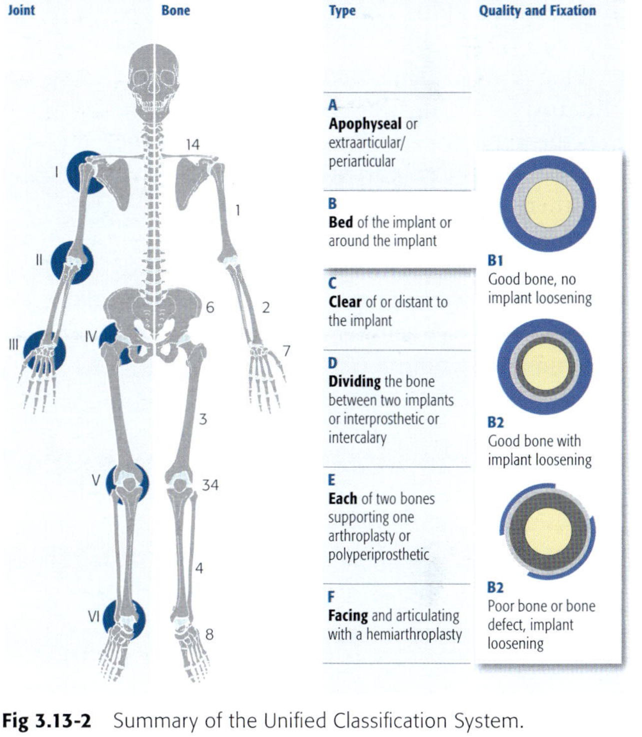


**Fig 3.13-2** Summary of the Unified Classification System.

## 4 Preoperative planning

Preoperative planning involves strategies for both the operative procedure as well as the perioperative care for the patient as a whole. Once we have established the "personality of the fracture", we can set out planning the continued care of the patient. The fracture personality is derived from the patient's health status, the fracture pattern and bone quality, the surgical competency, and perioperative skills available.

We need to remember that frail patients with numerous comorbidities have different abilities to tolerate immobility and surgical delay, as noted previously in the case of native hip fracture. Part of the planning is assessing the rehabilitation requirements of the patient after surgery and to have these requirements in place postoperatively. Many older adults have prefracture functional challenges that only worsen after fracture.

## 5 Decision making

The goal of treatment is to allow the patient to return to their highest level function as soon as possible. Early pain-free motion and weight bearing is essential to support early functional care and therapy. Five essential questions need to be answered before embarking on treating a geriatric patient with a PPHF:

- What is the patient's medical and prefracture functional status?
- Is the implant loose or well fixed in the bone?
- Is the implant or bearing worn?
- Is there a possibility of infection?
- What is the quality of the bone?

Once the patient has been established as a candidate for surgery, the choice between revision arthroplasty or reduction and osteosynthesis can be made.

### 5.1 Operative versus nonoperative treatment

Nonoperative treatment is no longer recommended for type B and type C fractures because of the patient's inability to tolerate prolonged immobilization without a high risk of complications such as pulmonary infection, pressure ulceration, and death [14, 26, 27]. Moreover, the rates of nonunion after nonoperative management are high because of inadequate fracture stability and the variable presence of bone cement at the fracture site [27, 28]. With modern treatment strategies, nonoperative management is reserved only for patients who would not be able to tolerate surgery. Although operative intervention is thought to offer the best outcomes, controversy still exists regarding the preferred fixation technique and optimal management strategy, given the high stress location of these fractures and the prosthesis. Many types of implants are available to maintain the reduction, none of which has demonstrated superiority. It has become apparent that certain methods of internal fixation are unsuitable, such as the Mennen paraskeletal clamp, which can be associated with early catastrophic failure [29, 30] and the Parham bands which do not provide adequate fixation and can cause substantial bone resorption [14, 31].

### 5.2 Type B1 or B2?

Accurate assessment and confirmation of stem stability is the key to a good outcome after fracture fixation:

- Plain x-rays should be carefully examined for signs of a loose stem, specifically looking to identify continuous lucency at the cemented stem and the bone-cement interface.
- In acute fractures, a cement mantle fracture alone is not considered diagnostic of a loose stem. In contrast, fractures of the cement mantle before acute trauma are indicative of a loose stem.
- If any doubt exists, routine intraoperative stem stability tests are recommended prior to fixation [32]. This approach, however, requires more exposure of the joint for plating of the femur, adding potential for postoperative dislocation.
- If the distal aspect of the stem is exposed at the fracture site, it may be tested for instability by generation of shear force along the longitudinal axis between the prosthesis and the proximal bone fragment or cement. This can be performed with a pointed reduction forceps on the femur and a Kocher forceps grasping the stem tip.
- If such a maneuver is not possible, a formal arthrotomy and dislocation is necessary to gain adequate exposure to exclude instability.

## 5.3 Can we fix type B2 fractures?

There is some discussion about fixation of type B2 fractures, taking into account a possible subsidence of 1–2 cm.

In general internal fixation of Vancouver B2 and B3 fractures result in a high reoperation rate [4, 33]. Although the Vancouver Classification has been proven to be a useful and reliable guide for the surgical planning of periprosthetic fractures, important factors like the patient physiology (medial comorbidities, physical status) and the surgeons' experience are not reflected. Joestl et al [34] published the concept of internal "biological fixation" utilizing internal fixation as an alternative operative option for treatment of periprosthetic femoral fracture fixation with a loose stem. They reported no significant differences in the patient outcome measured by the Parker Mobility Score or operative time. However, most studies are retrospective case series with missing specific details like the type of the original implant used with missing information regarding the type of primary fixation. When treating fractures around cementless or cemented femoral prostheses the surgeon must understand the primary fixation principle, eg, in cementless stems if the primary fixation is proximal or distal and in cemented stems if the fracture occurred around a composite beam stem or shape-closed designs with bonding of the prosthesis-cement interface or a polished tapered or force-closed design with no bonding between the prosthesis and the cement. In case of a noncomminuted fracture around a polished tapered stem with an intact cement mantle, internal fixation following anatomical reduction can be a treatment option. A CT scan might help in these cases to analyze the fracture pattern and cement mantle integrity. Following internal fixation, the stem may subside a few millimeters until stability is reestablished in the intact cement mantle. In case of small cement deficiencies with no bone loss, a cement-in-cement revision technique is also an option. However, in both cases an anatomical reconstruction of the fracture is mandatory. Good results with this technique in fractures around a polished tapered stem have been reported [35, 36]. The literature nowadays is not absolutely conclusive as to which patients require stem revision and which ones will benefit from internal fixation only. Internal fixation of a loose stem is an option as a palliative procedure in immobile and severely ill patients except in case of a polished tapered stem with an intact cement mantle.

## 5.4 Should cortical strut allograft be used?

This is an ongoing discussion. Many arthroplasty surgeons still like to use cortical strut allograft but the incidence seems to be much lower than in the past. Technically, it works but there is significant soft-tissue stripping required. If surgeons think more stability is required, there are other methods available, such as double plating.

Historically, type B1 fractures were reduced using stainless steel cerclage wires with rigid dynamic compression plates, occasionally in combination with cortical allograft struts [18, 37–39]. The use of allograft struts is an alternative or adjunct fixation method. Strut grafts, in case of a stable prosthesis, may be used as the only means of stabilization with either a single strut or as a double strut complex in 90° or 180° to each other (or in combination with osteosynthesis). Strut grafts have the advantage of being a biological and osteoconductive technique, providing reduced stress shielding due to similar modulus of elasticity as the native bone, augmenting the host bone stock and strength after union [39–43]. Placing two strut grafts with three fixation points above and below the fracture have been shown to yield good outcomes [44, 45]. Combined plating with proximal cable fixation augmented with an anterior or medial strut graft may provide better stability than an allograft strut alone [41]. The disadvantages of strut grafts are their high cost, limited availability, increased danger of infection, and potential for transmitting infection. In addition, remodeling occurs subsequent to the initial incorporation of the strut graft, leading in turn to biomechanical weakness during the first 4–6 months following grafting.

As an alternative, plates that can accommodate cables and screws have been designed, such as the Ogden plate (construct), secured to the proximal fragment by heavy-duty cables and to the distal fragment by (nonlocking) cortical screws [28]. This construct has proven to be significantly stronger than two allograft struts with cables [46]. The relative ease, minimal morbidity, and stability of the technique with the Ogden plate made it popular, but its disadvantages included the potential for stress risers as a result of the transcortical screws, fractures below the plate, prosthetic loosening, and nonunion [28].

## 6 Surgical planning

Surgical planning includes the preferred procedure and preferably one or two backup procedures in case they are necessary so as to manage intraoperative complications that may occur:

- Fixation or arthroplasty? When operating on a periprosthetic fracture, the two main choices of treatment are either reduction and osteosynthesis, or revision arthroplasty. Each of these procedures may demand specialist capabilities beyond that of the treating surgeon, so either a specialist trauma or arthroplasty surgeon will need to be available if needed.
- Templating—the operation needs to be performed virtually prior to entering the operating room. Templates should be used to determine implant type, size and possible site of placement to maximize fixation, leg length, and offset.
- Preparing instruments and implants—part of the preoperative planning is verifying the availability of implants for all possible primary and backup procedures, if not immediately on hand, then available if required. Instruments that facilitate implant removal (cemented or cementless) should be available if there is a possibility of revision.

## 7 Periprosthetic fracture fixation

### 7.1 General aspects

Treatment of PPHFs is dependent on characteristics of the fracture such as fracture location, bone stock, prosthesis stability, as well as patient's age, medical comorbidities, and surgeon experience. Optimal management around a stable femoral prosthesis has not been conclusively established.

Historically, treatment has included nonoperative strategies such as protected weight bearing, traction, and casting or bracing. Nonoperative treatment of unstable fractures has resulted in prolonged inpatient admission and recumbency, which is associated with delayed mobilization and higher nonunion and malunion rate [47].

Modern operative fixation techniques have largely replaced nonoperative ones except for protected weight bearing in highly selected cases. Operative management through internal fixation provides optimal fracture reduction, and a superior biological local environment for healing due to biomechanical stability; this leads ultimately to early mobilization and shorter in-hospital stay [7], while also affording a reduction in systemic and local complications such as malunion and nonunion [48].

Fractures associated with a stable femoral stem can be managed effectively with osteosynthesis principles, which most orthopedic surgeons are familiar with, where stabilization of the fracture with plates, screws, cerclage wires, nails, strut grafts, or a combination is recommended. The goals of surgery should be fracture union, prosthetic stability, and anatomical alignment in terms of axis, rotation, and length, as well as return to preinjury function.

The patient's final outcome depends on fracture union, implant stability, early functional recovery, and return to preinjury level of independence. Identifying the operative approach and confirming which implants are currently in situ, including the weight-bearing surface used, will facilitate preoperative planning.

Management of PPHFs includes some of the same core principles that apply to osteoporotic fracture fixation in general:

- Adequate preoperative planning, acknowledging that the extent and stability of the fracture, the degree of bone loss, and bone quality may not be fully appreciated until directly visualized.
- Operative approaches that minimize soft-tissue trauma, regardless of the fixation technique. Most important are attempts to preserve the blood supply to the fracture fragments and surrounding soft tissues by limiting operative dissection to the minimum needed for adequate reduction and fixation.
- Accurate fracture reduction is helpful to optimize healing, through either open or indirect means. In a simple fracture pattern, the fracture should be reduced as anatomically as possible with a fracture gap of less than 1–2 mm and in comminuted fractures, the fracture zone should be bridged with a plate or nail.
- Since the bone is almost always osteopenic/osteoporotic, fixation according to AO principles of relative stability as opposed to absolute stability is recommended, even in simple fractures with anatomical reduction.
- The use of robust implants with sufficient length and mechanical fixation is imperative for successful bone healing.
- Medical and nutritional therapy to optimize bone biology is essential (see chapter 1.10 Osteoporosis).

## 7.2 Fixation principles

Simple long oblique or spiral fractures can first be stabilized with cerclage wires or lag screws. Modern internal fixation is frequently achieved with locking plates, which can provide absolute and relative fracture stability. Locking plates potentially preserve the periosteal blood supply to the fractured bone, especially when minimally invasive surgery and indirect fracture reduction techniques are used [49]. This technique has the potential advantage of preserving the periosteal blood supply with minimal soft-tissue stripping, thereby reducing the risk of nonunion or failure. In conjunction with minimally invasive principles, soft-tissue dissection at the fracture site should be minimized. Failure to preserve the blood supply to the main fragments and to achieve adequate plate fixation at the level of the stem, as well as distally, can lead to catastrophic failure. The fixation at the plate ends, either proximal or distal, can most often be performed through a small open approach and is very unlikely to negatively impact the fracture healing process in between.

Plate length is an important consideration. In general, the plate cannot be too long. The following reasons to use a long plate include:

- By increasing the plate length from the fracture zone, the lever arm and the pull-out strength is higher. This prevents the construct from fixation failure at the plate end like a pull-out of screws or breakage of cables.
- The plate must overlap the prosthesis by at least two to three cortical diameters to allow plate fixation with a minimum of four to five bicortical screws and cables. This is the minimal overlapping distance and is independent of the bridging length over the fracture site. Proximally, the lever arm can be extended by bending the plate over the GT or using special plates with hooks or attachment plates. This technique or implant selection can be important when fixing very proximal femoral fractures starting just distal to the GT.
- Distally, the plate should not end in the metaphyseal region due to the risk of a stress riser and a secondary fracture at this level, especially in osteoporotic bone. In patients with reduced bone quality, the whole femur should be protected with the plate extending distally over the lateral condyle.
- A long plate allows more options of fixation, eg, screws, cerclage wires, or locking attachment plates, especially if the bone quality is poor, as is sometimes judged intraoperatively.
- Long plates can facilitate the restoration of the femoral axis and their application in a minimally invasive technique.

Plate fixation technique is crucial for success in PPHF. The combination of poor proximal fixation in osteoporotic bone with an intramedullary (IM) device and associated difficult screw placement is problematic for the geriatric patient, for whom partial weight bearing (PWB) is impossible.

The plate fixation proximally around the stem can be achieved with either screws, cerclage wires (with and without using locking eyelet attachments), or locking attachment plates. Constructs with proximal screws, even unicortical in combination with cerclage wires, result in significantly more stable fixation than constructs with cerclages alone (so-called Ogden construct). The main benefit of using screws in the proximal fragment over cerclage wires alone is the benefit of additional rotational stability in combination with less soft-tissue disruption [50]. Furthermore, it has been shown that cables are better than wires and double-looped cerclage wires provide a better fixation stability compared to a single-looped cerclage [51]. Although the clinical results are comparable, there are biomechanical concerns that two allograft struts with cerclage wires alone are inferior to the combination of screws and cerclage wires [39, 46, 52]. Screw types can be conventional, (variable angle) locking, or flat-tipped unicortical locking screws. Conventional screws and (variable angle) locking screws might be inserted proximally in the greater trochanteric region or in the proximal fragment posterior to the stem where a 5–7 mm bone cortex or cement mantle allows good screw purchase [53]. When flat unicortical screws are used, care should be taken to avoid choosing excessively long screws since they may push against and loosen the stem or fail to engage in the plate properly. Another option for plate fixation around an implant is the locking attachment plate [54]. This plate typically locks into the standard long locking plate and facilitates insertion of up to four locking screws that bypass the stem anteriorly and posteriorly for bicortical purchase (**Fig 3.13-3**). Biomechanically, bicortical screw fixation using a locking attachment plate (LAP) improves proximal plate fixation in periprosthetic fractures and is superior to cerclage wires and unicortical screw combination [56]. Subtrochanteric placement of the LAP provides increased fixation strength compared to hook plate fixation in the GT [57].

The distal fixation of the plate either in the diaphyseal region or over the lateral condyle (in the case of a distally extended plate) can most often be easily achieved with at least eight cortices, preferably ten [58]. Locking screws in particular can improve fixation in osteopenic and osteoporotic bone [59]. If the plate ends in the diaphyseal region, either a unicortical or conventional screw at the most distal plate hole may be essential to avoid creation of stress risers and recurrent fracture (**Fig 3.13-4**) [60, 61]. Due to risk of pull-out, the use of unicortical screws in either the proximal or the distal segment is not recommended.

Inserting screws close to and far from the fracture site is advocated [62]. In simple transverse or short oblique fractures two to three screw holes over the fracture site should be omitted [63], and in comminuted fractures the bridging length

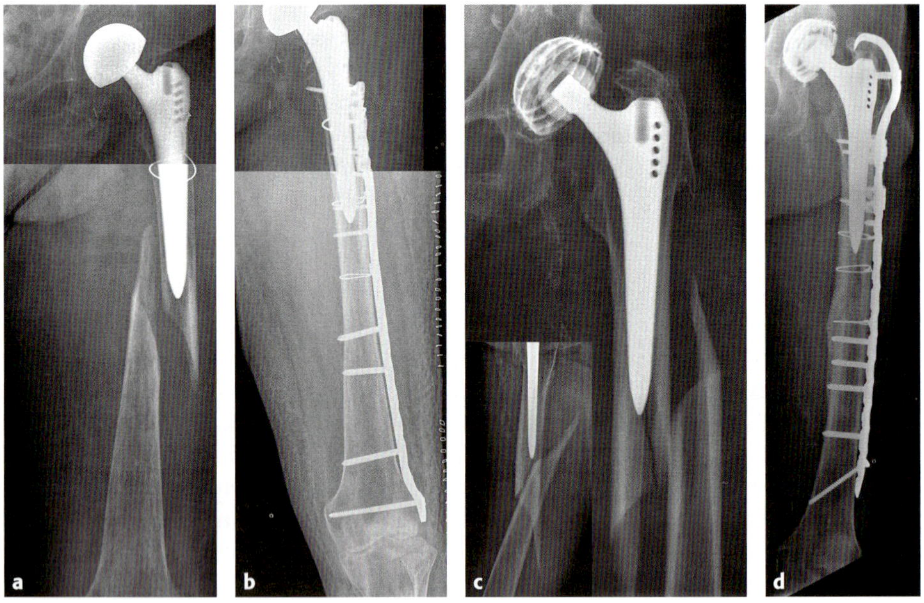

**Fig 3.13-3a–d** Two cases (A: **a–b**, B: **c–d**) of a simple displaced type B1 or C fracture where the general fixation principles for these kinds of fractures are shown.

1. In both cases, the fracture was reduced nearly anatomically and held with single wire loops; in case B (**c–d**) a closed reduction was not possible due to soft-tissue interposition posteriorly.
2. In both cases a long plate was chosen. In case A (**a–b**) the bone in the area of the greater trochanter was completely deficient. Due to the significant osteoporosis, the plate should not end in the metaphyseal area and was therefore bent distally over the lateral condyle. In case B (**c–d**) the hooked version of the plate increases the lever arm proximally. Due to the better bone quality, the plate ended in the distal diaphysis.
3. In both cases proximal fixation was completed with bicortical and flat-tipped unicortical screws together with cerclage wires and locking attachment plates.
4. Distal fixation was achieved in both cases with at least five bicortical screws. In case B (**c–d**) the most distal conventional screw decreases the risk of a stress riser and the oblique position of the screw increases the fixation strength by increasing the pull-out strength [55].

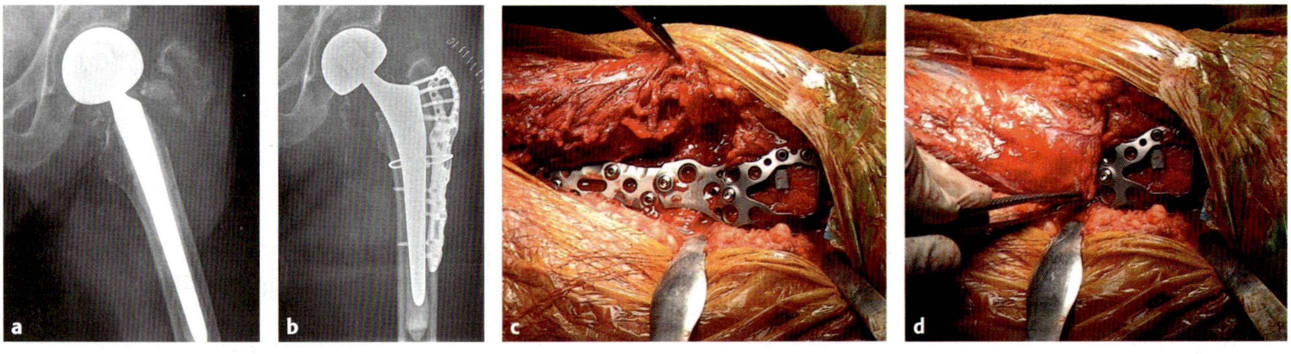

**Fig 3.13-4a–d** Displaced fracture of the greater trochanter (Unified Classification System IV.3.A1).

**a–b** Displaced fracture type A of the greater trochanter before and after fixation with a ring plate (eg, periprosthetic trochanter plate), extending distally with fixation around the stem.

**c–d** Intraoperative situs following open reduction and internal fixation using the ring plate. The posterior L-shaped detached vastus lateralis muscle is resutured over the plate at the end of the fracture fixation.

should be minimized by inserting the screws as close to the fracture site as possible, leaving at most four to five holes unoccupied.

Simple, long oblique or spiral fractures can first be stabilized with cerclage wires or cables. Plate-independent lag screws can also help maintain fracture reduction. Short oblique or transverse fractures can be treated with biplanar fixation on the anterior and lateral aspects with any combination of plates and cortical onlay grafts [64]. In the case of strut grafts, the graft should be sculpted with a burr to provide optimal intimate contact with the underlying native bone. Bone-graft substitute may also be used to enhance graft incorporation and facilitate healing for selected patients [41].

## 7.3 Type A fracture

### 7.3.1 Greater trochanter

Type A GT fractures include those involving the GT. Usually, these fractures are associated with reduced bone quality and are typically stable and minimally displaced, due to the composite tendons of the glutei and vastus muscles [65]. If there is any doubt, a CT scan can clarify if a fracture of the GT is a simple type A GT fracture or a spiral type B fracture, possibly compromising the stability of the stem. The treatment of nondisplaced fractures smaller than 1–2 cm is generally nonoperative, with PWBAT for 6–12 weeks [66, 67]. However, in most fragility fracture patients PWB is not possible, as they often lack the necessary upper-body strength, balance, and sometimes cognition to use forearm crutches and avoid full weight bearing (FWB).

Displaced fractures larger than 2 cm or a painful nonunion following nonoperative treatment of an undisplaced fracture may require fixation with operative methods. This depends on the size of the fragment (eg, involvement of the attachment of the abductors), patient condition (good previous mobility), and type of joint replacement (ie, THA with a head size smaller than 32 mm have a higher risk of hip dislocation in the absence of stabilizing abductors). The fixation methods are similar to those for trochanteric osteotomy, namely using wires, screws, cables, or specialized plates, eg, a hook or ring (cable) plate construct (**Fig 3.13-4**) [65]. Cable grip systems provide a more rigid fixation than cables alone and have lower rates of nonunion and trochanteric migration [65]. For additional fixation, the cable plate may be extended distally beyond the prosthesis to obtain bicortical screw fixation in the femur. In the absence of osteolysis of the GT, the surgeon should not mobilize the trochanter unless it is absolutely necessary and preferably keep the abductor-vastus sling in continuity. In the presence of osteolysis, stable fixation and fracture healing is difficult to achieve [68]. In such cases, operative treatment is warranted and should first address the underlying cause of osteolysis, eg, acetabular liner revision or any source of metallosis. The surgery should then include adjuvant cancellous allograft fill of the osteolytic lesion in conjunction with trochanteric fixation. The bone graft is usually well incorporated (**Fig 3.13-5**) [68].

### 7.3.2 Lesser trochanter

Type A LT fractures that involve the lesser trochanter are rare, usually representing avulsion fractures through osteoporotic bone or areas with osteolysis [69]. They must be carefully assessed because a fracture of the medial cortex may destabilize the prosthesis, necessitating operative intervention. A CT scan can determine if the fracture is isolated and the prosthesis is presumably stable. In this case nonoperative treatment is warranted, and close clinical and radiographic follow-up to monitor for prosthesis loosening is advised.

Operative treatment is necessary when the fracture compromises the stability of the prosthesis by involving distal extension and a large portion of the calcar region with medial buttress loss. In this case, treatment may include cerclage

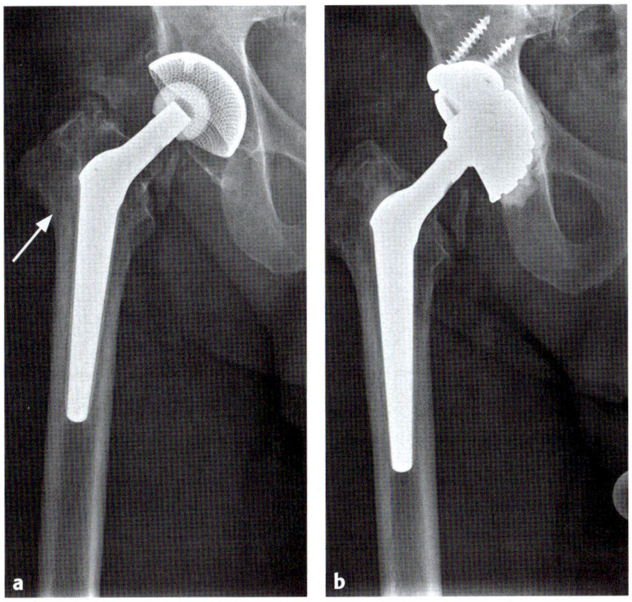


**Fig 3.13-5a–b** Hip AP preoperatively and 6 months postoperatively of a nondisplaced type A greater trochanteric (GT) fracture with a large amount of osteolysis due to acetabular wear. The acetabular shell was revised, the osteolysis in the GT removed, and the defect with allograft impacted. Since the abductor-vastus sling remained in continuity with no displacement, no additional fracture fixation was required.

wiring and revision if the prosthesis is deemed unstable, but only if bone stock is adequate (**Fig 3.13-6**). However, in the presence of osteolysis, revision surgery to a long diaphyseal-fitting stem is indicated to remove the particle debris generator [67, 68] with or without bone graft required to achieve stem stability [10].

## 7.4 Type B1 and type C fractures

A femoral fracture occurring around (at or just distal to) a well-fixed stable femoral stem is classified as a type B1 fracture and below the stem as a type C fracture. In most cases both require surgery. While most type B1 and proximal type C fractures are plated from proximal to distal, more distal type C fractures can either be plated or stabilized with a distally inserted retrograde IM nail on condition that there is at least 10 cm between the tip of the nail and the femoral stem [70].

The aims of fixation include fracture union with early FWB and mobilization of the patient so that hip and knee function are preserved [13]. Notable advances have been made regarding the reduction techniques and implants used for fixation of type B1 and type C fractures:

- Closed/indirect or open/direct accurate fracture reduction with restoration of length, axis, and rotation. For both techniques surgeons should use the least amount of dissection possible. A fracture reduction that results in the proximal fragment left in varus position must be avoided due to the high incidence of fixation failure (**Fig 3.13-7**) [71].
- Open or minimally invasive internal fixation has been further advanced.
- Cortical strut allograft or an additional plate based on the bone quality that is observed intraoperatively can be implemented to provide a more stable construct (**Fig 3.13-8**).

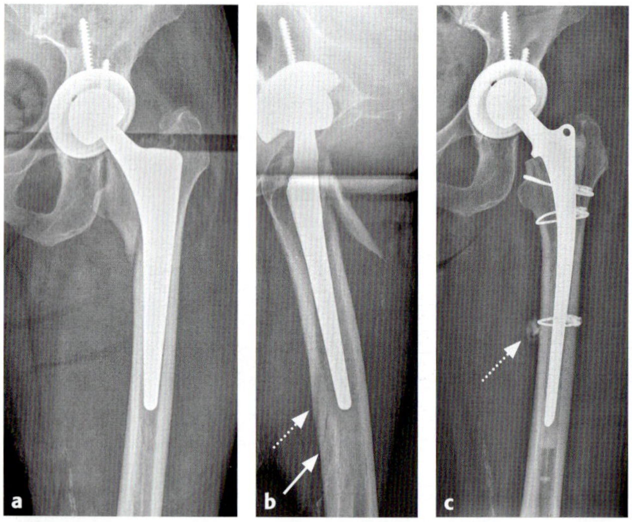


**Fig 3.13-6a–c** Preoperative (**a–b**) and postoperative (**c**) x-rays of a type B2 fracture. It is not an isolated type A2 fracture as the fracture is extending distally posteriorly. The two lines in the posterior cortex (**b**) represent a nutritional vessel (white arrow) and the spiral fracture extension distally (dotted arrow). The fracture is stabilized with cables and the loose stem revised to a cemented stem (an uncemented distally fluted, tapered stem would have been also an option). Even in the presence of an anatomical reduction and stable fixation (**c**), a small amount of cement protruded through the distal fracture site (arrow).

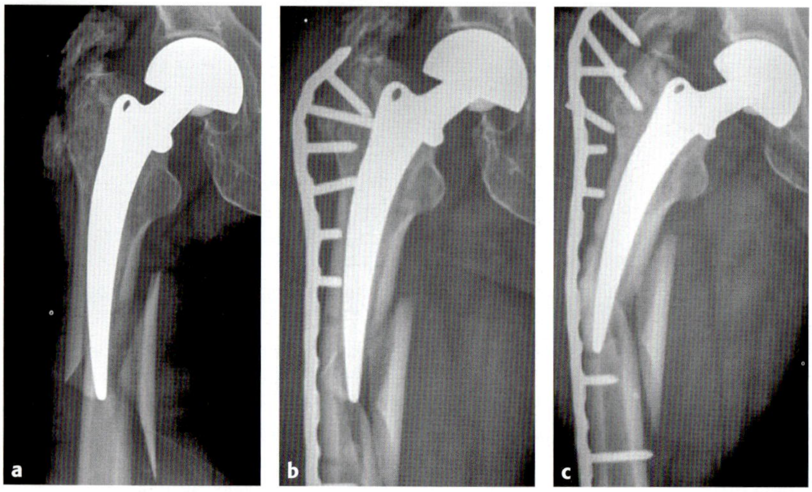


**Fig 3.13-7a–c** Fracture reduction with the proximal fragment in varus position and missing medial support must be avoided due to the high failure rate.

### 7.4.1 Minimally invasive plate osteosynthesis

Indications for a minimally invasive plate osteosynthesis (MIPO) technique are either minimally displaced, nondisplaced, or comminuted fractures. In minimally displaced fractures limited exposure of the fracture site with a single reduction clamp and gentle traction/rotation may be all that is necessary to achieve a near anatomical reduction with a fracture gap of less than 2 mm. The reduction can be maintained by either the clamp alone, cables/wires or plate-independent lag screws (**Fig 3.13-9**).

In an attempt to minimize the extent of soft-tissue dissection, MIPO technique is proposed, incorporating indirect reduction and percutaneous insertion of plates and screws (**Fig 3.13-10**) [72]. It is important that the biology of fracture healing is understood and accurate fracture reduction achieved.

In comminuted fractures an external fixator might help to maintain the overall length, axis, and rotation before a MIPO technique can be performed (**Fig 3.13-8**). In very unstable fracture patterns in osteoporotic bone, a medial buttress plate placed with an allograft strut or a second plate may be helpful (**Fig 3.13-8**). This technique is also particularly helpful when the distal fixation is limited because of a total knee replacement that has a box-type or stem-type design, allowing only unicortical screw fixation [73].

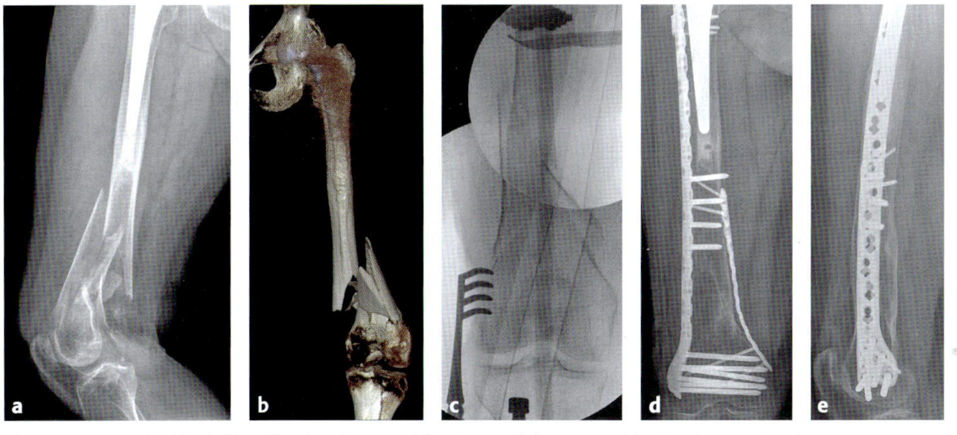

**Fig 3.13-8a–e** Unified Classification System IV.3.C type C fracture with distal comminution.

**a–c** Displaced and comminuted type C fracture in osteoporotic bone. The reduction can be achieved and temporarily maintained with an external fixator.

**d–e** Six months postoperative the fracture has healed after using minimally invasive fracture fixation with a long-spanning plate laterally and an additional medial plate for stability. The long plate was chosen so as to bypass the tip of the stem by at least twice the diameter diaphyseally and fixed with a locking attachment plate at the end. The hole just below the stem is from the Schanz screw from the external fixator, which had been used preoperatively for indirect fracture reduction.

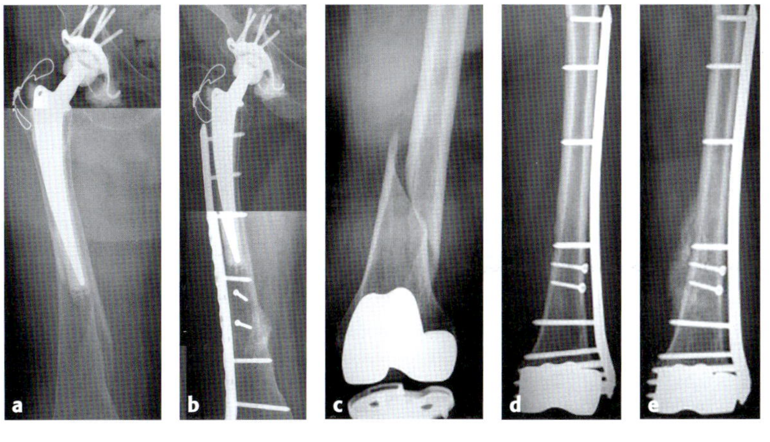

**Fig 3.13-9a–e** Preoperative and postoperative x-rays of a simple displaced type B1 fracture (**a–b**) and a simple supracondylar fracture (Unified Classification System V.3.B1, **c–e**). Both fractures have been reduced with minimally invasive techniques and the reduction maintained with two plate-independent lag screws. The purpose of the screws are only to hold the reduction ("approximation screws") and do not function as interfragmentary compression screws since the screws are turned one half turn backward after tightening and almost always become loose in osteoporotic bone. Cables would have the same effect. Following fracture reduction and fixation with plate-independent screws, a lateral-based locking plate in minimally invasive plate osteosynthesis technique was applied. Both fractures healed with callus formation.

Another MIPO technique to treat distal type C fractures is fixation with a retrograde nail. The main concern about the use of a nail relates to the possible creation of a stress riser between the tip of the nail and the femoral component [39]. If the distance between the two IM implants is less than twice the diameter of the femur, a protection bridge by at least two diameters is necessary (**Fig 3.13-11**).

### 7.4.2 Open reduction and internal fixation

If a near anatomical reduction for simple displaced fracture or in combination with a butterfly fragment/large intermediate fragment is not possible, open reduction with direct visualization and reduction of the fracture is indicated. Even with an open approach, limited incision length and periosteal stripping is warranted to decrease the amount of soft-tissue dissection and optimize fracture healing (**Fig 3.13-11**).

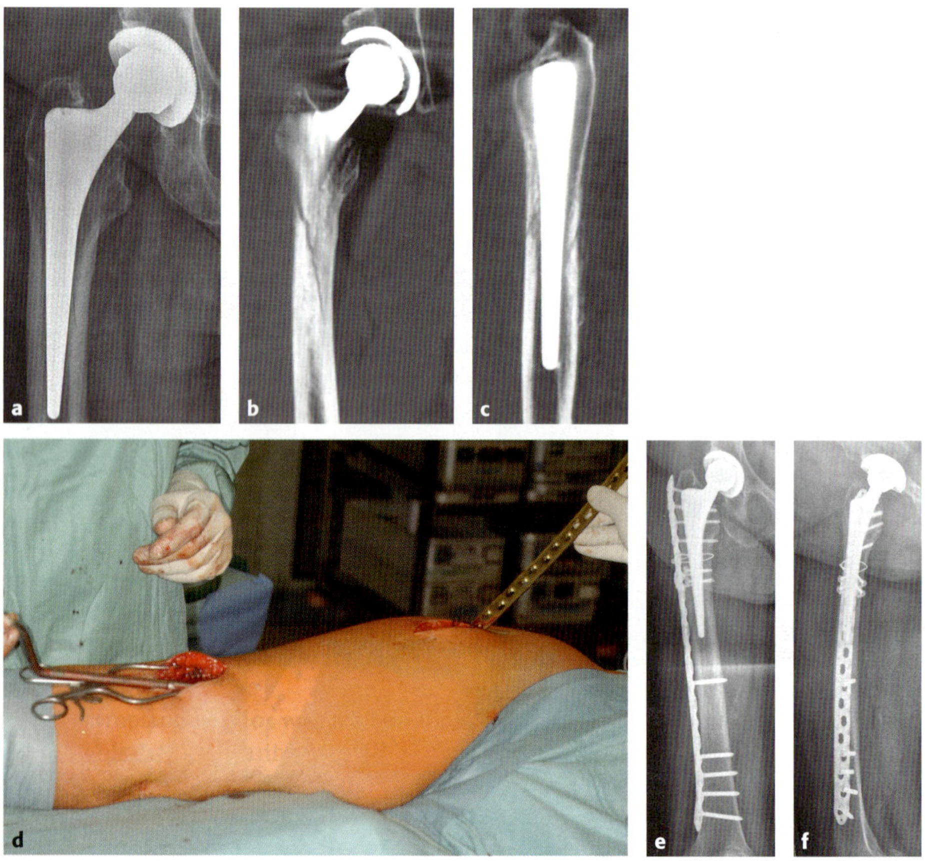

**Fig 3.13-10a–f** Unified Classification System IV.3.B1/B2 fracture.

**a–c** Preoperative x-ray (**a**) and computed tomographic scans (**b–c**) with a minimally displaced periprosthetic hip fracture (Vancouver type B1).

**d–f** Intraoperative clinical photograph (**d**) and postoperative x-rays (**e–f**). A long plate was used with a minimally invasive technique. The proximal fixation was achieved using conventional and locking screws, cables, and a locking attachment plate. For the distal fixation five bicortical locking screws were used. The stability of the stem can be questioned since the fracture location compromises the stability of the uncemented stem.

(Images courtesy of Prof Michael Blauth, University Department for Trauma Surgery Innsbruck, Austria.)

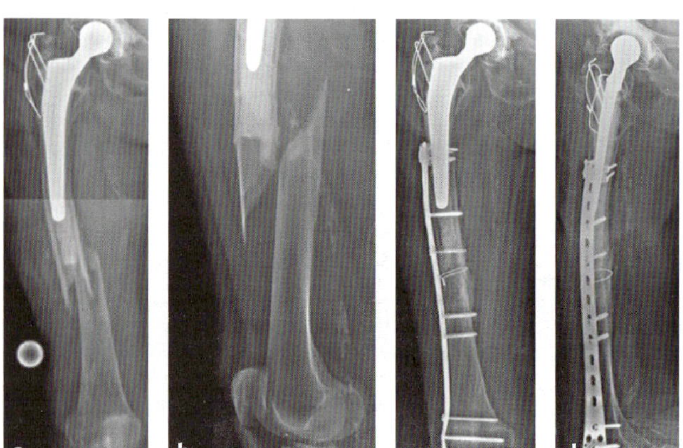

**Fig 3.13-11a–d** Preoperative AP (**a**) and lateral (**b**) x-rays. Six-month postoperative AP (**c**) and lateral (**d**) x-rays following open reduction and internal fixation of a type C fracture. Due to the posterior spike of the distal fragment, it was not possible to perform closed reduction. The fracture was first stabilized with a cerclage and then fixed with a plate from distal to proximal. The plate should be compressed to the bone distally over the condyle using a conventional screw. This improves rotational stability and reduces soft-tissue irritation of the iliotibial band [74]. The distal fixation was accomplished with additional locking screws. The stem was bypassed proximally with the plate by nearly twice the diameter of the femur and then fixed with screws and a locking attachment plate.

### 7.4.3 Interprosthetic fractures around stable prosthesis of the femur

Interprosthetic fractures are rare [75, 76] but challenging to manage since successful reduction and fixation are difficult to achieve with a hip and knee prosthesis in place and typically poor bone quality. The rehabilitation is also more problematic in frail, comorbid, and functionally limited older adults. However, the clinical results published using locking plates show satisfactory results [77–79].

Important factors are the type of prosthesis (eg, primary, revision, stemmed, cemented), fracture type (eg, simple, comminuted), local soft-tissue condition (eg, hypertrophic, scars), local bone quality, and the function of the joint arthroplasties (eg, stiff, painful). After considering these factors, the surgeon can choose the operative approach (ie, minimally invasive soft-tissue sparing) and the implants (ie, single or double plates/strut grafts). All the principles listed in topics 7.1 and 7.2 of this chapter also apply to treat interprosthetic fractures (**Fig 3.13-12**, **Fig 3.13-13**).

### 7.4.4 Revision arthroplasty in type B1 fractures

Revision arthroplasty for type B1 fractures is seldom warranted except in transverse fractures at the tip of a cemented stem just above the cement restrictor, also called the "problematic fracture". Although the fracture can usually

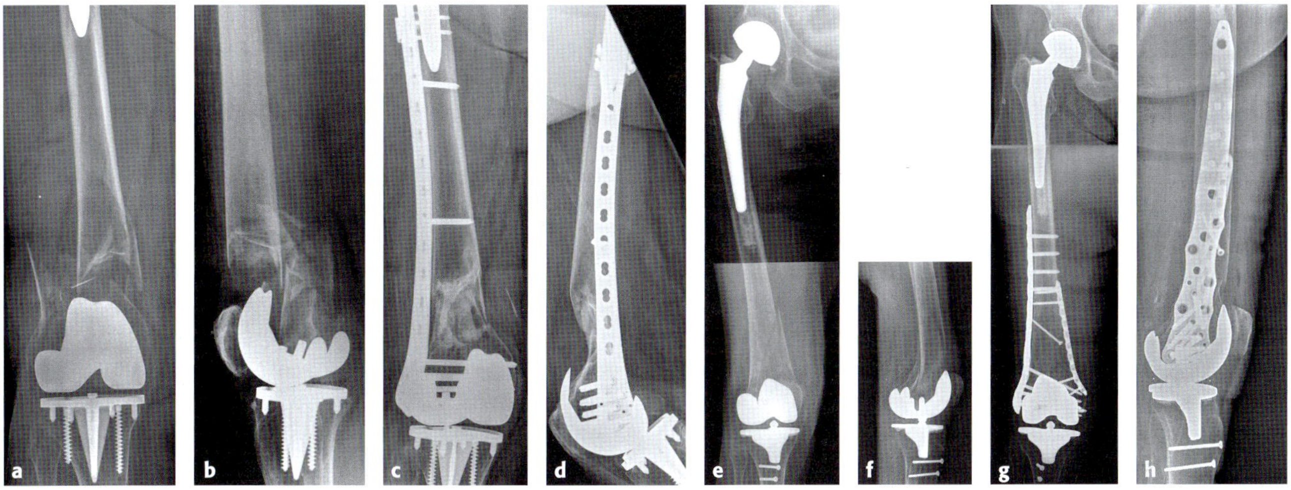

**Fig 3.13-12a–h** The appropriate plate length should attempt to prevent a secondary fracture between the plate end and the stem proximally by either overlapping the implant (**a–d**) or keeping a distance between the plate and the prosthesis (**e–h**) by at least two diameters or 6 cm [78, 80]. Depending on the fracture type and the bone quality, an additional plate/strut might be necessary to prevent a catastrophic failure of the construct (**g–h**).

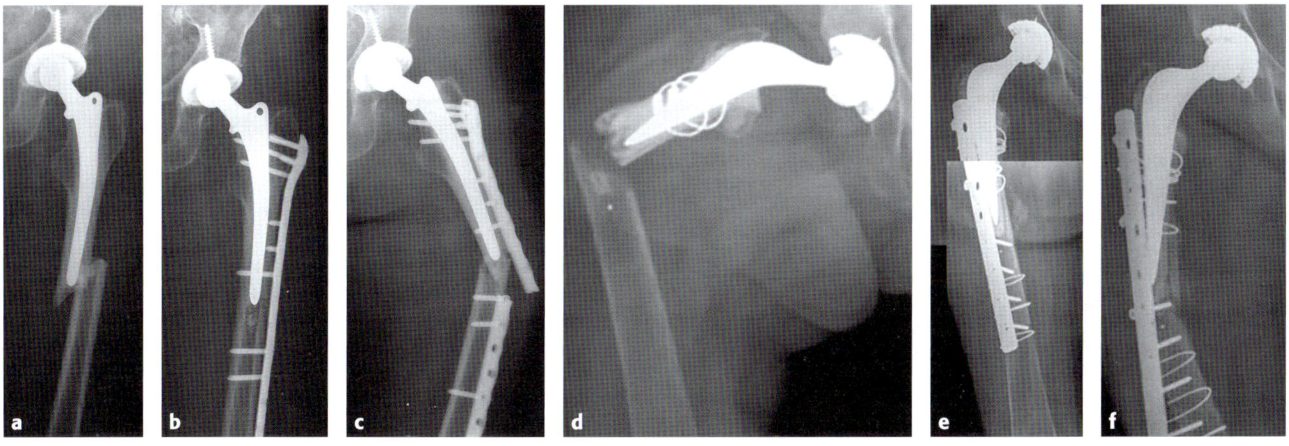

**Fig 3.13-13a–f** Two cases (A: **a–c**, B: **d–f**) of a "problematic fracture" between the tip of a cemented stem and the distal cement plug. In this situation the biology is compromised with an implant failure (**a–c**) and fixation failure (**d–f**).

be nearly anatomically reduced, the secondary healing factors remain problematic due to the vascular damage from the endomedullary cavity as well as the disrupted periosteum at the fracture site. These biological consequences can result in implant failure (**Fig 3.13-13**). In this situation additional treatment with allograft cortical struts or plate has been associated with a high likelihood of fracture union [41]. Alternatively, a primary revision arthroplasty should be considered (**Fig 3.13-14**) [81].

## 8 Revision arthroplasty

Once it has been established that the implant is not stable in the femoral canal or in the acetabular socket, the usual course of action is to perform a revision arthroplasty, revising the component or components that are affected. The vast majority of these fractures and revisions involve the femur. The acetabulum is more often revised for concomitant wear than for fracture. In very frail patients with low functional demands and expectations, a fracture around a loose stem may be fixed by osteosynthesis as long as there is adequate bone stock to support weight bearing.

For these reasons, preoperative bone quality needs to be assessed. If bone quality is poor, the procedure of choice is to bypass the defect with a long-stemmed prosthesis or a proximal femoral composite allograft. In cases of adequate bone quality, the fracture may be reduced to recreate an intact femoral tube with reduction and cerclage wire or cable fixation prior to inserting a distal femoral revision arthroplasty stem. It is also possible to first implant the femoral stem to its final position and then reconstruct the proximal femur around the implant with cable or wire cerclages. In older adults less emphasis is placed on reconstructing the bone, but strut grafts may be considered to improve stability. For sufficient fixation in the femoral diaphysis there needs to be at least 4–6 cm of interference fit of the distal stem in the diaphysis. The usual fixation method of the femoral stem is cementless; however, cemented fixation may be used if the diaphyseal bone is severely osteoporotic or metabolically inactive.

### 8.1 Implant selection

There are a number of possible types of implant that can be used in the management of these revisions: straight or curved monoblock stems, modular tapered stems, long cemented stems, mega tumor prostheses, and allograft composite implants. Choice of implant is typically based on the patient's bone morphology, the amount of bony comminution, quality of the bone, and surgeon's preference.

Some valuable technical tips are:

- When reaming and impacting the femoral stem, it is advisable to protect the intact diaphysis from fracture by placing a cerclage wire or cable around the intact proximal end of the distal fragment.
- When using cementless fixation with distal fixation, proper-sized implants must be used. Too small implants may result in axial instability with subsidence and/or rotatory instability of the implant.

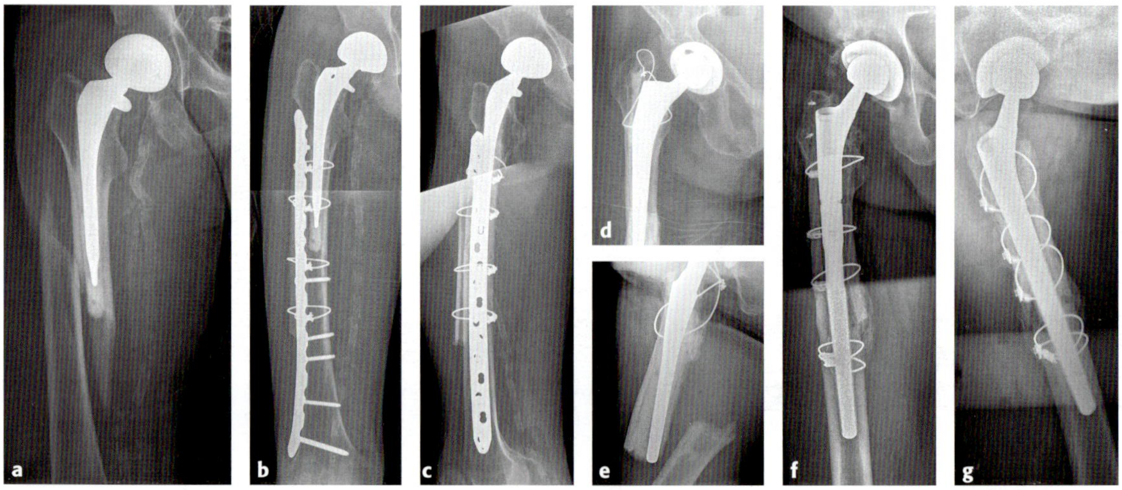


**Fig 3.13-14a–g** Alternatives to a single lateral plate osteosynthesis in "problematic fractures" include either enhanced fixation with a second implant like a strut graft or a plate (**a–c**), or a primary revision arthroplasty (**d–e**) is recommended. X-rays (**f–g**) were taken 1 year postoperatively.

- When using a long femoral implant, be sure that it is curved, as femoral bowing is often exaggerated in older adults. Straight and even curved implants may penetrate the distal cortex of a very bowed femur, causing a stress riser with risk for future fracture (**Fig 3.13-15**, **Fig 3.13-16**, **Fig 3.13-17**, **Fig 3.13-18**).

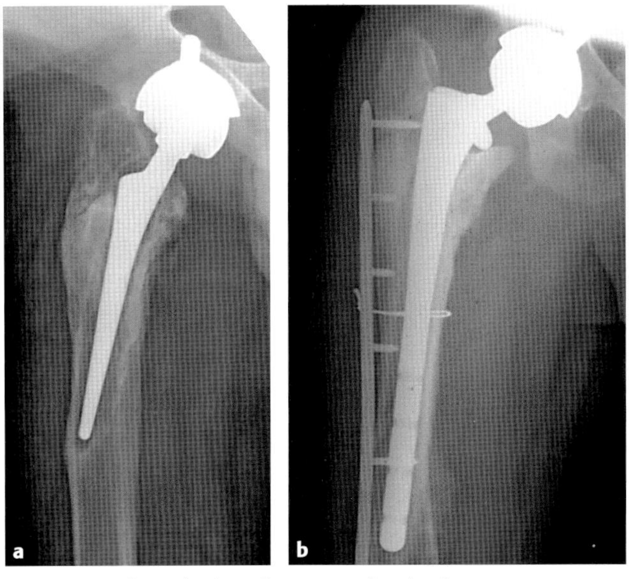


**Fig 3.13-15a–b** Selection of an appropriate implant.
**a** The x-ray showing a loose cementless femoral stem with varus displacement. This presents a hazard for femoral canal penetration and periprosthetic fracture at the time of revision surgery.
**b** Postoperative x-ray of the same patient after open reduction and internal fixation of intraoperative periprosthetic fracture that was propagated by femoral canal preparation.

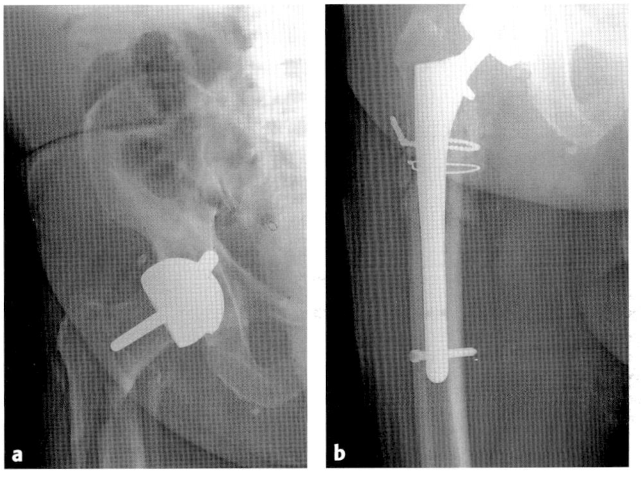


**Fig 3.13-16a–b** Atypical Vancouver type fracture.
**a** Periprosthetic fracture below a resurfacing hip arthroplasty (Vancouver type C fracture).
**b** Treated with reconstruction of the femoral "tube" and bypass of the reconstructed comminuted fracture with a cementless implant.

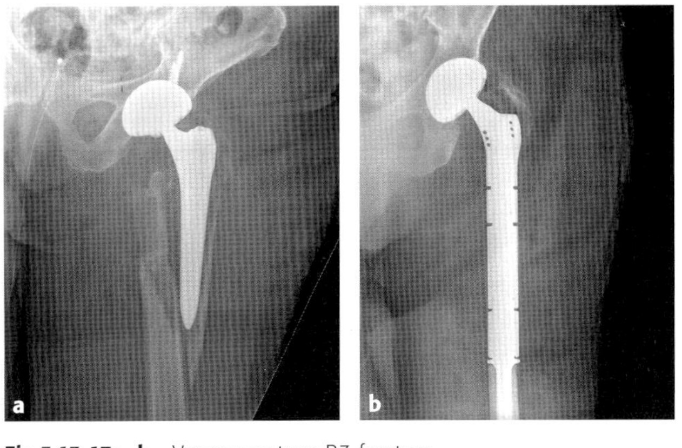


**Fig 3.13-17a–b** Vancouver type B3 fracture.
**a** Fracture around a femoral stem causing stem instability with poor remaining bone quality in the fractured segment.
**b** Fracture bypassed with a distal fixating long proximal femoral replacement stem.

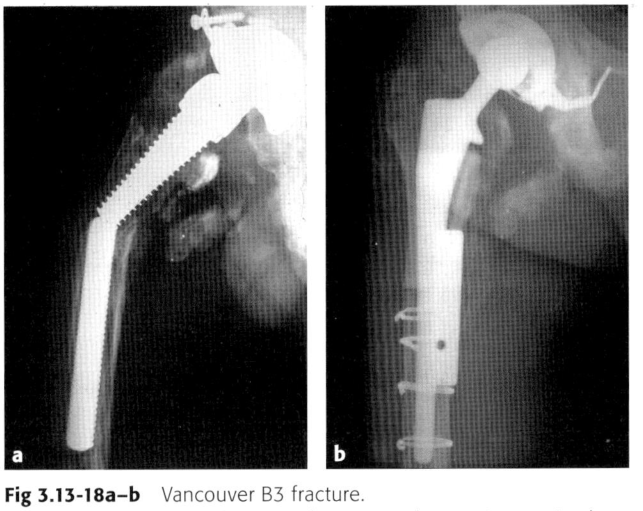


**Fig 3.13-18a–b** Vancouver B3 fracture.
**a** Fracture of femoral stem with associated extensive proximal femoral osteolysis and fracture.
**b** Reconstruction with proximal femoral allograft cemented onto a cementless stem that is fixed into the distal femur with a cementless scratch fit. The allograft host femoral junction is stabilized with a short plate.

## 9 Complications

The complications associated with these fractures may be divided into the two main categories medical and surgical.

### 9.1 Medical

As with native fragility fractures of the hip, there are many common medical complications for PPHF patients: atelectasis and pneumonia, pressure sores, urinary retention and infection, delirium, and venous thromboembolic disease. The best way to prevent these complications is early operative fracture stabilization to allow for early mobilization and adequate pain control. See chapters 1.7 Postoperative medical management and 1.8 Postoperative surgical management on postoperative care.

### 9.2 Surgical

Risk of operative complication is elevated due to comorbidities affecting bone quality, malnutrition, and overall frailty. The bone is often pathological due to osteoporosis; implant wear-associated osteolysis, and comminuted fractures. These mechanical and biological issues have an effect on fracture fixation and fracture union as evidenced by the high reoperation rate of 23% at 22 months [10]. The most common reasons for reoperation include nonunion of the fracture, failure of fixation, and surgical site infections. Other possible complications include dislocation of the hip and wound hematoma.

The mortality rates for open reduction and internal fixation (ORIF) are higher than for revision arthroplasty at 33% and 12%, respectively [10]. This may be because revision arthroplasty typically results in earlier weight bearing and more mobility than ORIF.

Inadequate fracture reduction may lead to early failure making accurate fracture reduction the priority over soft-tissue exposure [62].

## 11 References

1. **Berry DJ.** Epidemiology: hip and knee. *Orthop Clin North Am.* 1999 Apr;30(2):183–190.
2. **Duwelius PJ, Schmidt AH, Kyle RF, et al.** A prospective, modernized treatment protocol for periprosthetic femur fractures. *Orthop Clin North Am.* 2004 Oct;35(4):485–492, vi.
3. **Lindahl H.** Epidemiology of periprosthetic femur fracture around a total hip arthroplasty. *Injury.* 2007 Jun;38(6):651–654.
4. **Lindahl H, Garellick G, Regner H, et al.** Three hundred and twenty-one periprosthetic femoral fractures. *J Bone Joint Surg Am.* 2006 Jun;88(6):1215–1222.
5. **Masri BA, Meek RM, Duncan CP.** Periprosthetic fractures evaluation and treatment. *Clin Orthop Relat Res.* 2004 Mar(420):80–95.
6. **Abdel MP, Watts CD, Houdek MT, et al.** Epidemiology of periprosthetic fracture of the femur in 32 644 primary total hip arthroplasties: a 40-year experience. *Bone Joint J.* 2016 Apr;98-B(4):461–467.
7. **Franklin J, Malchau H.** Risk factors for periprosthetic femoral fracture. *Injury.* 2007 Jun;38(6):655–660.
8. **Zhu Y, Chen W, Sun T, et al.** Risk factors for the periprosthetic fracture after total hip arthroplasty: a systematic review and meta-analysis. *Scand J Surg.* 2015 Sep;104(3):139–145.
9. **Garbuz DS, Masri BA, Duncan CP.** Periprosthetic fractures of the femur: principles of prevention and management. *Instr Course Lect.* 1998;47:237–242.
10. **Greidanus NV, Mitchell PA, Masri BA, et al.** Principles of management and results of treating the fractured femur during and after total hip arthroplasty. *Instr Course Lect.* 2003;52:309–322.
11. **Mitchell PA, Greidanus NV, Masri BA, et al.** The prevention of periprosthetic fractures of the femur during and after total hip arthroplasty. *Instr Course Lect.* 2003;52:301–308.
12. **Khanuja HS, Vakil JJ, Goddard MS, et al.** Cementless femoral fixation in total hip arthroplasty. *J Bone Joint Surg Am.* 2011 Mar 2;93(5):500–509.
13. **Berry DJ.** Periprosthetic fractures associated with osteolysis: a problem on the rise. *J Arthroplasty.* 2003 Apr;18(3 Suppl 1):107–111.
14. **Fredin HO, Lindberg H, Carlsson AS.** Femoral fracture following hip arthroplasty. *Acta Orthop Scand.* 1987 Feb;58(1):20–22.
15. **Grammatopoulos G, Pandit H, Kambouroglou G, et al.** A unique peri-prosthetic fracture pattern in well fixed femoral stems with polished, tapered, collarless design of total hip replacement. *Injury.* 2011 Nov;42(11):1271–1276.
16. **Chevillotte CJ, Ali MH, Trousdale RT, et al.** Inflammatory laboratory markers in periprosthetic hip fractures. *J Arthroplasty.* 2009 Aug;24(5):722–727.
17. **Duncan CP, Masri BA.** Fractures of the femur after hip replacement. *Instr Course Lect.* 1995;44:293–304.
18. **Bethea JS 3rd, DeAndrade JR, Fleming LL, et al.** Proximal femoral fractures following total hip arthroplasty. *Clin Orthop Relat Res.* 1982 Oct;(170):95–106.
19. **Johansson JE, McBroom R, Barrington TW, et al.** Fracture of the ipsilateral femur in patients wih total hip replacement. *J Bone Joint Surg Am.* 1981 Dec;63(9):1435–1442.
20. **Kelley SS.** Periprosthetic Femoral Fractures. *J Am Acad Orthop Surg.* 1994 May;2(3):164–172.
21. **Duncan CP, Haddad FS.** The Unified Classification System (UCS): improving our understanding of periprosthetic fractures. *Bone Joint J.* 2014 Jun;96-B(6):713–716.

22. **Rayan F, Dodd M, Haddad FS.** European validation of the Vancouver classification of periprosthetic proximal femoral fractures. *J Bone Joint Surg Br.* 2008 Dec;90(12):1576–1579.
23. **Brady OH, Garbuz DS, Masri BA, et al.** The reliability and validity of the Vancouver classification of femoral fractures after hip replacement. *J Arthroplasty.* 2000 Jan;15(1):59–62.
24. **Vioreanu MH, Parry MC, Haddad FS, et al.** Field testing the Unified Classification System for peri-prosthetic fractures of the pelvis and femur around a total hip replacement: an international collaboration. *Bone Joint J.* 2014 Nov;96-B(11):1472–1477.
25. **Brady OH, Garbuz DS, Masri BA, et al.** Classification of the hip. *Orthop Clin North Am.* 1999 Apr;30(2):215–220.
26. **Haddad FS, Duncan CP.** Cortical onlay allograft struts in the treatment of periprosthetic femoral fractures. *Instr Course Lect.* 2003;52:291–300.
27. **Harrington IJ, Tountas AA, Cameron HU.** Femoral fractures associated with Moore's prosthesis. *Injury.* 1979 Aug;11(1):23–32.
28. **Zenni EJ Jr, Pomeroy DL, Caudle RJ.** Ogden plate and other fixations for fractures complicating femoral endoprostheses. *Clin Orthop Relat Res.* 1988 Jun;(231):83–90.
29. **Kamineni S, Ware HE.** The Mennen plate: unsuitable for elderly femoral peri-prosthetic fractures. *Injury.* 1999 May;30(4):257–260.
30. **Liu AM, Flores M, Nadarajan P.** Failure of Mennen femoral plate. *Injury.* 1995 Apr;26(3):202–203.
31. **Jones DG.** Bone erosion beneath partridge bands. *J Bone Joint Surg Br.* 1986 May;68(3):476–477.
32. **Corten K, Vanrykel F, Bellemans J, et al.** An algorithm for the surgical treatment of periprosthetic fractures of the femur around a well-fixed femoral component. *J Bone Joint Surg Br.* 2009 Nov;91(11):1424–1430.
33. **Khan T, Grindlay D, Ollivere BJ, et al.** A systematic review of Vancouver B2 and B3 periprosthetic femoral fractures. *Bone Joint J.* 2017 Apr;99-B(4 Supple B):17–25.
34. **Joestl J, Hofbauer M, Lang N, et al.** Locking compression plate versus revision-prosthesis for Vancouver type B2 periprosthetic femoral fractures after total hip arthroplasty. *Injury.* 2016 Apr;47(4):939–943.
35. **Quah C, Porteous M, Stephen A.** Principles of managing Vancouver type B periprosthetic fractures around cemented polished tapered femoral stems. *Eur J Orthop Surg Traumatol.* 2017 May;27(4):477–482.
36. **Solomon LB, Hussenbocus SM, Carbone TA, et al.** Is internal fixation alone advantageous in selected B2 periprosthetic fractures? *ANZ J Surg.* 2015 Mar;85(3):169–173.
37. **Partridge AJ, Evans PE.** The treatment of fractions of the shaft of the femur using nylon cerclage. *J Bone Joint Surg Br.* 1982;64(2):210–214.
38. **Tsiridis E, Narvani AA, Timperley JA, et al.** Dynamic compression plates for Vancouver type B periprosthetic femoral fractures: a 3-year follow-up of 18 cases. *Acta Orthop.* 2005 Aug;76(4):531–537.
39. **Parvizi J, Rapuri VR, Purtill JJ, et al.** Treatment protocol for proximal femoral periprosthetic fractures. *J Bone Joint Surg Am.* 2004;86-A Suppl 2:8–16.
40. **Brady OH, Garbuz DS, Masri BA, et al.** The treatment of periprosthetic fractures of the femur using cortical onlay allograft struts. *Orthop Clin North Am.* 1999 Apr;30(2):249–257.
41. **Haddad FS, Duncan CP, Berry DJ, et al.** Periprosthetic femoral fractures around well-fixed implants: use of cortical onlay allografts with or without a plate. *J Bone Joint Surg Am.* 2002 Jun;84-A(6):945–950.
42. **Mihalko WM, Beaudoin AJ, Cardea JA, et al.** Finite-element modelling of femoral shaft fracture fixation techniques post total hip arthroplasty. *J Biomech.* 1992 May;25(5):469–476.
43. **Wong P, Gross AE.** The use of structural allografts for treating periprosthetic fractures about the hip and knee. *Orthop Clin North Am.* 1999 Apr;30(2):259–264.
44. **Dennis MG, Simon JA, Kummer FJ, et al.** Fixation of periprosthetic femoral shaft fractures: a biomechanical comparison of two techniques. *J Orthop Trauma.* 2001 Mar-Apr;15(3):177–180.
45. **Wilson D, Frei H, Masri BA, et al.** A biomechanical study comparing cortical onlay allograft struts and plates in the treatment of periprosthetic femoral fractures. *Clin Biomech (Bristol, Avon).* 2005 Jan;20(1):70–76.
46. **Dennis MG, Simon JA, Kummer FJ, et al.** Fixation of periprosthetic femoral shaft fractures occurring at the tip of the stem: a biomechanical study of 5 techniques. *J Arthroplasty.* 2000 Jun;15(4):523–528.
47. **Somers JF, Suy R, Stuyck J, et al.** Conservative treatment of femoral shaft fractures in patients with total hip arthroplasty. *J Arthroplasty.* 1998 Feb;13(2):162–171.
48. **Rayan F, Konan S, Haddad FS.** Uncemented revision hip arthroplasty in B2 and B3 periprosthetic femoral fractures—A prospective analysis. *Hip Int.* 2010 Jan-Mar;20(1):38–42.
49. **Stoffel K, Sommer C, Kalampoki V, et al.** The influence of the operation technique and implant used in the treatment of periprosthetic hip and interprosthetic femur fractures: a systematic literature review of 1571 cases. *Arch Orthop Trauma Surg.* 2016 Apr;136(4):553–561.
50. **Fulkerson E, Koval K, Preston CF, et al.** Fixation of periprosthetic femoral shaft fractures associated with cemented femoral stems: a biomechanical comparison of locked plating and conventional cable plates. *J Orthop Trauma.* 2006 Feb;20(2):89–93.
51. **Lenz M, Perren SM, Richards RG, et al.** Biomechanical performance of different cable and wire cerclage configurations. *Int Orthop.* 2013 Jan;37(1):125–130.
52. **Rosenberg AG.** Managing periprosthetic femoral stem fractures. *J Arthroplasty.* 2006 Jun;21(4 Suppl 1):101–104.
53. **Serocki JH, Chandler RW, Dorr LD.** Treatment of fractures about hip prostheses with compression plating. *J Arthroplasty.* 1992 Jun;7(2):129–135.
54. **Kim MB, Cho JW, Lee YH, et al.** Locking attachment plate fixation around a well-fixed stem in periprosthetic femoral shaft fractures. *Arch Orthop Trauma Surg.* 2017 Sep;137(9):1193–1200.
55. **Stoffel K, Stachowiak G, Forster T, et al.** Oblique screws at the plate ends increase the fixation strength in synthetic bone test medium. *J Orthop Trauma.* 2004 Oct;18(9):611–616.
56. **Lenz M, Perren SM, Gueorguiev B, et al.** A biomechanical study on proximal plate fixation techniques in periprosthetic femur fractures. *Injury.* 2014 Jan;45(Suppl 1):S71–S75.
57. **Lenz M, Stoffel K, Kielstein H, et al.** Plate fixation in periprosthetic femur fractures Vancouver type B1-Trochanteric hook plate or subtrochanterical bicortical locking? *Injury.* 2016 Dec;47(12):2800–2804.
58. **Berlusconi M, Accetta R, Pascale V, et al.** Locking Compression Plates (LCP) for treatment of periprosthetic fractures of the hip [abstract]. *J Orthop Trauma.* 2004;18(Suppl. 9):S20–S21.
59. **Ricci WM, Bolhofner BR, Loftus T, et al.** Indirect reduction and plate fixation, without grafting, for periprosthetic femoral shaft fractures about a stable intramedullary implant. *J Bone Joint Surg Am.* 2005 Oct;87(10):2240–2245.

60. **O'Toole RV, Gobezie R, Hwang R, et al.** Low complication rate of LISS for femur fractures adjacent to stable hip or knee arthroplasty. *Clin Orthop Relat Res.* 2006 Sep;450:203–210.
61. **Kregor PJ, Stannard J, Zlowodzki M, et al.** Distal femoral fracture fixation utilizing the Less Invasive Stabilization System (L.I.S.S.): the technique and early results. *Injury.* 2001 Dec;32(Suppl 3):Sc32–47.
62. **Pike J, Davidson D, Garbuz D, et al.** Principles of treatment for periprosthetic femoral shaft fractures around well-fixed total hip arthroplasty. *J Am Acad Orthop Surg.* 2009 Nov;17(11):677–688.
63. **Stoffel K, Dieter U, Stachowiak G, et al.** Biomechanical testing of the LCP—how can stability in locked internal fixators be controlled? *Injury.* 2003 Nov;34(Suppl 2):B11–B19.
64. **Lenz M, Stoffel K, Gueorguiev B, et al.** Enhancing fixation strength in periprosthetic femur fractures by orthogonal plating-A biomechanical study. *J Orthop Res.* 2016 Apr;34(4):591–596.
65. **Jarit GJ, Sathappan SS, Panchal A, et al.** Fixation systems of greater trochanteric osteotomies: biomechanical and clinical outcomes. *J Am Acad Orthop Surg.* 2007 Oct;15(10):614–624.
66. **Pritchett JW.** Fracture of the greater trochanter after hip replacement. *Clin Orthop Relat Res.* 2001 Sep;(390):221–226.
67. **Lewallen DG, Berry DJ.** Periprosthetic fracture of the femur after total hip arthroplasty. Treatment and results to date. *J Bone Joint Surg Am.* 1997;79(12):1881–1890.
68. **Wang JW, Chen LK, Chen CE.** Surgical treatment of fractures of the greater trochanter associated with osteolytic lesions. *J Bone Joint Surg Am.* 2005 Dec;87(12):2724–2728.
69. **Brady OH, Kerry R, Masri BA, et al.** The Vancouver Classification of periprosthetic fractures of the hip: a rational approach to treatment. *Techniques in Orthopaedics.* 1999;14(2):107–114.
70. **Zuurmond RG, van Wijhe W, van Raay JJ, et al.** High incidence of complications and poor clinical outcome in the operative treatment of periprosthetic femoral fractures: an analysis of 71 cases. *Injury.* 2010 Jun;41(6):629–633.
71. **Tadross TS, Nanu AM, Buchanan MJ, et al.** Dall-Miles plating for periprosthetic B1 fractures of the femur. *J Arthroplasty.* 2000 Jan;15(1):47–51.
72. **Ricci WM, Bolhofner BR, Loftus T, et al.** Indirect reduction and plate fixation, without grafting, for periprosthetic femoral shaft fractures about a stable intramedullary implant. Surgical technique. *J Bone Joint Surg Am.* 2006 Sep;88(Suppl 1 Pt 2):275–282.
73. **Marsland D, Mears SC.** A review of periprosthetic femoral fractures associated with total hip arthroplasty. *Geriatr Orthop Surg Rehabil.* 2012 Sep;3(3):107–120.
74. **Stoffel K, Lorenz KU, Kuster MS.** Biomechanical considerations in plate osteosynthesis: the effect of plate-to-bone compression with and without angular screw stability. *J Orthop Trauma.* 2007 Jul;21(6):362–368.
75. **Kenny P, Rice J, Quinlan W.** Interprosthetic fracture of the femoral shaft. *J Arthroplasty.* 1998 Apr;13(3):361–364.
76. **Fink B, Fuerst M, Singer J.** Periprosthetic fractures of the femur associated with hip arthroplasty. *Arch Orthop Trauma Surg.* 2005 Sep;125(7):433–442.
77. **Ebraheim N, Carroll T, Moral MZ, et al.** Interprosthetic femoral fractures treated with locking plate. *Int Orthop.* 2014 Oct;38(10):2183–2189.
78. **Hou Z, Moore B, Bowen TR, et al.** Treatment of interprosthetic fractures of the femur. *J Trauma.* 2011 Dec;71(6):1715–1719.
79. **Mamczak CN, Gardner MJ, Bolhofner B, et al.** Interprosthetic femoral fractures. *J Orthop Trauma.* 2010 Dec;24(12):740–744.
80. **Walcher MG, Giesinger K, du Sart R, et al.** Plate positioning in periprosthetic or interprosthetic femur fractures with stable implants—a biomechanical study. *J Arthroplasty.* 2016 Dec;31(12):2894–2899.
81. **Schwarzkopf R, Oni JK, Marwin SE.** Total hip arthroplasty periprosthetic femoral fractures: a review of classification and current treatment. *Bull Hosp Jt Dis.* 2013;71(1):68–78.

# 3.14 Periprosthetic fractures around the knee

Frank A Liporace, Iain McFadyen, Richard S Yoon

## 1 Introduction

Periprosthetic fractures around the knee (PPKFs) present a difficult clinical scenario for the following reasons:

- They mostly affect older adults and are complicated by the increased prevalence of comorbidity, cognitive and functional impairments seen in this population; these nonoperative factors need to be addressed in order to maximize outcomes.
- They are associated with a higher risk of morbidity and mortality; definitive treatment must allow for early mobilization.
- Operative management of periprosthetic fractures is inherently associated with increased infection risk due to open operative history.
- Antecedent pain and/or a poorly functioning implant prior to periprosthetic fracture may indicate the need for an infection workup.
- They are complicated by the presence of a total knee arthroplasty (TKA) and the wide spectrum of components, implant wear status, and surrounding bone stock.
- The overall mechanical alignment must be evaluated prior to definitive treatment.
- Total knee arthroplasty components may be stable or unstable, in good or poor alignment, and with or without good surrounding bone stock.
- The wide variety of TKA components also adds difficulty, especially if revision is indicated. Some may be obsolete and no longer available.
- A concomitant proximal hip prosthesis or implant is not uncommon, adding further difficulty and frequently requiring alternative fixation strategies.
- There is no consensus on the ideal mode of fixation and/or treatment, and thus, several options exist.

Periprosthetic fractures around the knee require careful planning in order to achieve the goals of early mobilization, fracture healing, and continued long-term implant survivorship (ie, a stable implant rendering revision arthroplasty unnecessary). Treatment strategy depends on surgeon experience, skill level, and preference, but should also fall in line with several principles in order to achieve a desired clinical result. This chapter presents a comprehensive and pragmatic approach to the management of periprosthetic fractures around the knee, along with some helpful tips and tricks to avoid pitfalls and complications.

## 2 Epidemiology and etiology

The incidence of PPKF approaches 2.5% following primary TKA, with even higher rates following revision TKA [1–4]. The following patient factors contribute to the incidence of periprosthetic fractures [3]:

- Younger age (< 60 years) and older age (> 80 years) groups are at higher risk for PPKF.
- Comorbidities that lead to falls [5].
- Dementia, limited ambulatory status, or other neurological conditions.
- Bone quality is poor.
- Changes in bone quality secondary to altered femoral stress and strain following TKA have been reported to be important. Studies have noted significantly decreased bone mineral density about the distal femur following primary TKA [3, 6].
- In a more recent finite element analysis, Sun et al [7] noted a high concentration of stress located just proximal to the femoral implant, which may explain why supracondylar periprosthetic fractures are the most common fractures seen after total knee replacement [3, 6].
- Femoral notching of the anterior femoral cortex with the bone cuts for the femoral component has been implicated as a potential cause for subsequent supracondylar fracture. However, in large cohort studies, a correlation between femoral notching and periprosthetic fracture has not been identified [8, 9].

## 3 Diagnostics

Periprosthetic fractures following TKA are associated with morbidity and mortality rates comparable to those in hip fracture patients, and medical optimization must begin immediately upon admission [10]. A thorough history and physical examination along with the appropriate imaging modalities must be performed to formulate a treatment plan. Issues of frailty and potential problems with the original knee prostheses need to be considered.

### 3.1 Imaging

#### 3.1.1 Plain x-rays

Plain x-rays are the primary imaging modality for diagnosis and in guiding operative treatment. Adequate preimaging pain management including femoral nerve blockade, utilizing cross-table views to obtain the laterals, manipulating the uninjured extremity, and gently propping up the injured extremity helps to obtain the desired imaging. The following views help achieve this:

- True AP and lateral views along with oblique views are essential.
- Full-length orthogonal view of the ipsilateral femur and tibia to examine the proximal and distal extent of the fracture lines and to provide an estimate of overall alignment as well as the existence of any preexisting hardware. Some centers can only obtain long leg x-rays with patients standing. A CT scanogram can be a helpful method of obtaining this imaging with patients supine.
- A low AP view of the pelvis helps to judge overall leg lengths, especially if a hip implant is present.
- For those fractures extending well into the femoral diaphysis, contralateral x-rays may also be valuable in recreating appropriate femoral rotation. This can be done by taking a perfect AP view of the knee, moving up to the ipsilateral femur and taking an AP of the hip. The profile of the lesser trochanter (LT) can be used to match the version on the injured side.
- Previous serial x-rays of the affected implant should be acquired, whenever possible. Analyzing previous serial x-rays offers the best insight into potentially loose components (aseptic or septic). If serial x-rays are unavailable, at the very least, try and obtain the most recent follow-up x-ray, as it provides the most recent component alignment prior to fracture.

#### 3.1.2 Computed tomography

Advances in software may provide even more information out of computed tomographic (CT) scans than previously realized (**Case 1: Fig 3.14-1**) [11–13].

CASE 1

**Patient**

A 63-year-old man was struck by a car as he stepped off a curb sustaining a closed injury to his right knee. This happened 3 years after a total knee arthroplasty of the right knee.

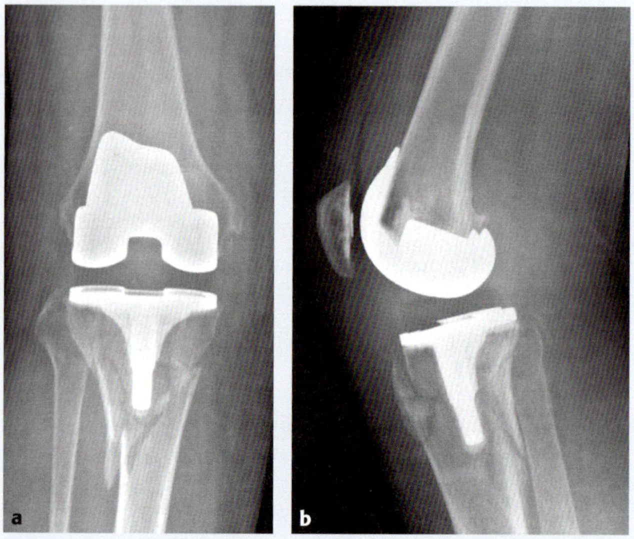

**Fig 3.14-1a–j** A 63-year-old man with a closed injury to his right knee.
**a–b** AP and lateral x-rays showing the periprosthetic fracture.

**Comorbidities**

- Hypertension

**Treatment and outcome**

The right lower extremity was neurovascularly intact. The AP (**Fig 3.14-1a**) and lateral (**Fig 3.14-1b**) x-rays of the knee exhibited a periprosthetic fracture about the tibial component. Further workup with computed tomography denoted a multiplanar fracture about the implant (**Fig 3.14-1c–f**) with a notable coronal plane fracture across the tibial tubercle (**Fig 3.14-1f**). A dual incision approach utilized the previous midline incision, distally extended to fix the tubercle component (**Fig 3.14-1g–h**), followed by a laterally based incision over Gerdy's tubercle to assess the lateral tibial plateau. Orthogonal plate placement was performed, with a long lateral plate utilized to disperse the deforming forces inherent in a proximal third tibial fracture. The patient went on to uneventful healing (**Fig 3.14-1i–j**). Here, key points are not only to restore proper component alignment in relation to the femur, but similar to the setting of a primary total knee arthroplasty (TKA), the final examination of TKA stability and tracking should be performed. Assuming the gaps were properly balanced prior to the fracture, lack of needing to upsize or downsize the liner is a crude measure of appropriate fracture reduction.

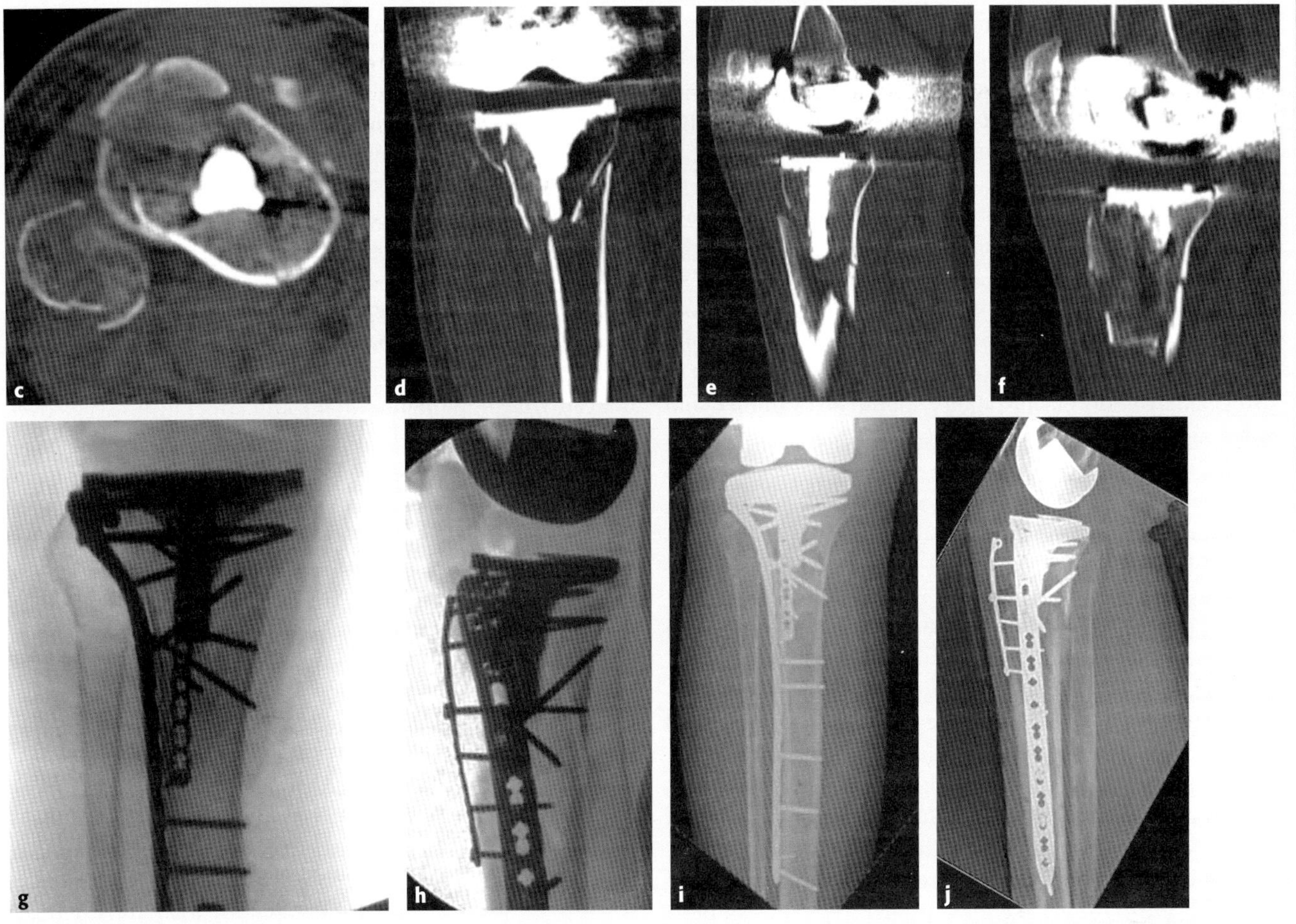


**Fig 3.14-1a–j (cont)** A 63-year-old man with a closed injury to his right knee.
**c–f** Computed tomographic scans denoting a multiplanar fracture about the implant with a notable coronal plane fracture across the tibial tubercle.
**g–h** The dual incision approach, utilizing the previous midline incision and distally extending to fix the tubercle component, followed by a laterally based incision over Gerdy's tubercle to assess the lateral tibial plateau.
**i–j** The orthogonal plate placement with a long lateral plate.

Despite metal artifact (ie, distortion of image quality caused by metal interference during scanning), conventional CT can offer:

- Better fracture characterization than plain x-rays in regard to the extent of fracture and degree of comminution.
- Reconstructed images in different planes to better assess specific fracture line locations.
- Highly sensitive and specific information regarding osteolytic pockets about the implant when combined with standard metal artifact reduction protocols [13].

Compiled 3-D reconstructions can also provide improved fracture pattern visualization. Dual-energy CT (DECT), a relatively new technology, has proven especially useful in reducing beam-hardening artifact created by metal implants [11, 12]. Ferrara et al [11] utilized DECT in order to reduce metal artifact and calculate TKA component position with subsequent clinical correlation. The authors reported DECT as a highly reproducible and accurate tool to assess TKA component position. Pessis et al [12] utilized the technology to recreate the DECT images into virtual monochromatic spectral images. In other words, images similar to plain x-rays were recreated but with a significantly higher degree of characterization, with information obtained from the DECT, and with additional metal artifact subtraction. While this new technology is on the cutting edge, its clinical availability and application needs further investigation.

### 3.1.3 Magnetic resonance imaging

Similar to CT, advances in magnetic resonance imaging (MRI) software and design sequences have provided greater ability to suppress metal artifact and characterize surrounding soft tissue and osteolysis about a TKA [14–16].

In the setting of periprosthetic fractures, however, MRI plays a limited role, mostly due to difficulty in performing the study in acutely unstable fracture patients. Subjecting an older patient to a confined loud area for a relatively long period is not a pragmatic approach to care, especially when the information obtained is comparable to that of CT [11]. Suspected ligamentous instability should be examined and addressed intraoperatively for TKA and does not typically require advanced imaging.

## 4 Classification

The purpose of classification systems is not only to help properly diagnose the injury but more important to help in guiding the optimal treatment choice. While some classification systems rarely do both, the most commonly applied systems for periprosthetic fractures about the femur are generally consistent in guiding the appropriate treatment based on the proper diagnosis. While some have attempted to classify periprosthetic fractures involving tibial and patellar components, these systems are largely not used in the clinical setting [17–20]. In general, proper treatment for periprosthetic fractures around the femoral, the tibial, and the patellar components are based on implant stability, the quality of the surrounding bone stock, and for the fractures about the patella, the status of the extensor mechanism.

### 4.1 Su classification

The Su classification [21] focuses primarily on fracture location in relation to the femoral component, which potentially aids in dictating treatment, but does not address implant stability and/or bone stock:

- Type I: Fracture is proximal to the femoral component.
- Type II: The fracture extends proximally with the origin at the proximal extent of the femoral component.
- Type III: Includes any fracture line seen within the femoral component.

In general, intact implants with fracture lines originating and/or extending proximally from the upper end of the femoral component can be treated with open reduction and internal fixation (ORIF), while a loose implant or fractures that are within the body of the femoral component should be considered for revision. However, while a general treatment algorithm can be applied, specific circumstances can yield different operative strategies.

### 4.2 Unified Classification System (UCS)

This classification system aims to unify classification systems used for periprosthetic fractures around various joint replacement components (eg, hip and knee) into a single system that can be universally applied to any periprosthetic fracture [22]:

- Type A: This is a fracture of an apophysis or protuberance of bone, eg, tibial tuberosityor greater trochanter in hips.
- Type B: This involves the bed supporting an implant, eg, fracture of the femoral shaft around an arthroplasty stem or fracture of the patella that has been resurfaced. This group can be subdivided into:
  - B1: Implant is well fixed.
  - B2: Implant is loose.
  - B3: Implant is loose and bone bed is poor quality because of osteolysis, comminution, or osteoporosis.
- Type C: Fracture is in the bone containing the implant but is distant from the implant.
- Type D: Fracture affects one bone that supports two replacements, eg, femur following hip and knee replacement (**Case 2: Fig 3.14-2**) or tibia following knee and ankle replacement.
- Type E: Involves two bones supporting one replacement, eg, fracture of femur and tibia after knee replacement ("floating knee replacement").
- Type F: Involves a joint surface that is not replaced but is directly articulating with an implant, eg, patellar fracture when the patella has not been resurfaced or acetabular fracture after hip hemiarthroplasty.

### Patient

A 73-year-old woman sustained low-energy falls 7 years and 5 years after a right total hip arthroplasty and total knee arthroplasty, respectively.

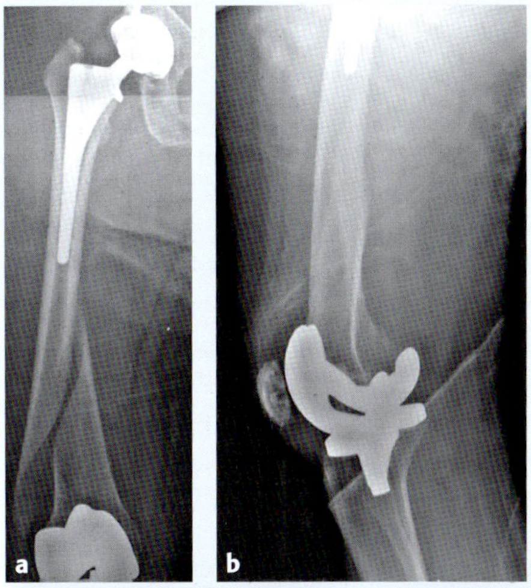

### Comorbidities

- Morbid obesity
- Hypertension
- Hyperlipidemia
- Type 2 diabetes mellitus

### Treatment and outcome

Initial workup and x-rays revealed a long, spiral, interprosthetic fracture (Unified Classification type D) between the two implants (**Fig 3.14-2a–b**). Decision making for definitive fixation relied heavily on early mobilization and immediate weight bearing. Lag screw fixation with lateral plate, along with a lateral plate alone was contemplated. However, due to the long extent of the fracture, the aforementioned options would not allow for immediate weight bearing. Thus, the decision was made to proceed with a combined retrograde nail and lateral locking plate combination that would allow for immediate weight bearing (**Fig 3.14-2c–h**). To allow for more stability without absolute rigidity, the reamed intramedullary nail was linked to the plate via the proximal and distal locking holes, forming a linked construct. The patient was made weight bearing as tolerated, and eventually there was uneventful healing (**Fig 3.14-2i–j**).

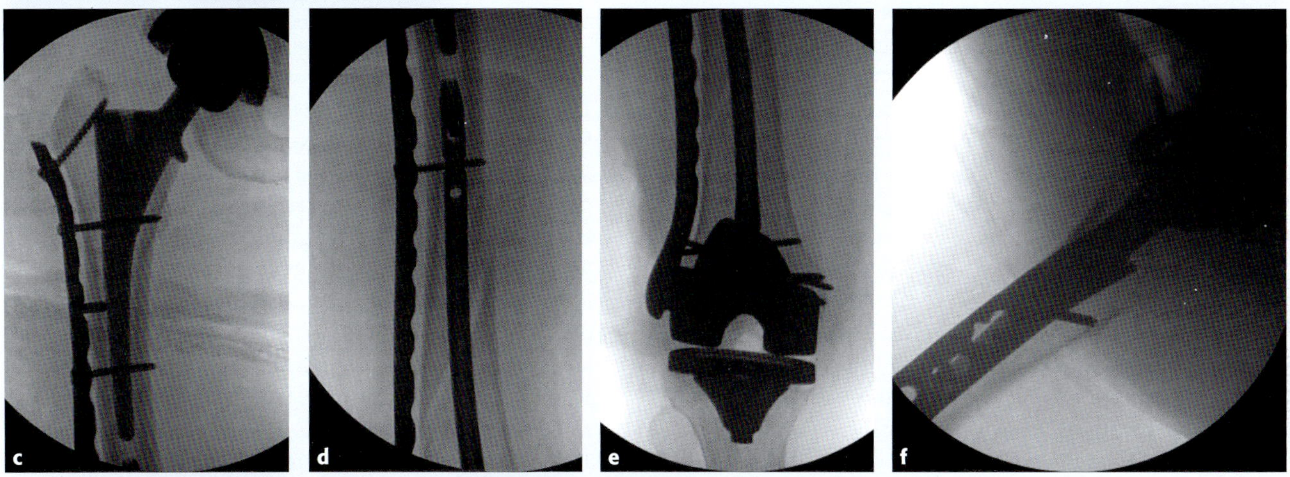

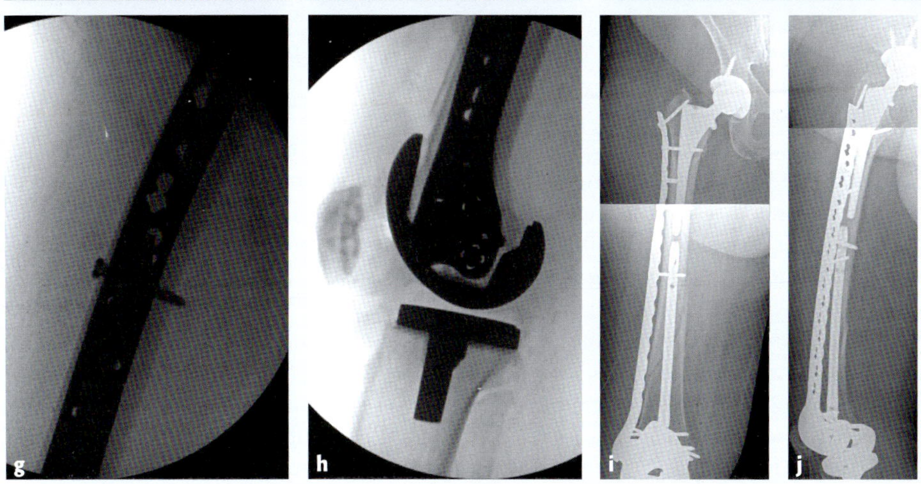

**Fig 3.14-2a–j** A 73-year-old woman with a long, spiral, interprosthetic fracture.

**a–b** X-rays showing the long spiral interprosthetic fracture between the two implants.

**c–h** Use of a combined retrograde nail and lateral locking plate combination, which allowed for immediate weight bearing.

**i–j** The reamed intramedullary nail was linked to the plate via the proximal and distal locking holes, forming a linked construct and allowing for more stability without absolute rigidity.

## 5 Decision making

For effective decision making, the basic treatment principles are as follows:

- Obtain as much information as possible about the articular design of the present implant. This will, for example, enable the surgeon to know when a posterior stabilized knee replacement will permit access for intramedullary fixation or not. Useful reference guides for this purpose have been published [23].
- Careful tissue handling and less invasive techniques should be performed whenever possible. Specific tools are available and helpful.
- Operative strategy must aim to achieve a stable construct. This includes spanning the entire femur to avoid stress risers and to distribute forces along a longer length.
- For fragility fracture patients (FFPs), there is no alternative to immediate mobilization with full weight bearing (FWB) and no external splints hindering mobility (see chapter 1.8 Postoperative surgical management).
- Assess the stability of the prosthetic joint replacement prior to surgery. In the absence of clear radiological evidence of loosening the concept of a "happy knee replacement" can be employed. If the patient had no preinjury problems with the knee replacement, and the x-rays do not show obvious loosening, then it is fairly safe to assume that the knee prosthesis is stable enough to be retained. An "unhappy knee replacement" (eg, pain, swelling, stiffness, poor function) should be regarded as possibly loose or unstable, and should be considered for revision. Here, this decision can be made intraoperatively by assessing the overall stability of the implant.
- Contingency plans need to be agreed preoperatively. Occasionally, despite good preoperative assessment, new information may become apparent during the procedure and the operative strategy needs to be adapted. For example, a presumed well-fixed implant may be identified as loose during surgery. A surgeon experienced in both trauma and arthroplasty would be well prepared to manage such a scenario if conversion from a fixation strategy to a joint replacement revision strategy is required (**Case 3: Fig 3.14-3**). Many trauma surgeons need to ask for assistance from arthroplasty colleagues in such a scenario.

Orthogeriatric care involves assessment of comorbidities and frailty that will help guide management and shared decision making with the patient and families [24, 25]. Frail older patients usually have delicate soft tissues and are prone to soft-tissue complications. Careful tissue handling and less invasive techniques are often required. The specifics are discussed in chapter 1.2 Principles of orthogeriatric surgical care.

### 5.1 Operative treatment

With few exceptions, periprosthetic fractures around the knee are managed operatively. The UCS classification can be used to outline, in general terms, the treatment options for periprosthetic fractures around the knee.

- Type A: if the apophysis or protuberance is displaced and is important to the function of the joint then it cannot be ignored and will require operative treatment. This is usually the case with avulsion of the tibial tuberosity or the poles of the patella.
- Type B: Management is usually determined by subtype:
  - Type B1 fractures can often be treated with fracture fixation techniques.
  - Type B2 fractures often require revision of the loose component often combined with fixation of the fracture using techniques such as long stem implants and cerclage fixation.
  - Type B3 fractures may require complex arthroplasty reconstruction techniques.
- Type C: the implant can often be "ignored" and fracture fixation performed using the principles outlined below.
- Type D: the fractures can be further analyzed by using a "block out analysis". In a fracture between a hip and a knee replacement, for example, block out the hip and assess the type of fracture present just for the knee. Ask it is a B or C type fracture. Repeat the process blocking out the knee and assessing the hip fracture. Then formulate a treatment plan following the general principles for whatever type of fracture is identified for each aspect of this "block out analysis".
- Type E: follow the same logic of a "block out analysis" as described for type D.
- Type F: if displaced, the fracture of an unsurfaced patella will usually require operative fixation.

### 5.2 Plate, nail, or revision arthroplasty?

Surgeons should remember that these techniques aim to employ relative stability and indirect fracture healing. Fixation should also enable early FWB. Initial assessment of the fracture location can aid in determining if fixation is possible. Very low fractures that run below the anterior flange are often associated with loose components and revision components should be on hand as backup. Frequently, component stability assessment is difficult to assess preoperatively and needs to be made intraoperatively. In periprosthetic TKA fractures, however, there is a lower incidence

**Patient**

A 78-year-old woman sustained a low-energy fall 16 years after a left total knee arthroplasty.

**Comorbidities**

- Hypertension
- Osteoporosis

**Treatment and outcome**

The x-rays revealed a periprosthetic fracture about both the femoral and tibial components (**Fig 3.14-3a–b**). Initially seen and evaluated at an outside institution, the treating surgeon, who was trauma trained but without an arthroplasty background, stabilized the distal femoral fracture in a good position to allow for healing (**Fig 3.14-3c–d**). Further questioning revealed symptoms of loosening prior to fracture, and on closer examination of the injury images, areas of osteolysis and loosening were likely the stress risers that caused an insufficiency fracture about the tibial component. Following stabilization, the patient was then referred to our senior author. Upon healing, the patient noted continued pain with weight bearing, and was revised on both the femoral and tibial sides with a retained lateral plate (albeit distal screws were removed). Five years following revision, the patient remains pain free, with full range of motion, and walking with a cane (**Fig 3.14-3e–f**).

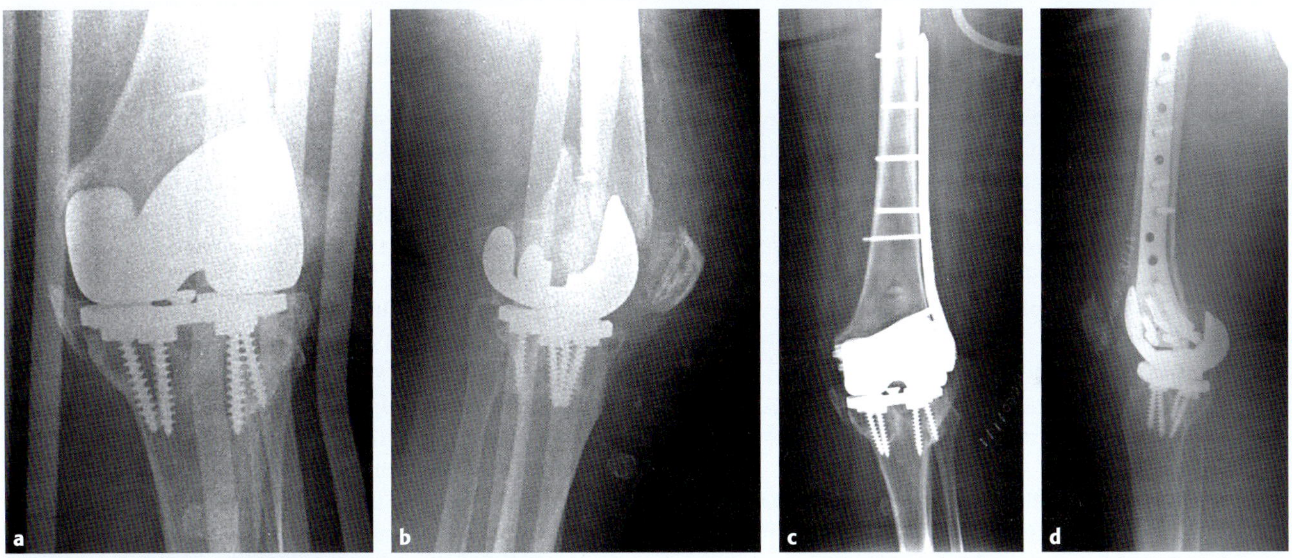


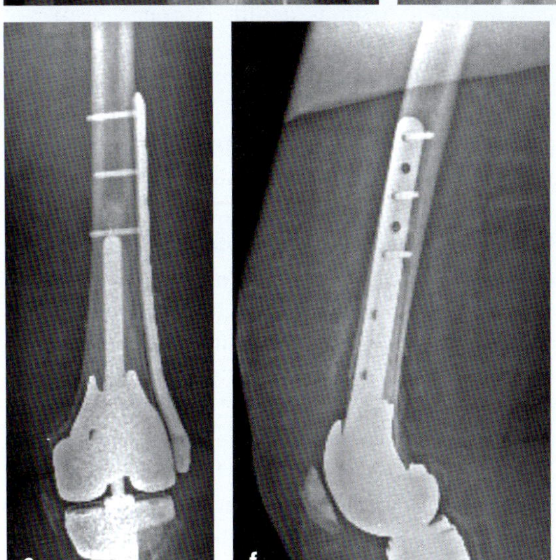


**Fig 3.14-3a–f** A 78-year-old woman with a periprosthetic fracture after a low-energy fall.
**a–b** X-rays revealing the periprosthetic fracture about both the femoral and tibial components.
**c–d** The distal femoral fracture was stabilized. Revision on both the femoral and tibial sides with a retained lateral plate.
**e–f** The implants at 5 years following revision, where the patient remained pain free and with full range of motion.

of needing revision as most fixation strategies are amenable to healing. Revision TKA or even distal femoral replacement (DFR) is reserved for the settings of obvious severe bone loss and/or lysis.

In regard to fixation, deciding between an intramedullary (IM) nail or a plate can be based on surgeon preference, the TKA design (posterior stabilized versus cruciate retaining), and preinjury range of motion (ROM). If the patient has limited ROM prefracture, reamed IM nailing may actually cause a malreduction since the appropriate starting point will not be possible. Fractures that are above the level of the metadiaphyseal junction are typically more amenable to either anterograde or retrograde IM nailing. At the level of the metaphyseal junction, surgeon preference usually can dictate plating or reamed IM nailing (if amenable).

### 5.3 Nonoperative treatment

Nonoperative treatment may be more appropriate for severely ill patients, those that have advanced dementia, are suffering from profound frailty and sarcopenia, and for patients who are chronically nonambulatory. Even in these patients, however, operative stabilization may be helpful for pain control, protecting soft tissues, and facilitating easier transfer and hygienic care; for the extremely frail patients, a definitive spanning external fixator can offer reasonable results.

## 6 Therapeutic options

### 6.1 Initial treatment in the emergency department

As with all FFPs, close attention to preoperative hydration, blood loss, and pain control is necessary. Assessment of nutrition, functional and cogntive status, and goals of care are important. Discharge planning should also be performed on admission. Preoperative optimization aims to achieve safe operative treatment, but is also important for achieving postoperative mobilization and avoidance of in-hospital complications (see chapter 1.4 Preoperative risk assessment and preparation). Pain control techniques should include careful use of analgesic medication in patients prone to adverse effects, the use of regional anesthetic techniques, and appropriate preoperative immobilization strategies (see chapter 1.12 Pain management). Traction is not usually required for PPKF but may be of benefit when the femur is shortened or severely displaced. With any immobilization, padding and protection of the skin to prevent pressure ulceration is critical.

### 6.2 Preoperative planning

Preoperative planning comprises positioning and operative details. When fracture fixation is indicated, preoperative planning should address the type and length of the implant. In the case of plate fixation, the number and location of screws must be determined. Since the operative approach depends on the fracture type and anticipated procedure, careful planning is required including reduction technique, placement of clamps and retractors, fixation techniques, positioning of fixation implants, and salvage options if problems are encountered.

### 6.3 Operating room setup and patient positioning

Good positioning and setup in the operating room can make the operation a more efficient process.

#### 6.3.1 Supine position

Typical setup includes a radiolucent flat table and the patient in the supine position. A small bump placed under the ipsilateral ischial tuberosity allows for a better-aligned limb in the operative field for improved visual orientation and an easier position for the operative surgeon. Large imaging with the image intensifier should be utilized and should come in from the contralateral side.

Skin preparation and draping should occur in the standard fashion, being sure to extend proximally to the anterior superior iliac spine (ASIS). Palpation of the ASIS and the ability to move the hip joint helps the surgeon identify anatomical landmarks to achieve correct alignment and rotation of the limb during surgery. An appropriately sized radiolucent knee triangle or rolled bump under the knee is useful to achieve adequate knee flexion and femoral curvature as described by Haidukewych et al [26].

#### 6.3.2 Lateral position

A stable lateral decubitus position of the patient is another viable alternative. The affected leg is freely draped and reduction can be performed with the C-arm underneath the table and an AP projection. The surgeon should make sure that the lateral projection of the femur is not interfered with by angulating the opposite leg. Minimally invasive plate osteosynthesis can be easily performed in this position.

## 6.4 Operative approaches

The approach takes into account the following fracture stabilization and fracture healing strategies:

- Fractures of the femoral shaft. These are ideally treated by indirect reduction and relative stability constructs. Less invasive surgery, indirect reduction techniques, relative stability, and indirect fracture healing are often appropriate for type C fractures separate from the prosthesis. The importance of utilizing biologically friendly approaches in order to provide the best environment for healing cannot be overemphasized.
- Fractures that may need conversion to revision arthroplasty. Anterolateral incisions can be converted to full open lateral parapatellar approaches for revision knee arthroplasty surgery.
- Fractures that require revision TKA from the outset. Either of the previous approaches can be used as well as more extensile approaches for more complex reconstructions (**Case 4: Fig 3.14-4**).
- Reamed intramedullary nailing may be possible for some prosthesis types and can be achieved using a standard anterior arthrotomy often utilizing part of the previous knee replacement incision.
- Patella fractures and avulsion of the tibial tubercle usually require direct approaches utilizing or extending the previous knee replacement.
- Tibial plateau fractures should be approached in a similar fashion to plateau fractures in the native knee joint. Fracture-specific incisions are preferable to midline incisions with extensive soft-tissue stripping. Particular care should be used when handling the anteromedial skin over the proximal tibia as wound problems in this region often lead to infection of the arthroplasty. Innovative approaches including posterior options may be required for tibial fractures distal to the TKA.

### 6.4.1 Lateral approach

Around the distal femur, a lateral or anterolateral incision is recommended for direct reduction and internal fixation. Submuscular plating should be performed using less invasive techniques to slide a plate up the lateral side of the femur using a small lateral distal window employing Gerdy's tubercle as a landmark [27]. It is rarely appropriate for an open reduction of the femoral shaft to be performed in older adults. Indications include placement of a lateral plate for supracondylar fractures with stable implants.

With an incision centered over the midaxis of the femur and lateral condyle, this approach can be extended distally by centering it over Gerdy's tubercle. Even in the most obese patient, Gerdy's tubercle can be readily found via the method described by Seigerman et al, which utilizes familiar anatomical landmarks (eg, interior pole of the patella, fibular head, and tibial tubercle) for localization [27].

If addressing an isolated fracture above a femoral component, a minimally invasive 3–4 cm incision can be utilized as a window to slide a locking plate proximally up the femur in order to minimize periosteal stripping and violating the vascular supply. Submuscular placement of the plate can be easily facilitated through this small incision with proximal screw fixation performed percutaneously to avoid an extensile incision.

If addressing a periprosthetic fracture around the tibial component, the incision can be extended distally, sliding anteriorly over Gerdy's tubercle in order to expose the joint line, and to facilitate a standard tibial plateau exposure for plate placement submuscularly under the anterior tibial muscle. In this case, an extensile distal extension is not required as for longer plates, and distal screw fixation can also be performed percutaneously.

### 6.4.2 Anterolateral approach with lateral parapatellar arthrotomy

Especially in procedures utilizing reamed IM nails, moving more anterior from the lateral incision can facilitate an easy lateral parapatellar arthrotomy that allows ready access to the joint line and the open box. This approach is typically more extensile, especially for reamed IM nailing, because knee flexion is required to visualize and utilize the correct starting point.

While the proximal portion of the approach remains the same as the lateral parapatellar approach for a native valgus knee, distally centering the incision and approach over Gerdy's tubercle will allow for access to the tibial component (if needed), as well as allowing for a large enough skin bridge if a medial approach to the tibia is required. While this approach readily facilitates access and application of reamed IM nails, it still allows for submuscular placement of a laterally based distal femoral locking plate, if needed. Finally, this approach can be converted to a fully fledged lateral parapatellar approach for a periprosthetic fracture requiring revision TKA or endoprosthetic replacement.

CASE 4

### Patient

A 72-year-old woman sustained a low-energy fall, approximately 16 years following a left total knee arthroplasty (TKA).

### Comorbidities

- Morbid obesity
- Osteoporosis
- Hypertension
- Hyperlipidemia

### Treatment and outcome

The x-rays initially revealed a subsided tibial component (**Fig 3.14-4a–b**) and fracture around the medial side. The patient and the family opted for nonoperative management, mainly due to the fact that the patient reported no issues or pain with the prosthesis prior to her fall. Three months after the injury, however, the patient reported persistent pain with weight bearing and progressive "bowing". Mechanical axis x-rays exhibited significant varus and axis deviation (**Fig 3.14-4c**). Opting for operative management, revision TKA was performed, and at the 4-year follow-up, the patient remained pain free and independent (**Fig 3.14-4d–f**).

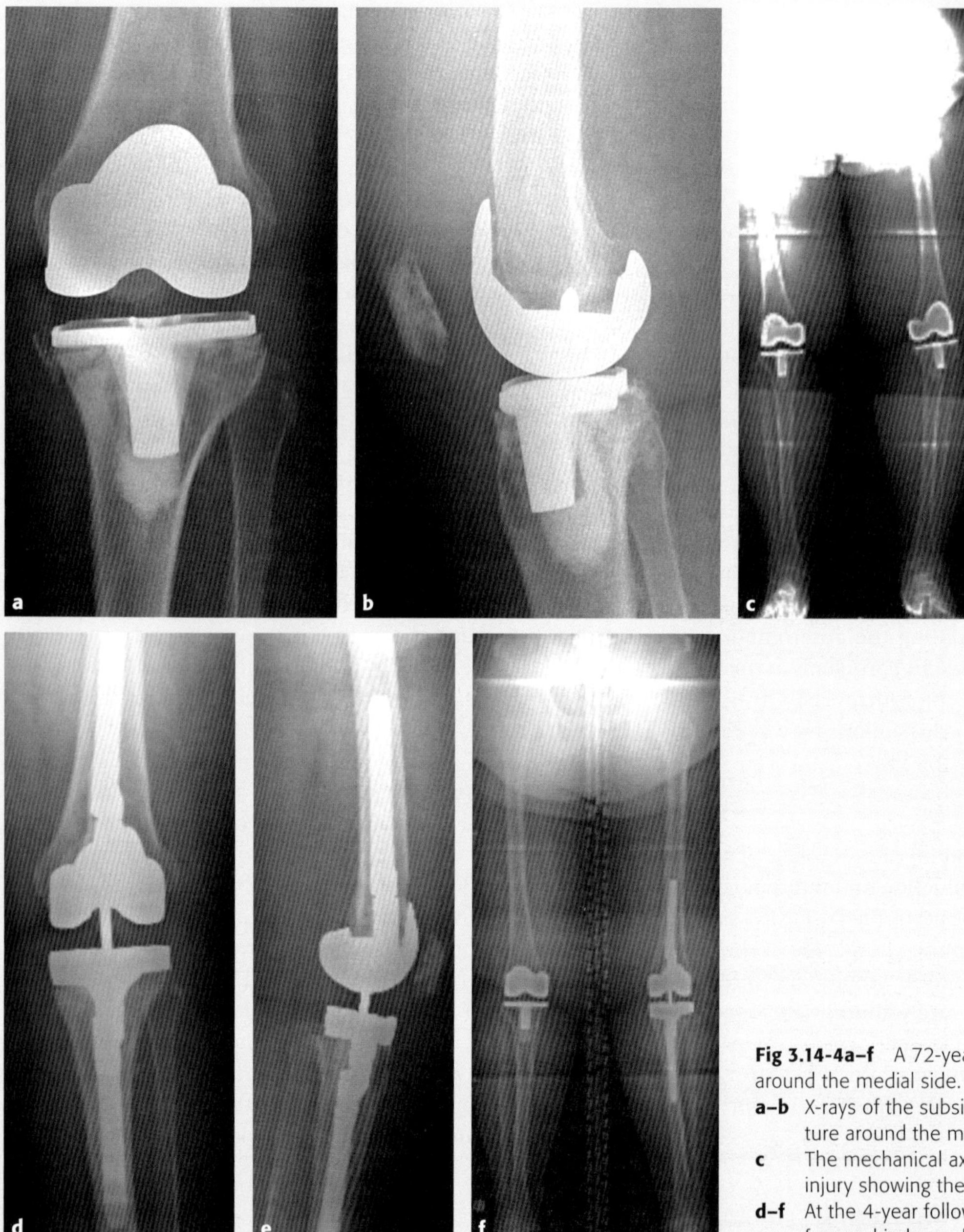


**Fig 3.14-4a–f** A 72-year-old woman with a fracture around the medial side.
**a–b** X-rays of the subsided tibial component and fracture around the medial side.
**c** The mechanical axis x-rays 3 months after the injury showing the varus and axis deviation.
**d–f** At the 4-year follow-up the patient remained pain free and independent.

### 6.5 Reduction

Whether the surgeon chooses to utilize a locking plate or retrograde nail, positioning and achieving indirect reduction is the key to any diaphyseal or extraarticular metaphyseal femoral periprosthetic fracture. Correcting the coronal plane deformity can be performed directly with large pointed reduction clamps and held with temporary K-wires. A femoral distractor can be helpful in obtaining appropriate length and correcting coronal plane deformity. Typically falling into valgus, indirect reduction techniques can also be utilized to correct coronal plane deformity [28]. By utilizing a bump and placing it proximal to the knee, under the fracture, the gastrocnemius muscle is relaxed relieving the primary deforming force, and helping to obtain the reduction in the sagittal plane [26, 29].

In the sagittal plane, it is important to avoid excessive flexion or extension of the fracture because doing so will result in malposition of the implant, causing TKA imbalance and possible nonunion of the fracture.

### 6.6 Locked plating

Consideration should be given to spanning the entire length of the bone and remove any notable stress risers in order to reduce the risk of fracture around the fixation implant in osteoporotic bone (**Case 5: Fig 3.14-5**, **Case 6: Fig 3.14-6**). With the reduction temporarily maintained, locked plating (LP) fixation should be placed in the distal fragment, making sure that it is parallel to the joint line as well as confirming appropriate plate placement in the sagittal plane. The plate should be provisionally fixed proximally with a temporary drill bit or another object flexible enough to allow for some plate movement. Next, placing the apex screw in a nonlocking fashion should bring the shaft to the plate, reducing the fracture. Reduction can also be obtained utilizing cerclage technique as an additional trick with care to not strip the vascularized periosteum.

Beware, however, that for plates that span the length of the femur, precontouring of the plate may be necessary in order to accommodate the native femoral bow as well as allowing

**CASE 5**

**Patient**

A 68-year-old woman with a history of left total knee arthroplasty revision (5 years prior to presentation), and 9 months out from a healed intertrochanteric hip fracture fixed with a sliding hip screw, presented to the emergency department after sustaining a fall from standing height.

**Comorbidities**

- Morbid obesity
- Type 2 diabetes mellitus
- Hypertension
- Hyperlipidemia
- Coronary artery disease

**Treatment and outcome**

The x-rays revealed an interprosthetic fracture extending from the femoral component proximally to the medial aspect of the sliding hip screw (**Fig 3.14-5a**). Already with a stemmed component in place, reamed intramedullary nailing was not an option, and the presence of the proximal side plate further complicated the reconstruction. Thus, the decision was made to remove the proximal implant and the span of the entire length of the femur to minimize further stress risers. The femoral head and neck were also protected with screw fixation as well as calcium phosphate void filler, placed in the area of the previous lag screw (**Fig 3.14-5b**).

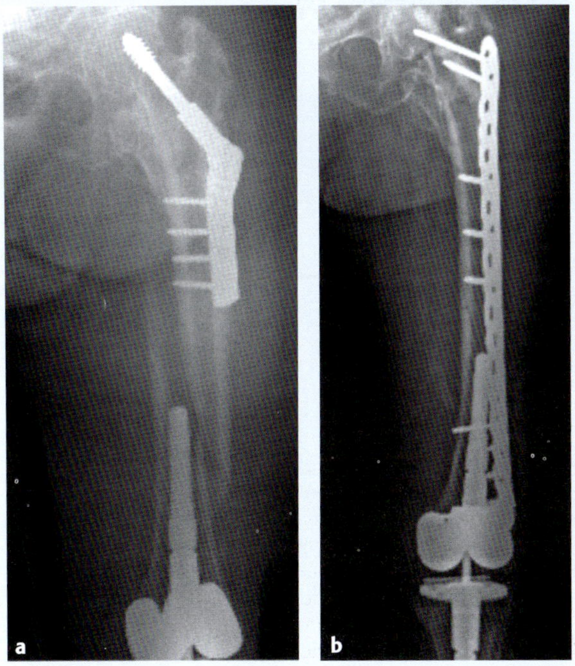


**Fig 3.14-5a–b** A 68-year-old woman with an interprosthetic fracture.
**a** The interprosthetic fracture extending from the femoral component proximally to the medial aspect of the sliding hip screw.
**b** The femoral head and neck were protected with screw fixation as well as calcium phosphate void filler in the area of the previous lag screw.

CASE 6

## Patient

An 84-year-old woman sustained a fall during transfer out of her wheelchair at her nursing home. This happened nearly 18 years following bilateral hybrid total hip arthroplasty (THA) and 12 years following bilateral total knee arthroplasty. A minimal ambulator, the patient presented in a considerable amount of pain.

## Comorbidities

- Hypertension
- Coronary artery disease
- Atrial fibrillation
- Osteoporosis

## Treatment and outcome

The x-rays showed bilateral, nearly symmetric distal femoral periprosthetic fractures (**Fig 3.14-6a–c**). Due to the patient's frailty with considerable medical comorbidities, minimally invasive lateral locking plates were placed, ensuring to span the proximal THA implants (**Fig 3.14-6d**).

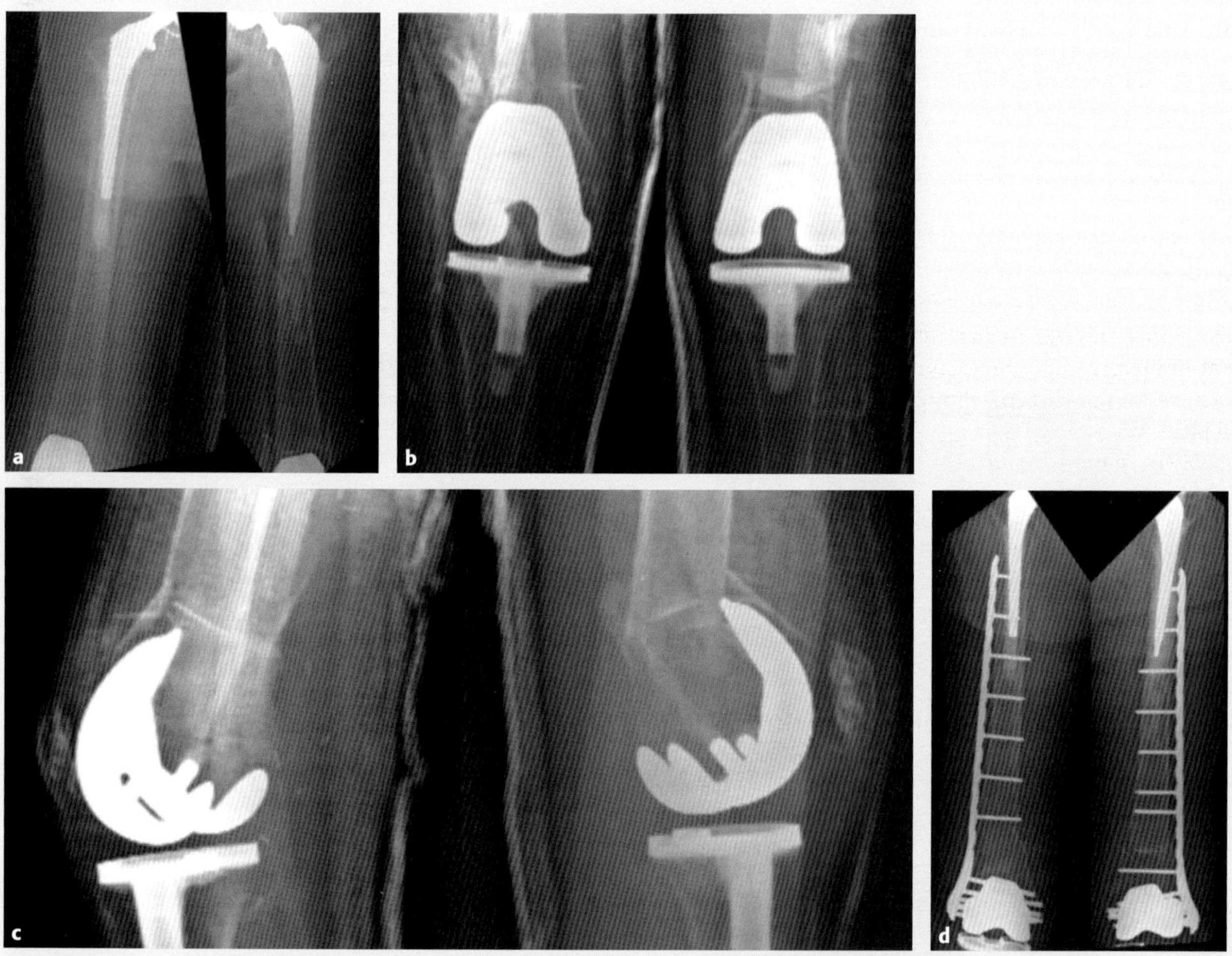


**Fig 3.14-6a–d** An 84-year-old woman with bilateral, nearly symmetric distal femoral periprosthetic fractures.
**a–c** X-rays of the bilateral distal femoral periprosthetic fractures.
**d** Minimally invasive lateral locking plates ensured spanning of the proximal total hip arthroplasty implants.

for placement of proximal screws around a proximal implant, if present. The ideal end point for the proximal end of the plate remains controversial. Extending past the innominate tubercle requires aforementioned custom bending, which may lead to soft-tissue irritation. Currently, plate length remains surgeon preference along with an option to splint the femoral neck with a screw angled to the head through the plate.

Finally, utilizing rigid fixation with only LP is not recommended. Locked plating fixation alone creates too rigid a construct, increasing risk of nonunion. Mixing in bicortical nonlocking screws with locking screws creates enough stability without creating too rigid a construct to promote motion. Appropriate screw placement depends on the fracture pattern (ie, simple versus comminuted), and if possible, increased stability can be obtained with interfragmentary lag screws and bicortical screws [30–34].

## 6.7 Intramedullary nailing

Reamed IM nailing is often possible for metaphyseal as well as diaphyseal fractures. New implant designs allow fixation or very distal fixation in the femur, and locking bolt or blade configurations enable adequate stability for early FWB.

When performing reamed IM nailing, obtaining the reduction prior to reaming is of paramount importance. Similarly, the aforementioned strategies can also be utilized to achieve reduction prior to guide wire placement and subsequent limited reaming. Remember the nail does reduce the fracture, so the surgeon should obtain reduction prior to nail placement. Here, sagittal plane deformity avoidance is probably even more important due to the abnormal starting point of the guide wire. Furthermore, using blocking (Poller) screws can aid in ideal guide wire and IM nail placement.

Service et al [35] examined the "ideal" starting point for reamed IM nailing and its influence by TKA component design. Although the ideal starting point for reamed IM nailing remains just anterior to the posterior cruciate ligament origin, many of the TKA components do not facilitate this starting point but offer a more posterior starting point instead that can cause undesired deformity. One must be cognizant of this abnormal starting point and compensate at the level of the fracture to ensure appropriate fracture reduction without compromising femoral component position in relation to the tibia. Varus/valgus malreduction can also occur with reamed IM nailing, and the surgeon must be aware of avoiding deformity as well. Femoral distractors and/or temporary K-wires can again be used here, with careful placement out of the plane of the nail. Furthermore, removing the polyethylene inlay of the prosthesis and/or using a cannulated guide can help avoid unwanted reaming/drilling and decrease foreign body debris.

Some reamed IM nail designs offer oblique locking screw options distally that can help facilitate out-of-plane fixation. Proximally, standard length locking screws can be utilized depending on the location of the target hole. Collinge et al [36] retrospectively analyzed more than 300 reamed IM nailings performed and arrived at a "best screw length" depending on the location of the proximal locking hole in relation to the LT:

- 1 cm proximal to LT = 36 mm
- At the level of the LT = 32 mm
- 1 cm distal to the LT = 32 mm

Proximally, the IM nail length should be maximized to avoid stress risers while not perforating. Due to limited lengths, the surgeon may be restricted by the manufacturer. Furthermore, length should be considered if an additional implant is required to splint the femoral neck; one disadvantage to reamed IM nailing is the lack of ability to protect the neck, if desired.

## 6.8 Rehabilitation

There is a lack of literature regarding specific rehabilitation protocols following treatment for periprosthetic fractures about the knee, but the primary goals are similiar to those for the typical hip fracture and arthroplasty patient, ie, early mobilization.

### 6.8.1 Partial weight bearing versus weight bearing as tolerated

There is no consensus regarding the best weight-bearing protocol following operative fixation of the distal femur [37–47]. No studies exist directly comparing partial weight bearing (PWB) to weight bearing as tolerated (WBAT) following ORIF of either the native or prosthetic femur, and the data comparing reamed IM nailing and ORIF still remains inconclusive [38, 39]. For periprosthetic fractures that are converted to a stable revision TKA or DFR, WBAT is the typically recommended and accepted protocol [40, 48]. Similarly, with today's technology, patients stabilized via reamed IM nailing are also typically allowed to WBAT with goals of immediate mobilization. In cases of severe comminution and poor bone quality, PWB use has been reported, albeit without data support [38, 44]. There is a real controversy regarding the ideal protocol in patients fixed with a lateral plate, where some proponents prioritize mobilization over the risk of construct failure and others are more conservative [2, 38, 42–45, 49–53]. For extensive discussion, see chapter 1.8 Postoperative surgical management.

With such a wide variation in postoperative rehabilitation protocols, the surgeon must rely on their own judgment and intraoperative findings to achieve specific goals:

- Create a stable construct to allow for immediate ROM and immediate mobilization out of bed.
- Aim to create a construct to allow for immediate WBAT, especially in frail patients who will benefit from early mobility.

Future studies are needed to address this area of controversy, where a general consensus can be helpful in allowing for data-supported immediate weight bearing for this population.

### 6.8.2 Continuous passive motion

The use of continuous passive motion (CPM) has waxed and waned over the past several years. While many surgeons still continue to utilize CPM as a part of their standard protocol, studies both in the arthroplasty and fracture literature have not demonstrated significant benefit [54–56]. Hill et al [55] conducted a randomized controlled trial (RCT) in patients who had just undergone stabilization of intraarticular knee fractures. While a significantly higher degree of flexion was noted in the CPM patients at 48 hours, no significant differences between the two groups were noted at any other time point over the year-long follow-up [55].

Most of the data regarding CPM stems from the arthroplasty literature and recent metaanalyses have yielded no benefit with higher cost [54, 56]. A recent prospective RCT conducted at a single institution not only yielded no clinical benefit in CPM use, but also noted a longer length of stay and hospital costs [56]. Chaudhry and Bhandari [54] conducted a metaanalysis, summarized data from over 20 level I studies and found no benefit to CPM use, leading to their moderate recommendation against its use.

## 6.9 Outcomes

Outcomes comparing LP and reamed IM nailing have been nearly equivocal [1, 57]. Most studies have been less valid study designs using retrospective databases, case series, and cohort comparisons that do not identify a clear superiority for either approach [1, 26, 44, 45, 47, 53, 57]. Without a level I prospective randomized trial, the published literature has reported conflicting data, depending on the analyzed series [38, 48, 53, 58–66].

Two recent metaanalyses yielded the highest level of evidence when comparing the two treatment modalities [1, 57]. Ristevski et al [1] included data from 44 studies and noted important differences between LP and reamed IM nailing outcomes. Specifically, while LP trended toward a higher nonunion rate compared to reamed IM nailing (8.8% versus 3.6%, $P = .08$), a significantly lower malunion rate was noted for LP compared to reamed IM nailing (7.6% versus 16.4%, $P = .02$). Utilizing more strict inclusion criteria, Li et al [57] performed a metaanalysis that only included six comparative studies that were determined to have the highest quality. The authors reported no significant differences in nonunion, malunion, or complication rates; the only notable difference was a significantly higher reoperation rate for the LP group, which echoed the results of the Ristevski study.

### 6.9.1 Failures and nonunions

Regardless of treatment modality, nonunions, malunions, infections, and subsequent failures are not an uncommon occurrence [1, 24, 25, 48, 57]. These are often complex, multimodal case scenarios that require careful planning and experienced hands. There is a paucity of literature that is limited to case reports and/or small series that often involve the use of salvage endoprostheses [67–69]. While revision arthroplasty components can be extremely helpful in these complex scenarios, their use is not the only option. Here, case examples are presented that outline unique problems, with specific technical tips and tricks to tackle the most difficult cases (**Case 7: Fig 3.14-7**, **Case 8: Fig 3.14-8**, **Case 9: Fig 3.14-9**, **Case 10: Fig 3.14-10**) [70].

## Patient

An 80-year-old man was struck by a car while crossing a street.

## Comorbidities

- Hypertension
- Obesity

## Treatment and outcome

A closed injury and neurovascularly intact, the x-rays revealed an isolated left distal femoral periprosthetic fracture (**Fig 3.14-7a–b**). Presenting to an outside institution, the initial treating surgeon recognized an open box configuration and decided to proceed with reamed intramedullary (IM) nailing (**Fig 3.14-7c–d**). While an open box can facilitate reamed IM nailing, it does not always mean that it is the appropriate fixation choice. This fracture pattern is relatively comminuted and very distal, which may not allow for proper fixation with distal locking screws alone. Furthermore, on careful analysis of the lateral images done by image intensification, an errant starting point will likely lead to aberrant nail placement, placing the femoral component into extension (**Fig 3.14-7d**). The patient was treated with protected weight bearing and followed up for 6 months. However, with continued pain, the patient was referred to the senior author for suspected nonunion. Infectious workup was negative and the patient's x-rays revealed a nonunion with malalignment of the femoral component in two planes (**Fig 3.14-7e–f**). An active octogenarian, the patient complained about the pain, and wanted to remain as active as he had been prior to the index injury. Decision was made to proceed with distal femoral replacement (DFR); at the time of surgery, the distal block was found to be in gross nonunion and in extension (**Fig 3.14-7g**). The distal fragment was removed in nearly one piece (**Fig 3.14-7h**) and once proper placement of the DFR was achieved, clinically appropriate alignment was noted (**Fig 3.14-7i**). The patient, 3 years following DFR, was active, independent, and pain free (**Fig 3.14-7j–k**).

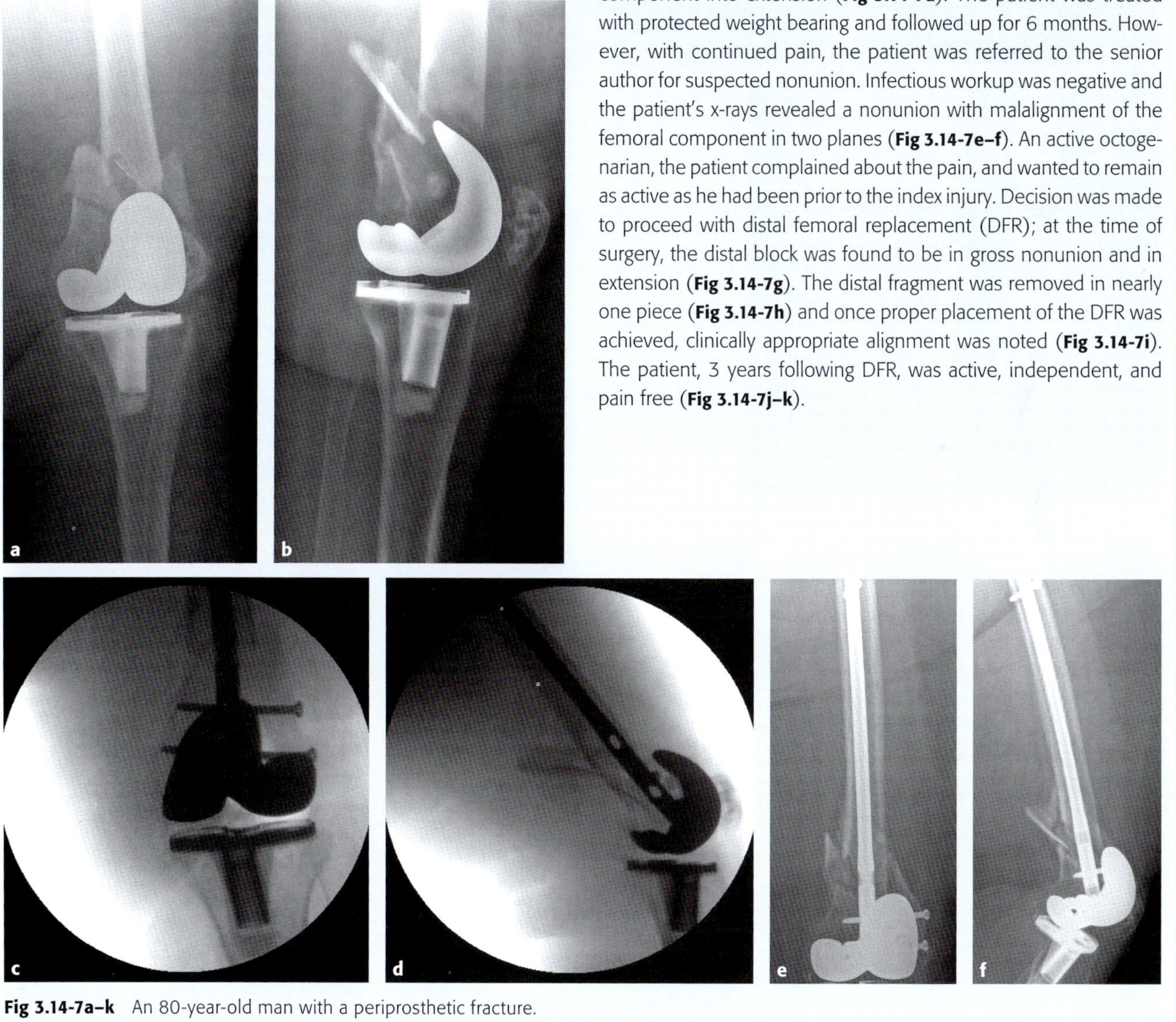


**Fig 3.14-7a–k** An 80-year-old man with a periprosthetic fracture.
**a–b** X-rays of the isolated left distal femoral periprosthetic fracture.
**c–d** Image intensification of the comminuted distal fracture. On analysis of the lateral images, an errant starting point will likely lead to aberrant nail placement, placing the femoral component into extension.
**e–f** X-rays of the nonunion with malalignment of the femoral component in two planes.

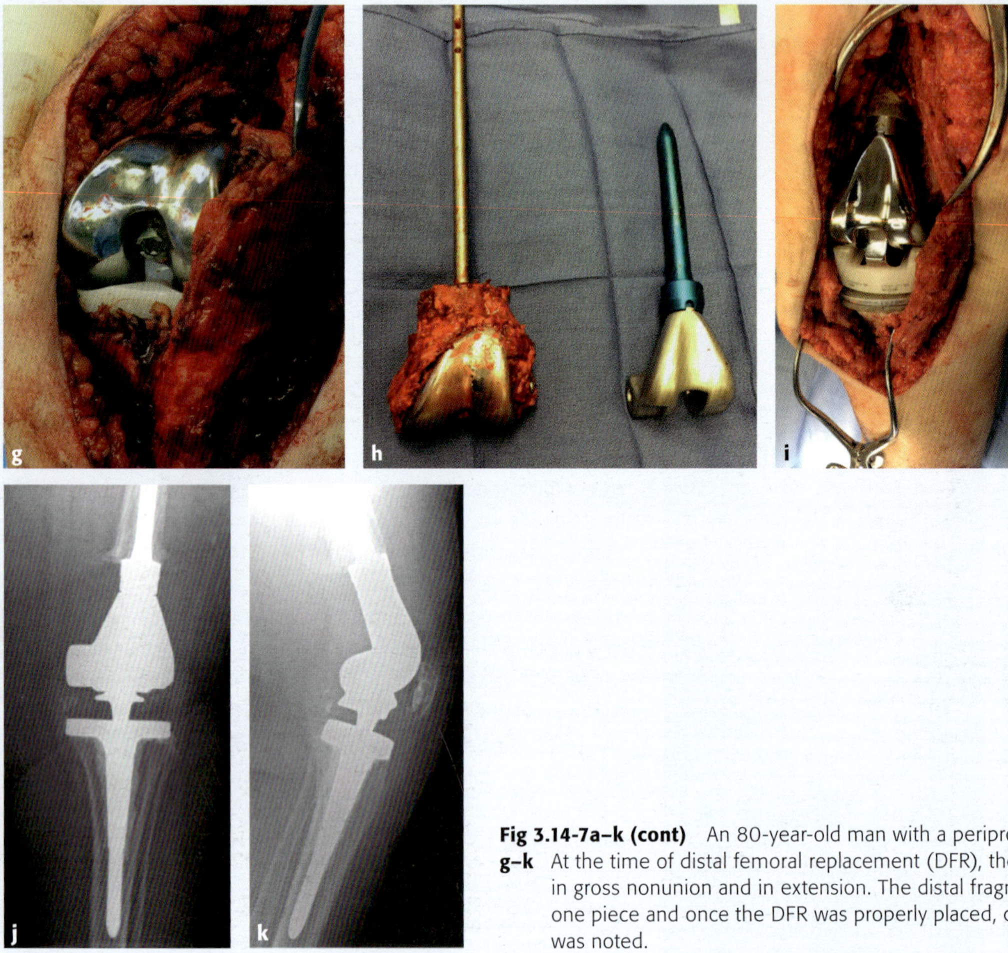

**Fig 3.14-7a–k (cont)** An 80-year-old man with a periprosthetic fracture.
**g–k** At the time of distal femoral replacement (DFR), the distal block was found to be in gross nonunion and in extension. The distal fragment was removed in nearly one piece and once the DFR was properly placed, clinically appropriate alignment was noted.

## Patient

A 59-year-old woman sustained a fall while hiking.

## Comorbidities

- Hypertension

## Treatment and outcome

Taken to a local hospital, x-rays had revealed a periprosthetic supracondylar femoral fracture, which was treated with reamed intramedullary (IM) nailing. Six months following discharge and return back home, the patient presented with persistent pain, inability to fully extend her knee, and limited functional ability. The x-rays revealed a nonunion, with reamed IM nails and with inappropriately placed locking screws in addition to the nail being left protruding within the femoral notch (**Fig 3.14-8a–b**). Exchange of nail, utilizing bone graft via reamer-irrigator-aspirator as well as iliac crest bone marrow aspiration, was performed. Further stability was provided via a linked lateral locking plate, which also spanned the entire femur and splinted the femoral neck (**Fig 3.14-8c**). Full range of motion returned immediately postoperatively, and at the 3-month follow-up, abundant callus was noted for a healed fracture (**Fig 3.14-8d–e**).

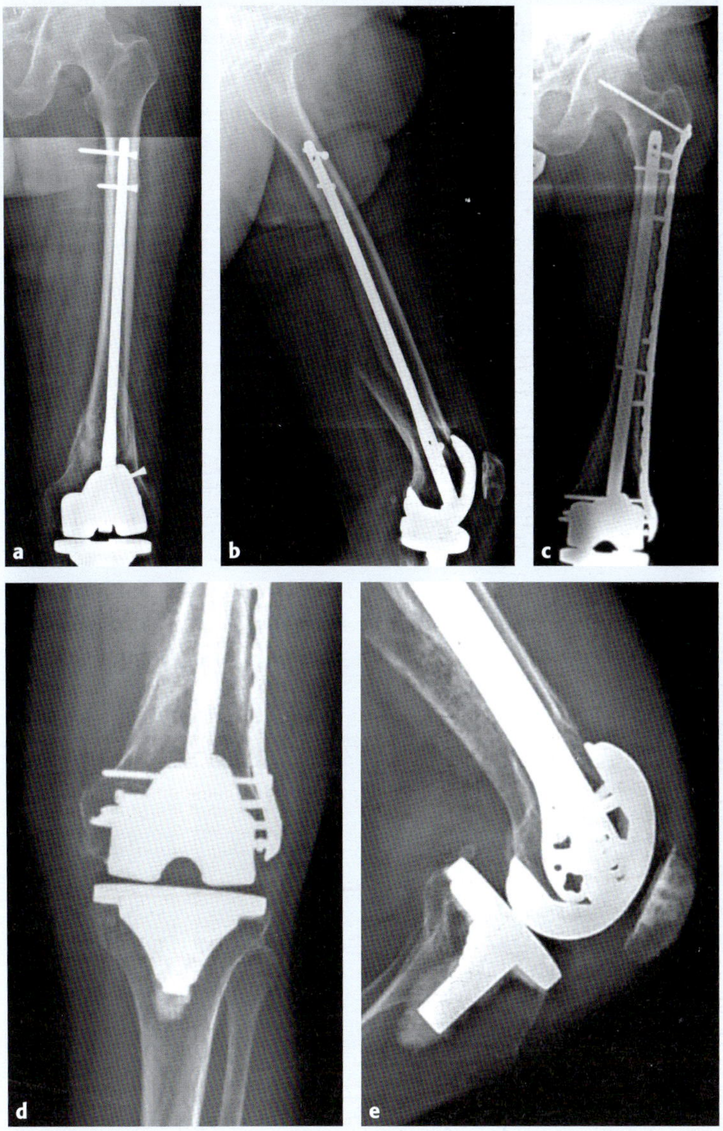


**Fig 3.14-8a–e** A 59-year-old woman with a periprosthetic supracondylar fracture of the femur.
**a–b** X-rays of the periprosthetic supracondylar femoral fracture treated with reamed intramedullary nailing. A nonunion resulted following inappropriately placed locking screws, and the nail was left protruding within the femoral notch.
**c** X-ray showing the linked lateral locking plate that spanned the entire femur and splinted the femoral neck.
**d–e** At the 3-month follow-up, abundant callus can be noted for a healed fracture.

CASE 9

### Patient

A 77-year-old man fell down stairs sustaining a supracondylar fracture above the femoral component (**Fig 3.14-9a–b**).

### Comorbidities

- Hypertension
- Smoker
- Coronary artery disease

### Treatment and outcome

When the patient returned to his index arthroplasty surgeon, several principles were violated in fixing this fracture, ie, extensive soft-tissue dissection was performed in order to cable and utilize a cat's claw, devitalizing crucial blood supply (**Fig 3.14-9c–d**). Furthermore, excessively rigid fixation over a short span was placed, with locking screws also placed in the fracture zone (**Fig 3.14-9e**). Unbalanced, rigid fixation over a short segment led to nonunion and hardware failure (**Fig 3.14-9f–g**). Upon failure, the patient was referred out and subsequently revised. All initial fixation was removed, anatomical axis restored, and with bone graft, a balanced linked construct with reamed intramedullary nailing and lateral plate was placed (**Fig 3.14-9h**). Applying the aforementioned principles, the patient went onto uneventful healing (**Fig 3.14-9i**).

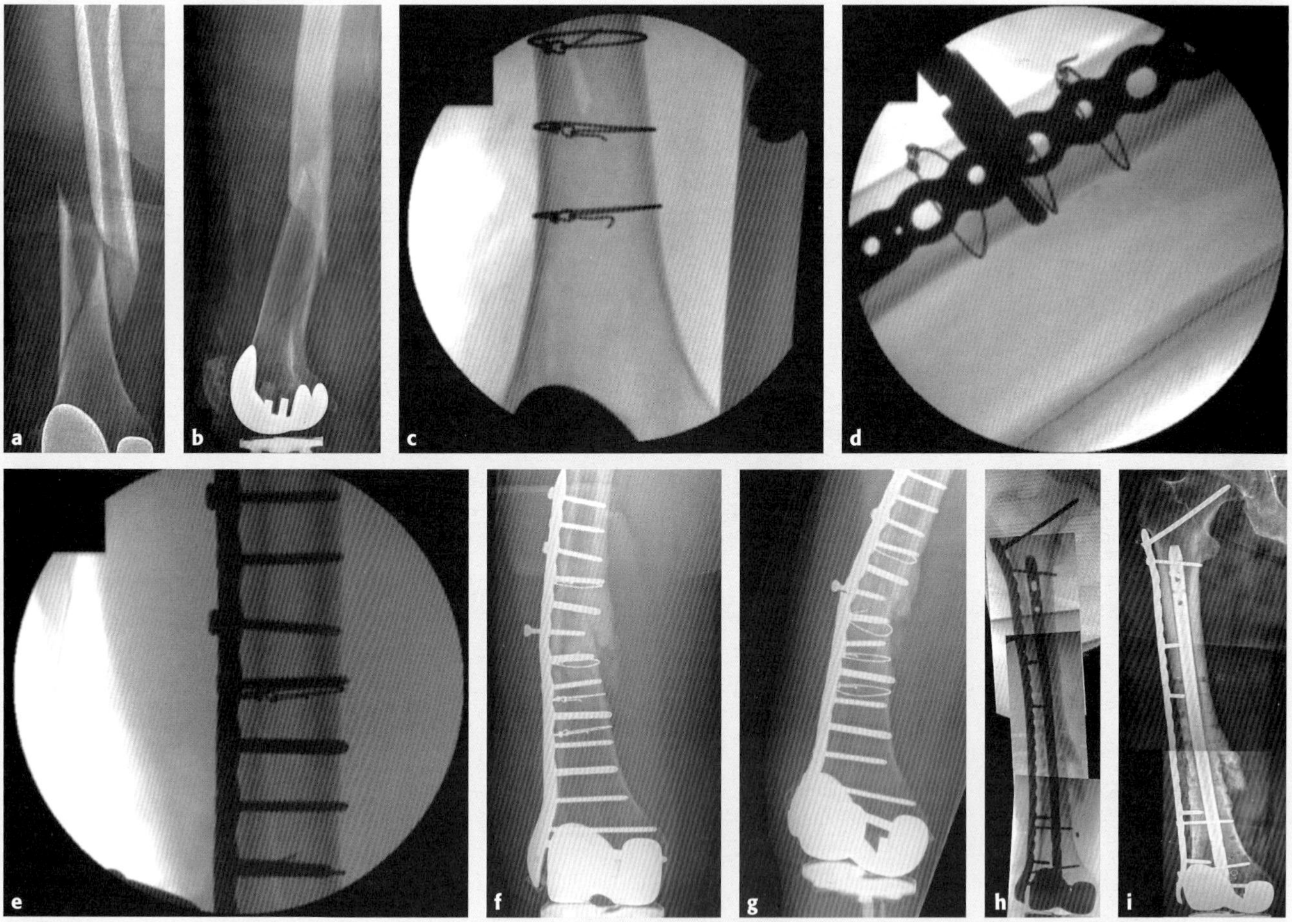


**Fig 3.14-9a–i** A 77-year-old man with a supracondylar fracture above the femoral component.
**a–b** X-rays showing the supracondylar fracture above the femoral component.
**c–d** Extensive soft-tissue dissection was performed to utilize a cat's claw, which devitalized blood supply.
**e** Excessively rigid fixation over a short span was placed, with locking screws also placed in the fracture zone.
**f–g** The nonunion and hardware failure was due to unbalanced, rigid fixation over a short segment.
**h** Removal of initial fixation, restoration of the anatomical axis, and with bone graft, placement of a balanced linked construct with reamed intramedullary nail and lateral plate.
**i** The fracture went onto uneventful healing.

## Patient

A 74-year-old man, who had sustained a distal femoral fracture 10 years prior to presentation, was treated for the fracture and subsequent nonunion with a total of five operations. Further history includes a fracture below a total hip arthroplasty stem on the same side.

## Comorbidities

- Obesity
- Hypertension
- Coronary artery disease

## Treatment and outcome

The patient presented as a nonambulator with persistent pain for a duration of 2.5 years (**Fig 3.14-10a–c**). Elevated inflammatory markers and bone biopsy confirmed an infected nonunion and the patient's initial stage was removal of all hardware, debridement, and placement of an antibiotic-coated locking plate (**Fig 3.14-10d–f**). Following 6 weeks of intravenous antibiotics, repeated biopsy and frozen negative, the antbiotic-coated plate was removed (**Fig 3.14-10g–h**) and definitive fixation included a linked construct between reamed intramedullary nailing and a lateral locking plate (**Fig 3.14-10i**). After not walking for 2.5 years, the patient was able to stand and began ambulating with a walker over the initial 6 weeks following definitive fixation. Three months following his final procedure, abundant callus was noted on the x-rays (**Fig 3.14-10j–l**) and at this point, he was ambulating with a rolling walker, pain free.

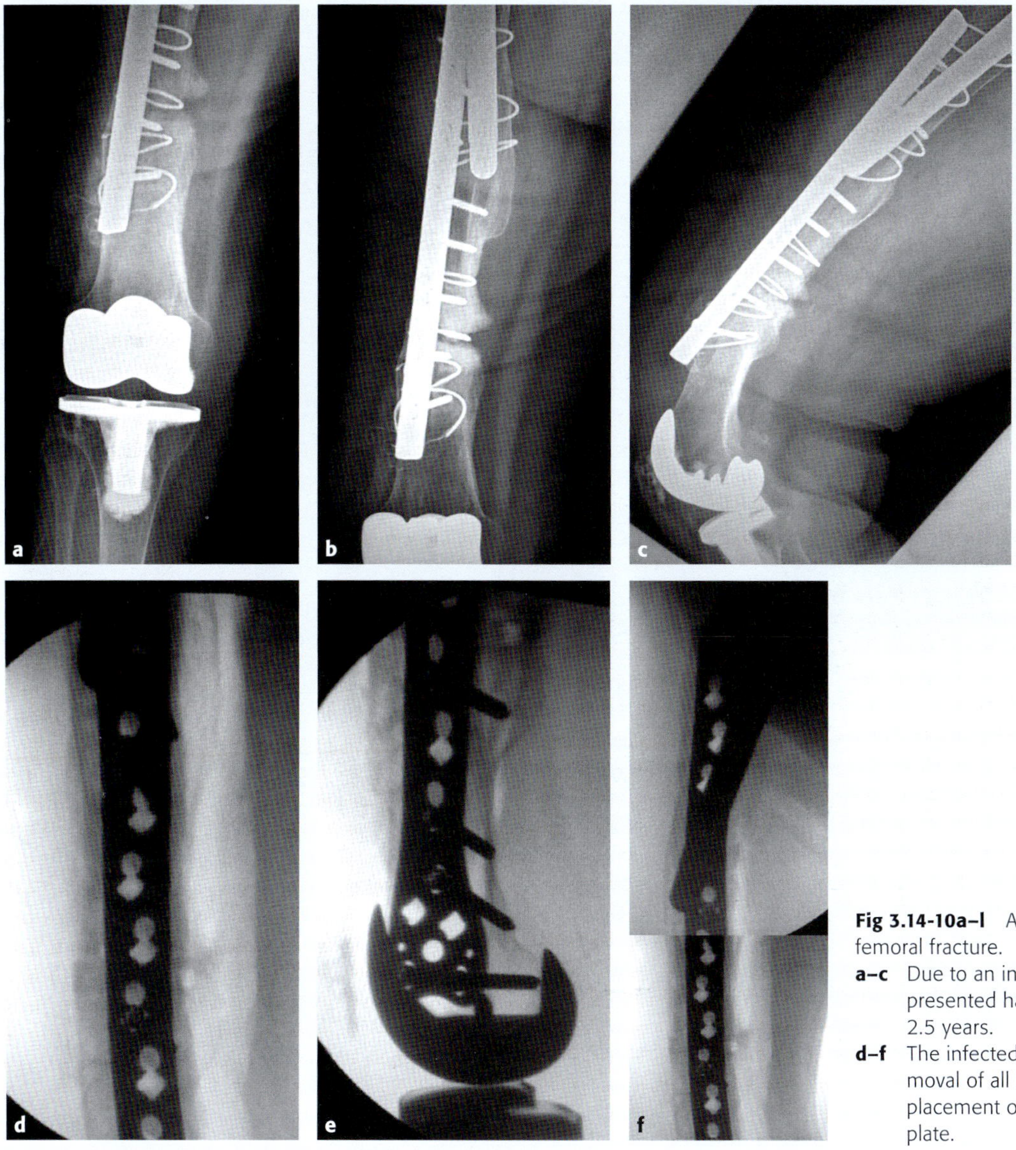


**Fig 3.14-10a–l** A 74-year-old man with a distal femoral fracture.

**a–c** Due to an infected nonunion, the patient presented having persistent pain for 2.5 years.

**d–f** The infected nonunion resulted in removal of all hardware, debridement, and placement of an antibiotic-coated locking plate.

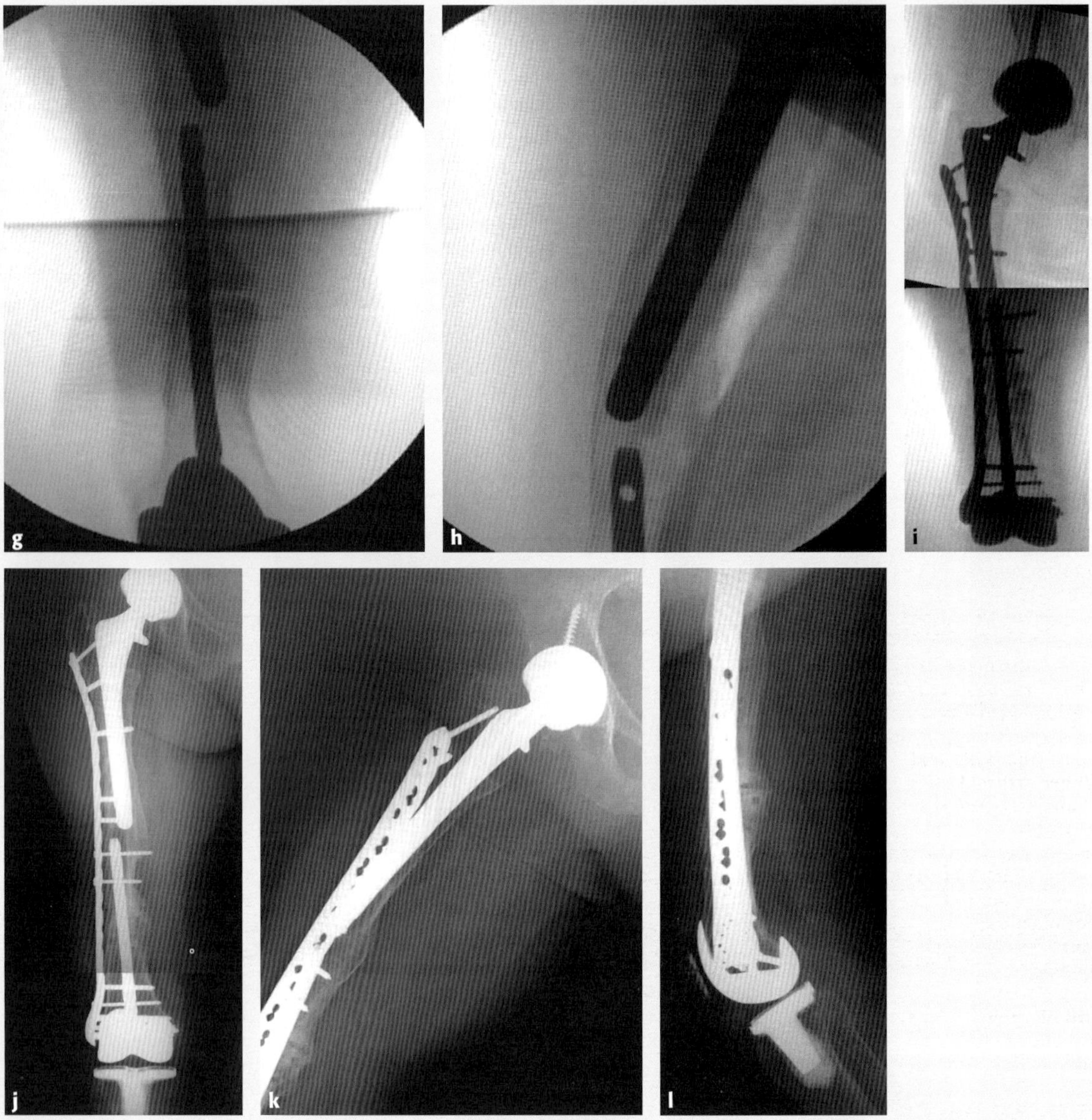


**Fig 3.14-10a–l (cont)** A 74-year-old man with a distal femoral fracture.

**g–i** The antbiotic-coated plate was removed and definitive fixation included a linked construct between reamed intramedullary nailing and a lateral locking plate.

**j–l** At the 3-month follow-up, abundant callus was noted.

## 8 References


1. **Ristevski B, Nauth A, Williams DS, et al.** Systematic review of the treatment of periprosthetic distal femur fractures. *J Orthop Trauma.* 2014 May;28(5):307–312.
2. **Rorabeck CH, Taylor JW.** Periprosthetic fractures of the femur complicating total knee arthroplasty. *Orthop Clin North Am.* 1999 Apr;30(2):265–277.
3. **Konan S, Sandiford N, Unno F, et al.** Periprosthetic fractures associated with total knee arthroplasty: an update. *Bone Joint J.* 2016 Nov;98-B(11):1489–1496.
4. **Della Rocca GJ, Leung KS, Pape HC.** Periprosthetic fractures: epidemiology and future projections. *J Orthop Trauma.* 2011 Jun;25(Suppl 2):S66–S70.
5. **Singh JA, Jensen M, Lewallen D.** Predictors of periprosthetic fracture after total knee replacement: an analysis of 21,723 cases. *Acta Orthop.* 2013 Apr;84(2):170–177.
6. **Mau-Moeller A, Behrens M, Felser S, et al.** Modulation and predictors of periprosthetic bone mineral density following total knee arthroplasty. *Biomed Res Int.* 2015;2015:418168.
7. **Sun ZH, Liu YJ, Li H.** Femoral stress and strain changes post-hip, -knee and -ipsilateral hip/knee arthroplasties: a finite element analysis. *Orthop Surg.* 2014 May;6(2):137–144.
8. **Ritter MA, Thong AE, Keating EM, et al.** The effect of femoral notching during total knee arthroplasty on the prevalence of postoperative femoral fractures and on clinical outcome. *J Bone Joint Surg Am.* 2005 Nov;87(11):2411–2414.
9. **Gujarathi N, Putti AB, Abboud RJ, et al.** Risk of periprosthetic fracture after anterior femoral notching. *Acta Orthop.* 2009 Oct;80(5):553–556.
10. **Bhattacharyya T, Chang D, Meigs JB, et al.** Mortality after periprosthetic fracture of the femur. *J Bone Joint Surg Am.* 2007 Dec;89(12):2658–2662.
11. **Ferrara F, Cipriani A, Rapisarda S, et al.** Assessment of implant position after total knee arthroplasty by dual-energy computed tomography. *Acta Radiol.* 2016 May;57(5):612–619.
12. **Pessis E, Campagna R, Sverzut JM, et al.** Virtual monochromatic spectral imaging with fast kilovoltage switching: reduction of metal artifacts at CT. *Radiographics.* 2013 Mar–Apr;33(2):573–583.
13. **Solomon LB, Stamenkov RB, MacDonald AJ, et al.** Imaging periprosthetic osteolysis around total knee arthroplasties using a human cadaver model. *J Arthroplasty.* 2012 Jun;27(6):1069–1074.
14. **Fritz J, Lurie B, Potter HG.** MR imaging of knee arthroplasty implants. *Radiographics.* 2015 Sep–Oct;35(5):1483–1501.
15. **Liebl H, Heilmeier U, Lee S, et al.** In vitro assessment of knee MRI in the presence of metal implants comparing MAVRIC-SL and conventional fast spin echo sequences at 1.5 and 3 T field strength. *J Magn Reson Imaging.* 2015 May;41(5):1291–1299.
16. **Vessely MB, Frick MA, Oakes D, et al.** Magnetic resonance imaging with metal suppression for evaluation of periprosthetic osteolysis after total knee arthroplasty. *J Arthroplasty.* 2006 Sep;21(6):826–831.
17. **Backstein D, Safir O, Gross A.** Periprosthetic fractures of the knee. *J Arthroplasty.* 2007 Jun;22(4 Suppl 1):45–49.
18. **Goldberg VM, Figgie HE 3rd, Inglis AE, et al.** Patellar fracture type and prognosis in condylar total knee arthroplasty. *Clin Orthop Relat Res.* 1988 Nov;(236):115–122.
19. **Keating EM, Haas G, Meding JB.** Patella fracture after post total knee replacements. *Clin Orthop Relat Res.* 2003 Nov;(416):93–97.
20. **Ortiguera CJ, Berry DJ.** Patellar fracture after total knee arthroplasty. *J Bone Joint Surg Am.* 2002 Apr;84-A(4):532–540.
21. **Su ET, Kubiak EN, Dewal H, et al.** A proposed classification of supracondylar femur fractures above total knee arthroplasties. *J Arthroplasty.* 2006 Apr;21(3):405–408.
22. **Duncan CP, Haddad FS.** The Unified Classification System (UCS): improving our understanding of periprosthetic fractures. *Bone Joint J.* 2014 Jun;96-B(6):713–716.
23. **Thompson SM, Lindisfarne EA, Bradley N, et al.** Periprosthetic supracondylar femoral fractures above a total knee replacement: compatibility guide for fixation with a retrograde intramedullary nail. *J Arthroplasty.* 2014 Aug;29(8):1639–1641.
24. **Streubel PN.** Mortality after periprosthetic femur fractures. *J Knee Surg.* 2013 Feb;26(1):27–30.
25. **Streubel PN, Ricci WM, Wong A, et al.** Mortality after distal femur fractures in elderly patients. *Clin Orthop Relat Res.* 2011 Apr;469(4):1188–1196.
26. **Haidukewych G, Sems SA, Huebner D, et al.** Results of polyaxial locked-plate fixation of periarticular fractures of the knee. Surgical technique. *J Bone Joint Surg Am.* 2008 Mar;90(Suppl 2 Pt 1):117–134.
27. **Donegan DJ, Seigerman DA, Yoon RS, et al.** Gerdy's tubercle: the lighthouse to the knee. *J Orthop Trauma.* 2015 Feb;29(2):e51–e53.
28. **Bolhofner BR, Carmen B, Clifford P.** The results of open reduction and Internal fixation of distal femur fractures using a biologic (indirect) reduction technique. *J Orthop Trauma.* 1996;10(6):372–377.
29. **Gebhard F, Kinzl L.** Femur, distal. In: Rüedi TP, Buckley RE, Moran CG, eds. *AO Principles of Fracture Management.* 2nd ed. Stuttgart, New York: Thieme Verlag; 2007: 787–799.
30. **Gautier E, Sommer C.** Guidelines for the clinical application of the LCP. *Injury.* 2003 Nov;34(Suppl 2):B63–B76.
31. **Gwinner C, Mardian S, Droge T, et al.** Bicortical screw fixation provides superior biomechanical stability but devastating failure modes in periprosthetic femur fracture care using locking plates. *Int Orthop.* 2015 Sep;39(9):1749–1755.
32. **Heyland M, Duda GN, Haas NP, et al.** Semi-rigid screws provide an auxiliary option to plate working length to control interfragmentary movement in locking plate fixation at the distal femur. *Injury.* 2015 Oct;46(Suppl 4):S24–S32.
33. **Mardian S, Schaser KD, Duda GN, et al.** Working length of locking plates determines interfragmentary movement in distal femur fractures under physiological loading. *Clin Biomech (Bristol, Avon).* 2015 May;30(4):391–396.
34. **Mardian S, Schmolz W, Schaser KD, et al.** Interfragmentary lag screw fixation in locking plate constructs increases stiffness in simple fracture patterns. *Clin Biomech (Bristol, Avon).* 2015 Oct;30(8):814–819.
35. **Service BC, Kang W, Turnbull N, et al.** Influence of femoral component design on retrograde femoral nail starting point. *J Orthop Trauma.* 2015 Oct;29(10):e380–e384.
36. **Collinge CA, Koerner JD, Yoon RS, et al.** Is there an optimal proximal locking screw length in retrograde intramedullary femoral nailing? Can we stop measuring for these screws? *J Orthop Trauma.* 2015 Oct;29(10):e421–e424.
37. **Bliemel C, Buecking B, Mueller T, et al.** Distal femoral fractures in the elderly: biomechanical analysis of a polyaxial angle-stable locking plate versus a retrograde intramedullary nail in a human cadaveric bone model. *Arch Orthop Trauma Surg.* 2015 Jan;135(1):49–58.

38. **Gliatis J, Megas P, Panagiotopoulos E, et al.** Midterm results of treatment with a retrograde nail for supracondylar periprosthetic fractures of the femur following total knee arthroplasty. *J Orthop Trauma.* 2005 Mar;19(3):164–170.
39. **Griffin XL, Parsons N, Zbaeda MM, et al.** Interventions for treating fractures of the distal femur in adults. *Cochrane Database Syst Rev.* 2015 Aug 13(8):CD010606.
40. **Jassim SS, McNamara I, Hopgood P.** Distal femoral replacement in periprosthetic fracture around total knee arthroplasty. *Injury.* 2014 Mar;45(3):550–553.
41. **Khursheed O, Wani MM, Rashid S, et al.** Results of treatment of distal extra: articular femur fractures with locking plates using minimally invasive approach–experience with 25 consecutive geriatric patients. *Musculoskelet Surg.* 2015 Aug;99(2):139–147.
42. **Kregor PJ, Hughes JL, Cole PA.** Fixation of distal femoral fractures above total knee arthroplasty utilizing the Less Invasive Stabilization System (L.I.S.S.). *Injury.* 2001 Dec;32(Suppl 3):SC64–SC75.
43. **Kregor PJ, Stannard J, Zlowodzki M, et al.** Distal femoral fracture fixation utilizing the Less Invasive Stabilization System (L.I.S.S.): the technique and early results. *Injury.* 2001 Dec;32(Suppl 3):SC32–SC47.
44. **Meneghini RM, Keyes BJ, Reddy KK, et al.** Modern retrograde intramedullary nails versus periarticular locked plates for supracondylar femur fractures after total knee arthroplasty. *J Arthroplasty.* 2014 Jul;29(7):1478–1481.
45. **O'Toole RV, Gobezie R, Hwang R, et al.** Low complication rate of LISS for femur fractures adjacent to stable hip or knee arthroplasty. *Clin Orthop Relat Res.* 2006 Sep;450:203–210.
46. **Ponzer S, Tidermark J, Tornkvist H.** Retrograde nailing of femoral fractures distal to a Moore prosthesis. *J Orthop Trauma.* 1998 Nov–Dec;12(8):588–591.
47. **Ricci WM, Borrelli J Jr.** Operative management of periprosthetic femur fractures in the elderly using biological fracture reduction and fixation techniques. *Injury.* 2007 Sep;38(Suppl 3):S53–S58.
48. **Saidi K, Ben-Lulu O, Tsuji M, et al.** Supracondylar periprosthetic fractures of the knee in the elderly patients: a comparison of treatment using allograft-implant composites, standard revision components, distal femoral replacement prosthesis. *J Arthroplasty.* 2014 Jan;29(1):110–114.
49. **Aldrian S, Schuster R, Haas N, et al.** Fixation of supracondylar femoral fractures following total knee arthroplasty: is there any difference comparing angular stable plate fixation versus rigid interlocking nail fixation? *Arch Orthop Trauma Surg.* 2013 Jul;133(7):921–927.
50. **Horneff JG 3rd, Scolaro JA, Jafari SM, et al.** Intramedullary nailing versus locked plate for treating supracondylar periprosthetic femur fractures. *Orthopedics.* 2013 May;36(5):e561–e566.
51. **Meyer C, Alt V, Schroeder L, et al.** Treatment of periprosthetic femoral fractures by effective lengthening of the prosthesis. *Clin Orthop Relat Res.* 2007 Oct;463:120–127.
52. **Moloney GB, Westrick ER, Siska PA, et al.** Treatment of periprosthetic femur fractures around a well-fixed hip arthroplasty implant: span the whole bone. *Arch Orthop Trauma Surg.* 2014 Jan;134(1):9–14.
53. **Ricci WM, Loftus T, Cox C, et al.** Locked plates combined with minimally invasive insertion technique for the treatment of periprosthetic supracondylar femur fractures above a total knee arthroplasty. *J Orthop Trauma.* 2006 Mar;20(3):190–196.
54. **Chaudhry H, Bhandari M.** Cochrane in CORR ((R)): continuous passive motion following total knee arthroplasty in people with arthritis (review). *Clin Orthop Relat Res.* 2015 Nov;473(11):3348–3354.
55. **Hill AD, Palmer MJ, Tanner SL, et al.** Use of continuous passive motion in the postoperative treatment of intra-articular knee fractures. *J Bone Joint Surg Am.* 2014 Jul 16;96(14):e118.
56. **Joshi RN, White PB, Murray-Weir M, et al.** Prospective randomized trial of the efficacy of continuous passive motion post total knee arthroplasty: experience of the hospital for special surgery. *J Arthroplasty.* 2015 Dec;30(12):2364–2369.
57. **Li B, Gao P, Qiu G, et al.** Locked plate versus retrograde intramedullary nail for periprosthetic femur fractures above total knee arthroplasty: a meta-analysis. *Int Orthop.* 2016 Aug;40(8):1689–1695.
58. **Althausen PL, Lee MA, Finkemeier CG, et al.** Operative stabilization of supracondylar femur fractures above total knee arthroplasty: a comparison of four treatment methods. *J Arthroplasty.* 2003 Oct;18(7):834–839.
59. **Chettiar K, Jackson MP, Brewin J, et al.** Supracondylar periprosthetic femoral fractures following total knee arthroplasty: treatment with a retrograde intramedullary nail. *Int Orthop.* 2009 Aug;33(4):981–985.
60. **Fulkerson E, Tejwani N, Stuchin S, et al.** Management of periprosthetic femur fractures with a first generation locking plate. *Injury.* 2007 Aug;38(8):965–972.
61. **Han HS, Oh KW, Kang SB.** Retrograde intramedullary nailing for periprosthetic supracondylar fractures of the femur after total knee arthroplasty. *Clin Orthop Surg.* 2009 Dec;1(4):201–206.
62. **Herrera DA, Kregor PJ, Cole PA, et al.** Treatment of acute distal femur fractures above a total knee arthroplasty: systematic review of 415 cases (1981-2006). *Acta Orthop.* 2008 Feb;79(1):22–27.
63. **Hoffmann MF, Jones CB, Sietsema DL, et al.** Outcome of periprosthetic distal femoral fractures following knee arthroplasty. *Injury.* 2012 Jul;43(7):1084–1089.
64. **Kolb W, Guhlmann H, Windisch C, et al.** Fixation of periprosthetic femur fractures above total knee arthroplasty with the less invasive stabilization system: a midterm follow-up study. *J Trauma.* 2010 Sep;69(3):670–676.
65. **Large TM, Kellam JF, Bosse MJ, et al.** Locked plating of supracondylar periprosthetic femur fractures. *J Arthroplasty.* 2008 Sep;23(6 Suppl 1):115–120.
66. **Tharani R, Nakasone C, Vince KG.** Periprosthetic fractures after total knee arthroplasty. *J Arthroplasty.* 2005 Jun;20(4 Suppl 2):27–32.
67. **Kress KJ, Scuderi GR, Windsor RE, et al.** Treatment of nonunions about the knee utilizing custom total knee arthroplasty with press-fit intramedullary stems. *J Arthroplasty.* 1993 Feb;8(1):49–55.
68. **Freedman EL, Hak DJ, Johnson EE, et al.** Total knee replacement including a modular distal femoral component in elderly patients with acute fracture or nonunion. *J Orthop Trauma.* 1995 Jun;9(3):231–237.
69. **Davila J, Malkani A, Paiso JM.** Supracondylar distal femoral nonunions treated with a megaprosthesis in elderly patients: a report of two cases. *J Orthop Trauma.* 2001 Nov;15(8):574–578.
70. **Liporace FA, Yoon RS, Frank MA, et al.** Use of an "antibiotic plate" for infected periprosthetic fracture in total hip arthroplasty. *J Orthop Trauma.* 2012 Mar;26(3):e18–e23.

# 3.15 Proximal tibia

Michael Götzen, Michael Blauth

## 1 Introduction

In the light of the increasing number of older adults with osteoporosis, treatment of proximal tibial fractures (PTFs) deserves new consideration. The increasing incidence, change in fracture types, new operative fixation techniques, perioperative risk, personal needs of the patient, and the general health conditions of the fragility fracture patient all demand a new way of thinking and approach for this type of injury.

Typically, geriatric PTFs present as lateral depression fractures caused by low-energy valgus stress in women. High-energy trauma in older patients presents as complex injury of the joint surface, the metaphysis, and the soft tissues. Preexisting muscle and skin atrophy often aggravate the situation. In this chapter, we discuss a new perspective on PTFs in the geriatric patient and present the available options. Poor bone quality should not be a limiting factor.

The proximal tibia is essential for weight bearing: 60% of body weight is transferred through the larger medial tibial condyle. The mechanical axis (Mikulicz line) of the leg crosses the knee joint approximately 2 mm medial to the intercondylar eminence. The anatomical axis of the knee joint has 5–6° valgus. In the older adult with preexisting varus or valgus axis deviations, altered forces are generated to the proximal tibial joint surface and may increase the risk of fracture [1]. Direct trauma to the knee joint is most commonly delivered to the lateral side, leading to a higher incidence of lateral proximal tibia fractures [2]. However, PTFs most commonly occur due to axial compression, in extension at the ventral rim of the plateau, and in flexion because of the roll-back of the femur at the dorsal rim [3]. Dorsal rim fractures are highly associated with knee dislocation and should be treated as unstable fractures.

## 2 Epidemiology and etiology

Kannus et al [4] investigated the incidence of osteoporotic knee fractures in a population of 100,000 people older than 59 years. They noted a dramatic increase of fractures from 1970 (218 per 100,000 women) until 1999 (685 per 100,000 women). Future predictions for 2020 and 2030 predict increases to 1,550 per 100,000 people (ie, women 1,250, men 300) and 2050 per 100,000 people (ie, women 1,700, men 350). Proximal tibial fractures have a bimodal fracture distribution, with increased incidence in older patients [5]. While they comprise 1% of all fractures in the overall population, they are responsible for up to 8% in adults older than 65 years [6]. From 2000 to 2007, the average age of patients with PTF increased from 48.9 to 56.0 years [7]. Both prevention and treatment of osteoporotic PTFs is an increasing priority.

## 3 Diagnostics

### 3.1 Clinical evaluation

Common reasons for a fall from standing height in older adults are frailty, sarcopenia, gait instability, and preexisting joint disorders. Sarcopenia has an incidence of 5–10% in people older than 65 and is a major cause for functional decline leading to falls and fractures [8]. Patients living in nursing homes with neurological comorbidities such as stroke or dementia often reach the hospital with some delay due to an inability to report the injury. Insufficiency fractures of the proximal tibia are often diagnosed with some delay resulting in secondary displacement [9–11], often requiring additional diagnostics (**Case 1: Fig 3.15-1**).

Comorbidities such as heart failure and venous insufficiency leading to soft-tissue edema are commonly encountered. Parchment skin due to long-term corticosteroid use is another common issue.

CASE 1

### Patient

An 86-year-old patient suffered a low-energy fall at home.

### Comorbidities

- Congestive heart failure
- Chronic kidney failure
- A recent deep vein thrombosis due to immobility

### Treatment and outcome

In the conventional x-rays, the trauma surgeon suspected an avulsion of the anterior cruciate ligament (**Fig 3.15-1a**). Computed tomographic scans showed the true extent of the fracture, which reached into the medial metaphysis (**Fig 3.15-1b**). Avoiding fracture displacement allowed for a percutaneous screw fixation. In order to gain a better screw purchase, the surgeon decided to augment the hollow metaphysis of the tibia with polymethylmethacrylate cement (**Fig 3.15-1c–d**).

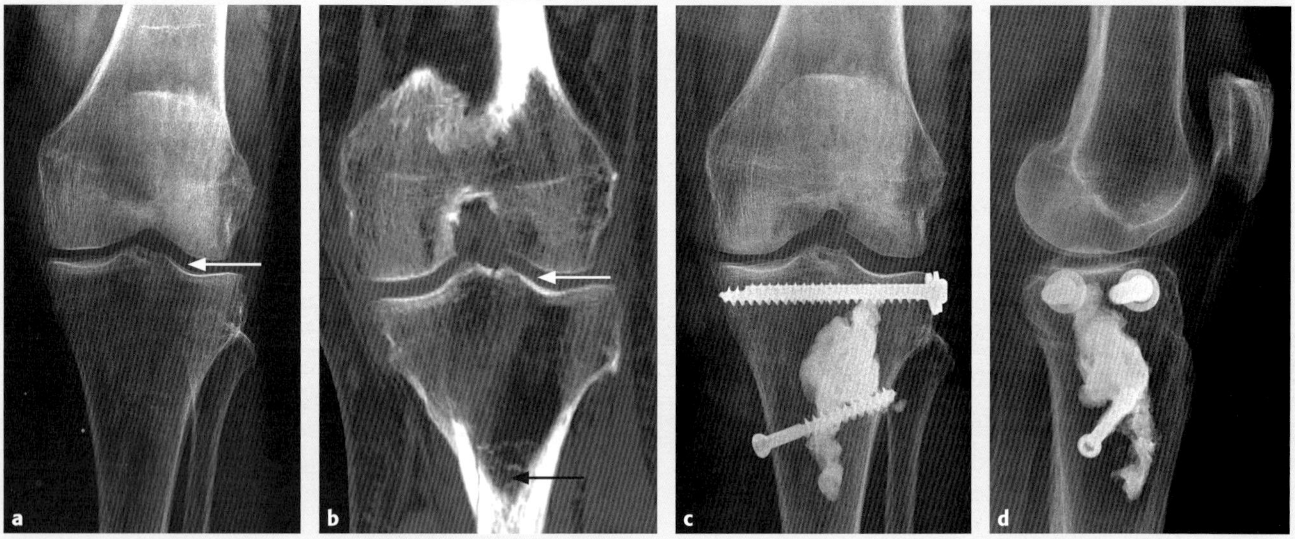


**Fig 3.15-1a–d** An 86-year-old patient with anterior cruciate ligament injury.
**a** X-ray of the anterior cruciate ligament fragment.
**b** Computed tomographic scan of the fracture going into the medial metaphysis.
**c–d** One-year postoperative x-rays of the polymethylmethacrylate-augmented tibial metaphysis.

Physical examination should follow this sequence:

- Inspection of the soft tissue, particularly in cognitively impaired geriatric patients or polytraumatized unconscious patients where verbal history is limited. Deformation of the knee, bruises, and pressure marks can help to understand the trauma mechanism.
- Peripheral neurovascular examination.
- Evaluation for compartment syndrome. This can occur in geriatric trauma patients taking antithrombotic or anticoagulant medications. Some case reports describe compartment syndromes triggered by spontaneous drug-induced bleeding [12–14].
- Examination of ligament stability and meniscal injuries:
  - The risk of ligament and meniscal injury is higher in high-energy trauma of young patients compared to geriatric patients where the osteoporotic bone has a higher risk of fracture [1, 15]. Ligament injuries in the young (< 60 years), after high-energy trauma constitutes 49–54% [16, 17] versus 5% [6] in older adults.
  - Valgus stress leading to lateral depression fractures have a higher risk of medial collateral ligament rupture [17, 18].
  - The risk of lateral meniscal tear in lateral depression fractures increases eightfold with displacement > 10 mm [15].
  - Anterior or posterior cruciate ligament rupture or avulsion in older adults are signs of higher instability, which require further evaluation of the neurovascular structures in the popliteal cavity.
- Swelling of the knee and evaluation of the soft-tissue envelope:
  - In case of a joint effusion, diagnostic and therapeutic knee puncture may be considered to relieve acute pain.
  - Soft-tissue edema and skin laceration may delay surgery.

### 3.2 Imaging

AP, lateral, oblique, and patella sunrise views of the knee joint are recommended. In case of unclear findings, further evaluation by means of computed tomographic (CT) scan or magnetic resonance imaging (MRI) should be added. Note that 6.3% of knee fractures are missed in emergency x-rays [19]:

- For CT scans a slice thickness of 1 mm is recommended [20, 21].
- Insufficiency fractures of the proximal tibia are often missed with plain x-rays and are best detected using MRI [9].

If surgery is indicated, CT scans are necessary for planning surgery. Most of the newer classification systems of the PTF are based on CT scan findings, which allow a better mapping of the fractured columns [20–22]:

- Three-dimensional reconstructions of the fragments allow a better preoperative planning of the approach and choice of osteosynthesis.
- Two-dimensional reconstructions of the fragments along the axis allow better estimation of fracture dislocation.

Concomitant soft-tissue injuries such as ligament avulsion or rupture can be best diagnosed using MRI [23, 24]. In case clinical examination of the knee stability is limited due to swelling, MRI imaging is strongly recommended preoperatively. The degree of ligament injury influences the timing of definitive surgery and the need for provisional stabilization [24].

### 3.3 Local bone quality

Cancellous and cortical bone decrease in the proximal tibia over time:

- Chen et al [25] identified reduction in trabecular number and thickness by means of high-resolution peripheral quantitative CT, showing a decrease in bone mineral density (BMD) of 4% per decade from 57–96 years.
- Cortical thickness of the tibia is typically smaller than at the proximal femur [25].
- Cortical porosity decreases over time [25].

## 4 Classification

The most popular classification systems for PTFs are in descending order the Schatzker [26], AO/OTA [27], and Hohl and Moore [28] classifications. First attempts to classify PTFs were made by Schatzker as early as 1979, which categorized six fracture patterns based on AP x-rays. The AO/OTA classification was strongly related to Schatzker's system but was part of a larger classification system for bone fractures, easier to remember and reproduce. The main difference between the two classifications is the addition of extraarticular fractures, type A. The Hohl and Moore classification is still often mentioned but has been outdated [29], perhaps due to its similarity to the Schatzker classification.

Characteristics of the Schatzker, AO/OTA, and Hohl and Moore classifications:

- Fractures are categorized into depression, monocondylar, or bicondylar fractures.
- All three systems are based on plain AP x-rays.
- Schatzker has the best interobserver and intraobserver reliability [29].

The wide availability of CT and 3-D fracture images has added to classification schemes of PTFs. While the Schatzker and AO/OTA classifications focus on the two condyles in AP view, shearing fractures of the dorsal rim of the tibial plateau are missed. Luo et al [22] first introduced the three-column classification system (**Fig 3.15-2**), which produces a more comprehensive evaluation with a high relevance for surgical decision making.

The three-column classification has the following advantages:

- Three-dimensional mapping of the proximal tibia.
- Better intraobserver reliability than Schatzker (0.810 versus 0.758) [20].
- A more comprehensive evaluation of the dorsal column fracture, which has a high incidence of 28.8% [21].
- Allows better surgical planning and operative positioning in the case of dorsal column involvement [22].

## 5 Decision making

### 5.1 Fracture dislocation or osteoporotic fracture?

It is essential to evaluate whether the knee is in stable or unstable condition.

In patients younger than 60 years, posteromedial rim fractures are highly associated with knee dislocation and ligamentous injuries. Tscherne and Lobenhoffer [30] found 96% of anterior cruciate ligament (ACL) injuries and 85% medial collateral ligament ruptures in this fracture type are unstable. In older adults the osteoporotic bone often fractures before ligament ruptures occur, but:

- Large posteromedial rim fractures should always be treated as unstable.
- Osteoporotic depression fractures at the posterolateral and central rim are not necessarily unstable.
- Additional avulsion fracture of the ACL is a clear sign for knee dislocation and instability [31].

Unstable fractures are typically associated with substantial soft-tissue swelling and should be treated in two stages. An external fixator until the time point of open reduction and internal fixation (ORIF) is usually necessary.

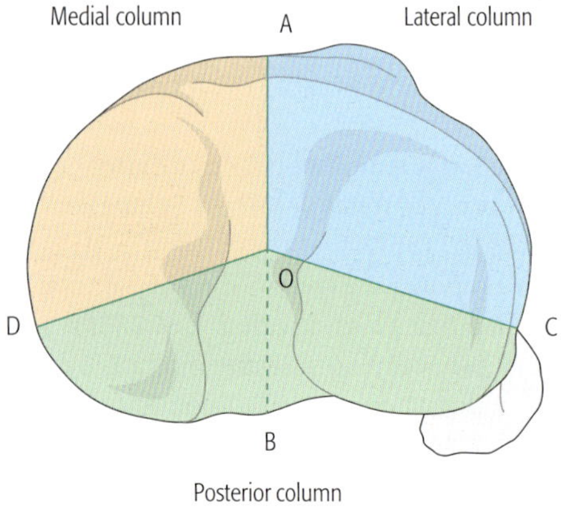


**Fig 3.15-2** Three-column classification according Luo et al [22]: Classification is made on transverse computed tomographic sections. The knee center (**O**) is connected with the anterior tuberosity (**A**), the posterior sulcus of the tibial head (**B**), the most anterior point of the fibular head (**C**), and the posterior medial ridge of the proximal tibia (**D**). The posterior column can be divided into a lateral and medial column indicated by the (**OB**) line.

### 5.2 Nonoperative versus operative treatment

In general, nondisplaced PTFs that are stable to varus and valgus stress can be treated nonoperatively. Ten degrees of varus axis deformity can be considered as unstable and requires operative treatment [32, 33]. Due to pain, clinical evaluation for ligamentous instability is difficult in acutely injured patients and can often result in further fracture displacement due to manipulation.

Minimally displaced depression fractures of the lateral proximal tibial plateau (zero-column, Schatzker III, AO/OTA 41B2.1), where the articular surface is maintained (depression ≤ 2 mm) and limb alignment is not disrupted, should be treated nonoperatively with a hinged brace or with a long leg cast in cognitively impaired or noncompliant patients [34–36]. However, one can question if the so-called critical size of 2 mm step-off for operative treatment is a relevant rule for older patients. Frail geriatric patients who are unable to tolerate surgery may require nonoperative treatment.

Segal et al [37] extended their indication of nonoperative treatment of lateral depression and split-depression fractures to 5 mm and had overall 95% of satisfactory results compared to operative treatment.

On the other hand, depression fractures tend to deteriorate in osteoporotic conditions because of bone voids. It might be reasonable to prevent varus or valgus deformation by prophylactic operative stabilization.

### 5.3 Operative approach

The operative approach can be based on the three-column classification.

#### 5.3.1 Zero-column fracture (Schatzker type III)

Pure depression fractures in the lateral proximal tibial plateau without involvement of the cortex are classified as zero-column fractures (**Fig 3.15-3a–b**). The operative approach can be made from lateral or medial via a small cortical window to elevate the depression (**Fig 3.15-3c–d**) [38–40]. In case of additional fixation, plate or screw osteosynthesis is performed from a lateral approach (**Fig 3.15-3e–f**) [38]. In osteoporotic bone, indirect elevation of the articular surface may not be possible or may be destructive. Balloon tibioplasty with subsequent augmentation is an alternative (**Fig 3.15-3g–h**).

### 5.3.2 One- and two-column fracture (Schatzker types I and II)

Simple lateral split or split-depression fractures usually involve the lateral anterior and/or the lateral posterior column and can be classified as one- or two-column fractures. The fracture can be best reached via a lateral straight incision in supine position. Voids or defects after joint reconstruction can be addressed with cement, bone substitutes, or allogenic bone grafting.

### 5.3.3 Two-column fracture (Schatzker type IV)

Medial condylar fractures usually involve the anteromedial and posteromedial column and are classified as the typical two-column fractures. Based on the two-column principle, an operative approach is possible in most cases from posteromedial to buttress the dorsal fragment with a plate, placing the patient in supine or prone position. The anteromedial fragment can be reached by medial subperiosteal dissection of the medial tibial rim and can also be addressed with a buttress plate [22].

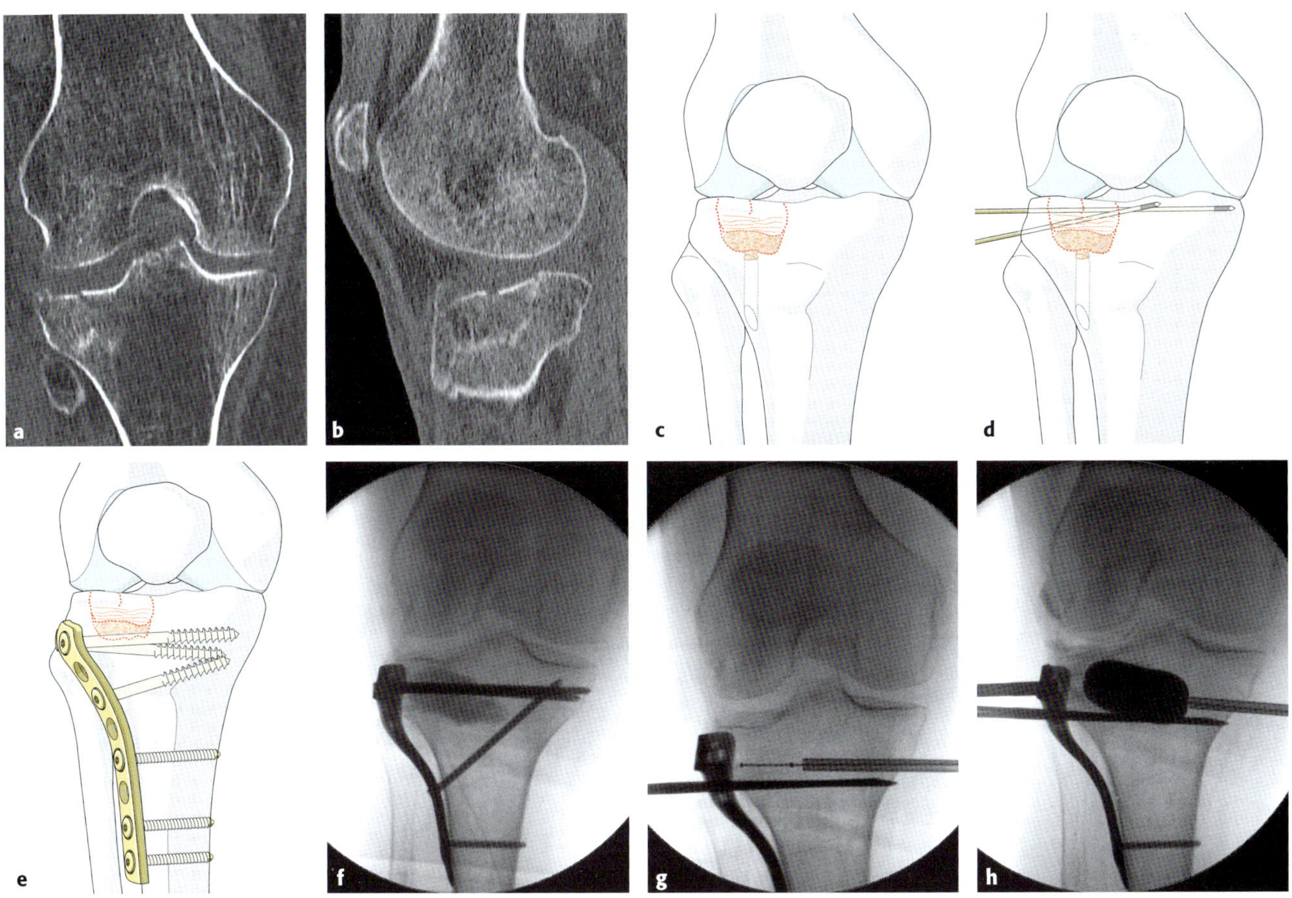


**Fig 3.15-3a–h** Operative approach to elevation and fixation of a depression fracture.

**a–b** Zero-column depression fracture.

**c–d** Elevation of the depression and filling of the subarticular void with polymethylmethacrylate.

**e–f** Lateral angular stable plate osteosynthesis.

**g–h** Elevation of the depression fracture with the help of a balloon tibioplasty percutaneously via a small cortical window medially.

### 5.3.4 Three-column fracture (Schatzker types V and VI)

Bicondylar fractures are often combined with a posterolateral fragment and thus classified as a three-column fracture (**Fig 3.15-4a–c**). Understanding and recognition of the additional dorsal fragment changes the recommendation from a single anterior approach to a double anterolateral and posteromedial incision (**Fig 3.15-4d–g**) [41, 42].

Some authors still recommend the single anterior incision, which may be useful in case of later salvage arthroplasty [43, 44]. However, we recommend a double incision (anterolateral and posteromedial), which allows better reconstruction of the joint surface and is associated with a lower risk of wound infections in critical soft-tissue conditions, leading to good results (**Fig 3.15-4h–i**) [45–47].

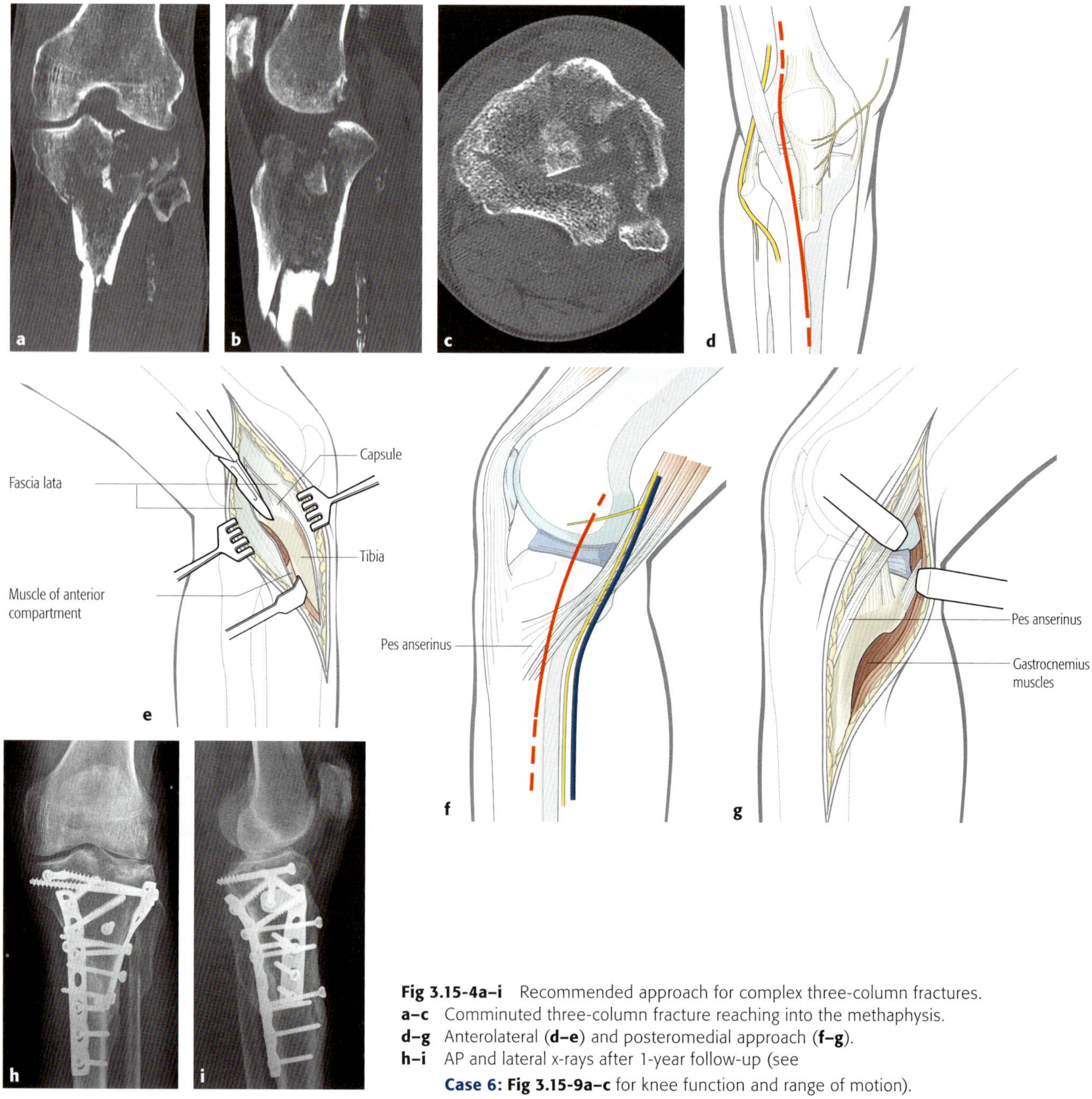


**Fig 3.15-4a–i** Recommended approach for complex three-column fractures.
**a–c** Comminuted three-column fracture reaching into the methaphysis.
**d–g** Anterolateral (**d–e**) and posteromedial approach (**f–g**).
**h–i** AP and lateral x-rays after 1-year follow-up (see **Case 6: Fig 3.15-9a–c** for knee function and range of motion).

## 6 Therapeutic options

### 6.1 Nonoperative treatment

The general recommendations for nonoperative treatment are:

- Immobilization with an adjustable hinged knee brace [3].
- Beginning with full extension during the first 2 weeks will help to decrease swelling, and starting early with range of motion (ROM) is essential to prevent contracture and muscle atrophy in frail geriatric patients [48, 49]. Continuous passive motion (CPM) may be used.
- Concomitant ligament injuries will increase the risk of knee contracture [50]. Twenty degrees of flexion contracture significantly influences gait velocity and stride length [51] and may lead to further falls in older adults.
- General recommendations are limited weight bearing for 6–8 weeks, although partial weight bearing may be impossible to achieve in older or cognitively impaired patients. Nonoperative treatment of lateral split and depression fractures in the young did not result in depressions greater than 2 mm [37]. No data are available for older cohorts.

### 6.2 External fixator and percutaneous reduction

The external fixator is the method of choice in cases of severe soft-tissue damage or vascular disease, which prevents primary ORIF surgery [52]. In older adults, soft-tissue edema and vascular disease can produce extensive swelling after low-energy trauma despite less severe fracture patterns (zero-, one-, or two-column, Schatzker types I–IV). In this situation using the external fixator may be considered. Fracture reduction can be performed percutaneously with minimal blood loss and without extensive soft-tissue exposure. Biomechanical studies support full weight bearing [53, 54]. No studies exist for osteoporotic bone.

### 6.3 Plate fixation with temporary external fixator

In comminuted bicondylar fractures of patients with poor bone stock, hybrid techniques of temporary external fixation to supplement the plate or screw fixation have been introduced as a promising new approach to allow immediate mobilization with weight bearing as tolerated (**Case 2: Fig 3.15-5**) [52, 55].

Ali et al [56] prospectively investigated 11 patients with an AO/OTA 41C2 or 3 fracture treated percutaneously with intrafragmentary screw fixation, followed by neutralization with a stable external fixator and early mobilization:

- Follow-up after 38 months
- 11 of 11 radiologically healed fractures
- 9 of 11 satisfactory results according to the Rasmussen score for postoperative knee function evaluation
- 2 of 11 revisions: one total knee arthroplasty (TKA), one corrective osteotomy
- 5 superficial pin-track infections, no deep infection

Krappinger et al [55] presented two cases of AO/OTA 41C3 fractures, which were initially stabilized with external fixation followed by additional internal fixation with anteromedial and anterolateral angular stable double plating after soft-tissue consolidation and external fixation for 8 weeks:

- Follow-up after 12 months
- 2 of 2 pain-free results
- ROM: 0–100°
- No radiographic progression of the preexisting significant osteoarthritis and no loss of reduction

### 6.4 Lateral locking plate

#### 6.4.1 Indication 1

Lateral locking plate fixation is also indicated for unicondylar, lateral or medial, PTFs (one- or two-column, Schatzker I, II, IV, AO/OTA 41B1, B3, C1) (**Case 3: Fig 3.15-6**) [70–72].

Gösling et al [73] performed biomechanical studies in cadaver bones with medial condylar fractures (Schatzker type IV, AO/OTA 41C1) instrumented with a lateral angular stable plate to double plating with a lateral buttress plate and a medial antiglide plate:

- No significant difference between the two techniques in regard to axial weight bearing.
- Maximum loading was 1,600 Newton (N), which showed plastic vertical subsidence of 1.1 mm in the single plate group versus 1.5 mm in the double plate group:
  - 1,600 N are approximately 163 kg which far exceeds a healthy body weight.
- Limitation of the study was the missing data with respect to bone quality or age of the specimens.

Gerich et al [52] reported a retrospective cohort with mean age of 69 years that showed the following poor results: ten split-depression fractures, two split fractures, and three bicondylar fractures were treated with ORIF and lateral angular stable locking plate. Loss of reduction had occurred in 13 of 15 cases.

In osteoporotic bone, additional implant augmentation with PMMA might improve these results [74].

CASE 2

## Patient

An 81-year-old woman sustained a comminuted bicondylar fracture of the left proximal tibial plateau (**Fig 3.15-5a–b**).

## Treatment and outcome

Temporary transarticular stabilization with a bridging external fixator was performed because of soft-tissue swelling; it was left in place until the swelling was reduced and soft tissue consolidated (**Fig 3.15-5c–d**). Open reduction and internal fixation was preformed after 2.5 weeks with reconstruction of the joint congruency via a single midline incision, open reduction, and defect filling with a fresh frozen bone allograft. A lateral undercontoured buttress plate combined with a medial antiglide plate was applied (**Fig 3.15-5e–f**). Due to the poor bone stock, the surgeon decided to continue using the external fixator in addition to plate osteosynthesis. The patient was mobilized with partial weight bearing (30 kg). The external fixator was finally removed after 3 months and full weight bearing was allowed.

At the 1-year follow-up, osseous consolidation, full knee extension, and 100° of flexion were achieved (**Fig 3.15-5g**). The patient was able to walk with one stick and live on her own. At the 2-year follow-up, the patient presented again with increasing pain. The x-rays showed osteonecrosis of the lateral proximal tibia with increasing valgus (**Fig 3.15-5h**).

## Discussion

A 2-staged procedure as proposed in this case is the gold standard for comminuted proximal tibial plateau fractures, with large soft-tissue damage after high-energy trauma [57, 58].

A midline approach was chosen in order to keep the external fixator in place and for better filling of the central defect with an allograft. However, it should be remembered that the risk of poor healing due to soft-tissue stripping and fragment devascularization is higher using a midline approach [52, 59]. Newer studies have shown that the timing of the definitive osteosynthesis has a higher influence on soft-tissue healing than the choice of approach [60, 61]. Nevertheless, a midline approach is no longer recommended.

Allograft bone was chosen to prevent donor site morbidity [62, 63]. Osteonecrosis occurred with subsidence of the laterocentral joint surface after 2 years (**Fig 3.15-5g–h**). Polymethylmethacrylate (PMMA) shows better results with regard to prevention of loss of reduction over time [64].

Angular stable plate fixation has shown good results to prevent loss of reduction. However, in osteoporotic bone, osteosynthesis failure is described frequently [6, 52, 65]. These results led to the decision to additionally maintain the external fixator, because the degree of comminution did not allow PMMA implant augmentation without the risk of cement leakage into the joint.

In this case the patient was allowed to partially bear weight and was mobilized with the help of two crutches. The importance of early mobilization for geriatric patients has been described in several studies to prevent complications related to immobilization [66, 67]. The 1-year follow-up showed satisfactory results with respect to bone healing, soft-tissue healing, and range of motion (**Fig 3.15-5g**). Unfortunately, osteonecrosis occurred after a 2-year follow-up. The mechanical axis of the leg was still maintained, which is the most important goal for complicated proximal tibial fractures (**Fig 3.15-5h**) [3, 68, 69]. Secondary total knee arthroplasty can now be considered after bone healing and maintained axial alignment.

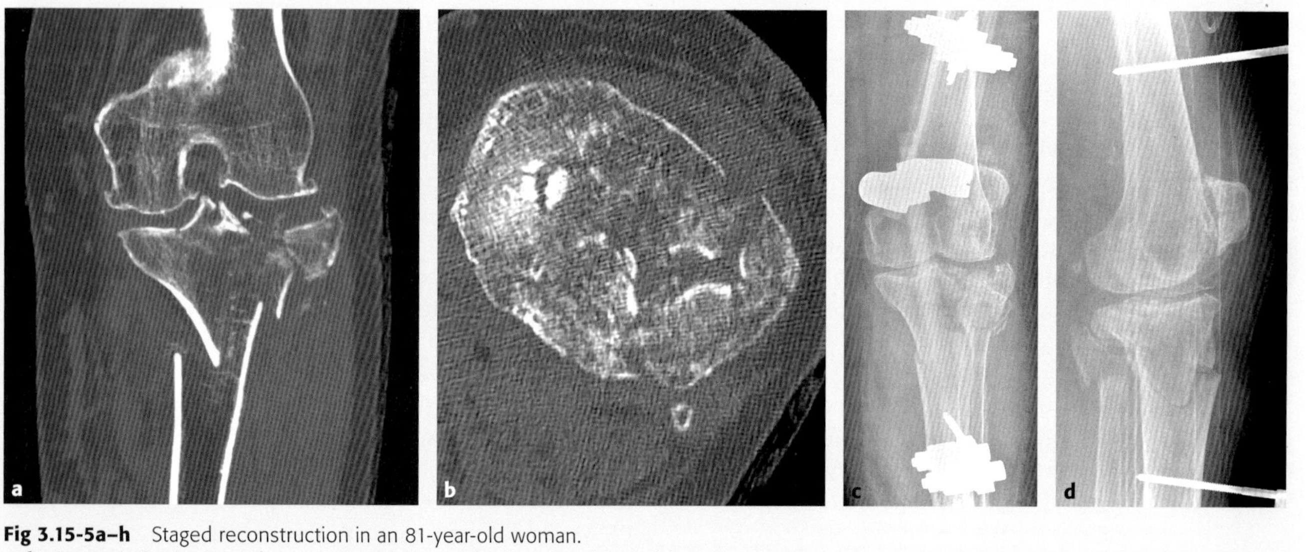


**Fig 3.15-5a–h** Staged reconstruction in an 81-year-old woman.
**a–b** Preoperative images of a comminuted bicondylar fracture of the left knee.
**c–d** X-rays showing bridging external fixator to stabilize the knee.

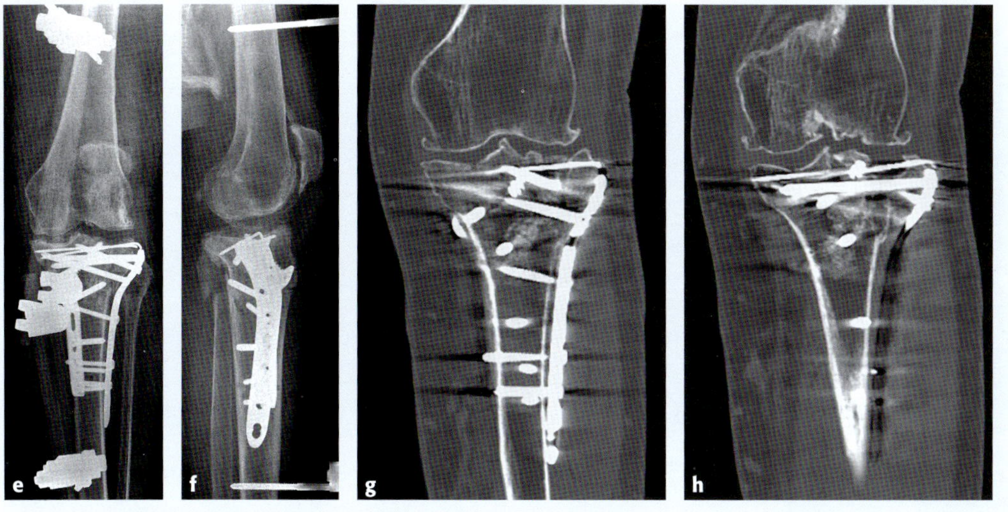


**Fig 3.15-5a–h (cont)** Staged reconstruction in an 81-year-old woman.
**e–f** Reconstruction following bone allograft.
**g** The 1-year follow-up without loss of reduction.
**h** A 2-year follow-up with laterocentral osteonecrosis but maintained leg axis.



### Patient

An 80-year-old woman was hit by a bicycle and fell from standing height. She sustained a split-depression proximal tibial fracture (PTF) (two-column, Schatzker type II, AO/OTA type 41B3) and an intraarticular distal radial fracture (DRF) (**Fig 3.15-6a–d**).

### Comorbidities

- Osteoporosis
- Diabetes
- Hypertension
- Epilepsy
- Polyneuropathy
- Peripheral arterial disease
- Internal carotid artery stenosis

### Treatment and outcome

She was treated with an angular stable lateral proximal tibial plate with polymethylmethacrylate (PMMA) augmentation of the proximal screws, via a minimally invasive plate osteosynthesis approach and a double plate osteosynthesis of the distal radius, volar and dorsal. The rehabilitation required a soft cast for the distal radius for 3 weeks. Mobilization of the left knee was allowed with weight bearing as tolerated (WBAT). Radiological follow-up showed no loss of reduction of the proximal tibial osteosynthesis after 3 months (**Fig 3.15-6e–f**).

### Discussion

Decision making for this case was based on a number of considerations. Due to her DRF, the use of crutches was limited. The surgeon decided on the most stable fixation of the radius using a double plate approach from palmar and volar for the distal radius. In the proximal tibia, he decided on a minimally invasive lateral approach in order to prevent further soft-tissue damage (peripheral arterial disease) and to augment the proximal screws of an angular stable lateral plate for the proximal tibia (**Fig 3.15-6e–f**).

Current practice often suggests limited weight bearing during the first 6–8 postoperative weeks for this fracture type treated with single lateral locking plate **[6, 75]**. In the older adult, WBAT should be the goal, because most geriatric patients are not able to partially bear weight. Goetzen et al **[74]** simulated a most unstable PTF (AO/OTA 41A3) in osteoporotic cadaveric bones and tested a biomechanically augmented angular stable plate osteosynthesis with good results. Increasing cyclic loading of the construct failed on average after 740 N (75.5 kg). Similar results were presented by Gosling et al **[73]**. Clinical studies are needed to investigate whether PMMA-augmented angular plates permit full weight bearing immediately after surgery.

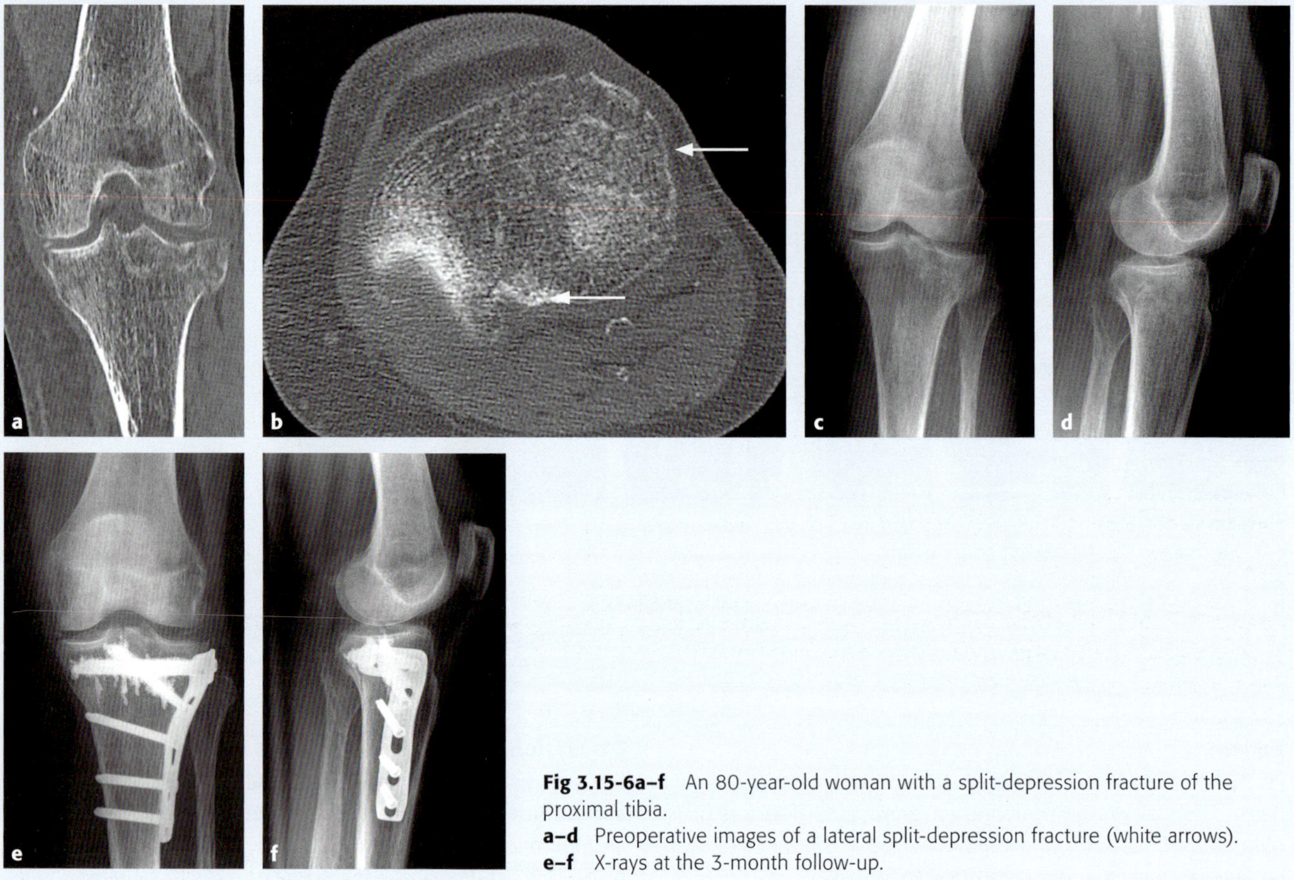


**Fig 3.15-6a–f** An 80-year-old woman with a split-depression fracture of the proximal tibia.
**a–d** Preoperative images of a lateral split-depression fracture (white arrows).
**e–f** X-rays at the 3-month follow-up.

### 6.4.2 Indication 2

Isolated lateral proximal tibial depression fractures (zero-column, Schatzker III, AO/OTA 41B2) should be treated with reduction of the tibial plateau and filling of the metaphyseal defect with either autogenous or allograft bone, calcium phosphate-based bone cement or PMMA (**Case 4: Fig 3.15-7**). Indications for surgery range between 2 and 5 mm of depression [37, 70]. In osteoporotic bone, additional plate fixation is recommended [38].

Mayr et al [38] compared in a biomechanical study in cadaveric bones, reduced depression fractures augmented with subcortical PMMA cement and additional screw raft fixation to subcortical PMMA augmentation and angular stable plate fixation. Their findings included:

- Plate fixation exhibited less subsidence at higher loads compared with screw raft fixation.
- Tests of the cement only, after plate and screw raft removal, showed the least effective results with additional subsidence of 1.3 mm and 1.9 mm, respectively, at 480 N (49 kg) of cyclic loading.

Russell and Leighton [76] compared autogenous bone graft with calcium phosphate-based bone cement in a prospective randomized trial (n = 120) of reduced and augmented metaphyseal defects. Their findings at 1 year included:

- Union rates and time to union between the two groups showed no significant difference.
- Subsidence was significantly higher in the autogenous bone graft group, which seemed to be inferior in respect to stability and donor side morbidity compared to calcium phosphate-based bone cement.

**Patient**

An 83-old-woman fell from a ladder and suffered an isolated lateral depression fracture (zero-column, Schatzker III) (**Fig 3.15-7a–c**).

**Comorbidities**

- Osteoporosis
- Hypercholesterolemia
- Urinary incontinence

**Treatment and outcome**

Surgery was performed 3 days after admission. She was treated with balloon tibioplasty reduction (abutted on two K-wires, which were inserted below the balloon to guarantee proximal expansion of the balloon), subarticular defect filling with polymethylmethacrylate (PMMA), and angular stable lateral plate osteosynthesis of the proximal tibia via a minimally invasive approach (**Fig 3.15-7d–f**). She was mobilized with the help of crutches with partial weight bearing (30 kg) for 8 weeks.

Radiographic follow-up after 3 months showed no subsidence of the joint surface (**Fig 3.15-7g**). The patient reached 120° of flexion and full extension and was able to walk without crutches after 3 months.

**Discussion**

The minimally invasive approach using balloon tibioplasty for reduction and defect filling with PMMA has shown good reduction results. The large surface of the balloon allows a gentle reduction of the fracture and decreases the risk of penetration into the joint [38, 39].

Defect filling with PMMA has the best biomechanical results. The discussion regarding which material should be used for bone void filling is of great interest; autogenous bone grafts from the iliac crest are currently the gold standard [76]. However, complications associated with graft harvest include prolonged pain at the iliac crest, wound infection, and numbness, which increases the morbidity, particularly in older adults [62, 63]. Alternatives, such as calcium phosphate-based bone cement or PMMA to replace the autogenous bone graft have been investigated [77, 78]. Calcium phosphate-based bone cement showed superior results with respect to resistance of subsidence compared to autogenous bone graft [79]. However, calcium phosphate cement is still inferior to PMMA with regard to biomechanical performance, handling ease [80], and is not capable of restoring reduction height over time [64]. Polymethylmethacrylate allows immediate mechanical strength, which is most important in order to mobilize geriatric patients.

Another point of interest is the discussion of plate osteosynthesis versus screw raft fixation. Biomechanical studies showed that augmented screws without additional lateral fixation will cut through the lateral cortex [38, 81]. Lateral locking plates should be applied in the older adult with thin cortical bone to reduce the risk for lateral screw cut-through.

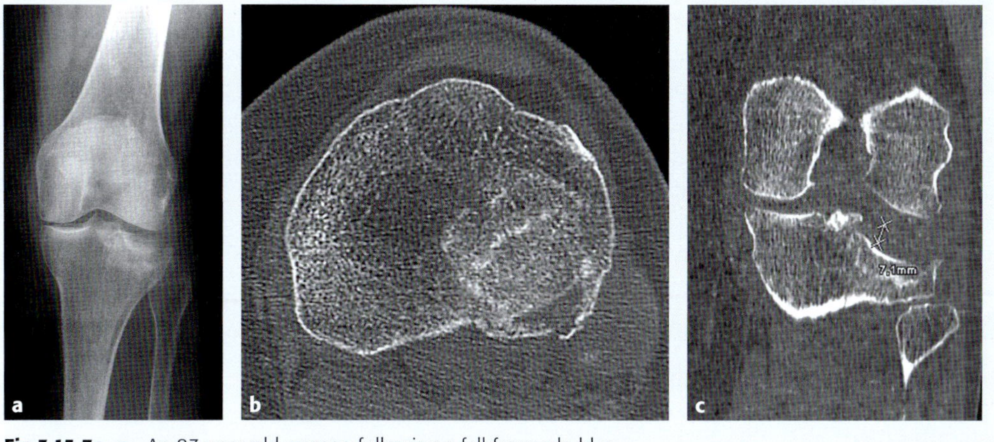


**Fig 3.15-7a–g** An 83-year-old woman following a fall from a ladder.
**a–c** Preoperative AP x-ray and computed tomographic scan of a depression fracture of the proximal laterodorsal tibia.

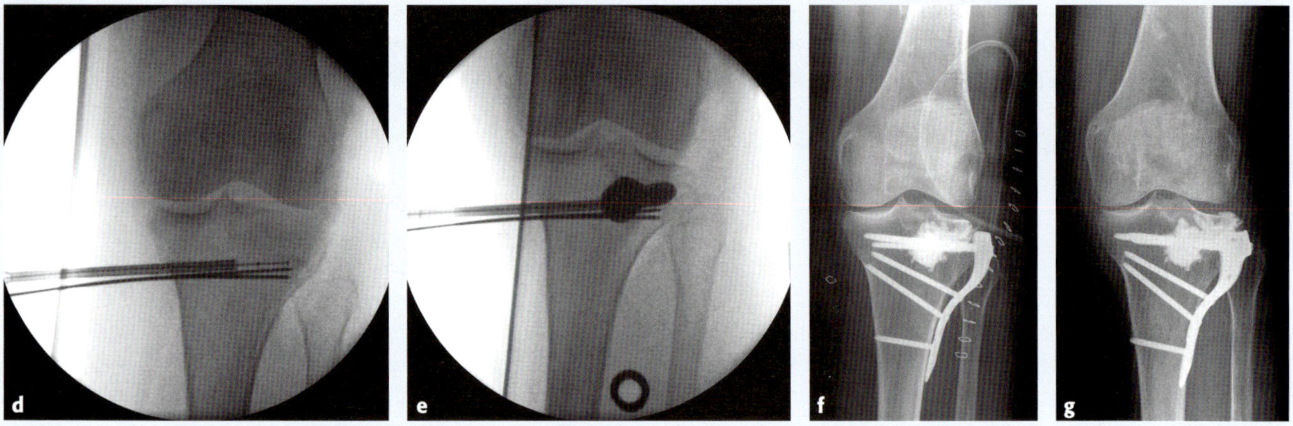


**Fig 3.15-7a–g (cont)** An 83-year-old woman following fall from ladder.
**d–e** Intraoperative images of the reduction by means of a balloon tibioplasty.
**f** Postoperative x-rays after tibioplasty with polymethylmethacrylate cement and osteosynthesis with an angular stable buttress plate.
**g** X-rays at a 3-month follow-up without loss of reduction.

### 6.4.3 Indication 3

Simple bicondylar and metaphyseal fractures may also be considered for single lateral locking plate fixation (**Case 5: Fig 3.15-8**) [82, 83]. In combination with PMMA augmentation, biomechanical studies have shown that single lateral locking plate fixation can be sufficient to stabilize comminuted extraarticular (AO/OTA 41A3) PTFs in osteoporotic bone [74]. In young patients, comminuted bicondylar fractures (Schatzker type VI) have been treated by Stannard et al [84] and Schütz et al [85] with acceptable results.

If fracture dislocation does not require a large open reduction, the surgical approach should be performed via a MIPO technique [73, 86–88]; a 6–8 cm long straight anterolateral incision is performed. The plate is slid down submuscularly without further violation of the distal soft tissue. The diaphyseal screws can be placed via stab incisions. Aiming devices such as the radiolucent handle of the less invasive stabilization system for PTFs are available to allow accurate percutaneous screw placement.

Goetzen et al [74] investigated biomechanically unstable PTFs (AO/OTA 41A3) in osteoporotic cadaveric bones treated with lateral locking plate with PMMA screw augmentation versus without PMMA augmentation:

- Average T-score of the bone was -3.6.
- There was a significantly higher axial loading until failure in the augmented group (14,792 load cycles) compared to the nonaugmented group (9,417 load cycles).

Stannard et al [84] published a prospective nonrandomized study of 25 intraarticular (Schatzker type V and VI) and 10 extraarticular PTFs treated with ORIF and single lateral locking plate via a MIPO approach. At 11 months the following results were noted:

- 1 of 32 fractures was a nonunion
- Mean ROM (extension-flexion): 2–110°
- 4.9% deep infections (open fractures)

Schütz et al [85] examined in a prospective nonrandomized study 12 intraarticular (AO/OTA 41C), 3 extraarticular PTFs (AO/OTA 41A), and 7 proximal tibial shaft fractures (AO/OTA 42) treated with ORIF and single lateral locking plate via a MIPO approach. Results at 12 months were:

- 1 of 20 fractures was a nonunion
- Mean ROM (extension-flexion): 0–105°
- One deep infection (open fracture)

### Patient

A 77-year-old patient suffered polytrauma in a car accident including an acetabular fracture of the posterior wall, a bicondylar proximal tibial fracture on the right side (three-column, Schatzker V) (**Fig 3.15-8a**), and multiple fractures of the ribs on both sides with contusion of the left kidney.

### Comorbidities

- Osteoporosis
- Diabetes
- Coronary heart disease

### Treatment and outcome

The posterior wall of the acetabulum was stabilized with plate fixation via a dorsal Kocher-Langenbeck approach. The proximal tibia was treated with a lateral angular stable plate via a minimally invasive plate osteosynthesis (MIPO) approach with augmented proximal screws (**Fig 3.15-8b**).

During rehabilitation, weight bearing as tolerated was allowed (**Fig 3.15-8c**). To obtain best range of motion in the right knee joint, continuous passive motion (CPM) was applied during hospitalization.

### Discussion

Decision making for this case was based on the following considerations. Hip arthroplasty and knee arthroplasty were discussed to allow early mobilization. Due to the combination of serial fractures of the ribs, kidney contusion, and the complex extremity fractures, bed rest was expected for at least 4–6 weeks. Mobilization of the knee was planned during the period of bed rest with the help of CPM. To obtain the necessary stability for passive mobilization, the surgeons decided on angular stable MIPO of the proximal tibia and augmentation of the proximal screws with polymethylmethacrylate.

In the current literature, there is agreement about treating Schatzker type V and VI fractures (two- or three-column) with double plating. Biomechanical studies have shown that double plating provides better stability than single plate fixation [89]. Good clinical results via a minimally invasive anterolateral and posteromedial incision have been reported [60, 90, 91]. However, double plating still remains more invasive than a single anterolateral MIPO approach. In this case of a geriatric patient suffering from diabetes and peripheral arterial disease, double plating is relatively contraindicated to prevent soft-tissue breakdown [59, 92]. Biggi et al [82] achieved sufficient stabilization of bicondylar proximal tibial fractures with a single lateral locking plate and augmentation with autogenous bone graft.

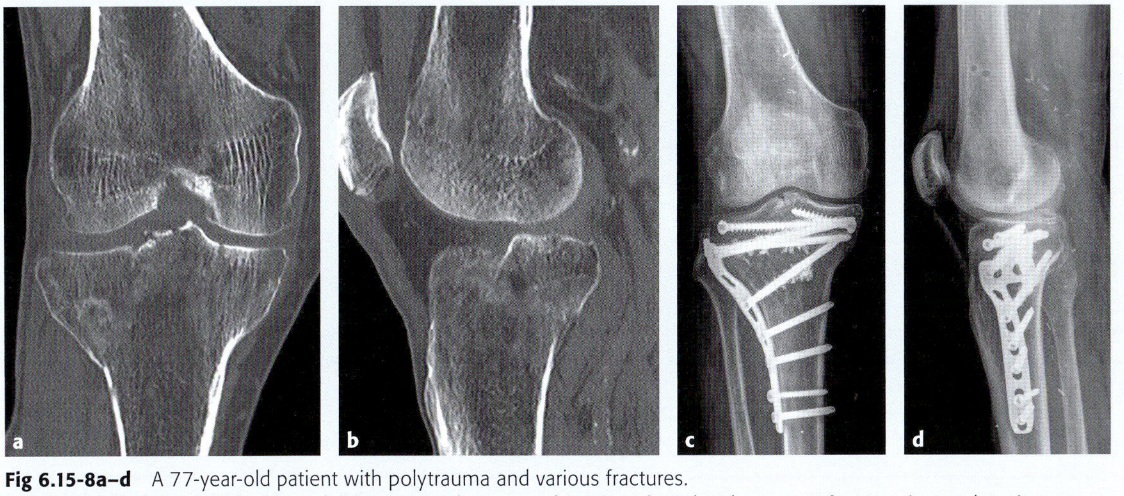


**Fig 6.15-8a–d** A 77-year-old patient with polytrauma and various fractures.
**a–b** Preoperative AP (**a**) and lateral (**b**) computed tomographic scan of a Schatzker type V fracture (two-column).
**c** Two-week postoperative x-ray with the staples still in.
**d** X-ray after 6 weeks without loss of reduction.

### 6.5 Bilateral double locking plate

Complex bicondylar PTFs (three-column, Schatzker V and VI, AO/OTA 41C) are typically treated by double plating (medial and lateral) (**Case 6: Fig 3.15-9**) [60, 91, 93–95]. In particular, in three-column fractures with posterior rim displacement, an additional posteromedial to the anterolateral approach is needed to address the dorsal fragment with a second or in some cases third posteromedial buttress plate [96, 97].

Higgins et al [98] compared in a biomechanical study of cadaveric bones cyclic loading of lateral only locked plating to medial and lateral nonlocked plating in simulated bicondylar PTFs. They found:

- Less subsidence in double plating, in particular of the medial condyle (0.78 mm), compared to lateral only locked plating (1.51 mm).
- No significant difference in maximum load between the two groups.

Neogi et al [99] published a prospective nonrandomized study (N = 61, AO/OTA type 41C) comparing double plating using a double incision approach (N = 29) versus lateral single locking plate (N = 32). They found at the 2-year follow-up:

- No significant difference in respect to healing.
- Significantly higher loss of reduction and alignment in single plating, ie, seven versus one in the double-plating group.
- ROM and clinical scoring were similar in both groups without a significant difference.
- Significantly higher infection rate in double plating, ie, six versus two.

Barei et al [92] radiographically investigated 23 cases with Schatzker type V and IV, treated with double incisions and medial and lateral plating. They found at the 59-month follow-up:

- 55% satisfactory reduction (≤ 2 mm step)
- 90% satisfactory coronal plane alignment (medial proximal tibial angle ≥ 87°)
- 68% satisfactory sagittal plane alignment (posterior proximal tibial angle ≥ 9°)

Wang et al [97] investigated retrospectively the clinical and radiographic outcome of 10 Schatzker type V and VI fractures treated with double incisions and medial and lateral plating. They found at the 26.5-month follow-up:

- ROM (extension-flexion): 2–110.5°
- 9 of 10 fractures with satisfactory reduction
- Mean Hospital for Special Surgery knee score was 92.7 points

**CASE 6**

**Patient**

An 84-year-old woman was admitted with a fracture dislocation (three-column fracture) of the proximal tibia after she fell off her bicycle (**Fig 3.15-9a–c**).

**Comorbidities**

- Osteoporosis

**Treatment and outcome**

On the day of admission an external fixator was placed; open reduction and internal fixation (ORIF) was performed via an anterolateral and posteromedial approach 1 week later. The metaphyseal void was filled with calcium phosphate-based bone cement. Due to the knee instability, the external fixator was retained for 8 weeks (**Fig 3.15-9d–f**). The 18-month follow-up showed satisfactory results. Range of motion reached 0–5–90° (**Fig 3.15-9g–i**). The knee was stable and the leg axis was achieved despite severe posttraumatic osteoarthritis (**Fig 3.15-9j–l**). Computed tomographic scans showed severe posttraumatic osteoarthritis at the lateral compartment of the joint surface. However, the patient was nearly pain free and able to walk by herself in the nursing home.

**Discussion**

This case report shows the typical 2-staged procedure for fracture dislocations. Use of the external fixator is mandatory in unstable fracture dislocations. Waiting for reduction of soft-tissue swelling is obligatory in such severe fractures before ORIF.

The restoration of the joint axis is the primary goal for older adults with such comminuted fractures so as to allow them to regain independent mobilization. Precise anatomical reduction is of minor importance and does not always correlate with clinical results. The analysis of 71 cases undergoing osteosynthesis of proximal tibial fractures showed no correlation between anatomical reduction and functional outcome after a 6-year follow-up [100].

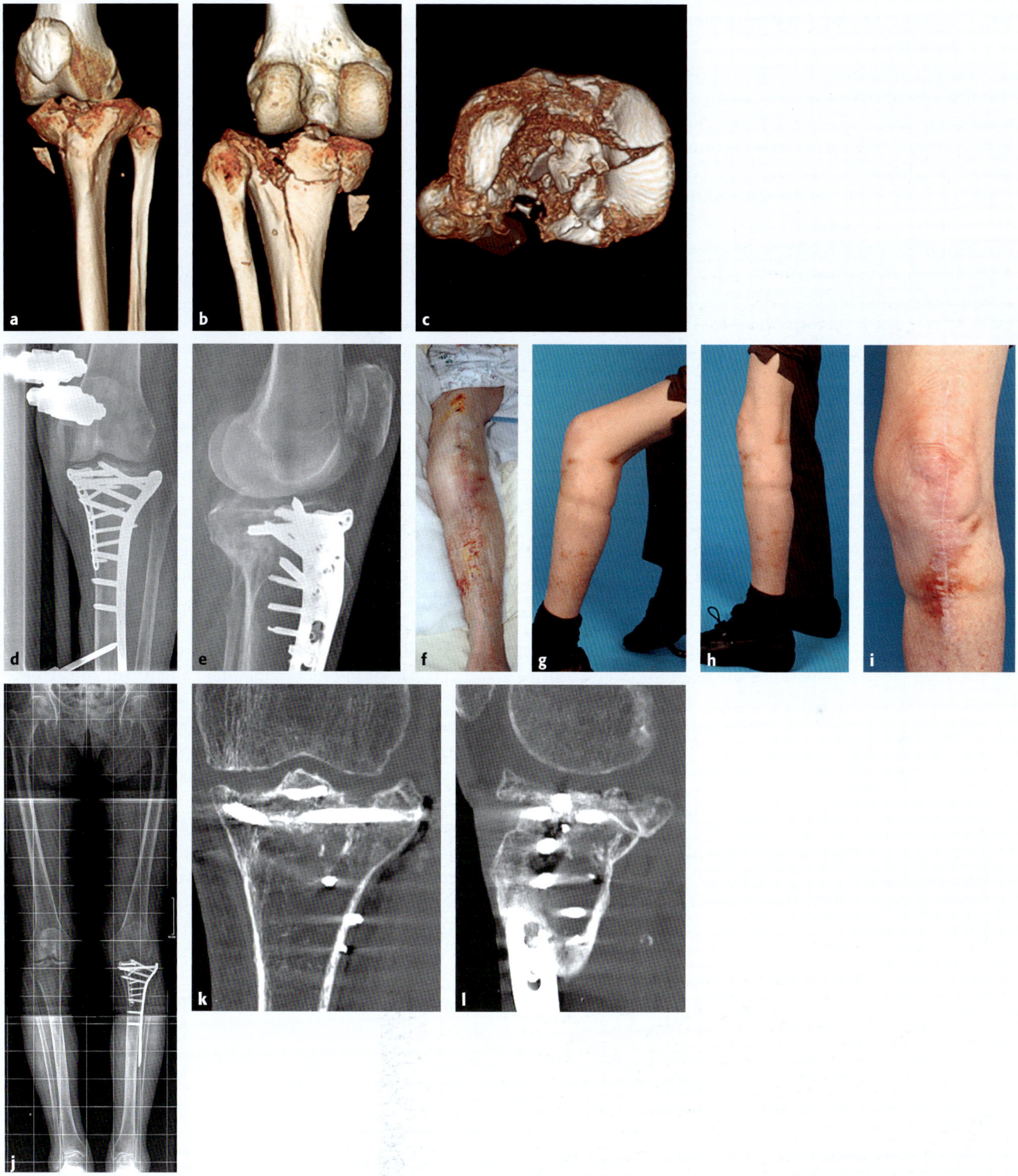

**Fig 3.15-9a–l** Comminuted proximal tibial fracture of an 84-year-old woman.
**a–c** Three-column fracture dislocation.
**d–f** Postoperative x-rays and clinical photograph after open reduction, internal fixation, and temporary fixator.
**g–i** Clinical photographs at the 18-month follow-up.
**j–l** X-rays at the 18-month follow-up.

### 6.6 Arthroscopy-assisted reduction and internal fixation

Arthroscopy-assisted reduction and internal fixation (ARIF) was first described in 1985 by Caspari et al [101]. Since then increasing clinical experience- and evidence-based results have been collected particularly in younger patients. It is not known if arthroscopic assistance is necessary in older adults. The main goal of ORIF in the older adult is to maintain knee axis. The risk of prolonged anesthesia requires a balance between attempting a precise anatomical reduction with ARIF and keeping the operative time short. Postoperative precise reduction may be achieved better with ARIF, however, maintenance of the reduction is only achieved with adequate application of bone graft or substitutes [102, 61].

Arthroscopy-assisted reduction and internal fixation is indicated and commonly used for Schatzker type I, II, and III fractures [103].

Advantages of ARIF:

- Allows more precise reduction under visual control [104–106].
- Arthroscopy-assisted reduction and internal fixation as opposed to ORIF achieves better anatomical reduction postoperatively, but no long-term data exist.
- Minimally invasive, without the need for large arthrotomy and transection of the meniscus [107].
- Diagnostic and treatment of intraarticular ligament [108] and meniscal [109] injuries.

Disadvantages of ARIF:

- Prolonged operative time, although Ohdera et al [104] found no significant difference for the surgery time between ARI and ORIF (126 minutes versus 131 minutes). These results may have been influenced by a selection bias.
- In the past, it was hypothesized that the risk of compartment syndrome may be triggered by the use of arthroscopy. Chan et al [110] had in 18 cases of ARIF 0 compartment syndromes in the young. Roerdink et al [111] also reported no compartment syndromes in a retrospective cohort of patients older than 55 years.

Whether clinical results of ARIF are better compared to ORIF is still under discussion. No prospective randomized study comparing the two techniques with respect to clinical outcome is currently available.

Roerdink et al [111] reported a retrospective cohort of 30 patients older than 55 years with Schatzker type I–VI fractures treated with ARIF and showed radiographically and clinically comparable results to younger patients. However, in 30% secondary displacement occurred after a 1-year follow-up. No arthroscopy-associated complications occurred and no serious infection was observed. Other findings at 3 years included:

- Radiological assessment:
  - Mean Rasmussen radiological score was 23.
- Clinical assessment:
  - Modified Rasmussen clinical score showed 12 excellent, 12 good, 3 fair, and 3 poor results.

### 6.7 Primary total knee arthroplasty

In fractures around the knee in geriatric patients, primary TKA is indicated for distal femoral fractures, because the distal femur has no direct attachment to the extensor and flexor tendons [112]. In complex PTFs (three-column, Schatzker V and VI, AO/OTA 41C) reattachment of the tuberosity and the biceps femoris tendons to the prosthesis is difficult and produces inferior functional results. For this reason fracture of the tuberosity must be seen as relative contraindication for primary TKA [112, 113]. Bicondylar fractures require at least additional plate fixation usually combined with long-stem prosthesis in order to maintain alignment and achieve enough purchase in the osteoporotic bone. Promising initial results in a small case series using this hybrid solution in Schatzker type V and VI fractures of older adults have been published by Vermeire et al (**Table 3.15-1**) [114].

Unicondylar fractures (one- or two-column, Schatzker type I, II, and IV) are similarly treated with tibial stems to maintain knee axis. Refixation of large condylar fragments with additional plate osteosynthesis and filling of osseous defects with PMMA or metal augments is recommended (**Case 7: Fig 3.15-10**) [114].

Primary TKA should be considered for active older patients suffering from osteoarthritis before the injury. Voids in depression fractures (zero-column, Schatzker III, AO/OTA B2) can be filled with PMMA cement or metal augments [112].

The complication rate with need for revision in primary arthroplasty of proximal tibial plateau fractures seems to be high ranging from 0% to 20%. **Table 3.15-1** shows the available results with respect to primary TKA in older adults after PTF. However, larger studies are urgently needed in order to compare primary TKA with primary osteosynthesis.

Complications with secondary TKA after primary osteosynthesis of the proximal tibia are even higher and range between 20% and 27% [113, 115]. This may be the reason why secondary conversion rate after primary osteosynthesis to TKA is still considerably low at 0–7.9% [6, 116, 117].

| Authors | Age, y | Number (N) | Follow-up | Results/knee score | Complications |
|---|---|---|---|---|---|
| Vermeire et al [114] | 73 (58–81) | Total N = 12: AO/OTA 41B1 (N = 1), B3 (N = 8), C3 (N = 3) | 31 months | Median KSS: 78 of 100; Functional score: 58 out of 100; 7 of 11 excellent, 1 of 11 fair, 2 of 11 poor | No revision |
| Parratte et al [118] | 80.5 (70–98) | Distal femoral fracture: N = 10<br>Tibial fracture: Total N = 16 AO/OTA 41B (N = 8) AO/OTA 41C (N = 8) | 16.2 months | Mean Parker Mobility Score: 6.2; 1.7 points less compared to preoperative score | Three revisions<br>Four prosthesis-related complications (avulsion of tubercle, infection, periprothtetic fracture, peroneal nerve palsy) Six medical complications |
| Schwarz et al [119] | 59–86 | PTF: Total N = 10 AO/OTA 41B3 (N = 8); AO/OTA 41C3 (N = 2) | 6 months | Mean KSS: 170 of 240 | Two revisions (infection) |
| Nourissat et al [120] | > 75 | PTF: Total N = 4 Schatzker V (N = 3); Schatzker IV (N = 1) | ≥ 24 months | Mean IKS: 69 of 100; IKS: 81 of 100 | No revision |

**Table 3.15-1** Results of primary total knee arthroplasty of proximal tibial fractures in older adults.
Abbreviations: IKS, International Knee Score; KSS, Knee Society Score [121]; PTF, proximal tibial fracture.

CASE 7

### Patient
A 71-year-old woman was hit by a car on the lateral left knee and sustained a lateral tibial condylar fracture with a large posterolateral rim fragment (two-column fracture) (**Fig 3.15-10a–b**).

### Treatment and outcome
One week after admission, soft-tissue swelling had improved allowing open reduction and internal fixation with a lateral nonlocking plate. The larger lateral metaphyseal void was filled with calcium phosphate bone cement. After an 18-month follow-up a conversion to total knee arthroplasty (TKA) was performed because of subsidence of the lateral joint surface and persistent pain; but tuberosity was healed (**Fig 3.15-10c–d**). The patient suffered from an iatrogenic peroneal palsy after surgery. The 1-year follow-up had a range of motion of 100–0–0°. The patient was pain free.

### Discussion
This case is representative of the inferior results of nonlocking plates. It is also recommended to use polymethylmethacrylate bone cement instead of calcium phosphate-based bone cement because of its biomechanically superior results. Polymethylmethacrylate can restore reduction longer than the bioresorbable calcium phosphate cement [64].

Using the metal cone allowed good restoration of the metaphysis. No loosening of the prosthesis or infection was investigated until loss of follow-up after 3 years (**Fig 3.15-10e–f**).

The iatrogenic peroneal palsy may be representative for the high complication rate after secondary TKA in proximal tibial fractures (20–27%) [113, 115].

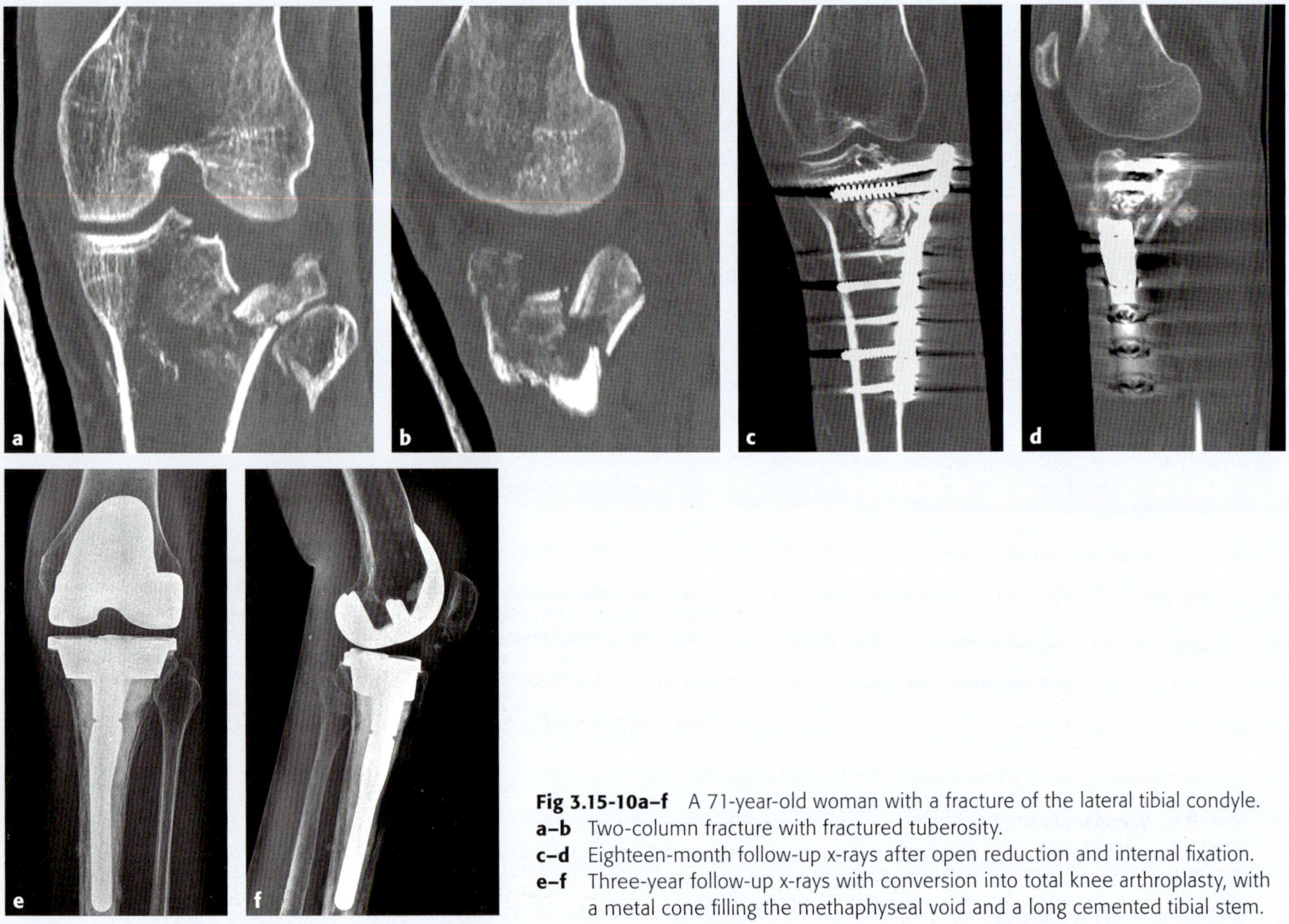


**Fig 3.15-10a–f** A 71-year-old woman with a fracture of the lateral tibial condyle.
**a–b** Two-column fracture with fractured tuberosity.
**c–d** Eighteen-month follow-up x-rays after open reduction and internal fixation.
**e–f** Three-year follow-up x-rays with conversion into total knee arthroplasty, with a metal cone filling the methaphyseal void and a long cemented tibial stem.

## 7 Risks and complications

General risk factors in older adults:

- Impaired cardiopulmonary status of the frail injured patient
- Reduced compliance with respect to PWB due to:
  - Cognitive disorders such as dementia
  - Musculoskeletal disorders, such as sarcopenia, paralysis in case of cerebral insults, and preexisting disorders of other joints
  - Decreased upper extremity strength
  - Impaired sensory and balance systems
- Anticoagulation-related increased bleeding leading to delayed surgery with prolonged bed rest

Fracture site complications:

- High rates of loss of reduction due to insufficient bone stock after ORIF 30–79% [52, 111, 116, 122]
- Polymethylmethacrylate implant augmentation reducing loss of reduction [74]
- Additional stability by hybrid fixations of temporary external fixator and ORIF
- Higher risk of soft-tissue break-down due to edema

Strategies to reduce complications include:

- Minimally invasive plate osteosynthesis techniques reducing soft-tissue damage
- Avoidance of large single midline approach if possible
- Use of external fixator in cases of highly unstable fractures without further impairment of the soft tissue

## 8 Prevention and future perspectives

Proximal femoral fracture risk can be predicted by means of the Fracture Risk Assessment tool [123] questionnaire and BMD measurements [124] (see chapter 1.10 Osteoporosis). A specific tool for fracture risk prediction of the proximal tibia is not yet available, but initial attempts are being investigated by finite element analysis of the tibia based on BMD measurements [125].

To date, BMD measurements of the proximal tibia have only been part of an experimental setting, whereas BMD measurements of the distal tibia are already in clinical use and have been validated to calculate fracture risk [126]. Beattie et al [127] used dual-energy x-ray absorptiometry scans to show that bone quality in the proximal femur is strongly related to that of the proximal tibia [127].

Gausden et al [128] correlated BMD in the distal femur with the clinical outcome after ORIF of PTFs in a geriatric group (> 65 years). Due to the appropriate use of augmentation with bone grafts, no correlation between BMD and subjective functional scores was found. No correlation between BMD and articular subsidence after 1-year follow-up was found.

## 9 References


1. **Koval KJ, Helfet DL.** Tibial plateau fractures: evaluation and treatment. *J Am Acad Orthop Surg.* 1995 Mar;3(2):86–94.
2. **Scolaro JA, Lee GC.** Tibial plateau fractures in the elderly. In: Pignolo RJ, Keenan MA, Hebela NM, eds. *Fractures in the Elderly. A Guide to Practical Management.* Totowa: Springer Science+Business Media, LLC; 2011:269–281.
3. **Rozell JC, Vemulapalli KC, Gary JL, et al.** Tibial plateau fractures in elderly patients. *Geriatr Orthop Surg Rehabil.* 2016 Sep;7(3):126–134.
4. **Kannus P, Niemi S, Palvanen M, et al.** Continuously rising problem of osteoporotic knee fractures in elderly women: nationwide statistics in Finland in 1970-1999 and predictions until the year 2030. *Bone.* 2001 Nov;29(5):419–423.
5. **Court-Brown CM, Caesar B.** Epidemiology of adult fractures: A review. *Injury.* 2006 Aug;37(8):691–697.
6. **Hsu CJ, Chang WN, Wong CY.** Surgical treatment of tibial plateau fracture in elderly patients. *Arch Orthop Trauma Surg.* 2001;121(1-2):67–70.
7. **Cowie J, Court-Brown C.** Focus On tibial fractures. Available at: https://pdfs.semanticscholar.org/0275/70da969f454f788d25a8f0ad7905724cad56.pdf. Accessed 2018.
8. **Morley JE, Anker SD, von Haehling S.** Prevalence, incidence, and clinical impact of sarcopenia: facts, numbers, and epidemiology-update 2014. *J Cachexia Sarcopenia Muscle.* 2014 Dec;5(4):253–259.
9. **Prasad N, Murray JM, Kumar D, et al.** Insufficiency fracture of the tibial plateau: an often missed diagnosis. *Acta Orthop Belg.* 2006 Oct;72(5):587–591.
10. **Cabitza P, Tamim H.** Occult fractures of tibial plateau detected employing magnetic resonance imaging. *Arch Orthop Trauma Surg.* 2000;120(5–6):355–357.
11. **Jarraya M, Hayashi D, Roemer FW, et al.** Radiographically occult and subtle fractures: a pictorial review. *Radiol Res Pract.* 2013;2013:370169.
12. **Beall S, Garner J, Oxley D.** Anterolateral compartment syndrome related to drug-induced bleeding. A case report. *Am J Sports Med.* 1983 Nov-Dec;11(6):454–455.
13. **Rancan M, Esser MP, Kossmann T, et al.** Acute anterior compartment syndrome following low energy non-contact injury. *ANZ J Surg.* 2004 Nov;74(11):1023–1024.
14. **Mendelson D, Kates S, Pacos J, et al.** Proximal tibia and fibula fragility fracture complicated by anticoagulation and demand-mediated myocardial infarction. *Geriatr Orthop Surg Rehabil.* 2011 May;2(3):110–116.
15. **Ringus VM, Lemley FR, Hubbard DF, et al.** Lateral tibial plateau fracture depression as a predictor of lateral meniscus pathology. *Orthopedics.* 2010 Feb;33(2):80–84.
16. **Stannard JP, Lopez R, Volgas D.** Soft tissue injury of the knee after tibial plateau fractures. *J Knee Surg.* 2010 Dec;23(4):187–192.
17. **Bennett WF, Browner B.** Tibial plateau fractures: a study of associated soft tissue injuries. *J Orthop Trauma.* 1994;8(3):183–188.
18. **Delamarter RB, Hohl M, Hopp E Jr.** Ligament injuries associated with tibial plateau fractures. *Clin Orthop Relat Res.* 1990 Jan(250):226–233.
19. **Wei CJ, Tsai WC, Tiu CM, et al.** Systematic analysis of missed extremity fractures in emergency radiology. *Acta Radiol.* 2006 Sep;47(7):710–717.
20. **Zhu Y, Yang G, Luo CF, et al.** Computed tomography-based Three-Column Classification in tibial plateau fractures: introduction of its utility and assessment of its reproducibility. *J Trauma Acute Care Surg.* 2012 Sep;73(3):731–737.
21. **Yang G, Zhai Q, Zhu Y, et al.** The incidence of posterior tibial plateau fracture: an investigation of 525 fractures by using a CT-based classification system. *Arch Orthop Trauma Surg.* 2013 Jul;133(7):929–934.
22. **Luo CF, Sun H, Zhang B, et al.** Three-column fixation for complex tibial plateau fractures. *J Orthop Trauma.* 2010 Nov;24(11):683–692.
23. **Kode L, Lieberman JM, Motta AO, et al.** Evaluation of tibial plateau fractures: efficacy of MR imaging compared with CT. *AJR Am J Roentgenol.* 1994 Jul;163(1):141–147.
24. **Markhardt BK, Gross JM, Monu JU.** Schatzker classification of tibial plateau fractures: use of CT and MR imaging improves assessment. *Radiographics.* 2009 Mar–Apr;29(2):585–597.
25. **Chen H, Zhou X, Fujita H, et al.** Age-related changes in trabecular and cortical bone microstructure. *Int J Endocrinol.* 2013;2013:213234.
26. **Schatzker J, McBroom R, Bruce D.** The tibial plateau fracture. The Toronto experience 1968–1975. *Clin Orthop Relat Res.* 1979 Jan-Feb(138):94–104.
27. **Müller M, Koch P, Nazarian S, et al.** *The Comprehensive Classification of Fractures of Long Bones.* Berlin: Springer; 1990.

28. **Hohl M, Moore TM.** *Articular fractures of the tibia. Surgery of the musculoskeletal system.* New York: Churchill Livingstone; 1990.
29. **Maripuri SN, Rao P, Manoj-Thomas A, et al.** The classification systems for tibial plateau fractures: how reliable are they? *Injury.* 2008 Oct;39(10):1216–1221.
30. **Tscherne H, Lobenhoffer P.** Tibial plateau fractures. Management and expected results. *Clin Orthop Relat Res.* 1993 Jul(292):87–100.
31. **Potocnik P, Acklin YP, Sommer C.** Operative strategy in postero-medial fracture-dislocation of the proximal tibia. *Injury.* 2011 Oct;42(10):1060–1065.
32. **Rasmussen PS.** Tibial condylar fractures. Impairment of knee joint stability as an indication for surgical treatment. *J Bone Joint Surg Am.* 1973 Oct;55(7):1331–1350.
33. **Lansinger O, Bergman B, Korner L, et al.** Tibial condylar fractures. A twenty-year follow-up. *J Bone Joint Surg Am.* 1986 Jan;68(1):13–19.
34. **Bohm ER, Tufescu TV, Marsh JP.** The operative management of osteoporotic fractures of the knee: to fix or replace? *J Bone Joint Surg Br.* 2012 Sep;94(9):1160–1169.
35. **DeCoster TA, Nepola JV, el-Khoury GY.** Cast brace treatment of proximal tibia fractures. A ten-year follow-up study. *Clin Orthop Relat Res.* 1988 Jun(231):196–204.
36. **Giannoudis PV, Tzioupis C, Papathanassopoulos A, et al.** Articular step-off and risk of post-traumatic osteoarthritis. Evidence today. *Injury.* 2010 Oct;41(10):986–995.
37. **Segal D, Mallik AR, Wetzler MJ, et al.** Early weight bearing of lateral tibial plateau fractures. *Clin Orthop Relat Res.* 1993 Sep(294):232–237.
38. **Mayr R, Attal R, Zwierzina M, et al.** Effect of additional fixation in tibial plateau impression fractures treated with balloon reduction and cement augmentation. *Clin Biomech (Bristol, Avon).* 2015 Oct;30(8):847–851.
39. **Mauffrey C, Roberts G, Cuellar DO, et al.** Balloon tibioplasty: pearls and pitfalls. *J Knee Surg.* 2014 Feb;27(1):31–37.
40. **Johnson EE, Timon S, Osuji C.** Surgical technique: Tscherne-Johnson extensile approach for tibial plateau fractures. *Clin Orthop Relat Res.* 2013 Sep;471(9):2760–2767.
41. **El-Alfy B, Ali KA, El-Ganiney A.** Bicondylar tibial plateau fractures involving the posteromedial fragment: morphology based fixation. *Acta Orthop Belg.* 2016 Aug;82(2):298–304.
42. **Bendayan J, Noblin JD, Freeland AE.** Posteromedial second incision to reduce and stabilize a displaced posterior fragment that can occur in Schatzker Type V bicondylar tibial plateau fractures. *Orthopedics.* 1996 Oct;19(10):903–904.
43. **Cho KY, Oh HS, Yoo JH, et al.** Treatment of Schatzker type V and VI tibial plateau fractures using a midline longitudinal incision and dual plating. *Knee Surg Relat Res.* 2013 Jun;25(2):77–83.
44. **Tejwani NC, Hak DJ, Finkemeier CG, et al.** High-energy proximal tibial fractures: treatment options and decision making. *Instr Course Lect.* 2006;55:367–379.
45. **Jiang R, Luo CF, Wang MC, et al.** A comparative study of Less Invasive Stabilization System (LISS) fixation and two-incision double plating for the treatment of bicondylar tibial plateau fractures. *Knee.* 2008 Mar;15(2):139–143.
46. **Stevens DG, Beharry R, McKee MD, et al.** The long-term functional outcome of operatively treated tibial plateau fractures. *J Orthop Trauma.* 2001 Jun-Jul;15(5):312–320.
47. **Horwitz DS, Bachus KN, Craig MA, et al.** A biomechanical analysis of internal fixation of complex tibial plateau fractures. *J Orthop Trauma.* 1999 Nov;13(8):545–549.
48. **Wong CH, Tan JL, Chang HC, et al.** Knee dislocations-a retrospective study comparing operative versus closed immobilization treatment outcomes. *Knee Surg Sports Traumatol Arthrosc.* 2004 Nov;12(6):540–544.
49. **Dittmer DK, Teasell R.** Complications of immobilization and bed rest. Part 1: Musculoskeletal and cardiovascular complications. *Can Fam Physician.* 1993 Jun;39:1428–1432, 1435–1437.
50. **Hegyes MS, Richardson MW, Miller MD.** Knee dislocation. Complications of nonoperative and operative management. *Clin Sports Med.* 2000 Jul;19(3):519–543.
51. **Cerny K, Perry J, Walker JM.** Adaptations during the stance phase of gait for simulated flexion contractures at the knee. *Orthopedics.* 1994 Jun;17(6):501–512; discussion 512–513.
52. **Gerich T, Blauth M, Witte F, et al.** Die Osteosynthese von Tibiakopffrakturen im höheren Alter. Eine Matched-pair-Analyse [Osteosynthesis of fractures of the head of the tibia in advanced age. A matched-pair analysis]. *Unfallchirurg.* 2001 Jan;104(1):50–56. German.
53. **Fleming B, Paley D, Kristiansen T, et al.** A biomechanical analysis of the Ilizarov external fixator. *Clin Orthop Relat Res.* 1989 Apr(241):95–105.
54. **Yilmaz E, Belhan O, Karakurt L, et al.** Mechanical performance of hybrid Ilizarov external fixator in comparison with Ilizarov circular external fixator. *Clin Biomech (Bristol, Avon).* 2003 Jul;18(6):518–522.
55. **Krappinger D, Struve P, Smekal V, et al.** Severely comminuted bicondylar tibial plateau fractures in geriatric patients: a report of 2 cases treated with open reduction and postoperative external fixation. *J Orthop Trauma.* 2008 Oct;22(9):652–657.
56. **Ali AM, Burton M, Hashmi M, et al.** Treatment of displaced bicondylar tibial plateau fractures (OTA-41C2&3) in patients older than 60 years of age. *J Orthop Trauma.* 2003 May;17(5):346–352.
57. **Dirschl DR, Del Gaizo D.** Staged management of tibial plateau fractures. *Am J Orthop (Belle Mead NJ).* 2007 Apr;36(4 Suppl):12–17.
58. **Tejwani NC, Achan P.** Staged management of high-energy proximal tibia fractures. *Bull Hosp Jt Dis.* 2004;62(1–2):62–66.
59. **Young MJ, Barrack RL.** Complications of internal fixation of tibial plateau fractures. *Orthop Rev.* 1994 Feb;23(2):149–154.
60. **Barei DP, Nork SE, Mills WJ, et al.** Complications associated with internal fixation of high-energy bicondylar tibial plateau fractures utilizing a two-incision technique. *J Orthop Trauma.* 2004 Nov–Dec;18(10):649–657.
61. **Papagelopoulos PJ, Partsinevelos AA, Themistocleous GS, et al.** Complications after tibia plateau fracture surgery. *Injury.* 2006 Jun;37(6):475–484.
62. **Kuik K, Putters TF, Schortinghuis J, et al.** Donor site morbidity of anterior iliac crest and calvarium bone grafts: A comparative case-control study. *J Craniomaxillofac Surg.* 2016 Apr;44(4):364–368.
63. **Seiler JG 3rd, Johnson J.** Iliac crest autogenous bone grafting: donor site complications. *J South Orthop Assoc.* 2000 Summer;9(2):91–97.
64. **Stubbs D, Deakin M, Chapman-Sheath P, et al.** In vivo evaluation of resorbable bone graft substitutes in a rabbit tibial defect model. *Biomaterials.* 2004 Sep;25(20):5037–5044.
65. **Biyani A, Reddy NS, Chaudhury J, et al.** The results of surgical management of displaced tibial plateau fractures in the elderly. *Injury.* 1995 Jun;26(5):291–297.

66. **Graf C.** Functional decline in hospitalized older adults. *Am J Nurs.* 2006 Jan;106(1):58–67, quiz 67–68.
67. **Adams SD, Cotton BA, McGuire MF, et al.** Unique pattern of complications in elderly trauma patients at a Level I trauma center. *J Trauma Acute Care Surg.* 2012 Jan;72(1):112–118.
68. **Burdin G.** Arthroscopic management of tibial plateau fractures: surgical technique. *Orthop Traumatol Surg Res.* 2013 Feb;99(1 Suppl):S208–S218.
69. **Tejwani NC.** *Fractures of the Tibia. A Clinical Casebook.* Cham: Springer International Publishing; 2016.
70. **Prat-Fabregat S, Camacho-Carrasco P.** Treatment strategy for tibial plateau fractures: an update. *EFORT Open Rev.* 2016 May;1(5):225–232.
71. **Hsieh CH.** Treatment of the posterolateral tibial plateau fractures using the anterior surgical approach. *Int J Biomed Sci.* 2010 Dec;6(4):316–320.
72. **Ehlinger M, Rahme M, Moor BK, et al.** Reliability of locked plating in tibial plateau fractures with a medial component. *Orthop Traumatol Surg Res.* 2012 Apr;98(2):173–179.
73. **Gosling T, Schandelmaier P, Marti A, et al.** Less invasive stabilization of complex tibial plateau fractures: a biomechanical evaluation of a unilateral locked screw plate and double plating. *J Orthop Trauma.* 2004 Sep;18(8):546–551.
74. **Goetzen M, Nicolino T, Hofmann-Fliri L, et al.** Metaphyseal screw augmentation of the LISS-PLT plate with polymethylmethacrylate improves angular stability in osteoporotic proximal third tibial fractures: a biomechanical study in human cadaveric tibiae. *J Orthop Trauma.* 2014 May;28(5):294–299.
75. **Vasanad GH, Antin SM, Akkimaradi RC, et al.** "Surgical management of tibial plateau fractures—a clinical study". *J Clin Diagn Res.* 2013 Dec;7(12):3128–3130.
76. **Russell TA, Leighton RK.** Comparison of autogenous bone graft and endothermic calcium phosphate cement for defect augmentation in tibial plateau fractures. A multicenter, prospective, randomized study. *J Bone Joint Surg Am.* 2008 Oct;90(10):2057–2061.
77. **Trenholm A, Landry S, McLaughlin K, et al.** Comparative fixation of tibial plateau fractures using alpha-BSM, a calcium phosphate cement, versus cancellous bone graft. *J Orthop Trauma.* 2005 Nov–Dec;19(10):698–702.
78. **Welch RD, Zhang H, Bronson DG.** Experimental tibial plateau fractures augmented with calcium phosphate cement or autologous bone graft. *J Bone Joint Surg Am.* 2003 Feb;85-A(2):222–231.
79. **Bajammal SS, Zlowodzki M, Lelwica A, et al.** The use of calcium phosphate bone cement in fracture treatment. A meta-analysis of randomized trials. *J Bone Joint Surg Am.* 2008 Jun;90(6):1186–1196.
80. **Lieberman IH, Togawa D, Kayanja MM.** Vertebroplasty and kyphoplasty: filler materials. *Spine J.* 2005 Nov–Dec;5(6 Suppl):305s–316s.
81. **Hofmann-Fliri L, Nicolino TI, Barla J, et al.** Cement augmentation of implants—no general cure in osteoporotic fracture treatment. A biomechanical study on non-displaced femoral neck fractures. *J Orthop Res.* 2016 Feb;34(2):314–319.
82. **Biggi F, Di Fabio S, D'Antimo C, et al.** Tibial plateau fractures: internal fixation with locking plates and the MIPO technique. *Injury.* 2010 Nov;41(11):1178–1182.
83. **Cole PA, Zlowodzki M, Kregor PJ.** Treatment of proximal tibia fractures using the less invasive stabilization system: surgical experience and early clinical results in 77 fractures. *J Orthop Trauma.* 2004 Sep;18(8):528–535.
84. **Stannard JP, Wilson TC, Volgas DA, et al.** Fracture stabilization of proximal tibial fractures with the proximal tibial LISS: early experience in Birmingham, Alabama (USA). *Injury.* 2003 Aug;34(Suppl 1):A36–42.
85. **Schütz M, Kaab MJ, Haas N.** Stabilization of proximal tibial fractures with the LIS-System: early clinical experience in Berlin. *Injury.* 2003 Aug;34(Suppl 1):A30–35.
86. **Musahl V, Tarkin I, Kobbe P, et al.** New trends and techniques in open reduction and internal fixation of fractures of the tibial plateau. *J Bone Joint Surg Br.* 2009 Apr;91(4):426–433.
87. **Gosling T, Schandelmaier P, Muller M, et al.** Single lateral locked screw plating of bicondylar tibial plateau fractures. *Clin Orthop Relat Res.* 2005 Oct;439:207–214.
88. **Cole PA, Zlowodzki M, Kregor PJ.** Compartment pressures after submuscular fixation of proximal tibia fractures. *Injury.* 2003 Aug;34(Suppl 1):A43–A46.
89. **Peindl RD, Zura RD, Vincent A, et al.** Unstable proximal extraarticular tibia fractures: a biomechanical evaluation of four methods of fixation. *J Orthop Trauma.* 2004 Sep;18(8):540–545.
90. **Prasad GT, Kumar TS, Kumar RK, et al.** Functional outcome of Schatzker type V and VI tibial plateau fractures treated with dual plates. *Indian J Orthop.* 2013 Mar;47(2):188–194.
91. **Oh CW, Oh JK, Kyung HS, et al.** Double plating of unstable proximal tibial fractures using minimally invasive percutaneous osteosynthesis technique. *Acta Orthop.* 2006 Jun;77(3):524–530.
92. **Barei DP, Nork SE, Mills WJ, et al.** Functional outcomes of severe bicondylar tibial plateau fractures treated with dual incisions and medial and lateral plates. *J Bone Joint Surg Am.* 2006 Aug;88(8):1713–1721.
93. **Yoo BJ, Beingessner DM, Barei DP.** Stabilization of the posteromedial fragment in bicondylar tibial plateau fractures: a mechanical comparison of locking and nonlocking single and dual plating methods. *J Trauma.* 2010 Jul;69(1):148–155.
94. **Jiang R, Luo CF, Zeng BF.** Biomechanical evaluation of different fixation methods for fracture dislocation involving the proximal tibia. *Clin Biomech (Bristol, Avon).* 2008 Oct;23(8):1059–1064.
95. **Lee MH, Hsu CJ, Lin KC, et al.** Comparison of outcome of unilateral locking plate and dual plating in the treatment of bicondylar tibial plateau fractures. *J Orthop Surg Res.* 2014 Jul 20;9:62.
96. **Wang Y, Luo C, Zhu Y, et al.** Updated three-column concept in surgical treatment for tibial plateau fractures—a prospective cohort study of 287 patients. *Injury.* 2016 Jul;47(7):1488–1496.
97. **Wang SQ, Gao YS, Wang JQ, et al.** Surgical approach for high-energy posterior tibial plateau fractures. *Indian J Orthop.* 2011 Mar;45(2):125–131.
98. **Higgins TF, Klatt J, Bachus KN.** Biomechanical analysis of bicondylar tibial plateau fixation: how does lateral locking plate fixation compare to dual plate fixation? *J Orthop Trauma.* 2007 May;21(5):301–306.
99. **Neogi DS, Trikha V, Mishra KK, et al.** Comparative study of single lateral locked plating versus double plating in type C bicondylar tibial plateau fractures. *Indian J Orthop.* 2015 Mar–Apr;49(2):193–198.
100. **van Dreumel RL, van Wunnik BP, Janssen L, et al.** Mid- to long-term functional outcome after open reduction and internal fixation of tibial plateau fractures. *Injury.* 2015 Aug;46(8):1608–1612.

101. **Caspari RB, Hutton PM, Whipple TL, et al.** The role of arthroscopy in the management of tibial plateau fractures. *Arthroscopy.* 1985;1(2):76–82.
102. **Hung SS, Chao EK, Chan YS, et al.** Arthroscopically assisted osteosynthesis for tibial plateau fractures. *J Trauma.* 2003 Feb;54(2):356–363.
103. **Siegler J, Galissier B, Marcheix PS, et al.** Percutaneous fixation of tibial plateau fractures under arthroscopy: a medium term perspective. *Orthop Traumatol Surg Res.* 2011 Feb;97(1):44–50.
104. **Ohdera T, Tokunaga M, Hiroshima S, et al.** Arthroscopic management of tibial plateau fractures—comparison with open reduction method. *Arch Orthop Trauma Surg.* 2003 Nov;123(9):489–493.
105. **Kayali C, Ozturk H, Altay T, et al.** Arthroscopically assisted percutaneous osteosynthesis of lateral tibial plateau fractures. *Can J Surg.* 2008 Oct;51(5):378–382.
106. **Bernfeld B, Kligman M, Roffman M.** Arthroscopic assistance for unselected tibial plateau fractures. *Arthroscopy.* 1996 Oct;12(5):598–602.
107. **Chen XZ, Liu CG, Chen Y, et al.** Arthroscopy-assisted surgery for tibial plateau fractures. *Arthroscopy.* 2015 Jan;31(1):143–153.
108. **Cetik O, Cift H, Asik M.** Second-look arthroscopy after arthroscopy-assisted treatment of tibial plateau fractures. *Knee Surg Sports Traumatol Arthrosc.* 2007 Jun;15(6):747–752.
109. **Ruiz-Iban MA, Diaz-Heredia J, Elias-Martin E, et al.** Repair of meniscal tears associated with tibial plateau fractures: a review of 15 cases. *Am J Sports Med.* 2012 Oct;40(10):2289–2295.
110. **Chan YS, Chiu CH, Lo YP, et al.** Arthroscopy-assisted surgery for tibial plateau fractures: 2- to 10-year follow-up results. *Arthroscopy.* 2008 Jul;24(7):760–768.
111. **Roerdink WH, Oskam J, Vierhout PA.** Arthroscopically assisted osteosynthesis of tibial plateau fractures in patients older than 55 years. *Arthroscopy.* 2001 Oct;17(8):826–831.
112. **Ries MD.** Primary arthroplasty for management of osteoporotic fractures about the knee. *Curr Osteoporos Rep.* 2012 Dec;10(4):322–327.
113. **Saleh KJ, Sherman P, Katkin P, et al.** Total knee arthroplasty after open reduction and internal fixation of fractures of the tibial plateau: a minimum five-year follow-up study. *J Bone Joint Surg Am.* 2001 Aug;83-A(8):1144–1148.
114. **Vermeire J, Scheerlinck T.** Early primary total knee replacement for complex proximal tibia fractures in elderly and osteoarthritic patients. *Acta Orthop Belg.* 2010 Dec;76(6):785–793.
115. **Gerich T, Bosch U, Schmidt E, et al.** Kniegelenkendoprothetik nach TibiakopffrakturenMittelfristige Ergebnisse einer Kohortenanalyse [Knee joint prosthesis implantation after fractures of the head of the tibia. Intermediate term results of a cohort analysis]. *Unfallchirurg.* 2001 May;104(5):414–419. German.
116. **Frattini M, Vaienti E, Soncini G, et al.** Tibial plateau fractures in elderly patients. *Chir Organi Mov.* 2009 Dec;93(3):109–114.
117. **Su EP, Westrich GH, Rana AJ, et al.** Operative treatment of tibial plateau fractures in patients older than 55 years. *Clin Orthop Relat Res.* 2004 Apr(421):240–248.
118. **Parratte S, Bonnevialle P, Pietu G, et al.** Primary total knee arthroplasty in the management of epiphyseal fracture around the knee. *Orthop Traumatol Surg Res.* 2011 Oct;97(6 Suppl):S87–S94.
119. **Schwarz N, Buchinger W, Mahring M, et al.** Unfallkrankenhaus. Knieendoprothese als Ersttherapie bei proximaler Tibiafraktur [Trauma hospital. Knee arthroplasty as primary therapy for proximal tibial fracture]. *Unfallchirurg.* 2008 Nov;111(11):928–932. German.
120. **Nourissat G, Hoffman E, Hemon C, et al.** Arthroplastie totale de genou pour fracture récente grave de l'épiphyse tibiale proximale chez le sujet âgé [Total knee arthroplasty for recent severe fracture of the proximal tibial epiphysis in the elderly subject]. *Rev Chir Orthop Reparatrice Appar Mot.* 2006 May;92(3):242–247. French.
121. **Insall JN, Dorr LD, Scott RD, et al.** Rationale of the Knee Society clinical rating system. *Clin Orthop Relat Res.* 1989 Nov(248):13–14.
122. **Ali AM, El-Shafie M, Willett KM.** Failure of fixation of tibial plateau fractures. *J Orthop Trauma.* 2002 May;16(5):323–329.
123. **Kanis JA, Johnell O, Oden A, et al.** FRAX and the assessment of fracture probability in men and women from the UK. *Osteoporos Int.* 2008 Apr;19(4):385–397.
124. **Kanis JA, McCloskey E, Johansson H, et al.** FRAX((R)) with and without bone mineral density. *Calcif Tissue Int.* 2012 Jan;90(1):1–13.
125. **Gislason MK, Coupaud S, Sasagawa K, et al.** Prediction of risk of fracture in the tibia due to altered bone mineral density distribution resulting from disuse: a finite element study. *Proc Inst Mech Eng H.* 2014 Feb;228(2):165–174.
126. **Popp AW, Senn C, Franta O, et al.** Tibial or hip BMD predict clinical fracture risk equally well: results from a prospective study in 700 elderly Swiss women. *Osteoporos Int.* 2009 Aug;20(8):1393–1399.
127. **Beattie KA, Boulos P, Duryea J, et al.** The relationships between bone mineral density in the spine, hip, distal femur and proximal tibia and medial minimum joint space width in the knees of healthy females. *Osteoarthritis Cartilage.* 2005 Oct;13(10):872–878.
128. **Gausden E, Garner MR, Fabricant PD, et al.** Do clinical outcomes correlate with bone density after open reduction and internal fixation of tibial plateau fractures. *Arch Orthop Trauma Surg.* 2017 Jun;137(6):755–760.

# 3.16 Tibial shaft

Björn-Christian Link, Philippe Posso, Reto Babst

## 1 Introduction

Tibial shaft fractures (TSFs) constitute one of the most common indications for surgery in trauma centers [1]. In the general population, most TSFs are the result of high-energy trauma, such as motor vehicle collisions, falls from a height, and sports-related collisions. Conversely, in older adults, TSFs occur predominantly in osteoporotic women following a low-energy fall [2].

As the population ages, the prevalence of osteoporosis and number of falls or risk for falls is on the rise. Nevertheless, some registries have noted a decrease in the incidence of TSF in older adults during the last decade [3].

Due to the mechanism of injury as well as the delicate soft-tissue envelope of the tibia, soft-tissue compromise is often a complicating factor. In the older population, this situation is even more pronounced:

- Medical comorbidities negatively impact the condition of the soft-tissue envelope.
- Vulnerability and impaired healing of the skin, subcutaneous tissue, and muscle can result in surgical site infection with more serious complications to follow. Trauma always results in a certain amount of stress to the soft tissues (first hit) as does surgery and possible complications (second hit).
- Meticulous soft-tissue handling techniques and dissection are of utmost importance. It is essential that reduction and osteosynthesis cause as little harm as possible, making minimally invasive plate osteosynthesis a preferred technique.
- An interdisciplinary team including a plastic surgeon, vascular surgeon, and dietician should address extensive soft-tissue damage.

Some important facts about TSFs:

- In the geriatric population, TSFs occur preponderantly in women following a low-energy fall from standing height.
- The incidence of compartment syndrome with TSFs is between 1.5% and 9% [4, 5].
- Compartment syndrome can result from the induced swelling (primary) or secondary to reperfusion syndrome.
- Intramedullary (IM) nail fixation is the preferred operative treatment in the general population; its high-load capacity allows for early weight bearing and its low invasiveness allows for minimal interaction with the skin and subcutaneous tissue around the fracture.
- Open fractures and fixations that do not use a nail are predictive factors for nonunion [3]. Optimizing fracture reduction is essential as greater diastases are associated with higher rates of nonunion [6].

## 2 Epidemiology and etiology

Tibial shaft fractures have an incidence of 17–22 per 100,000 population per year. They account for 2% of all fractures and 36.7% of all long bone fractures in adults making them the most common long bone fracture [2, 7].

Patient age-related fracture distribution displays two main demographic peaks: young men and older women. Incidence rates in women show a steady increase with patient age and reach their maximum at > 90 years of age at 36 per 100,000 per year. Incidence rates in men, however, decrease with patient age reaching a relatively stable level of around 13 per 100,000 per year from > 60 years of age [7]. The typical bimodal fracture distribution in young men and older women implies that osteoporosis is an underlying etiological factor in the geriatric population [2].

The traumatic etiology of TSFs varies significantly between countries. While in developing countries traffic accidents are the leading cause, in developed countries ground-level falls have become the most common mechanism [2, 7, 8]. This is probably due to differences in road safety, life expectancy, and the age distribution of the population.

Most TSFs are closed injuries. However, between 20% and 30% are open fractures. Open fractures are significantly associated with perioperative complications. Motor vehicle collisions are the most common cause of injury for open fractures (60%) [7]. In developed countries, pedestrians older than 65 years involved in motor vehicle collisions account for about 30% of TSFs and almost 60% of open TSFs.

The incidence of open fractures tends to rise with age in women, from 200 per million per year between the age of 60 and 69 years to over 525.7 per million per year over the age of 80 years. In men, the incidence of open fracture decreases linearly to reach 232.0 per million per year over the age of 90 years [9].

Interestingly, open TSFs increase with age in both women (351.6 per million per year in those ≥ 80 years versus 24.4 per million per year in those ≤ 65 years) and men (149.3 versus 31.5, respectively). About 60% of open TSFs in women older than 80 years are caused by a fall. The higher incidence of open fractures in women may partly be explained by the relatively thicker skin in men (1.8-fold, $P < .05$) [6]. Skin aging decreases collagen and elastin organization and skin thickness decreases from the fourth to fifth decade of life [10]. Furthermore, skin thickness is a predictor of bone density. Those two factors likely explain the increase in open TSF with age.

A major complicating factor is the development of compartment syndrome. This potentially devastating injury is often associated with tibial fractures. The incidence of compartment syndrome with TSFs is between 1.5% and 9% [4], in the general population [5], with little data available for older adults. Clement et al [3] reported a prevalence of 2.6% in 6 of 233 patients older than 65 years with TSFs. In those patients, all underwent four compartment fasciotomies and 3 of them (50%) developed deep infections. Compartment syndrome and fasciotomy was not associated with a higher mortality.

## 3 Diagnostics

The implication of comorbidities and medication on treatment decision are thoroughly described in chapters 1.1 Principles of orthogeriatric medical care and 1.4 Preoperative risk assessment and preparation. Special attention should be paid to the tetanus vaccine status, as immunity is often waning in this population.

### 3.1 Clinical evaluation

The affected leg and adjacent ankle and knee should be examined. In high-energy trauma, a systematic approach should be followed (eg, airway, breathing, circulation, disability, exposure/examination (ABCDE) following advanced trauma life support), with additional evaluation of common relevant geriatric conditions like chronic edema, arterial insufficiency, and degenerative joint disease. A thorough full body examination should exclude any concomitant fractures, contusions, and wounds (**Case 1: Fig 3.16-1**).

CASE 1

**Patient**

A 72-year-old woman presented following a motor vehicle collision. Upon workup by the trauma team, she was found to have an isolated open left distal tibial shaft fracture (TSF) (**Fig 3.16-1a–c**). She had a past medical history significant for a left Charcot hindfoot arthropathy and a previous left total knee arthroplasty.

**Comorbidities**

- Insulin-dependent diabetes
- Obesity
- Peripheral vascular disease

**Treatment and outcome**

The patient received immediate intravenous antibiotics, and her tetanus status was up to date. Initial operative management included irrigation and debridement and placement of an external fixator to stabilize the injury (**Fig 3.16-1d–e**). Given the nature of the open wound, the debridement involved excision of the fracture fragments that had been contaminated and devitalized at the time of injury (**Fig 3.16-1f–g**).

Multiple factors dictated the definitive management of this patient, including her medical comorbidities, proximal total knee implant as well as previous ipsilateral ankle and hindfoot fusion. To stabilize the leg and facilitate mobilization, the decision was made to proceed with a loadbearing hindfoot fusion nail, with the plan to return for later bone grafting once the soft tissues were stable and healed (**Fig 3.16-1h–i**).

**Key points**

- Older patients have multiple comorbidities, including diabetes and obesity, that may compound the healing and infection risks associated with open fractures. These need to be considered when making treatment decisions.
- Prior to orthopedic surgery, other conditions may also commonly impact treatment decisions in this patient population. While the typical treatment for this TSF may have involved a standard antegrade tibial intramedullary nail, the ipsilateral total knee arthroplasty and prior hindfoot/ankle autofusion made a hindfoot fusion nail an acceptable option.

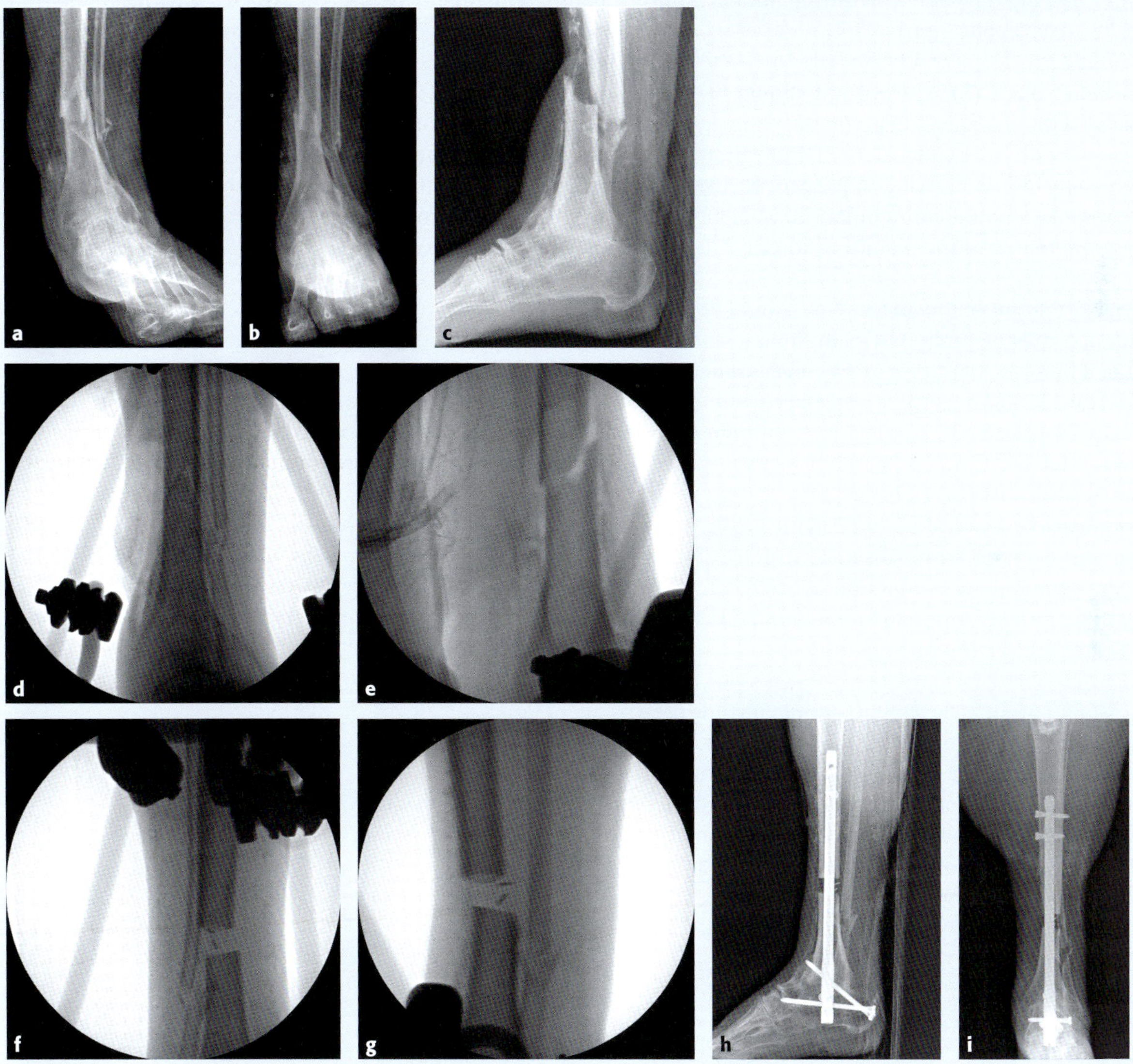


**Fig 3.16-1a–i** A 72-year-old woman with an isolated open fracture of the left distal tibial shaft.
**a–c** In addition to the left distal tibial shaft fracture, there is evidence in these views of the hindfoot and tibiotalar autoarthrodesis as a sequelae of previous Charcot arthropathy. Not visible in these x-rays is the ipsilateral total knee arthroplasty proximally.
**d–e** Intraoperative x-rays showing provisional alignment following placement of the external fixator.
**f–g** X-rays showing excised fracture fragments that were contaminated and devitalized at the time of injury.
**h–i** Postoperative x-rays showing the fixation with a hindfoot arthrodesis intramedullary nail.

(Case courtesy of Julie A Switzer and Herman Johal, authors of chapter 3.20 Polytrauma.)

The local skin status is critically important in suspected TSF. Any pathological finding should be photographed and documented. Skin compromise can result from both open and closed fractures. Any malalignment and areas under pressure from bony fragments should prompt timely restoration of alignment. A closed fracture can quickly convert to an open fracture resulting in full-thickness skin necrosis and impaired wound healing with catastrophic consequences. In cognitively impaired patients, repeated evaluations are advised, especially after moving the patient or during limb manipulation (eg, x-ray, cast application).

In case of primary open TSF, the wound should be thoroughly irrigated in the emergency department, photographed and documented (with ruler and patient identification), and covered with a wet sterile dressing to prevent further unnecessary manipulation and contamination. A radical debridement should follow in the operating room.

Motor and sensory status of the affected leg should be evaluated. Evaluation may be limited by pain, limb instability, and dementia, if present. Sensation in the tibial, saphenous, superficial peroneal, and deep peroneal nerves should be tested. In case of suspected polyneuropathy, a monofilament examination is advised.

Vascular examination is best done with both tactile pulse examination and Doppler scan. Absence of pulse should prompt a reposition and reexamination as well as further vascular investigation (eg, computed tomographic [CT] angiography, digital subtraction angiography).

General assessment of geriatric patients should include preinjury level of function, cognitive status, and recent functional trajectory, in addition to evaluating closely for cardiovascular and other comorbidities. For open fractures findings such as fracture contamination, length of skin tear, and proximal based flap should be assessed (**Table 3.16-1**) [11].

## 3.2 Compartment syndrome

Compartment syndrome is a well-known and feared complication of TSF. Tibial shaft fractures are the leading cause of acute compartment syndrome and are the primary etiology in 36% of all compartment syndromes. The incidence of compartment syndrome after TSF ranges from 1.5% to 11%. Patients with a TSF-associated compartment syndrome tend to be younger (ie, mean age 30 years) than those with compartment syndrome without TSF [12]. In the general population, open TSFs are not associated with a higher rate of compartment syndrome than closed TSFs. No data are specifically available for the geriatric population. It should be kept in mind that the older patient, because of tissue aging as well as confounding comorbidities, has diminished physiological reserves, prompting a need for rapid diagnosis and therapy. Further analyses are required to determine to what extent anticoagulation plays a role in the development of compartment syndrome in older adults [13].

| Significant findings | Present in older adult |
|---|---|
| Preexisting venous stasis | Yes/No |
| Pitting edema | Yes/No |
| CHF/CVD | Yes/No |
| Fracture comminution | Yes/No |
| Fracture contamination | Yes/No |
| Length of skin tear | < 1 cm, 1–5 cm, > 5 cm |
| Proximal based flap | Yes/No |
| Knows time of the day | 1 |
| Remembers recent events | 1 |
| Is picking, disorderly, restless | 0 |
| Pulls intravenous tubing, feeding tubes, catheters, etc | 0 |
| Easily or suddenly emotional | 0 |
| Sees/hears things which are not there | 0 |

**Table 3.16-1** Risk factors for assessing older adults; from Court-Brown, 2016: Musculoskeletal Trauma in the elderly [11]. Abbreviations: CHF, congestive heart failure; CVD, cardiovascular disease.

Generally, compartment syndrome can occur as a result of the induced swelling or secondary to reperfusion syndrome. Since cognitively impaired patients are unable to clearly communicate their pain, a low threshold of suspicion should always trigger an examination by an experienced surgeon. Physical examination may be supplemented by compartment pressure measurement.

When in doubt, fasciotomy of the affected compartments should be performed. A missed compartment syndrome has dramatic consequences for the patient, the surgeon, and the health system.

The rate of amputation for TSFs is low. Amputation is typically a result of severe soft-tissue trauma with neurovascular compromise, arterial injury, compartment syndrome, or infection. The Swedish National Patient Register reports an amputation rate of 3.6% in open tibial fractures [14], with age as a significant predictive factor.

### 3.3 Imaging

AP and lateral views of the tibia should be obtained with x-rays of the adjacent ankle (mortise and lateral views) and knee (AP, lateral, and patellar axial views). A suspected extension of the fracture line to the ankle or knee should prompt a CT scan. In cognitively impaired patients, any symptomatic or suspected region should be imaged. Any bone lesions suggesting a pathological fracture, malignancy, or osteomyelitis should be further investigated with CT scan and/or magnetic resonance imaging.

Interpretation of radiographic studies should include both fracture pattern classification and soft-tissue assessment. The spectrum of treatment modalities should be restricted and matched to the physiological reserves of the older, frail patient. The fracture pattern, its location, and the soft-tissue status will allow for a limited spectrum of treatment options with its specific pros and cons.

## 4 Classification

The AO/OTA Fracture and Dislocation Classification of tibial diaphyseal fractures is the generally accepted classification for this bone segment but is clinically inadequate without additional soft-tissue classification. This additional information is considered in the Gustilo classification for open fractures and the Tscherne classification for closed fractures. By itself, the AO/OTA Fracture and Dislocation Classification fails to predict treatment outcome. Further study with integration of soft-tissue grading is necessary and may help guide treatment and predict outcome.

### 4.1 AO/OTA Fracture and Dislocation Classification of tibial diaphyseal fractures

Tibial diaphysis corresponds to bone segment 42. The fracture morphology is then classified by type (A for simple, B for wedge, and C for multifragmentary). Each type consists of three groups describing the geometry of the fracture (1 for spiral, 2 for oblique [≥ 30°], and 3 for transverse [< 30°]). An accompanqing fibular fracture is coded separately, using the locations 2F1 (proximal), 2F2 (diaphyseal), or 2F3 (distal). This morphology of fibular fractures is further divided into types. In patients older than 65 years, a higher AO/OTA type is associated with a longer mean time to union (A: 20.5 weeks, B: 28.5 weeks, and C: 35 weeks, $P > .008$) and a higher rate of amputation (A: 1%, B: 5%, C: 6%), types B and C show higher nonunion rates (26% and 19% versus 3% in type A fractures) but does not predict a higher mortality rate [3].

### 4.2 Soft-tissue classification

Common geriatric findings of poor skin quality and common comorbidities, such as venous stasis, peripheral arterial disease, and hyperpigmentation disorders render interpretation of the skin more difficult. It is therefore recommended to consider the previous skin condition while deducing soft-tissue classification.

### 4.3 Gustilo classification for open fractures

The Gustilo classification is widely used and well established (**Case 2: Fig 3.16-2**). But it also carries a high degree of interobserver variability even among experienced surgeons [15]. Studies show higher rates of nonunions with higher Gustilo grades. Unfortunately, this classification fails to provide specific outcome data for treatments in the geriatric population.

CASE 2

**Patient**

An 86-year-old woman sustained an open fracture (Gustilo type II–IIIA; AO/OTA 42A1) of her right lower leg after a fall in her garden (**Fig 3.16-2a–c**).

**Comorbidities**

- Charlson Comorbidity Index 2
- Osteoporosis
- Sarcopenia
- Barthel Index 55/75
- Mild dementia

**Treatment and outcome**

Wound debridement, irrigation, reduction with a Weber clamp, and operative fixation 3 hours after admission with an expert tibial nail. Locking with angular stable locking system because of osteoporosis and closure of soft tissues (**Fig 3.16-2d–f**).

Uneventful healing of soft tissues and fracture. Recurrent swelling of the lower leg with expanded mobilization. Follow-up after 1 year showed good alignment despite the entry portal of the nail being too medial (**Fig 3.16-2g–h**).

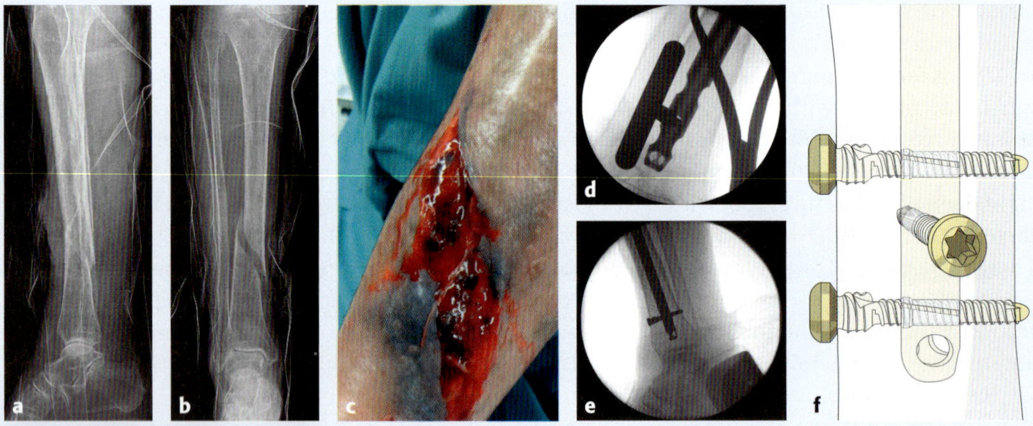


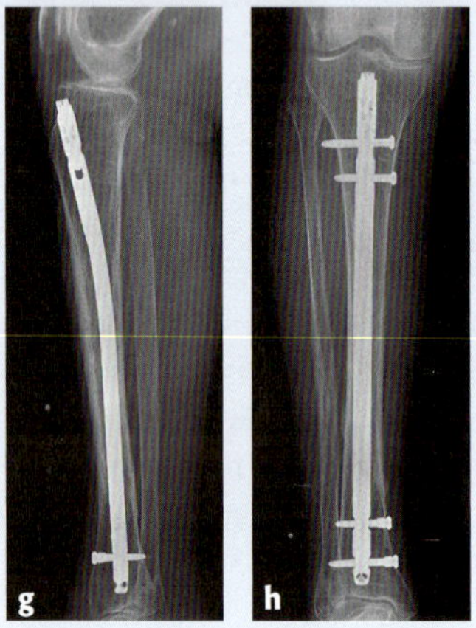


**Fig 3.16-2a–h** An 86-year-old woman with an open fracture.
**a–c** X-rays and clinical photograph showing open fracture of the lower leg.
**d–f** Nail fixation and locking of fracture.
**g–h** One-year follow-up x-rays.

(Case courtesy of University Department for Trauma Surgery Innsbruck, Austria.)

## 4.4 Tscherne classification for closed fractures

The Tscherne classification for closed fractures is well established. In patients older than 65 years, higher grades of soft-tissue injuries are associated with higher infection rates as well as longer times to union (16.9 weeks for Tscherne C0 and 25.8 weeks for Tscherne C3) [9].

## 5 Decision making

Clement et al [3] concluded that intramedullary (IM) nail fixation is the preferred treatment option in older adults, used in 58% of patients older than 65 years and 46% in patients older than 80 years. This fixation is both minimally invasive and permits early weight bearing [3].

However, in the metaphysis, some fractures are too distal or too proximal to be adequately stabilized by IM nail fixation and will require plate fixation. The fracture level at which plate fixation is recommended depends on the number of fixation screws that can be placed in the proximal or distal fragments, respectively. At least three multiplane screws are needed for IM nail fixation.

In open fractures, high degree of contamination and soft-tissue injury will require debridement and early stabilization with an external fixator before a definitive treatment with internal fixation can be achieved safely. Soft-tissue coverage may be limited due to poor vascular status or diabetes. Plastic reconstructive surgery or even amputation may be necessary in patients with limited healing potential due to their comorbidities.

The treatment of osteoporotic fractures implies an additional challenge due to the reduced holding power of implants and the fragile mechanical properties of the osteoporotic bone which mandate more indirect than direct reduction techniques.

The classic principles of anatomical reduction, interfragmentary compression, and long-spanning mechanical support can be supplemented by recent developments such as angular stability (in both plates and nails) as well as bone cement augmentation to increase holding power of fixation [16].

### 5.1 Nonoperative versus operative treatment

In a prospective study, Clement et al [3] noted that the proportion of TSFs treated with IM nail fixation is decreasing with age, with a solitary nonoperative treatment applied in 18% of patients > 65 years and in 30% of patients older than 80 years. This can be explained by an increasing proportion of older adults with bed-bound or wheelchair-bound disabilities, for whom early weight bearing cannot be achieved. However, 18% of patients treated nonoperatively seem to be a rather high rate in the authors' opinions and the influence of the healthcare system on treatment decisions needs to be considered in this context.

Randomized controlled trials (RCTs) comparing nonoperative treatment with IM nail fixation in displaced TSFs showed a significantly longer time to union, increased angular deformity, and shortening associated with nonoperative treatment [17]. In nondisplaced TSFs, IM nailing was shown to provide an improved functional and clinical outcome as well as more rapid return to work [18]. No RCTs focusing on the geriatric population are available. Indications for closed treatments include high anesthetic risk and low degree of displacement (angulation, rotation, and length). In his series of 780 patients treated with functional bracing, Sarmiento at al [19] reported that an age greater than 49 years is an independent predictor of longer time to union. In another study, Sarmiento et al [20] reported that most fractures healed with < 6° varus (90%), < 5° valgus (95%), < 6° apex anterior angulation (95%), and < 7° of apex posterior angulation.

Dementia and polyneuropathy reduce the ability to comply with activity restrictions and therapy treatments. These factors combined with the difficulty in identifying and communicating pain should be kept in mind if nonoperative treatment is considered, because of the risk of pressure ulcers due to cast immobilization.

The need for partial weight bearing (PWB) in nonoperative treatment of TSF is a limiting factor as well. Partial weight bearing is usually difficult to achieve because of diminished strength, balance, and cognition, as well as the additional risk of falls.

Because of the abovementioned risks associated with nonoperative treatment, operative treatment should be the first option for functionally intact patients. Nonoperative treatment should only be considered in patients with short life expectancy or bed- or wheelchair-bound patients with minimal risk for sequela of cast immobilization and the risk of irreversible functional decline with any limitations in weight-bearing status.

### 5.2 Open lower leg fractures

The types of open TSFs in older adults differ from those in the general population, with low-energy trauma due to simple falls as the predominant cause.

Open fractures pose an additional challenge in older adults. Alteration in skin resistance increases the risk of wounds and wound-healing complications. The fragile skin barrier coupled with an impaired immune system and increased lifetime exposure to antibiotics may additionally increase the problem of antibiotic-resistant infection [21].

The basic principles of treatment for open fractures in older adults are the same as in the general population and comprise early debridement, irrigation, and stabilization. The type of stabilization (temporary versus definitive and plate versus nail) depends on the extent of soft-tissue damage as well as the potential need for future vascular or reconstructive interventions.

The course of prophylactic antibiotic therapy should be discussed with infectious diseases specialists based on the Gustilo classification, kidney function, allergies, drug interactions, and history regarding potential microbial resistance [22].

Regarding definitive fixation, reamed IM nail fixation has been shown to be safe in low-grade open fractures in patients younger than 55 years [23]. In high-grade open fractures, conflicting results regarding infection rates have been reported. The use of an antibiotic-coated nail can further decrease the risk of local bone infection as supported by evidence from in vivo animal studies [24].

### 5.3 Nailing versus plating

Intramedullary nailing offers various advantages compared to plating. First, IM nails have a high-load capacity allowing for early weight bearing, which is important in older patients. Second, it avoids skin incision at the fracture site, another goal in this population. For these reasons, IM nail fixation is the preferred operative treatment in TSF when technically feasible. Nonetheless, RCTs comparing nailing versus plating showed increased nonunion, malunion, and malalignment in IM nail fixation with no increase in deep infection.

### 5.4 Other options

In heavily contaminated open fractures, external fixation can be a temporary or definitive treatment option.

## 6 Nonoperative treatment

Nonoperative treatment includes manipulation of displaced fractures and immobilization of the injured leg with a long leg cast or a functional brace (**Fig 3.16-3**). Because of skin fragility, special attention should be paid to padding and protecting bony prominences during crafting of the cast or molding of the brace.

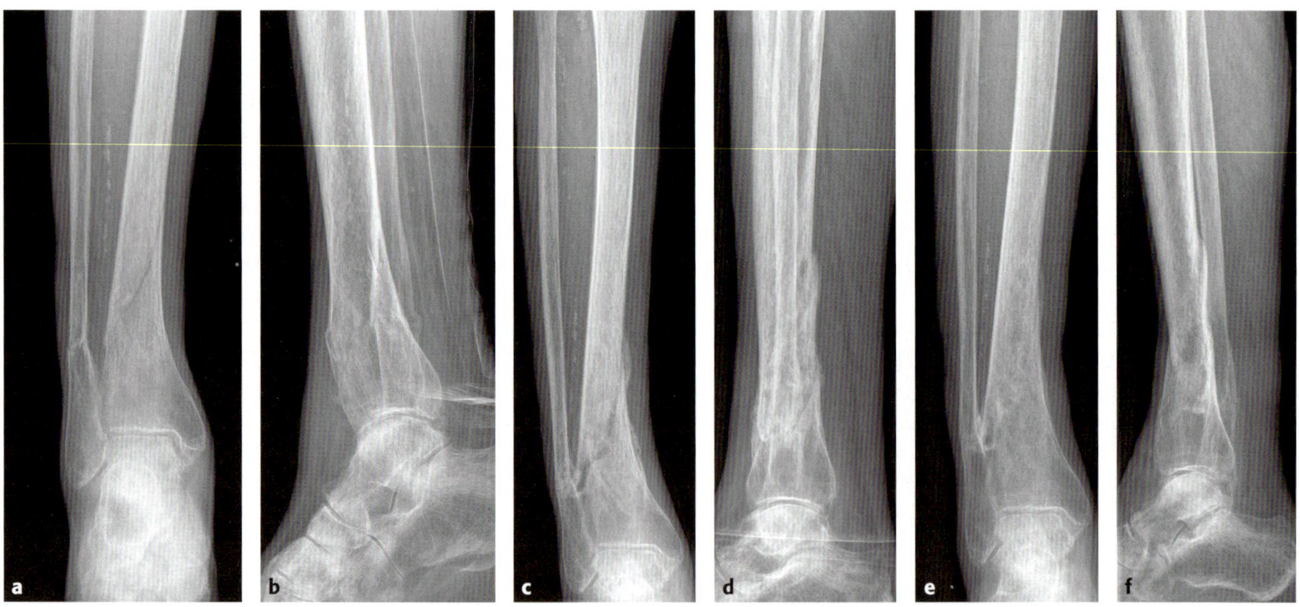


**Fig 3.16-3a–f** Nonoperative treatment of a nondisplaced metaphyseal tibial fracture associated with a Weber A fracture of the distal fibula in a 90-year-old woman.
**a–b** X-rays at the time of diagnosis.
**c–d** X-rays 12 weeks after treatment with cast.
**e–f** X-rays 7 months after treatment with cast.

## 7 Intramedullary nailing

### 7.1 Approaches

Medial parapatellar, tendon-splitting, suprapatellar as well as semiextended lateral or medial approaches are described (**Fig 3.16-4**).

The medial parapatellar approach can be problematic in finding a suitably lateral insertion point. An excessively medial entry point results in valgus deformity in proximal TSF. The anatomy of the patient has to be studied well before choosing this approach.

The tendon-splitting approach avoids the aforementioned difficulty. In the older patient, adipose tissue can be sparse and great care is necessary to avoid damage to the patellar tendon. In proximal TSFs, the inability to control the entry angle of the guide wire near the patella carries a risk of an excessive posterior angulation with subsequent displacement during nail insertion.

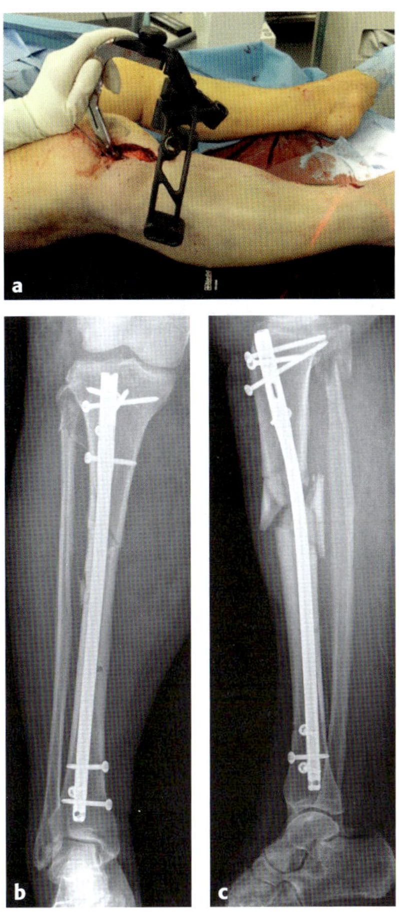

**Fig 3.16-4a–c** Approach for intramedullary (IM) nailing.
**a** Semiextended, extraarticular approach for IM nailing.
**b–c** Postoperative x-rays.

The suprapatellar approach allows for semiextended positioning of the knee. The authors recommend 30° flexion in both hip and knee with foam support under the knee. This approach is a good option for proximal TSFs, as it allows a more posterior entry point to avoid recurvatum of the proximal fragment caused by the nail curvature. Evidence regarding the risk of retropatellar cartilage injury is disputed and might play a small role in geriatric patients [25, 26]. On the other hand, the suprapatellar approach is intraarticular and carries the risk of septic arthritis, especially in open fractures. Studies are ongoing to address this concern [27].

To avoid the risk of cartilage injury and the risks associated with the arthrotomy of the suprapatellar approach, Kubiak et al [28] proposed a semiextended extraarticular approach. This approach can be done either laterally or medially to the patella, following the path of least resistance depending on patient anatomy. The cornerstone of this approach is careful preparation of the superficial retinaculum, release of the inferior deep retinacular bands and preservation of the synovium over the trochlea. This approach is of particular interest in more proximal TSFs.

In all approaches, the entry point of the nail is vital. Obtaining a true AP of the knee is essential, as slight misalignment of the C-arm can induce an excessively lateral or medial insertion point.

### 7.2 Nail diameter

In older adults, the IM canal is wider and a larger nail diameter may be required (11–13 mm) [11]. Intramedullary reaming should be 1–2 mm more than the nail diameter. Decreased vascularity of the cortices can be expected.

### 7.3 Interlocking

It is recommended to place the distal interlocking screws first, allowing for gentle backstrokes that increase bony contact to ideally decrease the nonunion rate. In the osteoporotic bone of older adults, more interlocking screws are advised than for younger patients. In more proximal fractures, at least three interlocking screws should be placed, and in distal fractures, multiplane screws are advised. If reduction is difficult to maintain or if sufficient purchase cannot be obtained with conventional interlocking screws, angular stable locking screws (eg, angular stable locking system) can be used, although evidence is limited [18]. Additional reduction and retention plates may be necessary.

### 7.4 Postoperative care

Early postoperative mobilization under physical therapy guidance with quick transition to full weight bearing is advised. Optimization of nutritional status, avoidance of iatrogenic harm, and careful management of comorbidities are essential for recovery.

## 8 Plating

Plating may offer better reduction in more distal or proximal diaphyseal fractures (**Fig 3.16-5**). However, the cost-effectiveness of plating and associated PWB should be kept in mind, especially in patients with multiple fractures or cognitive impairment. Minimally invasive plating techniques should be considered, as these techniques decrease soft-tissue damage and presumably rates of nonunion. In frail patients with atrophic skin due to long-term corticosteroid use, anatomical low-profile plates are preferred to minimize soft-tissue compromise from the inserted implant (**Case 3: Fig 3.16-6**).

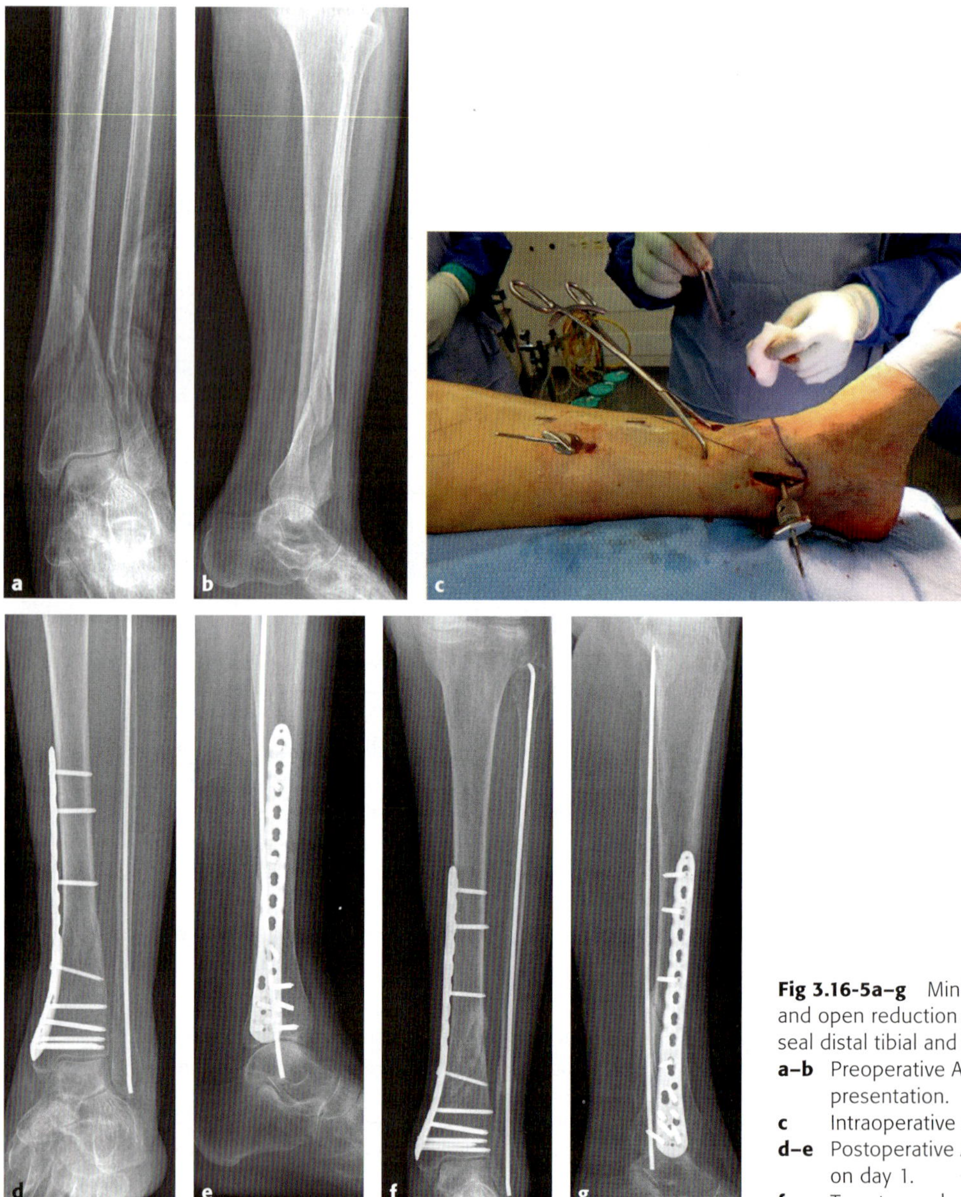

**Fig 3.16-5a–g** Minimally invasive plate osteosynthesis and open reduction and internal fixation of a metaphyseal distal tibial and fibular fracture.

- **a–b** Preoperative AP (**a**) and lateral (**b**) x-ray presentation.
- **c** Intraoperative clinical photograph.
- **d–e** Postoperative AP (**d**) and lateral (**e**) x-rays on day 1.
- **f–g** Twenty-week postoperative follow-up x-rays.

**Patient**

A 99-year-old woman with tibial and fibular shaft fractures.

**Comorbidities**

- Dementia
- Renal insufficiency (glomerular filtration rate 33 mL/min/1.73 m$^2$)
- Peripheral artery disease stage IIb on the left side with diffuse arteriosclerosis and single artery perfusion (fibular artery)
- Arterial hypertension
- Normochromic normocytic anemia

**Treatment and outcome**

Open reduction and internal fixation was used to fix the tibial and fibular shaft fractures with a subsequent development of full-thickness skin necrosis (**Fig 3.16-6a–e**).

Four weeks after initial plating, the plate was removed and the intramedullary nail inserted (**Fig 3.16-6f–g**). X-rays taken 6 months postoperatively are shown in **Fig 3.16-6h–i**.

Free flap coverage was not possible due to poor vascular status, therefore local flaps and negative-pressure wound therapy had to be used (**Fig 3.16-6j–k**).

Almost all skin defects could be closed except for one which remained open. The patient was able to walk on a walker with full weight bearing and without pain (**Fig 3.16-6l–n**).

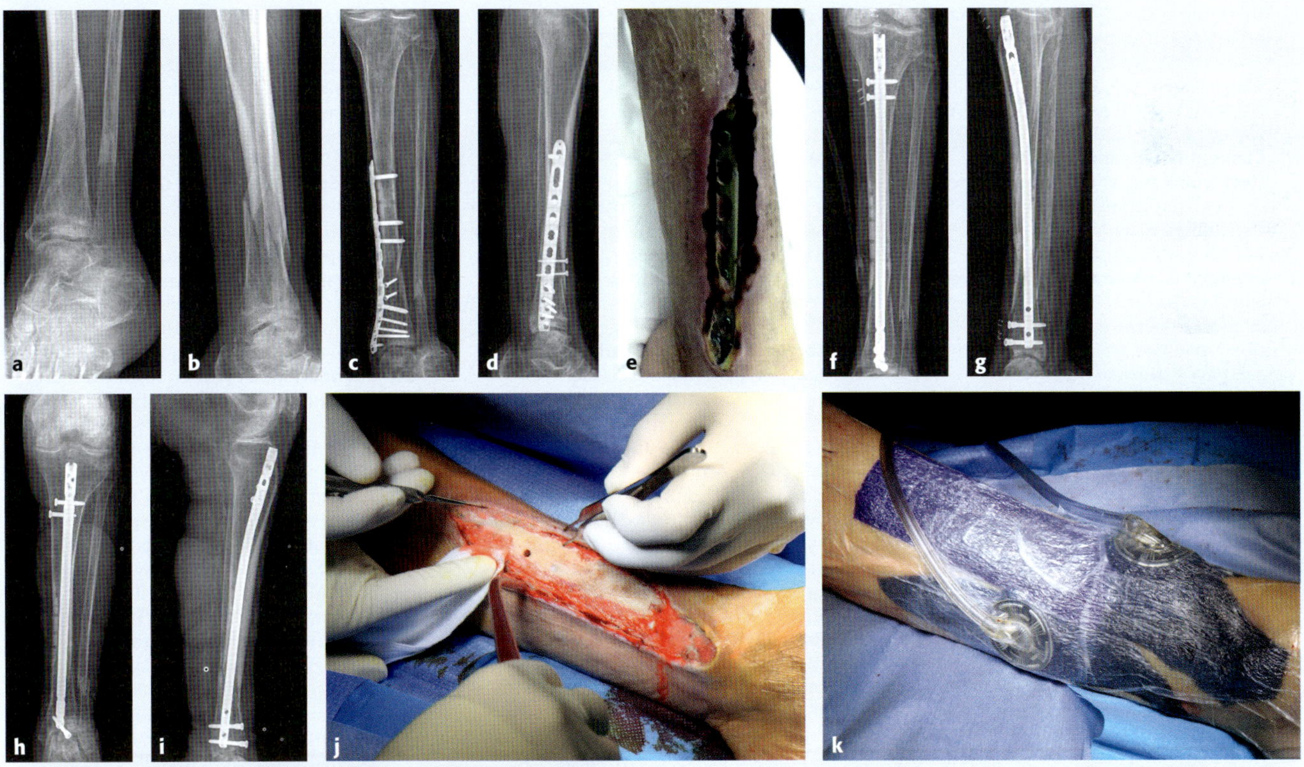

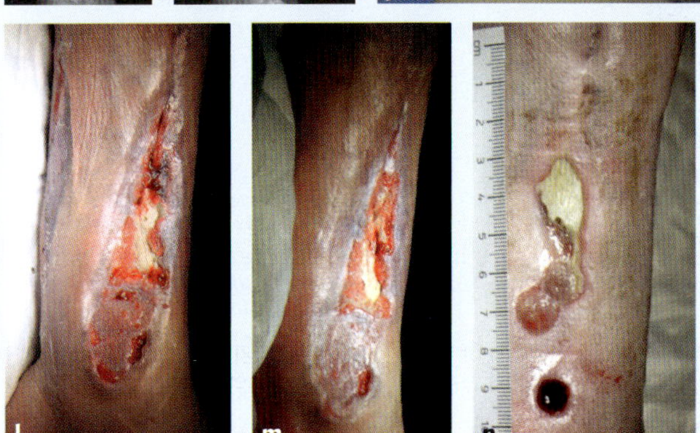

**Fig 3.16-6a–n** A 99-year-old woman with fractures of the tibial and fibular shaft.

**a–b** X-rays of initial presentation.
**c–d** Postoperative x-rays on day 2.
**e** Full thickness skin necrosis.
**f–g** Postoperative x-rays after plate removal and intramedullary nail fixation 4 weeks after initial plating.
**h–i** Six-month postoperative x-rays.
**j–k** Local flap coverage and negative-pressure wound therapy (NPWT).
**l–n** Clinical photographs showing the lower leg 7 weeks after conducting NPWT (**l**), 9 weeks of NPWT (**m**), and 5 months after NPWT (**n**).

## 9 External fixation

External fixation is often indicated for open fractures, either as a temporary measure to allow for preoperative debridement, or as a primary definitive treatment. External fixation can be very difficult to tolerate for frail, cognitively impaired patients, so the need for PWB, additional nursing care, and a higher infection risk should be kept in mind.

## 10 Nonunion

Clement et al [3] noted a 10% incidence of nonunion in TSFs in older adults. Patients older than 80 years did not have higher rates of nonunion compared to patients between 65 and 80 years of age. In this study, open fractures and fixations that do not use a nail were predictive factors for nonunion [3]. Optimizing fracture reduction is essential as greater diastasis is associated with higher rates of nonunion [6].

## 11 References

1. **Busse JW, Morton E, Lacchetti C, et al.** Current management of tibial shaft fractures: a survey of 450 Canadian orthopedic trauma surgeons. *Acta Orthop.* 2008 Oct;79(5):689–694.
2. **Court-Brown CM, Caesar B.** Epidemiology of adult fractures: A review. *Injury.* 2006 Aug;37(8):691–697.
3. **Clement ND, Beauchamp NJ, Duckworth AD, et al.** The outcome of tibial diaphyseal fractures in the elderly. *Bone Joint J.* 2013 Sep;95-B(9):1255–1262.
4. **Shadgan B, Pereira G, Menon M, et al.** Risk factors for acute compartment syndrome of the leg associated with tibial diaphyseal fractures in adults. *J Orthop Traumatol.* 2015 Sep;16(3):185–192.
5. **Allmon C, Greenwell P, Paryavi E, et al.** Radiographic predictors of compartment syndrome occurring after tibial fracture. *J Orthop Trauma.* 2016 Jul;30(7):387–391.
6. **Fong K, Truong V, Foote CJ, et al.** Predictors of nonunion and reoperation in patients with fractures of the tibia: an observational study. *BMC Musculoskelet Disord.* 2013 Mar 22;14:103.
7. **Weiss RJ, Montgomery SM, Ehlin A, et al.** Decreasing incidence of tibial shaft fractures between 1998 and 2004: information based on 10,627 Swedish inpatients. *Acta Orthop.* 2008 Aug;79(4):526–533.
8. **Grecco MAS, Prado Junior ID, Rocha MA, et al.** Estudo epidemiológico das fraturas diafisárias de tíbia [Epidemiology of tibial shaft fractures]. *Acta Ortopédica Brasileira.* 2002 Oct/Dec;10(4). Available at: http://www.scielo.br/scielo.php?script=sci_arttext&pid=S1413-78522002000400002&lng=en&nrm=iso&tlng=en. Accessed 2017. Portuguese.
9. **Court-Brown CM, Biant LC, Clement ND, et al.** Open fractures in the elderly. The importance of skin ageing. *Injury.* 2015 Feb;46(2):189–194.
10. **Uitto J.** The role of elastin and collagen in cutaneous aging: intrinsic aging versus photoexposure. *J Drugs Dermatol.* 2008 Feb;7(2 Suppl):S12–S16.
11. **Court-Brown C, McQueen M, Swiontkowski MF, et al.** *Musculoskeletal trauma in the elderly.* Boca Raton: CRC Press; 2016.
12. **McQueen MM, Gaston P, Court-Brown CM.** Acute compartment syndrome. Who is at risk? *J Bone Joint Surg Br.* 2000 Mar;82(2):200–203.
13. **Kurmis AP.** Diagnosing acute lower-limb compartment ayndrome in the older population: a clinical conundrum. *Clin Geriatrics.* 2008:29.
14. **Tampe U, Weiss RJ, Stark B, et al.** Lower extremity soft tissue reconstruction and amputation rates in patients with open tibial fractures in Sweden during 1998–2010. *BMC Surg.* 2014 Oct 16;14:80.
15. **Brumback RJ, Jones AL.** Interobserver agreement in the classification of open fractures of the tibia. The results of a survey of two hundred and forty-five orthopaedic surgeons. *J Bone Joint Surg Am.* 1994 Aug;76(8):1162–1166.
16. **Roth SE, Kreder H, Stephen D, et al.** Biomechanical stability of intramedullary nailed high proximal third tibial fractures with cement augmented proximal screws. *J Orthop Trauma.* 2005 Aug;19(7):457–461.
17. **Hooper GJ, Keddell RG, Penny ID.** Conservative management or closed nailing for tibial shaft fractures. A randomised prospective trial. *J Bone Joint Surg Br.* 1991 Jan;73(1):83–85.
18. **Obremskey WT, Cutrera N, Kidd CM.** A prospective multi-center study of intramedullary nailing vs casting of stable tibial shaft fractures. *J Orthop Traumatol.* 2017 Mar;18(1):69–76.
19. **Sarmiento A, Gersten LM, Sobol PA, et al.** Tibial shaft fractures treated with functional braces. Experience with 780 fractures. *J Bone Joint Surg Br.* 1989 Aug;71(4):602–609.
20. **Sarmiento A, Sharpe FE, Ebramzadeh E, et al.** Factors influencing the outcome of closed tibial fractures treated with functional bracing. *Clin Orthop Relat Res.* 1995 Jun(315):8–24.
21. **Yoshikawa TT.** Antimicrobial resistance and aging: beginning of the end of the antibiotic era? *J Am Geriatr Soc.* 2002 Jul;50(7 Suppl):S226–S229.
22. **Rodriguez L, Jung HS, Goulet JA, et al.** Evidence-based protocol for prophylactic antibiotics in open fractures: improved antibiotic stewardship with no increase in infection rates. *J Trauma Acute Care Surg.* 2014 Sep;77(3):400–407; discussion 407–408; quiz 524.
23. **Bhandari M, Guyatt G, Tornetta P 3rd, et al.** Randomized trial of reamed and unreamed intramedullary nailing of tibial shaft fractures. *J Bone Joint Surg Am.* 2008 Dec;90(12):2567–2578.
24. **Schmidmaier G, Lucke M, Wildemann B, et al.** Prophylaxis and treatment of implant-related infections by antibiotic-coated implants: a review. *Injury.* 2006 May;37(Suppl 2):S105–S112.
25. **Sanders RW, DiPasquale TG, Jordan CJ, et al.** Semiextended intramedullary nailing of the tibia using a suprapatellar approach: radiographic results and clinical outcomes at a minimum of 12 months follow-up. *J Orthop Trauma.* 2014 Aug;28(Suppl 8):S29–S39.
26. **Zamora R, Wright C, Short A, et al.** Comparison between suprapatellar and parapatellar approaches for intramedullary nailing of the tibia. Cadaveric study. *Injury.* 2016 Oct;47(10):2087–2090.
27. **Zelle BA.** Intramedullary nailing of tibial shaft fractures in the semi-extended position using a suprapatellar portal technique. *Int Orthop.* 2017 Sep;41(9):1909–1914.
28. **Kubiak EN, Widmer BJ, Horwitz DS.** Extra-articular technique for semiextended tibial nailing. *J Orthop Trauma.* 2010 Nov;24(11):704–708.

# 3.17 Ankle

Christian CMA Donken, Michael HJ Verhofstad

## 1 Introduction

Ankle fractures (AFs) in older adults are among the most common injuries and present trauma surgeons with multiple unique problems:

- Ankle fractures in older adults are a predictor of osteoporotic fractures [1] but can also be the result of osteoporosis treatment with bisphosphonates [2].
- Geriatric patients more often present with unstable fractures, predominantly pronation-abduction stage III, supination-external rotation stage IV, and pronation-external rotation stage IV [3]. These severe injuries are often accompanied by articular cartilage damage, influencing functional outcome [4].
- Ankle fractures have an increased risk of complications after surgery [5–7]. Patients with diabetes, peripheral vascular disease, type C fractures, tobacco use, and those who reside in nursing homes have increased risk for wound infections (up to 4%), resulting in reduced functional recovery [8, 9]. Poor soft-tissue conditions require delicate handling.
- Obesity is common in older adults. Although it has been suggested that a larger soft-tissue envelope might protect against wound-healing complications in obese patients with open AFs, it has never been shown, and instead a trend towards increased complications exists. There is no literature support for a unique treatment approach in obese patients with AFs [10].
- Osteoporosis is commonly present in the aged population. Bone mass, quality, and bone mineral density of the cortical layer are the main factors, which affect the purchase of screws in bone [11]. Poor bone quality is vulnerable during fracture reduction, drilling, and screw insertion.

## 2 Epidemiology and etiology

The incidence of AF is anticipated to increase over the next 20 years, especially in women. The incidence of AFs in patients older than 60 years in 2000 was 1,545 per 100,000 people per year and is expected to increase by 319% in 2030 [12, 13]. The majority of patients continue to have symptoms and functional limitations one year after the injury [14, 15]. Octogenarians are at a high risk for poor functional recovery and loss of autonomy. Additional risk factors for poor functional outcomes include inadequate surgical reduction, two or more comorbidities, and female gender [16].

## 3 Open ankle fractures

Open AFs in geriatric patients are associated with high morbidity and increased mortality [17]. These injuries usually result from low-energy trauma, whereas in young patients open fractures are often the result of high-energy trauma. This difference might explain why older patients have surprisingly fewer wound complications in open fractures than young patients [18]. Although the medial and lateral malleoli lie subcutaneously, most wound problems are seen at the medial side of the ankle because the foot almost invariably dislocates laterally. This holds true for open as well as closed AFs (**Case 1: Fig 3.17-1**).

CASE 1

**Patient**

A 71-year-old man fell from his bike and sustained a Gustilo grade 2 medial open bimalleolar type C left ankle fracture dislocation (**Fig 3.17-1a–b**). A few centimeters proximal to the obvious fibular fracture, a second fracture (fissure) was present.

**Comorbidities**

- Morbid obesity (body mass index 45)
- Type 2 diabetes mellitus
- Peripheral polyneuropathy
- Obstructive sleep apnea syndrome
- Hypertension
- Pulmonary embolism
- Ischemic heart disease treated with coronary artery bypass grafting and percutaneous transluminal coronary angioplasty

**Treatment and outcome**

After reduction, surgery was performed the same day. The medial wound was cleaned and fixed with a tension band technique. The fibula was fixed with two lag screws and a locking compression plate with locking screws (**Fig 3.17-1c–d**). The postoperative x-rays show some angulation of the proximal fibular fissure at the most proximal screw. During surgery, the second fissure was observed with image intensification. No longer plate was inserted, because the patient was planned for nonweight-bearing plaster postoperatively due to the open wound and obesity. The syndesmosis was unstable and fixed with a tricortical screw approximately 6 cm above the joint space. Literature supports a screw lower than 4 cm above the joint; single tricortical screws above 4 cm are associated with poorer results [19]. Two weeks after surgery, the medial wound had healed and 50% weight bearing in a plaster was allowed for another 6 weeks. Complete union was achieved. X-rays show a broken syndesmotic screw (**Fig 3.17-1e**). The medial tension band was removed 9 months after the initial operation, because of pain in that area.

**Discussion**

Despite severe comorbidities and a severe injury, good functional outcome can be achieved if immediate and aggressive surgery is performed to clean and close the joint and to support the soft tissues. Fibular length is restored using a solid plate, but congruency of the ankle joint is secured with a positioning screw.

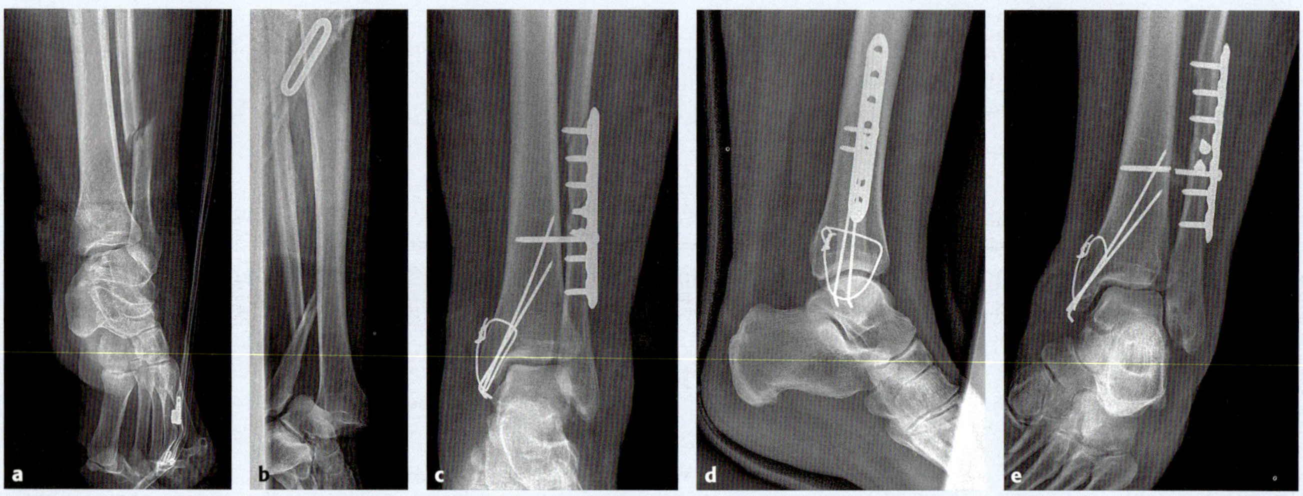


**Fig 3.17-1a–e** A 71-year-old man with a Gustilo grade 2 medial open bimalleolar type C fracture dislocation.
**a–b** Injury AP (**a**) and lateral (**b**) views of fracture dislocation.
**c** Postoperative AP x-ray after open reduction and internal fixation (ORIF) showing the second more proximal fracture.
**d** Postoperative lateral view after ORIF.
**e** X-ray showing the broken syndesmotic screw.

## 4 Emergency treatment

In case of severe medial skin problems in a closed dislocated fracture, prompt reduction of the ankle joint is required to improve perfusion of the medial skin. In such cases, operative fixation of the fibula alone with or without delayed fixation of the medial malleolus must be considered. However, in open fractures, a proper wash out and debridement of the (medial) wound with fracture reduction and fixation to reduce the amount of dead space is indicated, regardless of age (**Case 2: Fig 3.17-2**).

## Patient

A 70-year-old woman sustained a Gustilo grade 2 open ankle fracture with a medial transverse fracture and a lateral multifragmentary injury (**Fig 3.17-2a–b**). The fracture could not be classified according to Lauge-Hansen.

## Comorbidities

- Severe osteoporosis

## Treatment and outcome

Patient was treated with immediate washout of the joint, debridement, and immediate internal fixation. Due to the specific fracture pattern, the medial and posterior malleolus were repaired first with a tension band and lag screw respectively. Finally, the lateral malleolus was fixed. First, anatomical reconstruction of the malleolar/articular piece using 1.8/2.4 mm compression screws, followed by bridging the fibular fracture using a locking distal radial plate (1.8/2.4 mm screws). Despite the posterior malleolar screw, an additional positioning screw was inserted to support the bridging plate (**Fig 3.17-2c–f**). A plaster of Paris cast was placed for 1 week to facilitate soft-tissue healing. Partial weight bearing began after soft-tissue healing was uneventful. X-rays were made after 5 weeks (**Fig 3.17-2g–h**) and 5 months (**Fig 3.17-2i–l**).

## Discussion

Uneventful healing and functional recovery. The patient has full range of motion and walks without pain. Implant removal after 6 months was necessary due to local plate irritation.

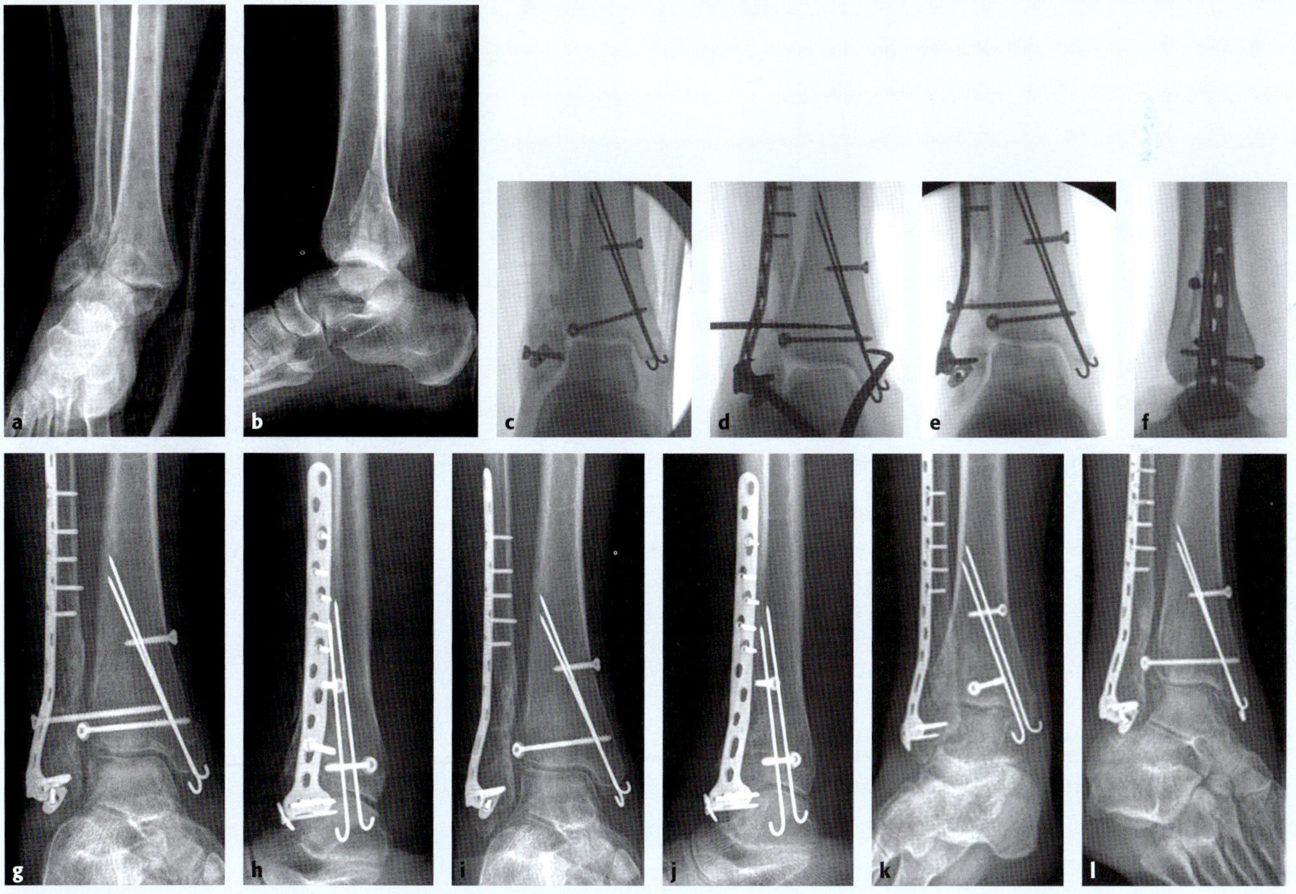

**Fig 3.17-2a–l** A 70-year-old woman with a Gustilo grade 2 open fracture with a medial transverse fracture and a lateral multifragmentary fracture pattern.
**a–b** AP (**a**) and lateral (**b**) views of the injury.
**c** Anatomical reconstruction of the lateral malleolar/articular piece using compression screws.
**d** Bridging the fibular fracture using a locking distal radial plate.
**e** Insertion of an additional positioning screw to support the bridging plate.
**f** Placement of a posterior malleolar screw.
**g–h** AP (**g**) and lateral (**h**) views 5 weeks postoperative.
**i–l** Mortise (**i**), lateral (**j**), oblique (**k**), and AP (**l**) views after 5 months.

## 5 Diagnostics

### 5.1 Clinical evaluation

History and physical examination are the first diagnostic steps in clinical evaluation. However, the reliability of typical clinical signs and symptoms in older adults can be reduced due to physical and cognitive comorbidities, polypharmacy, or other factors. Hematoma formation can be more extensive due to anticoagulant use, but on the other hand, the discriminative power of pain can be reduced due to peripheral neuropathy (eg, in diabetes), use of analgesics, or cognitive impairment. Especially in older adults, one must realize that tenderness at the medial malleolus might be absent despite injury of the (deep) deltoid ligament fibers. Health status and preinjury functional performance may influence the type of operative treatment but cannot serve as an excuse for suboptimal operative treatment. The goal of treatment should be to restore the patient back to the same level of mobility and independence. Treatment of older frail patients with AFs is often challenging and time-consuming but important work (**Case 3: Fig 3.17-3**).

CASE 3

#### Patient

An 88-year-old woman fell while standing up from her chair. She sustained a fracture dislocation pronation-abduction stage III injury, which was treated immediately with surgery (**Fig 3.17-3a–b**). Both ankles were significantly swollen due to peripheral edema.

#### Comorbidities

- Hypertension
- Polyneuropathy
- Atrial fibrillation
- Benign paroxysmal positional vertigo
- Slowly growing meningioma

#### Treatment and outcome

The lateral malleolus was fixed with an 8-hole locking compression plate. Due to the multifragmentary zone, adequate fibular length could only be estimated. The medial malleolus was fixed with two K-wires (**Fig 3.17-3c–d**). The treating surgeon reported very poor bone quality during surgery. A plaster cast was applied to facilitate wound healing. Within 1 month, all hardware was removed because of an infection, and an external fixator was placed (**Fig 3.17-3e**). One week later, vascular reconstruction was unsuccessful. Plastic surgery was consulted. Despite intensive wound care and antibiotics, union could not be achieved. Both medial (**Fig 3.17-3f**) and lateral (**Fig 3.17-3g**) fractures were visible through open infected wounds with pus, and a below-knee amputation was performed 6 weeks after injury. The patient died 6 months later.

#### Discussion

In these multimorbid patients, perfect anatomical bony reconstruction is not the treatment goal. Complications often result in a horrible scenario. The treatment goal is to prevent complications like these above. Initial definitive external fixation, even with a ring fixator, and better diagnostics of the vascular status could have avoided the catastrophic outcome.

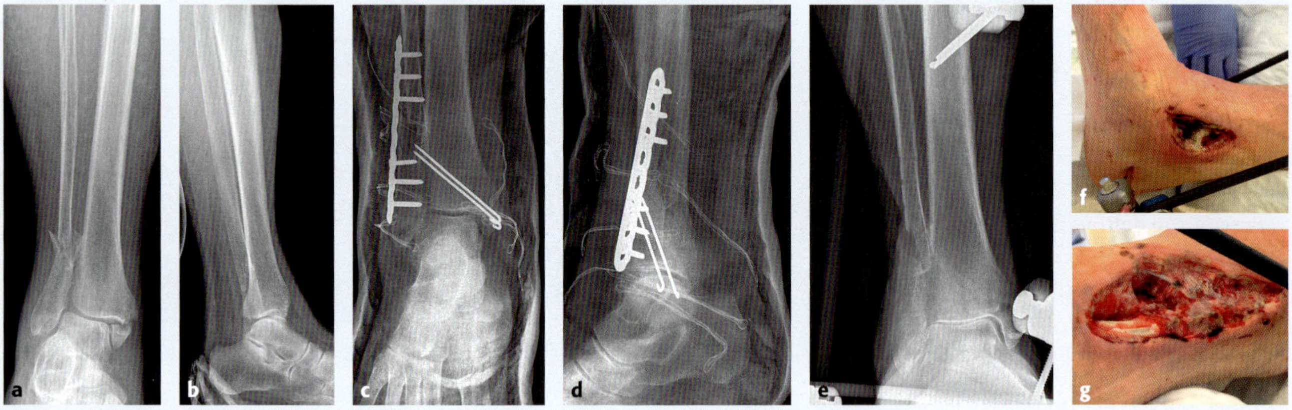

**Fig 3.17-3a–g** An 88-year-old woman with a displaced pronation-abduction stage III injury.
**a–b** AP (**a**) and lateral (**b**) views of the injury.
**c–d** AP (**a**) and lateral (**d**) views showing the early postoperative result.
**e** Postoperative x-ray after conversion to external fixation.
**f** Medial wound.
**g** Lateral wound.

## 5.2 Imaging

Clinical signs that justify radiographic investigations are summarized in the Ottawa ankle rules [20]: if the patient has pain or tenderness over the posterior 6 cm or tip of the medial or lateral malleolus, pain or tenderness over the navicular bone or base of the fifth metatarsal, or is unable to take four steps, an x-ray of the painful area is indicated. Because of the reduced reliability of physician exam findings, plain x-rays should be performed liberally and consist of AP, lateral, and mortise views. Mortise views with the ankle in 15–20° internal rotation are important to judge tibiotalar congruity [21, 22].

## 5.3 Stress views

Stress x-rays are often considered in light of the difficulty in identifying instability in nonstress x-rays [23]. Cadaver studies have shown that dorsiflexion combined with external rotation are the best stress position to detect medial ligament rupture [24]. A medial clear space of more than 5 mm probably reflects a rupture of the deep deltoid ligament fibers best. It must be noted that medial tenderness is not always accompanied with a deltoid ligament rupture leading to medial clear space widening in ankle stress x-rays [25]. Alternatively, gravity stress views can be used [26].

## 5.4 Computed tomography and magnetic resonance imaging

The deep fibers of the deltoid ligament are the key structures that prevent lateral dislocation and external rotation of the talus [27, 28]. The problem with ankle injuries is the "invisible medial injury" of the deltoid ligament. The short and less elastic fibers can be ruptured, resulting in external rotation or lateral dislocation of the talus, whereas the longer, superficial ligaments are not. There is no literature that justifies the acceptance of more (medial) joint space widening in osteoporotic AFs than in the highly active young patient.

Several diagnostic findings and tools to investigate the integrity of the deltoid ligament have been studied (eg, presence of a hematoma, external rotation, or gravity stress x-rays, medial clear space widening, ultrasound examination, arthroscopic examination, and magnetic resonance imaging [MRI]). None of these tools has been proven reliable enough to be adopted as an accepted best practice [29].

Magnetic resonance imaging seems to be the best diagnostic test to diagnose rupture of the deep [30] and anterior [31] deltoid ligament fibers. Its sensitivity is estimated 80% and specificity 100% compared to operative exploration. Magnetic resonance imaging can diagnose syndesmotic injury as predicted with the Lauge-Hansen classification [32, 33]. Radiographic images can be used for a rough estimate of the size of the posterior fragment, but a computed tomographic (CT) scan is superior in evaluating the type of fracture, extension to the medial malleolus, the degree of impaction, and osteochondral lesions [34, 35]. Preoperative CT scans influence the operative plan in up to 24% [36] and are often helpful prior to posterior malleolar fixation [3]. More frequent use of CT scans may be appropriate in older adults, as osteoporosis results in more atypical fracture patterns.

## 5.5 Instability and displacement

As noted above, the integrity of both the medial and posterior pillars is important. Bi- and trimalleolar fractures are clearly unstable injuries, visible on plain x-rays. But in isolated lateral malleolar fractures, stability is much more difficult to assess. A lateral shift of the talus of more than 2 mm is considered to reflect an unstable joint and is a widely accepted indication for operative reduction and fixation of the fibular fracture [37]. However, such a cut-off point is a simplification of reality. A lateral talar dislocation of only 1 mm is believed to lead to a substantial reduction of the contact area between talus and tibia [38], which results in excessive peak loads to the joint. Moreover, one must realize that the dislocation as seen on a plain x-ray might not be the maximum dislocation that can occur during weight bearing. Any displacement leads to a certain instability of the ankle joint. The same holds true for associated posterior malleolar fractures. Peak contact stress and instability may lead to secondary loss of cartilage, which in turn increases the risk of posttraumatic arthritis. Scientific proof supporting a statement that "the patient is too old to develop osteoarthritis" does not exist. On the contrary, older adults might be more susceptible to posttraumatic arthritis due to a thinner layer of cartilage. Malalignment and slight joint instability can result in symptomatic osteoarthritis in a relatively short period of time.

Joint stability results from bony joint configuration and ligamentous support. Energy creating a fracture can compromise both joint configuration and ligamentous stability. In theory, more energy leads to more damage, which results in more instability. On the other hand, young and healthy bone is able to absorb more energy than osteoporotic bone without the occurrence of a fracture. The energy that remains after fracturing of the bone determines the extent of soft-tissue injury.

## 6 Classification

### 6.1 Lauge-Hansen classification

With experimental studies, Lauge-Hansen classified malleolar fractures according to their injury pattern [33]. Using experimental cadaver studies, Lauge-Hansen offered more insight into the various fracture mechanisms and developed a classification system that is still broadly used today.

The Lauge-Hansen classification has been a matter of debate in the past. Some authors claim a poor correlation between trauma mechanism and MRI or other radiographic findings [39, 40]. Nevertheless, the 17 different stages within the Lauge-Hansen classification describe almost all AFs. The Lauge-Hansen classification describes the trauma mechanism via the position of the ankle and the direction of the injury force. Five categories are described: supination-adduction, supination-external rotation, pronation-abduction, pronation-external rotation, and pronation-dorsiflexion (axial loading). The axial loading injury, better known as the pilon fracture, will not be covered in this chapter. Each mechanism category is further subdivided based on severity (**Table 3.17-1**). The classification is useful for a grounded and balanced treatment protocol. For instance, the theoretical distinction between the supination-external rotation stages II–III and supination-external rotation stage IV AFs can provide the basis for choosing operative or nonoperative treatment.

### 6.2 Weber classification

The Weber classification is an anatomical classification that considers the level of the fracture of the fibula (**Table 3.17-2**) [41]. Unlike the Lauge-Hansen classification, it does not take medial and posterior injury into account, nor does it describe the trauma mechanism. This makes the Weber classification easier to use than the Lauge-Hansen classification, but less descriptive and specific.

### 6.3 AO/OTA classification system

The trauma mechanism injury classification of Lauge-Hansen and the anatomical classification of Danis and Weber [41, 42] have been combined in the AO/OTA Fracture and Dislocation Classification system [43].

| Type of injury<br>Foot position/direction of force | Stage | Pathology |
|---|---|---|
| Supination-adduction | I | Transverse fracture of the fibula at or distal to the level of the tibiofibular joint/ tear of collateral ligaments |
| | II | Vertical oblique fracture of the medial malleolus/tear of the deltoid ligament |
| Supination-external rotation | I | Disruption of the anterior tibiofibular ligament or an avulsion of its tibial attachment (Tillaux fracture) or fibular attachment (Wagstaffe-Le Fort fracture) |
| | II | Spiral oblique fracture of the distal fibula. The fracture line runs from distal anterior to proximal posterior at a variable distal from the tibiotalar joint |
| | III | Disruption of the posterior tibiofibular ligament or fracture of the posterior malleolus |
| | IV | Fracture of the medial malleolus or rupture of the deltoid ligament |
| Pronation-abduction | I | Transverse fracture of the medial malleolus or rupture of the deltoid ligament |
| | II | Rupture of the anterior and posterior syndesmotic ligaments or avulsion fracture of their insertion(s) |
| | III | Short oblique fracture of the fibula 0.5–1 cm above the distal articular surface of the tibia |
| Pronation-external rotation | I | Transverse fracture of the medial malleolus or disruption of the deltoid ligament |
| | II | Disruption of the anterior tibiofibular ligament may avulse its tibial attachment (Tillaux fracture) |
| | III | High oblique spiral fibular fracture. No fracture is less than 2.5 cm above the tibiotalar joint. The fracture pattern runs from proximal anterior to distal posterior. The fibula may fracture proximally at the neck (Maisonneuve fracture) |
| | IV | Rupture of the posterior tibiofibular ligament or avulsion fracture of the posterolateral tibia |
| Pronation-dorsiflexion/pilon fracture | I | Fracture of the medial malleolus |
| | II | Fracture of the anterior margin of the tibia |
| | III | Supramalleolar fracture of the fibula |
| | IV | Transverse fracture of the posterior tibial surface |

**Table 3.17-1** The Lauge-Hansen classification.

| Type | Fracture description |
|---|---|
| A | Fibular fracture below the level of the syndesmosis |
| B | Spiral oblique fibular fracture starting ventral at the level of the tibiotalar joint running proximally dorsal, leaving the syndesmosis intact |
| C | Fibular fracture above the level of the syndesmosis, and may be as high as just below the fibular head (Maisonneuve fracture) |

**Table 3.17-2** The Weber classification.

## 7 Decision making

The ultimate goal is to restore pretraumatic functional status. Functional independence for older adults depends strongly on mobility and AFs are a serious threat to long-term mobility and independence. Whereas treatment in a mobile octogenarian living an independent life should almost certainly involve surgery, a similar fracture in a wheelchair- or bed-bound patient can be treated with a plaster cast. Decision making in older adults requires more patient-specific treatments than in younger patients.

### 7.1 Operative versus nonoperative treatment

In current practice, most Weber A fractures are treated nonoperatively and most Weber C fractures are treated by open anatomical reduction and internal fixation. The remainder (roughly 50%) of all AFs consists of Weber B fractures, which are treated with or without surgery. The Lauge-Hansen and Weber classification systems cannot assess the intrinsic stability of all AFs, which is considered an additional determinant for the type of treatment.

There is some variation in practice over the use of nonoperative measures in AFs; some consider precise anatomical reconstruction essential to prevent posttraumatic osteoarthritis, while others believe nonoperative measures are sufficient. The tendency for operative intervention increases with the number of malleoli fractures, but depending on location, a wide range (14–72%) in the frequency of operative repair has been reported in the US [44].

There is controversy regarding the treatment of frail adults with osteoporosis and comorbidities that increase the risk of operative complications [5]. In 2012, the authors of this chapter published a Cochrane review about operative versus nonoperative treatment for AFs in adults [45], suggesting that there is insufficient high-quality evidence to conclude that operative or nonoperative treatment results in superior long-term outcomes. Only one of the four included studies specifically considered older patients [37]. This study included 36 patients with a mean age of 66 years, randomized to closed reduction or operative treatment. Operatively treated patients had a higher functional outcome score and range of motion after 2 years and a better anatomical reduction. The nonoperative group showed more loss of reduction. However, there was no intention-to-treat analysis where 11 patients did not participate.

Since this Cochrane review, there have been no new randomized controlled trials (RCTs) to inform the management of AFs in geriatric patients. Currently, anatomical reduction and stable internal fixation is recommended, if the soft tissues around the ankle and the patient's health are not surgical contraindications.

### 7.2 Stable versus unstable injury

There is no "true" definition for an unstable AF, but we know medial joint space widening is indicative of mortise displacement. Understanding the trauma mechanism according to Lauge-Hansen is essential for adequate treatment [33]. Ankle mortise incongruity is poorly tolerated and leads to abnormal loads on the articular cartilage [38]. The apparent long-term advantage of anatomical restoration relevant for younger patients may not be realized for older adults due to shorter life expectancy. The development of end-stage osteoarthritis can take up to 20 years [46], although some disabling changes can develop within 1 year [47]. There is a tendency towards nonoperative treatment in geriatric patients, even with fracture patterns that would demand operative treatment in younger patients. It is not clear if the time course and outcomes of nonoperative treatment are clearly understood; it is possible that osteoarthritis may develop more quickly in older adults, making exact reduction even more important than in young patients. This dilemma stresses the need for personalized decision making.

Historically, a prolonged period of immobilization and nonweight bearing was advised for osteoporotic fractures. However, deficits in coordination, baseline impaired mobility and reduced arm strength required for the use of crutches increase the risk of falling and often limit nonweight-bearing rehabilitation. Such functional immobilization in older adults can lead to catastrophic complications including pressure sores, sarcopenia, joint stiffness, and permanent loss of function (see chapter 1.8 Postoperative surgical management).

Long-term outcomes may be irrelevant to patients in the last months to years of life, but even poor short-term outcomes may have a significant negative impact on the lives of older adults. Direct operative stabilization can facilitate enhanced postoperative mobilization and recovery. Most authors agree that standard internal fixation techniques are recommended in patients younger than 80 years [48] and open reduction and internal fixation (ORIF) is superior to closed reduction [49–54], as claimed by Makwena et al [37]. However, chronological age alone should not dictate treatment selection in geriatric patients but should be based on preinjury functional status and comorbidity. From a mechanical point of view, operative fixation of fractures in osteoporotic bone requires a larger contact area between bone and implant. This implies that at least an equal amount of implant contact is needed as in young patients to maintain reduction and fixation. Generally, in operative treatment of AFs in geriatric patients, there is little room for error and a meticulous operative technique is important [55, 56].

## 8 Therapeutic options

The authors of this chapter performed a systematic search for relevant articles in the Medline and Embase databases from the year 2000, identifying 394 potentially relevant articles that were all screened for possible use in this chapter. This yielded 55 relevant articles, which are referenced throughout this chapter.

### 8.1 Nonoperative treatment

If the ankle mortise is stable and congruent, unimalleolar fibular fractures in mobile older patients can be best treated nonoperatively. Operatively treated patients show better radiographic alignment but no better functional outcome [57]. The outcomes of a nonoperative approach cannot be determined from a simple x-ray or protocol only. Pain, pretraumatic physical and mental health, local soft-tissue injury, and socioeconomic status of the patient are important additional determinants. The goal of nonoperative treatment is to make life as comfortable as possible during the period of fracture healing. Early weight bearing during this period is preferred. For severe pain, a plaster cast can be an excellent analgesic, but unfortunately can be highly problematic in older adults. A simple lower leg cast can lead to catastrophic complications related to immobility. Once fracture-related pain and swelling have subsided, a plaster cast should be removed and replaced by a device that provides more comfort and allows weight-bearing mobilization. A high shoe or removable boot can be appropriate [58, 59]. Such a tailored therapy requires intensive follow-up, especially in the early phase. Immobilization should not exceed 4–5 weeks in healthy older adults, although there have been recommendations for longer non-weight bearing for patients with diabetes [60]. However, a recent paper suggested that the number of complications of nonoperative treatment exceeds those after surgery [61].

Nonoperative treatment is also indicated in wheelchair-bound or bedridden patients for both stable and unstable fractures simply because anatomical reduction of the ankle joint and internal fixation will not produce improvement in mobility or function. Although a plaster cast will reduce pain in the group of immobile patients, attention should be paid to local soft-tissue problems in this group, as these patients are often at exceptional risk for the development of pressure sores related to the cast. These patients not only develop outside-in skin problems due to the cast, but also dislocation of the fracture can result in inside-out skin problems, especially at the medial aspect of the ankle. A plaster cast immobilizing both ankle and knee might reduce this risk, but in this particular group minimally invasive surgical stabilization may be a better alternative (**Case 4: Fig 3.17-4**).

**CASE 4**

**Patient**

An 89-year-old woman fell while going to bed in her nursing home after consuming alcohol. Before this fall, she was able to walk with a walker inside the house. The patient used an orthopedic shoe because of preexisting drop foot.

X-rays after reduction (**Fig 3.17-4a–b**) show an atypical fracture configuration. The oblique lateral malleolar fracture fits a supination-external rotation injury (type B fracture), but they usually start anterior at the level of the joint space. This fracture is situated more proximally, suggesting a type C ankle fracture. But a typical type C fracture is horizontal or multifragmentary. The medial malleolar fracture in type B fractures is horizontal, whereas in type C fractures it is vertical. Medially, a small skin abrasion with severe edema was present (**Fig 3.17-4c–d**); sensation was absent due to known neuropathy.

**Comorbidities**

- Multiple myocardial infarctions with cardiac failure and atrial fibrillation
- Chronic obstructive pulmonary disease Gold 1
- Type 2 diabetes mellitus with peripheral polyneuropathy
- Hypertension
- Cerebrovascular accident
- Left total knee replacement complicated by pulmonary embolism
- Right total hip replacement
- Cataract surgery of both eyes
- Frequent falling
- Urinary incontinence

### Treatment and outcome

She was scheduled for delayed surgery but developed blisters on the heel, first and second toes, and medial malleolus. Wound healing was delayed because of occlusion of the superficial femoral artery requiring revascularization. Osteosynthesis was therefore cancelled. She left the hospital after 12 days. The fibular fracture healed in malunion before the wounds healed. Seven months after the accident the medial malleolus had developed a nonunion with tibiotalar incongruity (**Fig 3.17-4e–f**). Calcaneotalotibial arthrodesis with a hindfoot nail was considered, but not done because the patient had little pain when mobilizing in orthopedic shoes.

### Discussion

An acceptable functional result can be achieved in older patients with severe comorbidities because of reduced functional requirements. In young patients, this fracture configuration would be a clear indication for surgery.

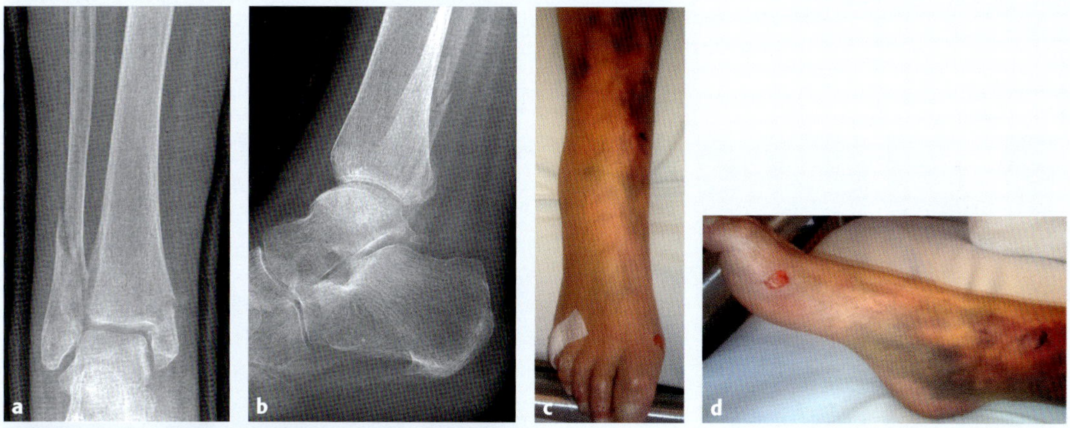


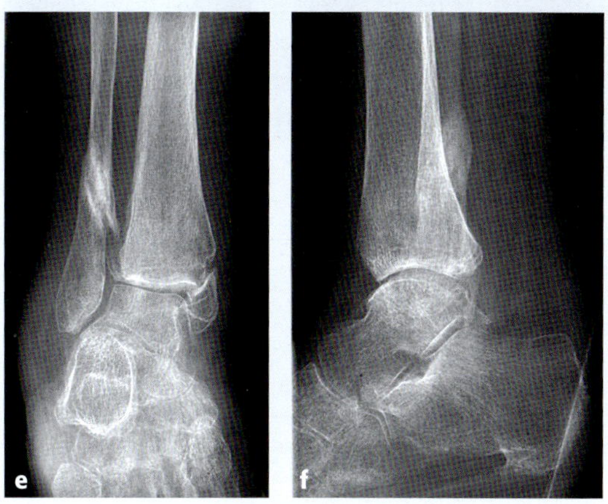


**Fig 3.17-4a–f** An 89-year-old woman with poor soft tissues in a type C fracture.
**a–b** AP (**a**) and lateral (**b**) views of the injury.
**c** AP view showing soft-tissue swelling and hematoma.
**d** Lateral view showing blisters, hematoma, and swelling.
**e** AP view showing medial nonunion 7 months after nonoperative treatment.
**f** Lateral view showing fibular union 7 months after nonoperative treatment.

## 8.2 Primary treatment in unstable fractures

The incidence of posttraumatic soft-tissue compromise is high due to several risk factors. First, older skin is atrophic making it more prone to injury. Second, in unstable AFs, the skin is easily torn at the time of dislocation. The skin directly covering the medial malleolus is at highest risk. It lacerates relatively easily, immediately resulting in a grade 2 open AF. Since most AFs are supination-external rotation injuries, anteromedial skin problems are common. Third, in both closed and open unstable fractures skin perfusion around the medial malleolus is diminished due to microvascular disruptions. Skin ischemia may not only result in posttraumatic or postsurgical skin necrosis, but also in postoperative wound infections. Prevention of a second ischemic insult to the soft tissues surrounding the medial malleolus is of utmost importance. Finally, hematoma formation in older adults can be extensive, particularly in the presence of anticoagulation (**Case 5: Fig 3.17-5**).

CASE 5

### Patient

An 86-year-old woman fell in the gutter while walking and talking to a friend. She sustained a displaced closed bimalleolar right ankle fracture dislocation, which was reduced in the emergency department (**Fig 3.17-5a–b**). A plaster cast was applied. Five days later she presented to the fracture clinic with secondary displacement and threatened skin with poor skin perfusion (**Fig 3.17-5c–d**).

### Comorbidities

- Hypertension
- Cerebrovascular accident
- Hemiarthroplasty of the left hip because of fracture

### Treatment and outcome

The fracture was reduced in the operating room and fixed with an external fixator with Schanz screws in the distal tibia, calcaneus, and base of the first metatarsal bone (**Fig 3.17-5e–f**). Despite reduction, the patient developed skin ulcers with progressive infection while taking antibiotics (**Fig 3.17-5g**). Vascular analysis showed diffuse atherosclerosis without operative vascular reconstruction being possible. The patient was scheduled for below-knee amputation. She refused surgery and died 3 weeks later.

### Discussion

Unstable ankle joints frequently redislocate in a plaster cast. In this case surgical stabilization was performed after such a redislocation. Immediate operative stabilization, eventually with a joint spanning external fixation, might have prevented this sad course.

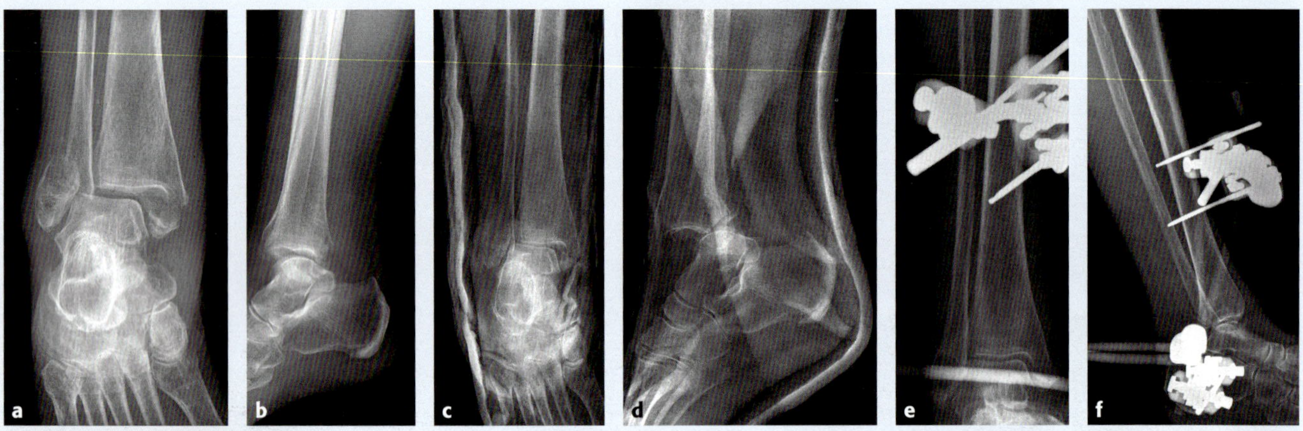


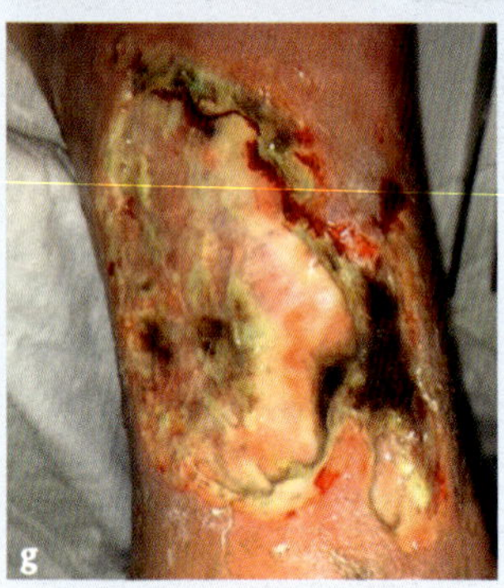


**Fig 3.17-5a–g** An 86-year-old woman with a displaced closed bimalleolar fracture.
**a–b** AP (**a**) and lateral (**b**) views of the injury.
**c–d** AP (**c**) and lateral (**d**) views showing secondary dislocation in a plaster cast after 5 days.
**e** AP view showing postoperative x-ray after external fixation.
**f** Lateral view with external fixation.
**g** Severe anterior ankle skin ulcers.

For these reasons, the surgeon should have a low threshold to apply an immediate joint-spanning external fixator in older adults with unstable AFs, and wait until the soft tissues have recovered enough to allow for definitive surgery. The severity of soft-tissue injury is often underestimated in this situation. Only in select cases is provisional treatment with a plaster cast prior to definitive surgery feasible. Immediate ORIF should be reserved for the expert surgeon and patients with a high-pressure hematoma (to prevent skin necrosis).

### 8.3 Fibular fixation—locking plate, nonlocking plate, or screws

Controversy exists whether contoured locking plates provide improved fixation strength in osteoporotic distal fibular fractures [62–67]. A metaanalysis on experimental studies by Dingemans et al [68] did not reveal a biomechanical benefit of locking plates. Fixation of simple oblique supination-external rotation fractures with a conventional lag screw and a neutralizing one-third tubular plate, or a dorsally applied antiglide plate yield similar fixation strength [69]. However, locking plates are presumably beneficial to multifragmentary fractures in osteoporotic bone [62, 70]. When compared to less bulky standard one-third tubular plates, standard small fragment locking plates can be associated with increased wound complications [71]. Less prominent and contoured plates with locking options can reduce this problem (**Case 6: Fig 3.17-6**).

CASE 6

**Patient**

A 74-year-old man fell from a ladder and sustained a Gustilo grade 2 open bimalleolar type B ankle fracture (**Fig 3.17-6a–c**).

**Comorbidities**

- Angina pectoris with percutaneous cardiac intervention
- Hypertension and a possible stroke or cerebrovascular ischemia history (transient cerebral ischemia attack).

**Treatment and outcome**

He was brought to the operating room for a wound washout, fixation, and wound closure. A small fragment locking compression plate was used for the fixation of the lateral malleolus. The distal fragment was fixated with a single angular stable screw, whereas both conventional and angular stable screws were used proximally. The medial malleolus was fixed with one K-wire and one partially threaded screw (**Fig 3.17-6d–e**). A plaster was applied until wound healing with frequent wound inspections. Wound and bone healing were uneventful. The patient was very happy and functioning well.

**Discussion**

Direct rigorous wound cleaning and a stable fixation of the lateral malleolus yielded a good result.

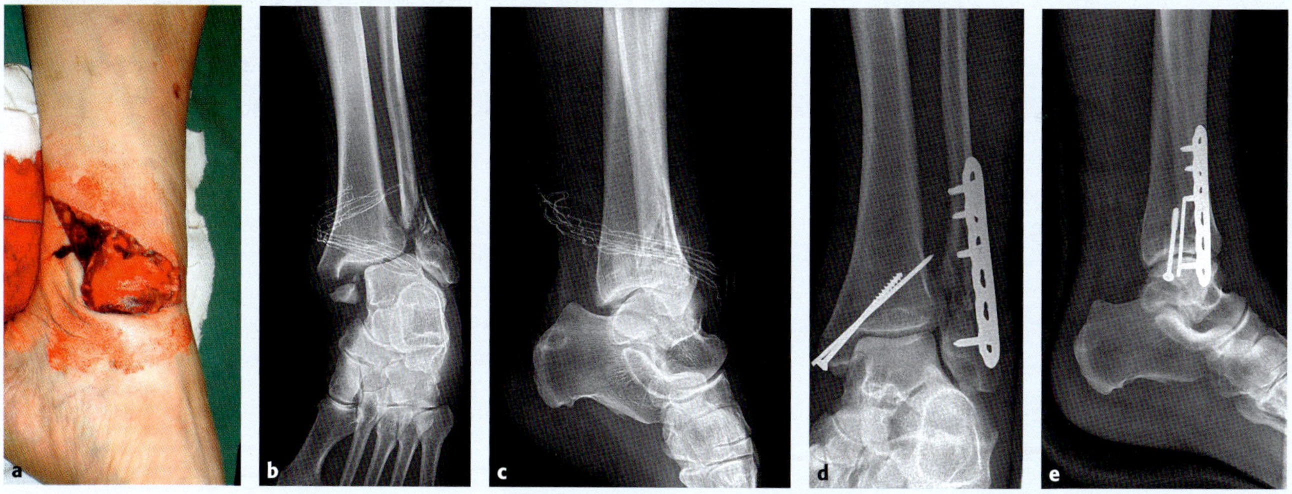


**Fig 3.17-6a–e** A 74-year-old man with a Gustilo grade 2 open bimalleolar type B fracture.
**a** Medial wound in the emergency department.
**b–c** AP (**b**) and lateral (**c**) views of the injury.
**d–e** AP (**d**) and lateral (**e**) views showing the postoperative result.

In cases of supination-external rotation injury, the plate should be positioned over the proximal apex of the fracture, the posterior aspect of the fibula; this effectively neutralizes the shear forces (antiglide principle) on the fracture to secure a stable construct (**Case 7: 3.17-7**) [72]. A posteriorly applied plate compressed with bicortical screw(s) also reduces the risk of iatrogenic joint perforation and the degree of implant irritation as compared to a laterally applied plate [56]. After the proper positioning of an appropriately sized plate, secured by at least one nonlocking bicortical screw, construct stability can be improved with locked head screws.

CASE 7

### Patient

A 78-year-old woman was involved in a high-energy motor vehicle collision, sustaining a distal radial fracture, 12 rib fractures, and a left bimalleolar fracture and possible posterior malleolar fracture (**Fig 3.17-7a–b**). No computed tomographic (CT) scan was obtained. Despite epidural anesthesia and pulmonary physiotherapy, pneumonia developed. Surgery was rescheduled twice due to poor soft tissues with blisters at the side of the incisions. The patient was operated after 20 days.

### Comorbidities

- Invasive breast cancer requiring lumpectomy, radiotherapy, and hormonal therapy
- Percutaneous cardiac intervention
- Diabetes mellitus type 2
- Hysterectomy due to clear cell carcinoma

### Treatment and outcome

Twenty days after the accident, a one-third tubular bridging plate was placed with some cortical and locking screws in the lateral malleolus. The medial malleolus was fixed using two relatively short partially threaded screws with washer. The surgeon noticed the screws had little grip, which is indicative of severe osteoporosis. The syndesmosis was not tested during surgery. Image intensification at operation shows a blurry but congruent distal tibiofibular joint (**Fig 3.17-7c–d**). But postoperative x-rays show slowly increasing lateralization of the talus (**Fig 3.17-7e–f**). The medial wound dehisced and became infected. Hardware at the medial malleolus was removed 3 months after stabilization (**Fig 3.17-7g–h**) and the infection was treated with antibiotics. This led to a chronic bone infection with constant pain (Visual Analog Scale 4/10) confirmed on nuclear leukocyte scan 5 months after surgery. Patient declined any further intervention.

### Discussion

This case stresses that one should be extremely careful in older patients with comorbidities. A preoperative CT scan can provide valuable information on both the exact fracture configuration and the bone quality. Single-shot surgery without any compromise or revision by an experienced surgeon is prerequisite. A critical evaluation of technical execution in this case reveals that the reduction of the lateral malleolus is fair, but fixation is not rigid enough. The plate is placed too anterior, forcing the screws in a medial direction. Therefore, screws are short. A more posterior position of a stronger and longer plate would direct the screws anteriorly and improve the mechanical support. Reduction of the medial malleolus appears fair as well, but like in the previous case, the compression screws are too short. At this level of the metaphysis, no screw purchase is experienced in osteoporotic bone. They should be exchanged immediately for longer ones reaching the lateral cortex of the tibia. An additional support of a cerclage wire or a regular tension band can provide sufficient strength to neutralize the pull force of the deltoid ligament.

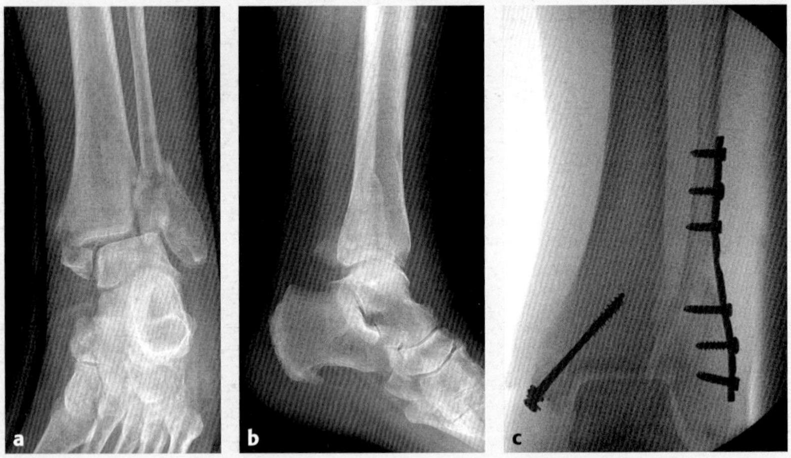


**Fig 3. 17-7a–h** A 78-year-old woman with a bi- or trimalleolar fracture after a high-energy trauma.
**a–b** AP (**a**) and lateral (**b**) views of the injury.
**c** AP image intensifier view showing a blurry syndesmosis.

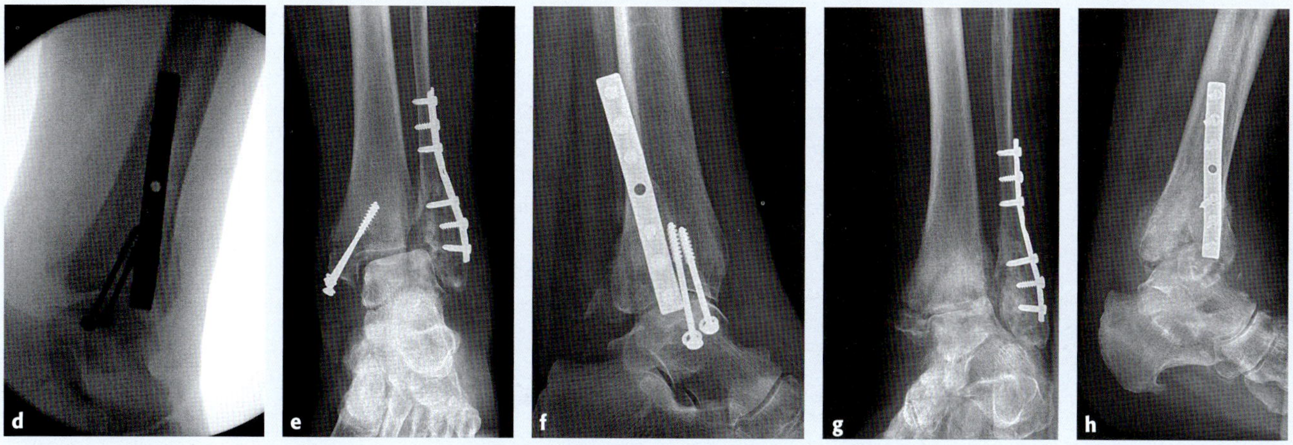


**Fig 3. 17-7a–h (cont)** A 78-year-old woman with a bi- or trimalleolar fracture after a high-energy trauma.
**d** Lateral image intensifier view suggesting a posterior malleolar fracture.
**e** Postoperative x-ray showing an incongruent ankle joint.
**f** Postoperative lateral view with suspicion of a posterior malleolar fracture.
**g** AP view after hardware removal of the medial malleolus because of infection 3 months after prior surgery.
**h** Lateral view after medial hardware removal showing destruction of the ankle joint.

The incision should be at the posterior border of the fibula. Distal from the lateral malleolus the incision can be curved anteriorly to allow tension-free exposure of the bone. Despite the presence of tissue swelling and/or a plate and screws, the skin can be closed tension-free. Once healed, the patient will not be limited by the atrophic scar in this functional area. A posterolateral approach also allows a direct exposure of the lateral 40% of the posterior malleolus [73]. Of course, the surgeon should be aware of the presence of the sural nerve posterior to the incision. A pure lateral incision straight to the bone is not advocated, as it is more prone to impaired wound healing, especially if the plate is positioned laterally or even anterolaterally. The surgeon should also be familiar with variations in the course of the superficial peroneal nerve. This structure is at a considerable risk for iatrogenic injury in a straight lateral or anterolateral operative approach. In more than 15% of patients, it crosses the distal fibula from posterior to anterior [74, 75]. Neurotmesis will often result in a painful neuroma.

Plate position must also respect the peroneal tendon groove distally to prevent irritation of these tendons, especially in posteriorly placed plates [76]. Several authors advocate minimally invasive percutaneous extraperiostally plate osteosynthesis (MIPPO) in type B and C fractures to prevent wound complications, but this requires special surgical expertise regarding indirect fracture reduction [77, 78]. To date there is no RCT comparing ORIF versus MIPPO in AFs. Open anatomical reduction and internal fixation remains the gold standard, and the majority of skin complications may be prevented with a posterolateral operative approach.

Lag screws alone reduce the amount of hardware laterally and thus the risk of soft-tissue irritation. Although this technique can yield good results in oblique supination-external rotation fractures [79, 80], it is not recommended in osteoporotic bone. If the "implant holding capacity" of the bone is reduced, an increased bone-implant interface is required to obtain a safe construct (**Case 8: Fig 3.17-8**).

CASE 8

### Patient

A 90-year-old woman was found in the morning by a care provider in the nursing home. Presumably she had fallen out of the chair in her room. She sustained a closed supination-external rotation stage IV fracture dislocation (**Fig 3.17-8a–b**). The dislocation was reduced by the ambulance paramedics.

### Comorbidities

- Severe dementia
- Congestive heart failure and atrial fibrillation
- Transient cerebral ischemic attacks
- Venous insufficiency
- Femoral neck fracture in the past

### Treatment and outcome

Nonoperative therapy with a plaster cast was started (**Fig 3.17-8c–d**). After 10 days, dorsal dislocation of the foot was observed (**Fig 3.17-8e–f**). Although her cardiopulmonary status was bad, it was decided to perform an open reduction and internal fixation. She could only be operated in a semi-sitting position. The lateral malleolus was reduced and fixed first. Because the purchase of the screws was poor, the surgeon used both a reconstruction plate and a one-third tubular plate. The fibula was fixed to the tibia with multiple screws, none having good purchase. It was hard to subsequently reduce the medial malleolus. Together with the talus, there was a continuous tendency to dislocate dorsally. Despite a compression screw, K-wire, and a buttress plate, there was still a tendency to dislocate. Therefore, an additional tension band using a nonresorbable suture wire was applied anteriorly, as reflected by the AP screw with washer on the x-rays taken the day after surgery (**Fig 3.17-8g–h**). All these efforts did not prevent redislocation of the ankle joint as shown on the images after 6 weeks (**Fig 3.17-8i–j**). No further surgery was performed. The patient died 3 months later.

### Discussion

Both decision making and the technical execution of surgery on ankle fractures in older adults can be challenging. The use of multiple locking plates in various directions and fixation to the tibia are good options if the bone quality is bad. This patient would have benefited from a more extensive exposure to elucidate the reason of nonreduction of the medial malleolus and talus. The posterior redislocation of the talus emphasizes the importance of achieving sound fixation of the posterior malleolus to prevent redislocation. However, cardiac limitations did not allow optimal positioning of the patient on the operating table.

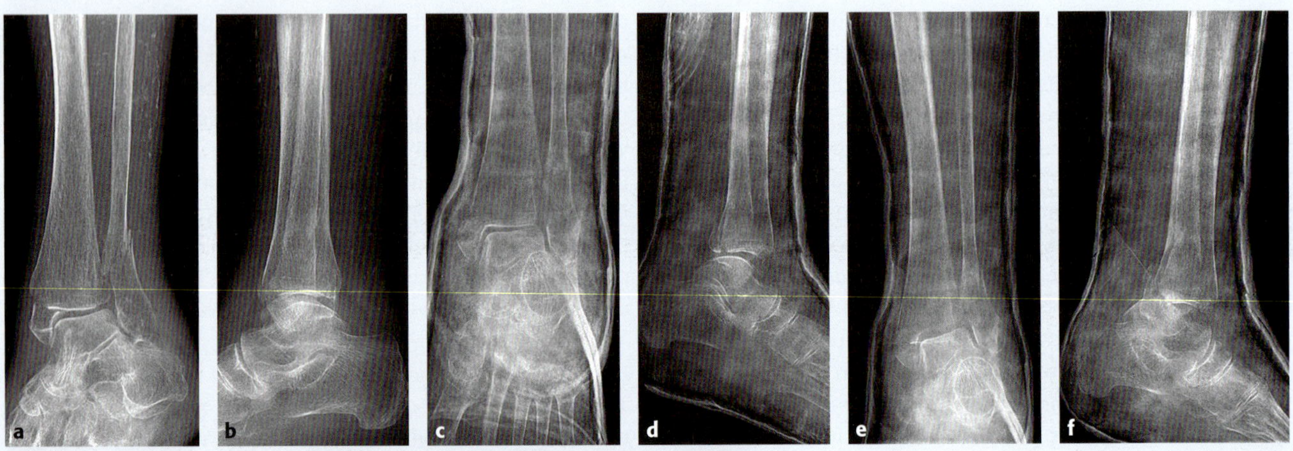

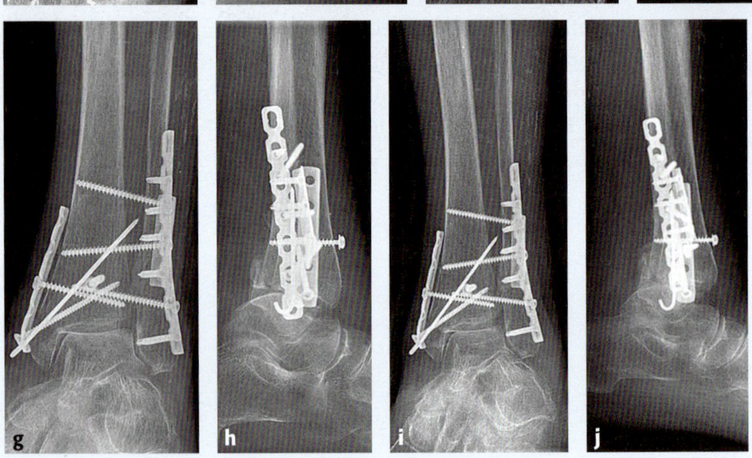

**Fig 3.17-8a–j** A 90-year-old woman with a closed supination-external rotation stage IV fracture dislocation.
**a–b** AP (**a**) and lateral (**b**) views of the injury.
**c–d** AP (**c**) and lateral (**d**) views in a plaster cast.
**e** AP view showing talar tilt after 10 days.
**f** Lateral view showing dorsal dislocation of the foot after 10 days.
**g** Postoperative AP view showing both a reconstruction plate and a one-third tubular plate. The fibula was fixed to the tibia with multiple screws. Medial using a buttress plate and K-wires.
**h** Postoperative lateral view confirming a tendency of dorsal dislocation of the foot.
**i–j** AP (**i**) and lateral (**j**) views 6 weeks after surgery.

### 8.4 Fibular fixation—intramedullary nails

Nailing of a fibular fracture is a new option and advocated by some in osteoporotic AFs. It seems a safe and minimally invasive option for unstable fractures when locking screws are used [81]. It produces few wound complications, provides a (rotational) stable construct, and good functional outcome [82, 83]. Besides small surgical incisions, it also leaves the fracture hematoma intact and does not require soft-tissue stripping. The number of soft-tissue complications after an intramedullary (IM) nail may be less than after plate osteosynthesis [84]. This could be particularly relevant to older adults with poor soft-tissue condition. However, it can be difficult to properly reduce length and rotation of the fracture, since the fracture is not open. The use of an IM fibular nail in spiral fractures "asking" for a posterior antiglide plate has not yet been investigated but seems illogical from a conceptual point of view. More research is needed to reveal the best design and positioning of an IM nail and appropriate surgical indications (**Case 9: Fig 3.17-9, Case 10: Fig 3.17-10**).

**CASE 9**

**Patient**

An 89-year-old woman had a fall at home sustaining a Gustilo grade 2 open trimalleolar fracture (Lauge-Hansen supination-external rotation stage IV) (**Fig 3.17-9a–b**).

**Comorbidities**

- Hypertension
- Alzheimer
- Chronic obstructive pulmonary disease Gold 3

**Treatment and outcome**

After an immediate washout and reduction of the joint, osteosynthesis was performed. Due to the very atrophic skin, an indirect reduction of the fibular fracture and internal fixation with a fibular nail was chosen. Note the very distal locking option into the tibia penetrating the distal tibiofibular joint. Due to the multifragmentary nature of the medial malleolus, multiple K-wires were used to give base to tension band wiring (**Fig 3.17-9c–d**). The postoperative x-rays were taken 3 days after surgery. To support soft-tissue healing, a plaster back slab was given (**Fig 3.17-9e–f**). Unfortunately, the patient died after 3 weeks due to heart failure and bilateral pneumonia. No local complications had been observed.

**Discussion**

This case shows the use of a fibular nail. Good indirect reduction and anatomical fixation is possible, but a fibular nail is not a solution for the most delicate soft-tissue problems always occurring at the medial side of the ankle.

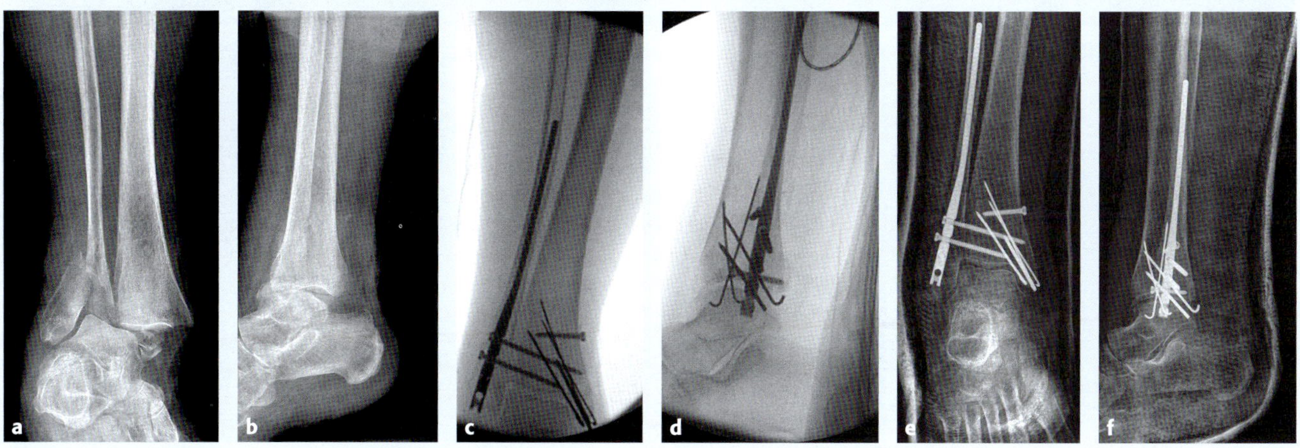


**Fig 3.17-9a–f** An 89-year-old woman with a Gustilo grade 2 open trimalleolar fracture.
**a–b** AP (**a**) and lateral (**b**) views of the injury.
**c** AP image intensifier view of a fibular nail and medial K-wires for tension band wiring.
**d** Lateral image intensifier view of a fibular nail and perpendicular K-wires for tension band wiring.
**e–f** Postoperative AP (**e**) and lateral (**f**) x-rays in a plaster cast for wound healing.

CASE 10

## Patient

A 67-year-old woman fell while walking. She sustained a Gustilo grade 2 open ankle fracture (Lauge-Hansen pronation-external rotation stage IV) (**Fig 3.17-10a–b**).

## Comorbidities

- No comorbidities known at presentation

## Treatment and outcome

Initial treatment consisted of immediate lavage of the ankle joint, wound debridement, screw osteosynthesis of the medial malleolus, wound closure, and a joint-spanning external fixator (**Fig 3.17-10c–d**). After 6 days, the external fixator was exchanged for a minimal exposure fibular intramedullary nail (**Fig 3.17-10e**). X-rays after 6 weeks showed good congruency of the ankle joint and position of fracture fragments. The joint space was adequate (**Fig 3.17-10f–g**). One year after trauma the fractures had healed, but traumatic arthritic changes were developing explaining the patient's pain. As a result of cartilage loss, the fibula impinged to the lateral side of the talus, resulting in lateralization and widening of the distal tibiofibular joint (**Fig 3.17-10h–i**). Four years after surgery both pain and osteoarthritic changes had progressed, but the patient refused arthrodesis (**Fig 3.17-10j–k**).

## Discussion

Pronation-external rotation injuries have a poor prognosis, especially in older adults. A staged procedure is feasible to minimize the risk of a bacterial arthritis. Despite a good tibiotalar alignment and the absence of infectious complication, severe posttraumatic osteoarthritis developed in this case. However, this cannot be attributed to the use of a fibular nail.

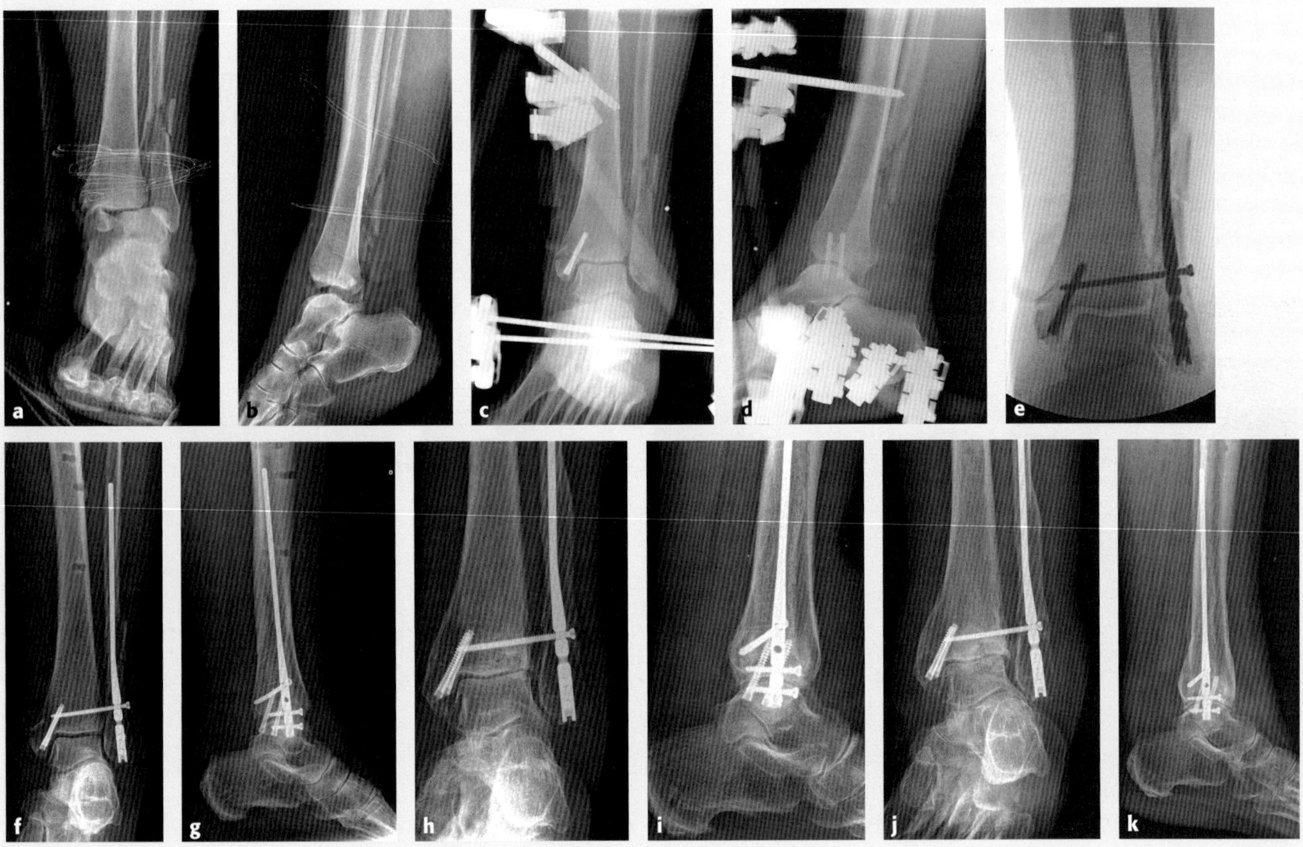


**Fig 3.17-10a–k** A 76-year-old woman with a Gustilo grade 2 open fracture.
**a–b** AP (**a**) and lateral (**b**) views of the injury.
**c–d** AP (**c**) and lateral (**d**) views after external fixation.
**e** Image intensification during conversion to a fibular nail and medial screws. The chosen medial screws are much too short. Ideally, they penetrate the opposite cortex.
**f–g** AP (**f**) and lateral (**g**) views showing congruent joint after 6 weeks.
**h** AP view showing traumatic arthritis with lateral impingement 1 year after surgery.
**i** Lateral view one year after surgery.
**j** AP view showing progression of traumatic arthritis 4 years postoperative.
**k** Lateral view 4 years after surgery.

### 8.5 Syndesmotic positioning screw

In older adults, the syndesmosis is less often injured because osteoporotic bone fails earlier than the ligamentous syndesmotic bands and membrane. Therefore, fractures are most often seen below the level of the syndesmosis and screws that aim to position a reconstructed fibula to the tibia are not typically required. However, syndesmotic screws can be used to add extra stability to a reconstructed osteoporotic fibular shaft, and the tibia can be used as an extra medial anchor. In general, syndesmotic screws penetrating four cortices provide more stability than bicortical fibular screws in osteoporotic fibular fractures (**Case 11: Fig 3.17-11**) [85].



**Patient**

A 79-year-old woman sustained a closed trimalleolar fracture dislocation after a fall at home (**Fig 3.17-11a–b**).

**Comorbidities**

- Type 2 diabetes mellitus
- Cataract
- Polymyalgia rheumatica for which the patient used prednisone
- Diverticulitis
- Previous operative reconstruction of left quadriceps rupture
- Hypertension
- Chronic obstructive pulmonary disease

**Treatment and outcome**

Due to poor soft tissues, surgery was delayed for 12 days. A one-third tubular plate was used to fix the fibular fracture. The medial malleolus was fixed with two partially threaded cancellous screws. The tibiotalar stability was still considered insufficient at testing. This fits better to a pronation-abduction stage III injury than a supination-external rotation stage IV fracture. A syndesmotic screw was placed (**Fig 3.17-11c–d**). Wound closure was difficult due to the remaining soft-tissue swelling. Postoperatively, the lateral incision dehisced, which resolved with local wound care. After healed fractures, the patient has pain while walking but uses no assistive devices.

**Discussion**

Although fixation would be more rigid with a locking compression plate, in this case a less bulky one-third tubular locking plate was used. Nevertheless, wound closure was difficult. In general, syndesmotic screws penetrating four cortices provide more stability [85] and should be placed at least below the level of the fracture.

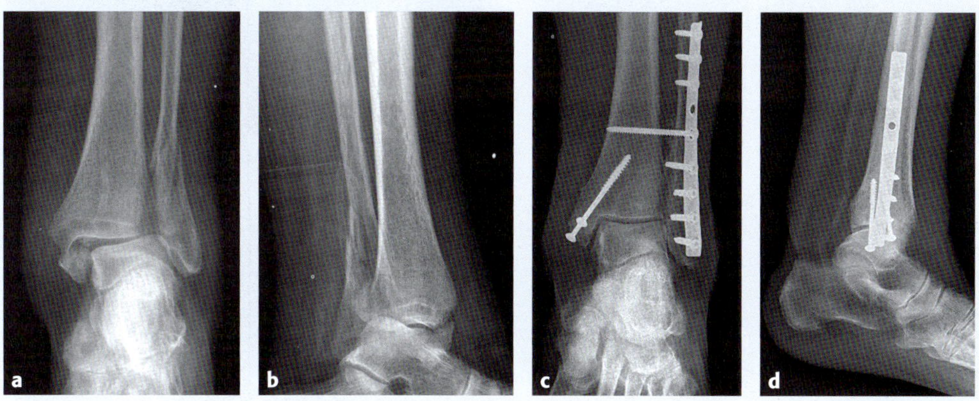


**Fig 3.17-11a–d** A 79-year-old woman with a trimalleolar fracture.
**a–b** AP (**a**) and lateral (**b**) views of the injury.
**c–d** Postoperative AP (**c**) and lateral (**d**) views.

### 8.6 Medial malleolar fixation

For medial malleolar fractures, the geometry of the fracture should be taken into account. Transverse fractures can be best treated with tension bands, with less need for revision surgery compared to lag screws. Even with small fragments, K-wires can often be placed and the tension band wire can be wrapped around the K-wires and deltoid ligament, and fixed in a figure-of-eight fashion. Oblique fractures can be treated with lag screws perpendicular to the fracture line. In these cases, long screws penetrating the lateral tibial cortex provide more stability than partially threaded cancellous screws ending in the metaphyseal bone of the distal tibia [86, 87]. Particularly in osteoporotic fractures, partially and incompletely threaded screws are preferred since a smaller drill diameter can be used for the distal part. The use of washers is mandatory in osteoporotic bone to provide compression. Vertical fractures require additional stabilization because of shear forces and show superior outcomes with buttress plating [88]. Vertical shear fractures in supination-adduction injuries are often accompanied with tibial plafond impaction cartilage lesions. Such lesions need disimpaction and, in osteoporotic bone, subchondral support (**Case 12: Fig 3.17-12**, **Case 13: Fig 3.17-13**).

CASE 12

## Patient

An 82-year-old man on a bike was hit by a car going at 60 km/h (37 mph). His left leg was trapped under the car. His only injury was a displaced bimalleolar pronation-abduction stage III fracture dislocation combined with a high fissure of the fibular shaft. This second fibular injury was judged as a direct impact injury, which required no surgery (**Fig 3.17-12a–b**).

## Comorbidities

- Alcohol abuse with liver steatosis
- Atrial fibrillation
- Glaucoma
- Cholecystectomy

## Treatment and outcome

The same day, the multifragmental fibular fracture was bridged with a one-third tubular plate. The oblique medial malleolar fracture was percutaneously secured with two relatively short partially threaded cancellous bone screws with washer. Intraoperatively, no diastasis was observed, but the postoperative x-rays showed insufficient compression of the medial fragment (**Fig 3.17-12c–e**). There was also some fibular shortening indicating instability. After 9 months, both fibular fractures had healed, but the medial malleolus had not (**Fig 3.17-12f–g**). The whole fibula was tender to palpation; there was still some edema and the patient required use of a stick for longer distances.

## Discussion

The final functional and radiographic outcome was not optimal. The x-rays show slight fibular shortening, lateralization of the talus, and a medial malleolus nonunion. Several explanations are possible. First, a 2-stage fibular fracture can be accompanied by an interosseous membrane rupture all the way up to the proximal fracture. The syndesmosis was neither tested nor fixed during surgery. Secondly, a one-third tubular plate is flexible, particularly if it is used as a bridging plate. The widening of the distal tibiofibular joint might have been prevented with the use of positioning screw(s) and/or a stronger plate. At the medial malleolus, the fracture appears not to be anatomically reduced. Interposition of a soft tissue is possible since fixation was percutaneously performed. Moreover, both medial screws are too short. At this level of the metaphysis the screw holding capacity in the older patient is low. Open and meticulous anatomical reduction combined with fully threaded screws penetrating the lateral cortex of the tibia would presumably have prevented the occurrence of this nonunion [86, 87]. Also, in this case there is severe osteoporosis (wide fibular canal with very thin cortex).

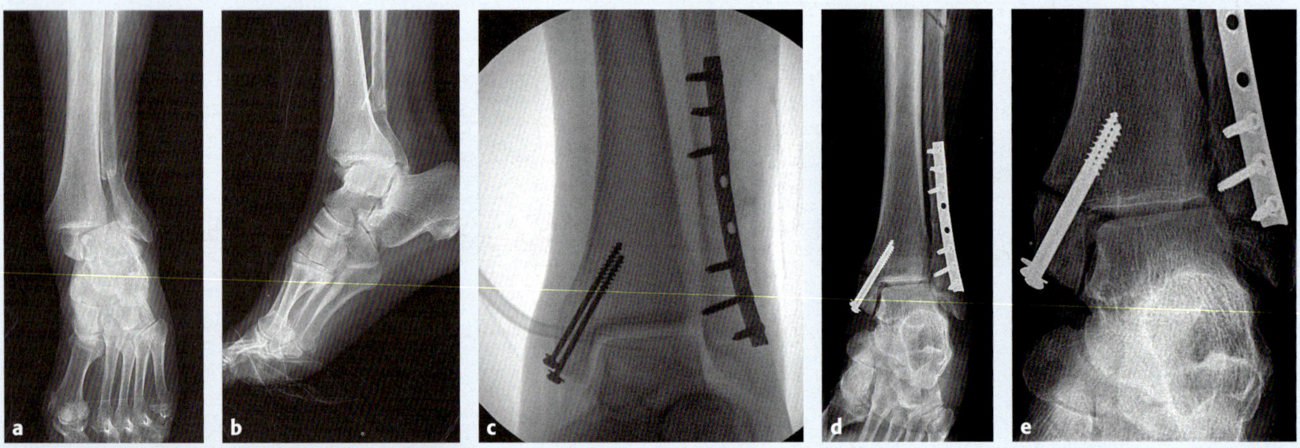


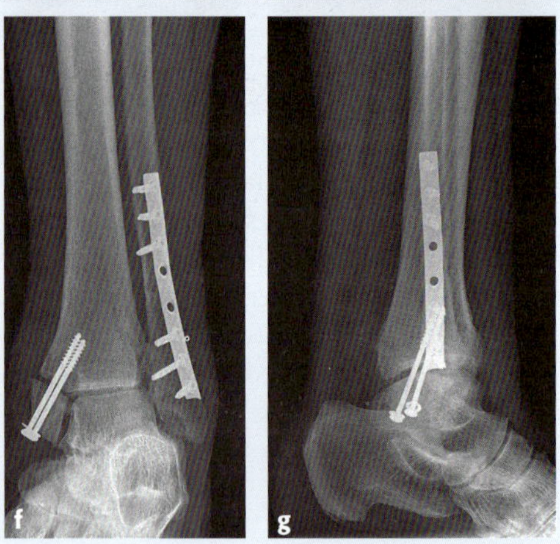


**Fig 3.17-12a–g** An 82-year-old man with a displaced bimalleolar pronation-abduction stage III fracture dislocation combined with a high fissure of the fibular shaft.
**a–b** AP (**a**) and lateral (**b**) views of the injury.
**c** Image intensification with a congruent joint.
**d** Postoperative AP view showing the high fibular fissure.
**e** Insufficient medial malleolar compression.
**f** Suggestion of fibular shortening.
**g** Lateral postoperative view.

### Patient

A 72-year-old woman fell while riding her bike and sustained an ipsilateral multifragmentary calcaneal fracture and a trimalleolar fracture dislocation (**Fig 3.17-13a–e**). Medial skin perfusion was compromised. Despite reduction by the paramedics, the initial x-ray at the emergency department showed a dislocated trimalleolar fracture. Closed reduction was performed and a plaster cast was applied.

### Comorbidities

- Curatively treated lymph node
- Positive breast cancer

### Treatment and outcome

Surgery was delayed 2 weeks due to poor soft tissues (**Fig 3.17-13f–g**). Medially, only K-wires were placed because of blisters. Laterally, a lag screw with neutralization plate was placed (**Fig 3.17-13h–i**). The calcaneal fracture was treated with nonweight-bearing plaster cast for 8 weeks. After removal of the medial K-wires, the patient could walk with orthopedic shoes using a walker (**Fig 3.17-13j–k**). The authors recommended primary external fixation and delayed percutaneous calcaneal fixation in this case. Now, there was a malunion of the medial malleolus and a widened hindfoot due to the calcaneal fracture, for which the patient used orthopedic shoes. Fortunately, she reported being pain free 9 months after surgery. Follow-up was limited to 1 year.

### Discussion

The primary concern is to reduce the fracture adequately in the prehospital setting in order to prevent soft-tissue problems, which influence treatment options. External fixation should play a central role in initial management.

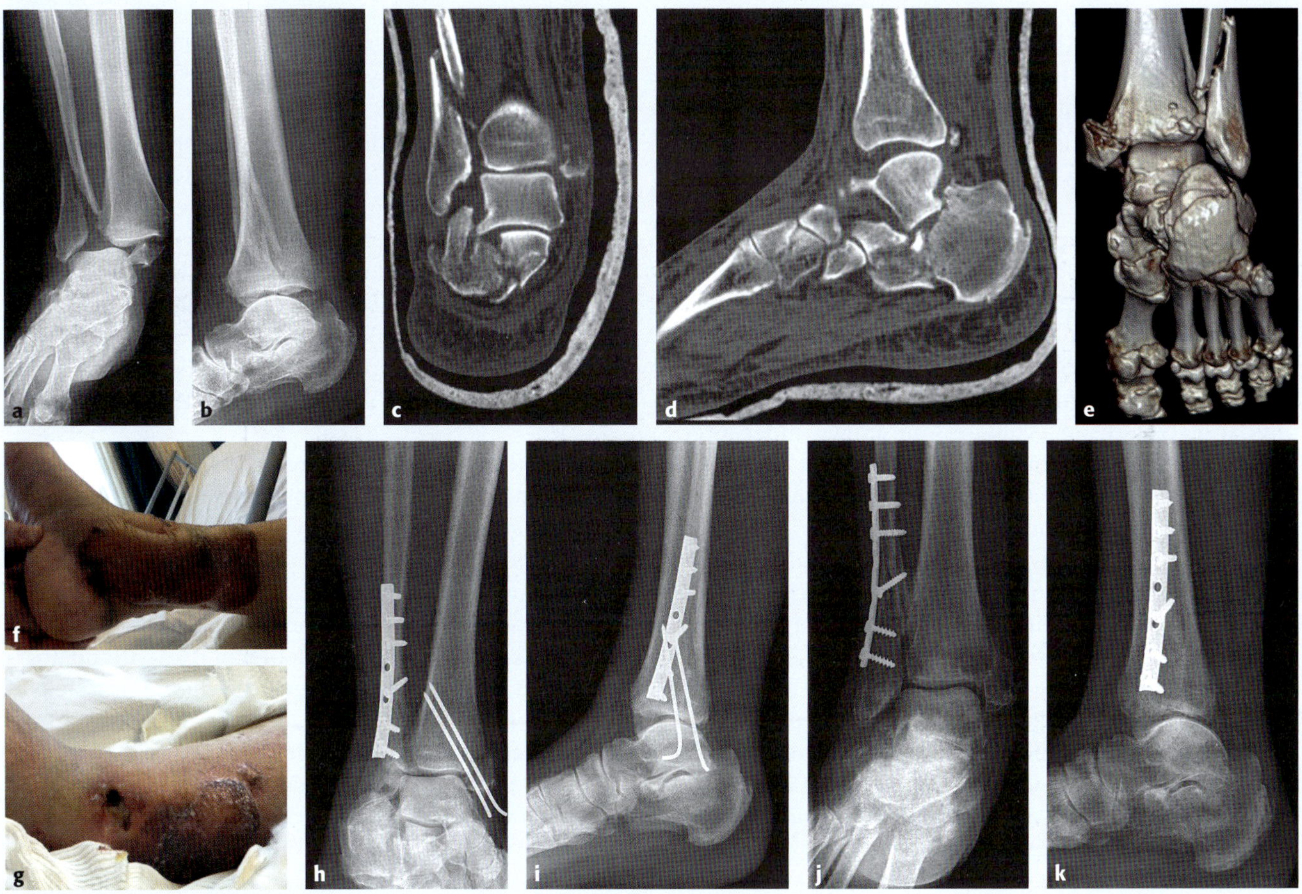


**Fig 3.17-13a–k** A 72-year-old woman with an ipsilateral multifragmentary calcaneal fracture and a trimalleolar fracture dislocation.
**a–b** AP (**a**) and lateral (**b**) views of the injury.
**c–d** Coronal (**c**) and sagittal (**d**) slices of computed tomography (CT) showing the calcaneal fracture.
**e** Three-dimensional CT reconstruction with dislocation of the hindfoot.
**f** Medial view showing severe soft-tissue swelling.
**g** Skin ulcer next to the blisters.
**h–i** Postoperative AP (**h**) and lateral (**i**) views after surgery of the ankle.
**j–k** AP (**j**) and lateral (**k**) views 1 year after surgery.

### 8.7 Posterior malleolar fixation

Whereas the criteria for and technique of fixation of a posterior malleolar fracture has not been a topic of interest in the past, recent biomechanical insights have demonstrated it is an important anatomical structure for proper function of the ankle joint. Assessment of the magnitude and shape of the fragment on plain lateral x-rays is unreliable since the fracture is not in line with the radiation beam. Assessment of the specific fracture configuration should be performed using a CT scan. Both Haraguchi and Bartonicek have described a classification system for posterior malleolar fractures based on CT scans [35, 89].

In displaced articular fractures of the posterolateral lip, one should have a low threshold for anatomical reduction and stable internal fixation. In the past, indirect reduction by maximum extension of the foot and the subsequent placement of a percutaneous AP lag screw was a widely accepted technique. However, the biomechanical, radiographic, and functional results of this technique appear inferior to a direct reduction and posterior-to-anterior fixation of the posterior malleolus with a lag screw with or without buttress plate [90, 91]. For posterolateral fractures, a single incision posterior to the fibula is advised for the exposure of both the lateral and posterior malleolar fracture [3, 92, 93]. This is best performed with the patient in a lateral decubitus or prone position. In the interval between the flexor and peroneal tendons, the posterior malleolus can easily be exposed. In this way, the fragment can be fixed with a one-third tubular plate and some compression screws under direct visualization of the fracture resulting in perfect anatomical congruity of the tibial plafond, rather than a single anterior screw that is not rotationally stable, particularly in osteoporotic bone. This strategy is less indicated in small shell-type fractures that do not involve the articular surface, but these are only a minority of the posterior fractures (14%) [89].

Another reason to fix the posterior malleolus is because the posterior syndesmotic ligament is attached to it. Proper anatomical reduction and stable fixation of this fragment improves stability of the lateral malleolus and adequately stabilizes the ankle mortise according to the Lauge-Hansen principles. This strategy may replace the use of positioning screws [94, 95]. However, in osteoporotic bone, an additional positioning screw may be required to secure the posterior-to-anterior fixation of the posterior malleolus.

### 8.8 Hindfoot nail, Steinman pin, or primary arthrodesis

The tibiotalar-calcaneal nail (hindfoot nail) allows for immediate mobilization with minimal risk for wound complications [96, 97], because its entry point is away from the fracture site and injured soft-tissue envelope. The nail is fixed with percutaneous locking screws above (distal tibia) and below (talus and/or calcaneus) the fracture site, providing a rigid construct. Prefracture mobility status can be achieved after removing the nail [98, 99].

A hindfoot nail is considered a salvage procedure for patients older than 80 years of age with more than two comorbidities and poor local soft-tissue status who cannot tolerate revision surgery. Inserting the nail damages the articular cartilage of calcaneus, talus, and tibia in the weight-bearing area. The nail is also used for arthrodesis in osteoarthritis. A systematic review showed an amputation rate of 1.5% after using a hindfoot nail in 613 patients [100].

The use of the much thinner Steinmann pin from plantar to the distal tibia as definitive care is considered obsolete. The Steinmann pin is not stable in the proximal metaphysis and shaft of the tibia. Moreover, it does not provide any rotational stability, unlike the hindfoot nail. Secondary dislocation is frequently encountered. From that point of view, an antegrade pin from the medial aspect of the distal tibia into the talus provides more stability. But like crossing Steinmann pins, it is still not a recommended treatment.

Primary arthrodesis can be an option in Gustilo grade 3 open multifragmentary fractures. A fibulectomy and tibial osteotomy removing approximately 1 cm of the distal tibia can be performed through a lateral incision to facilitate wound closure. Subsequently, osseous fixation can be achieved with a plate (95° blade plate or preshaped locking plate), external fixation [101], or hindfoot nail [102]. Although arthrodesis is considered a salvage procedure, it is a helpful treatment for local soft tissue, sometimes followed by a lengthy aftertreatment in case of delayed union or nonunion. Although arthrodesis can be done arthroscopically with percutaneous screws from anterior or posterior [103], this technique completely depends on the "implant holding capacity" of the tibia and talus. In osteoporotic AFs, this is obviously reduced.

### 8.9 External fixation

External fixation is always a good option for damage-control surgery. It provides a window for soft tissues to recover from the initial trauma before open reduction and definitive internal fixation is performed. However, in patients with poor skin condition or severe soft-tissue injury, external fixation can be an attractive option for definitive care. Pin-tract sites tend to get infected despite laborious pin-tract care. Operative ring fixation has shown to be successful in older adults with diabetes, peripheral vascular disease, and an unstable AF [104]. This can be used as a weight-bearing construct. Consolidation of the fracture should be tested before pin removal. In cases of delayed union, the bars/rings can be secured again.

### 8.10 Augmentation

In cases of severe osteoporosis, bone augmentation should be considered. This can facilitate direct postoperative weight bearing in a removable brace. Assal et al described good outcomes in 36 patients with type B fractures treated with augmented internal fixation using an IM wire, lateral plate, and screw augmentation with polymethylmethacrylate (PMMA) [19]. Treatment of infection is difficult when PMMA is in situ. Moreover, it is not biocompatible and highly exothermic inducing local osteonecrosis if not touching a metallic implant, which acts as a heat sink. A biomechanical study showed no difference in construct strength with or without augmentation in osteoporotic AF [85]. Based on current literature, standard augmentation has not yet gained general acceptance for osteoporotic AFs.

## 9 Aftertreatment

The ultimate goals of fracture treatment of older patients are early mobilization and pain control. Physical performance rapidly decreases in immobilized geriatric patients. Patients should be out of bed and into a chair as soon as possible to support good pulmonary function and prevent the occurrence of complications such as pressure ulcers, atelectasis, pneumonia, and muscle wasting. Patients should be encouraged to get out of the chair and mobilize (ie, stand and walk), with a walking aid if needed. Partial or non-weight bearing is often impossible in geriatric patients. Injury to the lower extremity affects mobility. Early and intensive rehabilitation in older adults can be as important as the management of the injury itself. Whereas in young patients the justification of an operative treatment is often a long-term benefit, in older adults the short-term advantages are important as well. Therefore, an osteosynthesis in the lower extremity should be performed in such a way that a plaster cast is not needed and immediate weight bearing is possible. In general, this requires more instead of less metal, as compared to young patients.

In the early phase after trauma or surgery, adequate analgesia is essential and consultation of a geriatrician can be helpful. The risk of falls and a second fracture should be assessed (see chapter 1.11 Sarcopenia, malnutrition, frailty, and falls), not only by bone densitometry and subsequent medical treatment of osteoporosis when appropriate (see chapter 1.10 Osteoporosis). Review of the patient's medication regimen, environment, and vision are essential. A physiotherapist not only provides tips, tricks, and walking aids, but also helps provide safety during exercise. A proper aftertreatment of AFs in geriatric patients is intensive and should be organized as such.

## 10 References

1. **Giannini S, Chiarello E, Persiani V, et al.** Ankle fractures in elderly patients. *Aging Clin Exp Res.* 2013 Oct;25(Suppl 1):S77–S79.
2. **Murray JC, Audet MC, Bedard M, et al.** Bilateral distal fibula fractures in a woman on long-term bisphosphonate therapy. *Osteoporos Int.* 2016 Feb;27(2):833–836.
3. **Zwipp H, Amlang M.** Frakturversorgung des oberen Sprunggelenks im hohen Lebensalter [Treatment of fractures of the ankle in the elderly]. *Orthopade.* 2014 Apr;43(4):332–338. German.
4. **Stufkens SA, Knupp M, Horisberger M, et al.** Cartilage lesions and the development of osteoarthritis after internal fixation of ankle fractures: a prospective study. *J Bone Joint Surg Am.* 2010 Feb;92(2):279–286.
5. **SooHoo NF, Krenek L, Eagan MJ, et al.** Complication rates following open reduction and internal fixation of ankle fractures. *J Bone Joint Surg Am.* 2009 May;91(5):1042–1049.
6. **SooHoo NF, Eagan M, Krenek L, et al.** Incidence and factors predicting pulmonary embolism and deep venous thrombosis following surgical treatment of ankle fractures. *Foot Ankle Surg.* 2011 Dec;17(4):259–262.
7. **Zaghloul A, Haddad B, Barksfield R, et al.** Early complications of surgery in operative treatment of ankle fractures in those over 60: a review of 186 cases. *Injury.* 2014 Apr;45(4):780–783.
8. **Korim MT, Payne R, Bhatia M.** A case-control study of surgical site infection following operative fixation of fractures of the ankle in a large U.K. trauma unit. *Bone Joint J.* 2014 May;96-B(5):636–640.
9. **Olsen JR, Hunter J, Baumhauer JF.** Osteoporotic ankle fractures. *Orthop Clin North Am.* 2013 Apr;44(2):225–241.
10. **Strauss EJ, Frank JB, Walsh M, et al.** Does obesity influence the outcome after the operative treatment of ankle fractures? *J Bone Joint Surg Br.* 2007 Jun;89(6):794–798.
11. **Thiele OC, Eckhardt C, Linke B, et al.** Factors affecting the stability of screws in human cortical osteoporotic bone: a cadaver study. *J Bone Joint Surg Br.* 2007 May;89(5):701–705.
12. **Court-Brown CM, McBirnie J, Wilson G.** Adult ankle fractures—an increasing problem? *Acta Orthop Scand.* 1998 Feb;69(1):43–47.
13. **Kannus P, Palvanen M, Niemi S, et al.** Increasing number and incidence of low-trauma ankle fractures in elderly people: Finnish statistics during 1970–2000 and projections for the future. *Bone.* 2002 Sep;31(3):430–433.
14. **Nilsson G, Jonsson K, Ekdahl C, et al.** Outcome and quality of life after surgically treated ankle fractures in patients 65 years or older. *BMC Musculoskelet Disord.* 2007 Dec 20;8:127.
15. **Davidovitch RI, Walsh M, Spitzer A, et al.** Functional outcome after operatively treated ankle fractures in the elderly. *Foot Ankle Int.* 2009 Aug;30(8):728–733.
16. **Gauthé R, Desseaux A, Rony L, et al.** Ankle fractures in the elderly: Treatment and results in 477 patients. *Orthop Traumatol Surg Res.* 2016 Jun;102(4 Suppl):S241–S244.
17. **Toole WP, Elliott M, Hankins D, et al.** Are low-energy open ankle fractures in the elderly the new geriatric hip fracture? *J Foot Ankle Surg.* 2015 Mar–Apr;54(2):203–206.
18. **Ovaska MT, Madanat R, Honkamaa M, et al.** Contemporary demographics and complications of patients treated for open ankle fractures. *Injury.* 2015 Aug;46(8):1650–1655.
19. **Schepers T, van der Linden H, van Lieshout EM, et al.** Technical aspects of the syndesmotic screw and their effect on functional outcome following acute distal tibiofibular syndesmosis injury. *Injury.* 2014 Apr;45(4):775–779.
20. **Stiell IG, McKnight RD, Greenberg GH, et al.** Implementation of the Ottawa ankle rules. *JAMA.* 1994 Mar 16;271(11):827–832.
21. **Donken CC, Verhofstad MH, Edwards MJ, et al.** Use of an acrylic mold for mortise view improvement in ankle fractures: a feasibility study. *The Journal of Foot and Ankle Surgery.* 2011;50(5):525–528.
22. **Takao M, Ochi M, Naito K, et al.** Computed tomographic evaluation of the position of the leg for mortise radiographs. *Foot Ankle Int.* 2001 Oct;22(10):828–831.
23. **Sanders DW, Tieszer C, Corbett B.** Operative versus nonoperative treatment of unstable lateral malleolar fractures: a randomized multicenter trial. *J Orthop Trauma.* 2012 Mar;26(3):129–134.
24. **Park SS, Kubiak EN, Egol KA, et al.** Stress radiographs after ankle fracture: the effect of ankle position and deltoid ligament status on medial clear space measurements. *J Orthop Trauma.* 2006 Jan;20(1):11–18.
25. **DeAngelis NA, Eskander MS, French BG.** Does medial tenderness predict deep deltoid ligament incompetence in supination-external rotation type ankle fractures? *J Orthop Trauma.* 2007 Apr;21(4):244–247.
26. **Michelson JD, Varner KE, Checcone M.** Diagnosing deltoid injury in ankle fractures: the gravity stress view. *Clin Orthop Relat Res.* 2001 Jun(387):178–182.
27. **McCullough CJ, Burge PD.** Rotatory stability of the load-bearing ankle. An experimental study. *J Bone Joint Surg Br.* 1980 Nov;62-B(4):460–464.
28. **Rasmussen O.** Stability of the ankle joint. Analysis of the function and traumatology of the ankle ligaments. *Acta Orthop Scand Suppl.* 1985;211:1–75.
29. **Stufkens SA, van den Bekerom MP, Knupp M, et al.** The diagnosis and treatment of deltoid ligament lesions in supination-external rotation ankle fractures: a review. *Strategies Trauma Limb Reconstr.* 2012 Aug;7(2):73–85.
30. **Warner S, Garner M, Fabricant P, et al.** The Diagnostic Accuracy of Mortise Radiographs and MRI in Predicting Deltoid Ligament Ruptures in Supination External Rotation Ankle Fractures. *Foot and Ankle,* paper #89. Available at: http://ota.org/media/238884/Session-6.pdf. Accessed 2016.
31. **Lee TH, Jang KS, Choi GW, et al.** The contribution of anterior deltoid ligament to ankle stability in isolated lateral malleolar fractures. *Injury.* 2016 Jul;47(7):1581–1585.
32. **Hermans JJ, Wentink N, Beumer A, et al.** Correlation between radiological assessment of acute ankle fractures and syndesmotic injury on MRI. *Skeletal Radiol.* 2012 Jul;41(7):787–801.
33. **Lauge Hansen N.** *Ankelbrud. Genetisk diagnose og reposition: experimental-chirurgiske og radiografiske undersøgelser, repositionsforsøg i kliniken. [Genetic diagnose of reposition].* Dissertation. Copenhagen: University of Copenhagen; 1942. Danish.
34. **Buchler L, Tannast M, Bonel HM, et al.** Reliability of radiologic assessment of the fracture anatomy at the posterior tibial plafond in malleolar fractures. *J Orthop Trauma.* 2009 Mar;23(3):208–212.

35. **Bartonicek J, Rammelt S, Kostlivy K, et al.** Anatomy and classification of the posterior tibial fragment in ankle fractures. *Arch Orthop Trauma Surg.* 2015 Apr;135(4):505–516.
36. **Black EM, Antoci V, Lee JT, et al.** Role of preoperative computed tomography scans in operative planning for malleolar ankle fractures. *Foot Ankle Int.* 2013 May;34(5):697–704.
37. **Makwana NK, Bhowal B, Harper WM, et al.** Conservative versus operative treatment for displaced ankle fractures in patients over 55 years of age. A prospective, randomised study. *J Bone Joint Surg Br.* 2001 May;83(4):525–529.
38. **Ramsey PL, Hamilton W.** Changes in tibiotalar area of contact caused by lateral talar shift. *J Bone Joint Surg Am.* 1976 Apr;58(3):356–357.
39. **Nielson JH, Gardner MJ, Peterson MG, et al.** Radiographic measurements do not predict syndesmotic injury in ankle fractures: an MRI study. *Clin Orthop Relat Res.* 2005 Jul(436):216–221.
40. **Kwon JY, Chacko AT, Kadzielski JJ, et al.** A novel methodology for the study of injury mechanism: ankle fracture analysis using injury videos posted on YouTube.com. *J Orthop Trauma.* 2010 Aug;24(8):477–482.
41. **Weber BG.** *Die Verletzungen des oberen Sprunggelenkes.* 2nd ed. Bern: H. Huber; 1972. German.
42. **Danis R.** Les fractures malléolaires. In: Danis, R. *Théorie et pratique de l'ostéosynthèse.* Paris: Masson; 1949:133–165. French.
43. **Meinberg E, Agel J, Roberts C, et al.** Fracture and Dislocation Classification Compendium—2018. *J Orthopaed Trauma.* 2018 Jan;32(Suppl 1).
44. **Koval KJ, Lurie J, Zhou W, et al.** Ankle fractures in the elderly: what you get depends on where you live and who you see. *J Orthop Trauma.* 2005 Oct;19(9):635–639.
45. **Donken CC, Al-Khateeb H, Verhofstad MH, et al.** Surgical versus conservative interventions for treating ankle fractures in adults. *Cochrane Database Syst Rev.* 2012 Aug;15(8):CD008470.
46. **Horisberger M, Valderrabano V, Hintermann B.** Posttraumatic ankle osteoarthritis after ankle-related fractures. *J Orthop Trauma.* 2009 Jan;23(1):60–67.
47. **Berkes MB, Little MT, Lazaro LE, et al.** Articular congruity is associated with short-term clinical outcomes of operatively treated SER IV ankle fractures. *J Bone Joint Surg Am.* 2013 Oct;95(19):1769–1775.
48. **Varenne Y, Curado J, Asloum Y, et al.** Analysis of risk factors of the postoperative complications of surgical treatment of ankle fractures in the elderly: A series of 477 patients. *Orthop Traumatol Surg Res.* 2016 Jun;102(4 Suppl):S245–S248.
49. **Wronka KS, Salama H, Ramesh B.** Management of displaced ankle fractures in elderly patients—is it worth performing osteosynthesis of osteoporotic bone? *Ortop Traumatol Rehabil.* 2011 May-Jun;13(3):293–298.
50. **Srinivasan CM, Moran CG.** Internal fixation of ankle fractures in the very elderly. *Injury.* 2001 Sep;32(7):559–563.
51. **Pagliaro AJ, Michelson JD, Mizel MS.** Results of operative fixation of unstable ankle fractures in geriatric patients. *Foot Ankle Int.* 2001 May;22(5):399–402.
52. **Herscovici D Jr, Scaduto JM.** Management of high-energy foot and ankle injuries in the geriatric population. *Geriatr Orthop Surg Rehabil.* 2012 Mar;3(1):33–44.
53. **Shivarathre DG, Chandran P, Platt SR.** Operative fixation of unstable ankle fractures in patients aged over 80 years. *Foot Ankle Int.* 2011 Jun;32(6):599–602.
54. **Strauss EJ, Egol KA.** The management of ankle fractures in the elderly. *Injury.* 2007 Sep;38(Suppl 3):S2–9.
55. **Ehrenfreund T, Haluzan D, Dobric I, et al.** Operative management of unstable ankle fractures in the elderly: our institutional experience. *Injury.* 2013 Sep;44(Suppl 3):S20–S22.
56. **McKean J, Cuellar DO, Hak D, et al.** Osteoporotic ankle fractures: an approach to operative management. *Orthopedics.* 2013 Dec;36(12):936–940.
57. **Pakarinen HJ, Flinkkil TE, Ohtonen PP, et al.** Stability criteria for nonoperative ankle fracture management. *Foot Ankle Int.* 2011 Feb;32(2):141–147.
58. **Zeegers AV, Van Raay JJ, van der Werken C.** Ankle fractures treated with a stabilizing shoe. *Acta Orthop Scand.* 1989 Oct;60(5):597–599.
59. **Bazarov I, Peace RA, Lagaay PM, et al.** Early Protected Weightbearing After Ankle Fractures in Patients With Diabetes Mellitus. *J Foot Ankle Surg.* 2017 Jan–Feb;56(1):30–33.
60. **Rosenbaum AJ, Dellenbaugh SG, Dipreta JA, et al.** The management of ankle fractures in diabetics: results of a survey of the American Orthopaedic Foot and Ankle Society membership. *Foot Ankle Spec.* 2013 Jun;6(3):201–205.
61. **Lovy AJ, Dowdell J, Keswani A, et al.** Nonoperative Versus Operative Treatment of Displaced Ankle Fractures in Diabetics. *Foot Ankle Int.* 2017 Mar;38(3):255–260.
62. **Zahn RK, Jakubietz M, Frey S, et al.** A locking contoured plate for distal fibular fractures: mechanical evaluation in an osteoporotic bone model using screws of different length. *J Appl Biomech.* 2014 Feb;30(1):50–57.
63. **White NJ, Corr DT, Wagg JP, et al.** Locked plate fixation of the comminuted distal fibula: a biomechanical study. *Can J Surg.* 2013 Feb;56(1):35–40.
64. **Lo EY, Tseng SS, Christiansen BA, et al.** Locking versus nonlocking construct in an osteoporotic, segmental fibula defect model. *Orthopedics.* 2013 Oct 01;36(10):e1262–e1268.
65. **Davis AT, Israel H, Cannada LK, et al.** A biomechanical comparison of one-third tubular plates versus periarticular plates for fixation of osteoporotic distal fibula fractures. *J Orthop Trauma.* 2013 Sep;27(9):e201–e207.
66. **Kim T, Ayturk UM, Haskell A, et al.** Fixation of osteoporotic distal fibula fractures: A biomechanical comparison of locking versus conventional plates. *J Foot Ankle Surg.* 2007 Jan-Feb;46(1):2–6.
67. **Minihane KP, Lee C, Ahn C, et al.** Comparison of lateral locking plate and antiglide plate for fixation of distal fibular fractures in osteoporotic bone: a biomechanical study. *J Orthop Trauma.* 2006 Sep;20(8):562–566.
68. **Dingemans SA, Lodeizen OA, Goslings JC, et al.** Reinforced fixation of distal fibula fractures in elderly patients; A meta-analysis of biomechanical studies. *Clin Biomech (Bristol, Avon).* 2016 Jul;36:14–20.
69. **Bariteau JT, Fantry A, Blankenhorn B, et al.** A biomechanical evaluation of locked plating for distal fibula fractures in an osteoporotic sawbone model. *Foot Ankle Surg.* 2014 Mar;20(1):44–47.
70. **Zahn RK, Frey S, Jakubietz RG, et al.** A contoured locking plate for distal fibular fractures in osteoporotic bone: a biomechanical cadaver study. *Injury.* 2012 Jun;43(6):718–725.
71. **Schepers T, Van Lieshout EM, De Vries MR, et al.** Increased rates of wound complications with locking plates in distal fibular fractures. *Injury.* 2011 Oct;42(10):1125–1129.
72. **Schaffer JJ, Manoli A 2nd.** The antiglide plate for distal fibular fixation. A biomechanical comparison with fixation with a lateral plate. *J Bone Joint Surg Am.* 1987 Apr;69(4):596–604.

73. **Assal M, Dalmau-Pastor M, Ray A, et al.** How to Get to the Distal Posterior Tibial Malleolus? A Cadaveric Anatomic Study Defining the Access Corridors Through 3 Different Approaches. *J Orthop Trauma.* 2017 Apr;31(4):e127–e129.
74. **Darland AM, Kadakia AR, Zeller JL.** Branching patterns of the superficial peroneal nerve: implications for ankle arthroscopy and for anterolateral surgical approaches to the ankle. *J Foot Ankle Surg.* 2015 May–Jun;54(3):332–337.
75. **Blair JM, Botte MJ.** Surgical anatomy of the superficial peroneal nerve in the ankle and foot. *Clin Orthop Relat Res.* 1994 Aug(305):229–238.
76. **Weber M, Krause F.** Peroneal tendon lesions caused by antiglide plates used for fixation of lateral malleolar fractures: the effect of plate and screw position. *Foot Ankle Int.* 2005 Apr;26(4):281–285.
77. **Pires RE, Mauffrey C, de Andrade MA, et al.** Minimally invasive percutaneous plate osteosynthesis for ankle fractures: a prospective observational cohort study. *Eur J Orthop Surg Traumatol.* 2014 Oct;24(7):1297–1303.
78. **Siegel J, Tornetta P 3rd.** Extraperiosteal plating of pronation-abduction ankle fractures. *J Bone Joint Surg Am.* 2007 Feb;89(2):276–281.
79. **Tornetta P 3rd, Creevy W.** Lag screw only fixation of the lateral malleolus. *J Orthop Trauma.* 2001 Feb;15(2):119–121.
80. **McKenna PB, O'Shea K, Burke T.** Less is more: lag screw only fixation of lateral malleolar fractures. *Int Orthop.* 2007 Aug;31(4):497–502.
81. **Bugler KE, Watson CD, Hardie AR, et al.** The treatment of unstable fractures of the ankle using the Acumed fibular nail: development of a technique. *J Bone Joint Surg Br.* 2012 Aug;94(8):1107–1112.
82. **Rajeev A, Senevirathna S, Radha S, et al.** Functional outcomes after fibula locking nail for fragility fractures of the ankle. *J Foot Ankle Surg.* 2011 Sep-Oct;50(5):547–550.
83. **Lee YS, Huang HL, Lo TY, et al.** Lateral fixation of AO type-B2 ankle fractures in the elderly: the Knowles pin versus the plate. *Int Orthop.* 2007 Dec;31(6):817–821.
84. **White TO, Bugler KE, Appleton P, et al.** A prospective randomised controlled trial of the fibular nail versus standard open reduction and internal fixation for fixation of ankle fractures in elderly patients. *Bone Joint J.* 2016 Sep;98-B(9):1248–1252.
85. **Panchbhavi VK, Vallurupalli S, Morris R.** Comparison of augmentation methods for internal fixation of osteoporotic ankle fractures. *Foot Ankle Int.* 2009 Jul;30(7):696–703.
86. **King CM, Cobb M, Collman DR, et al.** Bicortical fixation of medial malleolar fractures: a review of 23 cases at risk for complicated bone healing. *J Foot Ankle Surg.* 2012 Jan-Feb;51(1):39–44.
87. **Ricci WM, Tornetta P, Borrelli J Jr.** Lag screw fixation of medial malleolar fractures: a biomechanical, radiographic, and clinical comparison of unicortical partially threaded lag screws and bicortical fully threaded lag screws. *J Orthop Trauma.* 2012 Oct;26(10):602–606.
88. **Ebraheim NA, Ludwig T, Weston JT, et al.** Comparison of surgical techniques of 111 medial malleolar fractures classified by fracture geometry. *Foot Ankle Int.* 2014 May;35(5):471–477.
89. **Haraguchi N, Haruyama H, Toga H, et al.** Pathoanatomy of posterior malleolar fractures of the ankle. *J Bone Joint Surg Am.* 2006 May;88(5):1085–1092.
90. **O'Connor TJ, Mueller B, Ly TV, et al.** "A to p" screw versus posterolateral plate for posterior malleolus fixation in trimalleolar ankle fractures. *J Orthop Trauma.* 2015 Apr;29(4):e151–156.
91. **Bennett C, Behn A, Daoud A, et al.** Buttress Plating Versus Anterior-to-Posterior Lag Screws for Fixation of the Posterior Malleolus: A Biomechanical Study. *J Orthop Trauma.* 2016 Dec;30(12):664–669.
92. **Choi JY, Kim JH, Ko HT, et al.** Single Oblique Posterolateral Approach for Open Reduction and Internal Fixation of Posterior Malleolar Fractures With an Associated Lateral Malleolar Fracture. *J Foot Ankle Surg.* 2015 Jul-Aug;54(4):559–564.
93. **Helmy N, Meyer DC, Vienne P, et al.** The posterolateral approach for the treatment of trimalleolar fractures. *Techniques in Foot & Ankle Surgery.* 2012;11(4):189–193.
94. **Miller AN, Carroll EA, Parker RJ, et al.** Posterior malleolar stabilization of syndesmotic injuries is equivalent to screw fixation. *Clin Orthop Relat Res.* 2010 Apr;468(4):1129–1135.
95. **Jonas SC, Young AF, Curwen CH, et al.** Functional outcome following tibio-talar-calcaneal nailing for unstable osteoporotic ankle fractures. *Injury.* 2013 Jul;44(7):994–997.
96. **Al-Nammari SS, Dawson-Bowling S, Amin A, et al.** Fragility fractures of the ankle in the frail elderly patient: treatment with a long calcaneotalotibial nail. *Bone Joint J.* 2014 Jun;96-B(6):817–822.
97. **O'Daly BJ, Harty JA, O'Malley N, et al.** Percutaneous Gallagher nail stabilisation for fragility ankle fracture. *European Journal of Orthopaedic Surgery & Traumatology.* 2010;20(8):651–655.
98. **Lemon M, Somayaji HS, Khaleel A, et al.** Fragility fractures of the ankle: stabilisation with an expandable calcaneotalotibial nail. *J Bone Joint Surg Br.* 2005 Jun;87(6):809–813.
99. **Jehan S, Shakeel M, Bing AJ, et al.** The success of tibiotalocalcaneal arthrodesis with intramedullary nailing--a systematic review of the literature. *Acta Orthop Belg.* 2011 Oct;77(5):644–651.
100. **Kugan R, Aslam N, Bose D, et al.** Outcome of arthrodesis of the hindfoot as a salvage procedure for complex ankle pathology using the Ilizarov technique. *Bone Joint J.* 2013 Mar;95-B(3):371–377.
101. **Crespo AM, Rautenberg AF, Siev N, et al.** Fibulectomy, tibial shortening, and ankle arthrodesis as an alternative treatment of nonhealing wounds following open ankle fracture in compromised elderly adults. *Foot Ankle Int.* 2015 Jan;36(1):103–107.
102. **Roussignol X.** Arthroscopic tibiotalar and subtalar joint arthrodesis. *Orthop Traumatol Surg Res.* 2016 Feb;102(1 Suppl):S195–203.
103. **DiDomenico LA, Brown D, Zgonis T.** The use of Ilizarov technique as a definitive percutaneous reduction for ankle fractures in patients who have diabetes mellitus and peripheral vascular disease. *Clin Podiatr Med Surg.* 2009 Jan;26(1):141–148.
104. **Assal M, Christofilopoulos P, Lubbeke A, et al.** Augmented osteosynthesis of OTA 44-B fractures in older patients: a technique allowing early weightbearing. *J Orthop Trauma.* 2011 Dec;25(12):742–747.

# 3.18 Atypical fractures

Chang-Wug Oh, Joon-Woo Kim

## 1 Introduction

Bisphosphonate (BP) therapy has been widely used for management of osteoporosis and has been shown to reduce the risk of vertebral and femoral neck fractures in postmenopausal osteoporotic patients. The use of BPs is also extended to metabolic bone diseases including Paget's disease, hypercalcemia due to a variety of causes, and skeletal metastases from cancer.

Long-term suppression of bone remodeling may impair microdamage repair and alter the biomechanical properties of bone. Overmineralization may have deleterious effects on bone quality, elasticity, and resistance in the long term. Long-term oversuppression of bone turnover with BPs has generated many reports of spontaneous peripheral fractures [1–4]. These so-called atypical femoral fractures occur after minimal trauma and have a distinct pattern and radiographic appearance when compared with typical osteoporotic fractures (**Case 1: Fig 3.18-1**). Although the subtrochanteric femoral location is the usual site of these atypical fractures, other weight-bearing sites have also been affected, including tibia, ulna, and other bones [5, 6].

In this chapter, we mainly describe atypical fractures of the femur that have been widely reported and are clinically important.

## 2 Epidemiology and etiology

All current evidence indicates that the atypical femoral fracture (AFF) represents a rare subset of subtrochanteric and femoral shaft fractures. The atypical femoral fracture has been associated with various factors, including Asian ethnicity, the use of BPs, glucocorticoids, and proton pump inhibitors, as well as medical conditions including rheumatoid arthritis, diabetes mellitus, or vitamin D deficiency.

Long-term use of BPs represents a relevant risk factor:

- The American Society for Bone and Mineral Research (ASBMR) task force reported an incidence of 2 per 100,000 cases per year after 2 years of BP use, increasing to 78 per 100,000 cases per year after 8 years of use [4].
- Almost 40% of patients who sustained a subtrochanteric or femoral shaft fracture had used BPs for a significantly longer period than subjects who sustained an intertrochanteric or femoral neck fracture.
- However, there has been no statistically significant increase in the risk of subtrochanteric femoral fracture in patients treated with BPs for as long as 10 years.

Therefore, there is a lack of specificity for associating BP use only with AFFs.

There have been several studies speculating about the etiology. It is likely multifactorial, although no specific underlying mechanism has been demonstrated.

Bisphosphonates inhibit osteoclast function and induce osteoclast apoptosis, and thus, they increase bone mineral density and suppress bone turnover. It has been suggested that this change in bone metabolism produces hypermineralized bone that is more brittle and therefore more susceptible to low-energy or stress fractures.

CASE 1

### Patient

A 61-year-old woman suffered a subtrochanteric fracture of the right femur after slipping and falling in her kitchen. Bisphosphonates had been used in this patient for more than 5 years to treat osteoporosis.

### Comorbidities

- Osteoporosis

### Treatment and outcome

After the patient had suffered a subtrochanteric fracture of the right femur, a periosteal reaction was seen on the lateral cortex of the left femur, at the same level of the fracture as on the right femur (**Fig 3.18-1a**). Intramedullary nailing was performed in both femurs (**Fig 3.18-1b–c**). Fracture healing was achieved on the right femur, and the previous stress reaction disappeared on the left femur (**Fig 3.18-1d–e**).

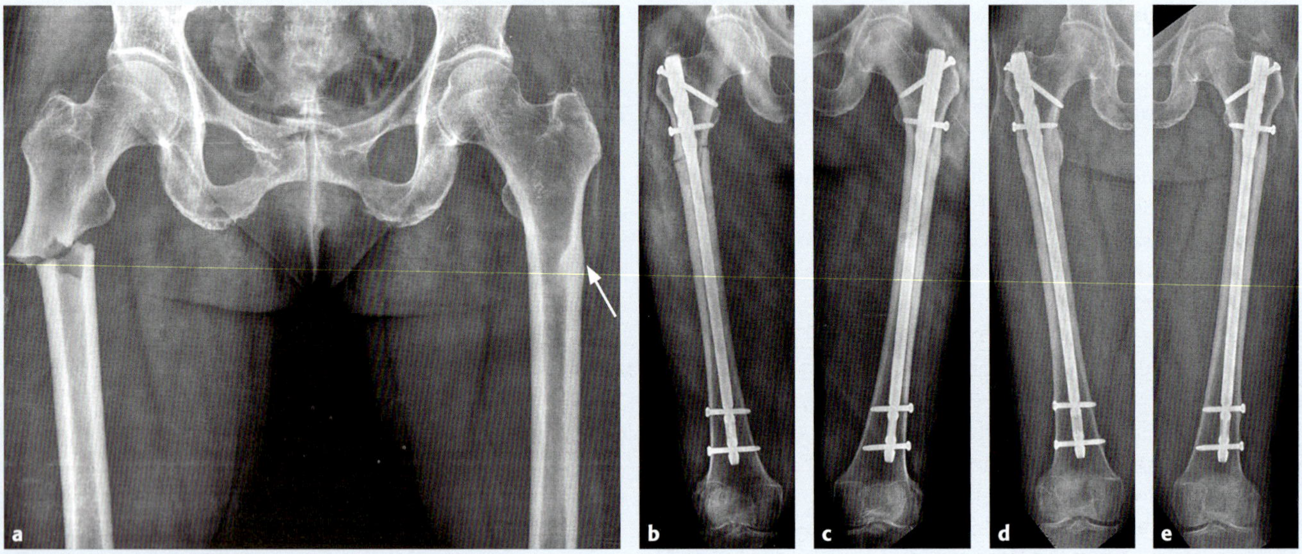


**Fig 3.18-1a–e** A 61-year-old woman with a subtrochanteric fracture of the right femur.
**a** The arrow localizing the periosteal reaction seen on the lateral cortex of the left femur was at the same height as the right femoral fracture.
**b–c** Intramedullary nailing was performed in both femurs.
**d–e** The fracture on the right femur had healed and the previous stress reaction on the left femur had disappeared.

Recently, it has been suggested that there may be an association between proximal or diaphyseal femoral geometry and the presence of AFFs. Hagen et al [7] reported that an association between varus proximal femoral geometry and a propensity to sustain AFFs in patients taking long-term BP therapy existed. Sasaski et al [8] also found that a significant increase in the lateral and anterior bow of the femur was associated with low-energy femoral shaft fractures. These patients were taking medications for osteoporosis but not exclusively BPs. The alteration of femoral geometry may result in an imbalance in strains and develop an AFF partly for biomechanical reasons.

## 3 Localization

Atypical fractures usually affect the femur as described. However, these fractures may also occur in other long bones including the tibia, ulna, clavicle, and pedicles of vertebrae [9–11]. Particularly in a patient taking long-term BPs, long bones with weight-bearing function may be susceptible to fractures,. In that situation, prompt investigation should be performed with x-rays and other modalities.

Recently, BP-induced periprosthetic fractures of the femur have been reported. As a high proportion of older osteoporotic patients are undergoing hip replacement, arthroplasty surgeons should consider the possibility of AFFs in patients receiving long-term BPs who present with thigh pain despite a well-fixed femoral component.

## 4 Diagnostics

It is inappropriate to screen all patients with prolonged BP treatment for AFFs, as the incidence is low and the actual incidence of abnormal radiographic features in the entire patient population taking BPs is unknown. The ASBMR defined AFF as atraumatic or low-trauma fractures located in the subtrochanteric region or femoral shaft [4]. The diagnosis of AFF specifically excludes high-trauma fractures, fractures of the femoral neck, intertrochanteric fractures with spiral subtrochanteric extension, pathological fractures associated with primary or metastatic bone tumors, and periprosthetic fractures.

### 4.1 Clinical symptoms

It seems to be important to raise awareness of prodromal symptoms of atypical fractures to facilitate the early diagnosis of an incomplete lesion. The development of groin or thigh pain in a patient on long-term BP treatment should raise the index of suspicion of an AFF. If the patient is at high risk, the same applies but for other reasons such as rheumatoid arthritis, diabetes, or the use of glucocorticoid therapy. As AFFs may represent stress fractures that progress over time, the pain in the thigh may be the only clinical symptom in incomplete fractures. It often comes with severe and constant pain in the lateral area of the affected hip and/or radiating to the knee area. Usually with this prodromal pain, the complete fracture develops with low-energy trauma, such as an injury caused by the equivalent to a fall from a standing height or less.

### 4.2 Imaging

#### 4.2.1 Plain x-rays

Characteristic radiographic features of AFFs are as follows:

- There is no comminution.
- There is a transverse fracture line at the point of origination in the lateral cortex.
- As the fracture propagates across the diaphysis to the medial cortex, the orientation may become more oblique and when it becomes complete, a prominent medial "spike" may be present.
- Focal or diffuse periosteal reaction of the lateral cortex surrounding the region where the fracture initiated. This reaction may appear as cortical "beaking" or "flaring" adjacent to a discrete transverse lucent fracture line, or as focal thickening of the lateral cortex.
- Focal and diffuse endosteal reactions near the fracture site. This focal cortical thickening represents cortical hypertrophy and may be unilateral or bilateral.
- Generalized cortical thickening.

Incomplete lesions can often convert to complete or displaced fractures by low-energy mechanisms, when a preceding history of thigh pain has been present in the ipsilateral extremity. Therefore, it is important to find the precursor lesion, which may need preventive treatment. Koh et al [12] described the presence of the "dreaded black line" (ie, a form of transverse radiolucency) indicative of increased risk of developing a complete insufficiency fracture. This line was interpreted as accumulated, partially healed microdamage.

#### 4.2.2 Magnetic resonance imaging

As radiographic findings alone may not be sufficient to support preventive measures, magnetic resonance imaging (MRI) or technetium (Tc) bone scintigraphy should be considered if a stress fracture is suspected. Magnetic resonance imaging findings of an incomplete AFF are often visible before they become evident on plain x-rays and they include:

- An incomplete cortical stress reaction that has been detected [13].
- A prominent or complete line from the outer to the inner border of the lateral cortex, which seems to be the precursor of the lesion on plain x-rays.
- Serial axial and coronal MRIs may reveal intracortical damage or the presence of bone marrow edema in contrast with only focal cortical protrusion or a faint transverse line on plain x-rays.

If these findings are associated with thigh pain, it can have the potential to develop into a complete fracture.

#### 4.2.3 Bone scintigraphy

Three-phase skeletal scintigraphy with Tc-99m methylene diphosphonate can identify incomplete AFFs. Focal tracer uptake may be shown at the lesion (**Case 2: Fig 3.18-2**). It is particularly useful to find the lesion of the contralateral side when a complete fracture has developed. In incomplete lesion, focal tracer uptake may be shown at the lesion. Also, mild uptake in multifocal endosteal thickening of the lateral femoral diaphysis can be noted, which is diagnostic of a BP-associated AFF in the femoral shaft.

CASE 2

### Patient

A 53-year-old woman had thigh pain for 3 months, which progressively increased over the course of time. She had a medical history of rheumatoid arthritis and use of corticosteroids (**Fig 3.18-1a–b**).

### Comorbidities

- Rheumatoid arthritis

### Treatment and outcome

The patient's thigh pain progressively increased. There was visible thickening of the lateral cortex of the femur as well as a localized lesion in the subtrochanteric area (**Fig 3.18-2a–b**). A so-called "dreaded black line" was detected at the lateral cortex of the subtrochanteric area, which was shown on magnetic resonance imaging to be a stress reaction. Therefore, a prophylactic fixation was recommended to this patient (**Fig 3.18-2c–d**). On the day of admission for planned surgery, the patient had a fracture after falling and suffered a subtrochanteric fracture at the same height as the previously diagnosed area (**Fig 3.18-2e**). Intramedullary nailing was performed (**Fig 3.18-2f–g**) resulting in healing 6 months postoperative (**Fig 3.18-2h–i**).

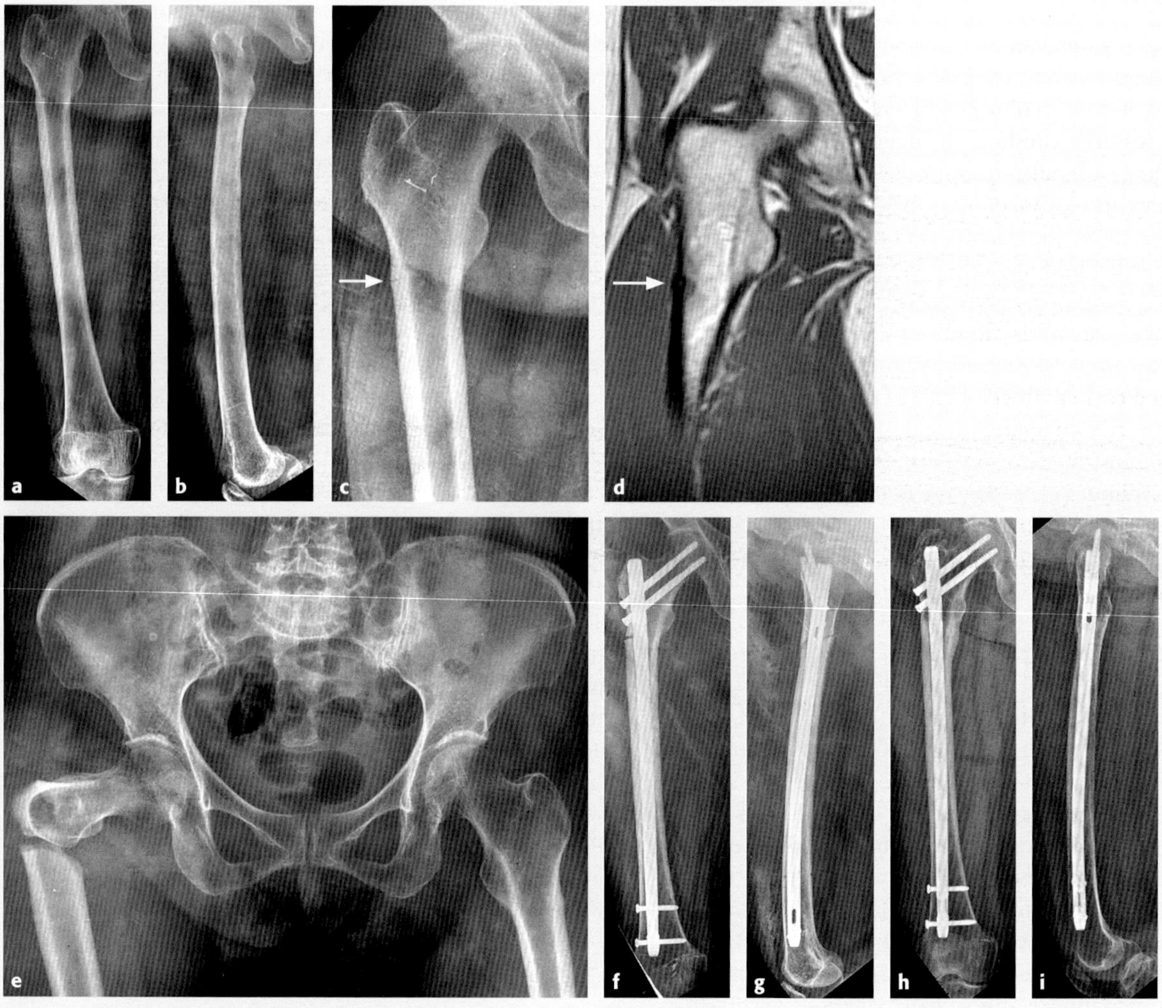


**Fig 3.18-2a–i** A 53-year-old woman with thigh pain.
**a–b** The x-rays showing thickened lateral cortex of the femur and localized lesion in the subtrochanteric area.
**c–d** The magnified view (**c**) showing the dreaded black line seen at the lateral cortex of the subtrochanteric area. Magnetic resonance imaging showed a stress reaction (**d**).
**e** The subtrochanteric fracture at the same height as the previously diagnosed area.
**f–g** Intramedullary nailing was performed.
**h–i** Satisfactory healing after 6 months.

## 5 Classification

The original ASBMR case definition divided these characteristics into major and minor features and differentiated between complete and incomplete AFFs. All major features are required to satisfy the case definition of AFF. None of the minor features are required but have sometimes been associated with these fractures.

Major features include:

- Location in the subtrochanteric region and diaphysis of the femur
- Association with no or minimal trauma
- Transverse or short oblique configuration
- Lack of comminution
- Incomplete lesion involving only the lateral cortex
- Complete lesion extending through both cortices and may have a medial spike, as in the case of a short oblique fracture, for instance

Minor features include:

- Localized periosteal reaction or beaking of the lateral cortex
- Generalized cortical thickening of the femoral shaft
- History of prodromal pain
- Bilateral fractures
- Delayed healing
- Associations with certain drugs, such as BPs, glucocorticoids, and proton pump inhibitors
- Associations with medical conditions, such as diabetes, rheumatoid arthritis, and vitamin D deficiency

## 6 Therapeutic options

Management of patients with AFFs includes fracture fixation as well as medical management.

### 6.1 Medical management

Once an AFF is diagnosed, discontinuation of the BP medication must be considered. Typical osteoporotic and atypical fracture risk can help guide decision making, using the Fracture Risk Assessment tool and bone turnover markers [14]. For patients at low risk of osteoporotic fracture, BPs can be discontinued. Patients should nevertheless take daily calcium and vitamin D supplements. For patients with a high risk of fracture, BP treatment may be continued beyond 5 years. Alternatively, denosumab or teriparatide may be provided if BP is discontinued, although it is not clear if denosumab perpetuates the risk of AFF. For patients at moderate risk of fracture, the management plan can be further divided on the basis of the bone turnover state (low turnover and high turnover states). Patients at moderate risk of fracture and in a low turnover state can be managed in a fashion that is similar to those at low risk of fracture. However, those patients at moderate risk but in a high turnover state should be managed as if they have high risk of fracture. Regardless of the decision on BP medication, all patients should receive calcium and vitamin D supplementation. Recombinant parathyroid hormone (eg, teriparatide) should also be considered, especially as there is evidence to suggest that teriparatide improves bone turnover and microarchitecture in patients on long-term alendronate treatment. Furthermore, teriparatide enhances and accelerates fracture healing by increasing callus formation and mechanical strength. It is also known that teriparatide shortened the time to healing in patients with osteoporotic fractures. Therefore, teriparatide may be beneficial to enhance fracture healing in patients with AFF. Since these considerations are highly individualized, consultation with a specialist in osteoporosis therapy is strongly recommended.

Careful surveillance of patients with an AFF is needed because of high frequency of bilateral involvement [15]. Radiographic images of the contralateral femur must be evaluated for evidence of any suspicious lesion. Technetium-99m bone scintigraphy or MRI should be considered if a stress fracture is suspected.

### 6.2 Treatment of incomplete fractures

A period of nonoperative therapy may be considered if there is an incomplete fracture with no or minimal pain:

- Partial weight bearing with use of a cane, crutches, or a walker
- Avoidance of strenuous activity
- The use of teriparatide
- Close monitoring, as the failure rate is known to be high with nonoperative treatment

In a study by Ha et al [16], no patient had spontaneous healing or resolution of pain during the follow-up period. Prophylactic fixation with intramedullary (IM) nailing in incomplete lesions is recommended when:

- Moderate to severe pain is present.
- Persistent or worsening pain after a period of nonoperative treatment occurs.
- Progression of the fracture line is observed on serial x-ray or other imaging modalities (**Case 3: Fig 3.18-3**) [17, 18].

CASE 3

### Patient

A 70-year-old woman had thigh pain in her left leg for 6 months. She had been administered bisphosphonates for more than 3 years.

### Treatment and outcome

The cortex was thickened from the subtrochanteric level to the shaft (**Fig 3.18-3a–b**). On a bone scan, focal, increased uptake was noted, which was shown as a stress reaction, and there was also an incomplete fracture noted at the lateral cortex (**Fig 3.18-3c–d**). Prophylactic intramedullary nailing was performed and the bisphosphonate medication discontinued (**Fig 3.18-3e–f**). After 8 months, the patient was free of thigh pain and the previous lesion at the subtrochanteric area had also disappeared (**Fig 3.18-3g–h**).

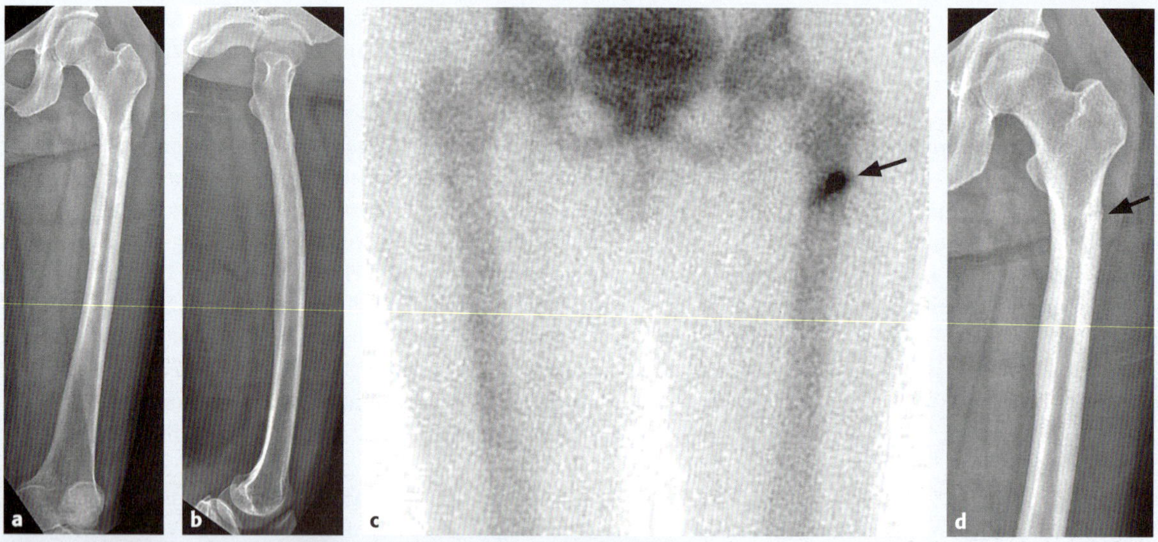

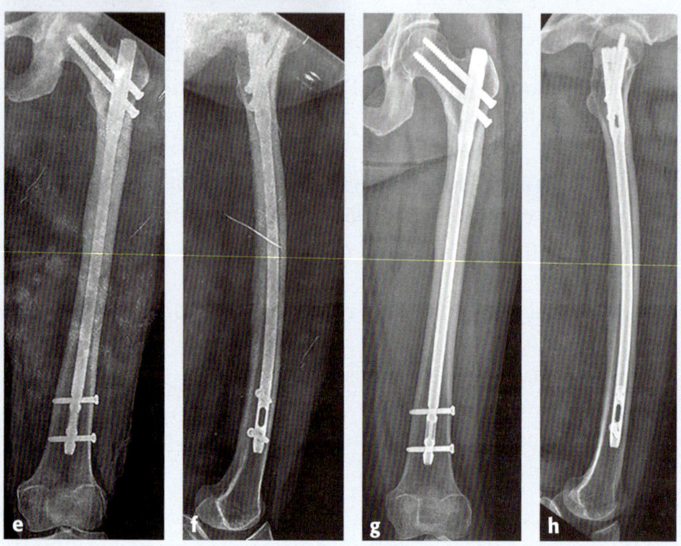

**Fig 3.18-3a–h** A 70-year-old woman with thigh pain for half a year.
**a–b** The x-ray showing the thickened cortex from the subtrochanteric level to the shaft.
**c–d** The arrows point to an incomplete fracture at the lateral cortex.
**e–f** The x-rays showing intramedullary nailing performed prophylactically.
**g–h** Disappearance of previous lesion at the subtrochanteric area 8 months postoperative.

## 6.3 Treatment of complete fractures

### 6.3.1 Intramedullary nailing

Nailing is a preferred method of fixation for AFFs. Sometimes, IM nailing of these femoral fractures could be impractical for subtrochanteric as well as diaphyseal fractures. The thickened cortices, which essentially trumpet from the metaphyseal trochanteric region to the thick diaphyseal cortex, make standard reconstruction nailing difficult as the increased proximal diameter of the nail results in iatrogenic fracture of a brittle cortex.

Excessive bowing of the femoral shaft is an obstacle for IM nailing. These features may lead to inadvertent fractures (**Case 4: Fig 3.18-4**), malreduction, or impaired fracture healing.

**Patient**

A 67-year-old woman suffered a diaphyseal fracture of the right femur after a fall. According to her medical history, she had been taking bisphosphonate for more than 3 years.

**Treatment and outcome**

The patient suffered a transverse-to-oblique configuration of fracture without comminution (**Fig 3.18-4a–b**), so antegrade intramedullary nailing was performed. An inadvertent butterfly fragment occurred at the lateral aspect, probably because of a mismatch between the radius of nail and exaggerated anterolateral bowing of the femur (**Fig 3.18-4c–d**). After 6 months, satisfactory healing was achieved (**Fig 3.18-4e–g**).

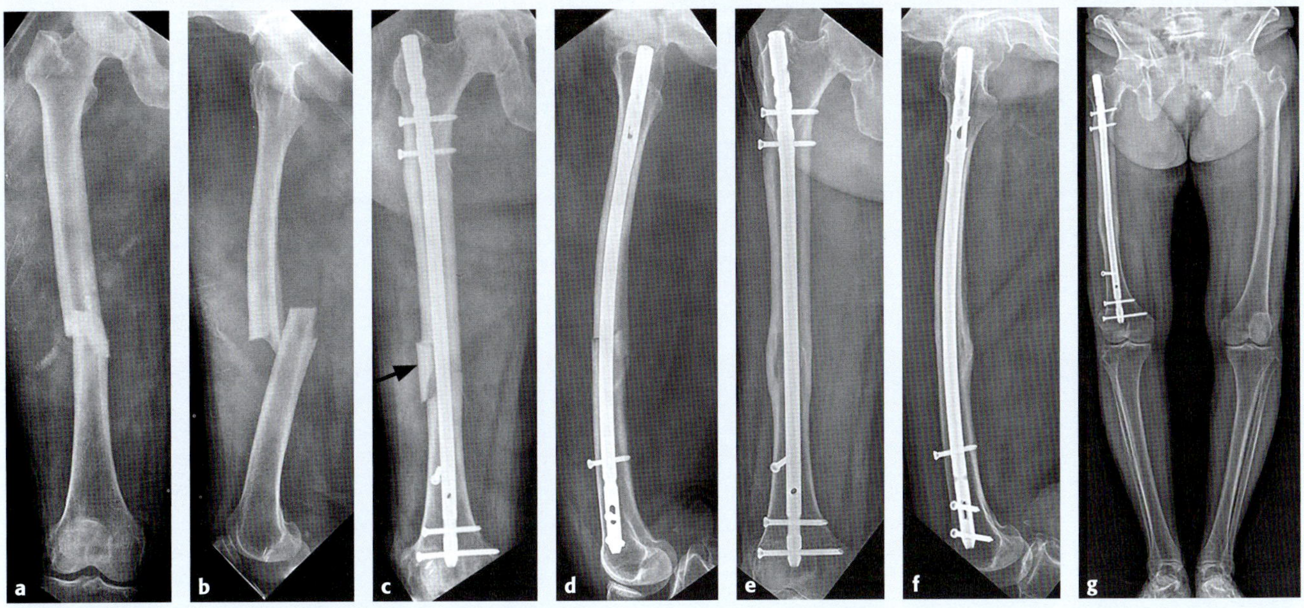


**Fig 3.18-4a–g** A 67-year-old woman with a diaphyseal fracture of the right femur.
**a–b** X-rays of the transverse-to-oblique fracture configuration.
**c–d** X-rays showing the butterfly fragment at the lateral aspect (arrow in **c**).
**e–g** X-rays showing satisfactory healing after 6 months but with slightly different bowing to the uninjured left femur.

The standard IM nails can be chosen to fix AFFs. But, there may be a chance of femoral neck or trochanteric fractures, as these osteoporotic patients have an elevated risk of fragility fractures (**Case 5: Fig 3.18-5**). To prevent a possible fragility fracture, a cephalomedullary nail can be chosen. Also, the distal interlocking fixation of a nail is important because of the thin cortex in the distal femur. For this reason, it may be better to use more than two screws in the distal fixation of the nail (**Case 6: Fig 3.18-6**). The angular stable locking system, a newly designed screw, may also help to have a secure fixation serving the same purpose.

Generally, IM reaming with sharp cutter heads up to 2 mm more than the desired diameter of the nail is recommended. This procedure is thought to ease insertion of the nail in the bowed bone and to promote healing. Evidence is sparse (see chapter 3.11 Femoral shaft, **Fig 3.11-1**).

As the other subtrochanteric fractures, AFF should not be fixed in a varus reduction. From the increased tension stress to this region, varus with the lateral gap may delay or impair the healing of the fracture.

CASE 5

## Patient

A 74-year-old woman complained about progressive pain in her left thigh.

## Treatment and outcome

The patient had a medical history of treating an atypical femoral fracture of the right femur (**Fig 3.18-5a–c**). Standard antegrade intramedullary (IM) nailing was performed to prevent complete fracture (**Fig 3.18-5d–e**). Three years after surgery, the patient still complained about intermittent thigh pain. The x-rays showed no abnormal findings except for persistent thickening of the lateral cortex of the femur (**Fig 3.18-5f–g**).

A femoral neck fracture with minimal trauma occurred near the dreaded black line on the midshaft, which was the previous lesion. The authors suppose that this neck fracture could have been prevented if a cephalomedullary rather than standard IM nail had been used (**Fig 3.18-5h–i**). Bipolar arthroplasty was performed. But the plate fixation was also used to prevent a fracture of incomplete lesion at the diaphysis (**Fig 3.18-5j–k**).

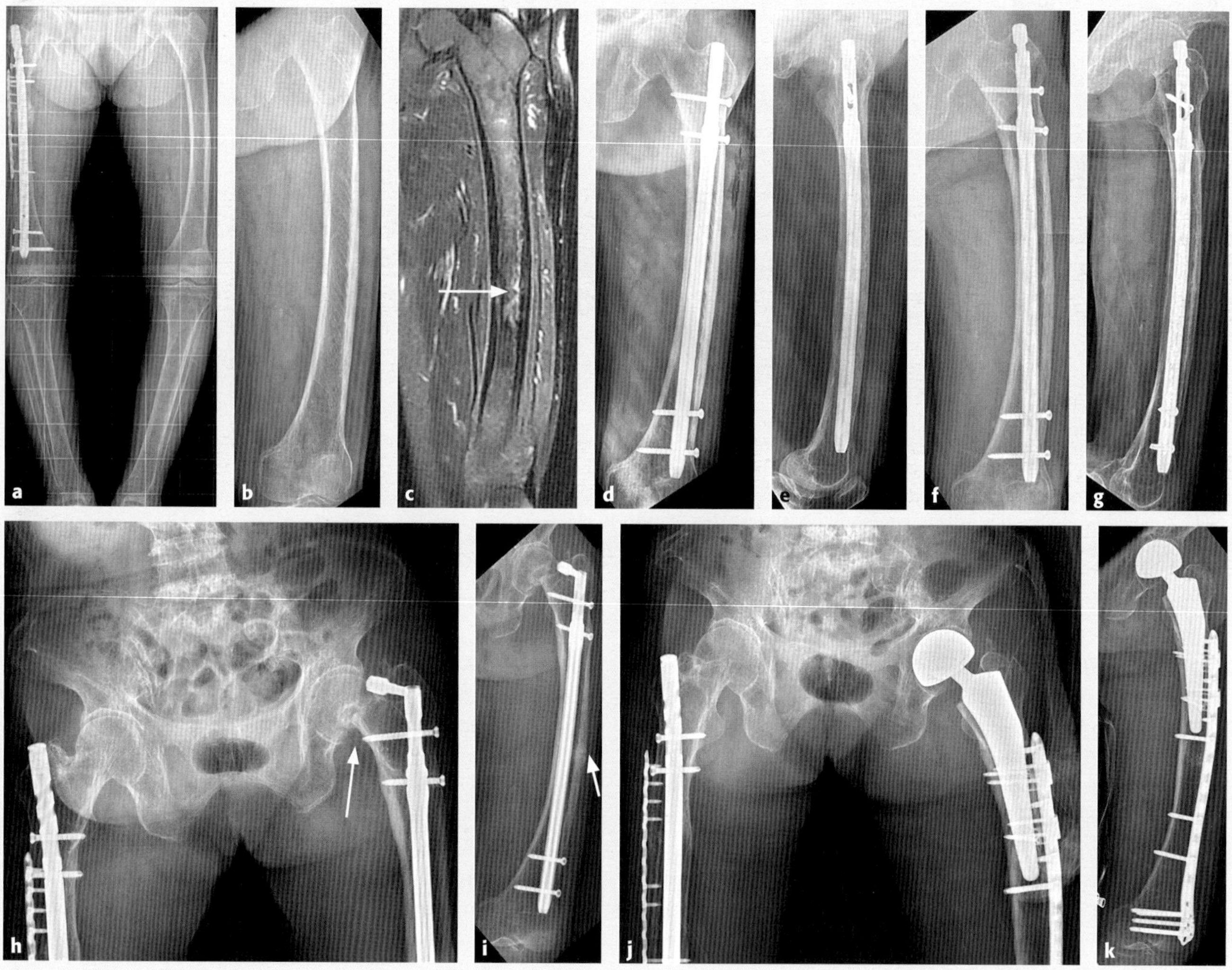


**Fig 3.18-5a–k** A 74-year-old woman with progressive pain in her left thigh.
**a–c** The x-rays showing the exaggerated curve and thickened lateral cortex of the left femur. Magnetic resonance imaging showing the multiple stress lesions at the lateral endosteum (arrow in **c**).
**d–e** Standard antegrade intramedullary nailing was performed.
**f–g** The 3-year postoperative x-rays showing no abnormal findings except for persistent thickening of the lateral cortex of the femur.
**h–i** The x-rays showing a femoral neck fracture with minimal trauma. The dreaded black line (white arrow in **i**) is shown on the midshaft, which was the previous lesion.
**j–k** Bipolar arthroplasty with plate fixation.

CASE 6

**Patient**

A 64-year-old woman developed a subtrochanteric fracture of the right femur after having taken bisphosphonates for 5 years (**Fig 3.18-6a–b**).

**Treatment and outcome**

Cephalomedullary nailing was performed, using three interlocking screws at the distal side to secure fixation (**Fig 3.18-6c–d**). Successful healing was achieved 10 months postoperatively (**Fig 3.18-6e–f**).

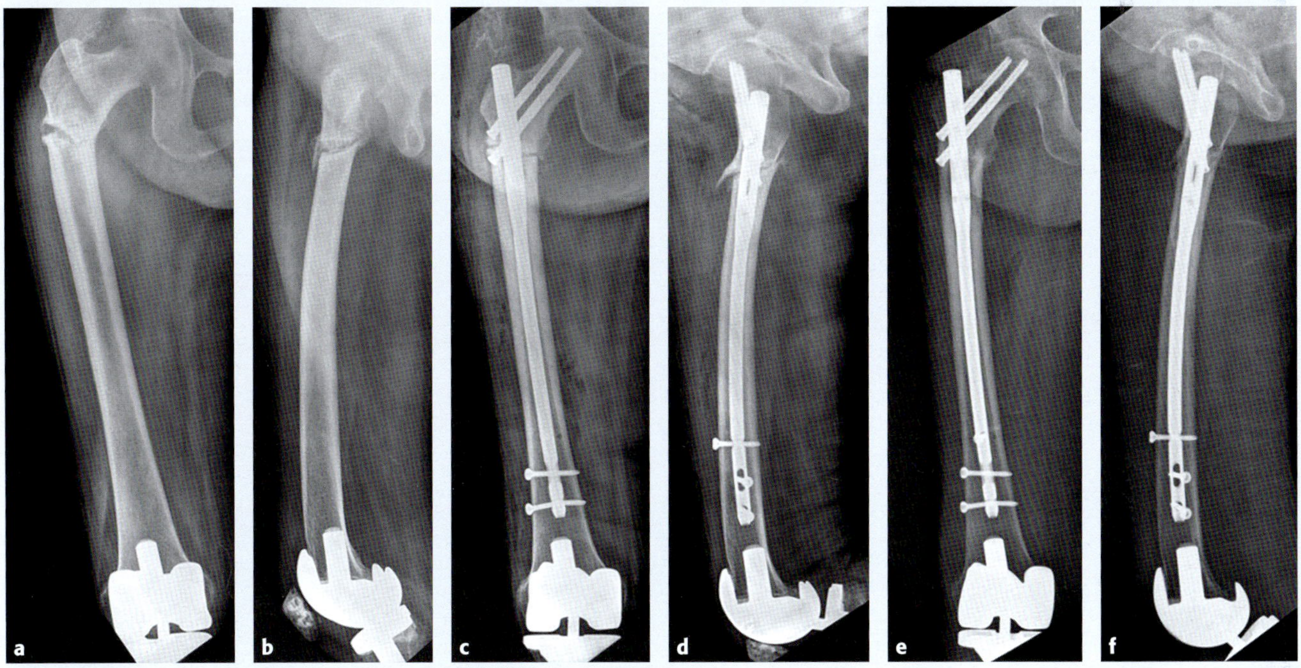


**Fig 3.18-6a–f** A 64-year-old woman with a subtrochanteric fracture of the right femur.
**a–b** The x-ray showing a subtrochanteric fracture of the right femur.
**c–d** The three interlocking screws at the distal side were used to secure fixation in cephalomedullary nailing.
**e–f** Successful healing occurred 10 months after surgery.

### 6.3.2 Plate fixation

Plate fixation may be justified if nailing is technically not feasible, especially with severe, anterolateral bowing of the femur. However, there was a high rate of implant failure resulting in a high rate of reoperation. This may be likely attributable to a short lever arm of the implant, a varus moment arm, and dependence on intramembranous healing inhibited by BPs (**Case 7: Fig 3.18-7**).

In postoperative outcomes of AFF, several studies report that a large proportion of the patients required revision surgery and suffered implant failure. The reason is thought to be associated with slow healing and prolonged postoperative immobility (**Case 8: Fig 3.18-8**) [17, 19].

CASE 7

### Patient

A 70-year-old woman had thigh pain in her left side for several months.

### Treatment and outcome

The thickened cortex of the femur was visible on the x-ray, and the bone scan showed a focal, hot uptake at the diaphysis. On the standing x-rays, the patient showed severe anterolateral bowing of both femurs (**Fig 3.18-7a–c**). Due to bowing, plate fixation was performed and the plate was bent to adjust the curvature. However, 5 days postoperative a fracture developed at the proximal end of the plate. Nailing had to be performed as a revision procedure (**Fig 3.18-7d–f**). The fracture was healed successfully 10 months after surgery, but there remained a difference in bowing of the femur compared to the uninjured side (**Fig 3.18-7g–i**).

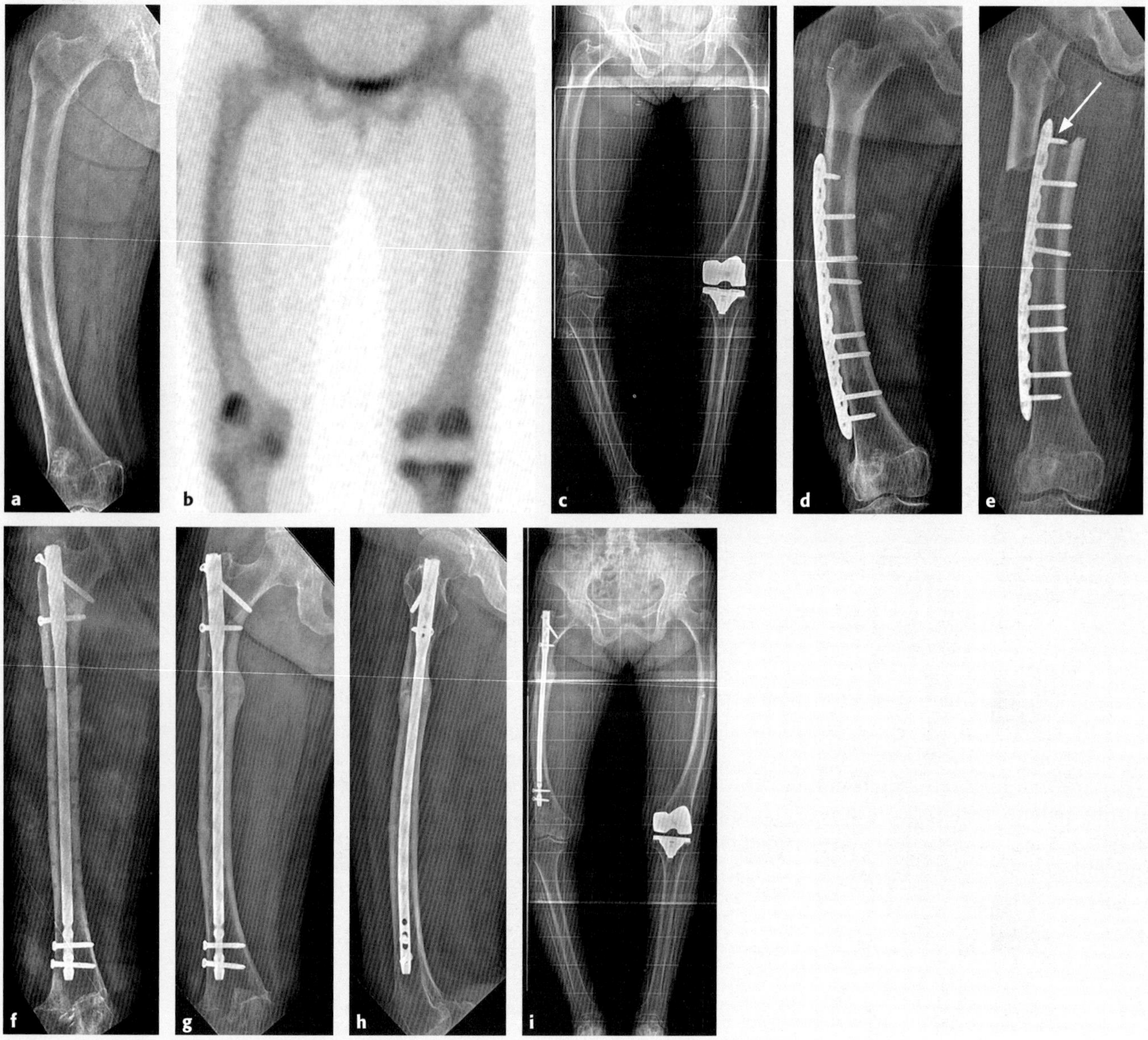


**Fig 3.18-7a–i** A 70-year-old woman with pain in her left thigh.
**a–c** X-rays showing the thickened cortex of the femur and the severe anterolateral bowing of both femurs. The bone scan showing a hot uptake in the midshaft area.
**d–f** X-rays showing plate fixation, with the plate being bent to adjust the curvature. A fracture at the proximal end of the plate after 5 days rendered nailing as a revision procedure necessary.
**g–i** Successful healing after 10 months with the difference in bowing of the femur compared to the uninjured side.

## Patient

A 75-year-old woman suffered an atypical fracture of the right femur.

## Treatment and outcome

There was an exaggerated curve and thickened lateral cortex of the left femur (**Fig 3.18-8a–b**). Good reduction was achieved with antegrade intramedullary nailing (**Fig 3.18-8c–d**). Nine months after surgery, the patient had persistent pain while walking. The fracture was not healed with hypertrophic callus and the distal screws were loosened (**Fig 3.18-8e–f**). A larger diameter nail was used after reaming for the revision procedure. Also, screws of angular stable locking system were fixed to further stabilize the distal fixation (**Fig 3.18-8g–h**). Successful healing was achieved 6 months postoperatively (**Fig 3.18-8i–k**).

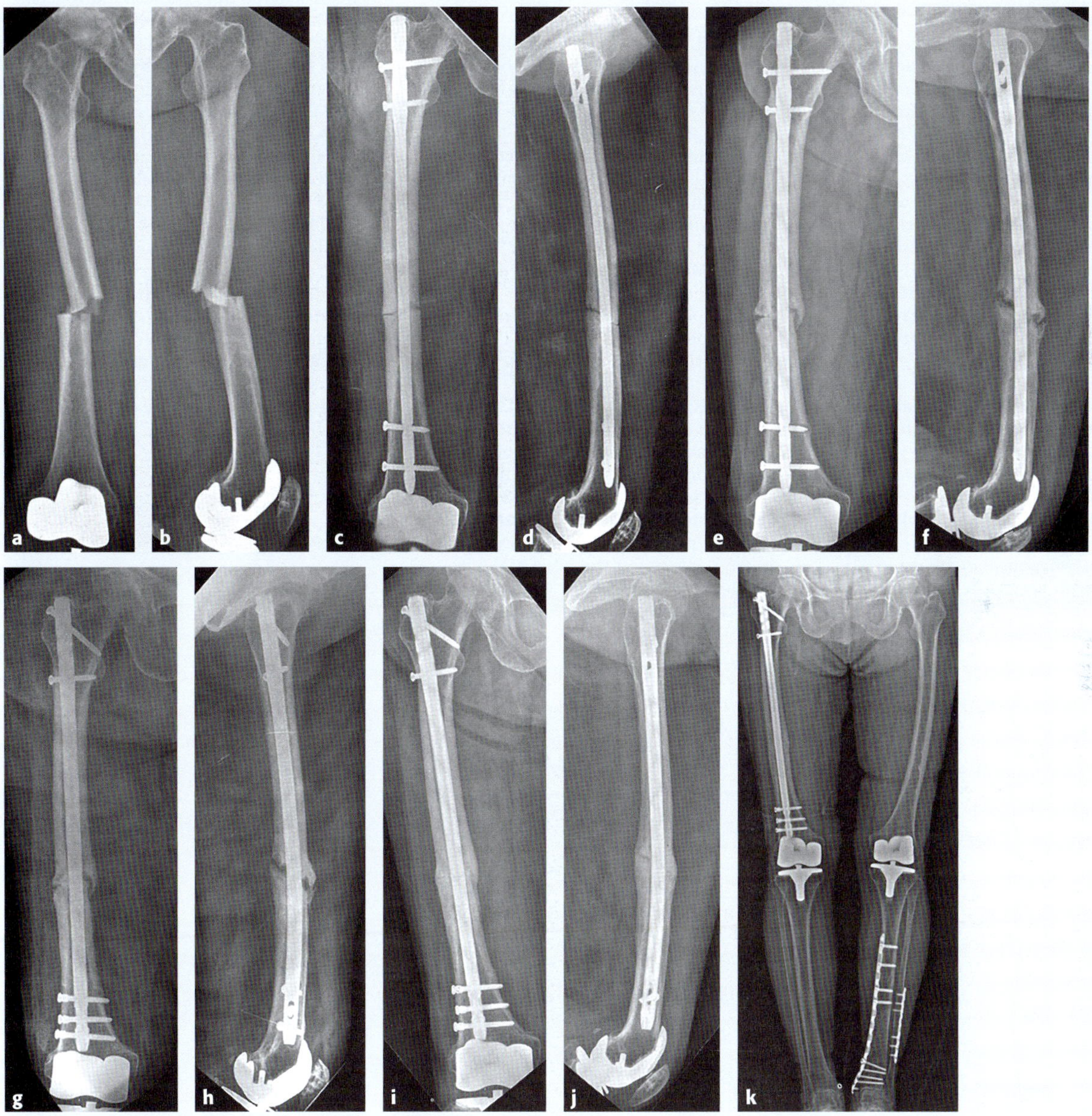


**Fig 3.18-8a–k** A 75-year-old woman with an atypical femoral fracture.
**a–b** X-rays showing the exaggerated curve and thickened lateral cortex of the left femur.
**c–d** Antegrade intramedullary nailing resulted in good reduction.
**e–f** Nine-month postoperative x-rays showing the unhealed fracture with hypertrophic callus and loosened distal screws.
**g–h** Revision procedure with a larger diameter nail used after reaming. Screws of an angular stable locking system were fixed to create further stability to the distal fixation.
**i–k** Successfully healed fracture at 6 months postoperatively.

## 7 References

1. **Goh SK, Yang KY, Koh JS, et al.** Subtrochanteric insufficiency fractures in patients on alendronate therapy: a caution. *J Bone Joint Surg Br.* 2007 Mar;89(3):349–353.
2. **Neviaser AS, Lane JM, Lenart BA, et al.** Low-energy femoral shaft fractures associated with alendronate use. *J Orthop Trauma.* 2008 May–Jun;22(5):346–350.
3. **Park-Wyllie LY, Mamdani MM, Juurlink DN, et al.** Bisphosphonate use and the risk of subtrochanteric or femoral shaft fractures in older women. *JAMA.* 2011 Feb 23;305(8):783–789.
4. **Shane E, Burr D, Abrahamsen B, et al.** Atypical subtrochanteric and diaphyseal femoral fractures: second report of a task force of the American Society for Bone and Mineral Research. *J Bone Miner Res.* 2014 Jan;29(1):1–23.
5. **Chiang GS, Koh KW, Chong TW, et al.** Stress fracture of the ulna associated with bisphosphonate therapy and use of walking aid. *Osteoporos Int.* 2014 Aug;25(8):2151–2154.
6. **Tan SH, Saseendar S, Tan BH, et al.** Ulnar fractures with bisphosphonate therapy: a systematic review of published case reports. *Osteoporos Int.* 2015 Feb;26(2):421–429.
7. **Hagen JE, Miller AN, Ott SM, et al.** Association of atypical femoral fractures with bisphosphonate use by patients with varus hip geometry. *J Bone Joint Surg Am.* 2014 Nov 19;96(22):1905–1909.
8. **Sasaki S, Miyakoshi N, Hongo M, et al.** Low-energy diaphyseal femoral fractures associated with bisphosphonate use and severe curved femur: a case series. *J Bone Miner Metab.* 2012 Sep;30(5):561–567.
9. **Bjorgul K, Reigstad A.** Atypical fracture of the ulna associated with alendronate use. *Acta Orthop.* 2011 Dec;82(6):761–763.
10. **Cross MB, Nam D, van der Meulen MC, et al.** A rare case of a bisphosphonate-induced peri-prosthetic femoral fracture. *J Bone Joint Surg Br.* 2012 Jul;94(7):994–997.
11. **El Rachkidi R, Sari-Leret ML, Wolff S.** Atypical bilateral pedicle fracture in long-term bisphosphonate therapy. *Spine (Phila Pa 1976).* 2011 Dec 15;36(26):E1769–E1773.
12. **Koh JH, Myong JP, Jung SM, et al.** Atypical femoral fracture in rheumatoid arthritis patients treated with bisphosphonates: a nested case-control study. *Arthritis Rheumatol.* 2016 Jan;68(1):77–82.
13. **Cheon SH, Oh CW, Lee JY, et al.** Early diagnosis of impending femoral insufficiency fractures by use of MRI: case report and review of the literature. *J Orthop Sci.* 2013 Sep;18(5):843–848.
14. **Unnanuntana A, Saleh A, Mensah KA, et al.** Atypical femoral fractures: what do we know about them?: AAOS Exhibit Selection. *J Bone Joint Surg Am.* 2013 Jan 16;95(2):e8 1–13.
15. **Capeci CM, Tejwani NC.** Bilateral low-energy simultaneous or sequential femoral fractures in patients on long-term alendronate therapy. *J Bone Joint Surg Am.* 2009 Nov;91(11):2556–2561.
16. **Ha YC, Cho MR, Park KH, et al.** Is surgery necessary for femoral insufficiency fractures after long-term bisphosphonate therapy? *Clin Orthop Relat Res.* 2010 Dec;468(12):3393–3398.
17. **Egol KA, Park JH, Prensky C, et al.** Surgical treatment improves clinical and functional outcomes for patients who sustain incomplete bisphosphonate-related femur fractures. *J Orthop Trauma.* 2013 Jun;27(6):331–335.
18. **Egol KA, Park JH, Rosenberg ZS, et al.** Healing delayed but generally reliable after bisphosphonate-associated complete femur fractures treated with IM nails. *Clin Orthop Relat Res.* 2014 Sep;472(9):2728–2734.
19. **Teo BJ, Koh JS, Goh SK, et al.** Post-operative outcomes of atypical femoral subtrochanteric fracture in patients on bisphosphonate therapy. *Bone Joint J.* 2014 May;96-B(5):658–664.

# 3.19 Chest trauma

Hans-Christian Jeske

## 1 Introduction

Chest trauma in geriatric patients has vastly higher morbidity and mortality compared to younger patients and represents a challenging problem for treating physicians [1]. This chapter describes the fundamentals of systemic pain control, important local and regional anesthesia techniques, and the rare indications for operative intervention.

## 2 Epidemiology and etiology

The prevalence of geriatric rib fractures is increasing due to an aging population with increased life expectancy. Over the last six decades, life expectancy in western countries has increased from 68.2 years to 78.7 years [2, 3], and it has been estimated that the geriatric population will represent 25% of the US population by 2030 [4], including a significant increase in those older than 85 years.

This demographic change is predictably associated with an increasing incidence of rib fractures. Today, thoracic trauma accounts for 10–15% of all trauma admissions [5]. This number is expected to rise, since 11.3% of ground-level falls in patients older than 90 years are estimated to result in rib fractures [6].

As noted throughout this text, geriatric patients require a multidisciplinary approach to reduce mortality and achieve optimal outcomes [7]. In equally severe traumas, the mortality rate in geriatric patients is approximately five times higher compared with younger patients [1, 8, 9]. Studies demonstrate a correlation between mortality and the number of broken ribs, ie, "severity of trauma" represented as higher "injury severity scores" [10]. The higher mortality rates in geriatric patients can partly be explained by decreased physiological reserves and increased frailty but is likely also due to undertreatment of pain.

## 3 Diagnostics

During the last decade, computed tomographic (CT) scans have been increasingly used for chest trauma patients rather than conventional x-rays; this was prompted in part by the increased sensitivity of CT scans compared to x-rays in detecting rib fractures [11, 12]. Kea et al [13] showed that 18.1% of trauma patients had fractures detected by CT scans but missed on conventional x-rays. It is important to note that these fractures are usually minor and nondisplaced and do not change the treatment protocol, rendering routine CT scanning for rib fractures of little benefit [13–16].

Up to 2% of malignancies in the US, such as malignant tumors (ie, sarcomas, breast cancer or leukemia etc), are estimated to be caused by CT radiation [17, 18]. While most members of the geriatric population might not live long enough to suffer consequences from this radiation, the additional information gained typically does not lead to a change in treatment only adding to higher costs and the burdens of incidental findings (eg, lung nodules and false positives for pulmonary embolism [PE]) [19]. A CT scan should only be ordered in severe thoracic trauma, polytrauma, and in patients with suspicion of pneumothorax or PE. In most patients, diagnostic plain x-rays are sufficient. Ultrasound is also a fast and cost-effective tool to evaluate rib fractures, especially in cases where the fracture has been seen on x-ray and the clinical symptoms are severe [20]. At the same time ultrasound can be used to guide an intercostal nerve block if necessary (**Fig 3.19-1**).

## 4 Therapeutic options

### 4.1 Pain treatment

When considering treatment options, physicians must account for specific issues unique to geriatric patients. The gold standard for patients suffering from broken ribs is nonoperative treatment with pain-adapted analgesia. Pain associated with rib fractures impairs respiratory function and increases pulmonary morbidity. Adequate pain control improves respiratory mechanics and decreases pulmonary complications such as atelectasis, pneumonia, and respiratory failure [8, 21, 22]. Unfortunately, geriatric chest trauma patients are often undertreated for pain, contributing to higher mortality rates [9, 23].

#### 4.1.1 Intravenous analgesics

Intravenous analgesics are usually required for initial pain control, with conversion to oral medication after a few days (see chapter 1.12 Pain management). Primary systemic analgesic treatment is outlined according to the World Health Organization *Treatment Guidelines on Pain* [24] and can serve as the analgesic foundation for rib fracture patients. In order to provide adequate analgesia, it is necessary to routinely monitor the patient's symptoms and response to medication. Geriatric patients in particular are often given inadequate analgesic treatment if not actively monitored. In practice, this can be achieved by routine pain assessment several times a day, using an appropriate and validated pain scale, eg, the Visual Analog Scale or Pain Assessment in Advanced Dementia scale for cognitively impaired patients (see chapter 1.12 Pain management). Analgesic medication dosing can be evaluated and adjusted as needed.

In general, patient-controlled analgesic systems are not appropriate for geriatric patients due to the high prevalence of dementia and delirium.

#### 4.1.2 Intercostal nerve blocks

Intercostal nerve blocks can be an effective adjuvant treatment for rib fracture pain and can minimize the doses and side effects of systemic opioids. Intercostal nerve blocks can be done as a single shot or continuous infusion. In comparative studies, the continuous intercostal block has achieved better outcomes than epidural anesthesia in terms of pneumonia and ventilation-dependent respiratory failure, and the placement is typically less time-consuming [25–27]. The intercostal block is easy and safe to perform and has only few adverse effects. In clinical practice, this is an alternative for physicians who do not use epidural anesthesia in their daily routine. In many older patients, epidural anesthesia is contraindicated due to chronic anticoagulant, antiplatelet therapy, or other bleeding tendencies.

The author prefers an ultrasound-guided block which, in addition to the obvious advantages in obese patients, enables high-quality visualization of fractured ribs and can thereby optimize the position of the block. A continuous block is also easy to perform and, in the author's experience, is ideally placed in patients with a high degree of pain on presentation, since these patients will otherwise require repeated injections. It is fairly easy to address two costal segments using only one skin puncture, by redirecting the needle while smoothly sliding from one subcostal space to the next. In this maneuver, sonographic guidance is also beneficial (**Fig 3.19-2**, **Fig 3.19-3**).

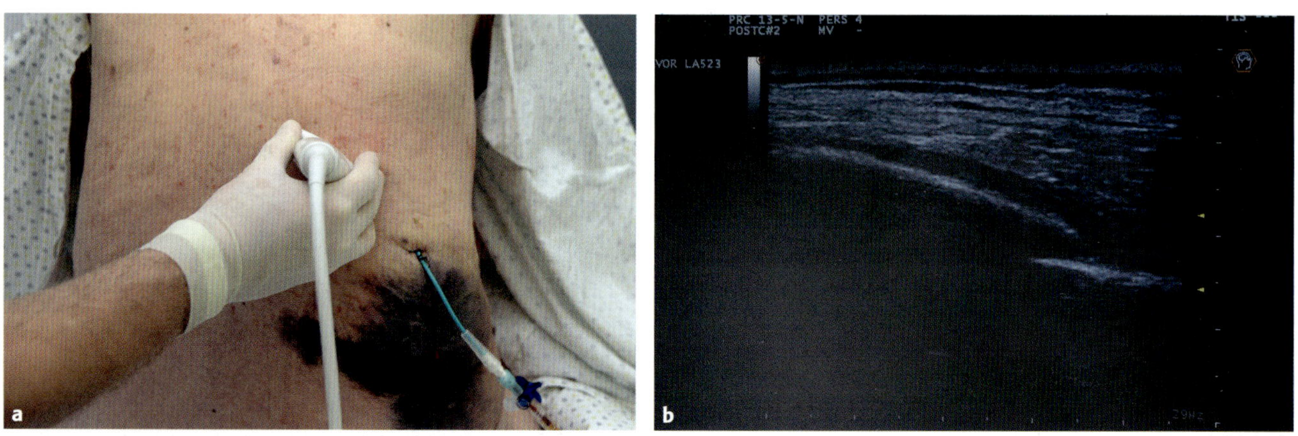

**Fig 3.19-1a–b** Diagnostic sonography (**a**). Rib fracture is seen on the monitor (**b**).

In the author's experience, a series of single-shot blocks over the first 3 days has shown to be effective. Recurrent pain after depletion of the local anesthesia is usually considered to be less intense than the initial pain. The application of the blocks can easily be repeated.

In summary, intercostal nerve blockade can be considered equally effective as epidural anesthesia in treating pain and can be safely performed as either continuous administration or repeated injections [28]. It is simple to apply and has no significant neurological complications, nausea, vomiting, dizziness, or epidural bleeding as observed in other measures such as thoracic epidural injection or intravenous patient-controlled opioid analgesia. The disadvantage of this treatment is that multiple injections are necessary in patients with multiple fractures, and the effect of a single injection may only last 6–8 hours [29, 30]. Potential complications of this procedure include iatrogenic pneumothorax, hemothorax, bleeding, and infection [31].

### 4.1.3 Epidural anesthesia

Epidural anesthesia is considered an effective but advanced analgesic treatment option in patients with multiple rib fractures for whom intercostal nerve blockade is inadequate for pain relief and pulmonary function. Epidural analgesia can be done as a single-shot measure or as a continuous infusion, enabling pain relief for days due to administration of local anesthesia via an epidural catheter system.

In some studies, epidural anesthesia was reported to show superior outcomes across multiple domains when compared to intravenous opioid analgesics [32–34], including increased respiratory tidal volumes, reduced inflammatory response [35, 36], and even decreased mortality, but the results of other studies are conflicting. These studies report worse outcomes of epidural anesthesia in patients with pulmonary comorbidities compared with patients treated with intravenous opioids [37]. In these studies, some older frail patients experienced additional complications associated with epidural anesthesia including urinary retention, headache, decreased respiratory function, infection, epidural hematoma and neurological injuries [8, 38].

A metaanalysis of randomized controlled trials using epidural analgesia in patients with traumatic rib fractures by Carrier et al [39] did not show significant benefits of epidural analgesia in terms of mortality, length of intensive care unit (ICU) time, or overall hospital stay. The authors [39] point out that there may be a reduction in the duration of mechanical ventilation with the use of thoracic epidural analgesia with local anesthetics.

Countering this is the evidence-based metaanalysis by Simon et al [40], who stated a level I recommendation for epidural anesthesia in patients with blunt chest trauma, including frail older adults. This metaanalysis maintained that epidural anesthesia significantly improves subjective pain perception and facilitates better pulmonary function tests as opposed to intravenous analgesia. Furthermore, this method of pain relief is associated with less respiratory depression, somnolence, and gastrointestinal symptoms than intravenous narcotics. Finally, epidural anaesthesia is considered to be a safer method in terms of complications, with low rates of permanent disability and negligible mortality. Epidural anesthesia requires the cooperation of a highly skilled anesthetist, as it is necessary to perform these blocks at a cervicothoracic spinal level, and can cause significant spinal injury if not performed properly. Epidural anesthesia is most

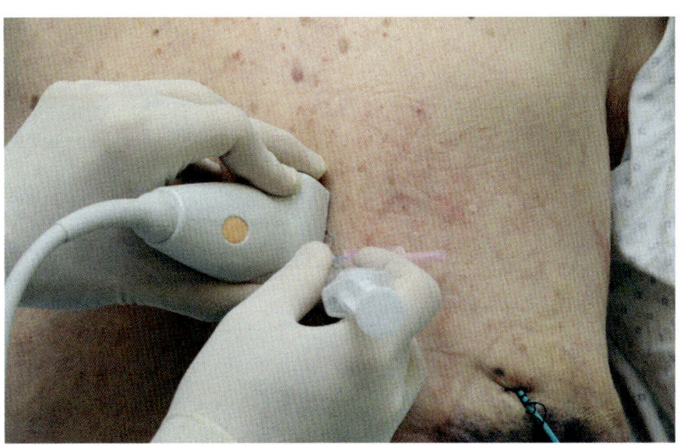

**Fig 3.19-2** Ultrasound-guided intercostal infiltration.

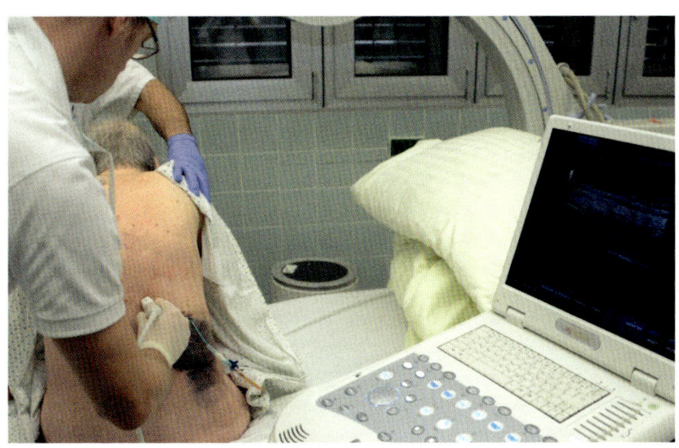

**Fig 3.19-3** Localizing rib fractures prior to administration of an intercostal block.

strongly indicated in severe cases with multiple bilateral rib fractures; for less severe cases, the author generally prefers intercostal nerve blockade.

### 4.2 Operative treatment

Concerning operative treatment of rib fractures, the data in literature is inconsistent. Some studies favor operative repair, while others show no benefit or even harm when compared to nonoperative treatment [41–43]. The author has performed plating of fractured ribs in only a small number of patients at his hospital (**Fig 3.19-4**). Surgery was performed after multidisciplinary consultation and consensus [7]. In practice, operative intervention was most commonly the result of inadequate respiratory function despite maximal nonoperative treatment. For the few flail chest patients the author treated with this operation, this measurement rapidly improved the patients' respiratory situation [7]. Although it has not been recommended as first-line treatment, it remains an important option in the difficult treatment of flail chest syndrome patients.

The author has treated only a few selected patients with open reduction and internal fixation (ORIF). The case, which was previously published by Zegg et al [7], is an example of a patient who was treated with this operative technique (**Case 1: Fig 3.19-5**).

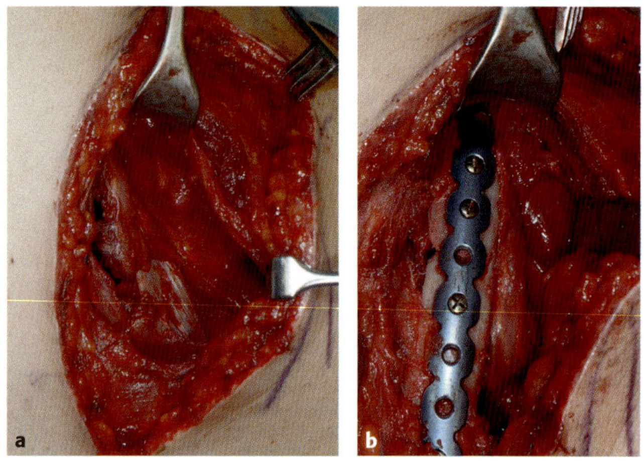


**Fig 3.19-4a–b** Fractured rib prior to plating (**a**). Plating with angular stable system after open reduction (**b**).

**CASE 1**

#### Patient

An 87-year-old woman, who was crushed against a wall by a bull, was transferred to the author's clinic after initial stabilization from a local hospital in October 2010.

#### Treatment and outcome

She had sustained bilateral rib fractures, including 1 to 10 on the right, with segmental fractures 2 to 10 and 1 to 8 on the left. Additional complications were severe and included a hemopneumothorax, pulmonary hemorrhage, massive subcutaneous emphysema, laceration of the thoracic diaphragm, liver laceration, compression fractures of the third and eighth thoracic vertebrae, and hemorrhagic shock (Injury Severity Score 1/4 41). On arrival at the clinic, the patient was intubated and mechanically ventilated (biphasic positive airway pressure [BIPAP]: level 19/10 mbar, time high 2.0/low 2.0 seconds, FiO2 1/41.0, PaO2 1/449 mm Hg, PaCO2 1/433 mm Hg) and treated with morphine and midazolam analgesia. After primary stabilization in the emergency department, she received four chest tubes on the right side, one on the left, and recombinant factor VIIa (6 mg) to stop hemorrhage of the lung. After initial treatment, she was transferred to the intensive care unit (ICU). Four days after arrival and after multidisciplinary consultation with physicians from the anesthesia, trauma surgery, intensive care, and acute geriatric departments, the patient received operative stabilization of three ribs on the right side, as seen in **Fig 3.19-5**.

After surgery, rapid improvement of the respiratory situation was noticed within hours. Following operative stabilization, augmented ventilation with BIPAP was successful within 1 day. Due to primary lack of vigilance and atelectasis of the lower lobe of the right lung requiring bronchoscopic treatment, weaning was delayed and extubation was not performed until day 13. Stable hemodynamics requiring mild support with vasopressors did not change over time. She was discharged from the ICU after 21 days. The patient was transferred back to the hospital near her hometown where she was discharged 2 weeks after admission.

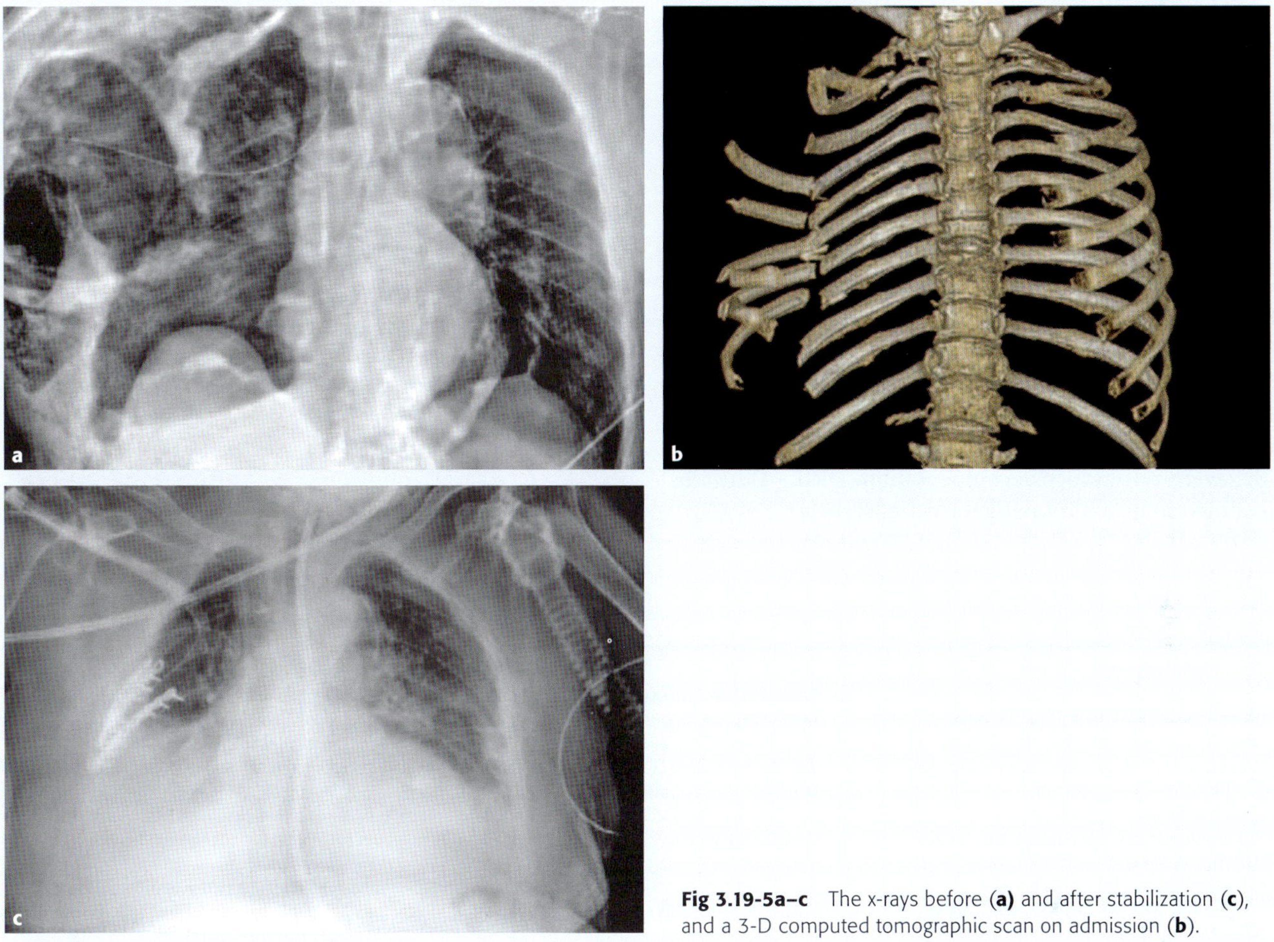

**Fig 3.19-5a–c** The x-rays before (**a**) and after stabilization (**c**), and a 3-D computed tomographic scan on admission (**b**).

## 5 Chest tube and "pigtail"

Heng et al [44] stated in a study that 5–10% of patients sustaining severe blunt thoracic trauma or 25% of all polytraumatized patients are in need of pleural decompression (ie, insertion of chest tubes) [45]. The indication for pleural decompression is hemodynamic or respiratory impairment due to pneumothorax, hemothorax or pneumohaemothorax [46]. In polytraumatized patients, these conditions should be addressed as early as possible before the patient begins to show signs of cardiopulmonary decompensation. This can be done using an anterior Monaldi approach in the midclavicular line (second intercostal space) or a lateral Bülau approach in the midaxillary line (fourth intercostal space).

Another factor to be considered is the size of thoracic drainage tube to use. Traditionally, large-sized drains have been recommended in thoracic trauma [47]. The reasoning here is that due to Pascal's physical law, a drain with a larger caliber would be able to drain more fluid than a smaller one. In the clinical setting however, this does not seem to be the case. Smaller drains simply drain enough fluid for what is needed, and drains that are clotted with blood seem to become obstructed regardless of their diameter [48].

In several recent studies [48–50], the 14 French (F) scale "pigtail" catheter has been shown to drain pneumothorax, hemothorax, hemopneumothorax, and tension pneumothorax as efficiently as 32–40F catheters, suggesting that less invasive smaller drains can be considered.

## 6 Flail chest syndrome

Patients with flail chest syndrome are an extraordinary challenge that may occasionally need operative stabilization of the fractured ribs [41]. Flail chest syndrome leads to a paradoxical motion of the chest in respiration, caused by thoracic instability due to rib fractures. These patients are prone to respiratory decompensation, their analgesic treatment is more difficult, and their overall mortality has been reported to be as high as 16% [51]. Optimal analgesic treatment may be supported with noninvasive positive pressure ventilation, but in some cases this will still be complicated by respiratory decompensation [51]. In this situation, intubation and mechanical ventilation is necessary. In some patients with severe respiratory decompensation, ORIF of the ribs has shown to be a life-saving measure [52, 53].

## 7 Acknowledgments

The author of this chapter acknowledges the contributions of Dr Michael Zegg, Dr Rebecca Schöpf, and Prof Michael Blauth for their thoughtful comments and input, which has substantially improved this chapter.

## 8 References

1. **Bergeron E, Lavoie A, Clas D, et al.** Elderly trauma patients with rib fractures are at greater risk of death and pneumonia. *J Trauma.* 2003 Mar;54(3):478–485.
2. **Xu J, Murphy SL, Kochanek KD, et al.** Deaths: final data for 2013. *Natl Vital Stat Rep.* 2016 Feb 16;64(2):1–119.
3. **Kochanek KD, Murphy SL, Xu J, et al.** Deaths: final data for 2014. *Natl Vital Stat Rep.* 2016 Jun;65(4):1–122.
4. **Mandavia D, Newton K.** Geriatric trauma. *Emerg Med Clin North Am.* 1998 Feb;16(1):257–274.
5. **Flagel BT, Luchette FA, Reed RL, et al.** Half-a-dozen ribs: the breakpoint for mortality. *Surgery.* 2005 Oct;138(4):717–723; discussion 723–725.
6. **Bhattacharya B, Maung A, Schuster K, et al.** The older they are the harder they fall: injury patterns and outcomes by age after ground level falls. *Injury.* 2016 Sep;47(9):1955–1959.
7. **Zegg M, Kammerlander C, Schmid S, et al.** Multidisciplinary approach to lifesaving measures in the elderly individuals with flail chest injury with ORIF of rib fractures: a report of 2 cases. *Geriatr Orthop Surg Rehabil.* 2012 Dec;3(4):164–166.
8. **Bulger EM, Arneson MA, Mock CN, et al.** Rib fractures in the elderly. *J Trauma.* 2000 Jun;48(6):1040–1046; discussion 1046–1047.
9. **Knudson MM, Lieberman J, Morris JA Jr, et al.** Mortality factors in geriatric blunt trauma patients. *Arch Surg.* 1994 Apr;129(4):448–453.
10. **Stawicki SP, Grossman MD, Hoey BA, et al.** Rib fractures in the elderly: a marker of injury severity. *J Am Geriatr Soc.* 2004 May;52(5):805–808.
11. **Traub M, Stevenson M, McEvoy S, et al.** The use of chest computed tomography versus chest X-ray in patients with major blunt trauma. *Injury.* 2007 Jan;38(1):43–47.
12. **Tillou A, Gupta M, Baraff LJ, et al.** Is the use of pan-computed tomography for blunt trauma justified? A prospective evaluation. *J Trauma.* 2009 Oct;67(4):779–787.
13. **Kea B, Gamarallage R, Vairamuthu H, et al.** What is the clinical significance of chest CT when the chest x-ray result is normal in patients with blunt trauma? *Am J Emerg Med.* 2013 Aug;31(8):1268–1273.
14. **Korley FK, Pham JC, Kirsch TD.** Use of advanced radiology during visits to US emergency departments for injury-related conditions, 1998–2007. *JAMA.* 2010 Oct 06;304(13):1465–1471.
15. **Atzema C, Mower WR, Hoffman JR, et al.** Defining "therapeutically inconsequential" head computed tomographic findings in patients with blunt head trauma. *Ann Emerg Med.* 2004 Jul;44(1):47–56.
16. **Barrios C, Malinoski D, Dolich M, et al.** Utility of thoracic computed tomography after blunt trauma: when is chest radiograph enough? *Am Surg.* 2009 Oct;75(10):966–969.
17. **Brenner DJ, Hall EJ.** Risk of cancer from diagnostic x-rays. *Lancet.* 2004 Jun 26;363(9427):2192; author reply 2192–2193.
18. **Fazel R, Krumholz HM, Wang Y, et al.** Exposure to low-dose ionizing radiation from medical imaging procedures. *N Engl J Med.* 2009 Aug 27;361(9):849–857.
19. **Wiener RS, Schwartz LM, Woloshin S.** When a test is too good: how CT pulmonary angiograms find pulmonary emboli that do not need to be found. *BMJ.* 2013 Jul 02;347:f3368.
20. **Turk F, Kurt AB, Saglam S.** Evaluation by ultrasound of traumatic rib fractures missed by radiography. *Emerg Radiol.* 2010 Nov;17(6):473–477.
21. **Ziegler DW, Agarwal NN.** The morbidity and mortality of rib fractures. *J Trauma.* 1994 Dec;37(6):975–979.
22. **Easter A.** Management of patients with multiple rib fractures. *Am J Crit Care.* 2001 Sep;10(5):320–327; quiz 328–329.
23. **Quattromani E, Normansell D, Storkan M, et al.** Oligoanalgesia in blunt geriatric trauma. *J Emerg Med.* 2015 Jun;48(6):653–659.
24. **World Health Organization.** Treatment Guidelines on Pain. Available at: www.who.int/medicines/areas/quality_safety/guide_on_pain/en/. Accessed May 2017.
25. **Britt T, Sturm R, Ricardi R, et al.** Comparative evaluation of continuous intercostal nerve block or epidural analgesia on the rate of respiratory complications, intensive care unit, and hospital stay following traumatic rib fractures: a retrospective review. *Local Reg Anesth.* 2015;8:79–84.

26. **Mohta M, Verma P, Saxena AK, et al.** Prospective, randomized comparison of continuous thoracic epidural and thoracic paravertebral infusion in patients with unilateral multiple fractured ribs—a pilot study. *J Trauma.* 2009 Apr;66(4):1096–1101.
27. **Holcomb JB, McMullin NR, Kozar RA, et al.** Morbidity from rib fractures increases after age 45. *J Am Coll Surg.* 2003 Apr;196(4):549–555.
28. **Luketich JD, Land SR, Sullivan EA, et al.** Thoracic epidural versus intercostal nerve catheter plus patient-controlled analgesia: a randomized study. *Ann Thorac Surg.* 2005 Jun;79(6):1845–1849; discussion 1849–1850.
29. **Pedersen VM, Schulze S, Hoier-Madsen K, et al.** Air-flow meter assessment of the effect of intercostal nerve blockade on respiratory function in rib fractures. *Acta Chir Scand.* 1983;149(2):119–120.
30. **Hwang EG, Lee Y.** Effectiveness of intercostal nerve block for management of pain in rib fracture patients. *J Exerc Rehabil.* 2014 Aug;10(4):241–244.
31. **Rauchwerger JJ, Candido KD, Deer TR, et al.** Thoracic epidural steroid injection for rib fracture pain. *Pain Pract.* 2013 Jun;13(5):416–421.
32. **Zaw AA, Murry J, Hoang D, et al.** Epidural analgesia after rib fractures. *Am Surg.* 2015 Oct;81(10):950–954.
33. **Bulger EM, Edwards T, Klotz P, et al.** Epidural analgesia improves outcome after multiple rib fractures. *Surgery.* 2004 Aug;136(2):426–430.
34. **Wu CL, Jani ND, Perkins FM, et al.** Thoracic epidural analgesia versus intravenous patient-controlled analgesia for the treatment of rib fracture pain after motor vehicle crash. *J Trauma.* 1999 Sep;47(3):564–567.
35. **Moon MR, Luchette FA, Gibson SW, et al.** Prospective, randomized comparison of epidural versus parenteral opioid analgesia in thoracic trauma. *Ann Surg.* 1999 May;229(5):684–691; discussion 691–692.
36. **Mackersie RC, Karagianes TG, Hoyt DB, et al.** Prospective evaluation of epidural and intravenous administration of fentanyl for pain control and restoration of ventilatory function following multiple rib fractures. *J Trauma.* 1991 Apr;31(4):443–449; discussion 449–451.
37. **Kieninger AN, Bair HA, Bendick PJ, et al.** Epidural versus intravenous pain control in elderly patients with rib fractures. *Am J Surg.* 2005 Mar;189(3):327–330.
38. **Auroy Y, Narchi P, Messiah A, et al.** Serious complications related to regional anesthesia: results of a prospective survey in France. *Anesthesiology.* 1997 Sep;87(3):479–486.
39. **Carrier FM, Turgeon AF, Nicole PC, et al.** Effect of epidural analgesia in patients with traumatic rib fractures: a systematic review and meta-analysis of randomized controlled trials. *Can J Anaesth.* 2009 Mar;56(3):230–242.
40. **Simon BJ, Cushman J, Barraco R, et al.** Pain management guidelines for blunt thoracic trauma. *J Trauma.* 2005 Nov;59(5):1256–1267.
41. **Lafferty PM, Anavian J, Will RE, et al.** Operative treatment of chest wall injuries: indications, technique, and outcomes. *J Bone Joint Surg Am.* 2011 Jan 05;93(1):97–110.
42. **Ahmed Z, Mohyuddin Z.** Management of flail chest injury: internal fixation versus endotracheal intubation and ventilation. *J Thorac Cardiovasc Surg.* 1995 Dec;110(6):1676–1680.
43. **Nirula R, Allen B, Layman R, et al.** Rib fracture stabilization in patients sustaining blunt chest injury. *Am Surg.* 2006 Apr;72(4):307–309.
44. **Heng K, Bystrzycki A, Fitzgerald M, et al.** Complications of intercostal catheter insertion using EMST techniques for chest trauma. *ANZ J Surg.* 2004 Jun;74(6):420–423.
45. **Maybauer MO, Geisser W, Wolff H, et al.** Incidence and outcome of tube thoracostomy positioning in trauma patients. *Prehosp Emerg Care.* 2012 Apr–Jun;16(2):237–241.
46. **Aul A, Klose R.** Invasive Techniken in der Notfallmedizin. II. Präklinische Thoraxdrainage—Indikationen und Technik [Invasive techniques in emergency medicine. II. Preclinical thorax drainage—indications and technique]. *Anaesthesist.* 2004 Dec;53(12):1203–1210. German.
47. **Fitzgerald M, Mackenzie CF, Marasco S, et al.** Pleural decompression and drainage during trauma reception and resuscitation. *Injury.* 2008 Jan;39(1):9–20.
48. **Inaba K, Lustenberger T, Recinos G, et al.** Does size matter? A prospective analysis of 28–32 versus 36–40 French chest tube size in trauma. *J Trauma Acute Care Surg.* 2012 Feb;72(2):422–427.
49. **Kulvatunyou N, Joseph B, Friese RS, et al.** 14 French pigtail catheters placed by surgeons to drain blood on trauma patients: is 14-Fr too small? *J Trauma Acute Care Surg.* 2012 Dec;73(6):1423–1427.
50. **Rivera L, O'Reilly EB, Sise MJ, et al.** Small catheter tube thoracostomy: effective in managing chest trauma in stable patients. *J Trauma.* 2009 Feb;66(2):393–399.
51. **Dehghan N, de Mestral C, McKee MD, et al.** Flail chest injuries: a review of outcomes and treatment practices from the National Trauma Data Bank. *J Trauma Acute Care Surg.* 2014 Feb;76(2):462–468.
52. **Leinicke JA, Elmore L, Freeman BD, et al.** Operative management of rib fractures in the setting of flail chest: a systematic review and meta-analysis. *Ann Surg.* 2013 Dec;258(6):914–921.
53. **Slobogean GP, MacPherson CA, Sun T, et al.** Surgical fixation vs nonoperative management of flail chest: a meta-analysis. *J Am Coll Surg.* 2013 Feb;216(2):302–311.e1.

# 3.20 Polytrauma

Julie A Switzer, Herman Johal

## 1 Introduction

Older adults and, in particular those over 80 years (ie, the oldest old), are the most rapidly growing segment of the world population. They often still participate in a number of activities that render them at risk for high-energy injuries or polytrauma, including driving, cycling, and working at heights. Taken together, society can expect a continued increase in geriatric polytrauma, which requires an understanding of the unique aspects of standard adult trauma [1]:

- The interpretation of the literature regarding geriatric polytrauma is limited due to the lack of agreement on the age criteria and definition of "older" for these studies.
- Increased life expectancy, increased independence, and increasingly active lifestyles predispose older individuals to polytrauma.

## 2 Epidemiology and etiology

- Approximately 20–30% of all trauma occurs in individuals older than 35 years [2].
- Most polytrauma occurs in men until approximately the age of 70 years; after 70 years, women are more commonly injured. Although few studies have focused on older trauma patients, reports of Swiss, Belgian, and Australian trauma populations have estimated the number of older individuals who have sustained polytrauma to be between 9% and 41% [3–5].
- For older adults who sustain polytrauma, falls and motor vehicle accidents are the most common injury mechanisms and result in the highest mortality [6].
- Falls in older adults, even falls from a low height, have been shown to result in injuries of similar nature to those sustained by younger individuals in higher-energy accidents [3].
- In individuals younger than 55 years, the incidence of trauma is decreasing. However, in all age groups older than 55 years, the incidence of trauma is steadily increasing [8–11].
- Injury patterns in the older trauma patient are different than in the younger patient with substantially higher rates of fractures, greater morbidity, and higher mortality [1].

## 3 Specific injuries

The distribution and pattern of injuries are different in older patients than for younger cohorts; older patients are more likely to sustain closed head injuries, cervical spine injuries, and bony thoracic injuries, ie, rib, sternal, and/or clavicular fractures [12]. Additional common injuries include thoracic injuries, pelvic fractures, and extremity fractures [13, 14].

### 3.1 Closed head injuries

- Older trauma patients experience a higher rate of intracranial injuries compared to younger age groups [15], with reported rates ranging from 63% to 88% [9, 14].
- Severe closed head injury, defined as Glasgow Coma Scale (GCS) $\leq 8$, has been found to be a significant risk factor for death [12].

### 3.2 Spinal injuries

- Cervical spine injuries are common [16].
- Common spondyloarthritic conditions, such as spinal stenosis and diffuse idiopathic skeletal hyperostosis, predispose to more catastrophic injury.

### 3.3 Chest injuries, including clavicle, ribs, and sternum

- In blunt chest trauma, each individual rib fracture has been shown to contribute a 19% increase in mortality and a 27% increase in risk of pneumonia [17].
- Clavicle, pelvis, and spine injuries are associated with increased mortality [18].

### 3.4 Pelvic and acetabular injuries

- For a given pelvic fracture pattern, there is a greater mortality risk in older adults compared to a younger cohort [19].
- Lateral compression pelvic fracture patterns and anterior column acetabular fractures are more common [20].
- Friability of pelvic vessels in older adults may contribute to blood loss, morbidity, and mortality [21].

### 3.5 Lower extremity injuries

- The severity of lower extremity injuries sustained in motor vehicle injuries is significantly higher in older adults [15].

## 4 Triage

Since 1986, the American College of Surgeons Committee on Trauma has published guidelines for field trauma triage. Unfortunately, older individuals who have sustained polytrauma are less likely to be transported to a higher acuity or level I trauma center [22, 23]. This apparent lack of understanding of the urgency or acuity in multiply injured older adults occurs despite the publication of studies that have demonstrated improved outcomes when older patients are triaged to hospitals with dedicated trauma resources (**Case 1: Fig 3.20-1**) [24, 25].

CASE 1

**Patient**

A 76-year-old male driver involved in a motor vehicle collision suffered polytrauma and was initially triaged to a nearby level III trauma center. His injuries were identified as an intracranial hemorrhage, pelvic ring fracture, right distal radial fracture, and left tibial plateau fracture. The patient had a Glasgow Coma Scale of 7.

**Comorbidities**

- Hypertension
- Hypercholesterolemia

**Treatment and outcome**

At the level III trauma center, the patient was found to be hemodynamically unstable and underwent an emergent exploratory laparotomy, symphyseal plating, placement of a pelvic C-clamp, and pelvic packing (**Fig 3.20-1a–b**). The remainder of his fractures were splinted and the patient was subsequently transferred to a level I trauma center for further management.

AP and lateral x-rays were obtained for the distal radius indicating volar shear intraarticular distal radial fracture (AO/OTA 2R3B3) (**Fig 3.20-1c–d**). Given the unstable nature of this pattern in a polytrauma patient, operative treatment was undertaken.

In addition, the AP and lateral injury views of the left knee identify a partial articular lateral tibial plateau fracture (AO/OTA 41B1.1), which may be treated either operatively or nonoperatively given its minimal displacement (**Fig 3.20-1e–f**). However, because of its B-type pattern and associated injuries, the patient received definitive surgical stabilization.

Upon arrival at the level I trauma center, the patient underwent computed tomographic angiography, where no arterial bleeding was identified. Intraoperative images of transsacral screw placement, with the C-clamp still in place, were obtained. The C-clamp was adjusted to obtain and maintain reduction while posterior fixation was completed. Once fixation was achieved, the C-clamp was removed and repeat exploratory laparotomy was completed, which did not identify any further pelvic injury, but a grade II splenic laceration and a small bowel contusion were noted. Postoperative AP, inlet, and outlet x-rays showed restoration of the pelvic ring (**Fig 3.20-1g–h**). The orientation of the transsacral screws was perpendicular to the plane of the midsagittal sacral fracture.

Following pelvic fixation, minimally invasive plate osteosynthesis (MIPO) of the tibial plateau was completed using provisional K-wire fixation and subsequent interfragmentary screw placement across the articular surface, as well as buttress fixation at the apex of the fracture (**Fig 3.20-1i–j**).

Simultaneously with the tibial plateau, the contralateral volar sheer distal radial fracture was treated with buttress plating for the B-type articular fragment, and interfragmentary screw fixation for a proximal sagittal plane extension that was noted intraoperatively (**Fig 3.20-1k–l**).

**Key points**

- Geriatric trauma patients are more likely to have intracranial injuries, pelvic injuries, and upper and lower extremity injuries (see topic 2 in this chapter).
- Appropriate triage of multiply injured older adults to a level I trauma center may provide more rapid access to dedicated trauma resources and potentially avoid placement of temporizing devices such as the C-clamp.
- While many distal radial fractures in older adults may be treated nonoperatively, recognition of unstable patterns is important to an improved functional outcome.
- Adherence to MIPO principles helps to minimize the physiological burden of lengthy, extensive procedures.
- Frailty is highly correlated with mortality, in-hospital complications, and "adverse" discharge disposition in older trauma patients [26].
- The orthopedic injuries did heal, and the patient was working on mobilization, but recovery was slow due to his neurological injury.

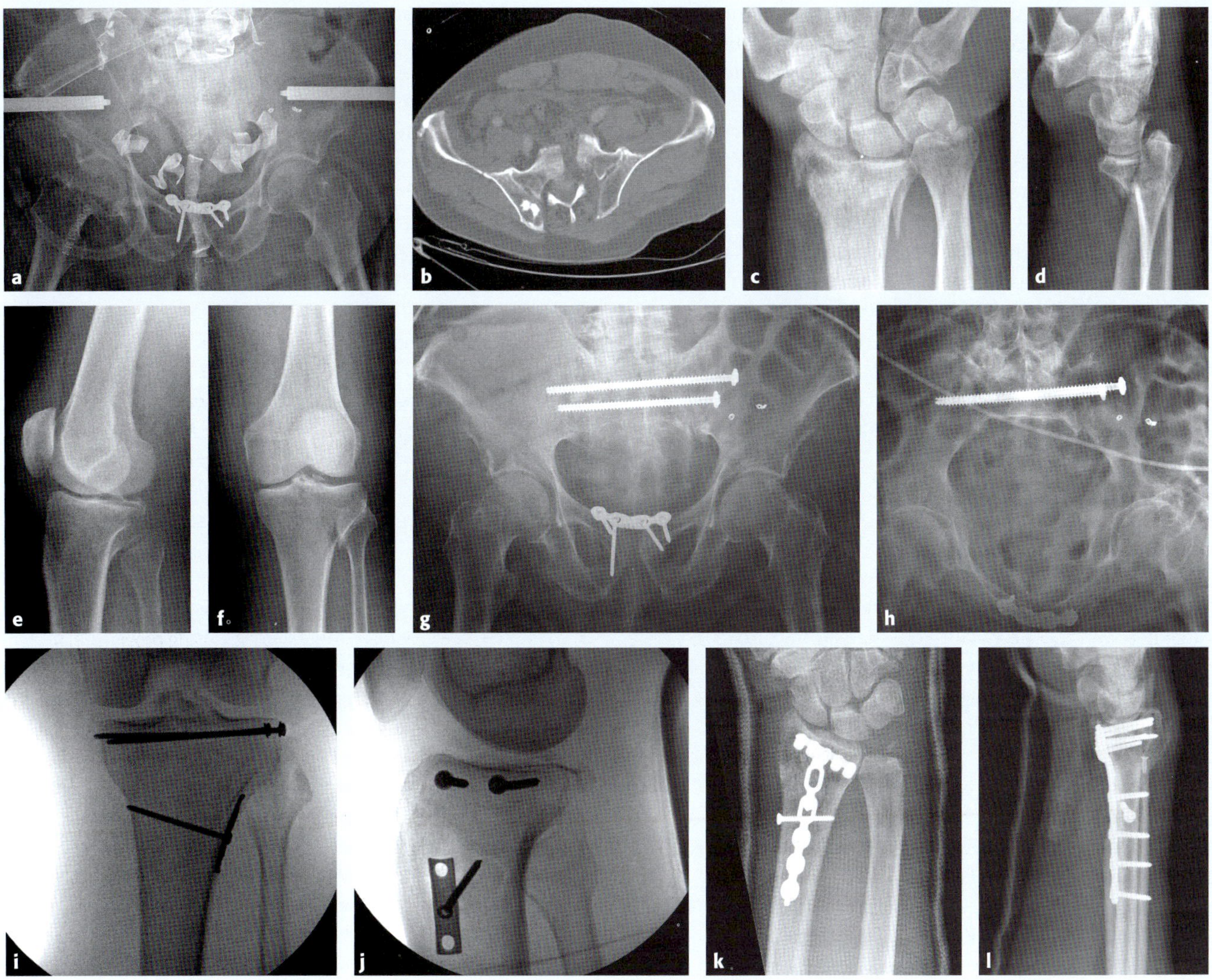


**Fig 3.20-1a–l** A 76-year-old man with intracranial hemorrhage and several fractures.
**a–b** AP x-ray and axial computed tomographic slice of an open book equivalent pelvic ring fracture.
**c–d** AP (**c**) and lateral (**d**) x-rays of a volar shear intraarticular distal radial fracture (AO/OTA 2R3B3).
**e–f** AP (**e**) and lateral (**f**) x-rays at the time of injury illustrating a partial articular lateral tibial plateau fracture (AO/OTA 41B1.1).
**g–h** Intraoperative AP, inlet, and outlet views showing restoration of the pelvic ring with transsacral screw placement and the C-clamp still in place. Note the orientation of the transsacral screws is perpendicular to the plane of the midsagittal sacral fracture.
**i–j** Intraoperative C-arm intensification images, AP (**i**) and lateral (**j**) views of the left proximal tibial plateau fracture reduction.
**k–l** Postoperative AP (**k**) and lateral (**l**) x-rays following right distal radial open reduction and internal fixation.

## 5 Resuscitation and comorbidities

Even though data has shown that aggressive rehydration and life support decrease mortality in the population, older polytraumatized individuals are often underresuscitated once they have reached the hospital. Goal-directed care in older polytrauma patients is therefore especially important. Invasive monitoring and aggressive resuscitation have been shown to decrease mortality [24, 27].

Older adults have lower total blood volume and cardiac output than younger adults, and a history of coronary artery disease or congestive heart failure are common. Both conditions can complicate resuscitation and anesthetic provision, if required:

- Higher resting preinjury blood pressure in older adults can mislead care providers into believing that patients are better resuscitated than they actually are.
- Renal insufficiency can significantly change pharmacokinetics of drugs important to resuscitation, increasing their physiological effects and toxicities.
- Pulmonary issues, such as chronic obstructive pulmonary disease, underlying pulmonary hypertension, and predisposition to pneumonia, can complicate management, especially if mechanical ventilation is warranted.

Preexisting neurological and cognitive conditions are common:

- Conditions such as Alzheimer's disease, Parkinson's disease, and a history of a cerebrovascular accident (stroke) can make communication challenging.
- Development of delirium is more common in polytrauma patients with "vulnerable brains" or dementia.

Osteoporosis, sarcopenia, and skin fragility contribute to infection risk and complications in older patients. Long-term medications, including beta-blockers, anticoagulants, corticosteroids, and angiotensin-converting enzyme inhibitors can interfere with evaluation and resuscitation efforts. Common previous orthopedic surgeries, such as total joint arthroplasty, can affect injury patterns and treatment plans.

CASE 2

### Patient

An 82-year-old male pedestrian was struck by a pick-up truck at 40 km/h (25 mph). He sustained right segmental tibial and fibular fractures with a concomitant tibial plateau fracture, a left distal femoral shaft fracture, right pubic rami fractures with right iliosacral disruption and an L5 transverse process fracture indicating translational instability of the left hemipelvis (**Fig 3.20-2a–d**).

### Comorbidities

- Alzheimer's dementia
- Coronary artery disease with prior by-pass grafting surgery
- Type 2 diabetes mellitus

### Treatment and outcome

External fixators were placed on the bilateral lower extremities initially for damage control and to maintain reasonable alignment. With significant swelling in the right leg, hematoma extraction and fasciotomy of the superficial posterior and lateral compartments was performed and closed 3 days postoperatively.

Bilateral external fixators were removed and open reduction and internal fixation of the tibial and femoral fractures were performed 7 days after placement of the external fixator. Pelvic fixation with iliosacral screws and anterior "pelvic bridge" was performed 13 days after initial presentation (**Fig 3.20-2e–h**).

### Key points

- Older adult pedestrians who are victims of motor vehicle accidents are more likely to sustain comminuted pelvic and lower extremity fractures than younger individuals [15, 30].
- It is important to establish goals of care with the patient and his or her family, if possible. Despite orthopedic solutions for his fractures, this patient had a traumatic brain injury as a result of the accident, and survived for just over 1 year following the accident. During this time, he remained ventilator-dependent and required parenteral nutrition.

## Discussion

There is a higher mortality risk for older polytrauma patients even with the same Injury Severity Score as for younger patients. Additionally, death from multiple injuries is more common in older than in younger trauma patients due to traumatic head injury and multisystem organ failure.

Early discussions with the family and patient, if possible, about the possibility of considerable disability, difficulty with activities of daily living, changes in residence or level of independence, and likelihood of death, are warranted. These often long but important discussions are best approached when possible by multiple members of the healthcare team (eg, surgeons, internal medicine and general medicine hospitalists, palliative care specialists, ancillary staff) providing the patient and family with a consistent message.

Additionally, common comorbidities and frailty, including osteoporosis, sarcopenia, and atrophic skin, render management more challenging. These comorbidities require geriatric comanagement to optimize outcomes. Medication management, comorbidity treatment, and disposition facilitation are maximized with geriatric team comanagement [31]. These findings echo the reports in the hip fracture literature of the importance of medical or geriatric comanagement in positively affecting outcomes for older orthopedic patients [32, 33].

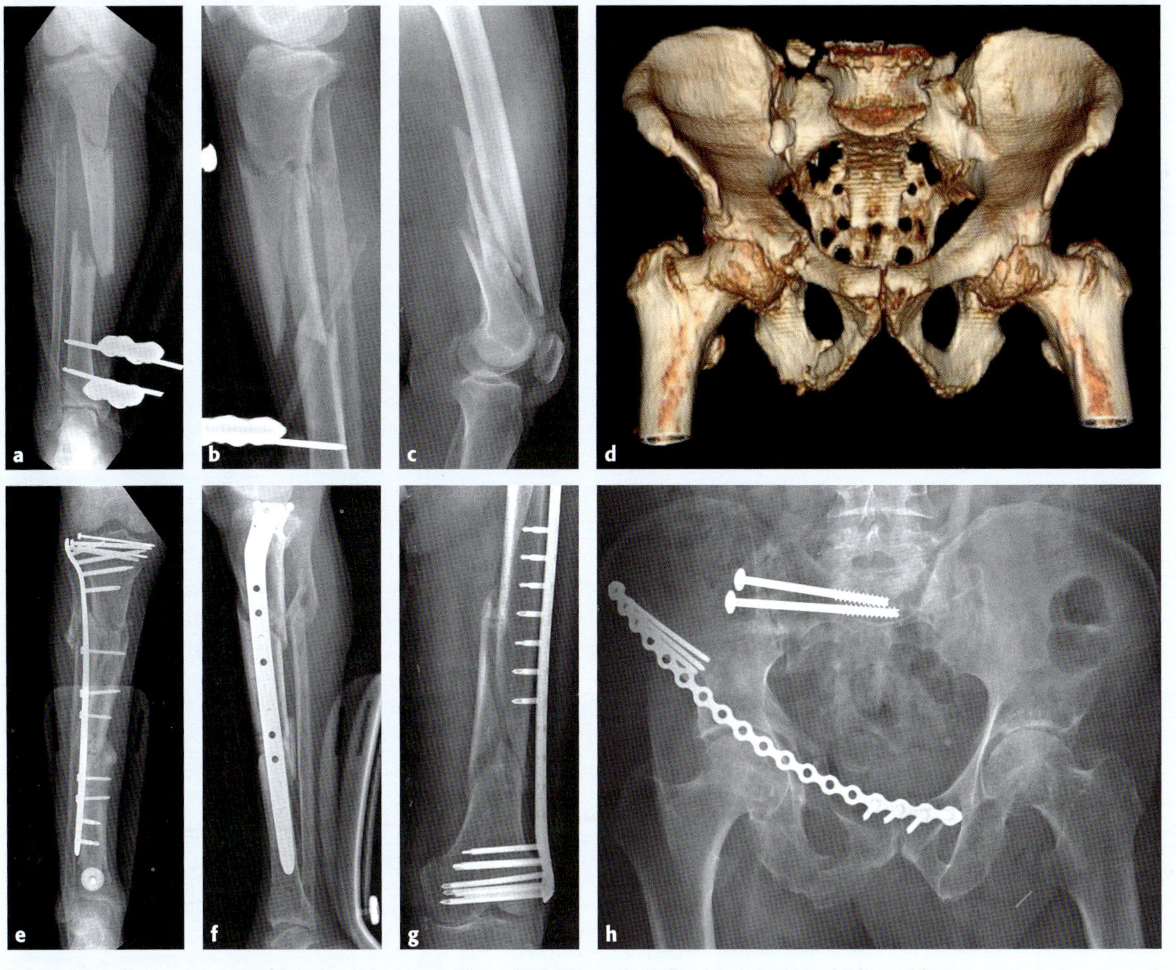


**Fig 3.20-2a–h** An 82-year-old male pedestrian with multiple fractures following a motor vehicle accident.
**a–b** AP (**a**) and lateral (**b**) views of the right segmental tibial and fibular fractures with concomitant tibial plateau fracture.
**c** Preoperative lateral x-ray illustrating the left distal femoral shaft fracture.
**d** A 3-D computed tomographic reconstruction illustrating right pubic rami fractures with right iliosacral disruption and L5 transverse process fracture.
**e–f** Postoperative AP (**e**) and lateral (**f**) x-rays demonstrating the results of open reduction and internal fixation (ORIF) of the right segmental tibial shaft and concomitant plateau fractures.
**g** Postoperative AP x-ray demonstrating the results of ORIF of the left distal femoral shaft fracture.
**h** AP x-ray showing pelvic fixation with iliosacral screws and anterior "pelvic bridge" performed 13 days after initial presentation.

## 6 Specific challenges

Polytrauma in older adults presents unique challenges (**Case 2: Fig 3.20-2**). However, the importance of adherence to the following tenets of adult trauma management are just as important in older adults as they are in younger ones:

- Primacy of ABCs of advanced trauma life support
- Avoidance of hypothermia
- Prevention of coagulopathy (ie, bleeding disorder)
- Emergent surgery to repair vital structures
- Nutritional supplementation
- Importance of orthopedic damage control [28, 29]
- Liberal use of temporary external fixation application as indicated
- Focus on comfort and mobilization

## 7 Therapeutic options

Treatment approaches to this population demand increased attention to the presence of decreased physiological reserve, blunted reactions to shock, and the presence of medications that may impair the patient's ability to respond to resuscitation and treatment attempts (**Case 3: Fig 3.20-3**, **Case 4: Fig 3.20-4**, **Case 5: Fig 3.20-5**, **Case 6: Fig 3.20-6**, **Case 7: Fig 3.20-7**).

CASE 3

### Patient

An 80-year-old woman fell about 4.6 m (15 feet) from a retaining wall while walking at night.

### Comorbidities

- Hypertension
- Asthma
- Dementia
- Prior cerebrovascular accident or stroke

### Treatment and outcome

Her injuries included a cervical burst fracture, a sternal fracture, and a pelvic fracture with disruption of the iliosacral joint (**Fig 3.20-3a–b**), with a bladder injury, and a left scapular fracture that was managed nonoperatively.

A postoperative AP x-ray of the pelvis after open reduction and internal fixation is shown in **Fig 3.20-3a–c**.

### Key points

- Sternal, clavicular, and rib fractures may be more common in older polytrauma patients. Each of these fractures is associated with increased mortality [17, 18], partly as a result of more central injuries in an individual who has little physiological reserve.
- In this case, the patient survived and thrived. Even in patients with similar Injury Severity Scores, older adults have higher rates of mortality. However, if the older patient survives the 3–6 months following the trauma, they can often expect to live independently and to function at a level similar to their preinjury level of activity [34].

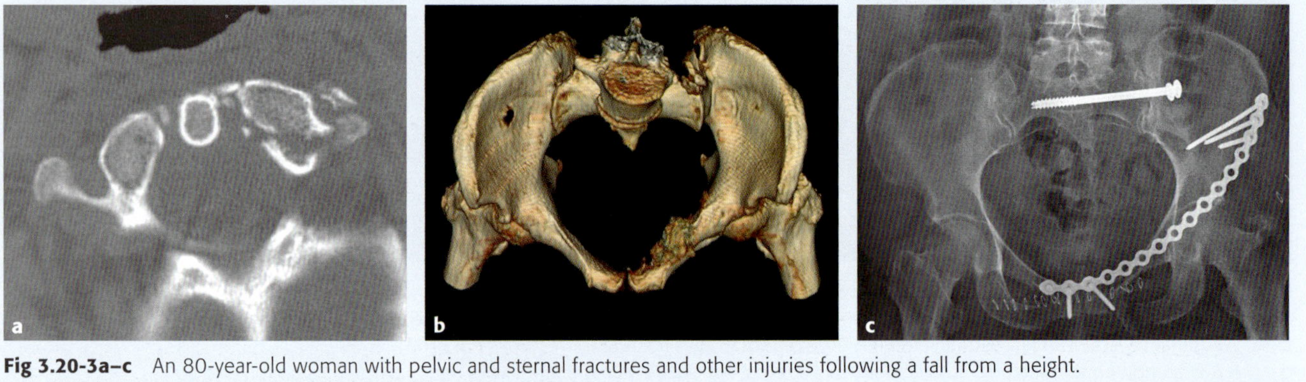


**Fig 3.20-3a–c** An 80-year-old woman with pelvic and sternal fractures and other injuries following a fall from a height.
**a** A 2-D computed tomographic (CT) axial slice illustrating the burst fracture.
**b** A 3-D CT reconstruction illustrating the sternal fracture, and pelvic (anterior rami) fracture including ipsilateral disruption of the iliosacral joint.
**c** Postoperative AP x-ray of the pelvis after stabilization by open reduction and internal fixation of both the anterior and posterior pelvic ring.

CASE 4

**Patient**

An 86-year-old woman involved in a vehicle rollover accident with prolonged extrication. She sustained a type III odontoid fracture with extension into C1 lateral mass, T1, T2, and T9 vertebral body fractures, multiple rib fractures, and a pneumothorax.

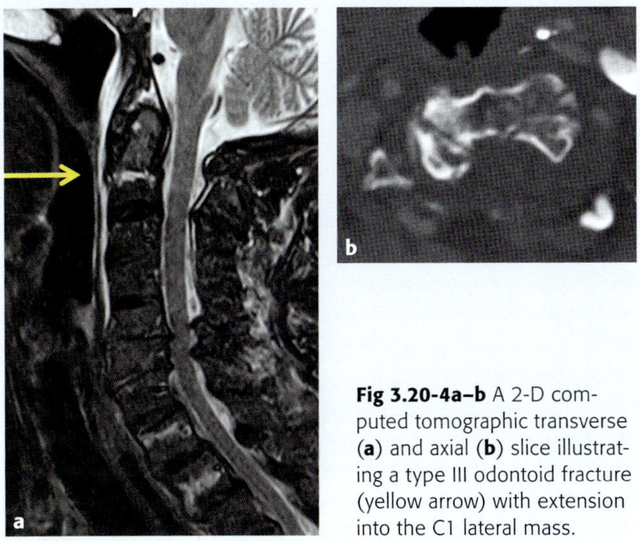


**Fig 3.20-4a–b** A 2-D computed tomographic transverse (**a**) and axial (**b**) slice illustrating a type III odontoid fracture (yellow arrow) with extension into the C1 lateral mass.

**Comorbidities**

- Chronic coronary artery disease with prior bypass surgery and aortic valve replacement
- Atrial fibrillation
- Hyperparathyroidism

**Treatment and outcome**

She was treated nonoperatively with a cervical neck brace with thoracic extension and went on to heal without neurological complications.

**Key points**

- Cervical spine injuries are more common in older trauma patients **[16]**.
- Thoracic injuries are predictive of worse outcome **[17, 18]**.
- In a study by Tashjian et al **[35]**, older adults with odontoid fractures who were treated with a halo vest had twice the rate of complications (nearly 70%) as those treated without a halo vest. Although halo vests are noted to be specifically associated with complications in the treatment of odontoid fractures in older adults, cervical orthoses in this population are also not benign.
- Degenerative changes in this patient's cervical spine, especially posterior osteophytes abutting the spinal cord at C4/5, present risk of devastating neurological injury.

CASE 5

**Patient**

A 72-year-old woman collided with a tree while driving. She sustained a right distal femoral fracture with intraarticular extension, bilateral patella fractures, and fractures of third to ninth right anterior ribs.

**Comorbidities**

- Coronary artery disease with stent placement
- Congestive heart failure
- Chronic obstructive pulmonary disease
- Atrial fibrillation
- Adrenal insufficiency
- Depression

**Treatment and outcome**

The x-rays of the right distal femur showed substantial metaphyseal comminution, shortening, and intraarticular involvement (**Fig 3.20-5a–b**). The right and left bilateral patellar fractures could also be clearly seen in the lateral views (**Fig 3.20-5b–c**).

A 2-D axial computed tomographic (CT) slice of the pelvis revealed what appeared to be a chronic left-sided sacral insufficiency fracture (**Fig 3.20-5d**). A knee-spanning external fixator was initially placed on the right. It was removed after 11 days and the distal femur was fixed with a variable angle locking plate. The right transversely fractured patella was fixed with two 4.0 mm cannulated screws, and the left patella fracture was fixed similarly with the addition of a modified tension band with 18-gauge wire through the cannulated screws.

**Figure 3.20-5e–f** shows open reduction and internal fixation of the right distal femoral and patellar fractures. The intraarticular aspect of the distal femoral fracture was reduced first. Then, the comminuted metaphyseal region was spanned with a long plate that allowed for locking technology. **Figure 3.20-5f** illustrates the left patellar open reduction and internal fixation construct incorporating the figure-8 tension band wiring technique.

A 2-D CT axial slice of the chest cavity illustrated that the third to ninth rib fractures on the right side resulted in decreased lung volume (**Fig 3.20-5g**). Consideration was made for treating a few of these rib fractures with plating. The patient was extubated within a few days of her injuries and so this intervention was not undertaken.

## Key points

- A focus on fracture and limb length, alignment, and rotation (following articular reduction) is paramount in all long-bone fracture treatment.
- Both the patellar and ipsilateral distal femoral fractures were approached through a midline anterior incision. This allowed for articular reduction of the distal femur as well as a direct approach to the extraarticular reduction and fixation of the patella.
- The chronic sacral fracture was indicative of her osteoporotic state. Her vitamin D, calcium, and parathyroid hormone levels were checked around the time of her injury. Her low vitamin D level was repleted with ergocalciferol (vitamin D2), 50,000 international units weekly for 3 weeks. Following vitamin D repletion, she was treated for her osteoporosis with teriparatide.

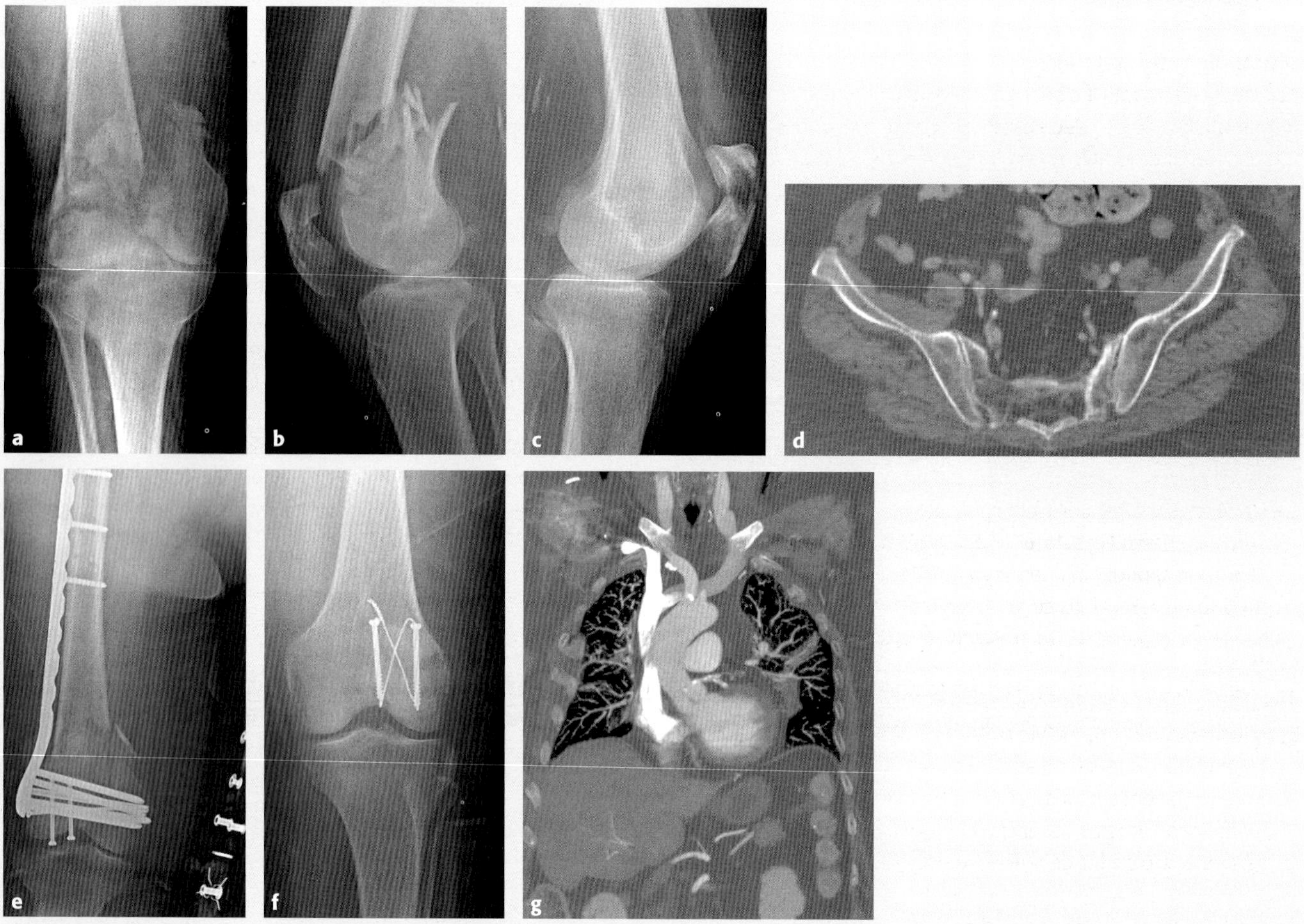


**Fig 3.20-5a–f** A 72-year-old woman with several fractures following a motor vehicle accident.

**a–b** AP (**a**) and lateral (**b**) x-rays of the right distal femur showing substantial metaphyseal comminution, shortening, and intraarticular involvement. The right patellar fracture can also be clearly seen in the lateral view (**b**).

**c** Lateral x-ray of the left patellar fracture.

**d** A 2-D axial computed tomographic (CT) slice of the pelvis illustrating left-sided sacral insufficiency fracture.

**e** Postoperative AP x-ray showing the right distal femoral and patellar fractures were fixed with open reduction and internal fixation (ORIF).

**f** Postoperative lateral x-ray of the left patellar fracture following ORIF.

**g** A 2-D CT axial slice of the chest cavity showing that the third to ninth rib fractures on the right side resulted in decreased lung volume.

**Patient**

A 79-year-old woman was hit by a motor vehicle. She suffered left-sided injuries, including left pneumothorax, left-sided combined pelvic ring and acetabular fracture, left tibial plateau fracture, and left ankle fracture.

**Comorbidities**

- Medical history significant for preexisting left hip pain (early osteoarthritis) requiring a cane for ambulation

**Treatment and outcome**

An advanced trauma life support protocol was initiated. The patient was intubated due to decreased oxygen saturation and received a chest tube. She was also placed in a pelvic binder and was resuscitated on the way to the operating room for damage-control treatment.

The initial AP pelvic x-rays show a combined left-sided pelvic ring injury and acetabular fracture before (**Fig 3.20-6a**) and after (**Fig 3.20-6b**) application of a pelvic binder. Note the reduction of the pelvic ring following application of the pelvic binder, which was an important step in preventing ongoing blood loss and increasing circulatory volume during the initial resuscitation of the patient.

Left AO/OTA C-type tibial plateau fracture and bimalleolar ankle fracture are shown **Fig 3.20-6c–d** and **Fig 3.20-6e–f**, respectively. As all of the orthopedic injuries were on the left side, each fracture needed to be taken into consideration during both initial and definitive management, as treatment of one would impact the rest.

The initial damage-control management of the patient included the external fixation of the pelvic ring and a spanning external fixation of the left tibial plateau and ankle. The preliminary skeletal stabilization of the patient's injuries allowed both ongoing resuscitation of the patient and time to better characterize the complex constitution of injuries and plan for definitive treatment.

Following external fixation procedures, complete pelvic radiographic imaging (**Fig 3.20-6g–k**) allowed better characterization of the combined pelvic ring and acetabular fractures. These showed that the pelvic ring was now well reduced and that the patient had a left-sided transverse, posterior wall acetabular fracture.

As the patient had a complex combined pelvic ring and acetabular fracture in addition to early osteoarthritis, a thorough discussion was had regarding the treatment options and expected outcomes. This led to the decision to proceed with staged internal fixation of the pelvic ring and a left total hip replacement.

The postoperative x-ray (**Fig 3.20-6l**) followed the removal of the pelvic external fixator, open reduction and internal fixation (ORIF) of the pubic symphysis, and percutaneous screw placement across the left sacroiliac joint. These showed anatomical restoration of the pelvic ring, which is important before proceeding to the management of the ipsilateral acetabular fracture.

The patient underwent left total hip arthroplasty for definitive treatment of the acetabular fracture (**Fig 3.20-6m**). Screws placed in the acetabular cup provided bridging stabilization across the transverse, posterior wall of the acetabular fracture, which would allow for instant mobilization and weight bearing across the hip. However, given the ipsilateral pelvic ring, tibial plateau, and ankle fractures, weight bearing would still be limited in this patient.

Computed tomographic images showed a bicondylar tibial plateau involvement with metadiaphyseal disruption (AO/OTA type C). Overall, there was minimal disruption at the articular surface with relatively large articular fracture fragments. Definitive fixation was carried out at 2 weeks postinjury once the soft-tissue envelope at the left lower leg was ready. Anatomical restoration of the articular surface and stabilization was performed using a large fragment, proximally locked, laterally based tibial plate (**Fig 3.20-6n**). Intraoperative images were taken following ORIF of the ipsilateral bimalleolar ankle fracture. Minimally invasive bridging fixation was used for the distal fibula due to the comminuted nature of the fracture and to limit soft-tissue dissection.

Length, alignment, and rotation as well as congruency at the ankle were restored (**Fig 3.20-6o**).

**Key points**

- The initial treatment and resuscitation of geriatric polytrauma patients is similar to that of younger adult patients, and damage-control principles are still applied as appropriate to facilitate their initial care.
- Careful planning is required in treating polytrauma patients, and injuries cannot be considered in isolation. Especially in this case, stabilization of the pelvic ring was carried out with definitive treatment for the acetabular fracture in mind.
- Due to an antecedent history of early osteoarthritis, and a thorough discussion of functional outcomes following either a total hip arthroplasty or ORIF for the acetabular fracture, arthroplasty was carried out for a definitive treatment.

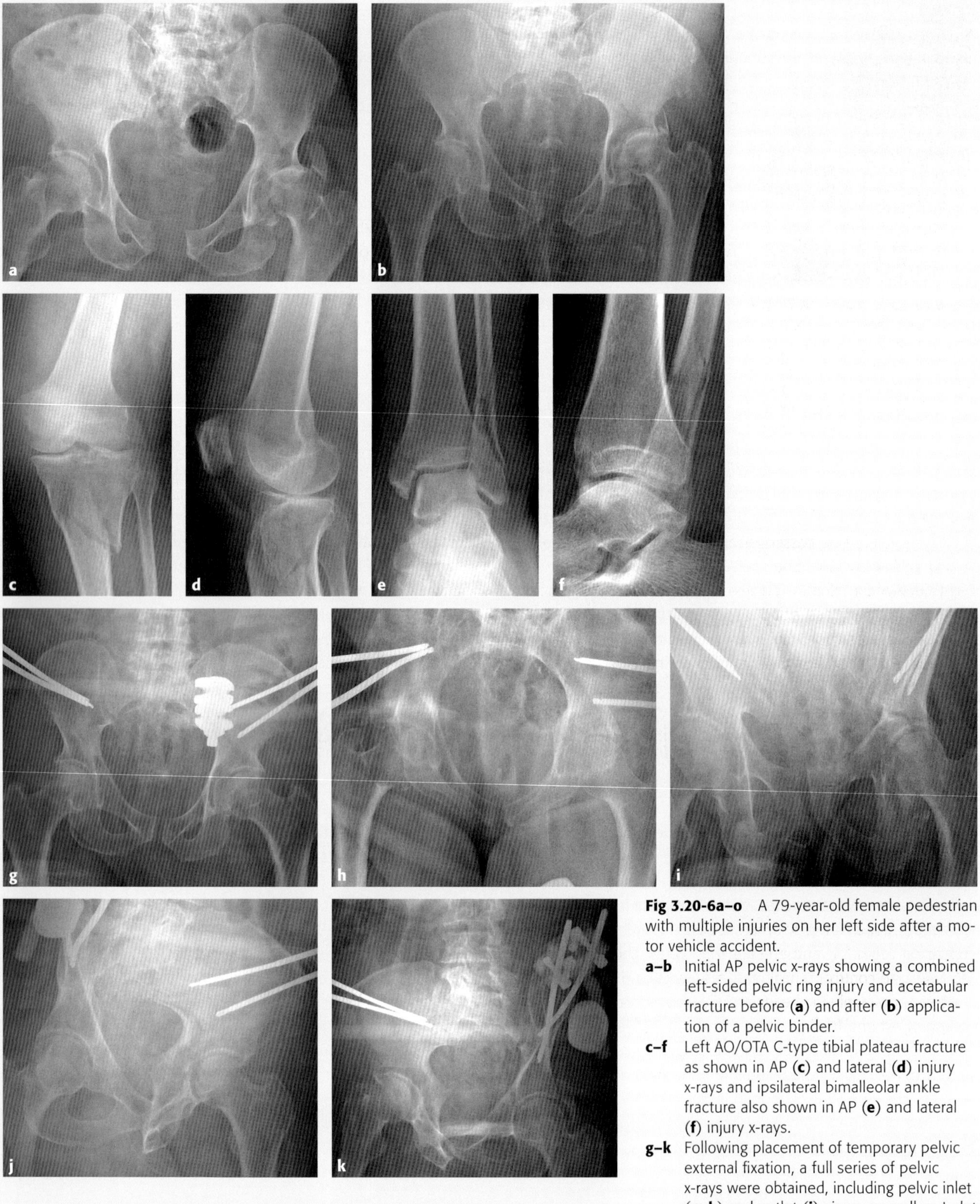


**Fig 3.20-6a–o** A 79-year-old female pedestrian with multiple injuries on her left side after a motor vehicle accident.

**a–b** Initial AP pelvic x-rays showing a combined left-sided pelvic ring injury and acetabular fracture before (**a**) and after (**b**) application of a pelvic binder.

**c–f** Left AO/OTA C-type tibial plateau fracture as shown in AP (**c**) and lateral (**d**) injury x-rays and ipsilateral bimalleolar ankle fracture also shown in AP (**e**) and lateral (**f**) injury x-rays.

**g–k** Following placement of temporary pelvic external fixation, a full series of pelvic x-rays were obtained, including pelvic inlet (**g–h**) and outlet (**i**) views, as well as Judet oblique views (**j–k**).

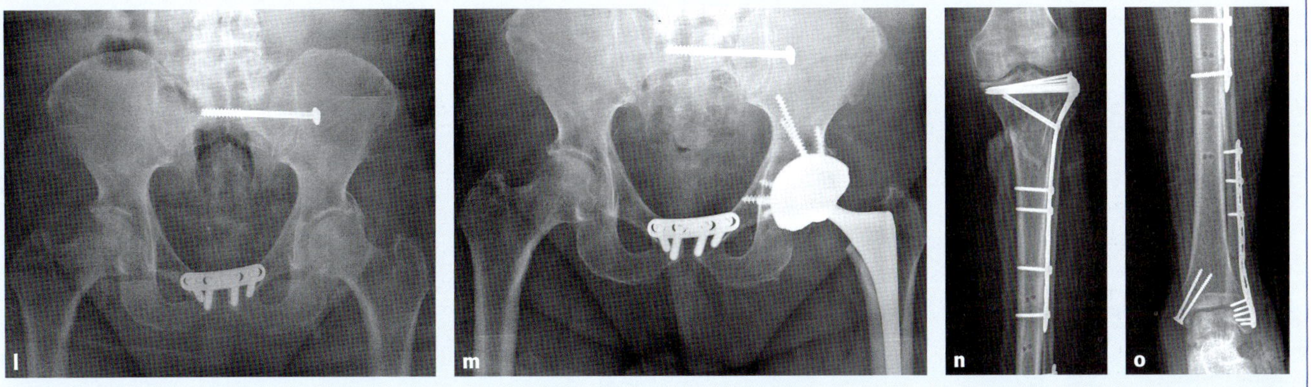


**Fig 3.20-6a–o (cont)** A 79-year-old female pedestrian with multiple injuries on her left side after a motor vehicle collision.
**l** Postoperative AP pelvis x-ray taken after removal of the pelvic external fixator, open reduction and internal fixation (ORIF) of the pubic symphysis, and percutaneous screw placement across the left sacroiliac joint.
**m** AP pelvis x-ray showing placement of a left total hip arthroplasty for definitive treatment of the acetabular fracture.
**n** Postoperative AP x-ray of the left tibia following ORIF.
**o** Postoperative AP x-ray of the left ankle following ORIF of both the medial and lateral malleoli and distal fibula.



### Patient

A 78-year-old female passenger on a motorcycle was involved in a motor vehicle collision. She presented to the trauma center with a right-sided pneumothorax, multiple rib fractures, and a liver laceration. Her orthopedic injuries included right open distal femoral and tibial plateau fractures (open floating knee) and left-sided open distal femoral fracture (**Fig 3.20-7a–c**). Her distal neurovascular examination to both lower extremities was intact, with strong peripheral pulses to her dorsalis pedis and posterior tibial arteries bilaterally.

### Comorbidities

- Chronic obstructive pulmonary disease
- Hypothyroid
- Osteoporosis

### Treatment and outcome

After initial resuscitation, chest tube placement, tetanus and antibiotic prophylaxis in the trauma bay, the patient was taken to the operating room for a trauma laparotomy, irrigation, debridement, and damage-control management for her lower extremity fractures. Placement of antibiotic beads and stabilization with bilateral knee-spanning external fixation facilitated repeated irrigation and debridement of the open wounds until the patient and soft tissues were ready for definitive stabilization.

Staged definitive stabilization was undertaken, beginning with the left distal femur. AP and lateral x-rays depicted anatomical restoration of the left distal femoral articular block with a locked lateral bridging plate.

Intraoperative images showed open reduction and internal fixation of both the distal femur and tibial plateau on the right side. The distal femur was initially stabilized with provisional K-wire fixation and interfragmental screws across the articular fragments, followed by placement of a lateral distal femoral locking plate. The tibial plateau fracture was stabilized using a long proximal tibial locking plate, with additional fixation placed at the diaphyseal fracture site. The alignment at the right femur (**Fig 3.20-7d**), the right tibia (**Fig 3.20-7e**), and the left femur (**Fig 3.20-7f**) was restored.

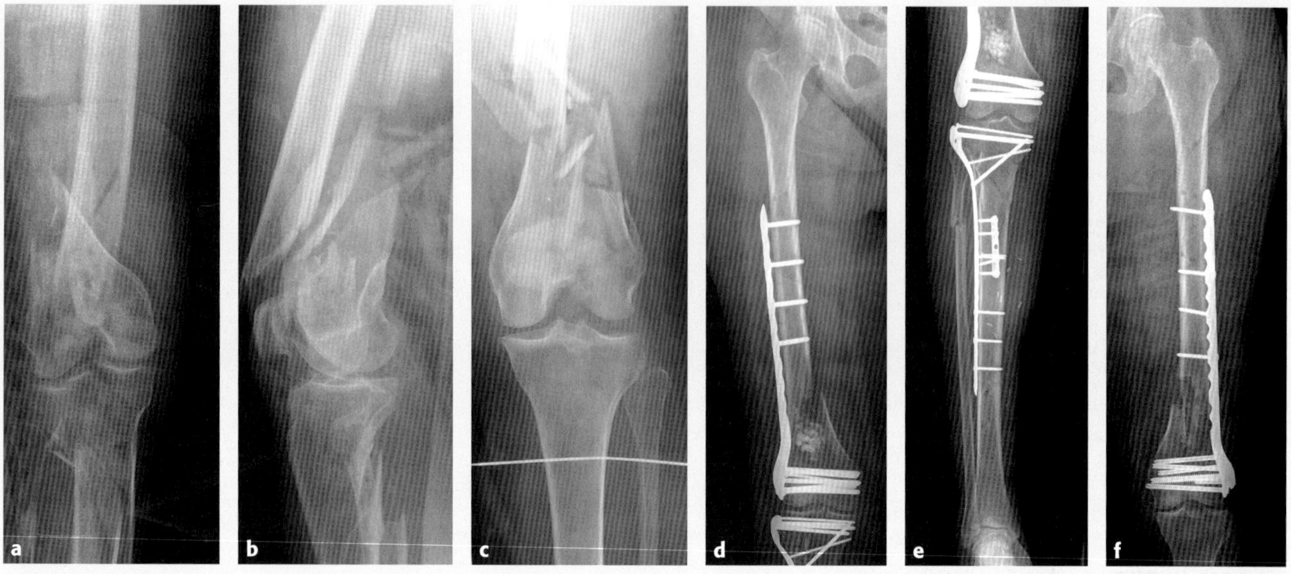


**Fig 3.20-7 a–f** A 78-year-old female polytrauma patient after a motorcycle versus motor vehicle collision.
**a–b** AP (**a**) and lateral (**b**) x-rays showing AO/OTA C-type fractures of the right distal femur and proximal tibial fracture with simple intraarticular splits.
**c** AP x-ray of the left distal femoral fracture.
**d–f** Postoperative AP x-rays of the bilateral lower extremities depicting restoration of alignment at the right femur (**d**), right tibia (**e**), and the left femur (**f**).

CASE 8

## Patient

A 90-year-old female driver who was struck broadside by another vehicle traveling at about 72 km/h (45 mph) sustained injuries including a sternal fracture, left rami fractures, bilateral sacral fractures, and pneumothorax.

## Comorbidities

- Hypercholesterolemia
- Hypertension
- Degenerative joint disease

## Treatment and outcome

The 2-D computed tomographic (CT) findings revealed a sternal fracture, left rami fractures, bilateral sacral fractures, and pneumothorax. Active extravasation was observed on CT angiogram in the left gluteal musculature and also in the pubic symphysis area, so the patient underwent emergent embolization.

A 3-D CT reconstruction was obtained to further evaluate the left rami fractures with symphyseal disruption and bilateral sacral fractures (**Fig 3.20-8a**) that are also seen on the 2-D CT axial slice (**Fig 3.20-8b**).

The patient was initially treated nonoperatively for her pelvic ring injuries (as well as her sternal fracture). However, at her first postinjury visit, her hemipelvis was noted to have migrated. Additionally, she was uncomfortable and, as a result of her pain, had essentially become bedridden.

Her operative risk was evaluated. Despite her age, she had few comorbidities. She was taken to the operating room for open reduction and internal fixation (ORIF).

**Figure 3.20-8c** shows a postoperative AP x-ray of the pelvis after ORIF stabilization of the anterior pelvic ring, using a bilateral internal fixator construct, which could be placed subcutaneously. An iliosacral and a transsacral screw were placed to stabilize the posterior ring injury.

Although she did well postoperatively, she experienced chest pain after a physiotheray session a few days following discharge and was diagnosed with a non-ST segment elevation myocardial infarction. She recovered and lived another 4 years.

**Key points**

- Minimally invasive fixation was employed for pelvic stabilization. One percutaneously placed 7.3 mm transsacral screw and one percutaneously placed 7.3 mm cannulated iliosacral screw were advanced through stab incisions and under image intensification.
- To minimize hardware prominence, occipital rods and pedicle screws, with 4.5 mm cortical screws for further augmentation, were used to create an internal fixator for her anterior pelvic disruption. She was allowed to bear weight as tolerated immediately following the pelvic surgery.

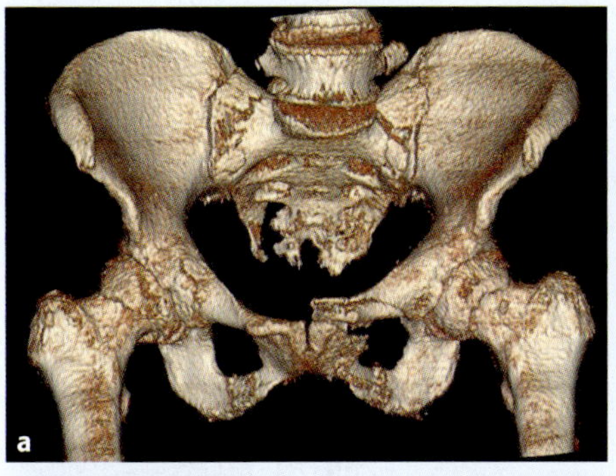

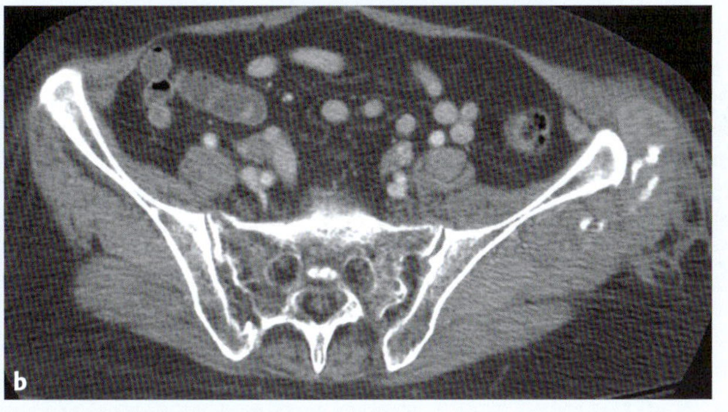

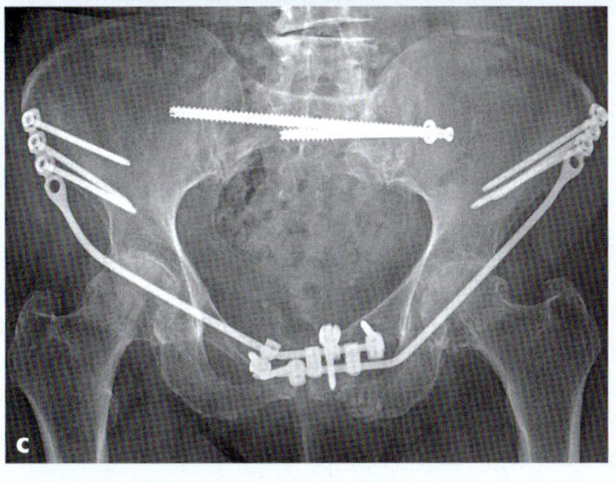

**Fig 3.20-8b–c** A 90-year-old woman with multiple fractures following a motor vehicle collision.
**a–b** A 3-D computed tomographic (CT) reconstruction illustrating left rami fractures with symphyseal disruption and bilateral sacral fractures (**a**), also seen on the 2-D CT axial slice (**b**).
**c** Postoperative AP x-ray of the pelvis following open reduction and internal fixation.

## 8 Outcomes

Mortality in older polytrauma patients correlates with ISS, frailty, comorbidities, and head and cervical spinal injuries. A GCS ≤ 8 and shock on presentation are also predictors of mortality [10].

Complications and, in particular infections, have been reported to occur at a significantly higher rate in older patients than in younger cohorts. In a study based on data from the National Trauma Data Bank, the total complication rate was 14%, whereas the complication rate in patients ≥ 65 years of age was 34% [36]. For patients with preexisting functional and cognitive decline, or expectations of severe posttreament disability, early investigation of goals of care with palliative care or other specialists is warranted.

## 9 Prevention

As in most cases of trauma-related injuries, prevention strategies are essential to decrease the individual and societal burdens of polytraumatized older adults.

- Older motor vehicle drivers are more likely to be women, to be struck at an urban intersection, and to be traveling < 97 km/h (< 60 mph) [37].
- In a study of geriatric trauma in Illinois, approximately 50% of patients tested positive for alcohol use and 12% tested positive for other illicit substances [38].
- Strategies for prevention should focus on fall prevention, safe vehicle operation, and prevention of impaired adults from engaging in high-risk and/or high-energy activities.

## 10 References


1. **Switzer JA, Gammon SR.** High-energy skeletal trauma in the elderly. *J Bone Joint Surg Am.* 2012 Dec 05;94(23):2195–2204.
2. **Davidson GH, Hamlat CA, Rivara FP, et al.** Long-term survival of adult trauma patients. *JAMA.* 2011 Mar 09;305(10):1001–1007.
3. **Marx AB, Campbell R, Harder F.** Polytrauma in the elderly. *World J Surg.* 1986 Apr;10(2):330–335.
4. **Broos PL, Stappaerts KH, Rommens PM, et al.** Polytrauma in patients of 65 and over. Injury patterns and outcome. *Int Surg.* 1988 Apr-Jun;73(2):119–122.
5. **Cox S, Morrison C, Cameron P, et al.** Advancing age and trauma: triage destination compliance and mortality in Victoria, Australia. *Injury.* 2014 Sep;45(9):1312–1319.
6. **Broos PL, D'Hoore A, Vanderschot P, et al.** Multiple trauma in elderly patients. Factors influencing outcome: importance of aggressive care. *Injury.* 1993 Jul;24(6):365–368.
7. **Sterling DA, O'Connor JA, Bonadies J.** Geriatric falls: injury severity is high and disproportionate to mechanism. *J Trauma.* 2001 Jan;50(1):116–119.
8. **American College of Surgeons.** National Trauma Data Bank (NTDB) Annual Report 2014. Available at: www.facs.org/~/media/files/quality programs/trauma/ntdb/ntdb annual report 2014.ashx. Accessed March 2017.
9. **Giannoudis PV, Harwood PJ, Court-Brown C, et al.** Severe and multiple trauma in older patients; incidence and mortality. *Injury.* 2009 Apr;40(4):362–367.
10. **Aldrian S, Koenig F, Weninger P, et al.** Characteristics of polytrauma patients between 1992 and 2002: what is changing? *Injury.* 2007 Sep;38(9):1059–1064.
11. **Cirera E, Perez K, Santamarina-Rubio E, et al.** Incidence trends of injury among the elderly in Spain, 2000–2010. *Inj Prev.* 2014 Dec;20(6):401–407.
12. **Zietlow SP, Capizzi PJ, Bannon MP, et al.** Multisystem geriatric trauma. *J Trauma.* 1994 Dec;37(6):985–988.
13. **Oreskovich MR, Howard JD, Copass MK, et al.** Geriatric trauma: injury patterns and outcome. *J Trauma.* 1984 Jul;24(7):565–572.
14. **Labib N, Nouh T, Winocour S, et al.** Severely injured geriatric population: morbidity, mortality, and risk factors. *J Trauma.* 2011 Dec;71(6):1908–1914.
15. **Siram SM, Sonaike V, Bolorunduro OB, et al.** Does the pattern of injury in elderly pedestrian trauma mirror that of the younger pedestrian? *J Surg Res.* 2011 May 01;167(1):14–18.
16. **Zusman NL, Ching AC, Hart RA, et al.** Incidence of second cervical vertebral fractures far surpassed the rate predicted by the changing age distribution and growth among elderly persons in the United States (2005–2008). *Spine.* 2013 Apr 20;38(9):752–756.
17. **Bulger EM, Arneson MA, Mock CN, et al.** Rib fractures in the elderly. *J Trauma.* 2000 Jun;48(6):1040–1046; discussion 1046–1047.
18. **Keller JM, Sciadini MF, Sinclair E, et al.** Geriatric trauma: demographics, injuries, and mortality. *J Orthop Trauma.* 2012 Sep;26(9):e161–e165.
19. **Dechert TA, Duane TM, Frykberg BP, et al.** Elderly patients with pelvic fracture: interventions and outcomes. *Am Surg.* 2009 Apr;75(4):291–295.
20. **Hill BW, Switzer JA, Cole PA.** Management of high-energy acetabular fractures in the elderly individuals: a current review. *Geriatr Orthop Surg Rehabil.* 2012 Sep;3(3):95–106.
21. **Henry SM, Pollak AN, Jones AL, et al.** Pelvic fracture in geriatric patients: a distinct clinical entity. *J Trauma.* 2002 Jul;53(1):15–20.
22. **Lane P, Sorondo B, Kelly JJ.** Geriatric trauma patients-are they receiving trauma center care? *Acad Emerg Med.* 2003 Mar;10(3):244–250.
23. **Ma MH, MacKenzie EJ, Alcorta R, et al.** Compliance with prehospital triage protocols for major trauma patients. *J Trauma.* 1999 Jan;46(1):168–175.
24. **Demetriades D, Karaiskakis M, Velmahos G, et al.** Effect on outcome of early intensive management of geriatric trauma patients. *Br J Surg.* 2002 Oct;89(10):1319–1322.
25. **Mann NC, Cahn RM, Mullins RJ, et al.** Survival among injured geriatric patients during construction of a statewide trauma system. *J Trauma.* 2001 Jun;50(6):1111–1116.
26. **Joseph B, Pandit V, Zangbar B, et al.** Superiority of frailty over age in predicting outcomes among geriatric trauma patients: a prospective analysis. *JAMA Surg.* 2014 Aug;149(8):766–772.
27. **Scalea TM, Simon HM, Duncan AO, et al.** Geriatric blunt multiple trauma: improved survival with early invasive monitoring. *J Trauma.* 1990 Feb;30(2):129–134; discussion 134–136.
28. **Nahm NJ, Como JJ, Wilber JH, et al.** Early appropriate care: definitive stabilization of femoral fractures within 24 hours of injury is safe in most patients with multiple injuries. *J Trauma.* 2011 Jul;71(1):175–185.
29. **Nahm NJ, Moore TA, Vallier HA.** Use of two grading systems in determining risks associated with timing of fracture fixation. *J Trauma Acute Care Surg.* 2014 Aug;77(2):268–279.
30. **Demetriades D, Murray J, Martin M, et al.** Pedestrians injured by automobiles: relationship of age to injury type and severity. *J Am Coll Surg.* 2004 Sep;199(3):382–387.
31. **Fallon WF Jr, Rader E, Zyzanski S, et al.** Geriatric outcomes are improved by a geriatric trauma consultation service. *J Trauma.* 2006 Nov;61(5):1040–1046.
32. **Friedman SM, Mendelson DA, Bingham KW, et al.** Impact of a comanaged Geriatric Fracture Center on short-term hip fracture outcomes. *Arch Intern Med.* 2009 Oct 12;169(18):1712–1717.
33. **Kates SL, Mendelson DA, Friedman SM.** The value of an organized fracture program for the elderly: early results. *J Orthop Trauma.* 2011 Apr;25(4):233–237.
34. **Battistella FD, Din AM, Perez L.** Trauma patients 75 years and older: long-term follow-up results justify aggressive management. *J Trauma.* 1998 Apr;44(4):618–623; discussion 623.
35. **Tashjian RZ, Majercik S, Biffl WL, et al.** Halo-vest immobilization increases early morbidity and mortality in elderly odontoid fractures. *J Trauma.* 2006 Jan;60(1):199–203.
36. **Min L, Burruss S, Morley E, et al.** A simple clinical risk nomogram to predict mortality-associated geriatric complications in severely injured geriatric patients. *J Trauma Acute Care Surg.* 2013 Apr;74(4):1125–1132.
37. **Clark DE.** Motor vehicle crash fatalities in the elderly: rural versus urban. *J Trauma.* 2001 Nov;51(5):896–900.
38. **McGwin G Jr, May AK, Melton SM, et al.** Recurrent trauma in elderly patients. *Arch Surg.* 2001 Feb;136(2):197–203.

# Index

Note: Information in figures and tables is indicated by *f* and *t*.

## A

# B

# C

# D

# E



# F

## G



## H



## I

# J



# K



# L



# M

## N



## O

# P

## Q



## R

# S



# T

# U



# V



# W



# X